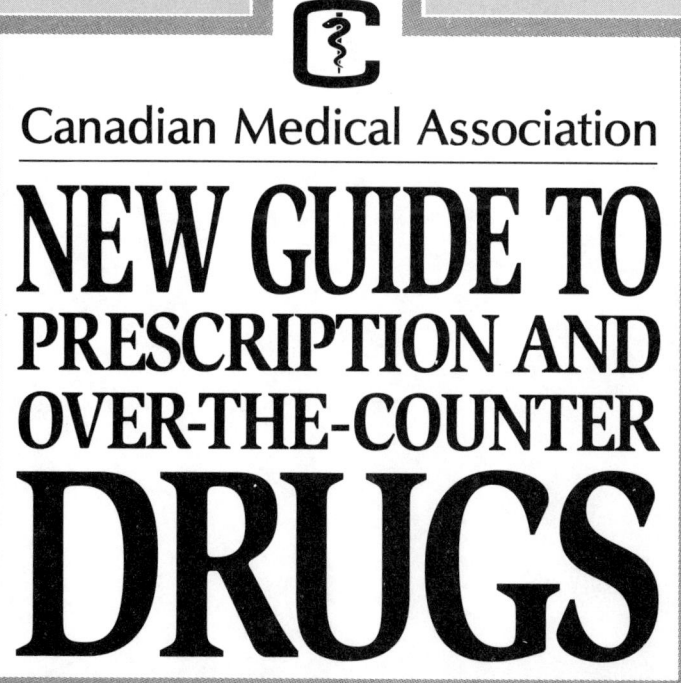

Canadian Medical Association

NEW GUIDE TO
PRESCRIPTION AND
OVER-THE-COUNTER
DRUGS

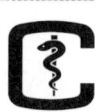

Canadian Medical Association

NEW GUIDE TO
PRESCRIPTION AND
OVER-THE-COUNTER
DRUGS

Co-Editors
Mark S. Berner, MD, CCFP(EM), FCFP
Gerald N. Rotenberg, BScPhm, FACA

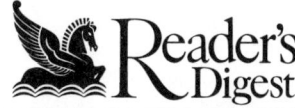

The Reader's Digest Association (Canada) Ltd.
Montreal

CANADIAN MEDICAL ASSOCIATION

President
Jack Armstrong, MD, FRCPC
Secretary-General
Léo-Paul Landry, MD
Executive Director
Barbara Drew
Director of Publications
Stephen Prudhomme
Editor-in-Chief
Bruce P. Squires, MD, PhD
Assistant Director, Publications
Brian Berube

Co-Editors
Mark S. Berner, MD, CCFP(EM), FCFP, *Montreal*;
Gerald N. Rotenberg, BScPhm, FACA, *Toronto*

Editorial Board (First Edition)
Pierre Biron, MD, MSc, *Montreal*; Jacques Bradwejn, MD,
FRCPC, *Toronto*; S. George Carruthers, MD, FRCPC,
Halifax; Gordon E. Johnson, PhD, *Saskatoon*; Ian W.D.
Henderson, MD, FRCSC, *Ottawa*; Keith L. MacCannell,
MD, PhD, *Calgary*; Edward L. Masson, MD, FCFP,
Toronto; Les Meissner, MD, FRCPC, *Montreal*; Paul A.
Mitenko, MD, FRCPC, *Nanaimo*; John Ruedy, MD,
Halifax; Edward M. Sellers, MD, PhD, FRCPC, *Toronto*;
Michael Spino, PharmD, *Toronto*; Bruce P. Squires, MD,
PhD, *Ottawa*

READER'S DIGEST

Senior Staff Editor Alice Philomena Rutherford
Associate Editor Anita Winterberg
Research Editor Wadad Bashour
Copy Editor Joseph Marchetti
Indexer Jane Broderick

DORLING KINDERSLEY LIMITED

SECOND EDITION
Senior Editor Edward Bunting
Editor Teresa Pritlove
Designer Anne Renel
Managing Editor Martyn Page
Managing Art Editor Bryn Walls
DTP Design Almudena Díaz, Raul López
Illustrations Karen Cochrane
Production Lauren Britton, Michelle Thomas

FIRST EDITION
Senior Editors Christopher Fayers, Cathy Meeus; **Project
Editor** Stephanie Jackson; **Editors** David Bennett, Marian
Broderick, Penny Gray, Christiane Gunzi, Terence Monaighan,
Jillian Somerscales; **Additional editorial assistance from**
Mike Darton, Ruth Swan, Susie Ward; **Managing Editor** Ruth
Midgley; **Managing Art Editor** Chez Picthall; **Designers** Gail
Jones, Laura Overton, Sandra Schneider; **Computer page
make-up** Peter Cooling, Rowena Feeny, Debra Lee;
Production Eunice Paterson

Edited and designed by Dorling Kindersley Limited
Copyright © 1996 Canadian Medical Association, Ottawa
and Dorling Kindersley Limited, London.

Published in Canada by
The Reader's Digest Association (Canada) Ltd.
215 Redfern Avenue
Montreal, Que. H3Z 2V9

CANADIAN CATALOGUING IN PUBLICATION DATA

Main entry under title:
Canadian Medical Association new guide to prescription
and over-the-counter drugs

2nd ed: Includes index. ISBN 0-88850-515-9

1. Drugs, Nonprescription – Popular works.
2. Drugs, Nonprescription – Handbooks, manuals, etc.
I. Berner, Mark S.
II. Rotenberg, Gerald N.
III. Canadian Medical Association.
IV. Reader's Digest Association (Canada).

RM301.12.C36 1996   615'.1   C95-900817-9

READER'S DIGEST and the Pegasus colophon are
trademarks of The Reader's Digest Association, Inc.

Reproduced by IGS, Bath, England
Printed by R. R. Donnelly, U.S.A.

96 97 98 99 / 5 4 3 2 1

WARNING
The information contained in this book is for reference
and education only and is not intended to be a substitute
for the advice of a physician. CMA assumes no
responsibility for liability arising from any error in or
omission from the book, or from the use of any
information contained in it.

PREFACE

Medical and pharmaceutical research continues apace and, in the last six years, drug therapy has changed significantly. While many of the stalwart medications remain, some have been replaced by newer, better drugs. Indeed, some 65 new profiles have been added to this edition to reflect progress in pharmaceutical research and in medical therapy. For many of the drugs that remain from the first edition, much more is now known about how they work and about their wanted and unwanted effects. This revised edition reflects that new knowledge.

While the revisions in the *CMA New Guide to Prescription and Over-the-Counter Drugs* bring the book up to date, they don't alter the purpose of the original: to inform Canadians about the beneficial effects – and the dangers – of drugs available in Canada. The prescription and over-the-counter drugs we take as part of medical therapy are beneficial only if we take them correctly. Even then, there may be unwanted effects. And occasionally, Canadians may intentionally or unintentionally abuse drugs.

The Canadian Medical Association has produced this book in the belief that an informed patient is better able to participate in the therapeutic process, whether self-initiated with over-the-counter drugs or physician supervised. The information in the drug profiles reinforces the information on the drug label and supplements the advice from your physician.

Although the *CMA New Guide to Prescription and Over-the-Counter Drugs* should continue to be helpful to physicians and their office staffs, to pharmacists, nurses, and other health-care workers, it is important to reemphasize that this book is not intended to be a comprehensive professional reference or textbook. It is intended, rather, to be a guide for the general public, to increase the average Canadian's knowledge of drugs, what they are prescribed for, how to take them, how they work, and what their side effects and possible drug interactions are. The aim is to develop a new "therapeutic alliance" between the physician, the patient, and the pharmacist. By increasing public knowledge through a book such as this and through physicians and pharmacists who encourage patients' questions and provide understandable answers, we can maximize the benefits of drugs and minimize the problems they cause.

The CMA wishes to acknowledge the dedication and commitment of both Dorling Kindersley Limited of London, England, and The Reader's Digest Association (Canada) Limited, whose continuing collaboration makes this ambitious project possible. Our gratitude to the co-editors, Dr. Mark Berner and Gerald Rotenberg, who guided the revision; and special thanks to Roger Korman, general manager of IMS Canada, who kindly provided Canadian drug sales statistics, and to the consultants for this second edition: Dr. Ross Davies, Dr. George Fodor, Dr. Paul Grof, Dr. Lyall Higginson, Dr. Robert Jackson, Eva Janecek, Dr. Peter Jessamine, Dr. Jean Maroun, Dr. Les Meissner, Dr. Maurice Mishkel, Dr. Carl Nimrod, Dr. Teik Ooi, Dr. Dilip Patel, Dr. John Peachey, Dr. Anita Pedvic-Leftick, Dr. Robert Peterson, Dr. Hyman Rabinovitch, Dr. Robert Rivington, Dr. Ray Saginur, Dr. Shailendra Verma, Dr. Gary Victor, and Dr. Oleg Zadorozny.

Jack Armstrong, MD, FRCPC
President
Canadian Medical Association

CONTENTS

Introduction   8

1 UNDERSTANDING AND USING DRUGS

What are drugs?   12

How drugs are classified   13

How drugs work   14

Methods of administration   17

Drug treatment in special risk groups   20

Drug dependence   23

Managing your drug therapy   25

2 DRUG FINDER INDEX

Color identification guide   34

Index of medications   49

3 MAJOR DRUG GROUPS

Brain and nervous system   90

Respiratory system   103

Heart and circulation   107

Gastrointestinal tract   118
Muscles, bones and joints   127
Allergy   135
Infections and infestations   138
Hormones and endocrine system   152
Nutrition   160
Malignant and immune disease   164
Reproductive and urinary tracts   170
Eyes and ears   179
Skin   184

4 A – Z OF DRUGS

A – Z of medical drugs   194
A – Z of vitamins and minerals   518
Drugs of abuse   531
Food additives   539

5 GLOSSARY AND INDEX

Glossary   546
General index   552

DRUG POISONING EMERGENCY GUIDE 574

INTRODUCTION

The *Canadian Medical Association New Guide to Prescription and Over-the-Counter Drugs* has been planned and written to provide clear information and practical advice on drugs and medicines in a way that can be readily understood by a non-medical reader. The text reflects current medical knowledge and standard medical practice in Canada. It is intended to complement and reinforce the advice of your physician.

How the book is structured

The book is divided into five parts. The first part, Understanding and Using Drugs, provides a general introduction to the effects of drugs and gives general advice on practical questions such as the administration and storage of drugs. The second part, the Drug Finder Index, provides the means of locating information on specific drugs. Part 3, Major Drug Groups, will help you to understand the uses and mechanisms of action of the principal classes of drugs. Part 4, the A-Z of Drugs, consists of detailed profiles of commonly prescribed drugs, and also includes special profiles on vitamins and minerals, drugs of abuse, and food additives. Part contains a glossary of drug-related terms and a general index.

Finding your way into the book

The information you require, whether on the specific characteristics of an individual drug or on the general effects and uses of a group of drugs, can be easily obtained without prior knowledge of the medical names of drugs or drug classification through one of the two indexes: the Drug Finder Index or the General Index. The diagram on the facing page shows how you can access informatio throughout the book on the subject concerning yo from each of these starting points.

1 UNDERSTANDING AND USING DRUGS

The introductory part of the book, Understanding and Using Drugs, gives a grounding in the fundamental principles underlying the medical use of drugs. Covering such topics as the classification of drugs, mechanisms of action and the proper use of medications, it provides valuable background information that backs up the more detailed descriptions and advice given in Parts 3 and 4. Read this section before seeking further specific information.

2 DRUG FINDER INDEX

This is composed of two elements. The Color Identification Guide contains photographs of over 250 brand-name tablets and capsules to help you identify medications. The Index of Medications helps you to find information on specific drugs.

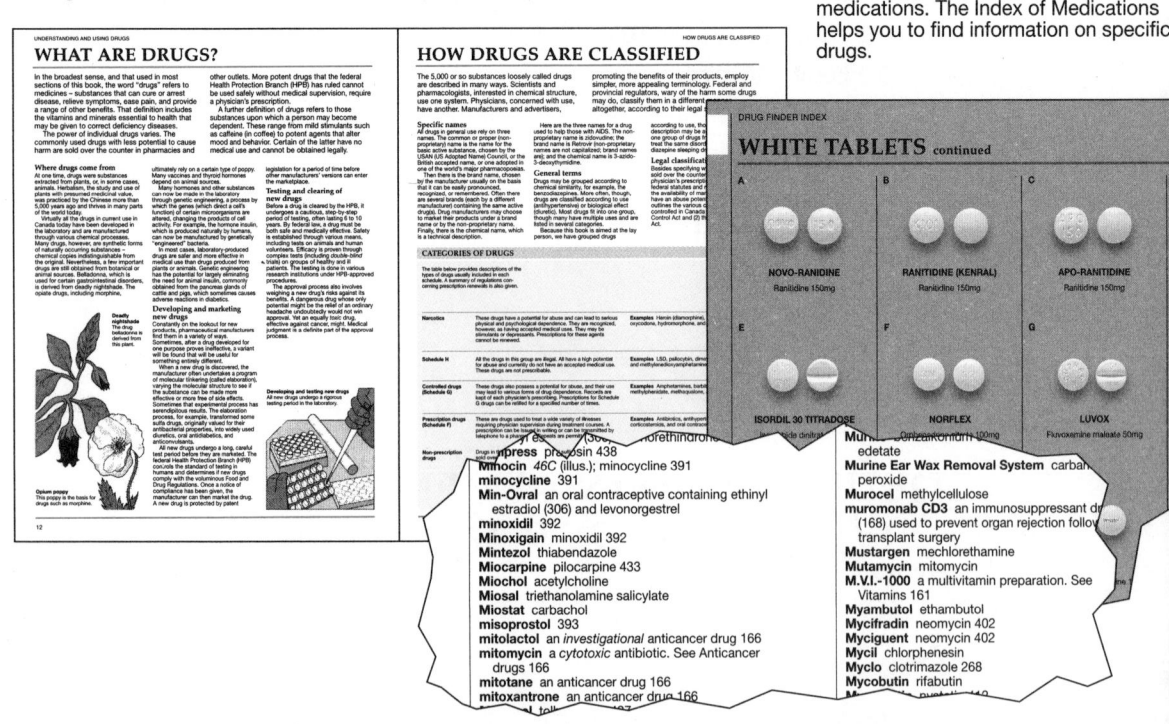

Finding your information

Whether you start by looking up an individual drug or a group of drugs, you will be led by cross-references to relevant information in all parts of the book.

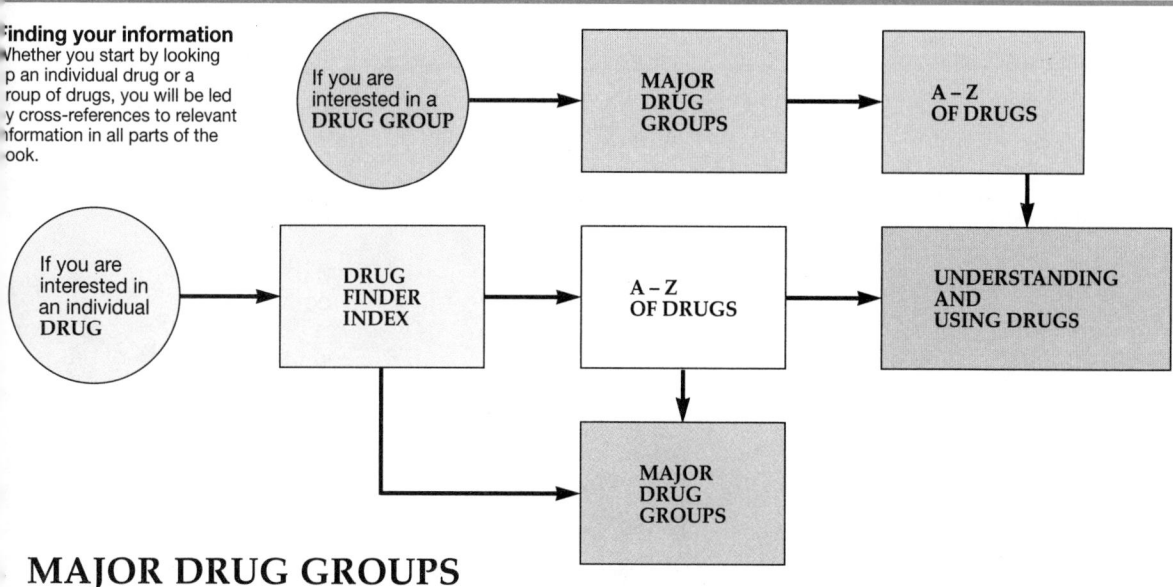

If you are interested in a **DRUG GROUP** → **MAJOR DRUG GROUPS** → **A – Z OF DRUGS**

If you are interested in an individual **DRUG** → **DRUG FINDER INDEX** → **A – Z OF DRUGS** → **UNDERSTANDING AND USING DRUGS**

MAJOR DRUG GROUPS

MAJOR DRUG GROUPS

...ubdivided into sections dealing with each body system (for example, heart and circulation) or major disease grouping or example, malignant and immune isease), this part of the book contains escriptions of the principal classes of drugs. Information is given on the uses, actions, effects, and risks associated with each group of drugs and is backed up by helpful illustrations and diagrams. Individual drugs in each group are listed to allow cross-reference to Part 4.

4 A – Z OF DRUGS

This part contains descriptions of individual drugs. The main listing includes 320 drug profiles written to standard format to help you find specific information quickly and easily. Cross-references to the relevant major drug groups are provided. Supplementary sections profile vitamins and minerals, drugs of abuse, and food additives.

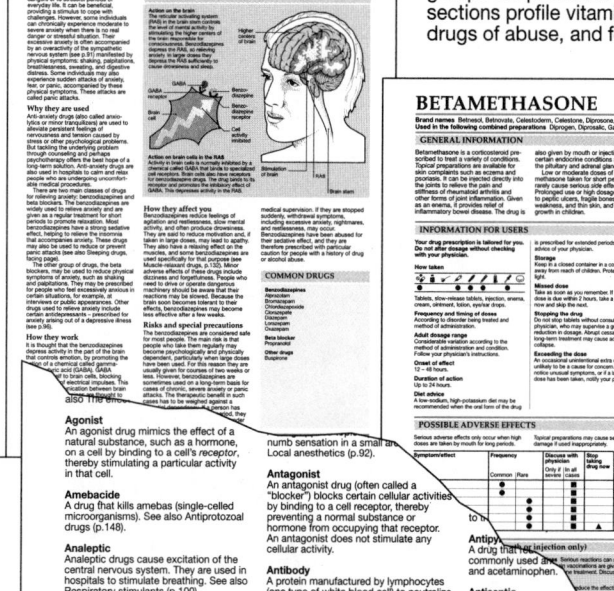

GLOSSARY AND INDEX

...he glossary explains technical words, rinted in italics in the text. The general dex enables you to look up references roughout the book.

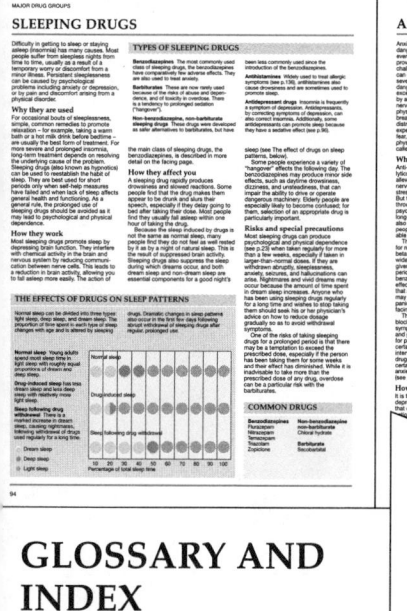

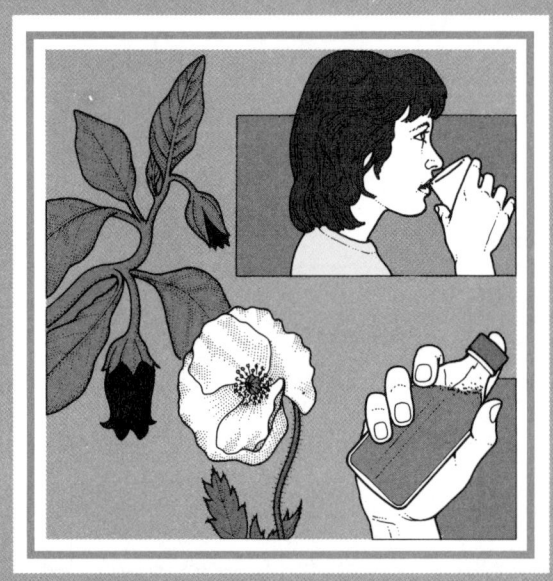

1

UNDERSTANDING AND USING DRUGS

WHAT ARE DRUGS?
HOW DRUGS ARE CLASSIFIED
HOW DRUGS WORK
METHODS OF ADMINISTRATION
DRUG TREATMENT IN SPECIAL RISK GROUPS
DRUG DEPENDENCE
MANAGING YOUR DRUG THERAPY

WHAT ARE DRUGS?

In the broadest sense, and that used in most sections of this book, the word "drugs" refers to medicines – substances that can cure or arrest disease, relieve symptoms, ease pain, and provide a range of other benefits. That definition includes the vitamins and minerals essential to health that may be given to correct deficiency diseases.

The power of individual drugs varies. The commonly used drugs with less potential to cause harm are sold over the counter in pharmacies and other outlets. More potent drugs that the federal Health Protection Branch (HPB) has ruled cannot be used safely without medical supervision, require a physician's prescription.

A further definition of drugs refers to those substances upon which a person may become dependent. These range from mild stimulants such as caffeine (in coffee) to potent agents that alter mood and behavior. Certain of the latter have no medical use and cannot be obtained legally.

Where drugs come from

At one time, drugs were substances extracted from plants, or, in some cases, animals. Herbalism, the study and use of plants with presumed medicinal value, was practiced by the Chinese more than 5,000 years ago and thrives in many parts of the world today.

Virtually all the drugs in current use in Canada today have been developed in the laboratory and are manufactured through various chemical processes. Many drugs, however, are synthetic forms of naturally occurring substances – chemical copies indistinguishable from the original. Nevertheless, a few important drugs are still obtained from botanical or animal sources. Belladonna, which is used for certain gastrointestinal disorders, is derived from deadly nightshade. The opiate drugs, including morphine,

ultimately rely on a certain type of poppy. Many vaccines and thyroid hormones depend on animal sources.

Many hormones and other substances can now be made in the laboratory through genetic engineering, a process by which the genes (which direct a cell's function) of certain microorganisms are altered, changing the products of cell activity. For example, the hormone insulin, which is produced naturally by humans, can now be manufactured by genetically "engineered" bacteria.

In most cases, laboratory-produced drugs are safer and more effective in medical use than drugs produced from plants or animals. Genetic engineering has the potential for largely eliminating the need for animal insulin, commonly obtained from the pancreas glands of cattle and pigs, which sometimes causes adverse reactions in diabetics.

Developing and marketing new drugs

Constantly on the lookout for new products, pharmaceutical manufacturers find them in a variety of ways. Sometimes, after a drug developed for one purpose proves ineffective, a variant will be found that will be useful for something entirely different.

When a new drug is discovered, the manufacturer often undertakes a program of molecular tinkering (called elaboration), varying the molecular structure to see if the substance can be made more effective or more free of side effects. Sometimes that experimental process has serendipitous results. The elaboration process, for example, transformed some sulfa drugs, originally valued for their antibacterial properties, into widely used diuretics, oral antidiabetics, and anticonvulsants.

All new drugs undergo a long, careful test period before they are marketed. The federal Health Protection Branch (HPB) controls the standard of testing in humans and determines if new drugs comply with the voluminous Food and Drug Regulations. Once a notice of compliance has been given, the manufacturer can then market the drug. A new drug is protected by patent

legislation for a period of time before other manufacturers' versions can enter the marketplace.

Testing and clearing of new drugs

Before a drug is cleared by the HPB, it undergoes a cautious, step-by-step period of testing, often lasting 6 to 10 years. By federal law, a drug must be both safe and medically effective. Safety is established through various means, including tests on animals and human volunteers. Efficacy is proven through complex tests (including *double-blind* trials) on groups of healthy and ill patients. The testing is done in various research institutions under HPB-approved procedures.

The approval process also involves weighing a new drug's risks against its benefits. A dangerous drug whose only potential might be the relief of an ordinary headache undoubtedly would not win approval. Yet an equally *toxic* drug, effective against cancer, might. Medical judgment is a definite part of the approval process.

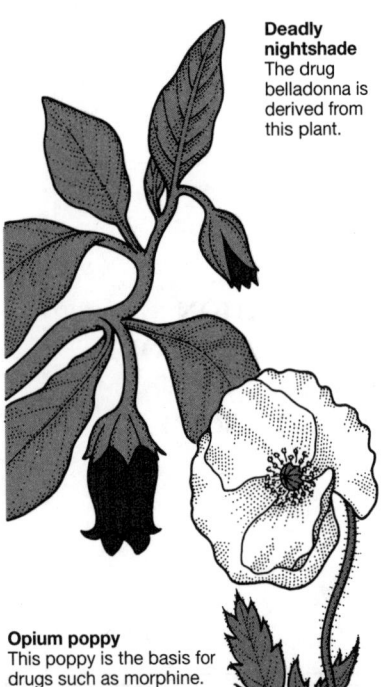

Deadly nightshade
The drug belladonna is derived from this plant.

Opium poppy
This poppy is the basis for drugs such as morphine.

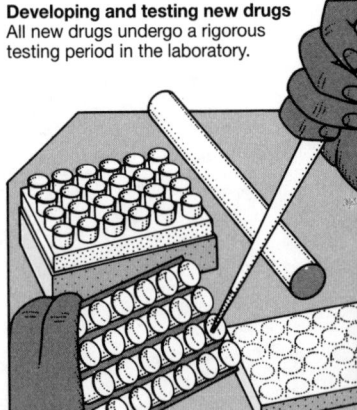

Developing and testing new drugs
All new drugs undergo a rigorous testing period in the laboratory.

HOW DRUGS ARE CLASSIFIED

The 5,000 or so substances loosely called drugs are described in many ways. Scientists and pharmacologists, interested in chemical structure, use one system. Physicians, concerned with use, have another. Manufacturers and advertisers, promoting the benefits of their products, employ simpler, more appealing terminology. Federal and provincial regulators, wary of the harm some drugs may do, classify them in a different manner altogether, according to their legal status.

Specific names

All drugs in general use rely on three names. The common or proper (non-proprietary) name is the name for the basic active substance, chosen by the USAN (US Adopted Name) Council, or the British accepted name, or one adopted in one of the world's major pharmacopoeias.

Then there is the brand name, chosen by the manufacturer usually on the basis that it can be easily pronounced, recognized, or remembered. Often there are several brands (each by a different manufacturer) containing the same active drug(s). Drug manufacturers may choose to market their products under a brand name or by the non-proprietary name. Finally, there is the chemical name, which is a technical description.

Here are the three names for a drug used to help those with AIDS. The non-proprietary name is zidovudine; the brand name is Retrovir (non-proprietary names are not capitalized; brand names are); and the chemical name is 3-azido-3-deoxythymidine.

General terms

Drugs may be grouped according to chemical similarity, for example, the benzodiazepines. More often, though, drugs are classified according to use (antihypertensive) or biological effect (diuretic). Most drugs fit into one group, though many have multiple uses and are listed in several categories.

Because this book is aimed at the lay person, we have grouped drugs according to use, though a chemical description may be added to distinguish one group of drugs from others used to treat the same disorder (e.g., benzo-diazepine sleeping drugs).

Legal classification

Besides specifying which drugs can be sold over the counter and which require a physician's prescription, provincial and federal statutes and regulations govern the availability of many substances which have an abuse potential. The table below outlines the various categories of drugs controlled in Canada by: (1) the Narcotic Control Act and (2) the Food and Drugs Act.

CATEGORIES OF DRUGS

The table below provides descriptions of the types of drugs usually included in each schedule. A summary of regulations concerning prescription renewals is also given.

Narcotics	These drugs have a potential for abuse and can lead to serious physical and psychological dependence. They are recognized, however, as having accepted medical uses. They may be stimulants or depressants. Prescriptions for these agents cannot be renewed.	**Examples** Heroin (diamorphine), morphine, codeine, oxycodone, hydromorphone, and meperidine.
Schedule H	All the drugs in this group are illegal. All have a high potential for abuse and currently do not have an accepted medical use. These drugs are not prescribable.	**Examples** LSD, psilocybin, dimethyltryptamine (DMT), and methylenedioxyamphetamine (MDA).
Controlled drugs (Schedule G)	These drugs also possess a potential for abuse, and their use may lead to various forms of drug dependence. Records are kept of each physician's prescribing. Prescriptions for Schedule G drugs can be refilled for a specified number of times.	**Examples** Amphetamines, barbiturates, methylphenidate, methaqualone, and diethylpropion.
Prescription drugs (Schedule F)	These are drugs used to treat a wide variety of illnesses requiring physician supervision during treatment courses. A prescription can be issued in writing or can be transmitted by telephone to a pharmacist. Repeats are permitted.	**Examples** Antibiotics, antihypertensive drugs, corticosteroids, and oral contraceptives.
Non-prescription drugs	Drugs in this category are considered sufficiently safe to be sold over the counter in pharmacies and other outlets. Most non-prescription drug products sold in pharmacies bear a DIN number, but similar preparations sold in other outlets carry a GP designation with a number following it. Although preparations of acetaminophen and ASA usually carry a DIN number, exceptions are made depending on the dosage, which allow some to be sold in outlets other than pharmacies.	**Examples** Laxatives, antacids, skin preparations, mild analgesics. (Small doses of codeine, a substance normally regarded as a narcotic drug, can be combined with other medications such as ASA and sold in pharmacies in limited quantities without a prescription.)

HOW DRUGS WORK

The vast array of drugs available to the modern physician has been developed, for the most part, in the last 50 years. Today, there are drugs that ease the painful symptoms of disease, drugs that make disorders like hypertension manageable, drugs that soothe inflammation, relieve anxieties, and bolster the body's natural defenses.

Before the discovery of the sulfa drugs in 1935, the physician's knowledge of drugs was limited. At that time, possibly only a dozen or so drugs had clear medical value. That, of course, has changed. Not only is an impressive variety of effective drugs now available, scientific knowledge in the drug field has virtually exploded.

Today's physician understands far better than his or her predecessors the complex actions of drugs in the body and the effects drugs can have on it, both beneficial and adverse. He or she can also recognize that some drugs interact harmfully with others, or with certain foods and alcohol.

DRUG ACTIONS

While the exact workings of some drugs are not fully understood, medical science provides clear knowledge as to what most of them do once they enter or are applied to the human body. Drugs, of course, serve different purposes, sometimes curing a disease, sometimes only alleviating symptoms. Their impact occurs in various parts of the anatomy. But although different drugs act in different ways, their actions generally fall into one of three categories.

Replacing chemicals that are deficient

To function normally, the body requires sufficient levels of certain chemical substances. These include vitamins and minerals, which the body obtains from food. A balanced diet usually supplies what is needed. But when deficiencies occur, various deficiency diseases result. Lack of vitamin C causes scurvy, lack of vitamin D leads to rickets, and iron deficiency causes anemia.

Other deficiency diseases arise from a lack of various *hormones*, chemical substances produced by glands which act as internal "messengers." Diabetes mellitus, Addison's disease, and hypo-thyroidism all result from deficiencies of different hormones.

Deficiency diseases are treated with drugs that replace the substances that are missing, or, in the case of some hormone deficiencies, with animal or synthetic replacements.

Interfering with cell function

Many drugs can change the way cells work by stimulating or reducing the normal level of activity. Vaccines, for example, function in this way by increasing the activity of the cells that produce the antibodies that fight invading organisms such as bacteria and viruses. Drugs that act in a similar manner are used in the treatment of a variety of conditions: hormone disorders, blood clotting problems, heart and kidney diseases.

Many such drugs do their work by altering the transmission system by which messages are sent from one part of the body to another.

A message – to contract a muscle, say – originates in the brain and enters a nerve cell through its receiving end. The message, in the form of an electrical impulse, travels the length of the nerve cell to the sending end. Here a chemical substance called a *neurotransmitter* is released, conducting the message across the tiny gap separating it from an adjacent nerve cell. That process is repeated until the message reaches the appropriate muscle.

Many drugs can alter this process, often by their effect on receptor sites on cells (see the box, left). Some drugs (*agonists*) intensify cell activity, while other drugs (*antagonists*) reduce activity in the cells.

Acting against invading organisms or abnormal cells

Many microorganisms are able to invade the body and cause infection. Some drugs destroy these microorganisms, either by preventing their multiplication or by killing them directly. Other drugs treat disease by killing abnormal cells – cancer cells, for example.

RECEPTOR SITES

Many drugs are thought to produce their effects by their action on special sites called receptors on the surface of body cells. Natural body chemicals such as *neurotransmitters* bind to these sites, initiating a response in the cell. Cells may have many types of receptors, each of which has an affinity for a different chemical in the body. Drugs may also bind to receptors, either adding to the effect of the body's natural chemicals and enhancing cell response (agonist drugs) or preventing such a chemical from binding to its receptor, and thereby blocking a particular cell response (antagonist drugs).

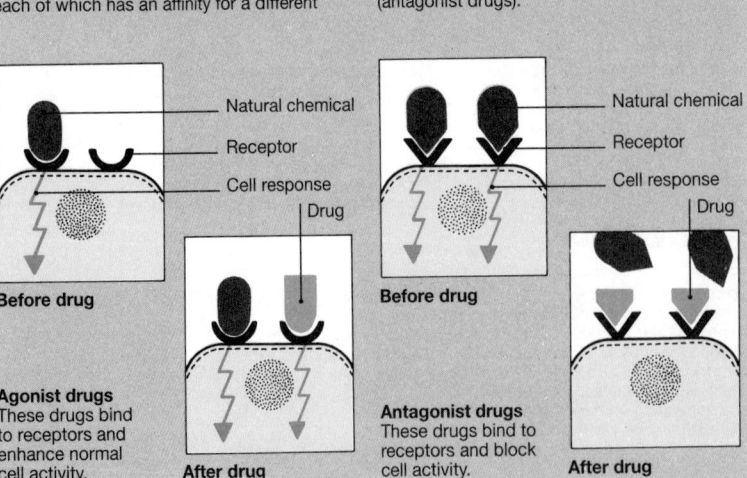

Natural chemical
Receptor
Cell response
Drug

Before drug

Agonist drugs
These drugs bind to receptors and enhance normal cell activity.

After drug

Natural chemical
Receptor
Cell response
Drug

Before drug

Antagonist drugs
These drugs bind to receptors and block cell activity.

After drug

THE EFFECTS OF DRUGS

Before a physician selects a drug to be used in the treatment of a sick person, he or she carefully weighs the benefits and the risks. Obviously, the physician expects a positive result from the drug, a cure of the condition or at least the relief of symptoms. At the same time, consideration has to be given to the risks, for all drugs are potentially harmful, some of them considerably more so than others.

Reaction time

Some drugs can produce rapid and spectacular relief from the symptoms of disease. Nitroglycerin frequently provides almost immediate relief for the pain of angina; other drugs can quickly alleviate the symptoms of an asthmatic attack. Conversely, some drugs take much longer to produce a response. It may, for example, require several weeks of treatment with an antidepressant drug before a person experiences maximum benefit. This can be worrisome unless the physician has warned of the possibility of a delay in the onset of beneficial effects.

Side effects

The side effects of a drug are the known and frequently experienced, expected reactions to a drug. The old concept of a drug as a "magic bullet" that could be targeted to a specific type of cell is now recognized as inaccurate. Whether a drug is taken by mouth, by injection, or by inhalation, it will be distributed throughout the body, and its effects are unlikely to be restricted to one particular type of tissue or organ.

For example, *anticholinergic* drugs, which are prescribed to relieve spasm in the wall of the intestine, may also affect the eyes, causing blurred vision; the mouth, causing dryness; and the bladder, causing the retention of urine. Such side effects may gradually disappear as the body becomes used to the drug. But if side effects persist, the dose of the drug may have to be reduced, or the time between doses may have to be increased.

DOSE AND RESPONSE

Not everyone responds in the same way to a drug, and in many cases the dose has to be adjusted to allow for such factors as the age, weight, or general heath of the patient. The dose of any drug should be sufficient to produce a beneficial response but not so great that it will cause excessive adverse effects. If the dose is too low, the drug may not have any effect, either beneficial or adverse; if it is too high, it will not produce any additional benefits and may produce adverse effects. The aim of drug treatment, therefore, is to achieve a concentration of drug in the blood or tissue that lies somewhere between the minimum effective level and the maximum safe concentration. This is known as the therapeutic range.

For certain drugs, such as digoxin, the therapeutic range is quite narrow, so the margin of safety/effectiveness is small. Other drugs, such as penicillin antibiotics, have a much wider therapeutic range.

Wide therapeutic range

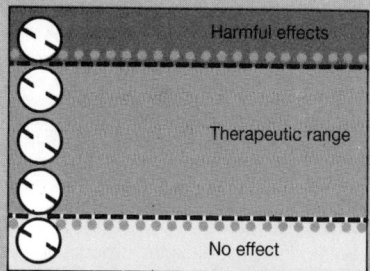

Dosage of drugs with a wide therapeutic range can vary considerably without altering the drug's effects.

Narrow therapeutic range

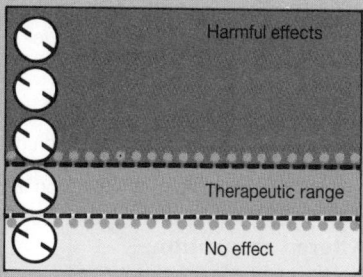

Dosage of drugs with a narrow therapeutic range has to be carefully calculated to achieve the desired effect.

The side effects of certain drugs, especially some anticancer drugs, can often be quite serious. Such drugs are administered because they may be the only agents available for the treatment of a disease that might otherwise prove fatal. However, all drugs, even the mildest, should be regarded as chemicals with a potential for producing serious, *toxic* reactions, especially if they are misused or abused.

Adverse reactions

Adverse reactions are unexpected, unpredictable reactions that are not related to the usual effects of a normal dose of a drug. Unpredictable drug reactions may be caused by conditions in the patient such as an allergy or a genetic disorder, like the absence of an *enzyme* that usually inactivates the drug. Common adverse reactions of this type include a rash, swelling of the face, or jaundice. They may also be due to interactions with other drugs. Unpredictable drug reactions usually necessitate withdrawal of the drug under medical supervision.

Beneficial vs. adverse effects

In evaluating the risk/benefit ratio of a drug which he or she may prescribe, a physician weighs the therapeutic benefit to the sick person against the possible adverse effects. For example, such side effects as nausea, headache, and diarrhea may result from taking an antibiotic. But they will certainly be considered acceptable risks if the problem is a life-threatening infection requiring immediate treatment. On the other hand, such side effects would be considered unacceptable for an oral contraceptive that is taken over a number of years by a healthy patient.

Because some people are more at risk from adverse drug reactions than others (particularly those with a history of drug allergy), the physician normally checks whether there is any reason why a particular drug should not be given (see Drug therapy in special risk groups, p.20).

PLACEBO RESPONSE

The word placebo – Latin for "I will please" – is used to describe any chemically inert substance given as a substitute for a drug. Any benefit gained from taking a placebo occurs because the person taking it believes that it will produce good results.

New drugs are almost always tested against a placebo preparation in clinical trials as a way to assess the efficacy of a drug before it is marketed. The placebo is made to look identical to the active preparation, and volunteers are not told whether they have been given the active drug or the placebo. Sometimes the physician is also unaware of which preparation an individual has been given. This is known as a *double-blind* trial. In this way, the purely placebo effect can be eliminated and the effectiveness of the drug determined more realistically.

Sometimes the mere taking of a medicine has a psychological effect that produces a beneficial physical response. This type of placebo response can make an important contribution to the overall effectiveness of a chemically active drug, and is most commonly seen with analgesics, antidepressants, and anti-anxiety drugs. Some people, known as placebo responders, are more likely to experience this sort of reaction than the rest of the population.

DRUG INTERACTIONS

When two different drugs are taken together, or when a drug is taken in combination with certain foods or with alcohol, this may produce effects different from those produced when the drug is taken alone. In many cases, this is beneficial, and physicians frequently make use of interactions to increase the effectiveness of a treatment. Very often, more than one drug may be prescribed to treat cancer or high blood pressure (hypertension).

Other interactions, however, are unwanted and may be harmful. They may occur not only between prescription drugs, but also between prescription and over-the-counter drugs. So it is important to read warnings on drug labels and tell your physician if you are taking any drug preparations – both prescription and over-the-counter – that the physician does not know about.

A drug may interact with another drug or with food or alcohol for a number of reasons. The main types of interaction are discussed below.

Altered absorption

Alcohol and some drugs (especially narcotics) slow down the digestive process that empties the stomach contents into the intestine. This may delay the absorption, and therefore the effect, of another drug taken at the same time.

Other drugs (for example, metoclopramide, an anti-emetic drug) may speed the rate at which the stomach empties and therefore may increase the rate at which another drug is absorbed and takes effect.

Some drugs also combine with another drug or a food in the intestine to form a compound that is not so readily absorbed. This occurs when tetracycline and iron tablets or antacids are taken together. Milk also reduces the absorption of certain drugs in this way.

Reduced absorption in the intestine

Absorption of drug (A) through the intestinal wall may be reduced if it combines with another drug (B).

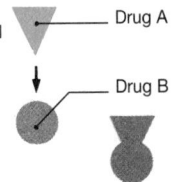

Drug A

Drug B

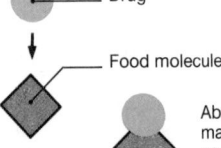

Drug

Food molecule

Absorption of a drug may be reduced if it combines with a food molecule.

EXAMPLES OF IMPORTANT INTERACTIONS

Adverse interactions between drugs may vary from a simple blocking of a drug's beneficial effect to a serious reaction between two drugs which may be life-threatening. Some of the more serious adverse interactions occur between the following:

Drugs that depress the central nervous system (sleeping drugs, narcotics, anti-histamines, and alcohol). The effects of two or more of these drugs in combination may be additive, causing dangerous oversedation.

Drugs that lower blood sugar levels and such drugs as sulfonamides and alcohol. The drug interaction increases the effect of blood sugar-lowering drugs, thus further depressing blood sugar levels.

Oral anticoagulants and other drugs, particularly ASA and antibiotics. Because these drugs may increase the tendency to bleed, it is essential to check the effects in every case.

Monoamine oxidase inhibitors (MAOIs). Many drugs (e.g., amphetamines, decongestants) and foods (e.g., cheese, pickled herring, red wine, beer, and chocolate) can produce a severe rise in blood pressure when taken with MAOIs. However, newer MAOIs have been developed which are much less likely to interact with food and drugs.

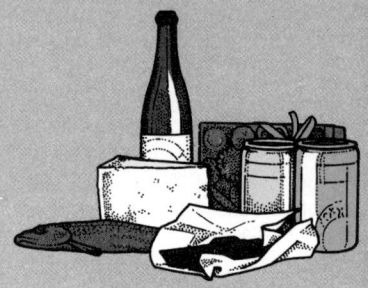

Enzyme effects

Some drugs increase the production of *enzymes* in the liver that break down drugs, while others may inhibit or reduce enzyme production. They therefore affect the rate at which other drugs are activated or inactivated.

Excretion in the urine

A drug may reduce the kidneys' ability to excrete another drug, thereby raising the level of the drug in the blood and increasing its effect.

Receptor effects

Drugs which act on the same *receptor* sites (p.14) sometimes redouble each other's stimulating effect on the body. Or they may compete with each other in occupying particular receptor sites. Naloxone, for instance, blocks the receptors used by narcotic drugs, thereby helping to reverse the effects of narcotic poisoning.

Similar effects

Drugs that produce similar effects (even though they do not act on the same receptor) may be given together so that a smaller dose of each is required, reducing the side effects of each. This is common practice in the treatment of high blood pressure, in giving anticancer drugs, and also in treating pain. Sometimes two antibiotics may be given simultaneously. Though their effects may be similar, the infecting organisms are less likely to develop resistance.

Reduced protein binding

Some drugs circulate around the body in the bloodstream with a proportion of the drug attached to the proteins of the blood plasma. The drug attached to plasma proteins is inactive. If another drug is taken, some of the second drug may also attach itself to the plasma proteins and displace the first drug, making more of the first drug active in the body.

Interaction between protein-bound drugs

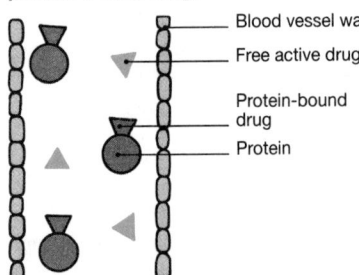

Blood vessel wall

Free active drug

Protein-bound drug

Protein

Protein-bound drug taken alone
Drug molecules that are bound to proteins in the blood are unable to pass into body tissues. Only free drug molecules are active.

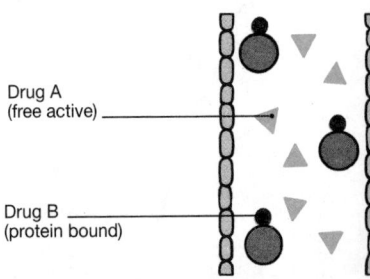

Drug A (free active)

Drug B (protein bound)

Taken with another protein-bound drug
If a drug (B) with a greater ability to bind with proteins is also taken, the first drug (A) is displaced, increasing the amount of active drug.

METHODS OF ADMINISTRATION

To be effective, the majority of drugs must be absorbed into the bloodstream in order to reach the site where their effects are needed. The method of administering a drug determines the route it takes to get into the bloodstream and the speed at which it is absorbed into the blood.

When a drug is meant to enter the bloodstream it is usually administered in one of the following ways: through the mouth or rectum, by injection, or inhalation. Drugs implanted under the skin or enclosed in a skin patch also enter the bloodstream. These are discussed under Slow-release preparations (p.18).

When it is unnecessary or undesirable for a drug to enter the bloodstream in large amounts, it may be applied *topically* so that its effect is limited mainly to the site of the disorder, such as the surface of the skin or mucous membranes (the

membranes of the nose, eyes, ears, mouth, vagina, or rectum). Drugs are administered topically in a variety of preparations, including creams, sprays, drops, and suppositories. Most inhaled drugs also have a local effect on the respiratory tract.

Very often, a particular drug may be available in different forms. Many drugs are available as tablets and injectable fluid. The choice between a tablet or an injection depends on a number of factors, including the severity of the illness, the urgency with which the drug effect is needed, the part of the body requiring treatment, and the patient's general state of health, in particular his or her ability to swallow.

The various routes of administration are discussed in greater detail below. For a description of the different forms in which drugs are given, see Drug forms (p.19).

ADMINISTRATION BY MOUTH

Giving drugs by mouth is the most frequently used method of administration. Most drugs that are given by mouth are absorbed into the bloodstream through the walls of the intestine. The speed at which the drug is absorbed and the amount of active drug that is available for use depend on several factors, including the form in which it is given (for example, as a tablet or a liquid) and

whether it is taken with food or on an empty stomach. If a drug is taken when the stomach is empty (before meals, for example) it may act more quickly than a drug that is taken after a meal when the stomach is full.

Some drugs (like antacids, which neutralize stomach acidity) are taken by mouth to produce a direct effect on the stomach or digestive tract.

Sublingual tablets
Tablets are available that are placed in the mouth but not swallowed. They are absorbed quickly into the bloodstream through the lining of the mouth, which has a rich supply of blood vessels. Both sublingual and buccal tablets act in this way. Sublingual tablets are placed under the tongue; buccal tablets are placed in the pouch between the cheek and teeth.

HOW DRUGS PASS THROUGH THE BODY

Most drugs taken by mouth reach the bloodstream by absorption through the small intestine wall. Blood vessels supplying the intestine then carry the drug to the liver where it may be broken down into a form that can be used by the body. The drug (or its breakdown product) then enters into the general circulation, which carries it around the body. It may pass back to the intestine before it is reabsorbed into the bloodstream. Some drugs are rapidly excreted via the kidneys; others may build up in fatty tissues in the body.

Certain insoluble drugs cannot be absorbed through the intestine and pass through the digestive tract unchanged. They are useful for treating bowel disorders, but if they are intended to have *systemic* effects elsewhere they must be given by intravenous injection.

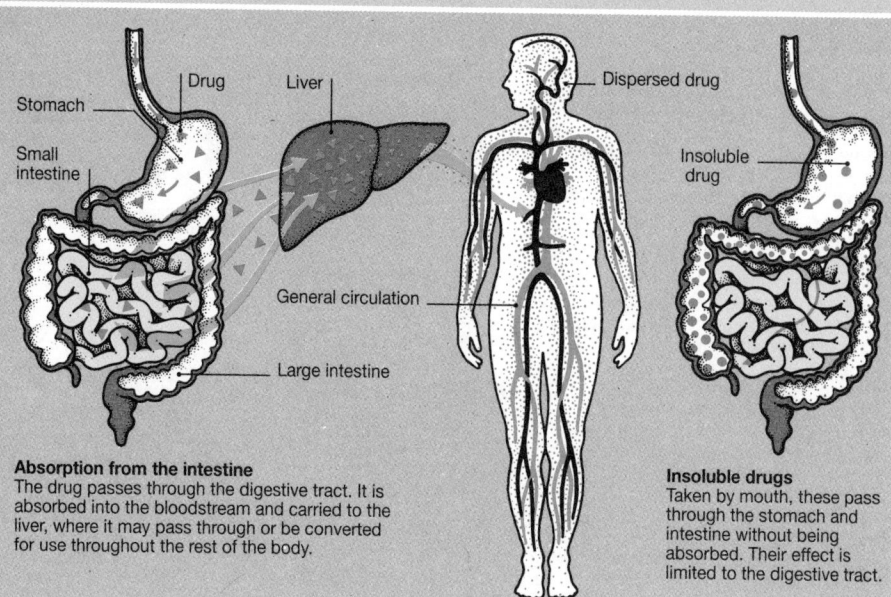

Absorption from the intestine
The drug passes through the digestive tract. It is absorbed into the bloodstream and carried to the liver, where it may pass through or be converted for use throughout the rest of the body.

Insoluble drugs
Taken by mouth, these pass through the stomach and intestine without being absorbed. Their effect is limited to the digestive tract.

RECTAL ADMINISTRATION

Drugs intended to have a *systemic* effect may be given in the form of suppositories inserted into the rectum, from where they are absorbed into the bloodstream. This method may be used to give drugs that might be destroyed by the stomach's digestive juices. It is also sometimes used to administer drugs to people who cannot take medication by mouth, such as those suffering from nausea and vomiting.

Drugs may also be given rectally for local effect, either as suppositories (to relieve hemorrhoids) or as enemas (for ulcerative colitis).

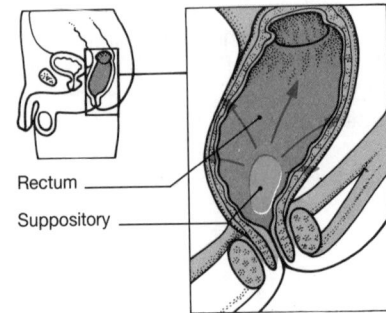

Rectal _____

Suppository _____

INHALATION

Drugs may be inhaled to produce a *systemic* effect or a direct local effect on the respiratory tract.

Gases to produce general anesthesia are administered by inhalation and are absorbed into the bloodstream through the lungs, producing a general effect on the body, particularly the brain.

Bronchodilators, used to treat certain types of asthma, emphysema, and bronchitis, are a common example of drugs administered by inhalation for their direct effect on the respiratory tract, although some of the active drug also reaches the bloodstream.

ADMINISTRATION BY INJECTION

Drugs may be injected into the body to produce a *systemic* effect. One reason for injecting drugs is the rapid response that follows. Other circumstances which call for injection are: a person's intolerance to a drug when taken by mouth; a drug's inability to resist inactivation by stomach acids (insulin is an example); the inability of the drug to pass through the intestinal walls into the bloodstream.

Drug injections may also be given to produce a local effect, as is often done to relieve the pain of arthritis.

The main types of injection – intramuscular, intravenous, and subcutaneous – are described in the illustration (see right). The type of injection depends on the nature of the drug and the condition being treated.

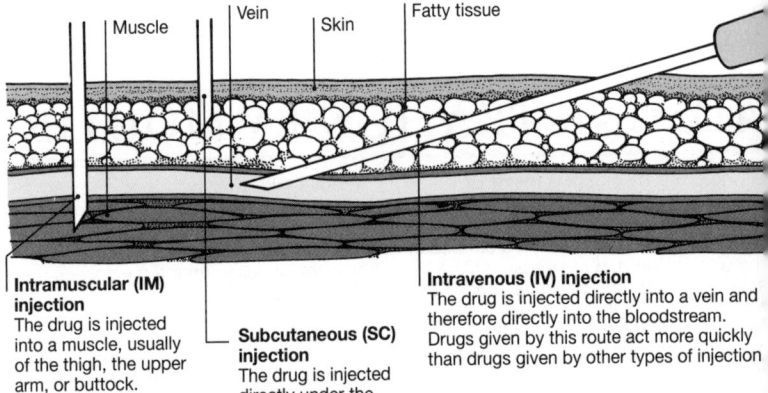

Muscle | Vein | Skin | Fatty tissue

Intramuscular (IM) injection
The drug is injected into a muscle, usually of the thigh, the upper arm, or buttock.

Subcutaneous (SC) injection
The drug is injected directly under the surface of the skin.

Intravenous (IV) injection
The drug is injected directly into a vein and therefore directly into the bloodstream. Drugs given by this route act more quickly than drugs given by other types of injection

TOPICAL APPLICATION

In treating localized disorders such as skin infections and nasal congestion, it is often preferable when a choice is available to prescribe drugs in a form that has a *topical*, or localized, rather than a *systemic* effect. The reason is that it is much easier to control the effects of drugs administered locally and to ensure that they produce the maximum benefit with minimum side effects.

Topical preparations are available in a variety of forms, from skin creams, ointments, and lotions to vaginal suppositories, inhalers, nasal sprays, and ear and eye drops. It is important when using topical preparations to follow instructions carefully, avoiding a higher dose than recommended or application for longer than necessary. This will help avoid adverse systemic effects caused by the absorption of larger amounts into the bloodstream.

SLOW-RELEASE PREPARATIONS

A number of disorders can be treated with drug preparations that have been specially formulated to release their active drug slowly over a given period of time. Such preparations may be beneficial when it is inconvenient for a person to visit the physician on a regular basis to receive treatment by injection, or when it is necessary to accurately control the release of small amounts of the drug into the body. Slow release of drugs can be achieved by *depot injections*, *transdermal patches*, slow-release capsules and tablets, and implants.

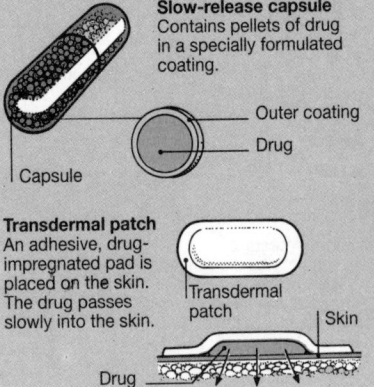

Slow-release capsule
Contains pellets of drug in a specially formulated coating.

Outer coating

Drug

Capsule

Transdermal patch
An adhesive, drug-impregnated pad is placed on the skin. The drug passes slowly into the skin.

Transdermal patch

Skin

Drug

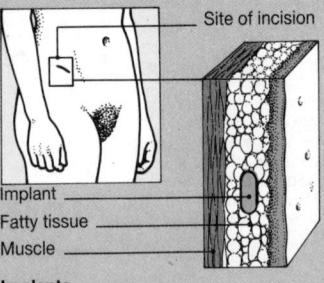

Site of incision

Implant
Fatty tissue
Muscle

Implants
A pellet containing the drug is implanted under the skin. By this rarely used method, a drug (usually a hormone) is slowly released into the bloodstream over a period of months.

DRUG FORMS

Most drugs are specially prepared in a form designed for convenience of administration. This helps to ensure that dosages are accurate and that taking the medication is as easy as possible. Other ingredients that, in most persons, have no therapeutic or adverse effect are sometimes added to flavor or color the medicine, or to improve its chemical stability, extending the period during which it is effective.

The more common drug forms are described in detail below.

Tablet

This contains the drug compressed into a solid dosage form, often round in shape. Other ingredients are added to the powder prior to compression, often including an agent to bind the tablet together (see right). In some tablets, the active drug is released slowly after the tablet has been swallowed whole, producing a prolonged (sustained) effect.

Capsule

The drug is contained in a cylindrically shaped gelatin shell that breaks open after the capsule has been swallowed, releasing the drug. Slow-release capsules contain pellets that dissolve in the gastrointestinal tract, releasing the drug slowly (facing page).

Liquids

Some drugs are available in liquid form, the active substance being combined in a solution, suspension, or emulsion with other ingredients – solvents, preservatives, and flavoring or coloring agents. Many liquid preparations should be shaken before use to ensure that the active drug is evenly distributed. If it is not, inaccurate dosages may result.

A mixture

A mixture contains one or more drugs, either dissolved to form a solution or suspended in a liquid (often water).

An elixir

An elixir is a solution of a drug, often highly flavored. It usually contains a high proportion of alcohol, plus sugar.

An emulsion

An emulsion is a drug dispersed in oil and water. An emulsifying agent is often included to stabilize the product.

A syrup

A syrup is a concentrated solution of sugar containing the active drug, with flavoring and stabilizing agents added.

Topical skin preparations

These are preparations designed for application to the skin and other surface tissues of the body. Preservatives are usually included to reduce the growth of

WHAT A TABLET CONTAINS

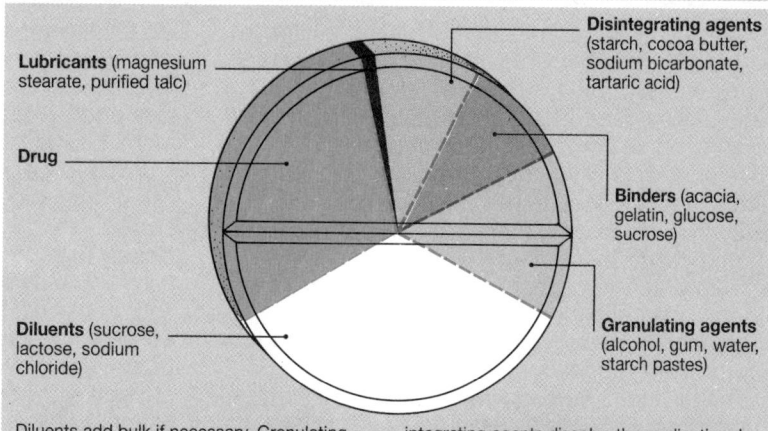

Disintegrating agents (starch, cocoa butter, sodium bicarbonate, tartaric acid)

Lubricants (magnesium stearate, purified talc)

Drug

Binders (acacia, gelatin, glucose, sucrose)

Diluents (sucrose, lactose, sodium chloride)

Granulating agents (alcohol, gum, water, starch pastes)

Diluents add bulk if necessary. Granulating agents and binders enable the ingredient to be formed into a tablet. Lubricants or a sugar coating ensure a smooth surface, and disintegrating agents dissolve the medication. In addition, coloring agents, dyes, and imprints are used to make the product recognizable. The proportions of each ingredient may vary.

bacteria. The most commonly used types of skin preparations are described below. For a more detailed discussion of the various preparations, see Bases for skin preparations, p.187.

A cream

A cream is a non-greasy preparation used to apply drugs to an area of the body or to cool or moisten the skin. It is less noticeable than an ointment.

An ointment

An ointment is a greasy preparation used to apply drugs to an area of the body, or as a protective or lubricant layer for dry skin conditions.

A lotion

A lotion is a solution or suspension applied to unbroken skin to cool and dry the area. Some are more suitable for use in hairy areas, since they are not as sticky as creams or ointments.

Injection solutions

Solutions for injections are sterile (germ-free) preparations of a drug dissolved or suspended in a liquid. Other agents (antioxidants) are often added to preserve the stability of the drug or to regulate the acidity or alkalinity of the solution. Most injectable drugs used today are packaged in sterile disposable syringes. This reduces chances of contamination. Certain drugs are still available in multiple-dose vials, and a chemical bactericide is added to prevent the growth of bacteria when the needle is reinserted through the rubber seal. For details on types of injection, see Administration by injection, facing page.

Suppository

A suppository is a solid, bullet-shaped dosage form specially designed for easy insertion into the rectum (rectal suppository) or vagina (vaginal suppository). It contains a drug and an inert (chemically inactive) substance that is often derived from cocoa butter or another type of vegetable oil. The active drug is gradually released in the rectum or vagina as the suppository dissolves at body temperature.

Eye drops

A sterile drug solution (or suspension) dropped behind the eyelid to produce an effect on the eye.

Ear drops

A solution (or suspension) containing a drug introduced into the ear by dropper. Ear drops are usually given to produce an effect on the outer ear canal.

Nasal drops/spray

A solution of a drug, usually in water, for introduction into the nose to produce a local effect.

Inhalers

Aerosol inhalers contain a solution or suspension of a drug under pressure. A valve mechanism ensures the delivery of the recommended dosage when the inhaler is activated. A mouthpiece fixed to the device facilitates inhalation of the drug as it is released from the canister. The correct technique is important; printed instructions should be followed carefully. Aerosol inhalers are used for respiratory conditions such as asthma (see also p.104).

DRUG THERAPY IN SPECIAL RISK GROUPS

Different people may respond in different ways to drug treatment. Taking the same drug, one person may suffer adverse effects while another experiences none. However, physicians know that certain people are always more at risk from adverse effects when they take drugs; the reason is that in those people the body handles drugs differently, or the drug has an atypical effect. Those people at special risk include infants and children, women who are pregnant or breast-feeding, the elderly, and people with long-term medical conditions, especially those who have impaired liver or kidney function.

The reasons that such people may be more likely to suffer adverse effects are discussed in detail on the following pages. Others who may need special attention include those already taking regular medication who may risk complications when they take another drug. Drug interactions are discussed more fully on p.16.

When physicians prescribe drugs for special risk groups they take extra care to select appropriate medication, adjust dosages, and closely monitor the effects of treatment. If you think you may be at special risk, be sure to tell your physician in case he or she is not fully aware of your particular circumstances. Similarly, before using over-the-counter medications ask your physician or pharmacist about possible adverse effects or hazardous drug interactions.

INFANTS AND CHILDREN

Infants and children need a lower dosage of drugs than adults because children have a relatively low body weight. Moreover, because of differences in body composition, as well as the distribution and amount of body fat, and differences in the state of development and function of organs such as the liver and kidneys at different ages, children cannot simply be given a proportion of an adult dose as if they were small adults. Dosages need to be calculated in a more complex way, taking account of both age and weight. Although newborn babies often have to be given very small doses of drugs, older children may need relatively large doses of some drugs.

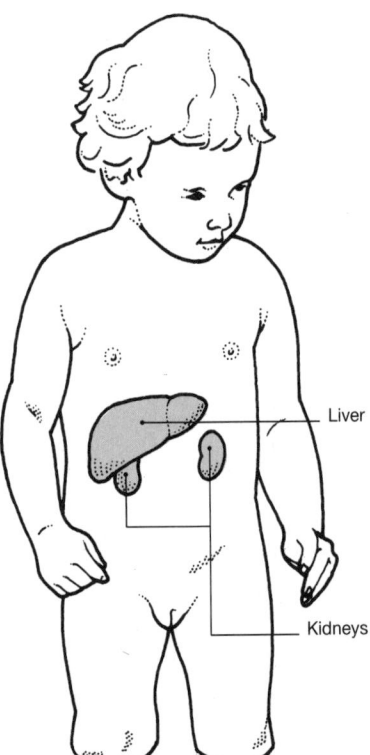

Liver

Kidneys

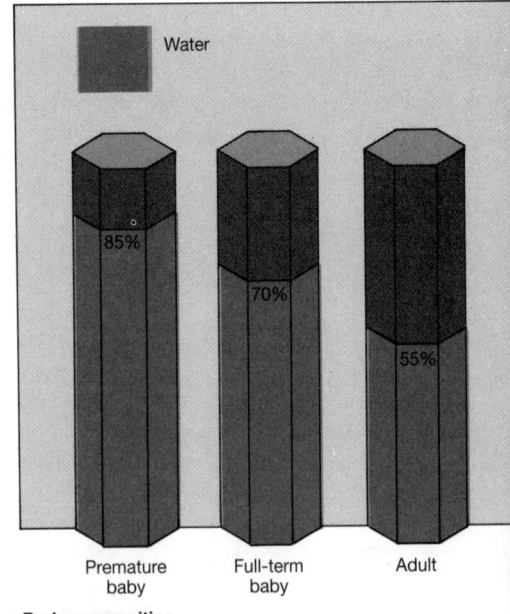

Water

85%

70%

55%

Premature baby

Full-term baby

Adult

The liver
The liver's enzyme systems are not fully developed when a baby is born. This means that drugs are not broken down as rapidly as in an adult, and may become dangerously concentrated in the baby's body. For this reason, many drugs are not prescribed for babies or are prescribed in very reduced doses. In older children, because the liver is relatively large compared to the rest of the body, some drugs may need to be given in proportionately larger doses.

The kidneys
During the first six months, a baby's kidneys are unable to excrete drugs as efficiently as those of an adult. This, too, may lead to a dangerously high concentration of a drug in the blood. The dose of certain drugs may therefore need to be reduced. Between one and two years of age, kidney function improves, and higher doses of some drugs may then be needed.

Body composition
The proportion of water in the body of a premature baby is about 85 per cent of its body weight, that of a full-term baby is 70 per cent, and that of an adult is only 55 per cent. This means that certain drugs are not as concentrated in an infant's body as in an adult's, and higher doses relative to weight may need be given initially.

PREGNANT WOMEN

Great care is needed during pregnancy to protect the fetus so that it develops into a healthy baby. Drugs taken by the mother can cross the placenta and enter the baby's bloodstream. With certain drugs, and at particular stages of pregnancy, there is a risk of developmental abnormalities, retarded growth, or problems affecting the newborn baby. In addition, some drugs may affect the health of the mother during pregnancy.

Many drugs are known to have adverse effects during pregnancy; others are known to be safe, but in a large number of cases there is no firm evidence to decide on risk or safety. **Therefore, the most important rule if you are pregnant or trying to conceive is to consult your physician before taking any prescribed or over-the-counter medication.** Drugs such as marijuana, nicotine, and alcohol should be avoided. Your physician will assess the potential benefits of drug treatment against any possible risks to decide whether or not a drug should be taken. This is particularly important if you need to take medication regularly for a chronic condition such as epilepsy, high blood pressure, or diabetes.

Drugs and the stages of pregnancy

Pregnancy is divided into three three-month stages called trimesters. Depending on the trimester in which they are taken, drugs can have different effects on the mother or the fetus or both. Some drugs may be considered safe during one trimester, but not during another. Physicians, therefore, sometimes need to substitute one medication for another given during the course of pregnancy.

The trimesters of pregnancy

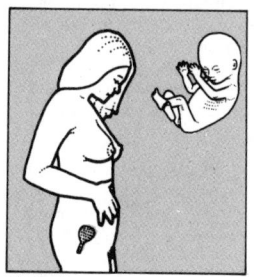 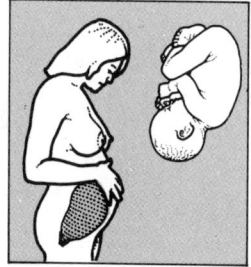 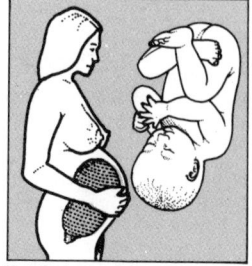

First trimester
During the first three months of pregnancy – the most critical period – drugs may affect the development of fetal organs, leading to congenital malformations. Very severe defects may result in miscarriage.

Second trimester
From the fourth through the sixth month some drugs may retard the growth of the fetus. This may also result in a low birth weight. Other drugs may affect neurological development.

Third trimester
During the last three months of pregnancy, some drugs may retard growth or may promote jaundice and/or bleeding. Some drugs may also affect labor, causing it to be premature, delayed, or prolonged.

How drugs cross the placenta
The placenta acts as a filter between the mother's bloodstream and that of the baby. It allows small molecules from nutrients to pass into the baby's blood, while preventing larger particles such as blood cells from doing so. Drug molecules are comparatively small and pass easily through the placental barrier.

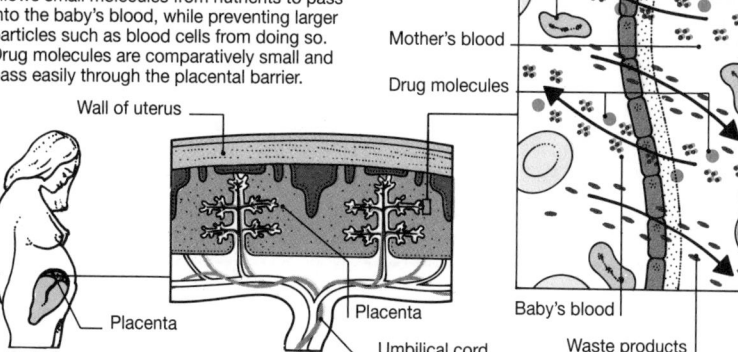

Nutrients
Blood cell
Mother's blood
Drug molecules
Wall of uterus
Placenta
Placenta
Umbilical cord
Baby's blood
Waste products

BREAST-FEEDING

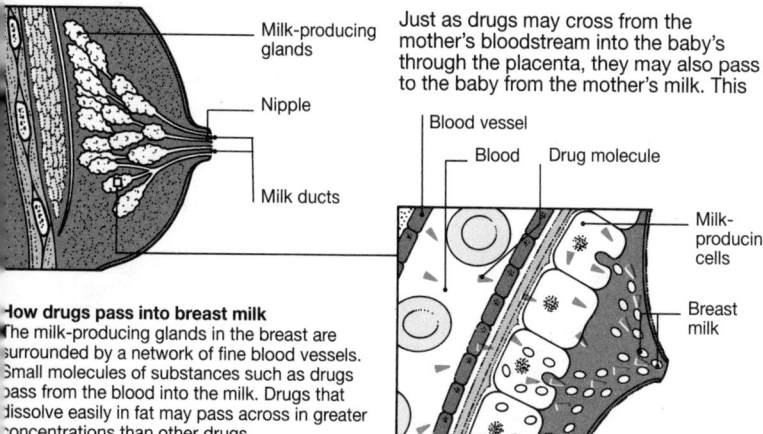

Milk-producing glands
Nipple
Milk ducts

Blood vessel
Blood   Drug molecule
Milk-producing cells
Breast milk

How drugs pass into breast milk
The milk-producing glands in the breast are surrounded by a network of fine blood vessels. Small molecules of substances such as drugs pass from the blood into the milk. Drugs that dissolve easily in fat may pass across in greater concentrations than other drugs.

Just as drugs may cross from the mother's bloodstream into the baby's through the placenta, they may also pass to the baby from the mother's milk. This means that a breast-fed baby will receive small doses of whatever drugs the mother is taking. In many cases this is not a problem, because the amount of drug that passes into the milk is too small to have any significant effect on the baby. However, some drugs can produce unwanted effects on the baby. Antibiotics may sensitize the infant and consequently prevent their use later in life. Sedative drugs may make the baby drowsy and cause feeding problems. Moreover, some drugs may reduce the amount of milk produced by the mother.

Physicians usually advise breast-feeding women to take only essential drugs. When a mother needs to take regular medication while breast-feeding, her baby may also need to be closely monitored for possible adverse effects.

THE ELDERLY

Older people are particularly at risk when taking drugs. This is partly due to the physical changes associated with aging, and partly to the need for some elderly people to take several different drugs at the same time. They may also be at risk because they may be unable to manage their treatment properly, or may lack the information to do so.

Physical changes

Elderly people have a greater risk of accumulating drugs in their bodies because the liver may be less efficient at breaking drugs down and the kidneys are less efficient at excreting them. Because of this, in some cases, the normal adult dose will produce side effects, where a reduced dose may be sufficient to produce a therapeutic effect without the side effects. (See also Kidney and liver disease, below.)

Older people tend to take more drugs than younger people – many take two or more drugs at the same time. Apart from increasing the number of drugs in their systems, taking more than one drug at a time can cause adverse drug interactions (see p.16).

As people grow older some parts of the body, such as the brain and nervous system, become more sensitive to drugs, thus increasing the likelihood of adverse reactions from drugs acting on those sites. A similar problem may occur due to changes in the body's ratio of body fat.

Although allergic reactions (see p.135) are rarely a function of age, changes in the immune system may account for some unexpected reactions.

Accordingly, physicians prescribe more conservatively for older people, especially those with disorders likely to correct themselves in time.

Incorrect use of drugs

Elderly people often suffer harmful effects from their drug treatment because they fail to take their medication regularly or correctly. This may happen because they have been misinformed about how to take it or receive vague instructions. Problems arise sometimes when elderly persons cannot remember whether they have taken the drug and take a double dosage (see Exceeding the dose, p.30). Problems may also occur because the person is confused; this is not necessarily due to senility, but can arise as a result of drug treatment, especially if an elderly person is taking a number of different drugs or a sedative drug.

All prescriptions dispensed for elderly patients should be especially clearly and fully labeled. Leaflets about the drug and its use are also helpful for the individual or the person taking care of him or her. Where appropriate, special containers with memory aids should be used for dispensing the medication in single doses.

Effect of drugs that act on the brain

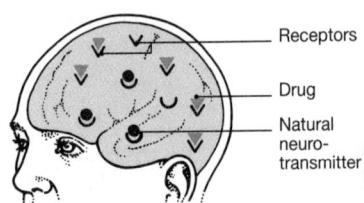

In young people
There are plenty of receptors to take up the drug as well as natural *neurotransmitters*.

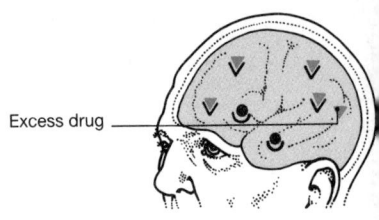

In older people
There are fewer receptors, so even a reduced drug dose may be excessive.

KIDNEY AND LIVER DISEASE

Long-term illnesses affect the way in which people respond to drug treatment. This is especially true of kidney and liver problems. The liver alters the chemical structure of many of the drugs that enter the body (see How drugs pass through the body, p.17) by breaking them down into simpler substances, while the kidneys excrete drugs in the urine. If the effectiveness of the liver or kidneys is interfered with or curtailed by illness, the effect of drugs on the individual can be marked. In most cases, people with kidney or liver disease will be prescribed a smaller number of drugs and in lower doses.

In addition, certain drugs may in rare cases damage the liver or kidneys. A physician may therefore be reluctant to prescribe such a drug to someone with already reduced liver or kidney function in order to avoid the risk of further damage.

Drugs and kidney disease

People with poor kidney function are at greater risk from drug side effects. There are two reasons for this. First, drugs build up in the system because smaller amounts are excreted in urine. Second, kidney disease can cause protein loss through the urine, which lowers the level of protein in the blood. Some drugs bind to blood proteins, and if there are fewer proteins, a greater proportion of drug becomes free and active in the body (see Effects of protein loss, left).

Drugs and liver disease

Severe liver diseases such as cirrhosis and hepatitis affect the way the body breaks down drugs. This can lead to a dangerous accumulation of certain drugs in the body. People suffering from these or similar liver diseases should consult their physician and pharmacist before taking any medication (including over-the-counter drugs) or alcohol. Many drugs must be avoided completely since they can cause coma in someone with a damaged or poorly functioning liver.

Effects of protein loss

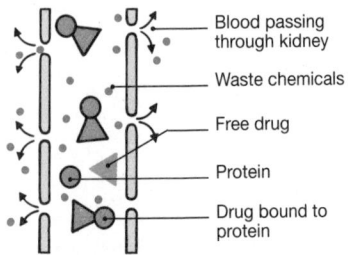

Normal kidney
Some drugs bind to proteins in the blood and are inactive; only free drugs affect the body.

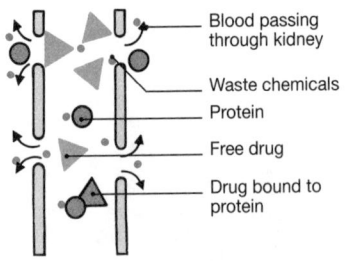

Damaged kidney
Loss of protein increases the amount of active drug, and therefore its overall effect.

DRUG DEPENDENCE

The term "drug dependence" applies far more widely than most people realize. It is usually thought of in association with use of illegal drugs like heroin or with excessive intake of alcohol. But many Canadians are dependent on other drugs, including stimulants – such as caffeine found in coffee and tea, and nicotine in tobacco – and certain prescription medicines, such as analgesics, sleeping drugs, and tranquilizers (anti-anxiety drugs).

Psychological and physical dependence

Drug dependence, implying a person's inability to control use of a substance with an abuse potential, is of two types. Psychological dependence is an emotional state of craving for a drug whose presence in the body has a desired effect or whose absence has an undesired effect. Physical dependence, which often includes psychological dependence, involves physiological adaptation to a drug or alcohol, characterized by severe physical disturbances – withdrawal symptoms – during a period of abstinence. Physical dependence on a drug is further characterized by a developing *tolerance* to the drug's effects; the line between tolerance and lethal dosage is sometimes extremely fine (see Drug tolerance, below).

Drug dependence, now widely preferred to the word addiction, is defined as the compulsive use of a substance resulting in physical, psychological, or social harm to the user, with continued use despite the harm.

Drugs that cause dependence

Many people who need to take regular medication worry that they may become dependent on their drugs. In fact, only a few groups of drugs produce physical dependence, most of them substances that alter mood or behavior. Such drugs include heroin and the narcotic analgesics (morphine, meperidine, and other similar drugs), sleeping drugs and anti-anxiety drugs (benzodiazepines and barbiturates), depressants (alcohol), and nervous system stimulants (amphetamines, cocaine, and nicotine). Consult the drug profile in Part 4 of this book to discover the dependence rating of any drug you are taking.

The use of nicotine in the form of tobacco and the controlled or uncontrolled use of narcotic analgesics invariably produce physical dependence if taken regularly over a period of time.

DRUG TOLERANCE

Drug tolerance occurs as the body adapts to the actions of a drug. Although people can develop a tolerance to many drugs, it is a dangerous characteristic of virtually all of the drugs of dependence. A person taking them needs larger and larger doses to achieve the original effect; as the dose increases, so do the risks of *toxic* effects and dependence.

The explanation of tolerance, still not fully understood, is highly complex. It stems from one (or both) of two actions. One is the liver increasing its capacity to break down and dispose of the drug, giving lower concentrations of it in the bloodstream and a shorter duration of action. The other potential action involves adaptation by the cells of the central nervous system, including the brain, to the drug, lowering responsiveness.

Brain tolerance can also lead to cross-tolerance, a person's tolerance to one drug leading to tolerance of similar drugs. For example, the regular drinker who can tolerate high levels of alcohol (a depressant) can have a dangerous tolerance to other depressants such as anti-anxiety drugs. While cross-tolerance raises problems, it does allow a substance with a less addictive potential to replace the original. The symptoms of alcohol withdrawal can thus be controlled by the anti-anxiety drug diazepam, which is also a depressant.

Tolerance to some drugs has its benefits. A person can develop tolerance to the side effects of a drug but remain responsive to its curative powers. Many people taking antidepressants find that unpleasant side effects slowly disappear, with the primary action of the drug continuing.

Increasing tolerance does, however, have its dangers. A person with a developed tolerance tends to increase dosage, sometimes to the toxic level.

Dosage and effect in drug tolerance
The chart below shows how some effects (these may be intended or unintended) of a fixed dose of tolerance-producing drugs gradually diminish over a period of time. If after this time the dose is significantly increased, the drug effect is restored. Remember, dosage of prescribed drugs should never be increased except on your physician's instructions.

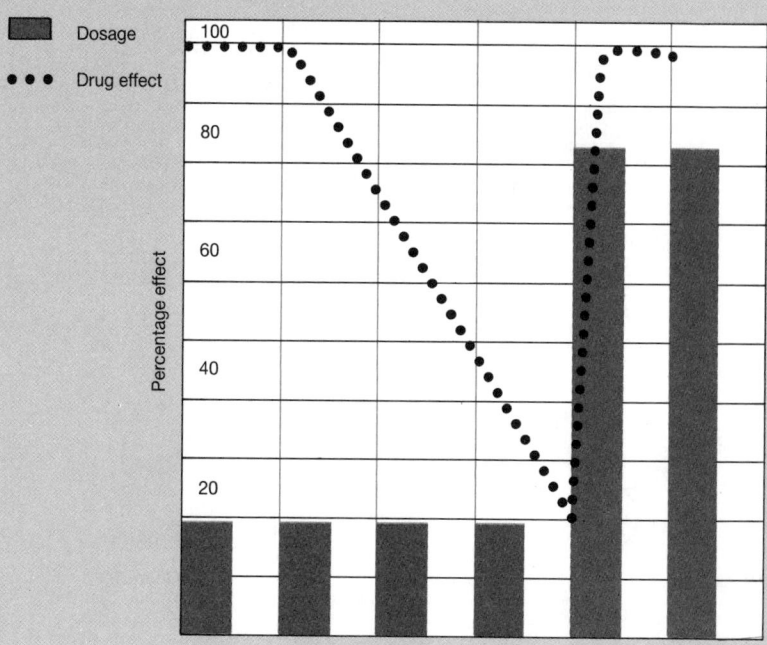

Dosage

Drug effect

Percentage effect

100

80

60

40

20

Time

DRUG DEPENDENCE continued

However, it is equally true that not all regular users of alcohol become alcoholics. There is much argument over the definition of an alcoholic. One definition is: A person who has experienced physical, psychological, social, or occupational impairment due to habitual, excessive consumption of alcohol.

Recognizing the dangers of drug dependence

Factors that determine the risk of developing physical dependence include the characteristics of the drug itself, the strength and frequency of doses, and the duration of use. However, the presence of these factors does not always result in dependence. Psychological and physiological factors unique to each individual also enter the equation, and there may be other, as yet unknown, factors involved. For example, when the use of narcotic analgesics is restricted to the immediate short-term relief of severe pain in a medical setting, long-term dependence is rare. Yet there is a high risk of physical dependence when narcotic analgesics, or other drugs of abuse, are taken for non-medical reasons. There is also risk in some cases of low-dose use when continued over a long period of time for chronic pain.

No one can say for sure just what leads an individual to drug-dependent behavior.

DRUG ABUSE

The term is defined as any use of drugs that causes physical, psychological, economic, legal, or social harm to the user, or to persons who may be affected by the user's behavior. Drug abuse commonly refers to taking drugs obtained illegally (such as heroin), but may also be used to describe the misuse of drugs generally obtainable legally (nicotine, alcohol), and to drugs obtainable through a physician's prescription only (everything from sleeping drugs and tranquilizers to analgesics and stimulants).

The abuse of prescription drugs deserves more attention than it usually receives. The practice can include the personal use of drugs left over from a previous course of treatment, the sharing with others of drugs prescribed for yourself, the deliberate deception of physicians, the forgery of prescriptions, and the theft of drugs from pharmacies. All of these practices can have dangerous consequences. Careful attention to the advice in the section on Managing your drug treatment (p.25) will help to avoid inadvertent misuse of drugs. The dangers associated with abuse of individual drugs are discussed under Drugs of abuse (pp.531 – 538).

> **Common drugs of abuse**
> Alcohol
> Amphetamines
> Amyl nitrite and similar drugs
> Cocaine (including "crack")
> Heroin
> LSD
> Marijuana
> Meperidine
> Mescaline
> Nicotine
> Phencyclidine
> Solvents

A person's physical and psychological makeup are thought to be factors, as well as his or her social environment, occupational pressures, and outlook on life. Motivation and setting play major roles.

The indiscriminate use of certain prescription drugs can also cause drug dependence. In this regard, barbiturate sleeping drugs, such as secobarbital and pentobarbital, are commonly cited as causative agents.

Benzodiazepines, which are much less likely to lead to a single fatal dose, have largely replaced them, though physicians discourage the use of any drug to induce sleep or calm anxiety for more than a few weeks. Appetite suppressants require close supervision. Similarly, amphetamines are now prescribed for fewer conditions than in the past because of the frequency with which they are abused.

Treating drug dependence

When a person is dependent on a drug, the cells in the body have adapted to a new chemical environment. To move someone from that condition to a drug-free state is a complex medical process. But a patient must become completely drug-free before long-term rehabilitation can occur.

The first step, detoxification, can take different forms. In cases of alcohol dependence, abstinence may often be abruptly imposed. With other substances the drug may be gradually withdrawn, or other safer substances substituted. There are, however, differing schools of thought, and some treatment centers argue for the abrupt cessation method of detoxification for substances besides alcohol.

Withdrawal can be mild or violent, and is occasionally fatal. Expert medical supervision is required.

For some patients, reducing alcohol or other drug use is appropriate.

Treatment to maintain a drug-free state or a lower and less hazardous level of drug use may involve psychotherapy, support groups, or the use of drugs such as disulfiram (Antabuse).

SYMPTOMS OF WITHDRAWAL

These can range from the mild (anxiety, sweating) to the serious (vomiting, confusion) to the extremely serious (seizures, coma). Alcohol withdrawal may be associated with delirium tremens, very occasionally fatal. Withdrawal from barbiturates can sometimes involve seizures and coma. But under medical guidance, withdrawal symptoms can be relieved with doses of the original drug, or with less addictive substitutes.

Withdrawal symptoms occur because the body has adapted to the action of the drug (see Drug tolerance, p.23). When a drug is continuously present, the body may stop the release of a natural chemical necessary to normal function, like endorphins (below).

Pain and heroin withdrawal

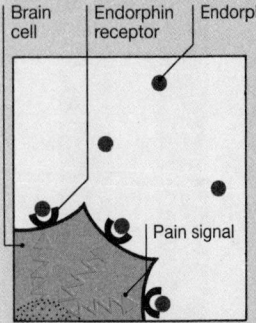

Normal brain
When no drug is present, natural substances called endorphins inhibit the transmission of pain signals.

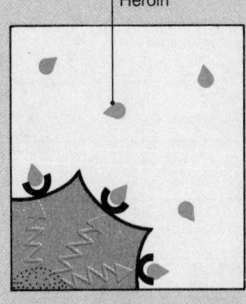

Effect of heroin
Heroin occupies the same receptors in the brain as endorphins and suppresses endorphin production.

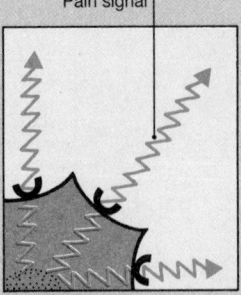

Heroin withdrawal
Abrupt withdrawal of heroin leaves the brain without a buffer to pain signals produced by even minor stimuli.

MANAGING YOUR DRUG THERAPY

A prescribed drug does not automatically produce a beneficial response. For a prescribed drug to have maximum benefit, it must be taken as directed by the physician. It is estimated that two out of every five people for whom a drug is prescribed do not take it properly, if at all. The reasons include failure to understand or remember instructions, fear of side effects, and lack of motivation, often arising after symptoms disappear.

It is your responsibility to take a prescribed drug at the correct time, and in the manner stipulated. To do this, you need to know where to obtain informa-

tion about the drug (see Questioning your physician, p.26) and to make certain that you understand the instructions.

The following pages describe the practical aspects of drug therapy, from filling a prescription and buying over-the-counter drugs to storing drugs and disposing of old medications safely. Problems caused by mismanaging drug therapy – overdosing, underdosing, or stopping the drug altogether – and long-term drug therapy are dealt with on pp.28 – 30. Information regarding specific drugs is given in Part 4.

OVER-THE-COUNTER DRUGS

Over-the-counter drugs are those for which a prescription is not required. They are sold in a variety of outlets (including supermarkets), although some are available only in pharmacies.

It is generally accepted that over-the-counter drugs are suitable for self-treatment and are unlikely to produce serious adverse reactions if taken as directed. But, as with all medicines, they can be harmful if they are misused. The ease with which they can be purchased is no guarantee of their absolute safety. For this reason, when using any over-the-counter medication, the same precautions should be taken as when using a prescription drug.

Using over-the-counter drugs

A number of minor ailments and problems, from coughs and colds to minor cuts and bruises, can be adequately dealt with by using over-the-counter medicines. However, be sure to read the directions on the label and follow them carefully, particularly those advising on dosage and on when to see your physician. Most over-the-counter drugs are clearly labeled. They may warn of conditions under which the drug should not be taken. These medications are for limited use. In general, if symptoms persist for more than a few days, consult your physician.

The pharmacist is usually a good source of information about over-the-counter drugs. He or she cannot make a diagnosis or a decision about therapy, but can tell what is suitable for your complaint. The pharmacist can also tell you when an over-the-counter drug will probably not be effective and can warn you if self-treatment or prolonged treatment is inadvisable.

It is particularly important to speak to your physician before buying over-the-

counter drugs for children. Some conditions, such as diarrhea in young children, should be treated only by a physician. Also, tell your pharmacist about any prescription drugs you are taking.

Buying over-the-counter medications

Various drugs are available over the counter, ranging from cough medicines to eye drops. Your pharmacist can often help you to select the appropriate medication.

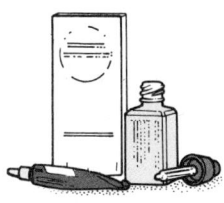

Eye preparations

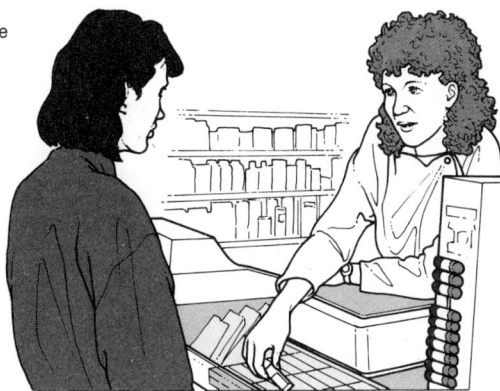

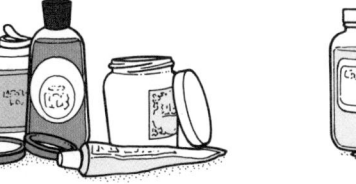

Medicated creams, lotions, and powders

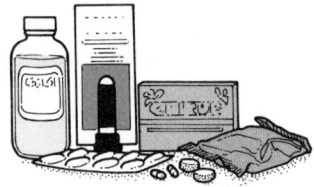

Cough and cold treatments

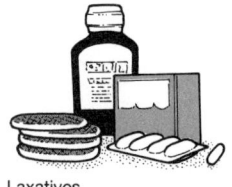

Laxatives

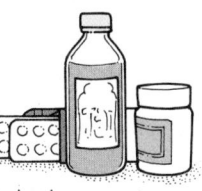

Analgesics

Antacids

PRESCRIPTION DRUGS

Conventional wisdom to the contrary, prescription drugs are not necessarily more potent or effective than over-the-counter drugs. The difference between the two, rather, reflects the policy of the Health Protection Branch of Health and Welfare Canada that over-the-counter drugs are safe and effective for self-medication for a limited time when taken as directed on the label, without the need for supervision by the physician.

When a physician prescribes a drug, he or she usually starts treatment at the normal dosage for the disorder being treated. The dosage may later be adjusted (lowered or increased) if the drug is not producing the desired effect or if there are adverse reactions, and the physician may also switch to an alternative drug that may be more effective.

Prescribing drugs

The federal Health Protection Branch acts to ensure the safety and effectiveness of all drugs marketed in Canada. In the interests of economy, most provinces have laws that require pharmacists to substitute lower-priced brands deemed to be interchangeable with the brands prescribed by physicians. In most instances this substitution does not lead to problems. However, since different manufacturers may formulate a drug product in different ways – even though the active ingredient is the same – two versions of the same drug may not always produce the same actions or take effect in the same amount of time. These are factors that a physician must consider before writing a prescription to give you the most effective drug for your disorder/condition. In certain situations the physician may decide to write "no substitution" on the prescription.

Therefore, if you are getting a prescription repeated, your new medication could be a different shape or color from your previous one. If you are at all concerned about the appearance of your medication, consult your pharmacist.

Cost to the patient may be important, but is secondary to medical considerations such as safety and effectiveness.

Filling your prescription

A trained and licensed professional, the pharmacist plays an important role in the health care system. He or she knows about drug actions, interactions, dosages, and potentially harmful side effects, and is a good source of information about over-the-counter drugs.

Many pharmacies keep a computerized profile of the drugs taken by regular clients. For that reason, it is highly advisable that you order all your prescription drugs from the same pharmacy.

If you take drugs prescribed by more than one physician, or by your dentist as well as your doctor, the pharmacy's profile calls attention to possible harmful interactions. Physicians do ask if you are taking other medicines, but the profile is a valuable additional safety measure.

Questioning your physician

Lack of information is the most common reason for drug failure. Responses like "the doctor is too busy to be bothered with a lot of questions" or "The doctor will think I'm stupid if I ask that" recur over and over. Be certain you understand the instructions for a drug before leaving the physician, and don't leave with any questions unanswered.

It is a good idea to make a list of the questions you may want to ask before your visit, and to make a few notes while

you are there about what you are told. It is not uncommon to forget some of the instructions your physician gives you during a consultation.

Know what you are taking

Although most of the important information you need will be written on the prescription and on the drug label, you should obtain any additional information as necessary from your physician or pharmacist.

Your physician should tell you the name of the drug he or she is prescribing, and exactly what condition or symptom the drug has been prescribed to treat.

As well as knowing the name of the drug prescribed, you should know what dose to take, how often to take it, and whether you should have your prescription refilled. Be certain you understand fully the instructions about how and when to take the drug (see also Taking your medication, facing page). For example, exactly how much is a teaspoonful, and does four times a day mean four times during the time you are awake, or four times in 24 hours? Ask your physician how long treatment should last; some drugs cause harmful effects if you stop taking them abruptly, or do not have beneficial effects unless the course is completed.

Risks and special precautions

All drugs have side effects (see The effects of drugs, p.15), and you should know what these are. Ask your physician what the possible adverse reactions of the drug are and what you should do if they occur. Also ask if there are any foods or other medications you should avoid during treatment and if you can drink alcohol while taking the drug.

Your prescription

Your prescription tells the pharmacist the type and amount of drug to supply, and gives the information that will appear on the container label. Some people like to read prescriptions, to compare instructions written by the physician with those on the label. If there are differences, you may discuss them with the pharmacist.

Most pharmacies include other facts on the drug label such as the name of the drug, the number of tablets or capsules in the container, and how or where the medication should be stored.

Drug name, strength, and amount to be dispensed

Special instructions

Patient's name and address

Physician's name and address

Drug name, strength, and amount to be dispensed

Physician's signature

Refill instructions

PRESCRIPTION TERMS

aa	of each	**pc**	after meals
ac	before meals	**PM**	evening
ad lib	freely	**po**	by mouth
AM	morning	**prn**	as needed
bid	twice a day	**qid**	four times
c	with		a day
cap	capsule	**stat**	at once
ext	for external use	**tab**	tablet
gtt	drops	**tid**	three times
h.s.	before bedtime		a day
i.c.	between meals	**top**	apply topically
mg	milligrams	**ut dict**	take as
mL	milliliter		directed
nocte	at night		
non rep	do not repeat		
o.u.	in each eye		

TAKING YOUR MEDICATION

Among the most important aspects of managing your drug therapy is knowing how often the medication is to be taken. On an empty stomach? With food? Mixed with something? Specific instructions on such points are given in the individual drug profiles in Part 4.

When to take your drugs

Certain drugs are taken only as necessary, when symptoms occur. Others are meant to be taken regularly at specified intervals. The prescription or label instructions can be confusing, however. For instance, does three times a day mean three times every eight hours out of 24 – at 8 a.m., 4 p.m., and midnight? Or does it mean take at three equal intervals during waking hours – morning, early afternoon, and bedtime? A patient must know just what the precise directions are. Either ask the physician when he or she writes the prescription, phone him or her (or the nurse) later, or ask your pharmacist. Try to take your dose at the recommended intervals; taking doses too close together increases the risk of side effects.

The actual time of day that you take a drug is generally flexible, so you can normally schedule your doses to fit your daily routine. This has the additional advantage of making it easier for you to remember to take your drugs. For example, if you are to take the drug three times during the day, it may be most convenient to take the first dose at 7 a.m., the second at 3 p.m., and the third at 11 p.m., while it may be more suitable for another person on the same regimen to take the first dose at 8 a.m., and so on. You must, however, establish with your pharmacist or your physician whether the drug should be taken with food, in which

Three times a day ?

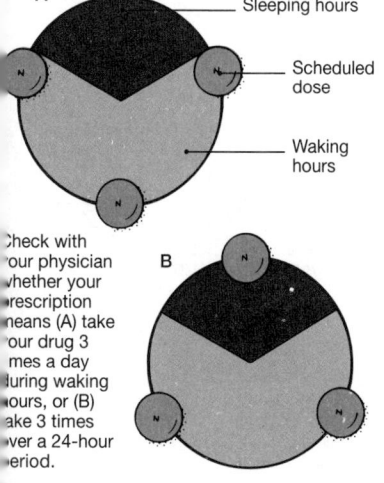

A — Sleeping hours
— Scheduled dose
— Waking hours

Check with your physician whether your prescription means (A) take your drug 3 times a day during waking hours, or (B) take 3 times over a 24-hour period.

TIPS ON TAKING MEDICINES

● Whenever possible, take capsules and tablets while standing, or at least when you are in an upright sitting position; take them with water, and drink both before and after swallowing the medication. If you take them when you are lying down, or without fluid, it is possible for capsules and tablets to become stuck in the esophagus. This can delay the action of the drug and may damage the esophagus.

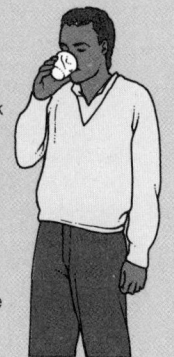

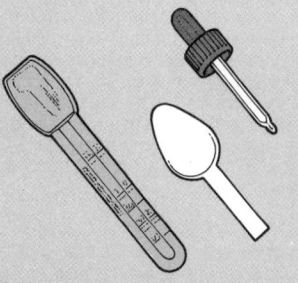

● Always measure your dose carefully, using a 5mL spoon when a teaspoonful is specified, or an accurate measure such as a dropper, children's medicine spoon, or oral syringe.

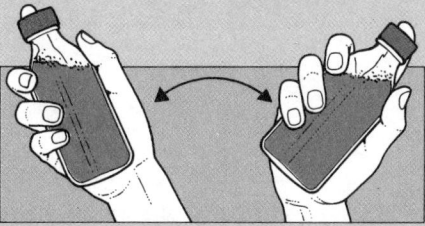

● When taking liquid medicines shake the bottle before measuring each dose, or you may give yourself improper dosages if the active substance has risen to the top or settled at the bottom of the bottle.

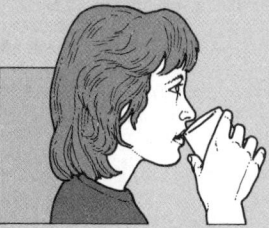

● A drink of cold water taken immediately after an unpleasantly flavored medicine will often hide the taste.

case you would probably need to take it with your breakfast, lunch, and dinner.

If you are taking several different medications, ask your physician or pharmacist if they can be taken together, or if they must be taken at different times in order to avoid any adverse effects or reduced effectiveness caused by an interaction.

How to take your drugs

If your prescription specifies taking your drug with food – or without food – it is very important to follow this instruction if you are to get the maximum benefit from your treatment.

Certain drugs such as ampicillin and captopril should be taken on an empty stomach (usually one hour before, or two hours after, meals) so they will be absorbed more quickly into the bloodstream; others, such as ibuprofen, metronidazole, and allopurinol, should be taken with food to avoid stomach irritation. Similarly, you should comply with any instructions to avoid particular foods. Milk and dairy products may inhibit the absorption of some drugs such as tetracycline; fruit juices can break down certain antibacterial drugs in the stomach and thereby decrease their effectiveness; alcohol is best avoided with all drugs. (See also Drug interactions, p.16.)

In some cases, when taking diuretics, for example, you may be advised to eat foods rich in potassium. But do not take potassium supplements unless you are advised to do so by your physician (see Potassium, p.524). If you use salt substitutes (all of which contain potassium), remember to tell your physician.

GIVING MEDICINES TO CHILDREN

A number of over-the counter medicines are specifically prepared for children. Many other medicines have labels that give both adult and children's dosages. For the purposes of drug labeling, anyone 12 years of age or under is considered a child.

When giving over-the-counter medicines to children you should follow the instructions on the label exactly and under no circumstances exceed the dosage recommended for a child. Never give a child even a small proportion of a medicine intended for adult use without the advice of your physician.

Never deceive your child about what you are giving, pretending that tablets are candy or that liquid medicines are soft drinks. Never leave a child's medicine within reach. He or she may be tempted to take an extra dose in order to hasten recovery.

MISSED DOSES

Missing a dose of your medication can be a problem only if you are taking the drug as part of a regular course of treatment. Although missing a drug dose is not uncommon, it is not a cause for concern in most cases. It may sometimes produce a recurrence of symptoms or a change in the action of the drug, so you should know what to do when you have forgotten to take your medication. For advice on individual medications, consult the drug profile in Part 4.

Additional measures

With some medications, the timing of doses depends on how long their actions last. When you miss a dose, the amount of drug in your body is lowered, and the effect of the drug may be diminished. You may therefore have to take other steps to avoid unwanted consequences. For example, if you are taking an oral contraceptive and forget to take one tablet, you should take one as soon as you remember, and for the rest of the cycle you should use a backup form of contraception.

If you miss more than one dose of any drug you are taking regularly, tell your physician. If you miss even one dose of insulin, consult your physician about how to continue treatment.

If you frequently forget to take your medication you should tell your physician. He or she may be able to simplify your treatment schedule by prescribing a multi-ingredient preparation that contains several drugs in one capsule, or a preparation that releases the drug slowly into the body over a period of time, and only needs to be taken once or twice daily.

REMEMBERING YOUR MEDICATION

If you take several different medications, it is useful to draw up a chart to remind yourself of when to take each preparation. This will also help anyone who looks after you, or a visiting physician unfamiliar with your treatment.

Furosemide (a diuretic to counter fluid retention), two 40mg tablets in the morning (small round tablets).

Spironolactone (another diuretic to counter the potassium loss caused by furosemide), one 50mg tablet in the morning (oval tablets).

The example given here is of a dosage chart made for an older woman suffering from arthritis and a heart condition who has trouble sleeping. Her physician has prescribed the following treatment:

Ibuprofen (for arthritis), three 400mg tablets daily with meals (large round tablets).

Nifedipine (to treat her heart condition), three 10mg capsules a day (one-color capsules).

Temazepam (a sleeping drug), one 15mg capsule at bedtime (two-color capsules).

Dosage chart

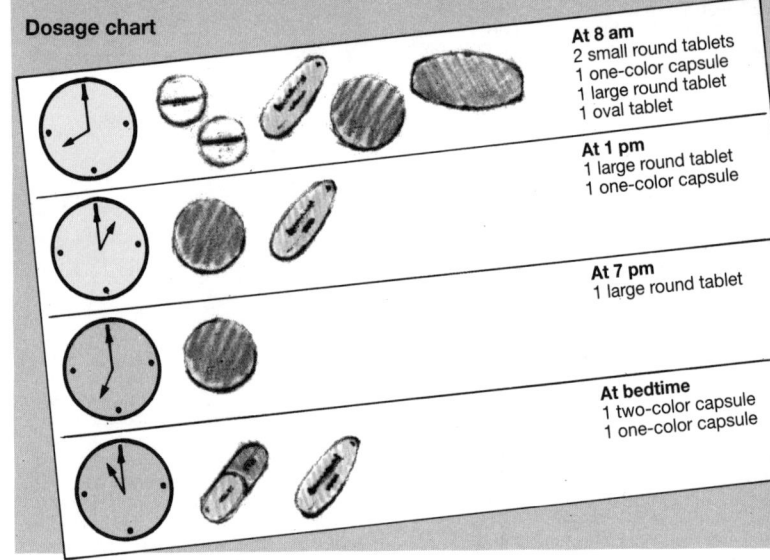

At 8 am
2 small round tablets
1 one-color capsule
1 large round tablet
1 oval tablet

At 1 pm
1 large round tablet
1 one-color capsule

At 7 pm
1 large round tablet

At bedtime
1 two-color capsule
1 one-color capsule

ENDING DRUG THERAPY

As with missed doses, ending drug therapy too soon can be a problem when you are taking a regular course of medications. With medication that you take as required, you can stop treatment as soon as you feel better.

Advice on stopping individual drugs is given in the drug profiles in Part 4. Some general guidelines to ending drug therapy are given below.

Risks of stopping too soon

Suddenly stopping drug therapy before completing your course of medication may cause the original condition to recur or lead to other complications, including withdrawal symptoms. Even if you begin to feel better, you still should not stop taking the drug unless your physician advises you to do so. People taking antibiotics often make this mistake. But the disappearance of the symptoms

does not necessarily mean that the infection is cured. The full course of treatment prescribed should always be followed.

Adverse effects

Do not stop taking a medication simply because it produces unpleasant side effects. Many side effects disappear or become bearable after a while. But if they do not, check with your physician who may want to reduce the dosage of the drug gradually or substitute another medication which does not produce the same side effects.

Gradual reduction

While many medications can be stopped suddenly, others must be reduced gradually to avoid a reaction when treatment ends. This is the case with long-term corticosteroid therapy (see right).

Phased reduction of corticosteroids

Corticosteroid drug

Natural adrenal hormone

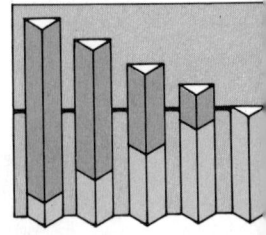

Normal hormone level

Corticosteroid drugs suppress production in the body of natural adrenal hormones. A phased reduction of the drug dosage allows levels of the natural hormones to revert to normal gradually.

STORING MEDICATIONS

Once you have completed a medically directed course of treatment, do not keep any unused medications. Other remedies for headaches, indigestion, and so forth should not be used if they show signs of deterioration or if their period of effectiveness has expired.

How to store medications

Over-the-counter and prescription medications should normally be stored in the container in which you purchased them. If you need to put them into other containers, say, special containers designed for the elderly, remember to keep the original container with the label and separate instructions for future reference. When visiting a foreign country, keep all medications in their original packaging.

Make certain that caps and lids are replaced and tightly closed after use; loose caps may leak and spill, or hasten deterioration of the drug.

Where to store medications

The majority of medications should be stored in a cool, dry place out of direct sunlight, even those in plastic containers or tinted glass. Room temperature is suitable for most drugs, away from sources of direct heat. A few medications should be stored in the refrigerator. Storage information for individual drugs is given in the drug profiles in Part 4.

All medications, including cough medicines, iron tablets, and oral contraceptives, should be kept out of the reach of children. If you are in the habit of keeping your medicines where you will see them as a reminder to take them, leave an empty medicine container out instead, and put the medicine itself safely out of reach.

Wall cabinets that can be locked are ideal for storing medications, as long as the cabinet itself is in a cool, dry place and not, as often happens, in the bathroom, which may be warm and humid.

WHEN TO DISPOSE OF MEDICATIONS

Old medications should be returned to the pharmacist for disposal. Always dispose of:

● ASA and acetaminophen tablets that smell of vinegar.

● Tablets that are chipped, cracked, or discolored, and capsules that have softened, cracked, or stuck together.

● Liquids that have thickened or discolored, or that taste or smell different in any way from the original product.

● Tubes that are cracked, leaky, or hard.

● Ointments and creams that have changed odor, or changed appearance by discoloring, hardening, or separating.

● Any liquid needing refrigeration that has been kept for over two weeks.

● Tablets or capsules over two years old.

LONG-TERM DRUG THERAPY

Many people may require regular, prolonged, or even lifelong therapy with one or more drugs. People suffering from chronic or recurrent disorders often need lifelong treatment with drugs to control symptoms or prevent complications. Antihypertensive agents for high blood pressure and insulin or oral antidiabetic drugs for diabetes mellitus are familiar examples. Many other disorders take a long time to cure; people with tuberculosis, for example, usually need at least six months' therapy with antituberculous drugs. Long-term treatment may also be necessary to prevent a condition from occurring, and will have to be taken for as long as the individual is at risk. Antimalarial drugs are a good example.

Possible adverse effects

You may worry that taking a drug for a long period will reduce its effectiveness or that you will become dependent on it. However, *tolerance* develops only with a few drugs; most drugs continue to have the same effect indefinitely. Similarly, taking a medication for more than a few weeks does not normally create dependence.

Changing drug therapy

If you are taking a medication regularly, you will need to know what to do if something else occurs to affect your health. If you wish to become pregnant, for example, you should ask your physician right away if it is preferable to continue on your regular medicine or switch to another less apt to affect your pregnancy. If you contract a new illness, for which an additional drug is prescribed,

your regular medication may be altered.

There are a number of other reasons for changing a drug. You may have had an adverse reaction, or an improved preparation may have become available.

Adjusting to long-term therapy

You should establish a daily routine for taking your medication in order to reduce the risk of a missed dose. Usually you should not stop taking your medication, even if there are side effects, without consulting your physician (see Ending drug treatment, facing page). If you become afraid of possible side effects from the drug, discuss these fears with your physician or pharmacist.

Many people deliberately stop their drugs because they feel well or their symptoms disappear. That can be dangerous, especially with a disease like hypertension which has no noticeable symptoms. Stopping treatment may lead to a recurrence or worsening of a disease. If you are uncertain about why you have to keep taking a medication, ask your physician.

Only a few drugs require an alteration in habits. Some drugs should not be taken with alcohol; with one or two drugs you should avoid certain foods. If you require a medication that makes you drowsy, you should not drive a car or operate dangerous equipment.

If you are taking a drug that should not be stopped suddenly or that may interact with other drugs, it is a good idea to carry a warning card or bracelet. Such information might be essential for emergency medical treatment in an accident.

Monitoring therapy

If you are on long-term therapy, you need to visit your physician for periodic checkups. He or she will check your underlying condition and monitor any adverse effects of treatment. Levels of the drug in the blood may be measured. With insulin, in addition to checks with the physician, you need to monitor blood or urine levels each day.

If a drug is known to cause damage to an organ, tests may be done to check the function of the organ. For example, blood and urine tests to check kidney function, or a blood count to check the bone marrow, may be indicated.

Medical checkups
Blood pressure is commonly checked in people on long-term drug therapy.

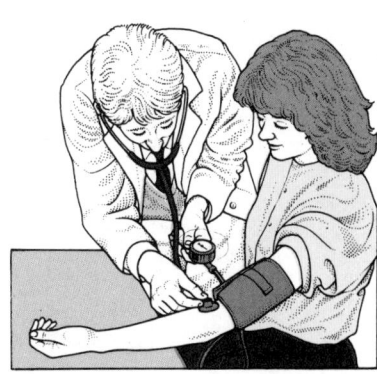

EXCEEDING THE DOSE

Most people associate drug overdoses with attempts at suicide or the fatalities and near fatalities brought on by abuse of street drugs. However, drug overdoses can also occur among people who deliberately or inadvertently exceed the stated dose of a drug that has been prescribed for them by their physician.

A single extra dose of most drugs is unlikely to be a cause for concern, although accidental overdoses can create anxiety in the individual and his or her family, and may cause overdose symptoms which appear in a variety of different forms.

Overdose of some drugs, however, is potentially dangerous even when the dose has been exceeded by only a small amount. Each of the drug profiles in Part 4 of this book gives detailed information on the consequences of exceeding the dose, symptoms to look out for, and what to do. Each drug has been given an overdose danger rating of low, medium, or high (described fully on p.196).

Taking an extra dose

People sometimes exceed the stated dose in the mistaken belief that by increasing dosage they will obtain more

Effects of repeated overdose
Repeated overdose of a drug over an extended period may lead to a buildup of high levels of the drug in the body, especially if liver or kidney function is reduced.

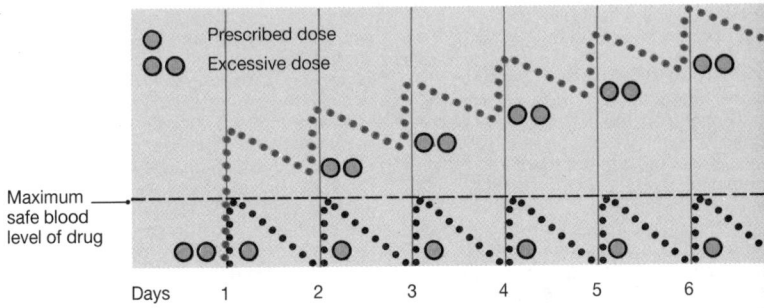

Prescribed dose
Excessive dose

Maximum safe blood level of drug

Days 1 2 3 4 5 6

immediate action or a more effective cure. This is a particular risk with *tolerance*-inducing drugs (see Drug dependence, p.23). Others exceed their dose accidentally, by miscalculating the amount or forgetting that the dose has already been taken.

Taking extra doses is often a problem in the elderly, who may repeat their dose through forgetfulness or confusion. This is

a special risk with medicines that cause drowsiness (see also p.22).

In some cases, especially when liver or kidney function is impaired, the drug builds up in the blood because the body cannot break down and excrete the extra dose quickly enough, so that symptoms of poisoning may result (see below left). Symptoms of excessive intake may not be apparent for many days.

When and how to get help

If you are not sure whether you have taken your tablets or medicine, think back and check again. If you honestly cannot remember, assume that you have missed the dose and follow the advice given in the individual drug profiles in Part 4 of the book. If you cannot find your drug there, consult your physician. Make a note to use some system in the future which will help you remember to take your medication.

If you are looking after an elderly person on regular medication who suddenly develops unusual symptoms such as confusion, drowsiness, or unsteadiness, consider the possibility of an inadvertent drug overdose and call the prescribing physician as soon as possible.

Deliberate overdose

While many cases of drug overdose are accidental or the result of a mistaken belief that increasing the dose will enhance the benefits of drug therapy, sometimes an excessive amount of a drug is taken with the intention of causing harm or even as a suicide attempt. Whether or not you think a dangerous amount of a drug has been taken, deliberate overdoses of this kind should always be brought to the attention of the physician. Not only is it necessary to ensure that no physical harm has occurred as a result of the overdose, but the psychological condition of a person who takes such action may indicate the need for additional medical help.

HOW DRUGS ACCUMULATE

In most people, the liver and kidneys are able to cope with an occasional extra dose of a drug. But if they are functioning below normal efficiency, excessive doses may accumulate in the body.

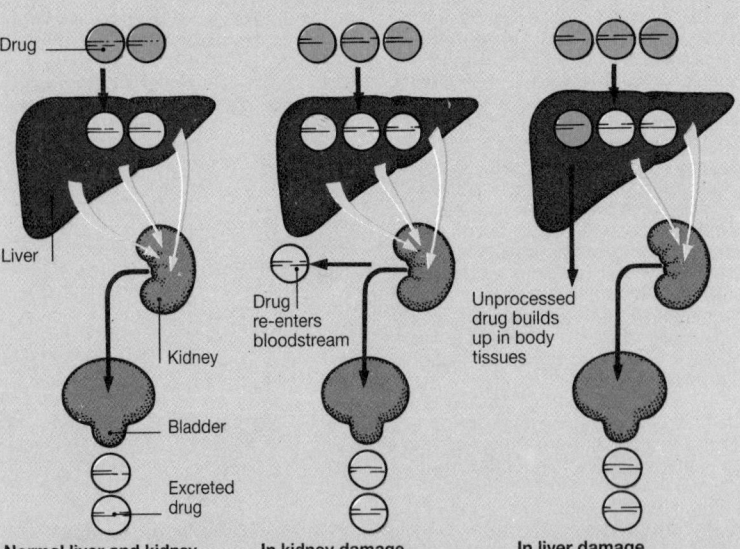

Drug

Liver

Drug re-enters bloodstream

Unprocessed drug builds up in body tissues

Kidney

Bladder

Excreted drug

Normal liver and kidney
Drugs taken by mouth are processed in the liver and later excreted by the kidneys.

In kidney damage
The kidneys cannot eliminate excess drug in the urine; drug levels in the blood may rise.

In liver damage
The liver cannot process the excess drug which may build up in the body tissues.

DOs AND DON'Ts

n this page you will find a summary of e most important practical points conerning the management of your drug erapy. The advice is arranged under general headings, explaining the safest methods of storing drugs and following treatment, whether it is a prescribed medication or an over-the-counter drug.

This information is equally applicable whether you are taking medication yourself or supervising the drug therapy of someone in your care.

the physician's office

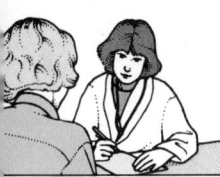

DO
● Tell your physician about any medications you are already taking, both prescription and over-the-counter.
● Tell your physician if you are pregnant, intending to become pregnant, or breast feeding.
● Tell your physician about any allergic reactions you have experienced to past drug treatments.
● Tell your physician if you have a current health problem, such as liver disease, or if you think you might be at risk from drug therapy for any other reason.

● Discuss your drug therapy with your physician and make sure you understand the reasons why you have been prescribed a particular drug and what benefits you can expect. People who do not understand the reasons for their treatment often fail to take their medication correctly.

DON'T
▼ Leave your physician's office without a clear understanding of how and when to take your medication.

the pharmacy

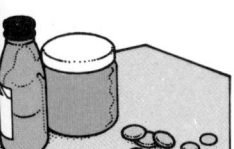

DO
● Ask your pharmacist's advice about over-the-counter drugs if you are not sure what you should buy, or if you think you may react adversely to a drug.
● Try to see the same pharmacist or use the same pharmacy to fill your regular prescriptions.
● Be sure you know the name of the drug you have been prescribed, and make sure you always receive the same brand of drug as you had previously if you are refilling a prescription.

● Make sure you understand what is on the drug label.
● Ask the pharmacist to put your medication in a container with an easy-to-remove cap if you have difficulty using child-resistant containers.

DON'T
▼ Send children to the pharmacy to get your medication for you.

ving medicines to ildren

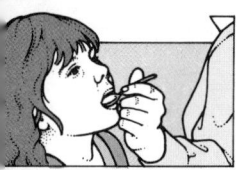

DO
● Check the dose on the label carefully before giving medicines to children.
● Make sure over-the-counter preparations you give to young children for viral infections or fevers of unknown cause do not contain ASA.

DON'T
▼ Pretend to children that medicinal preparations are candy or soft drinks.
▼ Give any medicines to children under the age of five, except on the advice of your physician.

king your medication

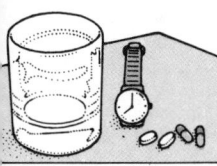

DO
● Make sure that your medication will not make you drowsy or otherwise affect your ability before you drive or perform difficult or dangerous tasks.
● Read the label carefully and do what it says. This is equally important with all types of creams and lotions as well as drugs taken by mouth.
● Finish the drug therapy your physician prescribes for you.
● Consult your physician for advice if you experience side effects.

DON'T
▼ Take any prescribed or over-the-counter drugs without first consulting your physician if you are pregnant or trying to conceive.
▼ Offer your medication to other people or take medication that has been prescribed for someone else (even if the symptoms are the same).

od, drink, d drugs of abuse

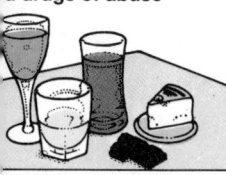

DO
● Check that it is safe to take alcohol with prescribed drugs, and that there are no foods you should avoid.

DON'T
▼ Take medication (except that prescribed by your physician), drugs of abuse, or alcohol if you are pregnant or trying to conceive. They may adversely affect the unborn baby.

oring medications

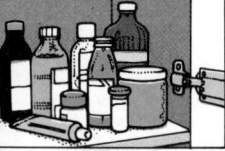

DO
● Take care to store medications in a cool, dry place and protect them from light or refrigerate them, if advised to do so.
● Keep all drugs – including seemingly harmless medications such as cough preparations – locked away out of the reach of children.
● Check your medicine chest regularly in case other members of the family have left their unwanted drugs in it, and to make sure that none of the normal supplies are out of date.

● Keep medications in their original containers with the original instructions to avoid confusion.

DON'T
▼ Hoard drugs at home. When you have stopped taking a prescribed drug, dispose of it unless it is part of your family first aid kit.

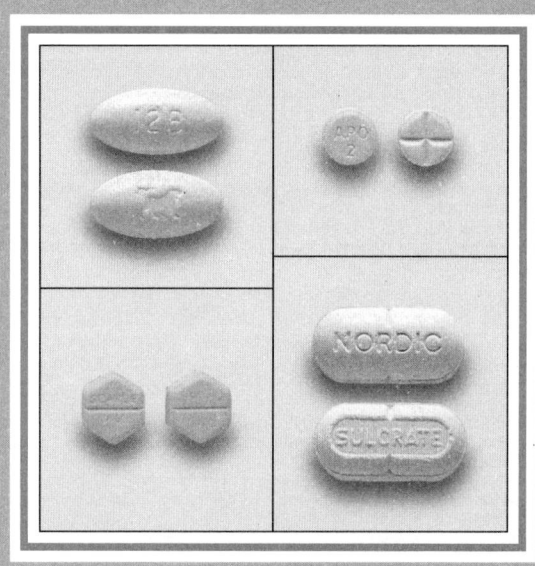

2

DRUG FINDER
INDEX

COLOR IDENTIFICATION GUIDE
INDEX OF MEDICATIONS

COLOR IDENTIFICATION GUIDE

The following pages contain photographs of 259 drug products. The guide is divided into two sections – tablets and capsules. These are arranged first according to their color groups, and secondly according to their size. The fact that a particular product is included in no way implies CMA endorsement of that brand over another similar product.

The products included on these pages represent a selection of the most popular drug products in use in Canada. Several dosage strengths of some of the more widely prescribed medications have been included. Each product is photographed approximately life-size. Beneath each photograph you will find the name of the tablet or capsule with details of its active ingredients and their amounts in grams (g) and milligrams (mg). The products are laid out in a grid format. Each entry can be located from the Index of Medications by reference to the page number and the letter in the top left-hand corner of each square of the grid.

To locate the photograph of a particular medication, consult the chart, which will direct you to the relevant color section. You will find an example of an entry in the section below.

HOW TO LOCATE YOUR MEDICATION

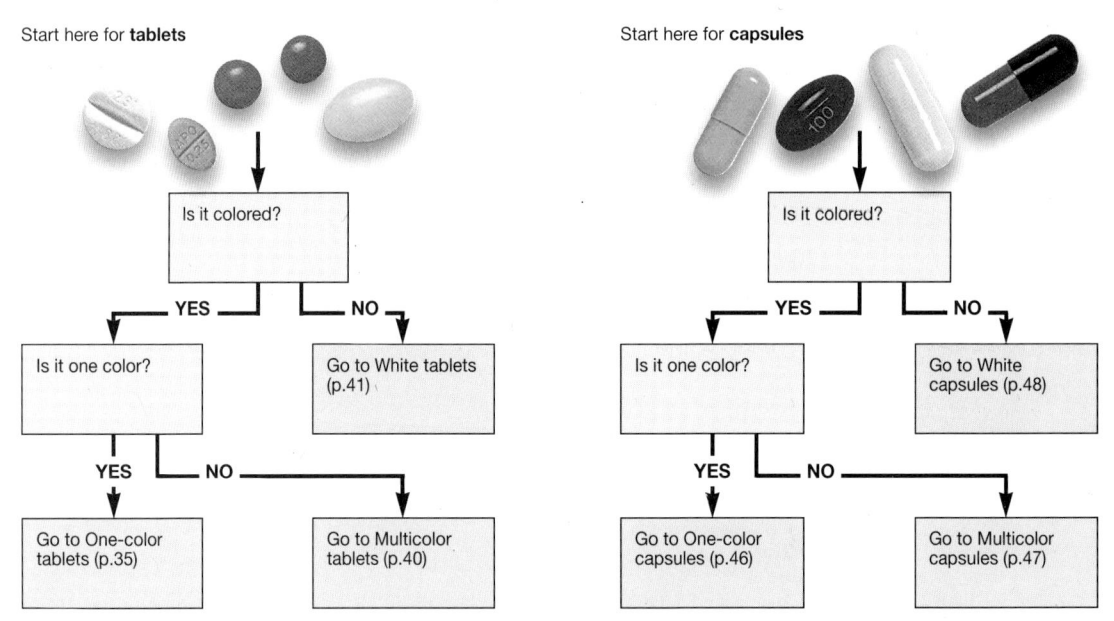

HOW TO UNDERSTAND THE ENTRIES

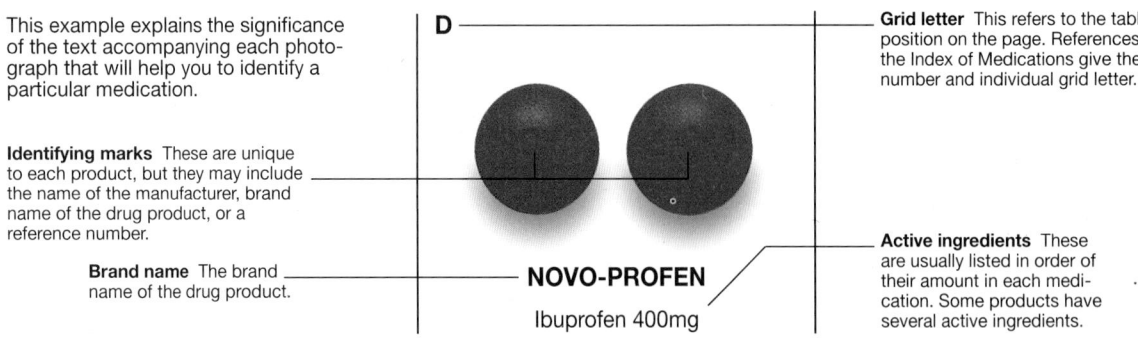

This example explains the significance of the text accompanying each photograph that will help you to identify a particular medication.

Identifying marks These are unique to each product, but they may include the name of the manufacturer, brand name of the drug product, or a reference number.

Brand name The brand name of the drug product.

Grid letter This refers to the tablet's position on the page. References in the Index of Medications give the page number and individual grid letter.

Active ingredients These are usually listed in order of their amount in each medication. Some products have several active ingredients.

NOVO-PROFEN

Ibuprofen 400mg

ONE-COLOR TABLETS

B

C

D

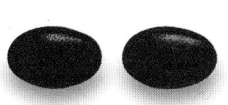
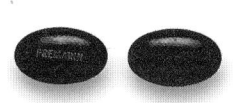
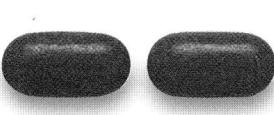
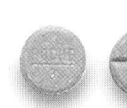

C.E.S.
Conjugated estrogens 0.625mg

PREMARIN
Conjugated estrogens 0.9mg

TRENTAL
Pentoxifylline 400mg

LECTOPAM
Bromazepam 3mg

F

G

H

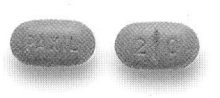
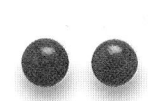
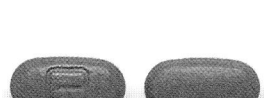
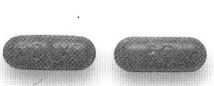

PAXIL
Paroxetine 20mg

LOZIDE
Indapamide hemihydrate 2.5mg

ERYTHROMID
Erythromycin 250mg

NOVO-METOPROL
Metoprolol tartrate 50mg

J

K

L

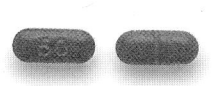
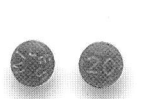
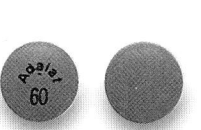
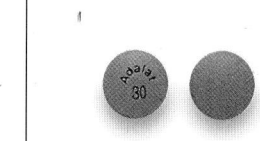

APO-METOPROLOL-L
Metoprolol tartrate 50mg

ADALAT PA 20
Nifedipine 20mg

ADALAT XL
Nifedipine 60mg

ADALAT XL
Nifedipine 30mg

N

O

P

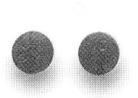
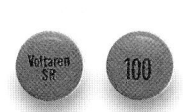
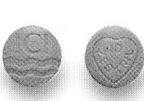
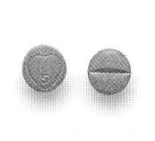

ADALAT PA 10
Nifedipine 10mg

VOLTAREN SR
Diclofenac sodium 100mg

ZESTRIL
Lisinopril 10mg

ZESTRIL
Lisinopril 5mg

R

S

T

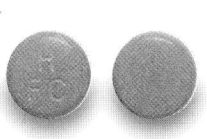
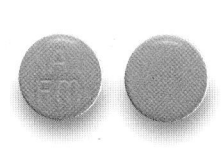
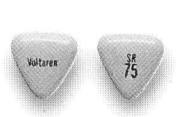
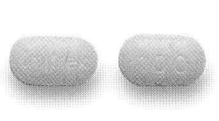

RENEDIL
Felodipine 5mg

PLENDIL
Felodipine 5mg

VOLTAREN SR
Diclofenac sodium 75mg

IMITREX
Sumatriptan 100mg

ONE-COLOR TABLETS continued

A

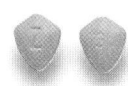

ZOCOR
Simvastatin 10mg

B

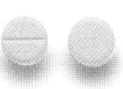

APO-HYDRO
Hydrochlorothiazide 25mg

C

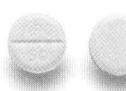

APO-HYDRO
Hydrochlorothiazide 50mg

D

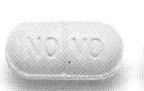

NOVO-NAPROX
Naproxen 375mg

E

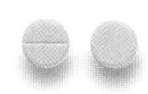

NOVO-HYDRAZIDE
Hydrochlorothiazide 25mg

F

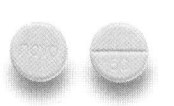

NOVO-HYDRAZIDE
Hydrochlorothiazide 50mg

G

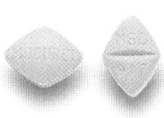

MODURET 50
Hydrochlorothiazide 50mg
Amiloride hydrochloride 5mg

H

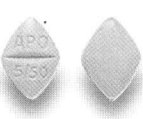

APO-AMILZIDE
Hydrochlorothiazide 50mg
Amiloride hydrochloride 5mg

I

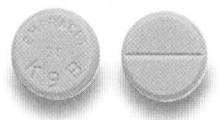

EMPRACET-30
Acetaminophen 300mg
Codeine phosphate 30mg

J

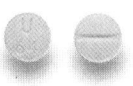

PROVERA
Medroxyprogesterone acetate
2.5mg

K

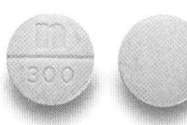

NADOPEN-V 500
Penicillin V potassium 300mg

L

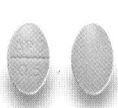

APO-ALPRAZ
Alprazolam 0.5mg

M

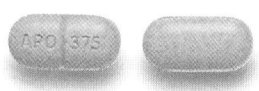

APO-NAPROXEN
Naproxen 375mg

N

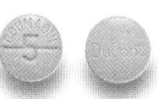

COUMADIN
Warfarin sodium 5mg

O

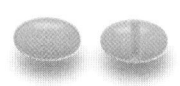

XANAX
Alprazolam 0.5mg

P

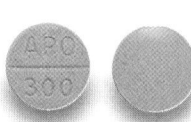

APO-ALLOPURINOL
Allopurinol 300mg

Q

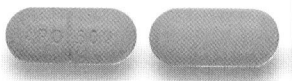

APO-CEPHALEX
Cephalexin 500mg

R

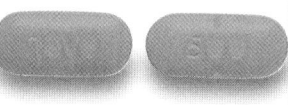

NOVO-LEXIN
Cephalexin 500mg

S

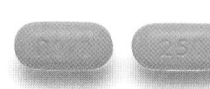

NOVO-LEXIN
Cephalexin 250mg

T

RIVOTRIL
Clonazepam 0.5mg

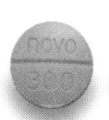 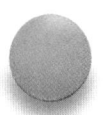

NOVO-PUROL

Allopurinol 300mg

B

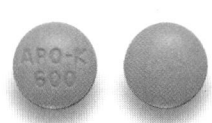

APO-K

Potassium chloride 600mg

C

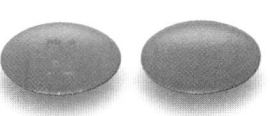

NOVASEN

Acetylsalicylic acid 650mg

D

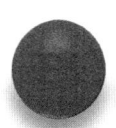 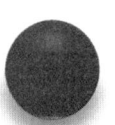

NOVO-PROFEN

Ibuprofen 400mg

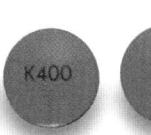

IBUPROFEN

Ibuprofen 400mg

F

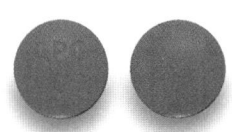

APO-IBUPROFEN

Ibuprofen 400mg

G

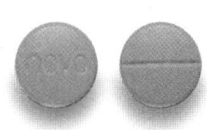

NOVO-PEN-VK-500

Penicillin V potassium 300mg

H

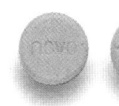 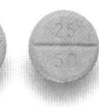

NOVO-TRIAMZIDE

Triamterene 50mg
Hydrochlorothiazide 25mg

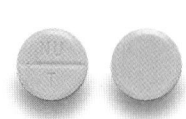

NU-TRIAZIDE

Triamterene 50mg
Hydrochlorothiazide 25mg

J

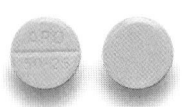

APO-TRIAZIDE

Triamterene 50mg
Hydrochlorothiazide 25mg

K

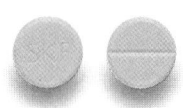

DYAZIDE

Triamterene 50mg
Hydrochlorothiazide 25mg

L

NOVOXAPAM

Oxazepam 15mg

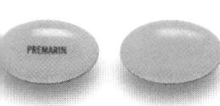

PREMARIN

Conjugated estrogens 1.25mg

N

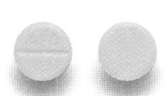

APO-OXAZEPAM

Oxazepam 15mg

O

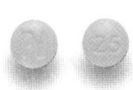

NOVO-TRIPTYN

Amitriptyline hydrochloride 25mg

P

FLEXERIL

Cyclobenzaprine hydrochloride
10mg

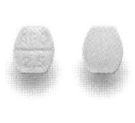

APO-ENALAPRIL

Enalapril maleate 2.5mg

R

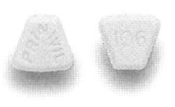

PRINIVIL

Lisinopril 10mg

S

VASOTEC

Enalapril maleate 2.5mg

T

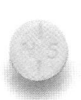

NOVO-DIPAM

Diazepam 5mg

ONE-COLOR TABLETS continued

A

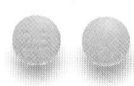

APO-AMITRIPTYLINE

Amitriptyline hydrochloride 25mg

B

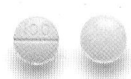

ELTROXIN

Levothyroxine sodium 100mcg

C

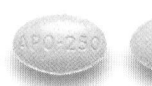

APO-NAPROXEN

Naproxen 250mg

D

NOVO-SEMIDE

Furosemide 40mg

E

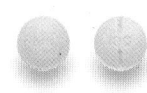

SYNTHROID

Levothyroxine sodium 100mcg

F

APO-DIAZEPAM

Diazepam 5mg

G

LANOXIN

Digoxin 0.125mg

H

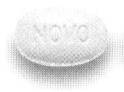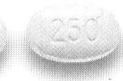

NOVO-NAPROX

Naproxen 250mg

I

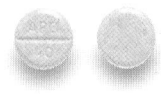

APO-FUROSEMIDE

Furosemide 40mg

J

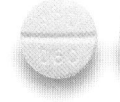

APO-DILTIAZ

Diltiazem hydrochloride 60mg

K

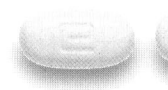

BIAXIN

Clarithromycin 250mg

L

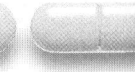

ISOPTIN SR

Verapamil hydrochloride 240mg

M

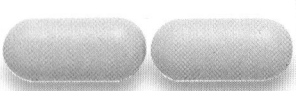

CALCIUM (NOVOPHARM)

Calcium 500mg
(as calcium carbonate 1,250mg)

N

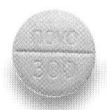

NOVO-CIMETINE

Cimetidine 300mg

O

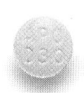

APO-DILTIAZ

Diltiazem hydrochloride 30mg

P

COUMADIN

Warfarin sodium 2.5mg

Q

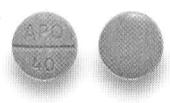

APO-PROPRANOLOL

Propranolol hydrochloride 40mg

R

ATIVAN SL

Lorazepam 0.5mg

S

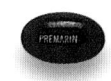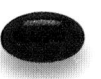

PREMARIN

Conjugated estrogens 0.3mg

T

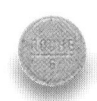

LECTOPAM

Bromazepam 6mg

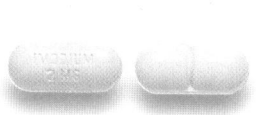

IMODIUM

Loperamide hydrochloride 2mg

B

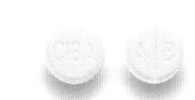

RITALIN

Methylphenidate hydrochloride 10mg

C

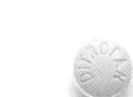

DITROPAN

Oxybutynin chloride 5mg

D

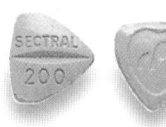

SECTRAL

Acebutolol 200mg

APO-AMITRIPTYLINE

Amitriptyline hydrochloride 10mg

F

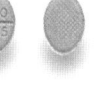

IMOVANE

Zopiclone 7.5mg

G

NOVO-TRIPTYN

Amitriptyline hydrochloride 10mg

H

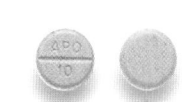

APO-DIAZEPAM

Diazepam 10mg

PROVERA

Medroxyprogesterone acetate 5mg

J

APO-TRIAZO

Triazolam 0.25mg

K

ANAPROX

Naproxen sodium 275mg

L

ELTROXIN

Levothyroxine sodium 150mcg

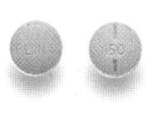

SYNTHROID

Levothyroxine sodium 150mcg

N

MEVACOR

Lovastatin 20mg

O

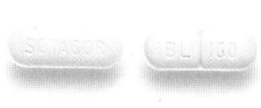

SOTACOR

Sotalol hydrochloride 160mg

P

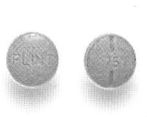

SYNTHROID

Levothyroxine sodium 75mcg

COUMADIN

Warfarin sodium 2mg

R

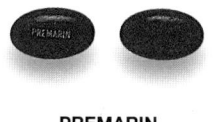

PREMARIN

Conjugated estrogens 0.625mg

S

NOVASEN

Acetylsalicylic acid 325mg

T

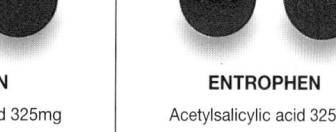

ENTROPHEN

Acetylsalicylic acid 325mg

ONE-COLOR TABLETS continued

A

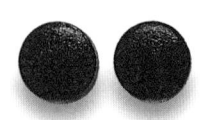

MSD E.C. ASA

Acetylsalicylic acid 325mg

B

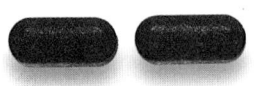

ASACOL

5-aminosalicylic acid 400mg

C

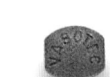

VASOTEC

Enalapril maleate 10mg

D

APO-ENALAPRIL

Enalapril maleate 10mg

E

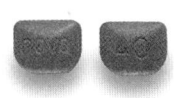

NOVO-FAMOTIDINE

Famotidine 40mg

F

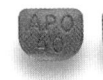

APO-FAMOTIDINE

Famotidine 40mg

G

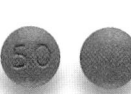

APO-AMITRIPTYLINE

Amitriptyline hydrochloride 50mg

H

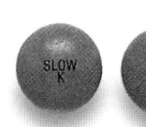

SLOW-K

Potassium chloride 600mg

I

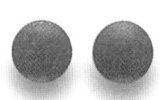

TEGRETOL CR

Carbamazepine 200mg

J

NOVO-DIFENAC

Diclofenac sodium 50mg

K

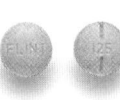

APO-DICLO

Diclofenac sodium 50mg

L

SYNTHROID

Levothyroxine sodium 125mcg

MULTICOLOR TABLETS

M

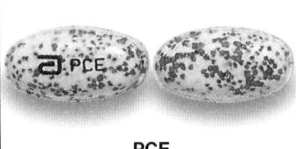

PCE

Erythromycin 333mg

N

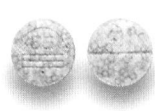

NITRONG SR

Nitroglycerin 2.6mg

O

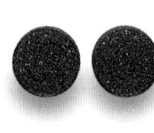

SENOKOT

Standardized sennosides 8.6mg

WHITE TABLETS

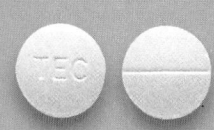

OXYCOCET

Oxycodone hydrochloride 5mg
Acetaminophen 325mg

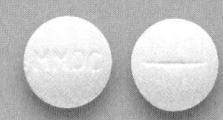

B

GLUCOPHAGE

Metformin hydrochloride 500mg

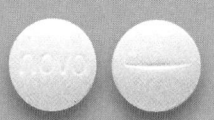

C

NOVO-METFORMIN

Metformin hydrochloride 500mg

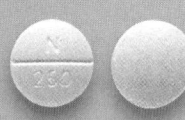

D

NOVO-NIDAZOL

Metronidazole 250mg

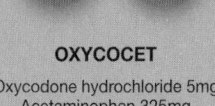

NOVO-TRIMEL

Sulfamethoxazole 400mg
Trimethoprim 80mg

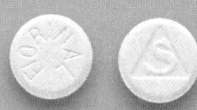

F

FIORINAL

Butalbital 50mg
Caffeine 40mg
Acetylsalicylic acid 330mg

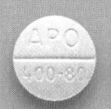 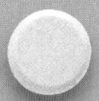

G

APO-SULFATRIM

Sulfamethoxazole 400mg
Trimethoprim 80mg

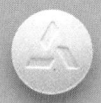 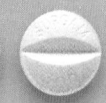

H

SURGAM SR

Tiaprofenic acid 300mg

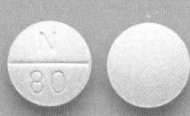

LENOL WITH CODEINE NO.3

Acetaminophen 300mg
Caffeine 15mg
Codeine phosphate 30mg

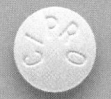 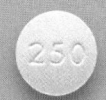

J

CIPRO

Ciprofloxacin 250mg

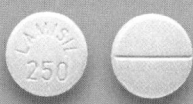

K

LAMISIL

Terbinafine 250mg

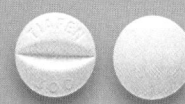

L

ALBERT TIAFEN

Tiaprofenic acid 300mg

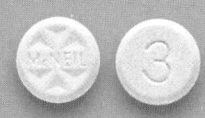

APO-ACETAMINOPHEN

Acetaminophen 500mg

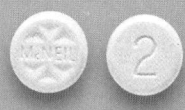

N

TYLENOL WITH CODEINE NO.2

Acetaminophen 300mg
Caffeine 15mg
Codeine phosphate 15mg

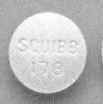

O

PRAVACHOL

Pravastatin sodium 20mg

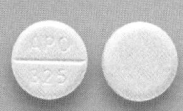

P

APO-ACETAMINOPHEN

Acetaminophen 325mg

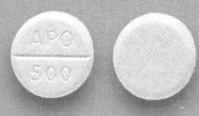

ARTHROTEC

Diclofenac sodium 50mg
Misoprostol 200mg

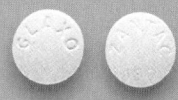

R

ZANTAC

Ranitidine 150mg

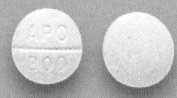

S

APO-PEN VK

Penicillin V potassium 300mg

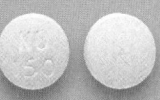

T

NU-RANIT

Ranitidine 150mg

WHITE TABLETS continued

A

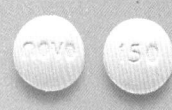

NOVO-RANIDINE

Ranitidine 150mg

B

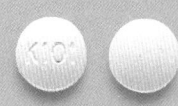

RANITIDINE (KENRAL)

Ranitidine 150mg

C

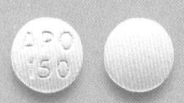

APO-RANITIDINE

Ranitidine 150mg

D

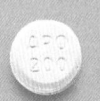

APO-CARBAMAZEPINE

Carbamazepine 200mg

E

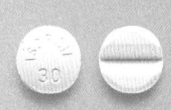

ISORDIL 30 TITRADOSE

Isosorbide dinitrate 30mg

F

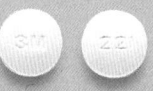

NORFLEX

Orphenadrine citrate 100mg

G

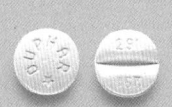

LUVOX

Fluvoxamine maleate 50mg

H

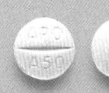

APO-ATENOL

Atenolol 50mg

I

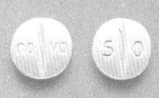

NOVO-ATENOL

Atenolol 50mg

J

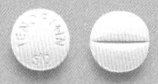

TENORMIN

Atenolol 50mg

K

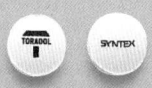

TORADOL

Ketorolac tromethamine 10mg

L

PREPULSID

Cisapride 10mg

M

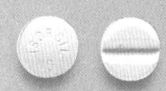

ISORDIL 10 TITRADOSE

Isosorbide dinitrate 10mg

N

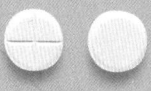

DIAMICRON

Gliclazide 80mg

O

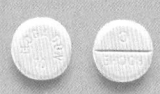

MOGADON

Nitrazepam 10mg

P

RIVOTRIL

Clonazepam 2mg

Q

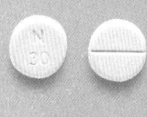

NOVOXAPAM

Oxazepam 30mg

R

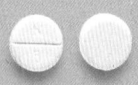

NOVO-PREDNISONE

Prednisone 5mg

S

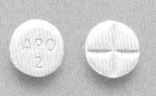

APO-BENZTROPINE

Benztropine mesylate 2mg

T

LANOXIN

Digoxin 0.25mg

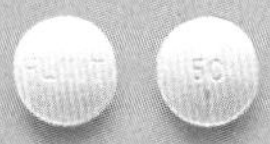

A

SYNTHROID

Levothyroxine sodium 50mcg

B

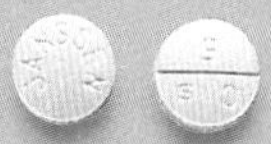

PREPULSID

Cisapride 5mg

C

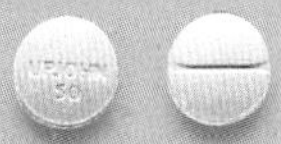

PROVERA

Medroxyprogesterone acetate 10mg

D

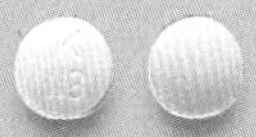

DOMPERIDONE (KENRAL)

Domperidone 10mg

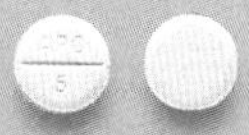

E

APO-PREDNISONE

Prednisone 5mg

F

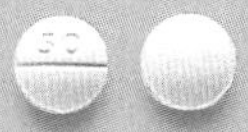

ELTROXIN

Levothyroxine sodium 50mcg

G

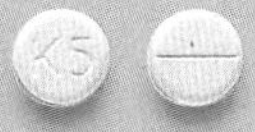

PREDNISONE (KENRAL)

Prednisone 5mg

H

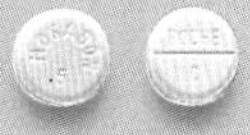

MOGADON

Nitrazepam 5mg

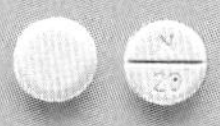

I

NOVO-SEMIDE

Furosemide 20mg

J

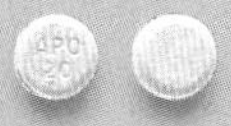

APO-FUROSEMIDE

Furosemide 20mg

K

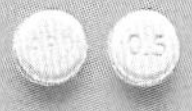

APO-LORAZEPAM

Lorazepam 0.5mg

L

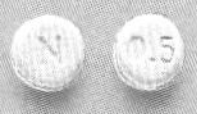

NOVO-LORAZEM

Lorazepam 0.5mg

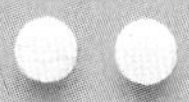

M

NITROSTAT

Nitroglycerin 0.3mg

N

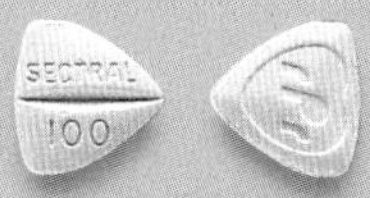

SECTRAL

Acebutolol 100mg

O

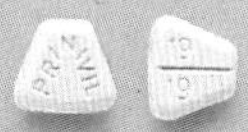

PRINIVIL

Lisinopril 5mg

P

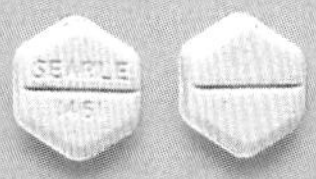

CYTOTEC

Misoprostol 200mcg

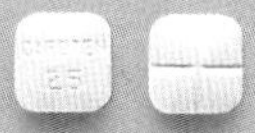

Q

CAPOTEN

Captopril 25mg

R

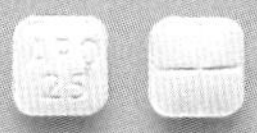

APO-CAPTO

Captopril 25mg

S

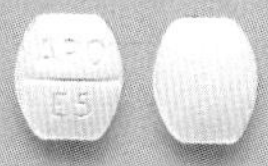

APO-ENALAPRIL

Enalapril maleate 5mg

T

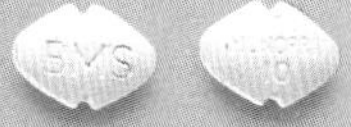

MONOPRIL

Fosinopril sodium 10mg

WHITE TABLETS continued

A

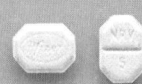

NORVASC

Amlodipine 5mg

B

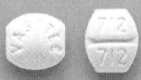

VASOTEC

Enalapril maleate 5mg

C

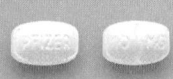

REACTINE

Cetirizine hydrochloride 10mg

D

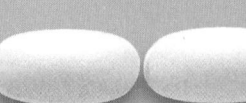

CLAVULIN-500

Amoxicillin 500mg
Clavulanate potassium 125mg

E

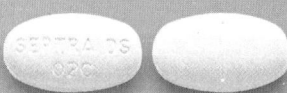

SEPTRA DS

Trimethoprim 160mg
Sulfamethoxazole 800mg

F

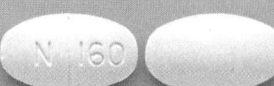

NOVO-TRIMEL DS

Trimethoprim 160mg
Sulfamethoxazole 800mg

G

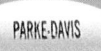 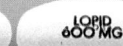

LOPID

Gemfibrozil 600mg

H

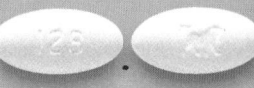

PONDOCILLIN

Pivampicillin 500mg

I

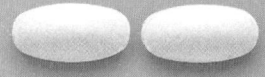

CLAVULIN-250

Amoxicillin 250mg
Clavulanate potassium 125mg

J

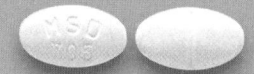

NOROXIN

Norfloxacin 400mg

K

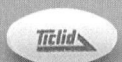

TICLID

Ticlopidine hydrochloride 250mg

L

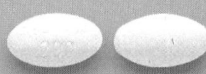

THEO-DUR

Theophylline 200mg

M

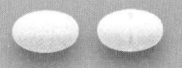

XANAX

Alprazolam 0.25mg

N

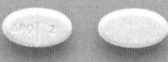

APO-LORAZEPAM

Lorazepam 2mg

O

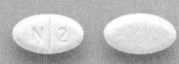

NOVO-LORAZEM

Lorazepam 2mg

P

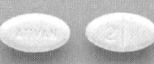

ATIVAN

Lorazepam 2mg

Q

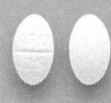

APO-ALPRAZ

Alprazolam 0.25mg

R

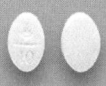

CLARITIN

Loratadine 10mg

S

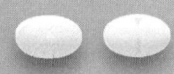

ALPRAZOLAM

Alprazolam 0.25mg

T

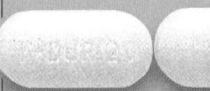

K-DUR 20

Potassium chloride 1,500mg

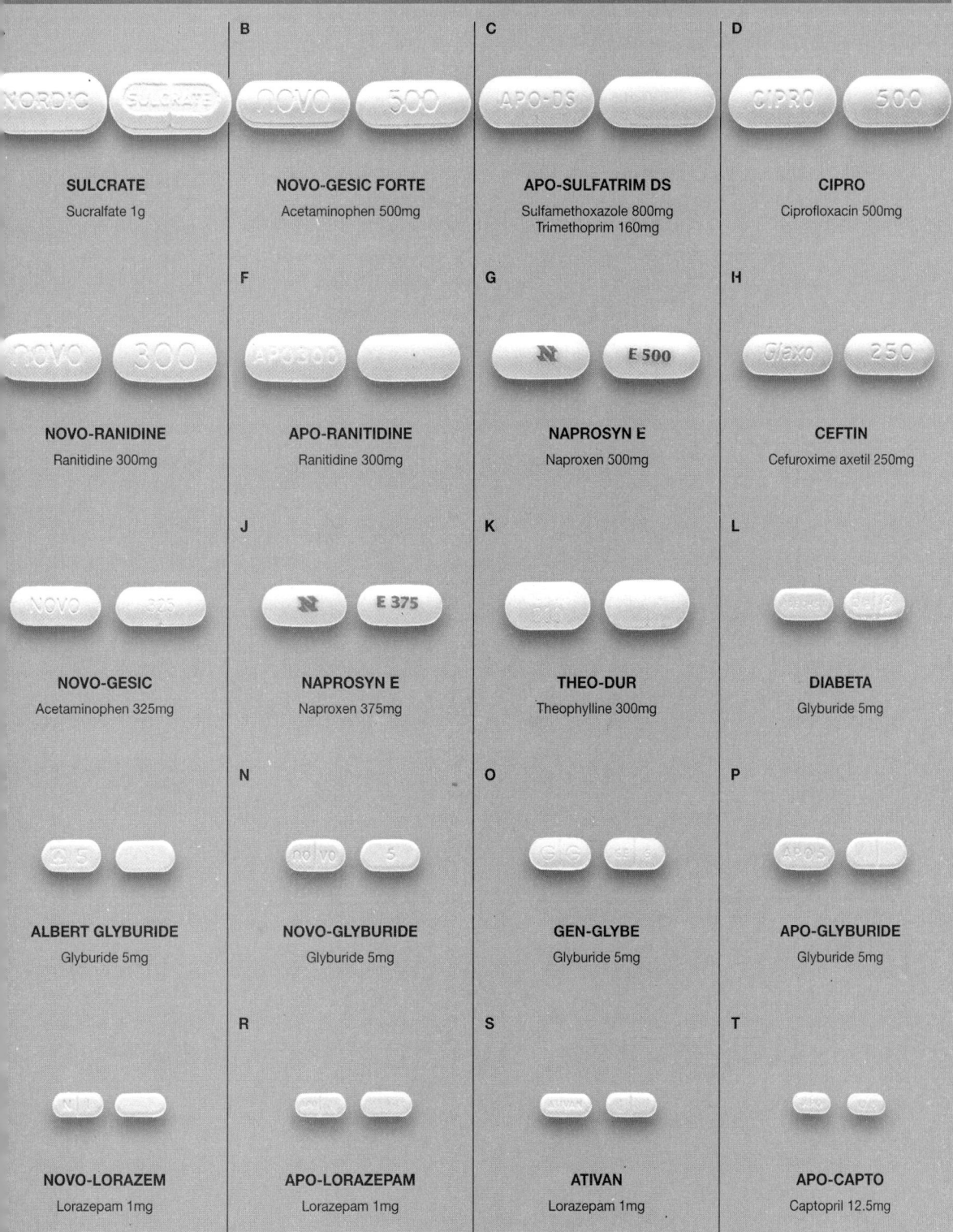

SULCRATE

Sucralfate 1g

B

NOVO-GESIC FORTE

Acetaminophen 500mg

C

APO-SULFATRIM DS

Sulfamethoxazole 800mg
Trimethoprim 160mg

D

CIPRO

Ciprofloxacin 500mg

NOVO-RANIDINE

Ranitidine 300mg

F

APO-RANITIDINE

Ranitidine 300mg

G

NAPROSYN E

Naproxen 500mg

H

CEFTIN

Cefuroxime axetil 250mg

NOVO-GESIC

Acetaminophen 325mg

J

NAPROSYN E

Naproxen 375mg

K

THEO-DUR

Theophylline 300mg

L

DIABETA

Glyburide 5mg

ALBERT GLYBURIDE

Glyburide 5mg

N

NOVO-GLYBURIDE

Glyburide 5mg

O

GEN-GLYBE

Glyburide 5mg

P

APO-GLYBURIDE

Glyburide 5mg

NOVO-LORAZEM

Lorazepam 1mg

R

APO-LORAZEPAM

Lorazepam 1mg

S

ATIVAN

Lorazepam 1mg

T

APO-CAPTO

Captopril 12.5mg

ONE-COLOR CAPSULES

A

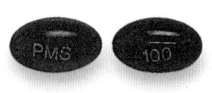

SOFLAX

Docusate sodium 100mg

B

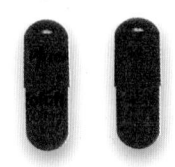

ZOLOFT

Sertraline hydrochloride 100mg

C

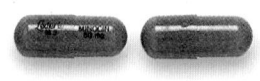

MINOCIN

Minocycline 50mg

D

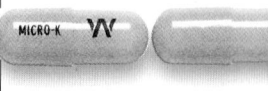

MICRO-K EXTENCAPS

Potassium chloride 600mg

E

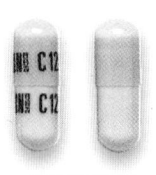

CARBOLITH

Lithium carbonate 300mg

F

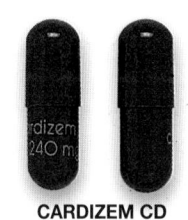

CARDIZEM CD

Diltiazem hydrochloride 240mg

G

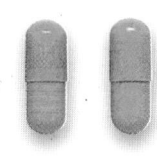

INDERAL-LA

Propranolol hydrochloride 80mg

H

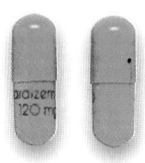

CARDIZEM CD

Diltiazem hydrochloride 120mg

I

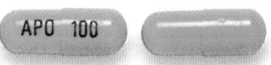

APO-DOXY

Doxycycline hyclate 100mg

J

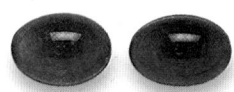

NOVO-CHLORHYDRATE

Chloral hydrate 500mg

K

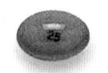

NOVO-HYDROXYZIN

Hydroxyzine hydrochloride 25mg

MULTICOLOR CAPSULES

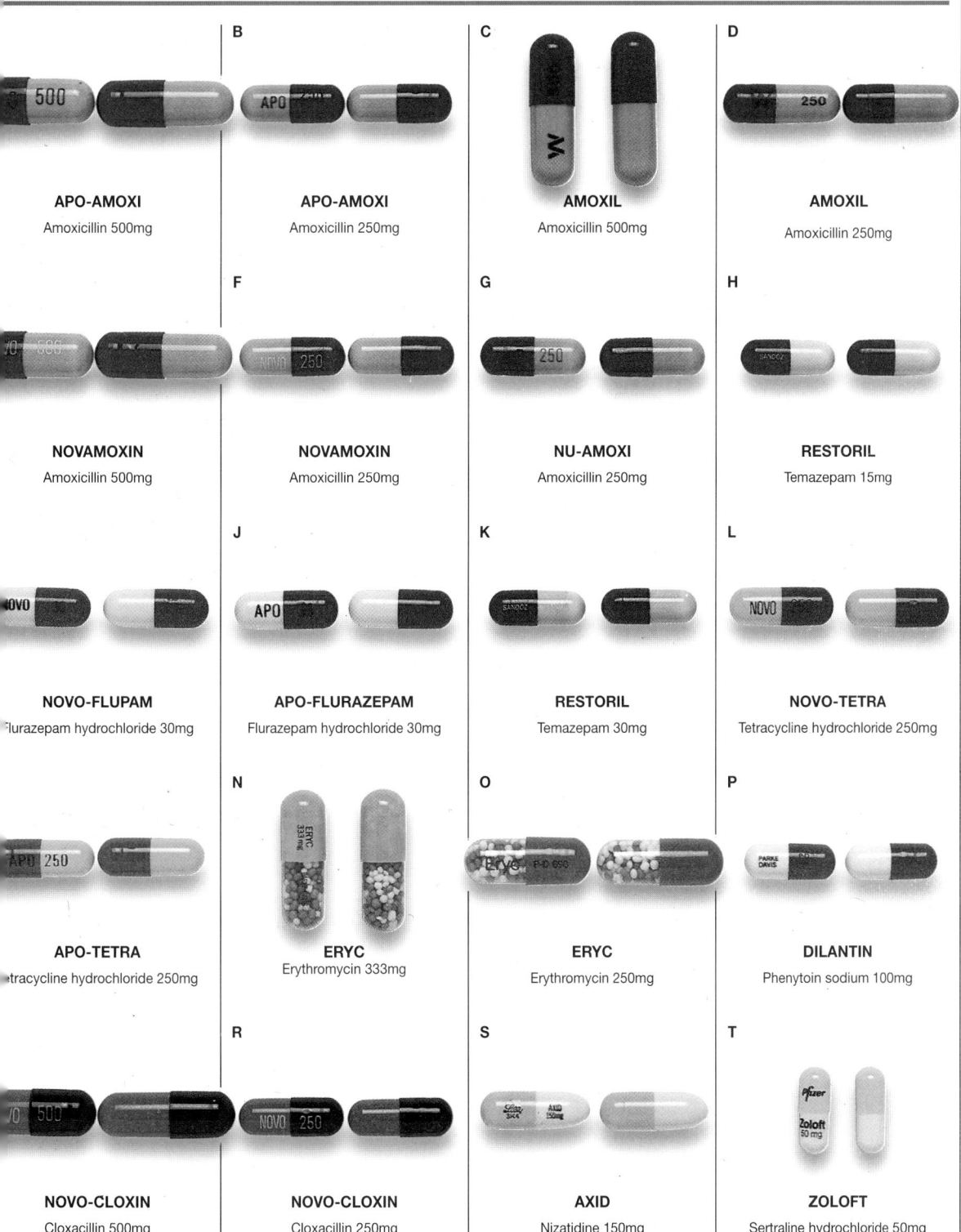

B

APO-AMOXI

Amoxicillin 500mg

APO-AMOXI

Amoxicillin 250mg

C

AMOXIL

Amoxicillin 500mg

D

AMOXIL

Amoxicillin 250mg

NOVAMOXIN

Amoxicillin 500mg

F

NOVAMOXIN

Amoxicillin 250mg

G

NU-AMOXI

Amoxicillin 250mg

H

RESTORIL

Temazepam 15mg

NOVO-FLUPAM

Flurazepam hydrochloride 30mg

J

APO-FLURAZEPAM

Flurazepam hydrochloride 30mg

K

RESTORIL

Temazepam 30mg

L

NOVO-TETRA

Tetracycline hydrochloride 250mg

APO-TETRA

Tetracycline hydrochloride 250mg

N

ERYC

Erythromycin 333mg

O

ERYC

Erythromycin 250mg

P

DILANTIN

Phenytoin sodium 100mg

NOVO-CLOXIN

Cloxacillin 500mg

R

NOVO-CLOXIN

Cloxacillin 250mg

S

AXID

Nizatidine 150mg

T

ZOLOFT

Sertraline hydrochloride 50mg

MULTICOLOR CAPSULES continued

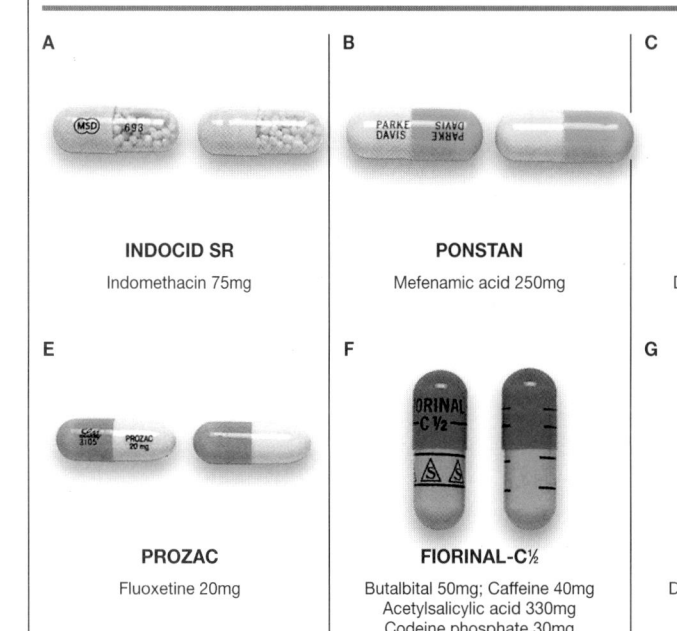

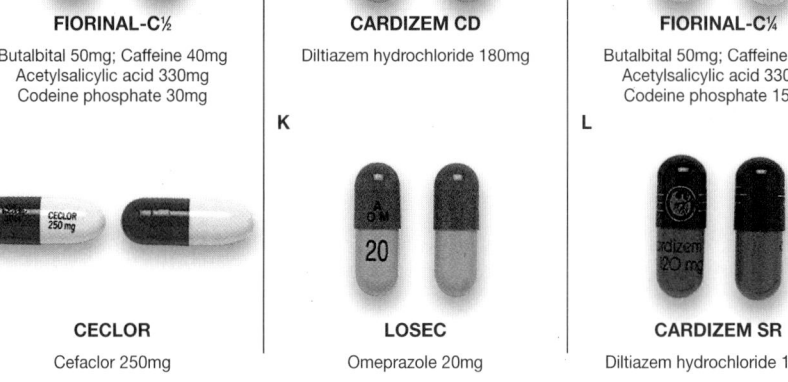

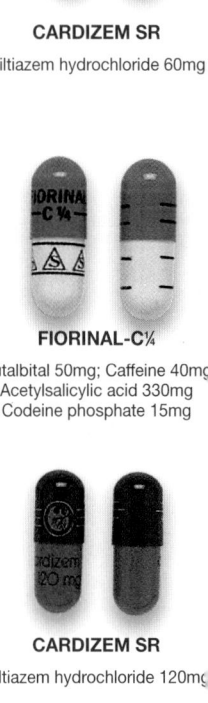

A

INDOCID SR

Indomethacin 75mg

B

PONSTAN

Mefenamic acid 250mg

C

CARDIZEM SR

Diltiazem hydrochloride 90mg

D

CARDIZEM SR

Diltiazem hydrochloride 60mg

E

PROZAC

Fluoxetine 20mg

F

FIORINAL-C½

Butalbital 50mg; Caffeine 40mg
Acetylsalicylic acid 330mg
Codeine phosphate 30mg

G

CARDIZEM CD

Diltiazem hydrochloride 180mg

H

FIORINAL-C¼

Butalbital 50mg; Caffeine 40mg
Acetylsalicylic acid 330mg
Codeine phosphate 15mg

I

NOVO-METHACIN

Indomethacin 25mg

J

CECLOR

Cefaclor 250mg

K

LOSEC

Omeprazole 20mg

L

CARDIZEM SR

Diltiazem hydrochloride 120mg

WHITE CAPSULES

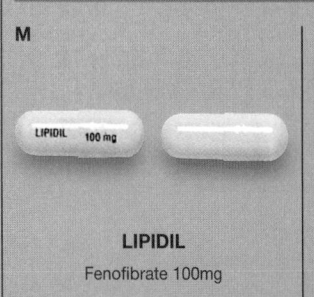

M

LIPIDIL

Fenofibrate 100mg

INDEX OF MEDICATIONS

his index contains the names of approximately ,500 individual drug products and substances. provides the entry point to the book for readers ho are interested in learning about a specific edication. There is no need for you to know efore using this index whether the name you ant to look up is a brand name or a non-roprietary name, or whether it is a prescription r over-the-counter product: all types of edications are listed.

What the index contains

ll major drug products, many less widely used reparations as well as vitamins and minerals re listed in the index. This comprehensive election of products is designed to reflect the ide diversity of agents available for the eatment and prevention of disease. It does not nply CMA endorsement of any of the drugs or roducts listed, nor does the exclusion of a articular product from the index indicate CMA sapproval.

How the entries are ordered

All entries are listed in alphabetical order. Brand-name products can be distinguished by their initial capital letter.

How the references work

References are either to the pages in Part 4 containing the drug profiles of each principal active ingredient, or to the section in Part 3 that describes the relevant drug group. Some entries for substances that have not been given a full-page profile contain a brief description. Where an entry for a brand-name product gives the name of the drug but no page number, go to the entry for that drug within the index, which will then direct you to further information as appropriate.

Color Identification Guide

Tablets and capsules that are pictured in the Color Identification Guide contain a reference in italic type to the page and grid letter where the photograph of that product may be found.

A

Abbokinase urokinase
Abenol acetaminophen 199
Accupril quinapril 455
Accutane isotretinoin 352
acebutolol 198
acecainide an anti-arrhythmic drug 112
aceclidine a *miotic* drug used in the treatment of glaucoma. See Drugs for glaucoma 180
acetaminophen 199
acetazolamide a carbonic anhydrase inhibitor diuretic. See Diuretics 111
Acetazone Forte chlorzoxazone and acetaminophen (199)
Acetazone Forte C8 chlorzoxazone, acetaminophen (199), and codeine (270)
acetic acid the acid found in vinegar. Used medically to inhibit infection in the vagina and in the ear
acetohexamide an oral antidiabetic drug. See Drugs used in diabetes 154
acetone a pharmaceutical solvent
acetophenazine a phenothiazine antipsychotic drug 97
Acetoxyl benzoyl peroxide 224
acetylcholine a chemical *neurotransmitter* that stimulates the parasympathetic nervous system

A

(91). Used as a *miotic* drug. See Drugs affecting the pupil 182
acetylcysteine a *mucolytic* agent. See Drugs to treat coughs 106
acetylsalicylic acid 200
Achrocidin tetracycline (489), salicylamide, caffeine, and chlorothen
Achromycin V tetracycline 489
Acilac lactulose 356
aclarubicin an *investigational* anticancer drug 166
Acnex a salicylic acid wash
Acnomel resorcinol and sulfur
Acnomel Acne Mask a salicylic acid cream
Acnomel B.P.5 benzoyl peroxide 224
acrisorcin an antifungal drug used in the treatment of tinea versicolor. See Antifungal drugs 150
acritretin an oral retinoid used to treat psoriasis
acrivastine a non-sedative antihistamine drug. See Antihistamines 136
acrosoxacin an antibacterial drug. See Antibacterial drugs 143
ACTH adrenocorticotropic hormone. See corticotropin
Acthar corticotropin
Acti-B$_{12}$ hydroxocobalamin
Actifed pseudoephedrine (450) and triprolidine
Actifed DM pseudoephedrine (450), triprolidine, and dextromethorphan (281)
Actifed Plus Extra Strength acetaminophen (199), pseudoephedrine (450), and triprolidine

ACTINAC – APO-CARBAMAZEPINE

A

Actinac chloramphenicol (249) hydrocortisone (338), sulfur, butoxyethyl nicotinate, and allantoin

Actiprofen ibuprofen 341

Activase tissue plasminogen activator 495

Acular ketorolac 355

acyclovir 201

Adalat PA *35J, 35M* (illus.); nifedipine 404

Adalat XL *35K, 35L* (illus.); nifedipine 404

Adasept Acne Gel triclosan, salicylic acid, and sodium thiosulfate

Adasept Cleanser triclosan

Adrenalin epinephrine 300

adrenocorticotropic hormone see corticotropin

Adrucil fluorouracil 317

Advil ibuprofen 341

Advil Cold Sinus ibuprofen (341) and pseudoephedrine (450)

Aerosporin polymyxin B

agar an emulsifying agent

Agarol Vanilla (or strawberry) liquids laxative preparations containing mineral oil, glycerin, and agar. See Laxatives 123

Agarol Plain a liquid laxative containing mineral oil, glycerin, and agar. See Laxatives 123

Agarol Tablets aloin and phenolphthalein

A-Hydrocort hydrocortisone 338

Akineton biperiden

Albalon-A Liquifilm naphazoline and antazoline

Albalon Liquifilm naphazoline

Albert Glyburide *45M* (illus.); glyburide 330

Albert Tiafen *41L* (illus.); tiaprofenic acid 492

albuterol see salbutamol

Alcaine proparacaine

alcohol, rubbing isopropyl alcohol. Used as a *rubefacient* and as a skin antiseptic. See Anti-infective skin preparations 187

alcometasone a topical corticosteroid for inflammatory skin disorders. See Topical corticosteroids 186

Alcomicin gentamicin 328

Aldactazide hydrochlorothiazide (336) and spironolactone (469)

Aldactone spironolactone 469

Aldomet methyldopa 384

Aldoril hydrochlorothiazide (336) and methyldopa (384)

alfacalcidol a vitamin D drug. See Vitamin D 529

Alfenta alfentanil

alfentanil a narcotic analgesic 93

algeldrate see aluminum hydroxide 204

alginic acid an antifoaming agent. See Antacids 120

Alka-Seltzer ASA (200), sodium bicarbonate, and citric acid (541)

Alkeran melphalan

allantoin a uric acid derivative. Applied *topically*, is said to encourage healing of minor wounds

Allerdryl diphenhydramine 290

Allernix diphenhydramine 290

allopurinol 202

allylestrenol a progestin drug. See Female sex hormones 159

A

aloin a stimulant laxative 123

Alomide lodoxamide

Alophen phenolphthalein

Alpha-Baclofen baclofen 221

Alpha Keri a mineral oil and lanolin bath additive for dry, itchy skin. See Antipruritic medications 185

Alpha-Lac lactulose 356

alphaprodine a narcotic analgesic 93

Alpha-Tamoxifen tamoxifen 480

alpha-tocopherol a form of vitamin E 529

Alphosyl allantoin and coal tar

alprazolam *44T* (illus.); alprazolam 203

alprostadil a drug used in congenital heart disease to keep open the blood vessels between the heart and lungs until surgery can be performed.

alseroxylon an antihypertensive drug 114

Altace ramipril

alteplase see tissue plasminogen activator (tPA) 495

altretamine an anticancer drug 166

aluminum acetate an *astringent* substance applied to soothe inflammation of the skin or outer ear canal. Also included in some rectal preparations. See Drugs for rectal and anal disorders 125

aluminum carbonate a drug used to reduce phosphate levels in the blood and occasionally used as an antacid. See Antacids 120

aluminum chloride an *antiperspirant*

aluminum hydroxide 204

Alupent orciprenaline 415

Alu-Tab aluminum hydroxide 204

alverine an antispasmodic drug used in the treatment of irritable bowel syndrome.

amantadine 205

Amatine midodrine

ambenonium a drug used to treat myasthenia gravis 133

Ambenyl codeine (270), diphenhydramine (290), bromodiphenhydramine, ammonium chloride, and guaiacolsulfonate

amcinonide a corticosteroid used in *topical* preparations to treat inflammatory skin disorders. See Topical corticosteroids 186

amdinocillin a penicillin antibiotic. See Antibiotics 140

Amesec aminophylline, ephedrine, and amobarbital

amethocaine a local anesthetic. See local anesthetics 92

amethopterin see methotrexate

Amicar aminocaproic acid

amikacin an aminoglycoside antibiotic 140

Amikin amikacin

amiloride 206

aminacrine an *antiseptic* dye used in *topical* preparations. See Anti-infective skin preparations 187

aminoacetic acid a substance occasionally used as an antacid 120

aminobenzoate potassium an antifibrotic agent used in the treatment of Peyronie's disease

A

aminobenzoic acid a chemical used in sun-screening preparations. See Sunscreens 191

aminocaproic acid a drug used to promote blood clotting. See Drugs that affect blood clotting 116

aminoglutethimide a drug used in the treatment of advanced breast cancer and Cushing's syndrome (an adrenal disorder). See Anticancer drugs 166

aminophylline 490

aminosalicylate sodium an antituberculous drug 144

aminothiadiazole an *investigational* anticancer drug 166

amiodarone 207

amitriptyline 208

amlodipine 209

ammoniated mercury an agent occasionally used in the treatment of skin conditions such as impetigo and dermatitis

ammonium chloride a drug used to increase the acidity of urine and to speed the excretion of certain poisons in the urine. Also used as an expectorant. See Drugs to treat coughs 106

amobarbital a barbiturate sleeping drug 94

amodiaquine an antimalarial drug not available in Canada. See antimalarial drugs 149

amoxapine a tricyclic antidepressant 96

amoxicillin 210

Amoxil *47C, 47D* (illus.); amoxicillin 210

amphetamine 533

Amphojel aluminum hydroxide 204

Amphojel 500 aluminum hydroxide (204) and magnesium hydroxide (370)

Amphojel Plus aluminum hydroxide (204), magnesium hydroxide (370), and simethicone

amphotericin B 211

ampicillin 212

Ampicin ampicillin 212

amrinone a drug used in the treatment of congestive heart failure

amsacrine an anticancer drug 166

AMSA-PD amsacrine

amyl nitrite a vasodilator drug formerly used in the treatment of angina, now considered a drug of abuse. See Nitrites 537

amylobarbitone see amobarbital

amylocaine a local anesthetic. See Local anesthetics 92

Amytal amobarbital

Anacin ASA (200) and caffeine

Anafranil clomipramine 264

anagrelide an *investigational* antiplatelet drug. See Drugs that affect blood clotting 116

Ana-Kit epinephrine (300) and chlorpheniramine (251)

Anandron nilutamide 405

Anapolon 50 oxymetholone

Anaprox *39K* (illus.); naproxen sodium 400

Anbesol Gel benzocaine (223) and phenol

Ancef cefazolin

Ancotil flucytosine

A

Ancrod an anticoagulant substance derived from Malayan pit viper venom. See Drugs that affect blood clotting 116

Andriol testosterone 488

Androcur cyproterone

Anectine succinylcholine

anetholtrithione a drug used to treat the oral symptoms of drug-induced dry mouth

Anexate flumazenil

anileridine a narcotic analgesic. See Analgesics 92

anisindione an anticoagulant drug. See Drugs that affect blood clotting 116

Ansaid flurbiprofen 321

ansamycin an *investigational* antibacterial drug related to rifampin 459

Antabuse disulfiram 294

antazoline a decongestant 105

Anthraforte anthralin 213

anthralin 213

Anthranol anthralin 213

Anthrascalp anthralin 213

antihemophilic factor a blood protein used to promote blood clotting in hemophilia. See Drugs that affect blood clotting 116

antipyrine an analgesic drug used in ear drops for outer ear inflammation. See Analgesics 92

Antivert meclizine (373) and niacin (523)

Anturan sulfinpyrazone 476

Anusol ointment and suppositories containing zinc sulfate (530) for the relief of anal irritation. See Drugs for rectal and anal disorders 125

Anusol-HC zinc sulfate (530) and hydrocortisone (338)

Anusol Plus pramoxine and zinc sulfate (530)

Anuzinc ointment and suppositories containing zinc sulfate (530) for the relief of anal irritation. See Drugs for rectal and anal disorders 125

APAP see acetaminophen

APL HCG 334

Apo-Acetaminophen *41M, 41P* (illus.); acetaminophen 199

Apo-Acetazolamide acetazolamide

Apo-Allopurinol *36P* (illus.); allopurinol 202

Apo-Alpraz *36L, 44Q* (illus.); alprazolam 203

Apo-Amilzide *36H* (illus.); amiloride (206) and hydrochlorothiazide (336)

Apo-Amitriptyline *38A, 39E, 40G* (illus); amitriptyline 208

Apo-Amoxi *47A, 47B* (illus.); amoxicillin 210

Apo-Ampi ampicillin 212

Apo-ASA ASA 200

Apo-Atenol *42H* (illus.); atenolol 215

Apo-Benztropine *42S* (illus.); benztropine 225

Apo-Bisacodyl bisacodyl 229

Apo-Bromocriptine bromocriptine 231

Apo-C ascorbic acid 528

Apo-Cal calcium carbonate 519

Apo-Capto *43R, 45T* (illus.); captopril 239

Apo-Carbamazepine *42D* (illus.); carbamazepine 240

APO-CEPHALEX – BENOXYL

A   **Apo-Cephalex** *36Q* (illus.); cephalexin 245
Apo-Chlorax chlordiazepoxide (250) and clidinium bromide
Apo-Chlordiazepoxide chlordiazepoxide 250
Apo-Chlorpropamide chlorpropamide 253
Apo-Chlorthalidone chlorthalidone 254
Apo-Cimetidine cimetidine 257
Apo-Clonidine clonidine 266
Apo-Clorazepate clorazepate 267
Apo-Cloxi cloxacillin 269
Apo-Diazepam *38F, 39H* (illus.); diazepam 282
Apo-Diclo *40K* (illus.); diclofenac 283
Apo-Diltiaz *38J, 38O* (illus.); diltiazem 287
Apo-Dimenhydrinate dimenhydrinate 288
Apo-Dipyridamole dipyridamole 292
Apo-Doxy *46I* (illus.); doxycycline 297
Apo-Enalapril *37Q, 40D, 43S* (illus.); enalapril 299
Apo-Erythro erythromycin 302
Apo-Erythro-ES erythromycin 302
Apo-Famotidine *40F* (illus.); famotidine 309
Apo-Ferrous Gluconate ferrous gluconate
Apo-Ferrous Sulfate ferrous sulfate
Apo-Fluphenazine fluphenazine 319
Apo-Flurazepam *47J* (illus.); flurazepam 320
Apo-Flurbiprofen flurbiprofen 321
Apo-Folic folic acid
Apo-Furosemide *38I, 43J* (illus.); furosemide 325
Apo-Gain minoxidil
Apo-Gemfibrozil gemfibrozil 327
Apo-Glyburide *45P* (illus.); glyburide 330
Apo-Guanethidine guanethidine
Apo-Haloperidol haloperidol 332
Apo-Hydralazine hydralazine 335
Apo-Hydro *36B, 36C* (illus.); hydrochlorothiazide 336
Apo-Hydroxyzine hydroxyzine 340
Apo-Ibuprofen *37F* (illus.); ibuprofen 341
Apo-Imipramine imipramine 343
Apo-Indomethacin indomethacin 345
Apo-ISDN isosorbide dinitrate 351
Apo-K *37B* (illus.); potassium chloride 524
Apo-Keto ketoprofen 354
Apo-Lorazepam *43K, 44N, 45R* (illus.); lorazepam 367
Apo-Meprobamate meprobamate 377
Apo-Methazide hydrochlorothiazide (336) and methyldopa (384)
Apo-Methyldopa methyldopa 384
Apo-Metoclop metoclopramide 387
Apo-Metoprolol metoprolol 388
Apo-Metoprolol-L *35I* (illus.); metoprolol 388
Apo-Metronidazole metronidazole 389
Apo-Nadol nadolol 398
Apo-Naproxen *36M, 38C* (illus.); naproxen 400
Apo-Nifed nifedipine 404
Apo-Nitrofurantoin nitrofurantoin 407
Apo-Oxazepam *37N* (illus.); oxazepam 417
Apo-Oxtriphylline oxtriphylline
Apo-Pen VK *41S* (illus.); penicillin V 425
Apo-Perphenazine perphenazine 428
Apo-Phenylbutazone phenylbutazone
Apo-Pindol pindolol 434

A   **Apo-Piroxicam** piroxicam 435
Apo-Prazo prazosin 438
Apo-Prednisone *43E* (illus.); prednisone 440
Apo-Primidone primidone 441
Apo-Propranolol *38Q* (illus.); propranolol 448
Apo-Quinidine quinidine 456
Apo-Ranitidine *42C, 45F* (illus.); ranitidine 458
Apo-Salvent salbutamol 461
Apo-Sulfamethoxazole sulfamethoxazole 474
Apo-Sulfatrim *41G* (illus.); sulfamethoxazole (474) and trimethoprim (507)
Apo-Sulfatrim-DS *45C* (illus.); sulfamethoxazole (474) and trimethoprim (507)
Apo-Sulfatrim Pediatric sulfamethoxazole (474) and trimethoprim (507)
Apo-Sulfinpyrazone sulfinpyrazone 476
Apo-Sulin sulindac 478
Apo-Tamoxifen tamoxifen 480
Apo-Terfenadine terfenadine 487
Apo-Tetra *47M* (illus.); tetracycline 489
Apo-Thioridazine thioridazine 491
Apo-Timol timolol 494
Apo-Timop timolol 494
Apo-Tolbutamide tolbutamide 497
Apo-Triazide *37J* (illus.); triamterene (502) and hydrochlorothiazide (336)
Apo-Triazo *39J* (illus.); triazolam 503
Apo-Trifluoperazine trifluoperazine 504
Apo-Trihex trihexyphenidyl 505
Apo-Trimip trimipramine 508
apraclonidine a drug used to control post-surgical intraocular pressure. See Drugs for glaucoma 180
Apresoline hydralazine 335
aprindine an anti-arrhythmic agent. See Anti-arrhythmic drugs 112
aprotinin an antifibrinolytic agent used to promote blood clotting. See Drugs that affect blood clotting 116
Aquasol A vitamin A 527
Aquasol A and D vitamin A (527) and vitamin D (52...
Aquasol E vitamin E 529
arachis oil refined peanut oil applied *topically* to treat scaly skin conditions
Aralen chloroquine
Aredia pamidronate
Arfonad trimethaphan
argipressin vasopressin 511
Aristocort triamcinolone 501
Aristoform triamcinolone (501) and clioquinol
Aristospan triamcinolone 501
Arlidin nylidrin
Arlidin Forte nylidrin
arnica an herbal preparation used to treat bruising. Widely employed in homeopathic medicine
Artane trihexyphenidyl 505
artemisinine an *investigational* antimalarial drug no... available in Canada 149
Arthrotec *41Q* (illus.); diclofenac (283) and misoprostol (393)
articaine a local anesthetic
Arvin ancrod

ASA 200

Asacol *40B* (illus.); mesalamine (also known as 5-aminosalicylic acid) 378

Asaphen ASA 200

Asasantine acetylsalicylic acid (200) and dipyridamole (292)

Ascofer ferrous ascorbate

ascorbic acid see vitamin C (528). See also A-Z of additives 540

Asendin amoxapine

Asmavent salbutamol 461

asparaginase a drug used to treat leukemia. See Anticancer drugs 166

Aspercreme a cream containing triethanolamine salicylate for relief of minor aches and pains

Aspergum a chewing gum preparation containing ASA 200

Aspirin ASA 200

astemizole 214

Atabrine quinacrine

Atarax hydroxyzine 340

Atasol acetaminophen 199

Atasol Forte acetaminophen 199

Atasol-8 acetaminophen (199) and codeine (270)

Atasol-15 acetaminophen (199) and codeine (270)

Atasol-30 acetaminophen (199) and codeine (270)

atenolol 215

Ativan *44P, 45S* (illus.); lorazepam 367

Ativan SL *38R* (illus.); lorazepam 367

atovaquone an antiprotozoal drug used to treat pneumocystis pneumonia 140

atracurium a drug used to relax the muscles in general anesthesia. See muscle-relaxant drugs 132

Atromid-S clofibrate

atropine an *anticholinergic* drug related to belladonna. Used in eye drops to dilate the pupil (182) and as *premedication* to dry secretions. It can also be inhaled as a bronchodilator 104

Atropisol atropine

Atrovent ipratropium bromide 348

attapulgite an antidiarrheal drug 122

Auralgan ear drops containing benzocaine (223) and antipyrine

auranofin 216

Aureomycin chlortetracycline

aurothioglucose a gold-based antirheumatic drug 129

AVC sulfanilamide

Aventyl nortriptyline 411

Avlosulfon dapsone

Axid *47S* (illus.); nizatidine 409

Ayercillin penicillin G 424

azacitidine an anticancer drug 166

azatadine 217

azathioprine 218

azidothymidine see zidovudine 516

azithromycin 219

azlocillin a penicillin antibiotic 140

Azmacort triamcinolone 501

Azo Gantrisin phenazopyridine (429) and sulfisoxazole (477)

AZT see zidovudine 516

aztreonam an *investigational* antibiotic 140

B

bacampicillin a penicillin antibiotic 140

Baciguent bacitracin 220

Bacitin bacitracin 220

bacitracin 220

baclofen 221

Bactigras chlorhexidine

Bactine benzalkonium chloride and lidocaine (360)

Bactrim sulfamethoxazole (474) and trimethoprim (507)

Bactrim DS sulfamethoxazole (474) and trimethoprim (507)

Bactroban mupirocin

Balminil Decongestant Syrup pseudoephedrine 450

Balminil DM dextromethorphan 281

Balminil Expectorant guaifenesin 331

Balnetar coal tar

Barriere dimethicone

Barriere-HC hydrocortisone (338) and silicone

Basaljel aluminum hydroxide 204

Beben betamethasone 227

Beclodisk beclomethasone 222

Becloforte beclomethasone 222

beclomethasone 222

Beclovent beclomethasone 222

Beclovent Rotacaps beclomethasone 222

Beconase beclomethasone 222

belladonna an *antispasmodic*, *anticholinergic* drug related to atropine

Bellergal belladonna, ergotamine (301), and phenobarbital (430)

Beminal a vitamin B complex preparation. See Vitamins 161

Beminal with C Fortis a vitamin B complex preparation with vitamin C. See Vitamins 161

Beminal 500 a vitamin B complex preparation. See Vitamins 161

Beminal Fortis Elixir a vitamin B complex preparation. See Vitamins 161

Benadryl diphenhydramine 290

Benadryl Decongestant diphenhydramine (290) and pseudoephedrine (450)

benazepril an ACE inhibitor 110

bendroflumethiazide a thiazide diuretic 111

Benemid probenecid 442

Ben Gay a *topical* preparation containing methyl salicylate and menthol used for the relief of joint and muscle pain

benoxinate a local anesthetic 92

Benoxyl benzoyl peroxide 224

BENSERAZIDE – CARBAMAZEPINE

B

benserazide a drug used to enhance the effect of levodopa (358) in the treatment of parkinsonism. See Drugs for parkinsonism 99

Bentylol dicyclomine

Benylin Codeine-D-E codeine (270), pseudoephedrine (450), and guaifenesin (331)

Benylin DM dextromethorphan 281

Benylin DM-D dextromethorphan (281) and pseudoephedrine (450)

Benylin DM-D-E dextromethorphan (281), pseudoephedrine (450), and guaifenesin (331)

Benylin DM-E dextromethorphan (281) and guaifenesin (331)

Benylin E guaifenesin

Benzac AC benzoyl peroxide 224

Benzac W benzoyl peroxide 224

Benzagel benzoyl peroxide 224

benzalkonium chloride a skin *antiseptic*. See Anti-infective skin preparations 187

benzathine penicillin G see penicillin G 424

benzethonium chloride a skin *antiseptic*. See Anti-infective skin preparations 187

benzhexol see trihexyphenidyl

benznidazole a drug used in the treatment of trypanosomiasis. See Antiprotozoal drugs 148

benzocaine 223

benzoic acid a *topical* antifungal drug 150. See also Food Additives 539

benzoin tincture an aromatic resin added to steam inhalations for the treatment of sinusitis and nasal congestion. See Decongestants 105

benzoyl peroxide 224

benzquinamide an anti-emetic drug 102

benztropine 225

benzydamine 226

benzyl alcohol a local anesthetic for *topical* application. See Local anesthetics 92

benzyl benzoate an antiparasitic agent used to treat scabies. See Drugs to treat skin parasites 188

benzylpenicillin see penicillin G 424

bephenium an anthelmintic drug 151

Berocca-C a vitamin B complex preparation with Vitamin C. See Vitamins 161

Berotec fenoterol 312

beta-carotene see vitamin A 527

Betacort betamethasone 227

Betaderm betamethasone 227

Betadine povidone-iodine

Betagan levobunolol

betahistine a *vasodilator* drug used in the treatment of Ménière's disease. See Vertigo and Ménière's disease 102

Betaloc metoprolol 388

Betaloc Durules metoprolol 388

betamethasone 227

Betaxin thiamine

betaxolol a beta blocker (109) used in the treatment of glaucoma. See Drugs for glaucoma 180

bethanechol a *parasympathomimetic* drug used to treat urinary retention. See Drugs used in urinary disorders 178

B

Betnesol betamethasone 227

Betnovate betamethasone 227

Betoptic eye drops containing betaxolol

bevantolol a beta blocker 109

Bewon thiamine

bezafibrate 228

Bezalip bezafibrate 228

Biaxin *38K* (illus.); clarithromycin 260

bicetonium a *topical antiseptic*

Bicillin penicillin G 424

BiCNU carmustine

bile salts substances derived from bile, sometimes included in combination preparations for the treatment of digestive disorders

Bioderm bacitracin (220) and polymyxin B

Bionet benzocaine (223) and bicetonium

biotin 519

biperiden an *anticholinergic* drug used in Parkinson's disease. See Antiparkinsonism drugs 99

Biquin Durules quinidine 456

bisacodyl 229

Bismed Liquid bismuth subsalicylate

Bismed Tablets bismuth subsalicylate and calcium carbonate

bismuth a metal whose salts are used to treat inflammatory diseases of the stomach and bowel. See Antidiarrheal drugs (122) and Drugs for rectal and anal disorders (125)

bisoprolol a beta blocker 109

bithionol an anthelmintic drug (151) and a *topical* anti-infective agent 187

bitolterol a *sympathomimetic bronchodilator* 104

Blenoxane bleomycin

bleomycin a cytotoxic antibiotic. See Anticancer drugs 166

Blephamide prednisolone (439) and sulfacetamide (473)

Bleph-10 sulfacetamide 473

Blocadren timolol 494

Bonamine meclizine 373

Bonefos clodronate

boric acid a skin and eye *antiseptic* now rarely used because of risk of excessive absorption through the skin

Boropak aluminum acetate and calcium acetate

Bradosol hexylresorcinol

Bretylate bretylium

bretylium an anti-arrhythmic drug 112

Brevibloc esmolol

Brevicon an oral contraceptive containing ethinyl estradiol (306) and norethindrone

Bricanyl terbutaline 485

Brietal methohexital

bromazepam 230

bromides a group of *sedative* drugs now used only rarely as anticonvulsant drugs 98

bromocriptine 231

bromodiphenhydramine an antihistamine 136

bromovinyldeoxyuridine an antiviral agent used to treat herpes simplex. See Antiviral drugs 145

brompheniramine 232
Bronalide flunisolide 315
Bronkaid Mistometer epinephrine 300
buclizine an antihistamine used for motion sickness. See anti-emetic drugs 102
budesonide 233
bufexamac a drug used to relieve skin inflammation
Bufferin ASA (200), magnesium carbonate, and dihydroxyaluminum
Bugs Bunny multivitamin and mineral supplement. See Vitamins 161
bumetanide 234
bupivacaine a long-lasting local anesthetic often used for epidural *anesthesia* during labor. See Local anesthetics 92
buprenorphine a narcotic analgesic 93
Burinex bumetanide
Buro-Sol aluminum acetate and benzethonium chloride
Buscopan scopolamine 463
buserelin a hormone used to treat prostate cancer. See Anticancer drugs 166
Buspar buspirone 235
buspirone 235
busulfan an alkylating agent used in the treatment of certain leukemias. See Anticancer drugs 166
butabarbital a barbiturate sleeping drug 94
butalbital a barbiturate sleeping drug (94) sometimes included in combined analgesic preparations
Butisol butabarbital
butoconazole a drug applied *topically* to treat vaginal thrush. See Antifungal drugs 150
butorphanol 236
butoxyethyl nicotinate a *topical vasodilator*
butyl aminobenzoate a local anesthetic (92) applied to the skin to relieve itching. See Antipruritics 185

C

Cafergot ergotamine (301) and caffeine
Cafergot-PB ergotamine (301), caffeine, and pentobarbital
caffeine a stimulant drug that is present in coffee, tea, and cola. It is sometimes added to *analgesic* medications. See Food additives 540
Caladryl diphenhydramine (290) and calamine
calamine an antipruritic substance used to soothe irritated skin. See Antipruritic medications 185
calamine lotion a *topical* preparation containing calamine and zinc oxide used to soothe irritated skin. See Antipruritic medications 185
calcifediol see vitamin D 529
Calcijex calcitriol
Calcilean heparin 333

C

Calcimar calcitonin
calcipotriol 237
Calcite 500 calcium carbonate 519
Calcite D-500 calcium carbonate (519) and vitamin D (529)
calcitonin a *hormone* produced by the thyroid gland used to treat bone disorders. See p.134
calcitriol see Vitamin D 529
calcium 519
calcium acetate see calcium 519
calcium carbimide a drug used to treat alcohol abuse
calcium carbonate *38M* (illus.); a calcium salt prescribed mainly as an antacid 120
calcium chloride see calcium 519
calcium citrate see calcium 519
calcium glubionate see calcium 519
calcium gluceptate see calcium 519
calcium gluconate see calcium 519
calcium iodide a calcium compound occasionally used as an *expectorant*
calcium lactate see calcium 519
calcium undecylenate see undecylenic acid
Calcium-Sandoz calcium 519
Caldesene Medicated Baby Powder calcium undecylenate
Calmurid carbamide
Calmurid HC carbamide and hydrocortisone (338)
Calmydone hydrocodone (337), etafedrine, and doxylamine
Calmylin Expectorant guaifenesin 331
Calmylin #1 dextromethorphan 281
Calmylin with Codeine codeine (270), diphenhydramine (290), and ammonium chloride
Calsan calcium carbonate 519
Caltine salcatonin
Caltrate calcium carbonate 519
cambendazole a drug used to treat strongyloidiasis. See Anthelmintic drugs 151
camphor a substance included in various *topical* preparations to relieve itching. See Antipruritic medications 185
Canesten clotrimazole 268
cannabis see marijuana 536
Canthacur cantharidin
Canthacur-PS cantharidin, podophyllin, and salicylic acid
cantharidin a drug applied *topically* to treat warts
Cantharone cantharidin
Cantharone Plus cantharidin, podophyllin, and salicylic acid
Capastat Sulfate capreomycin sulfate
Capoten *43Q* (illus.); captopril 239
capreomycin an antituberculous drug 144
capsaicin 238
captopril 239
caramiphen a cough suppressant. See Drugs to treat coughs 106
carbachol a *miotic* drug used to treat glaucoma. See Drugs affecting the pupil 182
carbamazepine 240

CARBAMIDE – COAL TAR

C

carbamide see urea

carbamide peroxide an agent used in drops for softening ear wax

carbaryl an antiparasitic agent used to treat head lice infestation. See Drugs to treat skin parasites 188

carbenicillin a penicillin antibiotic 140

carbenoxolone a licorice derivative used in the treatment of ulcers. See Anti-ulcer drugs 121

carbetapentane a cough suppressant. See Drugs to treat coughs 106

carbidopa a drug used to enhance the therapeutic effect of levodopa (358) in the treatment of Parkinson's disease. See Antiparkinsonism drugs 99

carbimide a drug similar to disulfiram 294

Carbocaine mepivacaine

carbocysteine a *mucolytic* decongestant

carbol-fuchsin an ingredient of Castellani's Paint

Carbolith *46E* (illus.); lithium 364

carboplatin an anticancer drug (166) similar to cisplatin

carboxymethylcellulose a bulk-forming laxative. See Laxatives 123

Cardene nicardipine

Cardioquin quinidine 456

Cardizem diltiazem 287

Cardizem-CD *46F, 46H, 48G* (illus.); diltiazem 287

Cardizem-SR *48C, 48D, 48L* (illus.); diltiazem 287

Cardura doxazosin

carfecillin a penicillin antibiotic 140

carisoprodol a drug used to treat muscle spasm. See muscle-relaxant drugs 132

carmustine an alkylating agent used in the treatment of tumors of the central nervous system and lymphatic system. See Anticancer drugs 166

carphenazine a phenothiazine antipsychotic drug 97

casanthranol a stimulant laxative 123

cascara a stimulant laxative 123

Castellani's Paint a mixture of carbol-fuchsin, phenol, resorcinol, acetone, and alcohol applied locally as an antifungal agent. See also Antifungal drugs 150

castor oil a stimulant laxative 123

Catapres clonidine 266

Catarase chymotrypsin

Ceclor *48J* (illus.); cefaclor 241

Cedocard-SR isosorbide dinitrate 351

CeeNU lomustine

cefaclor 241

cefadroxil a cephalosporin antibiotic 140

cefamandole a cephalosporin antibiotic 140

cefazolin a cephalosporin antibiotic 140

cefixime 242

Cefizox ceftizoxime

cefonicid a cephalosporin antibiotic 140

ceforanide a cephalosporin antibiotic 140

Cefotan cefotetan

cefotaxime a cephalosporin antibiotic 140

cefotetan a cephalosporin antibiotic 140

cefoxitin 243

ceftazidime a cephalosporin antibiotic 140

C

Ceftin *45H* (illus.); cefuroxime axetil 244

ceftizoxime a cephalosporin antibiotic 140

ceftriaxone a cephalosporin antibiotic 140

cefuroxime 244

Celestoderm-V betamethasone 227

Celestone betamethasone 227

Celestone-S betamethasone (227) and sulfacetamide (473)

Celestone Soluspan betamethasone 227

Cellufresh carboxymethylcellulose

Celluvisc carboxymethylcellulose

Celontin methsuximide

Centrum a multivitamin preparation plus minerals. See Vitamins 161

Centrum Forte a multivitamin preparation plus minerals. See vitamins 161

cephalexin 245

cephradine a cephalosporin antibiotic 140

Cephulac lactulose 356

Ceptaz ceftazidime

Cerevon ferrous succinate

Cerubidine daunorubicin

C.E.S. *35A* (illus.); conjugated estrogens 272

Cesamet nabilone

Cetamide sulfacetamide 473

cetirizine 246

cetrimide a skin *antiseptic*. See Anti-infective skin preparations 187

cetylpyridinium an *antiseptic* used in throat lozenges and mouthwashes

Ce-Vi-Sol ascorbic acid 540

charcoal activated charcoal is sometimes given to adsorb or inactivate poisons or drug overdoses that have been taken by mouth. It has also been used to treat diarrhea

Charcodote activated charcoal

chenodiol an *investigational* drug used to treat gallstones. See 126

Cheracol codeine (270), guaifenesin (331), and ammonium chloride

chlophedianol a cough suppressant. See Drugs to treat coughs 106

chloral hydrate 247

chlorambucil 248

chloramphenicol 247

chlorcyclizine an antihistamine 136

chlordiazepoxide 250

chlorhexidine a skin *antiseptic*. See Anti-infective skin preparations 187

chlormezanone an anti-anxiety drug 95

chlorobutanol a preservative

chloroform a general *anesthetic*

chloroguanide a drug used in the treatment of malaria. See Antimalarial drugs 149

Chloromycetin chloramphenicol 249

chlorophenothane see DDT

chloroprocaine a local anesthetic 92

Chloroptic chloramphenicol 249

chloroquine an antimalarial drug. See antimalarial drugs 149

chlorothen an antihistamine 136

C

chlorothiazide a thiazide diuretic 111

chlorotrianisene an estrogen drug used primarily to treat cancer. See Female sex hormones (159) and Anticancer drugs (166)

chloroxylenol a skin *antiseptic*. See Anti-infective skin preparations 187

chlorphenesin a *topical* antifungal agent. See Antifungal drugs 150

chlorpheniramine 251

chlorpromazine 252

chlorpropamide 253

chlorprothixene a phenothiazine antipsychotic drug 97

chlortetracycline a tetracycline antibiotic 140

chlorthalidone 254

Chlor-Tripolon chlorpheniramine 251

Chlor-Tripolon Decongestant Syrup chlorpheniramine (251) and phenylpropanolamine

Chlor-Tripolon Decongestant Tablets chlorpheniramine (251) and pseudoephedrine (450)

Chlor-Tripolon N.D. loratadine (366) and pseudoephedrine (450)

chlorzoxazone a muscle relaxant drug. See Muscle relaxant drugs 132

Choledyl oxtriphylline

Choledyl Expectorant oxtriphylline and guaifenesin (331)

Choledyl SA oxtriphylline

cholestyramine 255

choline magnesium trisalicylate a drug similar to ASA (200) used in arthritic conditions

choline salicylate a drug similar to ASA (200) used in pain-relieving mouth gels

choline theophyllinate see oxtriphylline

Choloxin dextrothyroxine

chorionic gonadotropin see Human chorionic gonadotropin 334

chromium 520

Chronulac lactulose 356

Chymodiactin chymopapain

chymopapain an *enzyme* used to treat sciatica

chymotrypsin an *enzyme* used in the treatment of cataracts

ciclopirox 256

Cidomycin gentamicin 328

cilastatin-imipenem an antibiotic 140

cilazapril an ACE inhibitor 110

Ciloxan ciprofloxacin 258

cimetidine 257

cinchocaine see dibucaine

cinnamates a drug used as a sunscreen 191

cinnarizine an antihistamine 136

cinoxacin a urinary tract *antiseptic*. See Antibacterial drugs 143

Cipro *41J, 45D* (illus.); ciprofloxacin 258

ciprocinonide a *topical* corticosteroid used to treat inflammatory skin disorders. See Topical corticosteroids 186

ciprofibrate a lipid-lowering drug 115

ciprofloxacin 258

cisapride 259

cisplatin an anticancer drug 166

Citanest-Forte epinephrine (300) and prilocaine

Citanest Plain prilocaine

citric acid 541

Citrocarbonate sodium bicarbonate and sodium citrate

Citro-Mag magnesium citrate

cladribine an anticancer drug 166

Claforan cefotaxime

clarithromycin 260

Claritin *44R* (illus.); loratadine 366

Claritin Extra loratadine (366) and pseudoephedrine (450)

clavulanic acid see potassium clavulanate

Clavulin-250 *44I* (illus.); amoxicillin (210) and potassium clavulanate

Clavulin-500 *44D* (illus.); amoxicillin (210) and potassium clavulanate

Clear Eyes naphazoline

Clearasil BP Plus benzoyl peroxide 224

clemastine an antihistamine 136

clidinium bromide an *antispasmodic* drug used in irritable bowel syndrome 122

Climacteron testosterone (488) and estradiol (304)

clindamycin 261

Clinoril sulindac 478

clioquinol a *topical* antibacterial and antifungal agent. See Anti-infective skin preparations 187

clobazam a benzodiazepine anticonvulsant drug. See Anticonvulsant drugs 98

clobetasol propionate 262

clobetasone butyrate a corticosteroid for *topical* application. See Topical corticosteroids 186

clocortolone a corticosteroid for *topical* application. See Topical corticosteroids 186

clodronate an agent used to treat high blood calcium in cancer patients

clofazimine a drug used in the treatment of leprosy 143

clofibrate a lipid-lowering drug 115

Clomid clomiphene 263

clomiphene 263

clomipramine 264

clonazepam 265

clonidine 266

clorazepate 267

Clotrimaderm clotrimazole 268

clotrimazole 268

cloves, oil of a substance applied *topically* as a home remedy for toothache

cloxacillin 269

clozapine an antipsychotic drug 97

Clozaril clozapine

Co Actifed codeine (270), triprolidine, and pseudoephedrine (450)

CoActifed Expectorant codeine (270), triprolidine, pseudoephedrine (450), and guaifenesin (331)

coal tar a substance included in many *topical* preparations for the treatment of psoriasis and dandruff. See Drugs for psoriasis (190) and Treatment for dandruff and hair loss 191

C

cobalt edetate an *antidote* used in cyanide poisoning

cocaine 534

codeine 270

cod liver oil oil obtained from the liver of cod that is rich in vitamin A (527) and vitamin D (529)

Cogentin benztropine 225

Colace docusate

colaspase see asparaginase

Colax-C docusate

Colax-S docusate

colchicine 271

Colestid colestipol

colestipol a lipid-lowering drug

colistin an antibiotic. See Antibiotics 140

collagenase an enzyme used to heal skin ulcers and burns

collodion a substance that dries to form a sticky film. It is used to protect broken skin. See Bases for skin preparations 187

colloidal oatmeal a preparation made from oats and used in *emollient* bath additives. See Antipruritics 185

Collyrium tetrahydrozoline, glycerin, boric acid, and sodium borate

Colpermin peppermint oil

Colprone medrogesterone

Coly-Mycin M colistin

Coly-Mycin Otic colistin, neomycin (402), and hydrocortisone (338)

Comalose-R lactulose 356

Combantrin pyrantel 452

Combipres clonidine (266) and chlorthalidone (254)

Complamin xanthinol niacinate

Compound W salicylic acid

Condyline podofilox

Congest conjugated estrogens 272

conjugated estrogens 272

Contac Allergy Formula terfenadine 487

Contac C chlorpheniramine (251) and phenylpropanolamine

Contac C Cold Care Formula acetaminophen (199), chlorpheniramine (251), dextromethorphan (281), and phenylpropanolamine

Contac Sinus Pain acetaminophen (199) and pseudoephedrine (450)

copper 520

Coptin trimethoprim (507) and sulfadiazine

Coradur isosorbide dinitrate 351

Cordarone amiodarone 207

Corgard nadolol 398

Coricidin ASA (200) and chlorpheniramine (266)

Coricidin "D" ASA (200), chlorpheniramine (251), and phenylpropanolamine

Coricidin "D" Long Acting chlorpheniramine (251) and phenylpropanolamine

Coricidin "D" Non-Drowsy Sinus Formula phenylpropanolamine and ASA (200)

Coricidin Sinus Headache Tablets acetaminophen (199), chlorpheniramine (251), and phenylpropanolamine

C

Coristex-DH phenylephrine (431) and hydrocodone (337)

Coristine-DH phenylephrine (431) and hydrocodone (337)

Coronex isosorbide dinitrate 351

Corsym chlorpheniramine (251) and phenylpropanolamine

Cortacet hydrocortisone 338

Cortamed hydrocortisone 338

Cortate hydrocortisone 338

Cortef hydrocortisone 338

Cortenema hydrocortisone 338

corticotropin a *hormone* released from the pituitary gland. See Drugs for pituitary disorders 157

Corticreme hydrocortisone 338

Cortifoam hydrocortisone 338

Cortiment hydrocortisone 338

cortisol see hydrocortisone 338

cortisone a corticosteroid 153

Cortisporin hydrocortisone (338), neomycin (402), polymyxin B, and bacitracin (220)

Cortoderm hydrocortisone 338

Cortone cortisone

Cortrosyn cosyntropin

Corynebacterium parvum a bacterium that stimulates the immune response and is used in the treatment of certain cancers. See Anticancer drugs 166

Corzide nadolol (398) and bendroflumethiazide

Cosmegen dactinomycin

CoSudafed codeine (270) and pseudoephedrine (450)

CoSudafed Expectorant codeine (270), pseudoephedrine (450), and guaifenesin (331)

cosyntropin a synthetic form of corticotropin used to diagnose the inadequate production of adrenal hormones. See Drugs for pituitary disorders 157

Cotazym pancrelipase

Cotridin triprolidine, codeine (270), and pseudoephedrine (450)

co-trimazine trimethoprim (507) and sulfadiazine

co-trimoxazole 273

Coumadin *36N, 38P, 39Q* (illus.); warfarin 514

Coversyl perindopril

Cozaar losartan potassium

Creon pancrelipase

Creo-Rectal diphenylpyraline, guaiacol, and camphor

cromolyn sodium 274

crotamiton an agent applied *topically* to treat scabies. See Drugs used to treat skin parasites 188

Crystapen penicillin G 424

C2 with Codeine ASA (200), codeine (270), and caffeine

Cuplex a lactic acid and salicylic acid gel

Cuprimine penicillamine 423

cyanocobalamin vitamin B_{12} 528

cyclacillin an antibiotic 140

cyclamate a non-caloric sweetener

cyclandelate a drug used to improve the blood supply to the limbs and brain. Sometimes prescribed to treat peripheral vascular disease and senile dementia. See Vasodilators 110
Cyclen an oral contraceptive containing norgestimate and ethinyl estradiol (306)
cyclizine an antihistamine used mainly as an anti-emetic. See Antihistamines (136) and Anti-emetic drugs (102)
cyclobenzaprine 275
Cyclocort amcinonide
Cyclogyl cyclopentolate
Cyclomen danazol 278
cyclomethicone a water-repelling agent used in skin cream
cyclomethycaine a local anesthetic 92
cyclopentamine a decongestant 105
cyclopentolate a *mydriatic* and *cycloplegic* drug See Drugs affecting the pupil 180
cyclophosphamide 276
cycloserine an antibiotic used to treat tuberculosis. See Antituberculous drugs 144
Cyclospasmol cyclandelate
cyclosporine 277
cyclothiazide a thiazide diuretic 111
Cyklokapron tranexamic acid
Cylert pemoline
cyproheptadine an antihistamine (136) that is also used to stimulate the appetite
cyproterone a synthetic sex *hormone* used in the treatment of cancer of the prostate gland. See Anticancer drugs 166
Cytadren aminoglutethimide
cytarabine a drug used in the treatment of leukemia. See Anticancer drugs 166
Cytomel liothyronine 362
Cytosar cytarabine
cytosine arabinoside see cytarabine
Cytotec *43P* (illus.); misoprostol 393
Cytovene ganciclovir
Cytoxan cyclophosphamide 276

D

dacarbazine a *cytotoxic* drug used in the treatment of malignant melanoma. See Anticancer drugs 166
dactinomycin a *cytotoxic* antibiotic. See Anticancer drugs 166
Dagenan sulfapyridine
Dairyaid lactase
Dalacin C clindamycin 261
Dalacin T clindamycin 261
Dalmane flurazepam 320
danazol 278

D

Dan-Gard zinc pyrithione
danthron a stimulant laxative 123
Dantrium dantrolene
dantrolene a muscle relaxant drug. See Muscle relaxant drugs 132
dapsone an antibacterial drug. See Antibacterial drugs 143
Daraprim pyrimethamine 454
Darvon-N propoxyphene 447
Darvon-N Compound propoxyphene (447), ASA (200), and caffeine
Darvon-N with ASA propoxyphene (447) and ASA (200)
daunorubicin a *cytotoxic* antibiotic. See Anticancer drugs 166
DDAVP desmopressin
ddC see zalcitabine
ddI see didanosine
DDS see dapsone
DDT a *topical* insecticide
Debrisan dextranomer
Decadron dexamethasone 280
Deca-Durabolin nandrolone 399
Declomycin demeclocycline
deferoxamine a *chelating* agent used in iron poisoning
Dehydral methenamine
dehydrocholic acid a laxative 123
dehydroemetine an antiprotozoal drug 148
Delatestryl testosterone 488
Delestrogen estradiol 304
Delfen a spermicidal foam. See nonoxynol-9
Delsym dextromethorphan 281
Deltasone prednisone 440
Demdec pseudoephedrine (450) and dextromethorphan (281)
demecarium a *miotic* drug used in the treatment of glaucoma. See Drugs for glaucoma 180
demeclocycline a tetracycline antibiotic. See Antibiotics 140
Demerol meperidine 376
Demulen an oral contraceptive containing ethinyl estradiol (306) and ethynodiol
Denorex coal tar, menthol, and chloroxylenol
Depakene valproic acid 510
Depen penicillamine 423
Depo-Medrol methylprednisolone 386
Depo-Medrol with Lidocaine methylprednisolone (386) and lidocaine (360)
Depo-Provera medroxyprogesterone 374
Depo-Testosterone testosterone 488
deprenyl see selegiline 464
Dequadin lozenges containing dequalinium
dequalinium an antifungal drug (150) used for mouth infections
Derma-Smoothe/FS fluocinolone 316
Dermasone clobetasol propionate 262
Dermoplast benzocaine (223), menthol, and benzethonium chloride
Dermovate clobetasol propionate 262
Dermoxyl benzoyl peroxide 224

DES – DROMOSTANOLONE

D

DES see diethylstilbestrol
Desenex undecylenic acid
deserpidine an antihypertensive drug 114
Desferal deferoxamine
desipramine 279
desmopressin a drug similar to vasopressin (511) for the long-term treatment of diabetes insipidus. See Drugs for pituitary disorders 157
desogestrel a progestin used in oral contraceptives (173). See Female sex hormones 159
desonide a corticosteroid used to treat inflammatory skin conditions. See Topical corticosteroids 186
desoximetasone a corticosteroid used to treat inflammatory skin conditions. See Topical corticosteroids 186
desoxycorticosterone a corticosteroid 153
Desquam-X benzoyl peroxide 224
Desyrel trazodone 499
dexamethasone 280
Dexasone dexamethasone 280
dexbrompheniramine an antihistamine 136
dexchlorpheniramine an antihistamine 136
Dexedrine dextroamphetamine
dexpanthenol a drug related to pantothenic acid (524). Used to relieve flatulence, and applied *topically* for various skin conditions such as burns and eczema
dextranomer a *topical* wound cleansing agent
dextroamphetamine an amphetamine. See Nervous system stimulants (100) and Amphetamines (533)
dextromethorphan 281
dextropropoxyphene see propoxyphene 447
dextrose a sugar often used to treat low blood sugar
dextrothyroxine a lipid-lowering drug 115
DHT see dihydrotachysterol
DiaBeta *45L* (illus.); glyburide 330
Diabinese chlorpropamide 253
diacetylmorphine see heroin 535
Diamicron *42N* (illus.); gliclazide 329
diamidine an antiprotozoal drug 148
diamorphine see heroin 535
Diamox acetazolamide
Diazemuls diazepam 282
diazepam 282
diazoxide an antihypertensive drug that is also used to treat hypoglycemia. See Drugs used in diabetes 154
dibucaine a local anesthetic 92
Dicetel pinaverium
dichloralphenazone a sedative drug similar to chloral hydrate 247
dichlorphenamide a carbonic anhydrase inhibitor used in the treatment of glaucoma 180
Diclectin doxylamine and pyridoxine, used to treat nausea and vomiting in pregnancy
diclofenac 283
dicloxacillin a penicillin antibiotic 140
dicyclomine an *anticholinergic*, *antispasmodic* drug used to treat irritable bowel syndrome. See Antidiarrheal drugs 122
didanosine 284

D

Didronel etidronate 307
dienestrol an estrogen drug. See Female sex hormones 159
diethylcarbamazine an anthelmintic drug 151
diethylpropion an appetite suppressant
diethylstilbestrol an estrogen drug. See Female sex hormones 159
diflorasone a *topical* corticosteroid used to treat inflammatory skin disorders. See Topical corticosteroids 186
Diflucan fluconazole 314
diflucortolone a *topical* corticosteroid used to treat inflammatory skin disorders. See Topical corticosteroids 186
diflunisal 285
difluoromethylornithine a drug used to treat protozoal infections and certain cancers. See Antiprotozoal drugs (148) and Anticancer drugs (166)
Digitaline digitoxin
digitalis a drug derived from foxglove leaves. See Digitalis drugs 108
digitoxin a digitalis drug. See Digitalis drugs 108
digoxin 286
dihydrocodeine a narcotic analgesic. See Analgesics 92
dihydroergotamine a drug used to treat migraine and cluster headaches. See Drugs used for migraine 101
dihydrotachysterol see vitamin D 529
dihydroxyaluminum an aluminum antacid. See Antacids 120
diiodohydroxyquin see iodoquinol
Dilantin *47P* (illus.); phenytoin 432
Dilantin with phenobarbital phenobarbital (430) and phenytoin (432)
Dilaudid hydromorphone 339
Dilaudid-HP hydromorphone 339
diloxanide an antiprotozoal drug used in the treatment of amebiasis. See Antiprotozoal drugs 148
diltiazem 287
Dimelor acetohexamide
dimenhydrinate 288
dimercaprol a *chelating* agent used to treat metal poisoning
dimercaptosuccinic acid an agent used in the treatment of lead poisoning
Dimetane brompheniramine 232
Dimetane Expectorant brompheniramine (232), guaifenesin (331), phenylephrine (431), and phenylpropanolamine
Dimetane Expectorant-C brompheniramine (232), phenylephrine (431), phenylpropanolamine, guaifenesin (331), and codeine (270)
Dimetane Expectorant-DC hydrocodone (337), brompheniramine (232), guaifenesin (331), phenylephrine (431), and phenylpropanolamine
Dimetapp brompheniramine (232), phenylephrine (431), and phenylpropanolamine
Dimetapp-A Sinus phenylephrine (431), acetaminophen (199), and phenylpropanolamine

D

Dimetapp-C brompheniramine (232), phenylephrine (431), phenylpropanolamine, and codeine (270)

Dimetapp-DM brompheniramine (232), dextromethorphan (281), phenylephrine (431), and phenylpropanolamine

Dimetapp Oral Infant Drops brompheniramine (232), phenylephrine (431), and phenylpropanolamine

dimethicone a water-repellent silicone-based substance used in barrier creams

dimethisoquin a local anesthetic 92

dimethothiazine an antihistamine 136

dimethyl sulfoxide a drug administered into the bladder to treat interstitial cystitis or applied to the skin to treat scleroderma

dimethyltubocurarine see metocurine

dinoprost a prostaglandin drug used to stimulate uterine contractions. See Drugs used in labor 177

dinoprostone 289

Diocaine proparacaine

Diocarpine pilocarpine 433

Diochloram chloramphenicol 249

dioctyl calcium sulfosuccinate see docusate

dioctyl sodium sulfosuccinate see docusate

Diodex dexamethasone 280

Diodoquin iodoquinol

Diogent gentamicin 328

Dionephrine phenylephrine 431

Diopred prednisolone 439

Dioptimyd prednisolone (439) and sulfacetamide (473)

Diorouge phenylephrine (431) and pheniramine

Diovol magnesium hydroxide (370) and aluminum hydroxide (204)

Diovol Ex aluminum hydroxide (204) and magnesium hydroxide (370)

Diovol Plus aluminum hydroxide (204), magnesium hydroxide (370), and simethicone

Dipentum olsalazine

diperodon a local anesthetic 92

diphenhydramine 290

diphenidol an anti-emetic drug 102

diphenoxylate 291

diphenylhydantoin see phenytoin 432

diphenylpyraline an antihistamine 136

dipivalyl epinephrine see dipivefrin

dipivefrin a drug related to epinephrine (300) used to reduce pressure inside the eye in the treatment of glaucoma 180

Diprogen betamethasone (227) and gentamicin (328)

Diprolene betamethasone 227

Diprosalic a skin preparation containing betamethasone (227) and salicylic acid

Diprosone betamethasone 227

dipyridamole 292

Disalcid salsalate

Disipal orphenadrine 416

disodium edetate see edetate disodium

disopyramide 293

disulfiram 294

dithranol see anthralin 213

Ditropan 39C (illus.); oxybutynin 418

divalproex an anticonvulsant drug 98

D

Dixarit clonidine 266

DMSO see dimethyl sulfoxide

Doan's Backache Pills magnesium salicylate

dobutamine a *sympathomimetic* drug that is injected to treat heart failure and, occasionally, shock

Dobutrex dobutamine

docusate calcium a laxative 123

docusate sodium a laxative 123

Dolobid diflunisal 285

domiphen an *antiseptic* included in sore throat lozenges

domperidone 43D (illus.); 295

Donnagel kaolin, pectin, atropine, hyoscyamine, and scopolamine (463)

Donnagel-MB kaolin and pectin

Donnagel-PG kaolin, pectin, and paregoric

Donnatal phenobarbital (430), atropine, hyoscyamine, and scopolamine (463)

dopamine a natural *neurotransmitter* used as a *sympathomimetic* drug in heart failure and shock

Dopram doxapram

Doryx doxycycline 297

Doss danthron and docusate

Dovonex calcipotriol 237

doxacurium a muscle relaxant drug 132

doxapram a respiratory stimulant. See Nervous system stimulants 100

Doxate-C docusate calcium

Doxate-S docusate sodium

doxazosin a drug used to treat hypertension (114), and to treat benign prostatic hyperplasia (178)

doxepin 296

Doxidan phenolphthalein and docusate calcium

Doxycin doxycycline 297

doxycycline 297

doxylamine an antihistamine 136

Drenison flurandrenolide

Drisdol ergocalciferol

Dristan chlorpheniramine (251), phenylpropanolamine, ASA (200), and caffeine

Dristan Formula P pyrilamine, ASA (200), caffeine, and phenylephrine (431)

Dristan Long Lasting Capsules chlorpheniramine (251) and phenylpropanolamine

Dristan Long Lasting Nasal Mist/Spray oxymetazoline 437

Dristan N.D. acetaminophen (199) and pseudoephedrine (450)

Dristan Nasal Mist phenylephrine (431) and pheniramine

Drixoral Day/Night Cold Relief System pseudoephedrine (450) and dexbrompheniramine

Drixoral N.D. pseudoephedrine 450

Drixoral Nasal Solution oxymetazoline 420

Drixoral Tablets pseudoephedrine (450) and dexbrompheniramine

Drixtab pseudoephedrine (450) and dexbrompheniramine

dromostanolone an androgenic drug used in rare cases to treat breast cancer. See Male sex hormones (158) and Anticancer drugs (166)

DRONABINOL– FIORINAL-C¼

D

dronabinol a drug derived from marijuana used primarily to treat nausea and vomiting induced by anticancer drugs. See Anti-emetic drugs 102

droperidol an anti-emetic drug similar to the phenothiazines. See Anti-emetic drugs 102

DTIC dacarbazine

Dulcolax bisacodyl 229

Duofilm a wart treatment containing salicylic acid and lactic acid in a collodion base

Duoforte 27 a salicylic acid wart remover in a collodion gel base

Duolube white petrolatum and mineral oil

Duonalc isopropyl alcohol

Duonalc-E ethyl alcohol

Duoplant salicylic acid, lactic acid, and formaldehyde

Duovent UDV fenoterol (312) and ipratropium bromide (348)

Durabolin nandrolone 399

Duragesic fentanyl

Duralith lithium 364

Duratears lanolin, petrolatum, and mineral oil

Duretic methylclothiazide

Duricef cefadroxil

Duvoid bethanechol

D-Vi-Sol vitamin D 529

Dyazide *37K* (illus.); hydrochlorothiazide (336) and triamterene (502)

Dycholium dehydrocholic acid

dyphylline a xanthine *bronchodilator* 104

Dyrenium triamterene 502

E

echothiophate a *miotic* drug used in the treatment of glaucoma 180

econazole 298

Ecostatin econazole 298

Ecotrin ASA 200

Ectosone Mild betamethasone 227

Ectosone Regular betamethasone 227

Ectosone Scalp Lotion betamethasone 227

Edecrin ethacrynic acid

edetate calcium disodium a *chelating* agent used to treat poisoning from lead and other metals

edetate disodium a *chelating* agent used to reduce calcium levels in the blood

edrophonium chloride a drug used to diagnose myasthenia gravis 133

EDTA see edetate disodium

EES-600 erythromycin 302

Efamol evening primrose oil

Effexor venlafaxine 512

Efudex fluorouracil 317

E

Elavil amitriptyline 208

Elavil Plus amitriptyline (208) and perphenazine (428)

Eldepryl selegiline 464

Eldisine vindesine

Eldopaque hydroquinone

Eldoquin hydroquinone

Elocom mometasone

Eltor 120 pseudoephedrine 450

Eltroxin *38B*, *39L*, *43F* (illus.); levothyroxine 359

Emcyt estramustine

emetine a drug used to treat amebiasis. See Antiprotozoal drugs 148

Emko a spermicidal vaginal foam containing nonoxynol-9 and benzethonium chloride

EMLA Cream/Patch lidocaine (360) and prilocaine

Emo-Cort hydrocortisone 338

Empracet-30 *36I* (illus.); acetaminophen (199) and codeine (270)

Emtec-30 acetaminophen (199) and codeine (270)

E-Mycin erythromycin 302

enalapril 299

encainide an anti-arrhythmic drug 112

Endantadine amantadine 205

Endocet oxycodone (419) and acetaminophen (199)

Endodan oxycodone (419) and ASA (200)

enflurane a general anesthetic

Enlon edrophonium chloride

enoxaparin a drug used to prevent blood clotting 116

Entacyl piperazine

Entex LA phenylpropanolamine and guaifenesin (331)

Entocort budesonide 233

Entozyme pancreatin. See Digestion of fats 126

Entrophen *39T* (illus.); ASA 200

enviroxime an *investigational* antiviral drug 145

ephedrine an oral decongestant 121

E-Pilo epinephrine (300) and pilocarpine (433)

Epi-Lyt glycerin and lactic acid lotion

Epimorph morphine 414

epinephrine 300

epinephryl borate an epinephrine-like drug. See epinephrine 300

EpiPen epinephrine 300

epirubicin a *cytotoxic* drug. See Anticancer drugs 166

Epival divalproex

epoprostenol an *investigational* vasodilator and antiplatelet drug. See Vasodilators (110) and Drugs that affect blood clotting (116)

Eprex erythropoietin 303

Equagesic ASA (200), ethoheptazine, and meprobamate (377)

Equanil meprobamate 377

Ergamisol levamisole

ergocalciferol see vitamin D 529

Ergodryl diphenhydramine (290), ergotamine (301), and caffeine

ergoloid mesylates a drug used occasionally to treat senile dementia

E

Ergomar ergotamine 301
ergometrine see ergonovine
ergonovine a uterine stimulant. See Drugs used in labor 177
ergotamine 301
Ergotrate Maleate ergonovine
Erybid erythromycin 302
ERYC *47N, 47O* (illus.); erythromycin 302
erythrityl tetranitrate a nitrate anti-angina drug. See Anti-angina drugs 113
Erythromid *35G* (illus.); erythromycin 302
erythromycin 302
erythropoietin 303
esdepallethrin a *topical* scabicide 188
esmolol a beta blocker 109
Estar coal tar
estazolam a benzodiazepine sleeping drug 94
esterified estrogens an estrogen preparation. See Female sex hormones 159
Estinyl ethinyl estradiol 306
Estrace estradiol 304
Estracomb estradiol (304) and norethindrone
Estraderm a transdermal preparation of estradiol 304
estradiol 304
estramustine an anticancer drug 166
estrogen a female sex hormone 159
estrone an estrogen preparation. See Female sex hormones 159
estropipate an estrogen drug. See Female sex hormones 159
etafedrine a decongestant 105
ethacrynate sodium a loop diuretic. See Diuretics 111
ethacrynic acid a loop diuretic. See Diuretics 111
ethambutol a drug used to treat tuberculosis 144
Ethamolin ethanolamine oleate
ethanolamine oleate a drug used to treat varicose veins
ethchlorvynol a sleeping drug 94
ethinyl estradiol 306
ethionamide a drug used to treat tuberculosis. See Antituberculous drugs 144
ethoheptazine a narcotic analgesic 93
ethopropazine a phenothiazine antiparkinsonism drug. See Antiparkinsonism drugs 99
ethosuximide an anticonvulsant drug 98
ethotoin an anticonvulsant drug 98
Ethrane enflurane
ethyl alcohol 532
ethylestrenol an anabolic steroid. See Male sex hormones 158
ethynodiol a progestin drug. See Female sex hormones 159
etidocaine a local anesthetic 92
etidronate 307
etodolac a non-steroidal anti-inflammatory drug 128
etofibrate an *investigational* lipid-lowering drug 115
etomidate a drug used for the induction of general anesthesia
etoposide an anticancer drug 166

E

Etrafon amitriptyline (208) and perphenazine (428)
etretinate 308
eucalyptus oil an antiseptic and expectorant
eucatropine an *anticholinergic mydriatic* drug. See drugs affecting the pupil 182
Euflex flutamide
Euglucon glyburide 330
Eumovate clobetasone butyrate
Eurax crotamiton
evening primrose oil an essential fatty acid supplement
Exdol-30 acetaminophen (199), caffeine, and codeine (270)
Ex-Lax phenolphthalein

F

famotidine 309
Famvir famciclovir
Fanciclovir an antiviral agent
Fansidar pyrimethamine (454) and sulfadoxine
Fastin phentermine
Feen-A-Mint phenolphthalein
Feldene piroxicam 435
felodipine 310
fenfluramine an appetite suppressant related to the amphetamines. See Nervous system stimulants 100
fenofibrate 311
fenoprofen a non-steroidal anti-inflammatory drug 128
fenoterol 312
fentanyl a narcotic analgesic (93) often used to induce general *anesthesia*
Fer-In-Sol ferrous sulfate
Fermentol pepsin
ferrous ascorbate an iron preparation. See Iron 522
ferrous fumarate an iron preparation. See Iron 522
ferrous gluconate an iron preparation. See Iron 522
ferrous succinate an iron preparation. See Iron 522
ferrous sulfate an iron preparation. See Iron 522
feverfew an herbal product used in migraine prophylaxis
Fibrepur psyllium 451
fibrinolysin a preparation containing plasmin, an agent that breaks down blood clots. Used *topically* to treat skin ulcers
filgrastim an agent used to decrease infection in selected cancer patients
finasteride 313
Fiorinal *41F* (illus.); ASA (200), butalbital, and caffeine
Fiorinal-C¼ *48H* (illus.); butalbital, caffeine, ASA (200), and codeine (270)

FLORINOL-C½ – HETACILLIN

F

Fiorinal-C½ *48F* (illus.); butalbital, caffeine, ASA (200), and codeine (270)
Flagyl metronidazole 398
Flagystatin metronidazole (398) and nystatin (412)
Flamazine silver sulfadiazine (466)
Flamazine C silver sulfadiazine (466) and chlorhexidine
Flarex fluorometholone
flavoxate a urinary antispasmodic and analgesic agent
Flaxedil gallamine
flecainide an anti-arrhythmic drug 112
Flexeril *37P* (illus.); cyclobenzaprine 275
Flintstones a multivitamin preparation. See Vitamins 161
floctafenine a non-steroidal anti-inflammatory drug 128
Flonase fluticasone 322
Florinef fludrocortisone
Florone diflorasone
Flovent fluticasone 322
Floxin ofloxacin
floxuridine an anticancer drug 166
Fluanxol flupenthixol
flubendazole an *investigational* anthelmintic drug 151
flucorolone a topical corticosteroid used to treat inflammatory skin conditions. See Topical corticosteroids 186
Fluclox flucloxacillin
flucloxacillin a penicillin antibiotic 140
fluconazole 314
flucytosine an antifungal drug 150
Fludara fludarabine
fludarabine an anticancer drug 166
fludrocortisone a corticosteroid 153
flumazenil a drug used to antagonize the effects of benzodiazepines
flumethasone a *topical* corticosteroid used to treat inflammatory skin disorders. See Topical corticosteroids 186
flunarizine a calcium channel blocker 113
flunisolide a corticosteroid mainly used to treat bronchial disorders. See Corticosteroids 153
fluocinolone 316
fluocinonide a *topical* corticosteroid used to treat inflammatory skin disorders. See Topical corticosteroids 186
fluocortin an *investigational* corticosteroid 153
Fluoderm fluocinolone 316
Fluonide fluocinolone 316
Fluor-A-Day sodium fluoride 521
fluoride 521
fluorometholone a corticosteroid drug mainly used *topically* to treat eye disorders. See Corticosteroids 153
Fluoroplex fluorouracil 317
fluorouracil 317
Fluothane halothane
Fluotic sodium fluoride 521
fluoxetine 318

F

fluoxymesterone an anabolic steroid 158
flupenthixol an antipsychotic drug 97
fluphenazine 319
flurandrenolide a *topical* corticosteroid used to treat inflammatory skin disorders. See Topical corticosteroids 186
flurazepam 320
flurbiprofen 321
fluspirilene an antipsychotic drug 97
flutamide an anti-androgen drug used to treat cancer of the prostate gland. See Anticancer drugs 166
fluticasone 322
Flutone diflorasone
fluvastatin a lipid-lowering agent 115
fluvoxamine 323
FML fluorometholone
FML Forte fluorometholone
FML-Neo fluorometholone and neomycin (402)
folic acid 521
folinic acid see leucovorin
Folvite folic acid 521
Forane isoflurane
formaldehyde a disinfectant and preservative
formestane an anticancer drug 166
Formula 44 dextromethorphan 281
Formula 44 D dextromethorphan (281) and pseudoephedrine (450)
Formula 44 E dextromethorphan (281) and guaifenesin (331)
Formula 44 M (Adult) dextromethorphan (281), pseudoephedrine (450), chlorpheniramine (251), and acetaminophen (199)
Formula 44 M (Pediatric) dextromethorphan (281), pseudoephedrine (450), and chlorpheniramine (251)
Fortamines 10 a multivitamin preparation. See Vitamins 161
Fortaz ceftazidime
fosinipril 324
framycetin a *topical* antibiotic used to treat eye, ear, nose, and skin infections. See Antibiotics 140
Freezone salicylic acid and zinc chloride
Frisium clobazam
Froben flurbiprofen 321
FSH follicle-stimulating hormone
Fucidin fusidic acid 326
FUDR floxuridine
Fulvicin P/G griseofulvin
Fulvicin U/F griseofulvin
Fungizone amphotericin B 211
furazolidone an antiprotozoal drug 148
furosemide 325
fusidic acid 326

G

gabapentin an anticonvulsant drug 98
gallamine a muscle-relaxant drug 132
Gamastan immune serum globulin. See Vaccines and immunization 146
Gamimune an immune globulin. See Vaccines and immunization 146
gamma benzene hexachloride see lindane 361
Gammabulin Immuno an immune globulin. See Vaccines and immunization 146
gamma globulin immune globulin. See Vaccines and immunization 146
ganciclovir an antiviral agent
Garamycin gentamicin 328
Garasone gentamicin (328) and betamethasone (227)
Garatec gentamicin 328
Gastrocote alginic acid, aluminum hydroxide (204), sodium bicarbonate, and magnesium hydroxide (370)
Gastrozepin pirenzepine
Gel "7" sodium fluoride 521
Gelusil magnesium hydroxide (370) and aluminum hydroxide (204)
gemfibrozil 327
Gen-Clobetasol clobetasol propionate
Gen-Glybe 450 (illus.); glyburide 330
Gen-Nifedipine nifedipine 404
Gentacidin gentamicin 328
gentamicin 328
gentian violet a dye used *topically* to treat skin infections. See Anti-infective skin preparations 187
Gen-Timolol timolol 494
Geopen carbenicillin
glibenclamide see glyburide 330
gliclazide 329
glipizide an oral antidiabetic drug. See Drugs used in diabetes 154
glucagon a pancreatic *enzyme* injected to treat hypoglycemia. See Drugs used in diabetes 154
Glucophage 41B (illus.); metformin 379
glutamic acid hydrochloride a gastric acidifier sometimes used to assist in digestion
glutaral a skin *antiseptic*. See Anti-infective skin preparations 187
glutethimide a sleeping drug 94
glyburide 330
glycerin an ingredient in cough mixtures (166), bases for skin preparations (187), laxative suppositories (123), and ear wax softening drops (183)
glycerol see glycerin
glyceryl guaiacolate see guaifenesin
glyceryl trinitrate see nitroglycerin
glycopyrrolate an *anticholinergic antispasmodic*. See Drugs for irritable bowel syndrome 122
Glysennid senna
gold sodium thiomalate a gold-based anti-rheumatic drug 129

G

GoLytely a preparation containing polyethylene glycol and salts of sodium and potassium that is used for cleaning the bowel before investigative procedures. See Laxatives 123
gonadotropin, human chorionic see HCG 334
goserelin an anticancer drug 166
gramicidin an aminoglycoside antibiotic for eye, ear, and skin infections 141
Gravergol dimenhydrinate (288), caffeine, and ergotamine (301)
Gravol dimenhydrinate 288
griseofulvin an antifungal drug 150
Grisovin-FP griseofulvin
growth hormone somatrem or somatropin. See Drugs for pituitary disorders 157
guaiacol an *expectorant* 106
guaiacolsulfonate an *expectorant* 106
guaifenesin 331
guanabenz a *sympatholytic* antihypertensive drug. See Antihypertensive drugs 114
guanethidine an antihypertensive drug. See Antihypertensive drugs 114
Gyne Cure tioconazole

H

Habitrol nicotine patch
Hair and Scalp a creme rinse conditioner containing zinc pyrithione
halazepam a benzodiazepine anti-anxiety drug 95
halcinonide a *topical* corticosteroid mainly used to treat inflammatory skin disorders. See Topical corticosteroids 186
Halcion triazolam 503
Haldol haloperidol 332
Haldol LA haloperidol 332
halobetasol a *topical* corticosteroid mainly used to treat inflammatory skin disorders. See Topical corticosteroids 186
halofenate a lipid-lowering drug 115
Halog halcinonide
haloperidol 332
haloprogin a drug used to treat fungal skin conditions. See Antifungal drugs 150
Halotestin fluoxymesterone
halothane a gas used to induce general *anesthesia*
HCG see human chorionic gonadotropin 334
Hemacort HC hydrocortisone (338) and zinc sulfate
Hepalean heparin 333
heparin 333
heroin 535
Herplex idoxuridine 342
Herplex-D idoxuridine 342
hetacillin a penicillin antibiotic 140

HETRAZAN – KEFLEX

H

Hetrazan diethylcarbamazine
Hexa-Betalin pyridoxine
hexachlorophene a skin *antiseptic*. See Anti-infective skin preparations 187
Hexadrol dexamethasone 280
Hexalen altretamine
hexamethylmelamine see altretamine
hexetidine an antiseptic used in mouthwashes
Hexifoam chlorhexidine
Hexit lindane 361
hexocyclium an *antispasmodic* drug. See Drugs for irritable bowel syndrome 122
hexylresorcinol a skin *antiseptic*. See Anti-infective skin preparations 187
H-F Antidote Gel calcium gluconate gel
Hibidil chlorhexidine
Hibitane chlorhexidine
Hip-Rex methenamine
Hismanal astemizole 214
histamethazine see meclizine 373
Histantil promethazine 446
Hivid zalcitabine
HMS Liquifilm medrysone
homatropine a *mydriatic* and *cycloplegic* drug used in certain eye conditions. See Drugs affecting the pupil 182
Honvol diethylstilbestrol
H₂ Oxyl benzoyl peroxide 224
human chorionic gonadotropin 334
human insulin 346
Humatrope somatropin
Humegon human gonadotropin
Humulin insulin 346
hyaluronidase an *enzyme* used in *topical* skin preparations to reduce bruising
hycanthone an anthelmintic drug 151
Hycodan hydrocodone 337
Hycomine hydrocodone (337), pyrilamine, phenylephrine (431), and ammonium chloride
Hydergine ergoloid mesylates
Hyderm hydrocortisone 338
hydralazine 335
Hydrea hydroxyurea
hydrochlorothiazide 336
hydrocodone 337
hydrocortisone 338
HydroDIURIL hydrochlorothiazide 336
hydrogen peroxide a skin *antiseptic*. See Anti-infective skin preparations 187
hydromorphone 339
hydrophilic ointment an oil-in-water emulsion used as a base for skin preparations 187
Hydropres hydrochlorothiazide (336) and reserpine
hydroquinone a drug used to bleach the skin
hydroxocobalamin see Vitamin B₁₂ 528
hydroxyamphetamine a *mydriatic* drug used to diagnose glaucoma. See Drugs affecting the pupil 182
hydroxychloroquine an antimalarial drug 149
hydroxydopamine an *investigational* drug used to treat glaucoma 180

H

hydroxyethylcellulose a substance used in artificial tear preparations 182
hydroxyprogesterone a progestin. See Female sex hormones 159
hydroxypropylcellulose a substance used in artificial tear preparations 182
hydroxypropylmethylcellulose a substance used in artificial tear preparations 182
hydroxyurea an anticancer drug 166
hydroxyzine 340
Hygeol sodium hypochlorite
Hygroton chlorthalidone 254
Hygroton-Reserpine chlorthalidone (254) and reserpine
hyoscine see scopolamine 463
hyoscyamine an *anticholinergic* drug used as an antispasmodic in irritable bowel syndrome (122) and in urinary incontinence 178
Hyperstat diazoxide
Hypertears Liquid polyvinyl alcohol
Hypotears Eye Ointment mineral oil and white petrolatum
Hytakerol dihydrotachysterol
Hytrin terazosin 483

I

ibuprofen *37E* (illus.); 341
ichthammol a substance used in skin preparations for the treatment of eczema
Idamycin idarubicin
Idarac floctafenine
idarubicin an anti-leukemic agent. See Anticancer drugs 166
I.D.M. Solution guaifenesin (331), potassium iodide, ephedrine, and mepyramine
idoxuridine 342
Ifex ifosfamide
ifosfamide an alkylating agent. See Anticancer drugs 166
Iletin insulin 346
Ilosone erythromycin 302
Ilotycin erythromycin 302
IMAP fluspirilene
IMAP Forte fluspirilene
Imdur isosorbide mononitrate 351
imipenem/cilastatin an antibiotic 140
imipramine 343
Imitrex *35T* (illus.); sumatriptan 479
immune serum globulin an *antibody* preparation injected to prevent certain infectious diseases. See Vaccines and immunization 146
Imodium *39A* (illus.); loperamide 365
Imovane *39F* (illus.); zopiclone 517

Imuran azathioprine 218
Inapsine droperidol
Incremin with Iron a vitamin B complex preparation with iron (522). See Vitamins 161
indapamide 344
Inderal propranolol 448
Inderal LA *46G* (illus.); propranolol 448
Inderide hydrochlorothiazide (336) and propranolol (448)
Indocid indomethacin 345
Indocid PDA indomethacin 345
Indocid SR *48A* (illus.); indomethacin 345
indomethacin 345
indoramin a *sympatholytic* antihypertensive drug 114
Indotec indomethacin 345
Infantol a multivitamin preparation. See Vitamins 161
Inflamase Forte prednisolone 439
Inflamase Mild prednisolone 439
INH see isoniazid 349
Inhibace cilazapril
Innovar droperidol and fentanyl
Inocor amrinone
inosiplex an antiviral drug (145) with possible stimulating effects on immune system activity
insulin 346
Intal cromolyn sodium 274
interferon 347
intrinsic factor a protein released in the gastrointestinal tract that is essential for the absorption of vitamin B_{12}. Intrinsic factor preparations may be administered when natural production is impaired
Intron A interferon 347
Intropin dopamine
iodinated glycerol an organic iodine preparation given orally as a mucolytic agent 105
iodine 522
iodochlorhydroxyquin see clioquinol
iodoquinol an antiprotozoal drug 148
Ionamin phentermine
Ionil benzalkonium chloride
Ionil-T benzalkonium chloride and coal tar
Ionil-T Plus coal tar
Iopidine apraclonidine
ipecac a drug in syrup form used to induce vomiting in the treatment of drug overdose and poisoning. It is also used as an *expectorant*. See Drug poisoning emergency guide (574) and Drugs to treat coughs (106)
ipratropium bromide 348
iron 522
Ismelin guanethidine
Ismelin-Esidrix guanethidine and hydrochlorothiazide (336)
Ismo isosorbide mononitrate 351
Isocaine mepivacaine
isoetharine an *adrenergic bronchodilator* 104
isoflurane a volatile liquid inhaled as a general anesthetic
isomeprobamate see carisoprodol
isoniazid 349
isoprenaline see isoproterenol

I

isoprinosine inosiplex
isopropamide an *anticholinergic antispasmodic* drug used to treat irritable bowel syndrome 122
isopropyl alcohol also known as rubbing alcohol. Used as a skin *antiseptic* 187
isoproterenol 350
Isoptin verapamil 513
Isoptin-SR *38L* (illus.); verapamil 513
Isopto Atropine atropine
Isopto Carbachol carbachol 182
Isopto Carpine pilocarpine 433
Isopto Homatropine homatropine
Isopto Tears hydroxypropylmethylcellulose
Isordil isosorbide dinitrate 351
Isordil 10 Titradose *42M* (illus.); isosorbide dinitrate 351
Isordil 30 Titradose *42E* (illus.); isosorbide dinitrate 351
isosorbide dinitrate/mononitrate 351
isotretinoin 352
Isotrex Gel isotretinoin 352
isoxsuprine a vasodilator (110) and uterine muscle relaxant (177)
Isuprel isoproterenol 350
itraconazole an antifungal drug 150
Iveegam immune serum globulin
ivermectin an *investigational* anthelmintic drug 151

J

Jectofer iron 522

K

Kalium Durules potassium chloride 524
kanamycin an aminoglycoside antibiotic 140
Kaochlor potassium chloride 524
Kaochlor-20 potassium chloride 524
kaolin an adsorbent substance used in certain types of poisoning and as an antidiarrheal 122
Kaon potassium gluconate 524
Kaopectate attapulgite
karaya gum a vegetable gum used as a bulk-forming laxative 123
Karidium sodium fluoride 521
K-Dur *44S* (illus.); potassium chloride 524
Keflex cephalexin 245

KEFUROX – MEDIPREN

K

Kefurox cefuroxime 244
Kefzol cefazolin
Kemadrin procyclidine 445
Kemsol dimethyl sulfoxide
Kenacomb nystatin (412), gramicidin (343), triamcinolone (501), and neomycin (402)
Kenalog triamcinolone 501
Keralyt salicylic acid gel
Ketalar ketamine
ketamine a drug given intravenously to induce general anesthesia
ketanserin an *investigational* antihypertensive drug 114
ketazolam a benzodiazepine anti-anxiety drug 95
ketoconazole 353
ketoprofen 354
ketorolac 355
ketotifen a drug used to treat asthma in children. See Bronchodilators 104
Kidrolase asparaginase
K-Lor potassium chloride 524
K-Lyte potassium citrate 524
K-Lyte/Cl potassium chloride 524
K-Med potassium chloride (524) and magnesium gluconate
K-Med 900 potassium chloride 524
Koffex DM dextromethorphan 281
K-10 potassium chloride 524
Kwellada lindane 361

L

labetalol a beta blocker drug
Lac-Hydrin ammonium lactate
Lacril methylcellulose
Lacri-Lube petrolatum and mineral oil
Lacrisert hydroxypropylcellulose
Lactaid lactase
lactase an *enzyme* that assists in the digestion of lactose
lactic acid an ingredient of some preparations for the treatment of warts. Also present in some *emollient* skin and vaginal preparations
lactose a constituent of milk sometimes used as a laxative (123) or diuretic (111)
Lactrase lactase
Lactulax lactulose 356
lactulose 356
Lamictal lamotrigine
Lamisil *41K* (illus.); terbinafine 484
lamotrigine an anticonvulsant drug 116
lanolin a fatty substance obtained from sheep wool and used as a base for *emollient* ointments and cosmetics. See Bases for skin preparations 187

L

Lanoxin *38G*, *42T* (illus.); digoxin 286
Lansoprazole an anti-ulcer drug 121
Lansoyl a mineral oil gel
Lanvis thioguanine
Largactil chlorpromazine 252
Lariam mefloquine
Larodopa levodopa 358
Lasix furosemide 325
Lasix Special furosemide 325
latamoxef a cephalosporin antibiotic 140
Lectopam *35D*, *38T* (illus.); bromazepam 230
Ledercillin VK penicillin V 425
Legatrin quinine 457
Lenoltec with Codeine acetaminophen (199) and codeine (270)
Lentaron formestane
Leritine anileridine
Lescol fluvastatin
leucovorin an injectable form of folic acid 521
Leukeran chlorambucil 248
leuprolide a hormonal anticancer drug 166
Leustatin cladribine
levamisole an agent used in the treatment of certai cases of malignant melanoma. See Anticancer drugs 166
levobunolol a beta blocker (109) used in the treatment of glaucoma. See Drugs for glaucoma 180
levocabastine 357
levodopa 358
Levo-Dromoran levorphanol
levomepromazine see methotrimeprazine 382
levonorgestrel a progestin used in oral contraceptives (173). See Female sex hormones 159
Levophed norepinephrine
levorphanol a narcotic analgesic 92
levothyroxine 359
Levsin hyoscyamine
Librax chlordiazepoxide (250) and clidinium bromide
Librium chlordiazepoxide 250
Lice-Enz pyrethrins and piperonyl butoxide
Lidecomb nystatin (412), fluocinonide, and neomycin (402)
Lidemol fluocinonide
Lidex fluocinonide
lidocaine 360
lidoflazine an anti-angina drug 129
Lidosporin Ear Drops lidocaine (360) and polymyxin B
lignocaine see lidocaine
Lincocin lincomycin
lincomycin a lincosamide antibiotic 142
lindane 361
Lioresal baclofen 221
liothyronine 362
Lipactin a *topical* gel with heparin (333) and zinc sulfate (530) used to treat cold sores
Lipidil *48M* (illus.); fenofibrate 311
liquid paraffin, liquid petrolatum see mineral oil

Liquifilm Forte polyvinyl alcohol
Liquifilm Tears polyvinyl alcohol
lisinopril 363
Lithane lithium 364
lithium 364
Lithizine lithium 364
Livostin levocabastine 357
Locacorten flumethasone
Locacorten-Vioform flumethasone and clioquinol
Locasalen flumethasone and salicylic acid
lodoxamide an anti-allergic agent
Loestrin an oral contraceptive containing ethinyl
  estradiol (306) and norethindrone
Loftran ketazolam
Lomotil Liquid diphenoxylate 291
Lomotil Tablets diphenoxylate (291) and atropine
lomustine an anticancer drug 166
Loniten minoxidil 392
loperamide 365
Lopid *44G* (illus.); gemfibrozil 327
Lopresor metoprolol 388
Loprox ciclopirox 256
loratadine 366
lorazepam 367
lorcainide an anti-arrhythmic drug 112
Lorelco probucol 115
Loroxide benzoyl peroxide 224
losartan an antihypertensive agent
Losec *48K* (illus.); omeprazole 413
Lotensin benazepril
Lotriderm betamethasone (227) and
  clotrimazole (268)
lovastatin 368
Lovenox enoxaparin
Loxapac loxapine 369
loxapine 369
Lozide *35F* (illus.); indapamide 344
Ludiomil maprotiline 371
Lugol's Solution see sodium iodide
Lupron leuprolide
Luvox *42G* (illus.); fluvoxamine 323
Lyderm fluocinonide
lypressin a synthetic form of the *hormone*
  vasopressin 511. See Drugs for diabetes insipidus
  157
Lysatec rt-PA alteplase
lysergic acid see LSD 535
Lysodren mitotane

M

Maalox aluminum hydroxide (204) and magnesium
  hydroxide (370)
Maalox GRF simethicone
Maalox Plus aluminum hydroxide (204), magnesium
  hydroxide (370), and simethicone

M

Maalox TC aluminum hydroxide (204) and
  magnesium hydroxide (370)
Macrobid nitrofurantoin 407
Macrodantin nitrofurantoin 407
mafenide an antibacterial drug applied *topically* to
  treat serious burns. See Anti-infective skin
  preparations 187
magaldrate an antacid drug that combines
  magnesium hydroxide (370) and aluminum
  hydroxide (204)
Maglucate magnesium gluconate
magnesium 523
magnesium alginate an antifoaming agent. See
  Antacids 120
magnesium carbonate an antacid 120
magnesium citrate a laxative 123
magnesium gluconate a magnesium salt used to
  treat deficiency. See Magnesium 523
magnesium hydroxide 370
magnesium oxide a laxative (123). See
  Magnesium 523
magnesium salicylate an oral analgesic
magnesium sulfate a stimulant laxative. See
  Magnesium 523
magnesium trisilicate an antacid 120
Magnolax magnesium hydroxide (370) and
  mineral oil
Majeptil thioproperazine
malathion a drug used to treat head lice and scabies
  infestation. See Drugs to treat skin parasites 188
Maltlevol a multivitamin preparation. See
  Vitamins 161
Maltlevol-M a multivitamin preparation plus iron. See
  Vitamins 161
Mandelamine methenamine
Mandol cefamandole
Manerix moclobemide 394
mannitol an osmotic diuretic 111
maprotiline 371
Marcaine bupivacaine
marijuana 536
Marvelon an oral contraceptive containing
  desogestrel and ethinyl estradiol (306)
Marzine cyclizine
Materna a multivitamin and mineral preparation. See
  Vitamins 161
Maxenal pseudoephedrine 450
Maxeran metoclopramide 387
Maxibolin ethylestrenol
Maxidex dexamethasone 280
Maxitrol dexamethasone (280), neomycin (402) and
  polymyxin B
mazindol an appetite suppressant. See Nervous
  system stimulants 100
mebendazole 372
mechlorethamine an alkylating agent. See
  Anticancer drugs 166
meclizine 373
Medihaler-Epi epinephrine 300
Medihaler-Ergotamine ergotamine 301
Medipren ibuprofen 341

MEDROGESTONE – MYSOLINE

M **medrogestone** a progestin drug. See Female sex hormones 159
Medrol methylprednisolone 386
medroxyprogesterone 374
medrysone a corticosteroid drug used mainly in *topical* eye preparations. See Corticosteroids 153
mefenamic acid 375
mefloquine an antimalarial drug 149
Mefoxin cefoxitin 243
Megace megestrol 166
Megacillin penicillin G 424
megestrol a female sex hormone (159) and anticancer drug (166)
Megral ergotamine (301), cyclizine, and caffeine
melarsoprol an antiprotozoal drug 148
Mellaril thioridazine 491
melphalan an alkylating agent for multiple myeloma. See Anticancer drugs 166
menadiol see vitamin K 530
menogaril an anticancer drug 166
menotropins a drug for infertility 176
menthol an alcohol prepared from mint oils, and used as an inhalation and *topical* antipruritic 185
mepacrine see quinacrine
meperidine 376
mephenytoin an anticonvulsant drug 98
mephobarbital a barbiturate anticonvulsant 98
mepivacaine a local *anesthetic* 92
meprobamate 377
Mepron atovaquone
meptazinol a narcotic analgesic drug 92
mepyramine see pyrilamine
mequitazine an *investigational* antihistamine 136
mercaptopurine an anticancer drug 166
Mercodol with Decapryn hydrocodone (337), etafedrine, sodium citrate, and doxylamine
mercury a poisonous metal, compounds of which are used as skin *antiseptics*. See Anti-infective skin preparations 187
Mersyndol with Codeine acetaminophen (199), codeine (270), and doxylamine
mesalamine 378
Mesasal mesalamine 378
M-Eslon morphine 395
mesna a drug used to reduce and prevent urinary tract toxicity caused by some anticancer drugs
mesoridazine a phenothiazine antipsychotic drug 97
Mestinon pyridostigmine 453
mestranol an estrogen drug. See Female sex hormones 159
Metamucil psyllium 451
Metandron testosterone 488
metaproterenol see orciprenaline 415
Meted Shampoo sulfur and salicylic acid
metformin 379
methadone a narcotic drug used to ease heroin withdrawal
methamphetamine an amphetamine nervous system stimulant 100
methandrostenolone an anabolic steroid 158

M **methaqualone** a non-barbiturate, non-benzodiazepine sleeping drug 94
methazolamide a carbonic anhydrase inhibitor diuretic (111) used primarily to treat glaucoma 180
methdilazine an antihistamine 136
methenamine a drug used to treat infections of the urinary tract. See Drugs used for urinary disorders 178
methicillin a penicillin antibiotic 140
methimazole an antithyroid drug 156
methocarbamol 380
methohexital a barbiturate drug used to induce general *anesthesia*
methotrexate 381
methotrimeprazine 382
methoxamine a drug to restore or maintain normal blood pressure during surgery. See Antihypertensive drugs 114
methoxsalen 383
methsuximide an anticonvulsant drug 98
methyclothiazide a thiazide diuretic 111
methylbenzethonium a skin *antiseptic*. See Anti-infective skin preparations 187
methyl-CCNU see semustine
methylcellulose a laxative (123), antidiarrheal drug (122), and artificial tear preparation 182
methyldopa 384
methylene blue a dye used in preparations for urinary tract infections 178
methylergonovine a uterine stimulant. See Drugs used in labor 177
methylformamide an *investigational* anticancer drug 166
methyl-glyoxalbis-guanylhydrazone an anticancer drug 166
methylparaben a preservative. See Food additives 539
methylphenidate 385
methylprednisolone 386
methyl salicyclate an analgesic in *rubefacient* preparations used to relieve muscle and joint pain
methylsulfoxide see dimethyl sulfoxide
methyltestosterone a testosterone drug. See Male sex hormones 158
methyprylon a non-barbiturate, non-benzodiazepine sleeping drug 94
methysergide a drug used to prevent migraine 101
Metimyd prednisolone (439) and sulfacetamide (473)
metoclopramide 387
metocurine a muscle-relaxant drug used in surgical procedures. See Muscle-relaxant drugs 132
metolazone a thiazide-like diuretic 111
Metopirone metyrapone
metoprolol 388
Metreton prednisone (440), chlorpheniramine (251), and vitamin C (528)
metrifonate an *investigational* anthelmintic drug 15
Metrodin urofollitropin
Metrogel metronidazole 389
metronidazole 389

M

Metubine Iodide metocurine
metyrapone a drug used to block production of adrenal *hormones* in Cushing's syndrome
metyrosine an antihypertensive drug 114
Mevacor *39N* (illus.); lovastatin 368
mexiletine an anti-arrhythmic drug. See Anti-arrhythmic drugs 112
Mexitil mexiletine
mezlocillin a penicillin antibiotic 140
Micatin miconazole 390
miconazole 390
Micro-K Extencaps *46D* (illus.); potassium chloride 524
Micro-K-10 Extencaps potassium chloride 524
Micronor norethindrone
Midamor amiloride 206
midazolam a benzodiazepine drug 94
midodrine a drug used to treat specific cases of low blood pressure
milrinone a drug used to treat heart failure. See Digitalis drugs 108
mineral oil used as a lubricant laxative (123) and in skin preparations 187
Minestrin 1/20 an oral contraceptive containing ethinyl estradiol (306) and norethindrone
Minipress prazosin 438
Minocin *46C* (illus.); minocycline 391
minocycline 391
Min-Ovral an oral contraceptive containing ethinyl estradiol (306) and levonorgestrel
minoxidil 392
Minoxigain minoxidil 392
Mintezol thiabendazole
Miocarpine pilocarpine 433
Miochol acetylcholine
Miosal triethanolamine salicylate
Miostat carbachol
misoprostol 393
mitolactol an *investigational* anticancer drug 166
mitomycin a *cytotoxic* antibiotic. See Anticancer drugs 166
mitotane an anticancer drug 166
mitoxantrone an anticancer drug 166
Mobenol tolbutamide 497
Mobiflex tenoxicam 482
moclobemide 394
Modecate fluphenazine 319
Moditen fluphenazine 319
Modulon trimebutine 506
Moduret 50 *36G* (illus.); amiloride (206) and hydrochlorothiazide (336)
Mogadon *42O, 43H* (illus.); nitrazepam 406
Moisturel an oil-in-water emulsion. See Bases for skin preparations 187
molindone an antipsychotic drug 97
molybdenum a mineral required in minute amounts in the diet. It is poisonous if ingested in large quantities.
mometasone a *topical* corticosteroid 130
Monistat miconazole 390
Monitan acebutolol 198

M

monobenzone a *topically* applied drug used to remove skin pigmentation in the treatment of severe vitiligo
Monopril *43T* (illus.); fosinopril 324
monosulfiram a drug used to treat scabies. See Drugs to treat skin parasites 188
moricizine an *investigational* phenothiazine drug used to treat abnormal heart rhythms. See Anti-arrhythmic drugs 112
morphine 395
Morphitec morphine 395
M.O.S. morphine 395
Motilium domperidone 295
Motrin ibuprofen 341
moxalactam a cephalosporin antibiotic 140
MS Contin morphine 395
MSD E.C. ASA *40A* (illus.); ASA 200
MS.IR morphine 395
Mucaine aluminum hydroxide (204), magnesium hydroxide (370), and oxethazaine
Mucomyst acetylcysteine
Multipax hydroxyzine 340
Multi-Tar Plus zinc pyrithione and coal tar
mupirocin 396
Murine benzalkonium chloride and disodium edetate
Murine Ear Wax Removal System carbamide peroxide
Murocel methylcellulose
muromonab CD3 an immunosuppressant drug (168) used to prevent organ rejection following transplant surgery
Mustargen mechlorethamine
Mutamycin mitomycin
M.V.I.-1000 a multivitamin preparation. See Vitamins 161
Myambutol ethambutol
Mycifradin neomycin 402
Myciguent neomycin 402
Mycil chlorphenesin
Myclo clotrimazole 268
Mycobutin rifabutin
Mycostatin nystatin 412
Mydfrin phenylephrine 431
Mydriacyl tropicamide
Myleran busulfan
Myochrysine gold sodium thiomalate
Myoflex triethanolamine salicylate
Myotonachol bethanechol
Mysoline primidone 441

NABILONE – NOVO-SUNDAC

N

nabilone a drug used to treat nausea and vomiting caused by anticancer drugs. See Anti-emetic drugs 102
nabumetone 397
nadolol 398
Nadopen-V 500 *36K* (illus.); penicillin 425
Nadostine nystatin 412
nafarelin a drug for the management of endometriosis. See Drugs used to treat menstrual disorders 172
nafcillin a penicillin antibiotic 140
naftifine a *topical* antifungal drug 150
Naftine naftifine
nalbuphine a narcotic analgesic 97
Nalcrom cromolyn sodium 274
Nalfon fenoprofen
nalidixic acid a quinolone antibiotic 141
naloxone an antidote to narcotic drug poisoning
naltrexone a drug for maintenance of opioid withdrawal. See Drug dependence 23
nandrolone 399
NAPAP see acetaminophen 199
naphazoline a *sympathomimetic* decongestant
Naphcon-A naphazoline and pheniramine
Naphcon Forte naphazoline
Naprosyn naproxen 400
Naprosyn E *45G*, *45J* (illus.); naproxen 400
naproxen sodium 400
Narcan naloxone
narcotine see noscapine
Nardil phenelzine
Nasacort triamcinolone 501
natamycin a drug used to treat fungal infections of the eye. See Antifungal drugs 150
Natulan procarbazine
Naturetin bendroflumethiazide
Navane thiothixene
Naxen naproxen 400
Nebcin tobramycin 496
nedocromil 401
nefazodone an antidepressant 96
NegGram nalidixic acid
Nembutal pentobarbital
Neo-Bex a vitamin B complex preparation plus vitamin C. See Vitamins 161
Neo-Cortef hydrocortisone (338) and neomycin (402)
Neo Decadron dexamethasone (280) and neomycin (402)
Neo-Estrone esterified estrogens
Neo-Medrol methylprednisolone (386) and neomycin (402)
neomycin 402
Neo-Pause testosterone (488) and estradiol (304)
Neosporin neomycin (402), polymyxin B, bacitracin (220), and gramicidin
neostigmine 403

N

NeoStrata HQ hydroquinone
Neotopic neomycin (402), polymyxin B, and bacitracin (220)
Neptazane methazolamide
Nerisone diflucortolone
Nesacaine chloroprocaine
netilmicin an aminoglycoside antibiotic 140
Netromycin netilmicin
Neuleptil pericyazine
Neupogen filgrastim
Neurontin gabapentin
Neutralca-S aluminum hydroxide (204) and magnesium hydroxide (370)
niacin 523
niacinamide see niacin 523
nicardipine a calcium channel blocker 113
Nicoderm nicotine 537
Nicorette nicotine 537
Nicorette Plus nicotine 537
nicotinamide see niacin 523
nicotinic acid see niacin 523
nicotinyl alcohol tartrate see niacin 523
Nicotrol nicotine 537
nicoumalone an anticoagulant drug. See Anti-coagulant drugs 116
NidaGel metronidazole 389
nifedipine 404
nifurtimox an antiprotozoal drug 148
nikethamide a respiratory stimulant 100
Nilstat nystatin 412
nilutamide 405
nimodipine a calcium channel blocker (113). See Drugs used for migraine 101
Nimotop nimodipine
Nipent pentostatin
Nipride sodium nitroprusside
niridazole an *investigational* anthelmintic drug 151
nitrazepam 406
Nitro-Dur nitroglycerin 408
nitrofurantoin 407
nitrofurazone a *topical* antibacterial drug (143). See Anti-infective skin preparations 187
Nitrogard-SR nitroglycerin 408
nitrogen mustard see mechlorethamine
nitroglycerin 408
Nitrol nitroglycerin 408
Nitrolingual Spray nitroglycerin 408
Nitrong nitroglycerin 408
Nitrong SR *40N* (illus.); nitroglycerin 408
Nitrostat *43M* (illus.); nitroglycerin 408
nitrous oxide a gas used to induce *anesthesia*. See Drugs used in labor 177
Nivea an oil-in-water emulsion. See Bases for skin preparations 187
Nix permethrin 427
nizatidine 409
Nizoral ketoconazole 353
Nolvadex tamoxifen 480
Nolvadex-D tamoxifen 480
nonoxynol-9 a spermicide used in contraceptive foams, creams, and gels

N

noradrenaline see norepinephrine
Norcuron vecuronium
norepinephrine a naturally occurring
neurotransmitter given to treat shock
norethindrone a progestin drug. See Female sex
hormones 159
norethisterone see norethindrone
norethynodrel a progestin drug. See Female
sex hormones 159
Norfemac bufexamac
Norflex *42F* (illus.); orphenadrine 416
norfloxacin 410
Norgesic ASA (200), orphenadrine (416), and
caffeine
Norgesic Forte ASA (200), orphenadrine (416),
and caffeine
norgestimate a progestin drug used in oral
contraceptives 173. See also Female sex
hormones 159
norgestrel a progestin drug. See Female sex
hormones 159
Norinyl 1/50 an oral contraceptive containing
mestranol and norethindrone
Norlutate norethindrone
Noroxin *44J* (illus.); norfloxacin 410
Noroxin Ophthalmic Solution norfloxacin 410
Norpace disopyramide 293
Norpace CR disopyramide 293
Norpramin desipramine 279
nortriptyline 411
Norvasc *44A* (illus.); amlodipine 209
noscapine a cough suppressant. See Drugs to treat
coughs 106
Novahistex C codeine (270) and phenylephrine (431)
Novahistex DH hydrocodone (337) and
phenylephrine (431)
Novahistex DH Expectorant hydrocodone (337),
guaifenesin (331), and phenylephrine (431)
Novahistex DM with Decongestant
dextromethorphan (281) and
pseudoephedrine (450)
Novahistex DM Expectorant with Decongestant
dextromethorphan (281), guaifenesin (331), and
pseudoephedrine (450)
Novahistex Expectorant with Decongestant
pseudoephedrine (450) and guaifenesin (331)
Novahistine Decongestant phenylephrine (431)
Novahistine DH hydrocodone (337) and
phenylephrine (431)
Novahistine DM Expectorant with Decongestant
dextromethorphan (281), guaifenesin (331), and
pseudoephedrine (450)
Novahistine DM with Decongestant
dextromethorphan (281) and
pseudoephedrine (450)
Novamilor amiloride (206) and
hydrochlorothiazide (336)
Novamoxin *47E, 47F* (illus.); amoxicillin 210
Novantrone mitoxantrone
Nova-Rectal pentobarbital
Novasen *37C, 39S* (illus.); acetylsalicylic acid 200

N

Novo-Alprazol alprazolam 203
Novo-Ampicillin ampicillin 212
Novo-Atenol *42I* (illus.); atenolol 215
Novo-AZT zidovudine 516
Novocain procaine
Novo-Capto captopril 239
Novo-Carbamaz carbamazepine 240
Novo-Chlorhydrate *46J* (illus.); chloral hydrate 247
Novo-Cimetine *38N* (illus.); cimetidine 257
Novo-Clopate clorazepate 267
Novo-Cloxin *47Q, 47R* (illus.); cloxacillin 269
Novo-Difenac *40J* (illus.); diclofenac 283
Novo-Diltazem diltiazem 287
Novo-Dipam *37T* (illus.); diazepam 282
Novo-Dipiradol dipyridamole 292
Novo-Doxepin doxepin 296
Novo-Doxylin doxycycline 297
Novo-Famotidine *40E* (illus.); famotidine 309
Novo-Flupam *47I* (illus.); flurazepam 320
Novo-Gesic *45B, 45I* (illus.); acetaminophen 199
Novo-Gesic-C8 acetaminophen (199), caffeine,
and codeine (270)
Novo-Gesic-C15 acetaminophen (199), caffeine,
and codeine (270)
Novo-Gesic-C30 acetaminophen (199), caffeine,
and codeine (270)
Novo-Glyburide *45N* (illus.); glyburide 330
Novo-Hydrazide *36E, 36F* (illus.);
hydrochlorothiazide 336
Novo-Hydroxyzin *46K* (illus.); hydroxyzine 340
Novo-Hylazin hydralazine 335
Novo-Keto-EC ketoprofen 354
Novo-Lexin *36R, 36S* (illus.); cephalexin 245
Novolin insulin 346
Novo-Lorazem *43L, 44O, 45Q* (illus.); lorazepam 367
Novo-Medopa methyldopa 384
Novo-Metformin *41C* (illus.); metformin 379
Novo-Methacin indomethacin 345
Novo-Metoprol *35H* (illus.); metoprolol 388
Novo-Naprox *36D, 38H* (illus.); naproxen 400
Novo-Nidazol *41D* (illus.); metronidazole 389
Novo-Pen-VK-500 *37G* (illus.); penicillin V 425
Novo-Peridol haloperidol 332
Novo-Pindol pindolol 434
Novo-Pirocam piroxicam 435
Novo-Prazin prazosin 438
Novo-Prednisone *42R* (illus.); prednisone 457
Novo-Profen *37D* (illus.); ibuprofen 341
Novo-Purol *37A* (illus.); allopurinol 202
Novo-Pyrazone sulfinpyrazone 476
Novo-Ranidine *42A, 45E* (illus.); ranitidine 458
Novo-Reserpine reserpine
Novo-Rythro Encap erythromycin 303
Novo-Salmol salbutamol 461
Novo-Selegiline selegiline 464
Novo-Semide *38D, 43I* (illus.); furosemide 325
Novo-Spiroton spironolactone 469
Novo-Spirozine-25 spironolactone (469) and
hydrochlorothiazide (336)
Novo-Sucralate sucralfate 472
Novo-Sundac sulindac 478

N

Novo-Tamoxifen tamoxifen 480
Novo-Tetra *47L* (illus.); tetracycline 489
Novo-Timol timolol 494
Novo-Triamzide *37H* (illus.); hydrochlorothiazide (336) and triamterene (502)
Novo-Trimel *41E* (illus.); sulfamethoxazole (474) and trimethoprim (507)
Novo-Trimel DS *44F* (illus.); sulfamethoxazole (474) and trimethoprim (507)
Novo-Triptyn *37O, 39G* (illus.); amitriptyline 208
Novoxapam *37L, 42Q* (illus.); oxazepam 417
Nozinan methotrimeprazine 382
Nu-Alpraz alprazolam 203
Nu-Amilzide amiloride (206) and hydrochlorothiazide (336)
Nu-Amoxi *47G* (illus.); amoxicillin 210
Nu-Ampi ampicillin 212
Nu-Atenol atenolol 215
Nubain nalbuphine
Nu-Cal calcium carbonate
Nu-Capto captopril 239
Nu-Cephalex cephalexin 245
Nu-Cimet cimetidine 257
Nu-Clonidine clonidine 266
Nu-Cloxin cloxacillin 269
Nu-Cotrimox co-trimoxazole 273
Nu-Diclo diclofenac 283
Nu-Diltiaz diltiazem 287
Nu-Hydral hydralazine 335
Nu-Indo indomethacin 345
Nu-Loraz lorazepam 367
Nu-Medopa methyldopa 384
Nu-Metop metoprolol 388
Numorphan oxymorphone
Nu-Nifed nifedipine 404
Nupercainal dibucaine
Nu-Pindol pindolol 434
Nu-Pirox piroxicam 435
Nu-Prazo prazosin 438
Nuprin ibuprofen 341
Nu-Prochlor prochlorperazine 444
Nu-Ranit *41T* (illus.); ranitidine 458
Nuromax doxacurium
Nu-Tetra tetracycline 489
Nu-Triazide *37I* (illus.); triamterene (502) and hydrochlorothiazide (336)
Nutrifer Plus a multivitamin and mineral preparation. See Vitamins 161
Nyaderm nystatin 412
nylidrin a drug used to improve blood flow to the limbs in peripheral vascular disease. See Vasodilators 110
Nyquil Liquid Nighttime Colds Medicine dextromethorphan (281), pseudoephedrine (450), doxylamine, and acetaminophen (199)
nystatin 412
Nytol diphenhydramine 290

O

Occlucort betamethasone 227
Occlusal salicylic acid
octoxynol a spermicide used in vaginal contraceptive creams
Ocuclear oxymetazoline 420
Ocudex dexamethasone 280
Ocufen flurbiprofen 321
Ocugram gentamicin 328
Ocusert Pilo pilocarpine 433
Ocuvite a multivitamin and mineral preparation. See Vitamins 161
oestradiol see estradiol 304
Oestrilin estrone
ofloxacin a quinolone antibiotic 141
Ogen estropipate 305
olsalazine a drug for ulcerative colitis 124
omeprazole 413
Omni-Tuss codeine (270), chlorpheniramine (251), ephedrine, phenyltoloxamine, and guaiacol
Oncovin vincristine
ondansetron 414
One A Day Advance Adult a multivitamin/mineral preparation. See Vitamins 161
One A Day Advance Fem a multivitamin/mineral preparation. See Vitamins 161
One-Alpha alfacalcidol
Onyvul urea
Opcon naphazoline
Opcon-A naphazoline and pheniramine
Ophthetic proparacaine
Ophtho-Chloram chloramphenicol 249
Ophthocort chloramphenicol (249), hydrocortisone (336), and polymyxin B
Ophtho-Sulf sulfacetamide 473
Ophtho-Tate prednisolone 439
Ophtrivin-A xylometazoline (515) and antazoline
opium a natural substance containing morphine (395). Opium, derived from the opium poppy, was formerly used in many medications. Highly addictive, opium is now seldom used, but its derivatives and synthetic versions of these (narcotics) are used as analgesics (92), cough suppressants (106), and antidiarrheal drugs (122)
Opticrom cromolyn sodium 274
Optimine azatadine 217
Oracort triamcinolone 501
Oramorph SR morphine 395
Orajel benzocaine 223
Orap pimozide
Orbenin cloxacillin 269
orciprenaline 415
Orifer-F a multivitamin and mineral preparation. See Vitamins 161
Orinase tolbutamide 497

Ornade chlopheniramine (251) and phenyl propanolamine and mineral preparation. See Vitamins 161

Ornade-A.F. chlorpheniramine (251) and phenylpropanolamine

Ornade-DM dextromethorphan (281), chlorpheniramine (251), and phenylpropanolamine

Ornade Expectorant chlorpheniramine (251), phenylpropanolamine, and guaifenesin (331)

ornidazole an antiprotozoal drug 148

orphenadrine 416

Oro-Clense CHX chlorhexidine

Ortho-Cept an oral contraceptive containing desogestrel and ethinyl estradiol (306)

Orthoclone OKT3 muromonab-CD3

Ortho 0.5/35 an oral contraceptive containing ethinyl estradiol (306) and norethindrone

Ortho 1/35 an oral contraceptive containing ethinyl estradiol (306) and norethindrone

Ortho 7/7/7 an oral contraceptive containing ethinyl estradiol (306) and norethindrone

Ortho 10/11 an oral contraceptive containing ethinyl estradiol (306) and norethindrone

Ortho-Novum 1/50 an oral contraceptive containing mestranol and norethindrone

Orudis ketoprofen 354

Orudis E ketoprofen 354

Oruvail ketoprofen 354

Os-Cal calcium carbonate 519

Os-Cal-D calcium carbonate (519) and vitamin D_3 (529)

Osmitrol mannitol

Ostac clodronate

Ostoforte vitamin D 529

Otrivin xylometazoline 515

ouabain see digitalis drugs 108

Ovol simethicone

Ovral an oral contraceptive containing ethinyl estradiol (306) and norgestrel

oxacillin a penicillin antibiotic 140

oxazepam 417

oxethazaine a local anesthetic (92) used in conjunction with antacids to treat reflux esophagitis. See Antacids 120

oxilapine see loxapine 369

Oxipor coal tar, benzocaine (223), and salicylic acid

oxprenolol a beta blocker 109

Oxsoralen methoxsalen 383

Oxsoralen-Ultra methoxsalen 383

oxtriphylline a xanthine *bronchodilator* drug 104

oxybenzone a sunscreening agent 191

oxybuprocaine see benoxinate

oxybutynin 418

oxychlorosene a *topical* antiseptic. See Drugs used for urinary disorders 178

Oxycocet *41A* (illus.); oxycodone (419) and acetaminophen (199)

Oxycodan acetylsalicylic acid (200) and oxycodone (419)

oxycodone 419

Oxyderm benzoyl peroxide 224

Oxy 5 Vanishing Formula benzoyl peroxide 224

oxymetazoline 420

oxymetholone an anabolic steroid 158

oxymorphone a narcotic analgesic 93

oxyphenbutazone a non-steroidal anti-inflammatory drug 128

oxyquinoline a preservative with antimicrobial properties used in *topical* preparations

oxytocin 421

P

PABA see aminobenzoic acid

paclitaxel an *antineoplastic* drug used to treat ovarian cancer 166

padimate-O a sunscreening agent. See Sunscreens 191

Palafer ferrous fumarate 522

Palafer CF ferrous fumarate (522), vitamin C (528), and folic acid (521)

Paludrine proguanil

pamabrom a weak diuretic (111) often combined with an analgesic to relieve premenstrual syndrome. See Drugs used to treat menstrual disorders 172

Pamergan meperidine (376) and promethazine (446)

pamidronate a drug used to treat high blood levels of calcium in cancer patients

Pamprin pamabrom, pyrilamine, and acetaminophen (199)

Pancrease pancrelipase

pancreatin a preparation of pancreatic *hormones*. See Agents used in disorders of the pancreas 126

pancrelipase a preparation of pancreatic *hormones*. See Agents used in disorders of the pancreas 126

pancuronium a drug used to produce muscle relaxation during general *anesthesia*

P & S Liquid Phenol phenol

P & S Plus coal tar and salicylic acid

P & S Shampoo salicylic acid and lactic acid

Panectyl trimeprazine

Panoxyl benzoyl peroxide 224

panthenol see pantothenic acid 524

Pantopon morphine (395) and opium

pantothenic acid 524

papaverine a smooth muscle relaxant. See Vasodilators 110

Papulex nicotinamide gel

para-aminobenzoic acid a sunscreening agent 191

paracetamol see acetaminophen 199

Parafon Forte acetaminophen (199) and chlorzoxazone

Parafon Forte C8 chlorzoxazone, codeine (270), and acetaminophen (199)

PARALDEHYDE – POLYVINYL ALCOHOL

P

paraldehyde an anticonvulsant drug 98
paramethadione an anticonvulsant drug 98
Paramettes Adults Complete a multivitamin and mineral preparation. See Vitamins 161
Paramettes 50+ Complete a multivitamin and mineral preparation. See Vitamins 161
Paramettes Teens a multivitamin and iron preparation. See Vitamins 161
Paraplatin carboplatin
paregoric a narcotic analgesic drug, also called camphorated opium tincture. See Antidiarrheal drugs 122
Parlodel bromocriptine 231
paroxetine 422
Parsitan ethopropazine
Parvolex acetylcysteine
PAS see aminosalicylate sodium
Pavulon pancuronium
Paxil *35E* (illus.); paroxetine 422
PCE *40M* (illus.); erythromycin 302
PCNU an *investigational* anticancer drug 167
PDF sodium fluoride
pectin a natural gelling agent included in some antidiarrheal medications
Pediatrix acetaminophen 199
Pediazole erythromycin (302) and sulfisoxazole (477)
Pedi-Dent sodium fluoride 521
pemoline a nervous system stimulant 100
Penbritin ampicillin 212
penbutolol a beta blocker 109
penfluridol an antipsychotic drug 97
Penglobe bacampicillin
penicillamine 423
penicillin G 424
penicillin V 425
Penntuss codeine (270) and chlorpheniramine (251)
Pentacarinat pentamidine
pentaerythritol tetranitrate a nitrate anti-angina drug 113
pentamidine an antiprotozoal (148) and anti-bacterial drug (143)
Pentamycetin chloramphenicol 249
Pentamycetin-HC chloramphenicol (249) and hydrocortisone (338)
Penta/3B a multivitamin preparation. See Vitamins 161
Penta/3B+C a multivitamin preparation. See Vitamins 161
Penta/3B Plus a multivitamin preparation. See Vitamins 161
Pentasa mesalamine 378
pentazocine a narcotic analgesic 93
pentetic acid an antidote used in certain types of radioactive isotope poisoning
pentobarbital a barbiturate sleeping drug 94
pentostatin an anticancer drug 167
Pentothal thiopental
pentoxifylline 426
Pentrax a coal tar shampoo
Pen-Vee penicillin V 425
Pepcid famotidine 309

P

peppermint oil used in medicine to treat indigestion and bowel spasm. See Drugs used for irritable bowel syndrome 122
pepsin a digestive *enzyme* used for the treatment of digestive disorders
Pepto-Bismol Liquid bismuth subsalicylate
Pepto-Bismol Tablets calcium carbonate and bismuth subsalicylate
Peptol cimetidine 257
Percocet acetaminophen (199) and oxycodone (419)
Percocet-Demi acetaminophen (199) and oxycodone (419)
Percodan ASA (200) and oxycodone (419)
Percodan-Demi ASA (200) and oxycodone (419)
pergolide an antiparkinsonism drug 99
Pergonal menotropins
Periactin cyproheptadine
Peri-Colace casanthranol and docusate
pericyazine an antipsychotic drug 93
Peridol haloperidol 332
perindopril an ACE inhibitor
Peritrate pentaerythritol tetranitrate
Permax pergolide
permethrin 427
Pernox sulfur and salicylic acid
perphenazine 428
Persantine dipyridamole 292
Persol benzoyl peroxide (224) and sulfur
Persol Forte benzoyl peroxide (224) and sulfur
Pertofrane desipramine 279
Peruvian balsam an ingredient of *topical* treatment for hemorrhoids. See Drugs for anal and rectal disorders 125
pethidine see meperidine
PETN see pentaerythritol tetranitrate
petrolatum see mineral oil
Pharmacal 500 calcium carbonate
Pharmorubicin epirubicin
Phazyme simethicone
phenacemide an anticonvulsant drug 98
phenacetin a nonnarcotic analgesic no longer used because of its adverse effects
Phenaphen with Codeine ASA (200), phenobarbital (430), and codeine (270)
Phenazo phenazopyridine 429
phenazocine a narcotic analgesic 93
phenazopyridine 429
phenelzine sulfate an MAOI used to treat depression. See antidepressant drugs 96
Phenergan promethazine (446)
Phenergan Expectorant Plain promethazine (446) and guaiacolsulfonate
Phenergan Expectorant with Codeine promethazine (446), guaiacolsulfonate, and codeine (270)
Phenergan VC Expectorant Plain promethazine (446), guaiacolsulfonate, and phenylephrine (431)
Phenergan VC Expectorant with Codeine promethazine (446), guaiacolsulfonate, phenylephrine (431), and codeine (270)

pheniramine an antihistamine 152

phenobarbital 430

phenol an *antiseptic* used in throat lozenges and sprays and some skin preparations. See Anti-infective skin preparations 187

phenolphthalein a stimulant laxative 123

phenoxybenzamine a *sympathomimetic* vasodilator used to treat hypertension. See Antihypertensive drugs 114

phenoxymethylpenicillin see penicillin V 425

phensuximide an anticonvulsant drug 98

phentermine an appetite suppressant similar to the amphetamines. See Nervous system stimulants 100

phentolamine an antihypertensive drug 114

phenylbutazone an NSAID. See Non-steroidal anti-inflammatory drugs 128

phenylephrine 431

phenylpropanolamine a decongestant. See Decongestants 105

phenyl salicylate a nonnarcotic analgesic similar to ASA 200

phenyltoloxamine an antihistamine 136

phenytoin 432

Phillips' Gelcaps magnesium hydroxide (370), docusate sodium, and phenolphthalein

Phillips' Milk of Magnesia magnesium hydroxide 370

pHisoHex hexachlorophene

pholcodine a cough suppressant. See Drugs to treat coughs 106

Phospholine Iodide echothiophate

phosphorus a mineral occasionally included in vitamin and mineral supplements. See Vitamins 161

Phyllocontin aminophylline

physostigmine a *miotic* drug used to treat glaucoma 180

phytomenadione see phytonadione

phytonadione a hemostatic drug used to prevent bleeding

pilocarpine 433

Pilopine HS pilocarpine 433

pimozide an antipsychotic drug (433) used to treat movement disorders

pinaverium a calcium channel antagonist used to treat irritable bowel syndrome 122

pindolol 434

piperacillin a penicillin antibiotic 140

piperazine an anthelmintic drug 151

piperazine estrone sulfate see estropipate

piperonyl butoxide a drug used in combination with pyrethrins to treat skin parasites 188

Piportil L4 pipotiazine

pipotiazine an antipsychotic drug 97

Pipracil piperacillin

pirenzepine an *anticholinergic* drug used to treat peptic ulcers. See Anti-ulcer drugs 121

pirmenol an anti-arrhythmic drug 112

piroxicam 435

Pitressin vasopressin 511

Pitrex tolnaftate 498

P

pivampicillin a penicillin antibiotic 140

pivmecillinam a penicillin antibiotic 140

pizotyline a drug used to prevent migraine headaches 101

Placidyl ethchlorvynol

Plaquenil hydroxychloroquine

Platinol cisplatin

Plendil *35R* (illus.); felodipine 310

plicamycin an anticancer drug (166) also used to treat hypercalcemia (abnormally high levels of calcium in the blood)

PMS-ASA ASA 200

PMS-Benztropine benztropine 225

PMS-Cholestyramine cholestyramine 255

PMS-Docusate Calcium docusate

PMS-Docusate Sodium docusate

PMS-Egozinc zinc sulfate

PMS-Fluphenazine fluphenazine 319

PMS-Hydromorphone hydromorphone 339

PMS-Isoniazid 349

PMS-Ketoprofen ketoprofen 354

PMS-Lactulose lactulose 356

PMS-Levazine amitriptyline (208) and perphenazine (428)

PMS-Levothyroxine Sodium levothyroxine 359

PMS-Lindane lindane 361

PMS-Loperamide Hydrochloride loperamide 365

PMS-Nylidrin nylidrin

PMS-Prochlorperazine prochlorperazine 444

PMS-Procyclidine procyclidine 445

PMS-Promethazine Syrup promethazine 446

PMS-Propranolol propranolol 448

PMS-Pyrazinamide pyrazinamide

PMS-Sulfasalazine sulfasalazine 475

PMS-Testosterone Enanthate testosterone 488

PMS-Trazodone trazodone 499

PMS-Trihexyphenidyl trihexyphenidyl 505

podifilox a drug used *topically* to treat genital warts

Podofilm podophyllin

podophyllin a drug used *topically* to treat warts

Polaramine dexchlorpheniramine

Polocaine mepivacaine

polycarbophil calcium a laxative 123

polyethylene glycol an emulsifying agent used in skin preparations and in certain preparations for clearing the bowel. See Bases for skin preparations (187) and Laxatives (123)

polymyxin B an antibacterial drug (143) mainly used *topically* to treat infections of the skin, eyes, and ears

Polysporin bacitracin (220), gramicidin, and polymyxin B

Polysporin Burn Formula polymyxin B, gramicidin, and lidocaine (360)

Polytopic bacitracin (220) and polymyxin B

Polytrim trimethoprim (507) and polymyxin B

Poly-Vi-Flor a mutivitamin preparation with fluoride. See Vitamins 161

polyvinyl alcohol an ingredient of artificial tear preparations

POLY-VI-SOL – RHOTRIMINE

P

Poly-Vi-Sol a multivitamin preparation. See
Vitamins 161
Ponderal fenfluramine
Pondimin fenfluramine
Pondocillin *44H* (illus.); pivampicillin 453
Ponstan *48B* (illus.); mefenamic acid 388
Pontocaine tetracaine 505
Potaba aminobenzoate potassium
potassium 524
potassium bicarbonate an antacid. See
Potassium 524
potassium chloride a salt. See Potassium 524
potassium citrate a drug that reduces the acidity,
thus relieving the discomfort caused by cystitis.
See Drugs used for urinary disorders (178) and
Potassium (524)
potassium clavulanate a substance given with
amoxicillin (231) to prevent inactivation and
increase the activity of the antibiotic against a
wider range of bacteria. See Antibiotics 156
potassium gluconate a potassium salt. See
potassium 524
potassium iodide an *expectorant;* also used to treat
thyrotoxicosis 172
potassium permanganate a skin *antiseptic*. See
Anti-infective skin preparations 187
Potassium-Sandoz potassium chloride and
potassium bicarbonate
povidone a dispersing and suspending agent
povidone-iodine a skin *antiseptic*. See Anti-
infective skin preparations 187
pralidoxime an antidote used in cases of poisoning
by certain pesticides
Pramox H.C. pramoxine and hydrocortisone (338)
pramoxine a local anesthetic 108
Pravachol *41O* (illus.); pravastatin 437
pravastatin 437
prazepam a benzodiazepine anti-anxiety drug 111
praziquantel an anthelmintic. See Anthelmintics 167
prazosin 438
Pred Forte prednisolone 439
Pred Mild prednisolone 439
prednisolone 439
prednisone 440
Prefrin phenylephrine 431
Prefrin-A phenylephrine (431) and pyrilamine
Premarin *35B, 37M, 38S, 39R* (illus.); conjugated
estrogens 272
prenalterol a *sympathomimetic* drug used to treat
heart failure
Prenavite a multivitamin preparation plus iron and
calcium. See Vitamins 161
prenylamine an anti-anginal drug 113
Prepidil Gel dinoprostone 289
Prepulsid *42L, 43B* (illus.); cisapride 259
Pressyn vasopressin 511
Prevacid lansoprazole
Prevex petrolatum and cyclomethicone
Prevex B betamethasone 227
Prevex Baby Diaper Rash Cream zinc oxide
Prevex HC hydrocortisone 338

P

prilocaine a local anesthetic 92
primaquine an antimalarial drug
Primaxim cilastatin/imipenem
primidone 441
Prinivil *37R, 43O* (illus.); lisinopril 363
Prinzide hydrochlorothiazide (336) and lisinopril (3
Priscoline tolazoline
Privine naphazoline 105
Pro-Air procaterol
Pro-Banthine propantheline
probenecid 459
probucol a lipid-lowering drug 115
procainamide 443
procaine a local anesthetic 92
Procan SR procainamide 443
procarbazine an anticancer drug 166
procaterol an adrenergic *bronchodilator* 104
prochlorperazine 444
procinonide a *topical* corticosteroid used to treat
inflammatory skin disorders. See Topical
corticosteroids 186
Proctofoam-HC hydrocortisone (338) and pramox
Proctosone hydrocortisone (338), neomycin (402)
and cinchocaine
Procyclid procyclidine 445
procyclidine 445
Procytox cyclophosphamide 276
Prodiem Plain psyllium 451
Prodiem Plus psyllium (451) and senna
Profasi HP human chorionic gonadotropin 334
Progestasert progesterone
progesterone a female sex hormone 159
Proglycem diazoxide
proguanil an antimalarial drug 149
Prolopa levodopa (358) and benserazide
Proloprim trimethoprim 507
Promani triclosan
Promatussin DM promethazine (446),
dextromethorphan (281), and
pseudoephedrine (450)
promazine a phenothiazine antipsychotic (97) anc
antiemetic drug (102)
promethazine 446
Prometrium progesterone. See Female sex
hormones 159
Pronestyl procainamide 443
Pronestyl SR procainamide 443
Propaderm beclomethasone 222
propafenone an anti-arrhythmic drug 112
propantheline an *anticholinergic antispasmodic* o
used to treat irritable bowel syndrome (122) and
urinary incontinence (178)
proparacaine a local anesthetic 92
Propine dipivefrin
propoxyphene 447
propranolol 448
propylene glycol a moisturizing agent used in sk
preparations 187
propylparaben a preservative added to skin
preparations
propylthiouracil 449

Propyl-Thyracil propylthiouracil 449
Proscar finasteride
Prosom estazolam
prostaglandin E₂ see dinoprostone 289
Prostigmin neostigmine 403
Prostin-E₂ dinoprostone 289
Prostin VR alprostadil
protirelin a drug used to test thyroid and pituitary
  function. See Drugs for thyroid disorders 156
Protopam Chloride pralidoxime
protriptyline a tricyclic antidepressant drug 96
Protropin growth *hormone* (somatrem)
Provera *36J, 39I, 43C* (illus.);
  medroxyprogesterone 374
Proviodine povidone-iodine
Prozac *48E* (illus.); fluoxetine 318
pseudoephedrine 450
Psorigel coal tar
psyllium 451
Pulmicort budesonide
Pulmophylline theophylline 490
Pulmorphan Expectorant dextromethorphan (281),
  guaifenesin (331), pheniramine, and
  phenylephrine (431)
Purinethol mercaptopurine
Purinol allopurinol 202
PVF K penicillin V 425
Pyopen carbenicillin
pyrantel 452
pyrazinamide an antituberculous drug 144
pyrethrins a drug used in combination with piperonyl
  butoxide to treat skin parasites 188
Pyribenzamine tripelennamine
Pyridium phenazopyridine 429
pyridostigmine 453
pyridoxine 525
pyrilamine an antihistamine 136
pyrimethamine 454
pyrvinium an anthelmintic drug 151

Q

quazepam a benzodiazepine sleeping drug 94
Quelicin Chloride succinylcholine
Questran cholestyramine 255
Questran Light cholestyramine 255
Quibron-T theophylline 490
Quibron-T/SR theophylline 490
quinacrine an antiprotozoal drug 148
quinalbarbitone see secobarbital
quinapril 455
Quinate quinidine 456
quinestrol an estrogen drug. See Female sex
  hormones 159

Q

quinfamide an *investigational* antiprotozoal drug 148
Quinidex quinidine 456
quinidine 456
quinine 457

R

Radiostol vitamin D 529
R & C pyrethrins and piperonyl butoxide
ramipril an ACE inhibitor 110
ranitidine 458
raubasine an antihypertensive drug 114
rauwolfia an antihypertensive drug 114
razoxane an *investigational* anticancer drug 166
Reactine *44C* (illus.); cetirizine 246
Rectocort hydrocortisone 338
Rectovalone tixocortol
Redoxon vitamin C 528
Redoxon-B a vitamin and mineral preparation.
  See Vitamins 161
Redoxon-Cal pyridoxine, vitamin D, vitamin C,
  and calcium
Refresh polyvinyl alcohol
Reglan metoclopramide 387
Regonol pyridostigmine 453
Regulex docusate sodium
Regulex-D danthron and docusate sodium
Relefact TRH protirelin
Renacidin a solution used to dissolve kidney
  stones
Renedil *35Q* (illus.); felodipine 310
reserpine an antihypertensive drug 114
resorcinol an ingredient of skin preparations for the
  treatment of acne, dermatitis, and fungal infections.
  See Anti-infective skin preparations 187
Restoril *47H, 47K* (illus.); temazepam 481
Resyl guaifenesin 331
Retin-A tretinoin 500
retinoic acid a derivative of vitamin A 527
Retisol-A tretinoin 500
Retrovir zidovudine 516
Revimine dopamine
Revitalose-C-1000 vitamin C
Rheumatrex methotrexate 381
Rhinalar flunisolide 315
Rhinaris polyethylene glycol and propylene glycol
Rhinaris-F flunisolide
Rhinocort Aqua budesonide 233
Rhinocort Turbuhaler budesonide 233
Rhodis ketoprofen 354
Rhoprolene betamethasone 227
Rhoprosone betamethasone 227
Rhotral acebutolol 198
Rhotrimine trimipramine 508

RIBAVIRIN – SODIUM THIOSULFATE

R   **ribavirin** a drug used in the prevention and treatment of certain viral infections. See Antiviral drugs 145

riboflavin 525

Ridaura auranofin 216

rifabutin an antibacterial agent 143

Rifadin rifampin 459

rifampicin see rifampin 459

rifampin 459

Rimactane rifampin 459

Rimso-50 dimethyl sulfoxide

Riopan magaldrate

Riopan Extra Strength magaldrate

Riopan Plus magaldrate and simethicone

Riopan Plus Extra Strength magaldrate and simethicone

Risperdal risperidone

risperidone an antipsychotic agent

Ritalin *39B* (illus.); methylphenidate 385

Ritalin SR methylphenidate 385

ritodrine 460

Rivotril *36T, 42P* (illus.); clonazepam 265

Robaxacet methocarbamol (380) and acetaminophen (199)

Robaxacet-8 methocarbamol (380), acetaminophen (199), and codeine (270)

Robaxin methocarbamol 380

Robaxisal ASA (200) and methocarbamol (380)

Robaxisal-C 1/8 ASA (200), methocarbamol (380), and codeine (270)

Robaxisal-C 1/4 ASA (200), methocarbamol (380), and codeine (270)

Robaxisal-C 1/2 ASA (200), methocarbamol (380), and codeine (270)

Robidone hydrocodone 337

Robidrine pseudoephedrine 450

Robinul glycopyrrolate

Robinul Forte glycopyrrolate

Robitussin guaifenesin 331

Robitussin A-C guaifenesin (331), pheniramine, and codeine (270)

Robitussin CF guaifenesin (331), dextromethorphan (281), and phenylpropanolamine

Robitussin DM dextromethorphan (281) and guaifenesin (331)

Robitussin PE guaifenesin (331) and pseudoephedrine (450)

Robitussin with Codeine guaifenesin (331), pheniramine, and codeine (270)

Rocaltrol calcitriol 529

R.O. Carpine pilocarpine 433

Rocephin ceftriaxone

R.O.-Dexsone dexamethasone 280

R.O.-Dry Eyes polyvinyl alcohol

R.O.-Eye Drops tetrahydrozoline

Rofact rifampin 459

Roferon-A interferon 347

Rogaine minoxidil 392

R.O.-Gentycln gentamicin

Rogitine phentolamine

R.O.-Naphz naphazoline

R   **Roniacol** nicotinyl alcohol tartrate

R.O.-Parcaine proparacaine

R.O.-Predphate Forte prednisolone 456

R.O.-Tropamide tropicamide

Roubac sulfamethoxazole (474) and trimethoprim (507)

Rovamycine spiramycin

Roxicet acetaminophen (199) and oxycodone (419

Roychlor potassium chloride 524

Royflex triethanolamine salicylate

Rubramin cyanocobalamin

Rynacrom cromolyn sodium 274

Rythmodan disopyramide 293

Rythmodan-LA disopyramide 293

Rythmol propafenone

S

Sabril vigabatrin

Salac salicylic acid cleanser

Salazopyrin sulfasalazine 475

salazosulfapyridine see sulfasalazine 475

salbutamol 461

salcatonin a drug for bone disorders 134

salicylamide a non-narcotic analgesic similar to ASA 200

salicylic acid a keratolytic drug applied *topically* to treat acne (189), dandruff (191), psoriasis (190) and warts

salicylazosulfapyridine see sulfasalazine 475

salicylsalicylic acid see salsalate

Saline from Otrivin sodium chloride

Salinex sodium chloride

Salinol polyethylene glycol and propylene glycol

salmeterol 462

Salofalk mesalamine 378

salsalate a non-steroidal anti-inflammatory drug 128

Sandimmune cyclosporine 277

Sandomigran pizotyline

Sandomigran DS pizotyline

Sanorex mazindol

Sans-Acne erythromycin (302) and ethyl alcohol

Sansert methysergide

Santyl collagenase

Sarna HC hydrocortisone 338

Sarna-P pramoxine, menthol, and camphor

SAS-500 sulfasalazine 475

Sastid salicylic acid and sulfur

Savlodil cetrimide and chlorhexidine

Savlon Hospital Concentrate chlorhexidine and cetrimide

Scabene esdepallethrin and piperonyl butoxide

Schamberg's Lotion zinc oxide, phenol, and menthol. See Antipruritic medications 185

scopolamine 463

Sebcur salicylic acid

Sebcur/T salicylic acid and coal tar

Sebulex salicylic acid and sulfur

Sebulon an antidandruff shampoo containing zinc pyrithione

Sebutone a shampoo containing coal tar, salicylic acid, and sulfur

Secaris propylene glycol and polyethylene glycol

secobarbital a barbiturate sleeping drug

Seconal secobarbital

Sectral *39D, 43N* (illus.); acebutolol 198

Selax docusate sodium

Seldane terfenadine 487

selegiline 464

selenium 526

selenium sulfide an agent included in antidandruff shampoos and applied to the skin for the treatment of tinea versicolor. See Treatment for dandruff and hair loss 191

Selexid pivmecillinam

Selsun selenium sulfide

semustine an alkylating agent. See Anticancer drugs 166

senna a stimulant laxative. See Laxatives 123

Senokot *40O* (illus.); senna

Senokot/S senna and docusate sodium

Septra sulfamethoxazole (474) and trimethoprim (507)

Septra DS *44E* (illus.); sulfamethoxazole (474) and trimethoprim (507)

Ser-Ap-Es hydralazine (335), hydrochlorothiazide (336), and reserpine

Serax oxazepam 417

Serc betahistine

Serentil mesoridazine

Serevent salmeterol

Seromycin cycloserine

Serophene clomiphene 263

Serpasil reserpine

Serpasil-Esidrix hydrochlorothiazide (336) and reserpine

sertraline 465

Serzone nefazodone

sevin see carbaryl

Shepard's Skin Cream an oil-in-water emulsion. See Bases for skin preparations 187

Sialor anetholtrithione

Sibelium flunarizine

silicone a water-repellent substance used in barrier creams

Silon zinc oxide and dimethicone

silver nitrate a *topical* antibacterial drug. See Anti-infective skin preparations 187

silver sulfadiazine 466

simethicone a silicone-based substance included as an antifoaming agent in many medications for the relief of excess gas and indigestion. See Types of antacids 120

S

simvastatin 467

Sinemet levodopa (358) and carbidopa

Sinemet CR levodopa (358) and carbidopa

Sinequan doxepin 296

Sintrom nicoumalone

Sinutab N.D. Daytime Formula acetaminophen (199) and pseudoephedrine (450)

Sinutab Nighttime Formula acetaminophen (199), chlorpheniramine (251), and pseudoephedrine (450)

Sinutab No Drowsiness acetaminophen (199) and pseudoephedrine (450)

Sinutab Regular acetaminophen (199), chlorpheniramine (251), and pseudoephedrine (450)

Sinutab SA acetaminophen (199), phenylpropanolamine, and phenyltoloxamine

Sinutab with Codeine acetaminophen (199), chlorpheniramine (251), pseudoephedrine (450), and codeine (270)

642 Tablets propoxyphene 447

692 Tablets propoxyphene (447), ASA (200), and caffeine

Sleep-Eze D diphenhydramine 290

Sleep-Eze D Extra Strength diphenhydramine 290

Slim Mint benzocaine (223) and methylcellulose

Slo-Bid theophylline 490

Slow-Fe ferrous sulfate 522

Slow-Fe-Folic ferrous sulfate (522) and folic acid (521)

Slow-K *40H* (illus.); potassium chloride 524

Slow-Trasicor oxprenolol

sodium common (table) salt. See Sodium 526

sodium ascorbate a form of vitamin C 528

sodium bicarbonate an antacid 120

sodium biphosphate a drug used to reduce high calcium levels in the blood, as a laxative, and to increase acidity of the urine. See Laxatives (123) and Drugs used for urinary disorders (178)

sodium borate a substance with weak *astringent* and antibacterial properties often included in mouthwashes and gargles

sodium cellulose phosphate an agent used for reducing abnormally high levels of calcium in the blood

sodium chloride common salt

sodium citrate an antacid. See Antacids 120

sodium cromoglycate see cromolyn sodium

sodium fluoride see fluoride 521

sodium hypochlorite a drug used *topically* as an *antiseptic* and as a disinfectant

sodium iodide a form of iodine used to treat thyrotoxicosis (156) and thyroid cancers

sodium nitrite an injectable antidote to cyanide poisoning

sodium nitroprusside a vasodilator 110

sodium salicylate a drug similar to ASA used to treat arthritic disorders. See Non-steroidal anti-inflammatory drugs 128

Sodium Sulamyd sulfacetamide 473

sodium thiosulfate a drug used *topically* to treat tinea infection of the skin, and given intravenously to treat cyanide poisoning

S

Soflax *46A* (illus.); docusate sodium
Sofracort framycetin, dexamethasone (280) and gramicidin
Soframycin Eye Drops/Ointment framycetin
Soframycin Nasal Spray framycetin, gramicidin, and phenylephrine (431)
Soframycin Ointment framycetin and gramicidin
Sofra-Tulle framycetin
Solaquin hydroquinone
Solaquin Forte hydroquinone
Solium chlordiazepoxide 250
Solu-Cortef hydrocortisone 338
Solugel benzoyl peroxide 224
Solu-Medrol methylprednisolone 386
Soluver salicylic acid
Soma carisoprodol
somatrem growth hormone
somatropin growth hormone
Somnol flurazepam 320
Somophyllin-12 theophylline 490
Sonacide glutaral
Sopamycetin chloramphenicol 249
Sopamycetin-HC chloramphenicol (249) and hydrocortisone (338)
Soriatene acritretin
Sotacor *390* (illus.); sotalol 468
sotalol 468
spectinomycin an antibiotic used to treat gonorrhea. See Antibiotics 140
Spectro Gram "2" chlorhexidine
Spectro Tar Antiseptic Shampoo chlorhexidine and coal tar
Spectro Tar Skin Wash coal tar
Spersacarpine pilocarpine 433
Spersadex dexamethasone 280
spiramycin an antibiotic 140
spironolactone 469
Sporanox itraconazole
SSD silver sulfadiazine 466
Stadol NS butorphanol 236
Statex morphine 395
Staticin erythromycin 302
Stelabid trifluoperazine (504) and isopropamide
Stelazine trifluoperazine 504
Stemetil prochlorperazine 444
Steri/Sol hexetidine
stibocaptate a drug used to eradicate blood fluke infections. See Anthelmintic drugs 151
stibogluconate a drug used to treat leishmaniasis. See Antiprotozoal drugs 148
StieVA-A tretinoin 500
Stievamycin erythromycin (302) and tretinoin (500)
stilboestrol see diethylstilbestrol
Streptase streptokinase 470
streptokinase 470
streptomycin 471
streptozocin a *cytotoxic* antibiotic. See Anticancer drugs 166
Stresstabs with Iron a multivitamin and mineral preparation. See Vitamins 161
Sublimaze fentanyl

S

Sucaryl cyclamate
succinylcholine a muscle-relaxant drug 132
sucralfate 472
Sucrets hexylresorcinol
Sudafed pseudoephedrine 450
Sudafed Cough and Cold Extra Strength pseudoephedrine (450), dextromethorphan (281), and acetaminophen (199)
Sudafed DM dextromethorphan (281) and pseudoephedrine (450)
Sudafed Expectorant guaifenesin (331) and pseudoephedrine (450)
Sudafed Sinus Extra Strength pseudoephedrine (450) and acetaminophen (199)
Sufenta sufentanil
sufentanil a narcotic analgesic 97
Sulcrate *45A* (illus.); sucralfate 472
Sulcrate Suspension Plus sucralfate 472
sulfabenzamide an antibacterial drug 143
sulfacetamide 473
Sulfacet-R sulfacetamide (473) and sulfur
sulfacytine a sulfonamide antibacterial agent (143) used to treat urinary tract infection
sulfadiazine a sulfonamide antibacterial drug 143
sulfadoxine a drug used in combination with pyrimethamine (454) in the prevention and treatment of malaria. See Antimalarial drugs 149
sulfaguanidine a sulfonamide antibacterial drug 14?
sulfamerazine a sulfonamide antibacterial drug 143
sulfamethazine a sulfonamide antibacterial drug 14?
sulfamethoxazole 474
sulfanilamide a sulfonamide antibacterial drug 143
sulfapyridine a sulfonamide antibacterial drug 143
sulfasalazine 475
sulfathiazole a sulfonamide antibacterial drug 143
Sulfex 10% sulfacetamide 473
sulfinpyrazone 476
sulfisoxazole 477
Sulfoxyl benzoyl peroxide (224) and sulfur
sulfur a *topical* antibacterial and antifungal agent used in preparations for acne (189) and dandruff (191)
sulindac 478
Sultrin sulfacetamide (473), sulfabenzamide, sulfathiazole, and urea
sumatriptan 479
Supeudol oxycodone 419
Suplevit a multivitamin and mineral preparation. See Vitamins 161
Supracaine tetracaine
Suprax cefixime 242
Suprefact buserelin
Supres methyldopa (384) and chlorothiazide
suramin an antiprotozoal (148) and anthelmintic drug (151)
Surbex-500 a multivitamin preparation. See Vitamins 161
Surbex-500 Plus Iron a multivitamin preparation plus iron 522. See Vitamins 161
Surbex-500 Plus Zinc a multivitamin preparation plus zinc 530. See Vitamins 161

Surfak docusate calcium
Surgam tiaprofenic acid 492
Surgam SR *41H* (illus.); tiaprofenic acid 492
Surmontil trimipramine 508
sutilains an enzyme compound used to heal skin ulcers and burns
suxamethonium see succinylcholine
Swiss One a multivitamin preparation plus minerals. See Vitamins 161
Symmetrel amantadine 205
Synacthen-Depot cosyntropin
Synalar fluocinolone 316
Synalar Bi-Otic fluocinolone (316), neomycin (402), and polymyxin B
Synamol fluocinolone 316
Synarel nafarelin
Syn-Captopril captopril 239
Syn-Diltiazem diltiazem 287
Synflex naproxen sodium
Syn-Flunisolide flunisolide 315
Syn-Nadolol nadolol 398
Synphasic an oral contraceptive containing ethinyl estradiol (306) and norethindrone
Syn-Pindolol pindolol 434
Synthroid *38E, 39M, 39P, 40L, 43A* (illus.); levothyroxine 359

T

217 Tablets ASA (200) and caffeine
217 Strong Tablets ASA (200) and caffeine
222 AF acetaminophen 199
222 Forte Tablets ASA (200), codeine (270), and caffeine
222 Tablets ASA (200), codeine (270), and caffeine
282 MEP ASA (200), caffeine, codeine (270), and meprobamate (377)
282 Tablets ASA (200), codeine (270), and caffeine
292 Tablets ASA (200), codeine (270), and caffeine
Tagamet cimetidine 257
talampicillin a penicillin antibiotic 140
Talwin pentazocine
Tambocor flecainide
Tamofen tamoxifen 480
Tamone tamoxifen 480
tamoxifen 480
Tanacet 125 feverfew
tannic acid an astringent
Tantaphen acetaminophen 199
Tantum benzydamine 226
Tapazole methimazole
Tardan salicylic acid and coal tar
Targel coal tar
Taro-Sone betamethasone 227

T

Tavist clemastine
Taxol paclitaxel
Tazidime ceftazidime
tazobactam a substance that increases the effectiveness of piperacillin
Tazocin piperacillin and tazobactam
Teardrops polyvinyl alcohol and povidone
Tears Naturale hydroxypropylmethylcellulose and dextran 70
Tears Plus polyvinyl alcohol and povidone
Tebrazid pyrazinamide
Tecnal ASA (200), caffeine, and butalbital
Tecnal C ASA (200), caffeine, codeine (270), and butalbital
Tedral phenobarbital (430), ephedrine, and theophylline (490)
Teejel choline salicylate
tegafur an antimetabolite anticancer drug 166
Tegison etretinate 308
Tegopen cloxacillin 269
Tegretol carbamazepine 240
Tegretol CR *40I* (illus.); carbamazepine 240
temazepam 481
Temposil calcium carbimide
Tempra acetaminophen 199
teniposide an anticancer drug 166
Tenoretic atenolol (215) and chlorthalidone (254)
Tenormin *42J* (illus.); atenolol 215
tenoxicam 482
Tensilon edrophonium chloride
Tenuate diethylpropion
Terazol terconazole 486
terazosin 483
terbinafine 484
terbutaline 485
terconazole 486
terfenadine 487
terpin hydrate an *expectorant*. See Drugs to treat coughs 106
Tersac triclosan and salicylic acid
Tersaseptic triclosan
Tersa-Tar coal tar
Tersa-Tar Mild coal tar
testosterone 488
tetrabenazene an *investigational* drug for the treatment of movement disorders
tetracaine a local *anesthetic*
tetrachloroethylene a drug used to treat hookworm infestations. See Anthelmintic drugs 151
tetracycline 489
Tetracyn tetracycline 489
tetrahydrozoline a decongestant used in nose drops and eye drops. See Decongestants 105
Texacort hydrocortisone 338
T/Gel coal tar
Theochron theophylline 490
Theo-Dur *44L, 45K* (illus.); theophylline 490
Theolair theophylline 490
Theolair-SR theophylline 490
theophylline/aminophylline 490
Theo-SR theophylline 490

THIABENDAZOLE – URSOFALK

T

thiabendazole an anthelmintic. See Anthelmintics 151

thiamine 527

thiamylal a barbiturate used in general *anesthesia*

thiethylperazine an anti-emetic drug 102

thimerosal a mercury compound with antimicrobial and *antiseptic* properties. See Anti-infective skin preparations 187

thioguanine an anticancer drug 167

thiopental a fast-acting barbiturate used to induce general *anesthesia*

thioproperazine an antipsychotic drug 97

thioridazine 491

thiotepa an alkylating agent. See Anticancer drugs 166

thiothixene an antipsychotic drug 97

thymoxamine a *miotic* drug used in the treatment of glaucoma. See Drugs for glaucoma 180

Thyro-Block potassium iodide

tiaprofenic acid 492

Ticar ticarcillin

ticarcillin a penicillin antibiotic used for septicemia and skin, genitourinary, and respiratory infections. See Antibiotics 140

Ticlid *44K* (illus.); ticlopidine 493

ticlopidine 493

Tilade nedocromil 401

Timentin ticarcillin and potassium clavulanate

Timolide hydrochlorothiazide (336) and timolol (494)

timolol 494

Timoptic timolol 494

Timpilo timolol (494) and pilocarpine (433)

Tinactin tolnaftate 498

tinidazole an antiprotozoal drug 148

tioconazole an antifungal drug. See Antifungal drugs 150

tissue plasminogen activator 495

tixocortol a drug used in the treatment of inflammatory bowel disease 124

tobramycin 496

Tobradex tobramycin (496) and dexamethasone (280)

Tobrex Ophthalmic tobramycin 496

tocainide an anti-arrhythmic drug 128

tocopherol see vitamin E 529

tocopheryl acetate a vitamin E drug. See vitamin E 529

Today Sponge nonoxynol-9

Toesen oxytocin 421

Tofranil imipramine 343

tolazoline a peripheral vasodilator 110

tolbutamide 497

Tolectin tolmetin

tolmetin a non-steroidal anti-inflammatory drug 128

tolnaftate 498

Tonocard tocainide

Topicaine benzocaine 223

Topicort desoximetasone

Topilene betamethasone 227

Topisone betamethasone 227

Topsyn fluocinonide

T

Toradol *42K* (illus.); ketorolac 355

Torecan thiethylperazine

Tracrium atracurium

Trandate labetalol

tranexamic acid an antifibrinolytic agent used to promote blood clotting 117

Transderm-Nitro nitroglycerin 408

Transderm-V scopolamine 463

Trans-Plantar salicylic acid

Trans•Ver•Sal salicylic acid

Tranxene clorazepate 267

Trasicor oxprenolol

Trasylol aprotinin

Travase sutilains

Travel Aid dimenhydrinate 288

Travel Tabs dimenhydrinate 288

trazodone 499

Trental *35C* (illus.); pentoxifylline 426

tretinoin 500

Triacomb triamcinolone (501), nystatin (412), neomycin (402), and gramicidin

Triadapin doxepin 296

Triaderm triamcinolone 501

Triamacort triamcinolone 501

triamcinolone 501

Triaminic-DM Expectorant dextromethorphan (28 guaifenesin (331), phenylpropanolamine, pheniramine, and pyrilamine

Triaminic-DM Nighttime dextromethorphan (281) chlorpheniramine (251), and pseudoephedrine (450)

Triaminic Expectorant guaifenesin (331), phenylpropanolamine, pyrilamine, and phenirami

Triaminic Expectorant DH hydrocodone (337), pheniramine, guaifenesin (331), phenylpropanolamine, and pyrilamine

Triaminicin pheniramine, pyrilamine, phenylpropanolamine, caffeine, and acetaminop (199)

Triaminicol DM dextromethorphan (281), phenylpropanolamine, pyrilamine, and pheniramine

Triaminic Tablets pheniramine, pyrilamine, and phenylpropanolamine

triamterene 502

Triavil amitriptyline (208), and perphenazine (428)

triazolam 503

trichloroacetic acid a *topical* preparation used to treat warts

triclocarban an antimicrobial agent with antibacterial and antifungal actions used in bar soap. See Anti-infective skin preparations 187

triclosan an antimicrobial agent used in bar soap and wound-cleansing products. See Anti-infecti skin preparations 187

Tri-Cyclen an oral contraceptive containing norgestimate and ethinyl estradiol (306)

Tridesilon desonide

Tridil nitroglycerin 408

trientine a *chelating* agent used to remove exces copper in Wilson's disease

T

triethanolamine salicylate a *topical* analgesic
triethylenetetramine see trientine
trifluoperazine 504
trifluridine an ophthalmic antiviral agent
trihexyphenidyl 505
Trikacide metronidazole 389
Trilafon perphenazine 428
Trilisate choline magnesium trisalicylate
trilostane a synthetic corticosteroid given to treat Cushing's syndrome. See Corticosteroids 153
trimazosin an antihypertensive drug 114
trimebutine 506
trimeprazine an antihistamine 136
trimethaphan a drug given to reduce blood pressure in an emergency. See Antihypertensive drugs 114
trimethoprim 507
trimipramine 508
Trinalin azatadine (217) and pseudoephedrine (450)
Trinsicon a multivitamin and iron preparation. See Vitamins 161
trioxsalen a psoralen drug used in PUVA treatment of psoriasis 190
tripelennamine an antihistamine 136
Triphasil an oral contraceptive containing ethinyl estradiol (306) and levonorgestrel
triprolidine an antihistamine 136
Triptil protriptyline
Triquilar an oral contraceptive containing ethinyl estradiol (306) and levonorgestrel
Trisoralen trioxsalen
Trisulfaminic pheniramine, pyrilamine, phenylpropanolamine, sulfadiazine, sulfamerazine, and sulfamethazine
Trisyn fluocinonide, procinonide, and ciprocinonide
Tri-Vi-Flor vitamins A, D, C, and fluoride (521). See Vitamins 161
Tri-Vi-Sol vitamins A, D, and C. See Vitamins 161
Tri-Vi-Sol with Fluoride vitamins A, D, C, and fluoride (521). See Vitamins 161
Trobicin spectinomycin
tropicamide a *mydriatic* drug. See Drugs affecting the pupil 182
Trosyd AF tioconazole
trypsin an *enzyme* formed in the intestine that is administered as a drug in the treatment of indigestion
Tryptan tryptophan
tryptophan a non-benzodiazepine, non-barbiturate drug with effects and risks similar to those of the barbiturates. See Sleeping drugs 94
T-Stat erythromycin (302) and ethyl alcohol
Tubarine tubocurarine
tubocurarine a drug used to relax muscles in general *anesthesia* 132
Tuinal secobarbital and amobarbital
Tums calcium carbonate
Tussaminic C codeine (270), phenylpropanolamine, pyrilamine, and pheniramine

Tussaminic DH hydrocodone (337), phenylpropanolamine, pyrilamine, and pheniramine
Tussionex hydrocodone (337) and phenyltoloxamine
222 AF acetaminophen 199
Tylenol acetaminophen 199
Tylenol Allergy Sinus Medication acetaminophen (199), pseudoephedrine (450), and chlorpheniramine (251)
Tylenol Cold Medication acetaminophen (199), dextromethorphan (281), chlorpheniramine (251), and pseudoephedrine (450)
Tylenol Sinus Medication acetaminophen (199) and pseudoephedrine (450)
Tylenol with Codeine no. 2 *41N* (illus.); acetaminophen (199), caffeine, and codeine (270)
Tylenol with Codeine no. 3 *41I* (illus.); acetaminophen (199), caffeine, and codeine (270)

U

Ulone chlophedianol
Ultradol etodolac
Ultra Mide 25 urea
UltraMOP methoxsalen 383
Ultraquin hydroquinone
Ultravate halobetasol
undecylenic acid an antifungal agent effective in tidea pedis (athlete's foot). See Antifungal drugs 150
Unipen nafcillin
Uniphyl theophylline 490
Univol magnesium hydroxide (370) and aluminum hydroxide (204)
urea a natural breakdown product of proteins excreted in the urine. It is included in skin preparations for the treatment of dry, scaling skin conditions
Urecholine bethanechol
Uremol urea
Uremol-HC hydrocortisone (338) and urea
Urisec urea
urofollitropin a drug to aid in the induction of ovulation. See Drugs for infertility 176
Uromitexan mesna
Urispas flavoxate
urokinase a thrombolytic drug. See Drugs that affect blood clotting 116
ursodeoxycholic acid see ursodiol
ursodiol 509
Ursofalk ursodiol 509

VALISONE – ZYLOPRIM

V

Valisone betamethasone 227
Valisone-G betamethasone (227) and gentamicin (328)
Valium diazepam 282
valproic acid 510
Vancenase beclomethasone 222
Vanceril beclomethasone 222
Vancocin vancomycin
vancomycin an antibiotic used mainly to prevent or treat endocarditis and other serious infections. See Antibiotics 140
Vanoxide-HC benzoyl peroxide (224) and hydrocortisone (338)
Vanquin pyrvinium
Vaponefrin epinephrine 300
Vaseline Petroleum Jelly a water-in-oil emulsion used to protect and lubricate dry skin
Vaseretic enalapril (299) and hydrochlorothiazide (336)
Vasocidin prednisolone (439) and sulfacetamide (473)
Vasocon naphazoline
Vasocon-A naphazoline and antazoline
vasopressin 511
Vasosulf sulfacetamide (473) and phenylephrine (431)
Vasotec *37S, 40C, 44B* (illus.); enalapril 299
Vasoxyl methoxamine
V-Cillin K penicillin V 425
vecuronium a muscle-relaxant drug 132
Velbe vinblastine
Velosulin insulin 346
Velvelan urea
venlafaxine 512
Ventodisk salbutamol 461
Ventolin salbutamol 461
Ventolin Rotacaps salbutamol 461
Vepesid etoposide
verapamil 513
Vermox mebendazole 372
Versed midazolam
Versel selenium sulfide
Viaderm-K.C. triamcinolone (501), neomycin (402), nystatin (412), and gramicidin
Vibramycin doxycycline 297
Vibra-Tabs doxycycline 297
Vicks Vaporub camphor, menthol, and eucalyptus oil
vidarabine a drug applied *topically* and administered *systemically* to treat viral infections. See Antiviral drugs 161
Videx didanosine 284
vigabatrin an anticonvulsant drug 98
viloxazine a nervous system stimulant 100
vinblastine an anticancer drug 166
vincristine an anticancer drug 166
vindesine an anticancer drug 166

V

Vioform clioquinol
Vioform-Hydrocortisone hydrocortisone (338) and clioquinol
Viokase pancrelipase
viprynium see pyrvinium
Vira-A vidarabine
Virazole ribavirin
Viroptic trifluridine
Viskazide pindolol (434) and hydrochlorothiazide (336)
Visken pindolol 434
Vitaday Forte a multivitamin and mineral preparation. See Vitamins 161
vitamin A 527
Vitamin A Acid tretinoin 500
vitamin B$_1$ see thiamine 527
vitamin B$_2$ see riboflavin 525
vitamin B$_6$ see pyridoxine 525
vitamin B$_{12}$ 528
vitamin C 528
vitamin D 529
vitamin E 529
vitamin K 530
Vivol diazepam 282
Volmax salbutamol 461
Voltaren diclofenac 283
Voltaren Ophtha diclofenac 283
Voltaren Rapide diclofenac 283
Voltaren SR *35N, 35S* (illus.); diclofenac 283
Vosol HC hydrocortisone (338), benzethonium chloride, and acetic acid
Vumon teniposide

W

warfarin 514
Warfilone warfarin 514
Wellferon interferon 347
Westcort hydrocortisone 338
Wigraine ergotamine (301), caffeine, and belladon
Winpred prednisone 440
witch hazel a soothing, mildly *astringent* agent us to alleviate irritation in genital and rectal areas
Wycillin penicillin G 424
Wydase hyaluronidase

X

Xanax *36O*, *44M* (illus.); alprazolam 203
xanthinol niacinate a lipid-lowering agent
X-Prep senna
X-Seb salicylic acid shampoo
X-Seb Plus salicylic acid and zinc pyrithione shampoo
X-Seb T salicylic acid and coal tar shampoo
X-Seb T Plus salicylic acid, coal tar, and menthol shampoo
Xylocaine lidocaine 360
Xylocaine Test Dose xylocaine (360) and epinephrine (300)
Xylocard lidocaine 360
xylometazoline 515

Y

Yocon yohimbine
yohimbine an antihypertensive drug 114
Yutopar ritodrine 460

Z

Zaditen ketotifen
zalcitabine a drug used in the treatment of HIV-infected patients
Zanosar streptozocin
Zantac *41R* (illus.); ranitidine 458
Zarontin ethosuximide
Zaroxolyn metolazone
Zephiran benzalkonium chloride
Zestoretic lisinopril (363) and hydrochlorothiazide (336)
Zestril *35O*, *35P* (illus.); lisinopril 363
Zetar coal tar
zidovudine 516
Zilactin tannic acid
Zinacef cefuroxime 244
Zinaderm zinc oxide
zinc 530
zinc chloride an astringent
Zincfrin phenylephrine (431) and zinc sulfate

Zincfrin-A naphazoline, antazoline, and zinc sulfate
zinc gluconate see zinc 530
Zincofax zinc oxide
zinc oxide an agent included in sunscreens (191) and in skin preparations for painful and itchy conditions such as ulcers, blisters, diaper rash, and hemorrhoids
zinc pyrithione an antimicrobial agent with antifungal and antibacterial properties that is used in the treatment of dandruff. See Treatment for dandruff and hair loss 191
zinc sulfate a mild *astringent* used in zinc supplement preparations 530
Zithromax azithromycin
ZNP zinc pyrithione
Zocor *36A* (illus.); simvastatin 467
Zofran ondansetron 414
Zoladex goserelin
Zoloft *46B*, *47T* (illus.); sertraline 465
zopiclone 517
Zostrix capsaicin 238
Zostrix H.P. capsaicin 238
Zovirax acyclovir 201
Z-Plus zinc pyrithione and menthol shampoo
Zyloprim allopurinol 202

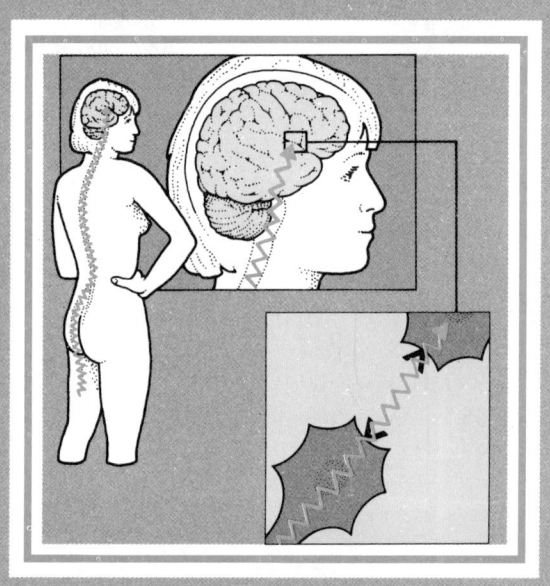

3

MAJOR DRUG GROUPS

BRAIN AND NERVOUS SYSTEM
RESPIRATORY SYSTEM
HEART AND CIRCULATION
GASTROINTESTINAL TRACT
MUSCLES, BONES, AND JOINTS
ALLERGY
INFECTIONS AND INFESTATIONS
HORMONES AND ENDOCRINE SYSTEM
NUTRITION
MALIGNANT AND IMMUNE DISEASE
REPRODUCTIVE AND URINARY TRACTS
EYES AND EARS
SKIN

BRAIN AND NERVOUS SYSTEM

Relying on billions of nerve cells (neurons), the brain is the supervisory center of the nervous system. Receiving electrochemical impulses from everywhere in the body, interpreting them and sending responsive signals back to various glands and muscles, the brain functions continuously as a switchboard for the human communications system. At the same time, it serves as the seat of emotions and mood, of memory, personality, behavior and thought. Extending from the brain is an additional cluster of nerve cells that forms the spinal cord. Together, these two elements compose the central nervous system.

Radiating from the central nervous system is the peripheral nervous system, which has three parts. One branches off the spinal cord and extends to muscles throughout the body. Another, in the head, links the brain to the eyes, ears, nose, and taste buds. The third is a semi-independent network called the autonomic, or involuntary, nervous system. This is the part of the nervous system that controls unconscious body functions such as breathing, digestion, and glandular activity (see facing page).

Signals traverse the nervous system by electrical and chemical means. Electrical impulses carry signals from one end of a neuron to the other. To cross the gap between neurons, chemical *neurotransmitters* are released from one cell to bind on to the *receptor* sites of nearby cells. *Excitatory* transmitters stimulate action; *inhibitory* transmitters reduce it.

What can go wrong

Disorders of the brain and nervous system can manifest themselves as illnesses with predominant physical impairments (for example: epilepsy, strokes) or as illnesses with predominant mental and emotional impairments (for example: schizophrenia or depression).

These illnesses can result from different types of disorders of the brain and nervous system. Death of neurons resulting from poor circulation can be the cause of paralysis; electrical disturbances of certain brain neurons produce the seizures of epilepsy. Temporary changes to blood circulation within and around the brain are thought to be the principal cause of migraine headaches. The exact brain disorder causing mental and emotional impairments such as schizophrenia or depression is not known. Nevertheless, scientific evidence indicates that a malfunction of neurons and neurotransmitters might be implicated. For example, there might be too much or too little neurotransmitter in a brain

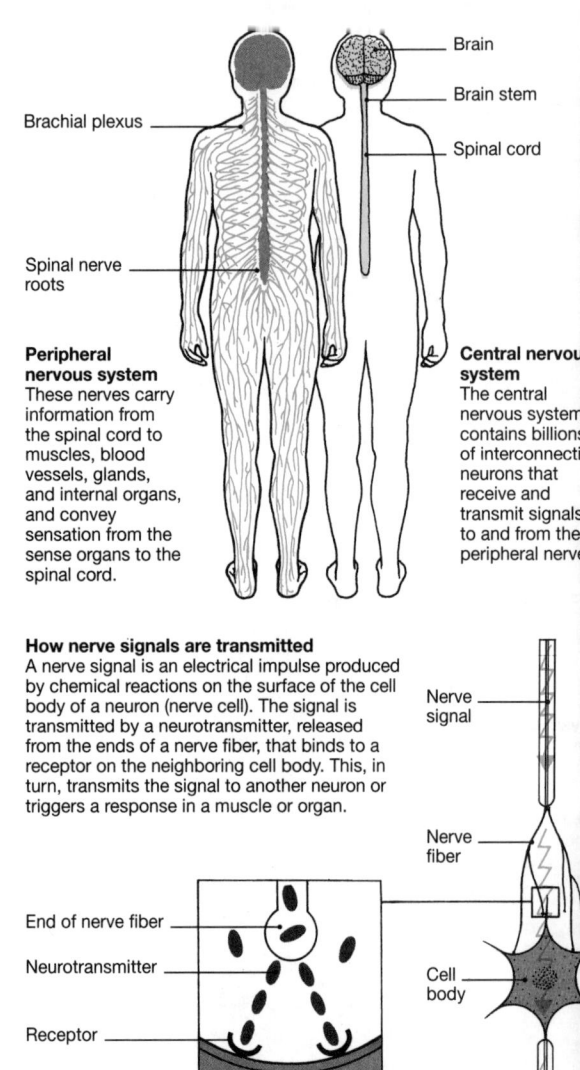

Peripheral nervous system
These nerves carry information from the spinal cord to muscles, blood vessels, glands, and internal organs, and convey sensation from the sense organs to the spinal cord.

Central nervou system
The central nervous system contains billions of interconnecti neurons that receive and transmit signals to and from the peripheral nerve.

How nerve signals are transmitted
A nerve signal is an electrical impulse produced by chemical reactions on the surface of the cell body of a neuron (nerve cell). The signal is transmitted by a neurotransmitter, released from the ends of a nerve fiber, that binds to a receptor on the neighboring cell body. This, in turn, transmits the signal to another neuron or triggers a response in a muscle or organ.

region or the neurons might be underactive, overactive, or poorly coordinated.

Why drugs are used

By and large, the drugs described in this section correct or modify the communication of the signal that traverse the nervous system. By doing so the can relieve symptoms or restore normal functioning and behavior. In some cases, such as anxiety and insomnia, drugs encourage the action of inhibitory neurotransmitters, lowering the level

AUTONOMIC NERVOUS SYSTEM

The autonomic, or involuntary, nervous system governs the actions of the muscles, of the organs, and glands. Such vital functions as heartbeat, salivation, and digestion continue without conscious direction, whether we are awake or asleep.

The autonomic system is divided into two parts, the effects of one generally balancing those of the other. The *sympathetic* nervous system has an *excitatory* effect. It widens the airways to the lungs, for example, and increases the flow of blood to the arms and legs. The *parasympathetic* system, by contrast, has an opposing effect. It slows the heart rate and stimulates the flow of the digestive juices.

Although the functional pace of most organs results from the interplay between the two systems, the muscles surrounding the blood vessels respond only to the signals of the sympathetic system. What decides between the constriction or dilation of the vessels is the relative stimulation of two sets of receptor sites: alpha sites and beta sites.

Neurotransmitters

The parasympathetic nervous system depends on the neurotransmitter acetylcholine to transmit signals from one cell to another. The sympathetic nervous system relies on epinephrine and norepinephrine, products of the adrenal glands that act as both hormones and neurotransmitters.

Drugs that act on the sympathetic nervous system

Drugs that stimulate the sympathetic nervous system are called adrenergics (or sympathomimetics, see chart). They either promote the release of epinephrine and norepinephrine or mimic their effects. Drugs which interfere with the action of the sympathetic nervous system are called sympatholytics. Alpha blockers act on alpha receptors; beta blockers act on beta receptors (see also Beta blockers, p.109).

Drugs that act on the parasympathetic nervous system

Drugs that stimulate the parasympathetic nervous system are called cholinergics (or parasympathomimetics), and drugs which oppose its action are called anticholinergics. Many drugs prescribed medically have anticholinergic properties (see chart, right).

Effects of stimulation of the autonomic nervous system

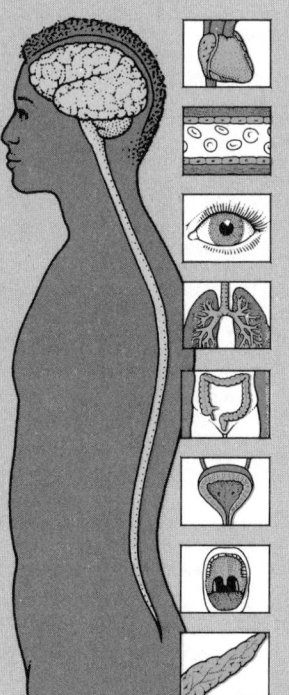

	Sympathetic	Parasympathetic
Heart	The rate and strength of the heartbeat are increased.	The rate and strength of the heartbeat are reduced.
Blood vessels in skin	These are constricted by stimulation of alpha receptors.	No effect.
Pupils	The pupils are dilated.	The pupils are constricted.
Airways	The bronchial muscles relax and widen the airways.	The bronchial muscles contract and narrow the airways.
Intestines	Activity of the muscles of the intestinal wall is reduced.	Activity of the muscles of the intestinal wall is increased.
Bladder	The bladder wall relaxes and the sphincter muscle contracts.	The bladder wall contracts and the sphincter muscle relaxes.
Salivary glands	Secretion of thick saliva increases.	Secretion of watery saliva increases.
Pancreas	Insulin secretion increases (beta receptors) or reduces (alpha receptors).	Insulin secretion is increased.

Drugs that act on the autonomic nervous system

	Sympathetic	Parasympathetic
Stimulated by		
Natural neurotransmitters	Epinephrine Norepinephrine	Acetylcholine
Drugs	Adrenergic drugs (including alpha agonists, beta agonists) Sympathomimetics	Cholinergic drugs Parasympathomimetics
Blocked by		
Drugs	Alpha blockers (antagonists) Beta blockers (antagonists)	Anticholinergic drugs

activity. In other disorders – depression is an example – the neurons are stimulated.

Drugs that act on the nervous system are also used for conditions that outwardly have nothing to do with nervous system disorders. Migraine headaches, for example, are often treated with drugs which cause the autonomic nervous system to send out signals constricting the dilated blood vessels that cause the migraine.

MAJOR DRUG GROUPS

Analgesics	Anticonvulsant drugs
Sleeping drugs	Antiparkinsonism drugs
Anti-anxiety drugs	Nervous system stimulants
Antidepressant drugs	Drugs used for migraine
Antipsychotic drugs	Anti-emetic drugs

ANALGESICS

Analgesics are drugs that relieve pain. For many disorders, the relief of pain is one of the most important aspects of treatment. Since pain is not a disease but a symptom, long-term relief depends on treatment of the underlying cause. For example, the pain of toothache can be relieved by drugs but can only be cured by appropriate dental treatment.

Damage to body tissue as a result of disease or injury is detected by nerve endings that transmit signals to the brain, where they are interpreted. The interpretation of these sensations can be affected by the psychological state of the individual, so that pain is worsened by anxiety and fear, for example. Often a reassuring explanation of the cause of discomfort can make pain easier to bear. Because of these psychological factors, sleeping drugs, anti-anxiety drugs, or antidepressants are sometimes prescribed in addition to, or instead of, analgesics, particularly in pain requiring many months of treatment.

Types of analgesics

Narcotics and non-narcotics are the two principal types of analgesics. Also, local anesthetics are commonly used to relieve pain (see below). Narcotics such as morphine are the most powerful analgesics but cause drowsiness. Non-narcotic drugs include ASA, acetaminophen, and non-steroidal anti-inflammatory drugs (NSAIDs) and may provide adequate pain relief without drowsiness.

Narcotics act directly on the brain and spinal cord to alter the perception of pain. They thus act like the endorphins, hormones naturally produced in the brain that stop the cell-to-cell transmission of pain sensation. Non-narcotics prevent stimulation of the nerve endings at the site of the pain.

When pain is treated under medical supervision, it is common to start with a non-narcotic, and if this provides inadequate relief, to change to a combination drug (a mixture of a mild narcotic and a non-narcotic). A strong narcotic may be used if the less powerful drugs are ineffective. More severe (e.g., post-operative) or long-lasting continuous pain may be treated by injections of narcotics.

When treating pain with an over-the-counter preparation, for example, taking ASA for a headache, you should seek medical advice if pain persists for longer than 48 hours, recurs, or is worse or different from previous pain.

Non-narcotic analgesics
ASA

Used for many years to relieve pain and reduce fever, ASA also reduces inflammation by blocking the production of chemicals such as prostaglandins that contribute to swelling and pain in inflamed tissue (see Action of analgesics, facing page). ASA is useful for the relief of headaches, toothaches, mild rheumatic pain, sore throat, and discomfort caused by feverish illnesses. Given regularly, it can also relieve the pain and inflammation of chronic rheumatoid arthritis (see Antirheumatic drugs, p.129).

ASA is often found in combination with other substances in a variety of medicines (see Cold remedies, p.106). Another use is in the treatment of some blood disorders, since an important effect of ASA is that it helps to prevent abnormal clotting of blood (see Drugs that affect blood clotting, p.116). For this reason, it is not suitable for people whose

SITES OF ACTION

Narcotic drugs (and possibly acetaminophen) act on the brain and spinal cord to reduce the perception of a painful stimulus. Non-narcotic drugs act at the site of pain to prevent the stimulation of nerve endings.

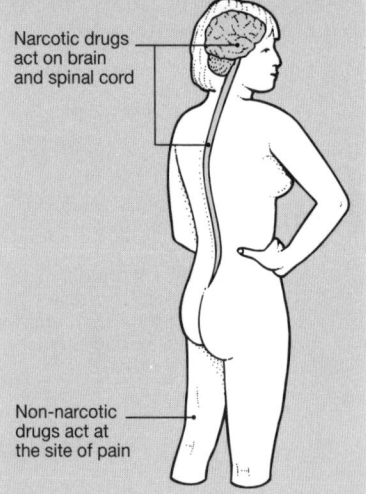

Narcotic drugs act on brain and spinal cord

Non-narcotic drugs act at the site of pain

ASA AND STOMACH IRRITATION

Regular ASA can irritate the stomach, but buffered or coated ASA preparations offer some protection against this. Buffered ASA is released in the stomach like regular ASA, but contains drugs that may reduce irritation. Coated preparations do not release ASA until in the small intestine.

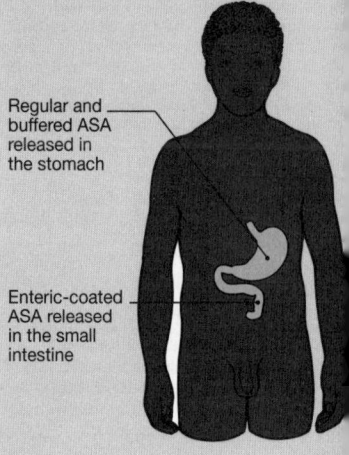

Regular and buffered ASA released in the stomach

Enteric-coated ASA released in the small intestine

blood does not clot normally.

ASA's major drawback is that it can cause irritation and even ulceration of th stomach and duodenum, possibly leadir to bleeding. For this reason it is best taken after a meal or with a full glass of water or milk. Specially formulated ASA preparations designed to avoid irritating the stomach are available, such as enteric-coated ASA. Although buffered ASA contains insufficient antacids to reduce the acidity of the stomach, some patients may experience less irritation. Enteric-coated ASA and certain special ASA capsules do not release the ASA until they have passed through the

LOCAL ANESTHETICS

These are used to prevent pain, usually in minor surgical procedures (for example, dental treatment and suturing lacerations). They can also be injected into the space around the spinal cord to numb the lower half of the body. This is called spinal or epidural anesthesia. Local anesthetics block the passage of nerve impulses at the site of administration, deadening all feeling at that site. They do not interfere with consciousness. Local anesthetics are usually given by injection, but they can also be applied to the skin to relieve pain caused by burns.

Local anesthetics occasionally cause the skin at the site of application to become red and itchy, and if high doses of the anesthetic enter the bloodstream it may cause a number of adverse effects – restlessness, nausea, anc tremors. Because such drugs may also lower blood pressure and disturb heart rhythm, they are given carefully to people with heart problems.

In order to restrict the anesthetic to the site of injection it is often given together with a vasoconstrictor drug such as epinephrine, which cuts down the blood supply at the site of injection and prevents the drug being carried away. This prolongs the action and minimizes the likelihood of side effects.

tomach and have entered the small
testine (see ASA and stomach irritation,
cing page). This delays absorption for
o to 4 hours, making it unsuitable for
eating conditions requiring prompt pain
lief. ASA in the form of soluble tablets,
ssolved in water before being taken, is
osorbed into the bloodstream quickly,
lieving pain faster than regular ASA
blets.

ASA is available in many formulations,
of which have a similar effect. But
ecause the amount of ASA in a tablet of
ch type varies, it is important to read
e packet for the correct dosage. ASA
ould not be given to children suffering
cute viral illnesses because its use has
en linked to Reye's syndrome, a
otentially fatal liver and brain disorder.

cetaminophen

his may act by reducing the production
prostaglandins in the brain. But, unlike
SA, it does not affect prostaglandin
oduction in the rest of the body and so
oes not reduce inflammation. Acetamin-
hen can be used for everyday aches
d pains, such as headaches, tooth-
he, and joint pains. It is given as a
uid for treating pain and reducing
ver in children. Acetaminophen is often
und in combination with other drugs
ch as decongestants and anti-
stamines in a variety of medicines (see
ld remedies, p.106).

It is one of the safest of all analgesics
en taken correctly. It does not usually
tate the stomach, and allergic reactions
e rare. However, an overdose can cause
vere and possibly irreversible liver dam-
e that may be fatal. For this reason it is
ed with caution for people with kidney
liver disease. Drinking large quantities
alcohol may increase its toxic potential.

on-steroidal anti-inflammatory
ugs (NSAIDs)

ese can relieve both pain and
ammation. NSAIDs are related to ASA
d also work by blocking the production
prostaglandins. They are most
mmonly used to treat muscle and joint
in and may also be prescribed for
enstrual period pain. Like ASA, NSAIDs
n irritate the stomach lining and they
e not usually given to people with
omach ulcers. For further information on
ese drugs, see p.128.

arcotic analgesics

ese are also called opioids and are rel-
ed to opium, an extract of poppy seeds.
ey act directly on several sites in the
ntral nervous system involved in pain
rception, and block the transmission of
n signals (see Action of analgesics,
ove). Because they act directly on the
rts of the brain where pain is perceived,
rcotics are the most effective analges-
and are used to treat the pain arising

ACTION OF ANALGESICS

Cause of pain
Damage to tissue (due to injury or
infection, for example) leads to
the production of mediator chemicals, which act on nerve endings
so that a signal is passed along a
series of nerve cells to the brain,
where the signal is interpreted as
pain by brain cells.

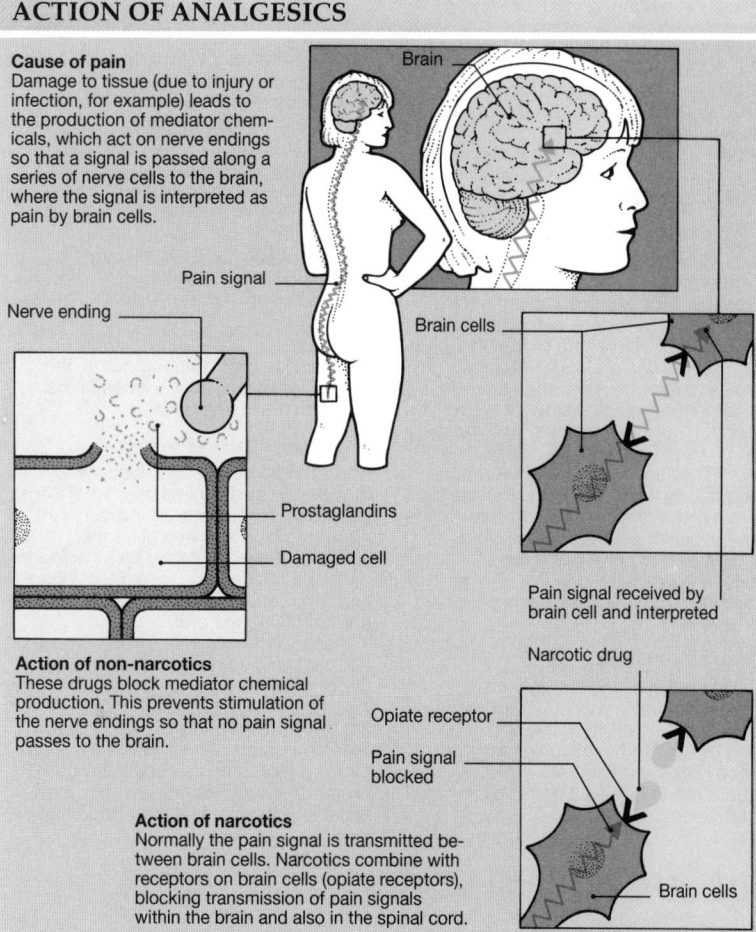

Brain

Pain signal

Nerve ending

Prostaglandins

Damaged cell

Brain cells

Pain signal received by
brain cell and interpreted

Narcotic drug

Opiate receptor

Pain signal
blocked

Brain cells

Action of non-narcotics
These drugs block mediator chemical
production. This prevents stimulation of
the nerve endings so that no pain signal
passes to the brain.

Action of narcotics
Normally the pain signal is transmitted between brain cells. Narcotics combine with
receptors on brain cells (opiate receptors),
blocking transmission of pain signals
within the brain and also in the spinal cord.

from surgery, serious injury, and disease.
Morphine is the best known narcotic
analgesic. Others include meperidine and
methadone. These powerful narcotics are
classified as controlled drugs because
they may produce euphoria, which can
lead to abuse and addiction. When they
are given under medical supervision to
treat severe pain for a few days the risk of
addiction is negligible.

Narcotic analgesics may cloud
consciousness and prevent clear thought.
Other drawbacks are that they can
produce drowsiness, nausea, vomiting,
constipation, and depressed breathing.
When taken in overdose, narcotics may
induce a deep coma and depress the
breathing mechanism to produce fatal
breathing difficulties.

In addition to the powerful narcotics,
there are less powerful drugs in this group
that are used to relieve mild to moderate
pain. They include codeine and
propoxyphene.

Combined analgesics

Mild narcotics, such as codeine, are often
found combined with non-narcotics, such
as ASA or acetaminophen. These
mixtures may combine the advantages of
analgesics that act on the brain with
those acting at the site of pain. When
given in sufficient doses (e.g., ASA 650mg
plus codeine 60mg), the combination is
more effective than either drug alone,
although it may also combine the side
effects of both.

COMMON DRUGS

Non-narcotics	Narcotics
Acetaminophen	Codeine
ASA	Meperidine
	Morphine
NSAIDs	Oxycodone
(see p.128)	Propoxyphene

SLEEPING DRUGS

Difficulty in getting to sleep or staying asleep (insomnia) has many causes. Most people suffer from sleepless nights from time to time, usually as a result of a temporary worry or discomfort from a minor illness. Persistent sleeplessness can be caused by psychological problems including anxiety or depression, or by pain and discomfort arising from a physical disorder.

Why they are used

For occasional bouts of sleeplessness, simple, common remedies to promote relaxation – for example, taking a warm bath or a hot milk drink before bedtime – are usually the best form of treatment. For more severe and prolonged insomnia, long-term treatment depends on resolving the underlying cause of the problem. Sleeping drugs (also known as hypnotics) can be used to reestablish the habit of sleep. They are best used for short periods only when self-help measures have failed and when lack of sleep affects general health and functioning. As a general rule, the prolonged use of sleeping drugs should be avoided as it may lead to psychological and physical dependence.

How they work

Most sleeping drugs promote sleep by depressing brain function. They interfere with chemical activity in the brain and nervous system by reducing communication between nerve cells. This leads to a reduction in brain activity, allowing you to fall asleep more easily. The action of

TYPES OF SLEEPING DRUGS

Benzodiazepines The most commonly used class of sleeping drugs, the benzodiazepines have comparatively few adverse effects. They are also used to treat anxiety.

Barbiturates These are now rarely used because of the risks of abuse and dependence, and of toxicity in overdose. There is a tendency to prolonged sedation ("hangover").

Non-benzodiazepine, non-barbiturate sleeping drugs These drugs were developed as safer alternatives to barbiturates, but have

been less commonly used since the introduction of the benzodiazepines.

Antihistamines Widely used to treat allergic symptoms (see p.136), antihistamines also cause drowsiness and are sometimes used to promote sleep.

Antidepressant drugs Insomnia is frequently a symptom of depression. Antidepressants, by correcting symptoms of depression, can also correct insomnia. Additionally, some antidepressants can promote sleep because they have a sedative effect (see p.96).

the main class of sleeping drugs, the benzodiazepines, is described in more detail on the facing page.

How they affect you

A sleeping drug rapidly produces drowsiness and slowed reactions. Some people find that the drug makes them appear to be drunk and slurs their speech, especially if they delay going to bed after taking their dose. Most people find they usually fall asleep within one hour of taking the drug.

Because the sleep induced by drugs is not the same as normal sleep, many people find they do not feel as well rested by it as by a night of natural sleep. This is the result of suppressed brain activity. Sleeping drugs also suppress the sleep during which dreams occur, and both dream sleep and non-dream sleep are essential components for a good night's

sleep (see The effect of drugs on sleep patterns, below).

Some people experience a variety of "hangover" effects the following day. The benzodiazepines may produce minor side effects, such as daytime drowsiness, dizziness, and unsteadiness, that can impair the ability to drive or operate dangerous machinery. Elderly people are especially likely to become confused; for them, selection of an appropriate drug is particularly important.

Risks and special precautions

Most sleeping drugs can produce psychological and physical dependence (see p.23) when taken regularly for more than a few weeks, especially if taken in larger-than-normal doses. If they are withdrawn abruptly, sleeplessness, anxiety, seizures, and hallucinations can arise. Nightmares and vivid dreams may occur because the amount of time spent in dream sleep increases. Anyone who has been using sleeping drugs regularly for a long time and wishes to stop taking them should seek his or her physician's advice on how to reduce dosage gradually so as to avoid withdrawal symptoms.

One of the risks of taking sleeping drugs for a prolonged period is that there may be a temptation to exceed the prescribed dose, especially if the person has been taking them for some weeks and their effect has diminished. While it inadvisable to take more than the prescribed dose of any drug, overdose can be a particular risk with the barbiturates.

THE EFFECTS OF DRUGS ON SLEEP PATTERNS

Normal sleep can be divided into three types: light sleep, deep sleep, and dream sleep. The proportion of time spent in each type of sleep changes with age and is altered by sleeping drugs. Dramatic changes in sleep patterns also occur in the first few days following abrupt withdrawal of sleeping drugs after regular, prolonged use.

Normal sleep Young adults spend most sleep time in light sleep with roughly equal proportions of dream and deep sleep.

Drug-induced sleep has less dream sleep and less deep sleep with relatively more light sleep.

Sleep following drug withdrawal There is a marked increase in dream sleep, causing nightmares, following withdrawal of drugs used regularly for a long time.

○ Dream sleep
● Deep sleep
◐ Light sleep

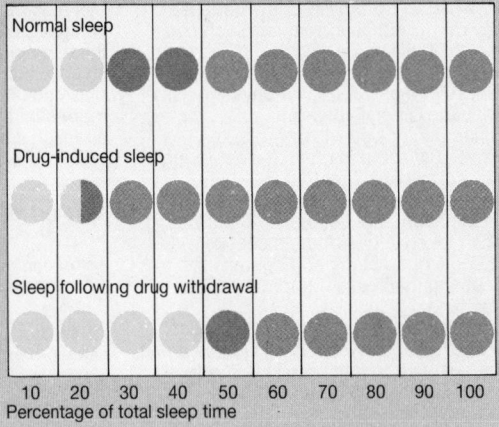

Normal sleep

Drug-induced sleep

Sleep following drug withdrawal

10 20 30 40 50 60 70 80 90 100
Percentage of total sleep time

COMMON DRUGS

Benzodiazepines
Flurazepam
Nitrazepam
Temazepam
Triazolam
Zopiclone

Non-benzodiazepine, non-barbiturate
Chloral hydrate

Barbiturate
Secobarbital

ANTI-ANXIETY DRUGS

Anxiety can be a normal reaction to real dangers or to stressful periods of everyday life. It can be beneficial, providing a stimulus to cope with challenges. However, some individuals can chronically experience moderate to severe anxiety when there is no real danger or stressful situation. Their excessive anxiety is often accompanied by an overactivity of the sympathetic nervous system (see p.91) manifested by physical symptoms: shaking, palpitations, breathlessness, sweating, and digestive distress. Some individuals may also experience sudden attacks of anxiety, fear, or panic, accompanied by these physical symptoms. These attacks are called panic attacks.

Why they are used

Anti-anxiety drugs (also called anxiolytics or minor tranquilizers) are used to alleviate persistent feelings of nervousness and tension caused by stress or other psychological problems. But tackling the underlying problem through counseling and perhaps psychotherapy offers the best hope of a long-term solution. Anti-anxiety drugs are also used in hospitals to calm and relax people who are undergoing uncomfortable medical procedures.

There are two main classes of drugs for relieving anxiety: benzodiazepines and beta blockers. The benzodiazepines are widely used to relieve anxiety and are given as a regular treatment for short periods to promote relaxation. Most benzodiazepines have a strong sedative effect, helping to relieve the insomnia that accompanies anxiety. These drugs may be used to reduce or prevent panic attacks (see also Sleeping drugs, facing page).

The other group of drugs, the beta blockers, may be used to reduce physical symptoms of anxiety, such as shaking and palpitations. They may be prescribed for people who feel excessively anxious in certain situations, for example, at interviews or public appearances. Other drugs used to relieve anxiety include certain antidepressants – prescribed for anxiety arising out of a depressive illness (see p.96).

How they work

It is thought that the benzodiazepines depress activity in the part of the brain that controls emotion, by promoting the action of a chemical called gamma-aminobutyric acid (GABA). GABA attaches itself to brain cells, blocking transmission of electrical impulses. This reduces communication between brain cells. Benzodiazepines are thought to increase the inhibitory effect of GABA on brain cells (see Action of benzodiazepines, above), thus preventing excessive brain activity, which causes anxiety.

ACTION OF BENZODIAZEPINES

Action on the brain
The reticular activating system (RAS) in the brain stem controls the level of mental activity by stimulating the higher centers of the brain responsible for consciousness. Benzodiazepines depress the RAS, so relieving anxiety. In larger doses they depress the RAS sufficiently to cause drowsiness and sleep.

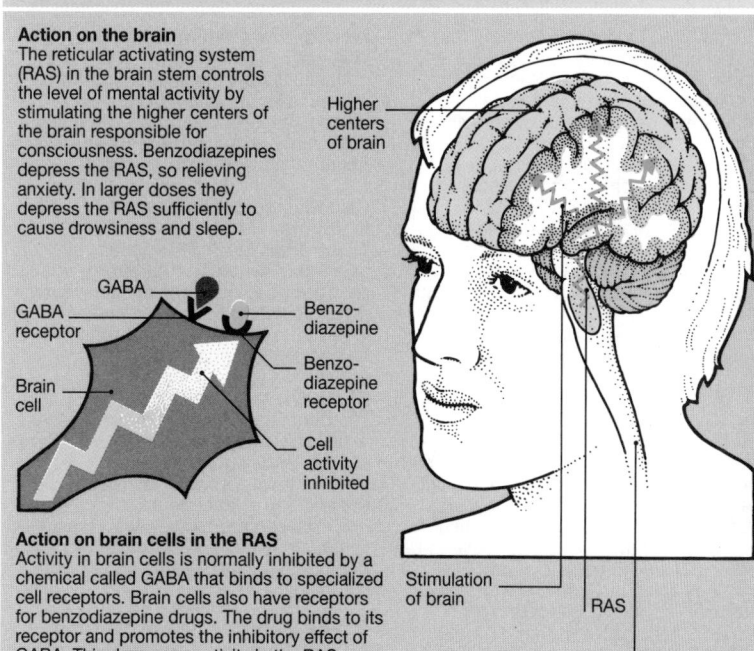

Higher centers of brain

GABA
GABA receptor
Brain cell

Benzo-diazepine
Benzo-diazepine receptor
Cell activity inhibited

Stimulation of brain
RAS
Brain stem

Action on brain cells in the RAS
Activity in brain cells is normally inhibited by a chemical called GABA that binds to specialized cell receptors. Brain cells also have receptors for benzodiazepine drugs. The drug binds to its receptor and promotes the inhibitory effect of GABA. This depresses activity in the RAS.

How they affect you

Benzodiazepines reduce feelings of agitation and restlessness, slow mental activity, and often produce drowsiness. They are said to reduce motivation and, if taken in large doses, may lead to apathy. They also have a relaxing effect on the muscles, and some benzodiazepines are used specifically for that purpose (see Muscle-relaxant drugs, p.132). Minor adverse effects of these drugs include dizziness and forgetfulness. People who need to drive or operate dangerous machinery should be aware that their reactions may be slowed. Because the brain soon becomes tolerant to their effects, benzodiazepines may become less effective after a few weeks.

Risks and special precautions

The benzodiazepines are considered safe for most people. The main risk is that people who take them regularly may become psychologically and physically dependent, particularly when large doses have been used. For this reason they are usually given for courses of two weeks or less. However, benzodiazepines are sometimes used on a long-term basis for cases of chronic, severe anxiety or panic attacks. The therapeutic benefit in such cases has to be weighed against a potential dependency. If a person has been taking them for a long period, they are normally withdrawn gradually under

medical supervision. If they are stopped suddenly, withdrawal symptoms, including excessive anxiety, nightmares, and restlessness, may occur. Benzodiazepines have been abused for their sedative effect, and they are therefore prescribed with particular caution for people with a history of drug or alcohol abuse.

COMMON DRUGS

Benzodiazepines
Alprazolam
Bromazepam
Chlordiazepoxide
Clorazepate
Diazepam
Lorazepam
Oxazepam

Beta blocker
Propranolol

Other drugs
Buspirone

ANTIDEPRESSANT DRUGS

Occasional moods of sadness or discouragement are normal and usually pass quickly. But more severe depression, accompanied by despair, lethargy, loss of sex drive, apathy, and poor appetite, may call for medical attention. Such depression can arise from the death of someone close, an illness, or sometimes from no apparent cause.

There are three main types of drugs used to treat depression: tricyclics, monoamine oxidase inhibitors, and selective serotonin reuptake inhibitors (see Types of antidepressants, below). Lithium, which is used to treat manic depression, is discussed under Antimanic drugs (facing page). Other antidepressants, such as maprotiline, have actions similar to those of the tricyclics.

Why they are used
Physicians usually avoid prescribing antidepressants when it is likely that the depression will soon pass. In such cases support and help in coming to terms with the cause is often more effective than drugs. Severe depression may be helped by antidepressants, which may have to be taken for many months or years. However, they can sometimes be withdrawn gradually after prolonged treatment without relapse occurring.

How they work
No one yet knows precisely how antidepressants produce their beneficial effect. However, research indicates that they can act on several types of neurons by either increasing or decreasing their electrical activity; these complex effects on neurons and their receptors seem to be related to their therapeutic effect.

Tricyclics
When neurotransmitters are released by neurons, they are normally taken up again into the cells. Tricyclics block this reuptake and also speed up or slow down the activity of receptors on brain neurons.

Monoamine oxidase inhibitors
These drugs block a brain enzyme that normally breaks down the neurotransmitters. Like tricyclics, MAOIs act on neurons, receptors, and neurotransmitters to produce an antidepressant effect (see Action of antidepressants, right).

Selective serotonin reuptake inhibitors
These drugs block the reuptake into neurons of a specific neurotransmitter, serotonin (see Action of antidepressants, right). Venlafaxine, a new antidepressant, inhibits the reuptake of both serotonin and norepinephrine.

How they affect you
The beneficial effect of antidepressants is usually noticeable after 10 to 14 days. But it may be six to eight weeks before you feel the full effect. However, within the first day of treatment some of the tricyclics can produce drowsiness and a variety of *anticholinergic* effects including dry mouth, blurred vision, and difficulty urinating.

Risks and special precautions
Tricyclics and MAOIs are dangerous in overdose: tricyclics can produce coma, cause seizures, and possibly fatal abnormal heart rhythms; MAOIs can also cause seizures and even death. Both are prescribed with caution for those with heart problems or epilepsy.

Monoamine oxidase inhibitors have numerous side effects because they deactivate enzymes in the body that normally break down certain chemicals (particularly tyramine) found in some foods. MAOIs taken with certain drugs or foods rich in tyramine (for example, cheese, meat or yeast extracts, and red wine) can produce a dramatic rise in blood pressure even two weeks after stopping the drug. A newer MAOI, moclobemide, is much less likely to lead to unwanted symptoms when taken with food, and restrictions in diet are not usually needed.

TYPES OF ANTIDEPRESSANTS

Tricyclics
Tricyclics are the most widely used group of antidepressants and usually the first to be tried. They are all equally effective but differ in the side effects they produce.

Monoamine oxidase inhibitors (MAOIs)
These are usually given to people who do not respond to the tricyclics, or for whom tricyclics are not suitable. MAOIs are effective in people who are anxious as well as depressed, or who suffer from panic attacks and phobias.

Selective serotonin reuptake inhibitors (SSRIs)
These increase the activity of the neurotransmitter serotonin. They often have fewer side effects than MAOIs or tricyclics, but may cause nausea.

COMMON DRUGS

SSRIs	Tricyclics
Fluoxetine	Amitriptyline
Fluvoxamine	Clomipramine
Paroxetine	Desipramine
Sertraline	Doxepin
	Imipramine
MAOIs	Nortriptyline
Moclobemide	
Phenelzine	**Other drugs**
Tranylcypromine	Maprotiline
	Trazodone

ACTION OF ANTIDEPRESSANTS

Normally brain neurons release quantities of excitatory chemicals (neurotransmitters) to act on neighboring neurons. In depression, this normal activity is disrupted. Neurons do not release neurotransmitters properly or neighboring neurons do not react normally to the effect of neurotransmitters on their receptors. Antidepressants correct these abnormalities.

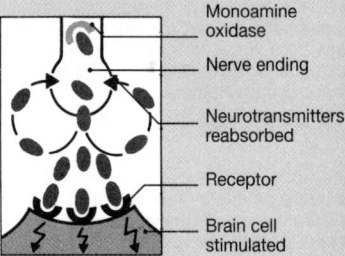

- Monoamine oxidase
- Nerve ending
- Neurotransmitters reabsorbed
- Receptor
- Brain cell stimulated

Normal brain activity
In a normal brain neurotransmitters are constantly being released, reabsorbed, and broken down.

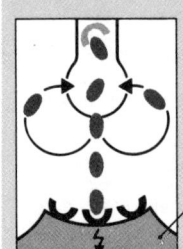

- Brain cell poorly stimulated

Brain activity in depression (one theory)
Fewer neurotransmitters than normal are released, leading to reduced stimulation.

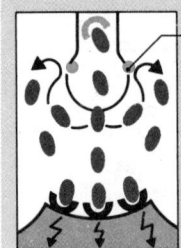

- Drug blocks reabsorption of neurotransmitter

Action of tricyclics and SSRIs (one theory)
Tricyclic and SSRI drugs increase the levels of neurotransmitters by blocking their reabsorption.

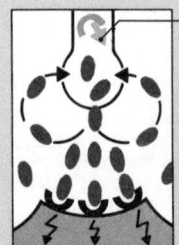

- Drug blocks enzyme

Action of MAOIs (one theory)
MAOIs increase the levels of neurotransmitters by blocking the action of the enzyme (monoamine oxidase) that breaks them down.

ANTIPSYCHOTIC DRUGS

"Psychosis" is a term used to describe mental disorders that prevent the sufferer from thinking clearly, recognizing reality, and acting rationally. These disorders include schizophrenia, manic depression, and paranoia. The precise causes of these disorders are unknown, although a number of factors, including stress, heredity, and brain injury, may be involved. Temporary psychosis can also arise as a result of alcohol withdrawal or the abuse of mind-altering drugs (see Drugs of abuse, p.531). A variety of drugs are used to treat psychotic disorders (see Common drugs, below), most of which have similar actions and effects. One exception is lithium, which is particularly useful for manic depression (see Antimanic drugs, right).

Why they are used

Because a person with a psychotic illness may recover spontaneously, a drug will not always be prescribed immediately. Long-term treatment is started only when normal life is seriously interfered with. Antipsychotic drugs also called major tranquilizers or neuroleptics) do not cure the underlying disorder but they can restore normal behavior.

The drug given to a particular individual depends on the nature of his or her illness and the side effects experienced. Drugs differ in the amount of sedation that they produce; the need for sedation also influences the choice.

Antipsychotics may also be given to calm or sedate a highly agitated or aggressive person, whatever the cause. Some antipsychotic drugs also have a powerful action against nausea and vomiting (see Anti-emetic drugs, p.102), and are sometimes used as premedication before surgery.

How they work

It is thought that some forms of mental illness are caused by an increase in communication between brain cells due to overactivity of a chemical called dopamine. This may disturb normal thought processes and produce abnormal behavior. Dopamine combines with *receptors* on the brain cells. Antipsychotics reduce the transmission of nerve signals by binding to these receptors, thus making the brain cells less sensitive to dopamine (see Action of antipsychotics, below).

How they affect you

By modifying abnormal behavior, the antipsychotics enable the sufferer to live outside of a mental institution, where psychotic patients were usually confined up until the 1950s.

Because antipsychotics depress the action of dopamine, they can disturb its balance with another chemical in the brain, acetylcholine. If that occurs, signs like those of parkinsonism can appear – for example, the expressionless face and shaky hands (see Antiparkinsonism drugs, p.99).

In those circumstances, a change in medication becomes necessary, or an additional drug may be prescribed to counteract the adverse effects of the antipsychotic.

Antipsychotics may also block the action of another neurotransmitter, norepinephrine. This lowers the blood pressure, especially when you stand up, causing dizziness. It may also prevent ejaculation.

Risks and special precautions

It is important to continue taking these drugs even if all symptoms have gone, because symptoms are controlled only by taking the prescribed dose.

ANTIMANIC DRUGS

Changes in mood are normal, but when a person's mood swings become grossly exaggerated, with peaks of elation or mania alternating with troughs of depression, they represent an illness called manic depression. This is usually treated with lithium, a drug that reduces the intensity of the mania, lifts the depression, and lessens the frequency of mood swings. Because it may take three weeks before the lithium starts to work, an antipsychotic may be prescribed with lithium at first to give immediate relief of symptoms.

Lithium can be toxic if levels of the drug in the blood rise too high. Checks on blood concentrations of lithium are therefore usually carried out regularly during treatment. Symptoms of lithium poisoning include blurred vision, twitching, vomiting, and diarrhea.

Because these drugs can have permanent as well as temporary side effects, the minimum necessary dosage is used. This is found by starting with a low dose and increasing it until symptoms are controlled. The dose is reduced gradually when drug treatment needs to be stopped.

The most serious long-term risk of antipsychotic treatment is a disorder known as *tardive dyskinesia*, which may develop after one to five years. This consists of repeated jerking movements of the mouth, tongue, and face, and sometimes the hands and feet.

Some physicians have suggested that periodic withdrawal of the drug for several months may reduce the severity of this condition, but the value of such "drug holidays" has not been proved.

How they are administered

Antipsychotics may be injected, or given as tablets, capsules, or syrup. They can also be given in the form of a *depot injection* that releases the drug slowly over several weeks. This is helpful for people who might forget to take their drugs or who might take an overdose.

COMMON DRUGS

Phenothiazine antipsychotics
Chlorpromazine
Methotrimeprazine
Perphenazine
Prochlorperazine
Thioridazine
Trifluoperazine

Antimanic drug
Lithium

Butyrophenone antipsychotic
Haloperidol

Other drugs
Clozapine
Loxapine
Pimozide
Risperidone

ACTION OF ANTIPSYCHOTICS

Brain activity is partly governed by the action of a chemical called dopamine, which transmits signals between brain cells. In psychotic illness the brain cells release too much dopamine, causing excessive stimulation. Antipsychotic drugs help to reduce the adverse effects of excess dopamine.

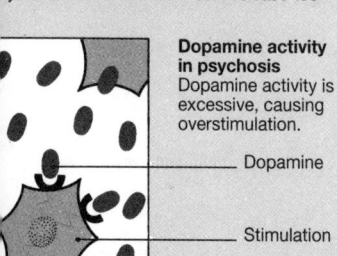

Dopamine activity in psychosis
Dopamine activity is excessive, causing overstimulation.

Dopamine

Stimulation

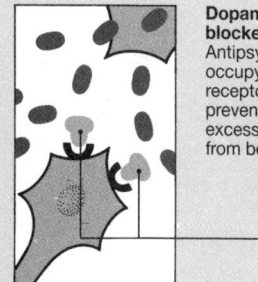

Dopamine activity blocked by drugs
Antipsychotic drugs occupy dopamine receptors and prevent the effects of excess dopamine from being felt.

Drug

ANTICONVULSANT DRUGS

Electrical signals from nerve cells in the brain are normally finely coordinated to produce smooth movements of arms and legs. But these signals can become paroxysmal and chaotic, and trigger the disorderly muscular activity and mental changes which are characteristic of a seizure (also called a fit or convulsion). The most common cause of seizures is the disorder known as epilepsy. However, seizures may also be brought on by outside stimuli – such as flashing lights – or caused by brain disease or injury, by the toxic effects of certain drugs, or, in young children, by a high temperature.

Anticonvulsant drugs are used to reduce the risk of a seizure and to stop one that is in progress.

Why they are used

Isolated seizures seldom require drug treatment, but anticonvulsant drugs are the usual treatment for controlling epileptic seizures. They permit epileptics to lead a normal life, reducing the possibility of brain damage, which can result from recurrent seizures.

ACTION OF ANTICONVULSANTS

Normally there is a relatively low level of electrical activity in the brain. In a seizure, excessive electrical activity builds up, causing uncontrolled stimulation of the brain. Anticonvulsant drugs have an inhibitory effect which neutralizes excessive electrical activity in the brain.

Normal brain activity

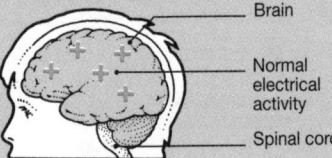

Brain

Normal electrical activity

Spinal cord

Brain activity in a seizure

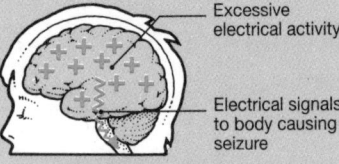

Excessive electrical activity

Electrical signals to body causing seizure

Drug action on brain activity

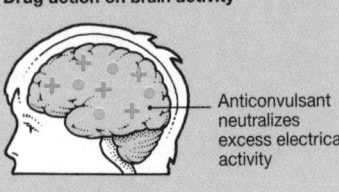

Anticonvulsant neutralizes excess electrical activity

Most people with epilepsy need to take anticonvulsants on a regular basis to prevent seizures. Usually a single drug is used, and treatment continues until there have been no attacks for at least two years. The particular drug prescribed depends on the kind of epilepsy (see Types of epilepsy, right). If one drug alone is not effective, a combination of drugs may be given. Even when under treatment a person can suffer seizures. A prolonged seizure can be halted by injection of diazepam or a similar drug.

How they work

Brain cells bring about body movement by a form of electrical activity which passes through the nerves to the muscles. In a seizure, excessive electrical activity starts in one part of the brain and spreads to other parts, causing uncontrolled stimulation of brain cells.

Most anticonvulsant drugs have an *inhibitory* effect on brain cells and damp down electrical activity, thus preventing the excessive buildup which causes a seizure (see Action of anticonvulsants, left).

How they affect you

Ideally, the only effect an anticonvulsant should have is to reduce or prevent seizures. Unfortunately, no drug prevents seizures without potentially affecting normal brain function, leading to poor memory, inability to concentrate, lack of coordination, and lethargy. It is important, therefore, to find a dosage that is sufficient to prevent seizures without causing unacceptable side effects. The dose has to be carefully tailored to the individual – there is no standard dose for anticonvulsants. It is usual to start with a low dose of a selected drug and to increase it gradually until a balance is achieved between the effective control of seizures and the occurrence of side effects, many of which wear off after the first few weeks of treatment. Blood tests to monitor levels of the drug in the body are usually carried out periodically. Finding the correct dose may take several months. It may sometimes be necessary to use more than one drug to adequately control seizures.

Risks and special precautions

Each anticonvulsant drug has its own specific adverse effects and risks. In addition, most of them affect the liver's ability to break down other drugs (see Drug interactions, p.16) and so may influence the action of other drugs you are taking. Physicians try to use the minimum number of anticonvulsants in any one person in order to reduce the risk of such interactions occurring.

People taking anticonvulsants need to be particularly careful to take their medication regularly as prescribed. If the levels of the anticonvulsant in the body

TYPES OF EPILEPSY

The selection of anticonvulsant drug depends on the type of epilepsy, although the individual's age and particular response to drug treatment are also important.

Tonic/clonic (grand mal) seizures This type of seizure is characterized by a warning sensation such as flashing lights or a noise, which is followed by a sudden loss of consciousness during which convulsions occur, and the sufferer may urinate uncontrollably or foam at the mouth. The seizure usually lasts for a few minutes only but it can occasionally last for up to an hour. Prolonged attacks are called status epilepticus.

The principal drugs used to prevent tonic/clonic seizures are phenytoin, phenobarbital, primidone, and carbamazepine. Physicians try to avoid prescribing phenytoin for young children because of its unpleasant side effects, such as overgrowth of the gums, acne, and increased body hair. These effects are less prominent in adults. Status epilepticus is usually treated by injection of a benzodiazepine drug such as diazepam.

Absence (petit mal) seizures This form of epilepsy most commonly affects children. The seizures consist of a momentary loss of consciousness, during which the child may seem to go blank. Convulsions do not occur. The following drugs are used for the prevention of this type of seizure: ethosuximide, valproic acid, and, less commonly, clonazepam.

Partial seizures There are a number of different variations of this form of epilepsy. Most partial seizures cause a sudden severe disturbance of the senses and/or muscle spasm without loss of consciousness. Phenytoin, phenobarbital, and carbamazepine are the drugs most commonly used to prevent partial seizures.

are allowed to fall suddenly, seizures are very likely to occur. The reason for this that without the inhibitory drug, there is little to stop the buildup of electrical activity that brings on seizures. Accordingly, the dose should not be reduced or the treatment stopped except on the advice of a physician. If, for any reason, treatment with anticonvulsants is to be stopped, the dose should be reduced gradually, usually over a period of months. People on anticonvulsant therapy are advised to carry an identification tag that gives full details their condition and treatment.

COMMON DRUGS

Carbamazepine	Lamotrigine
Clobazam	Phenobarbital
Clonazepam	Phenytoin
Diazepam	Primidone
Ethosuximide	Valproic acid
Gabapentin	Vigabatrin

ANTIPARKINSONISM DRUGS

Antiparkinsonism drugs are used in the treatment of parkinsonism. This is the general term used to describe shaking of the head and limbs, muscular stiffness, an expressionless face, and inability to control or initiate movement. It is caused by an imbalance between the chemicals dopamine and acetylcholine in the brain. These chemicals transmit nerve signals in the part of the brain that coordinates movement. They have opposing actions and are normally finely balanced. In parkinsonism there is a reduction in the action of dopamine, so that the effect of acetylcholine is increased.

Parkinsonism has a variety of causes, but the most common is degeneration of the dopamine-producing cells in the brain, known as Parkinson's disease. Other causes include the side effects of certain drugs, notably antipsychotics (see p.97), brain damage, and narrowing of the blood vessels to the brain.

Why they are used

Antiparkinsonism drugs can help to relieve the symptoms of parkinsonism, but they cannot cure the underlying cause of the chemical imbalance. The degeneration of brain cells in Parkinson's disease cannot be halted, although drugs can minimize symptoms of the disease for many years.

How they work

Antiparkinsonism drugs restore the balance between dopamine and acetylcholine. They fall into two main groups: those drugs that act by reducing the effect of acetylcholine (anticholinergic drugs) and those that act by boosting the effect of dopamine.

Anticholinergic drugs

Acetylcholine acts by combining with receptors on brain cells and stimulating them. Anticholinergic drugs combine with these receptors and prevent acetylcholine from binding to them. This reduces acetylcholine's relative overactivity and restores the balance with dopamine.

Drugs that boost the effect of dopamine

Dopamine levels in the brain cannot be boosted by giving dopamine directly because it is poorly absorbed through the digestive tract, and cannot pass from the bloodstream into the brain. Levodopa – the chemical from which dopamine is naturally produced in the brain – can be absorbed well through the digestive tract. It increases the level of dopamine and so restores the balance with acetylcholine. Because a high proportion of each dose of levodopa is broken down in the body before it reaches the brain, it is usually combined with a drug called carbidopa, which prevents this breakdown. Dopamine is broken down in the brain.

ACTION OF ANTIPARKINSONISM DRUGS

Normal movement depends on a balance in the brain between dopamine and acetylcholine, which combine with receptors on brain cells. In parkinsonism there is less dopamine, so that acetylcholine is relatively overactive. The balance between acetylcholine and dopamine may be restored by anticholinergic drugs, which combine with the receptors for acetylcholine and block acetylcholine's action on the brain cell or by dopamine-boosting drugs, which increase the level of dopamine activity in the brain.

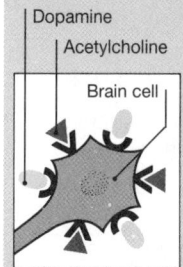

Normal chemical balance
Normally dopamine and acetylcholine are balanced.

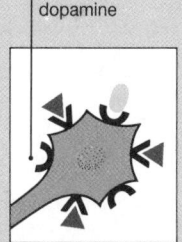

Chemical imbalance in parkinsonism
When dopamine activity is reduced, acetylcholine is overactive.

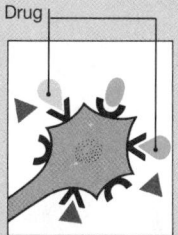

Action of anticholinergic drugs
Anticholinergic drugs displace acetylcholine and restore balance.

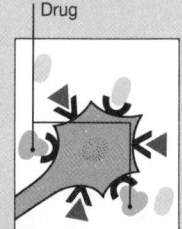

Action of dopamine-boosting drugs
These drugs increase dopamine activity and restore balance.

Amantadine (also used as an antiviral agent, see p.145) boosts the levels of dopamine in the brain by stimulating its release. Selegiline acts by inhibiting the breakdown of dopamine in the brain. Dopamine action can also be boosted by bromocriptine, which mimics the action of dopamine.

How they affect you

Each type of drug relieves some symptoms of parkinsonism better than others, although it is difficult to control symptoms in the more advanced stage of the disease. Anticholinergics improve stiffness more than shaking or the inability to initiate movement, and benefit is felt within a few days. They also reduce excessive salivation: dribbling is often a problem in Parkinson's disease.

Levodopa often produces a dramatic improvement in all symptoms. Side effects of levodopa include nausea, vomiting, and flushing. When given in excess it can also cause involuntary movements in the face and the body. Although these problems may be alleviated by reducing the dose, as the disease progresses it becomes increasingly difficult to give sufficient levodopa to improve symptoms without causing side effects. Also, in the later stage of the disease, the effect of each dose wears off before the next one is taken, and it may be necessary to take the drug more frequently.

Amantadine relieves all symptoms of parkinsonism in people with mild to moderate cases. It has few side effects but the beneficial effect may wear off over a few months. The most common side effects of bromocriptine and selegiline are the same as those produced by levodopa.

Choice of drug

The particular drug prescribed depends on both the severity of the disease and the potential adverse effects of the drug.

Anticholinergic drugs are often effective in the early stages of Parkinson's disease, when they may control symptoms adequately without any other antiparkinsonism drugs. They are often used to treat parkinsonism caused by antipsychotic drugs. If a person cannot take anticholinergic drugs because of their side effects, amantadine may be given. Levodopa is usually prescribed when the disease impairs walking. The effectiveness of levodopa usually wanes after two to five years; if this happens selegiline, bromocriptine, or amantadine may be prescribed as well. In newly diagnosed patients, selegiline may delay the need to begin therapy with levodopa. People who do not benefit from levodopa, or suffer side effects, may be given one of the other drugs.

COMMON DRUGS

Anticholinergic drugs	Dopamine-boosting drugs
Benztropine	Amantadine
Orphenadrine	Bromocriptine
Procyclidine	Levodopa
Trihexyphenidyl	Selegiline

NERVOUS SYSTEM STIMULANTS

A person's state of mental alertness varies throughout the day and is under the control of chemicals in the brain, some of which are depressant (causing drowsiness) and others that are stimulant (heightening awareness).

It is thought that an increase in the activity of the depressant chemicals may be responsible for a rare condition called narcolepsy, a tendency to fall asleep for no obvious reason. Nervous system stimulants are given to increase wakefulness. They include the amphetamines and related drugs, notably methylphenidate. Respiratory stimulants, including caffeine (found in coffee, tea, and cola), are used to improve breathing (see Respiratory stimulants, right).

Why they are used

In adults who suffer from narcolepsy these drugs can be used to stimulate the brain and prevent excessive drowsiness during the day. Stimulants do not cure narcolepsy, and since the disorder usually lasts throughout the sufferer's lifetime, they may have to be taken indefinitely. Nervous system stimulants are also occasionally given to hyperactive children with a short attention span.

Because reduced appetite is a side effect of amphetamines, they have also been used as part of the treatment for obesity. However, because of the risk of addiction, sometimes accompanied by paranoid delusions, this use is generally condemned (see Risks and special precautions, right).

Caffeine is sometimes added to analgesic preparations. Various reasons have been offered to justify this.

Unfortunately, apart from their use in narcolepsy, stimulants are not useful in the long term because the brain soon becomes tolerant to them. Unless the dose is increased, no stimulation is felt.

How they work

The level of wakefulness is controlled by a part of the brain stem called the reticular activating system (RAS). Activity here depends on the balance between chemicals, some of which are *excitatory* (including norepinephrine) and some *inhibitory* (such as gamma-aminobutyric acid). Stimulants promote the release of norepinephrine, increasing activity in the RAS and other parts of the brain, so raising the level of alertness.

How they affect you

In adults, central nervous system stimulants taken in the prescribed dose for narcolepsy increase wakefulness allowing normal concentration and thought processes to occur. They may also reduce appetite and cause tremors. In hyperactive children they reduce the general level of activity to a more normal level and increase the attention span.

RESPIRATORY STIMULANTS

Some stimulants (for example, aminophylline, theophylline and doxapram) act on the part of the brain – the respiratory center – that controls respiration. They are sometimes used in hospitals to help people who have difficulty breathing, mainly very young babies and adults with severe bronchitis.

Risks and special precautions

Some people, especially the elderly or those with previous psychiatric problems are particularly sensitive to stimulants and may experience adverse effects, even when the drugs are given in comparatively low doses. They are used with caution in children because they can retard growth if taken for prolonged periods. In a child, an excess of these drugs depresses the nervous system, producing drowsiness or possibly loss of consciousness. Palpitations may occur.

These drugs reduce the level of natural stimulants in the brain, so that after a few weeks' regular use a person may become physically dependent on them for normal function. If they are then abruptly withdrawn, the excess of natural inhibitory chemicals in the brain depresses activity in the central nervous system, producing withdrawal symptoms These may include lethargy, depression, and increased appetite.

If used by adults in excess or inappropriately, stimulants can produce over-activity in the brain, resulting in extreme restlessness, sleeplessness, and feelings of nervousness or anxiety. They also stimulate the sympathetic branch of the autonomic nervous system (see p.91), causing shaking, sweating, and palpitations. More serious risks of exceeding the prescribed dose are seizures and a disturbance in mental functioning that may result in delusions and hallucinations. Amphetamines have been abused; they are classified as controlled substances (see p.533).

COMMON DRUGS

Amphetamine
Dextroamphetamine

Respiratory stimulants
Aminophylline
Doxapram
Theophylline

Other drugs
Caffeine
Methylphenidate
Pemoline

ACTION OF NERVOUS SYSTEM STIMULANTS

Wakefulness is controlled by a part of the brain stem called the reticular activating system (RAS).

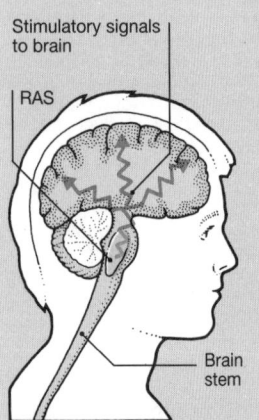

Stimulatory signals to brain

RAS

Brain stem

Normal brain activity
When the brain is functioning normally, signals from the RAS stimulate the upper parts of the brain, which control thought processes and alertness.

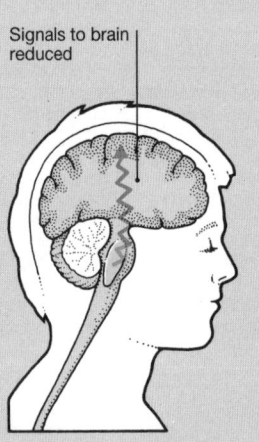

Signals to brain reduced

Brain activity in narcolepsy
In narcolepsy the level of signals from the RAS is greatly reduced.

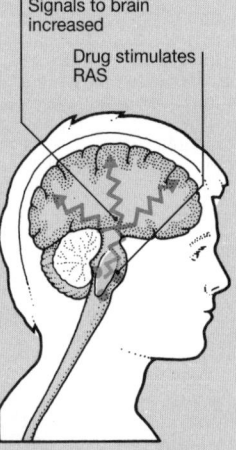

Signals to brain increased

Drug stimulates RAS

Normal brain activity restored
Central nervous system stimulants act on the RAS to increase the level of stimulatory signals to the brain.

DRUGS USED FOR MIGRAINE

Migraine is a term applied to recurrent severe headaches affecting only one side of the head and caused by changes in the blood vessels. Such headaches may be accompanied by nausea and vomiting and preceded by flashing lights or numbness and tingling in the arms. Occasionally, speech may be impaired, and the attack may be disabling. The exact cause of migraine is unknown, but an attack may be triggered by excitement, tension, shock, physical exertion, a blow to the head, some foods, and some drugs. Victims often have a family history of migraine.

Why they are used

Drugs are used either to relieve symptoms or to prevent attacks. Different drugs are used in each approach, but none cures the underlying disorder. However, the migraine can clear up spontaneously, and if you are taking drugs regularly to prevent attacks, your physician may recommend that you stop them after a few months to see whether this has happened.

In most people migraine headaches can be relieved by a mild analgesic such as ASA or acetaminophen, or a stronger one like codeine (see Analgesics, p.92). But because the migraine may be accompanied by nausea and vomiting, these drugs may not be absorbed sufficiently to provide relief. Thus suppository forms may be used. Preparations containing caffeine have been used for decades to suppress the headache when the early warning symptoms are present but before the pain is manifest. Drugs such as ergotamine or sumatriptan are given once the headache begins.

When attacks occur more often than once a month, daily drug therapy for a period of weeks or months with clonidine (an antihypertensive) or propranolol (a beta blocker) may be advised to prevent them.

Amitriptyline, an antidepressant, is sometimes prescribed regularly for a while to prevent migraine attacks, even in people who are not suffering from depression (see p.96).

Anxiety or depression which can accompany migraine may be treated with other drugs (see Anti-anxiety drugs, p.95, and Antidepressant drugs, p.96). Nausea and vomiting may be controlled with an anti-emetic drug (see p.102).

How they work

A migraine attack begins when blood vessels surrounding the brain constrict. This is thought to be caused by certain chemicals in food or produced in the body. Methysergide and propranolol block the effect of the chemicals on blood vessels and so prevent attacks. The next stage occurs when blood vessels in the scalp and around the

ACTION OF DRUGS USED FOR MIGRAINE

Migraine is caused by the action of chemicals in the bloodstream on blood vessels surrounding the brain and in the scalp. In the first stage of a migraine attack, the blood vessels surrounding the brain constrict, causing warning signs (below left). In the second stage, the blood vessels in the scalp dilate, causing a severe headache (below right).

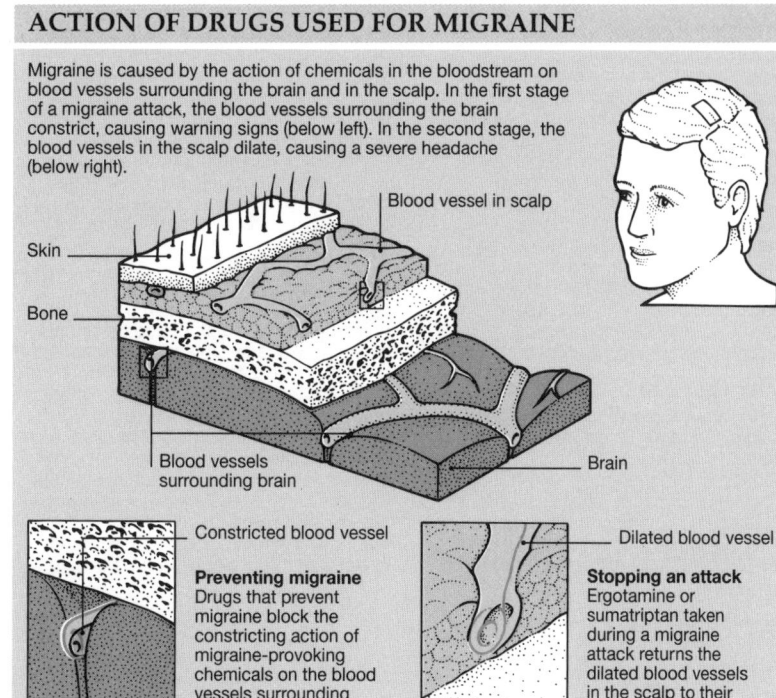

Blood vessel in scalp
Skin
Bone
Blood vessels surrounding brain
Brain

Constricted blood vessel

Preventing migraine
Drugs that prevent migraine block the constricting action of migraine-provoking chemicals on the blood vessels surrounding the brain.

Dilated blood vessel

Stopping an attack
Ergotamine or sumatriptan taken during a migraine attack returns the dilated blood vessels in the scalp to their normal size.

eyes dilate, releasing pain-producing chemicals called prostaglandins. ASA and acetaminophen relieve pain by blocking the production of prostaglandins, while codeine acts directly on the brain to alter the perception of pain (see Action of analgesics, p.93). Ergotamine and sumatriptan relieve pain by narrowing the dilated blood vessels.

How they affect you

All these drugs have their own side effects. Sumatriptan may cause chest tightness. Ergotamine may cause drowsiness, tingling sensations in the skin (paresthesia), cramps, weakness in the legs, and pain in the abdomen, arms, and legs.

For more information about the effects of propranolol, see Beta blockers, p.109, and for more information on the effects of analgesics, see p.92.

Risks and special precautions

Ergotamine should be used with caution if you have poor circulation because it can damage blood vessels through prolonged overconstriction. Frequent use can lead to dependence and numerous adverse effects, including headache. You should not take more than your physician advises in any one week. Ergotamine should not be used if you have an infection because it can restrict blood flow to the site of infection and delay recovery.

Sumatriptan should not be used if you are taking ergotamine or if you suffer from coronary heart disease, angina, or high blood pressure.

Methysergide can produce pain in the abdomen or lower back, and also shortness of breath due to an unusual type of damage to tissues.

How they are administered

Sumatriptan is normally taken in tablet form, but if an attack is getting worse and vomiting is present, it can be administered by a self-injection device. Dihydroergotamine, a drug similar to ergotamine, may be given by injection. Ergotamine may also be taken by aerosol inhalation, or as tablets to be dissolved under the tongue.

COMMON DRUGS

Drugs to relieve migraine	Drugs to prevent migraine
Acetaminophen	Amitriptyline
ASA	Clonidine
Codeine	Methysergide
Ergotamine	Pizotyline
Sumatriptan	Propranolol

ANTI-EMETIC DRUGS

Anti-emetic drugs are used to suppress vomiting and nausea. Vomiting (emesis) is a reflex action that protects the body by expelling harmful substances. Common causes of vomiting and nausea are digestive tract infection, pregnancy, motion sickness, and vertigo. They can also occur as a side effect of a medication, or drug or radiation therapy for cancer.

The main anti-emetic drugs are metoclopramide, domperidone, ondansetron, the antihistamines, and phenothiazine drugs, which are also used to treat mental illness (see Antipsychotic drugs, p.97). Nabilone, a marijuana derivative, may be used in cancer patients needing an anti-emetic.

Why they are used

Physicians usually diagnose the cause of vomiting before prescribing an anti-emetic because vomiting may be the reaction to infection, or to an abdominal condition that might require surgery. Suppressing vomiting and nausea may delay diagnosis, consequently delaying a needed operation. Anti-emetics are often taken to prevent motion sickness (antihistamines) and nausea resulting from other drug treatment (domperidone, metoclopramide, ondansetron, and phenothiazines), to suppress nausea in vertigo (see right), and occasionally to relieve severe vomiting in pregnancy (antihistamines and phenothiazines).

You should not take an anti-emetic drug for longer than a couple of days without consulting your physician.

How they work

Nausea and vomiting occur when a specialized part of the brain called the vomiting center is stimulated by signals which may arise from various points in the brain and body: from the digestive system, from the part of the brain that is responsible for consciousness, or from the inner ear. Signals may also arise from an area of the brain called the chemoreceptor trigger, which stimulates the vomiting (emetic) center if it detects any harmful substances present in the blood. Anti-emetic drugs may act at one or more of these places in the body. In

VERTIGO AND MÉNIÈRE'S DISEASE

VERTIGO AND MÉNIÈRE'S DISEASE

Vertigo is a spinning sensation in the head often accompanied by nausea and vomiting. It is usually caused by disease of the organ of balance in the inner ear. Anti-emetic drugs are prescribed to relieve symptoms with modest effect.

Ménière's disease is a disorder in which excess fluid builds up in the inner ear causing vertigo, noises in the ear, and gradual deafness. It is usually treated with an antihistamine, prochlorperazine, or an anti-anxiety drug (see p.95). A diuretic (see p.111) may also be given in order to reduce the excess fluid in the ear.

addition, these drugs may also promote the normal emptying of the stomach contents into the intestine (see Action of anti-emetics, below left).

How they affect you

In addition to reducing or preventing vomiting and nausea, most anti-emetics may make you feel drowsy. Certain non-sedating antihistamines (see p.137) may therefore be preferred for the prevention of motion sickness.

Because the antihistamines block the parasympathetic system (see p.91), they can produce many *anticholinergic* side effects, including dry mouth, blurred vision, and difficulty passing urine. Phenothiazine drugs – which also may produce anticholinergic side effects – ca produce dizziness.

Risks and special precautions

Because antihistamines can make you drowsy, it may not be advisable to drive or operate potentially dangerous machinery while taking them.

Phenothiazines and metoclopramide can produce uncontrolled movements o' the face and tongue, and for this reason they are used with caution in people who suffer from movement disorders such as *parkinsonism*.

COMMON DRUGS

Antihistamines
Dimenhydrinate
Meclizine
Promethazine

Phenothiazines
Fluphenazine
Perphenazine
Prochlorperazine
Promazine
Trifluoperazine

Other drugs
Domperidone
Metoclopramide
Nabilone
Ondansetron
Scopolamine

ACTION OF ANTI-EMETICS

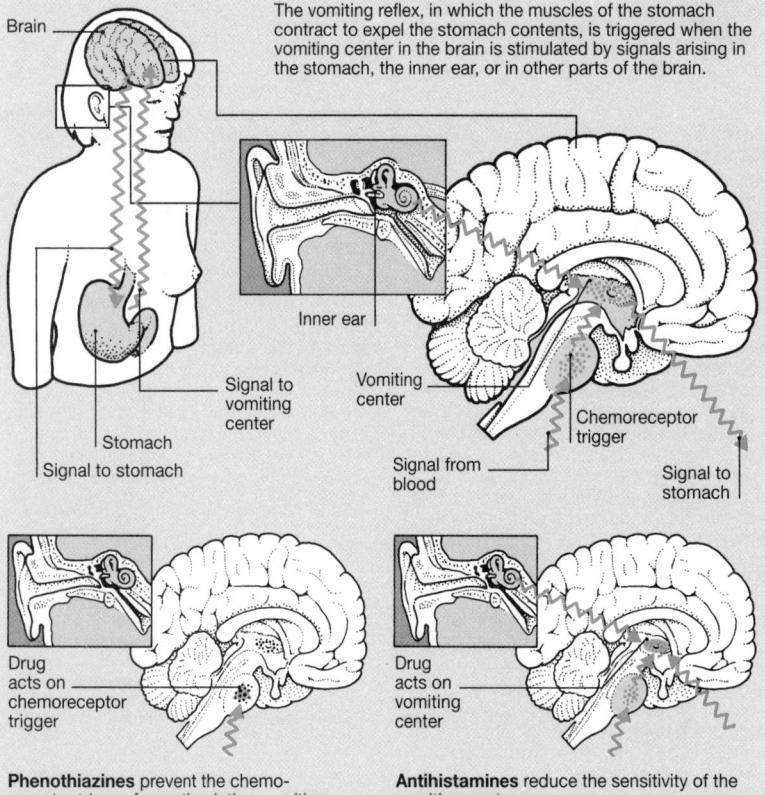

The vomiting reflex, in which the muscles of the stomach contract to expel the stomach contents, is triggered when the vomiting center in the brain is stimulated by signals arising in the stomach, the inner ear, or in other parts of the brain.

Brain

Inner ear

Signal to vomiting center

Vomiting center

Stomach

Signal to stomach

Signal from blood

Chemoreceptor trigger

Signal to stomach

Drug acts on chemoreceptor trigger

Drug acts on vomiting center

Phenothiazines prevent the chemoreceptor trigger from stimulating vomiting.

Antihistamines reduce the sensitivity of the vomiting center.

RESPIRATORY SYSTEM

Comprising the lungs and the passageways by which air reaches them, the respiratory system performs a vital function. Through the process of inhaling and exhaling air – breathing – the body is able to obtain necessary oxygen and expel carbon dioxide, the waste product of metabolism at the cellular level.

What can go wrong

Difficulty in breathing can arise in many ways including partial blockage of an airway by a physical object, damage to the alveoli (emphysema), and the destruction of lung tissue by tuberculosis or other diseases. The most common problems, however, occur because of allergic reactions (usually in the nasal passages), spasmodic contractions of the bronchi (asthma), or an infection. Most infections, usually viral or bacterial in nature, lead to inflammation of various parts of the airways, with consequent fever, irritation, coughing, and phlegm, a gooey combination of mucus and pus. Such inflammations carry the names of their location: rhinitis (nose), pharyngitis (throat), tonsillitis (tonsils), laryngitis (larynx), bronchitis (bronchial tubes) and pneumonia (lungs).

The respiratory system is also damaged by long-term exposure to tobacco smoke and other airborne impurities.

Why drugs are used

Drugs with a variety of actions are used to clear the air passages, soothe inflammation, and reduce the production of mucus. Many of these can be bought without a prescription as single-ingredient or combined-ingredient preparations, often with an analgesic.

Decongestants (p.105) reduce the swelling inside the nose, making it possible to breathe more freely. If the congestion is an allergic response, an antihistamine (p.136) is often used to relieve symptoms or to prevent attacks. Respiratory tract infections are usually treated with antibiotics.

Drugs that widen the bronchi – bronchodilators (p.104) – are used to relieve or prevent asthma attacks. The bronchodilators include drugs that relax the muscles surrounding the airways and those, such as corticosteroids (p.153), that widen the air passages by reducing inflammation of the mucous lining. These may also be of limited benefit in chronic respiratory problems.

A variety of drugs may be used to relieve coughs. Some of them make it easier to eliminate phlegm; others suppress coughing by inhibiting the cough reflex itself.

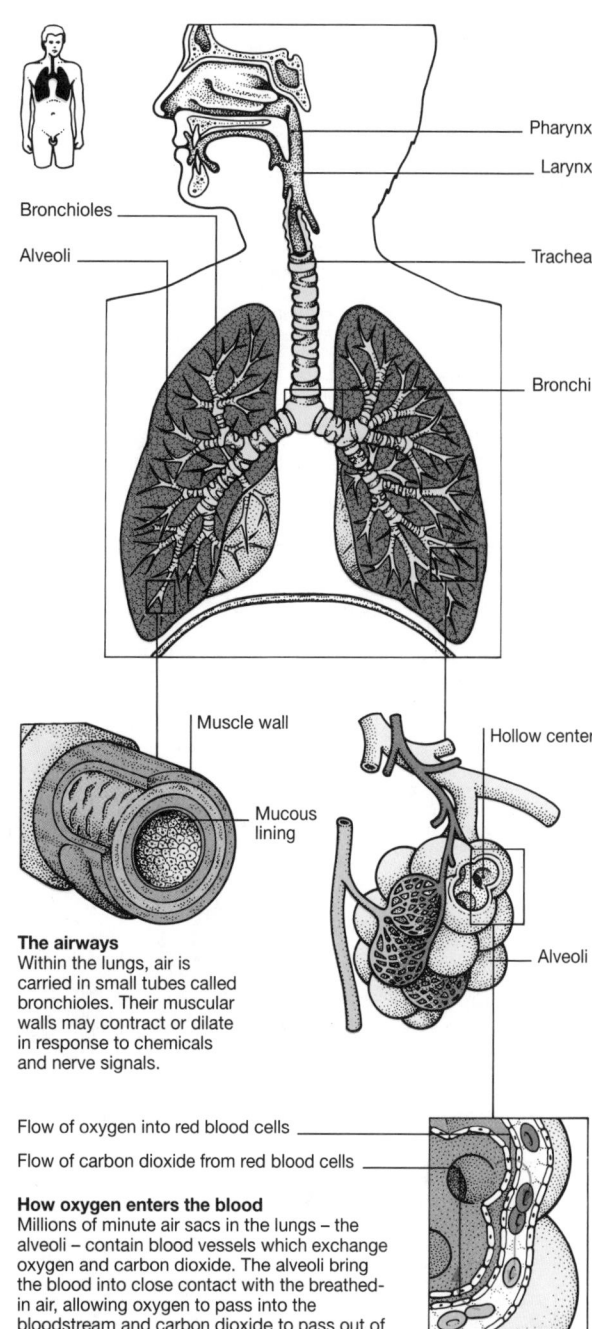

Pharynx

Larynx

Bronchioles

Alveoli

Trachea

Bronchi

Muscle wall

Hollow center

Mucous lining

Alveoli

The airways
Within the lungs, air is carried in small tubes called bronchioles. Their muscular walls may contract or dilate in response to chemicals and nerve signals.

Flow of oxygen into red blood cells

Flow of carbon dioxide from red blood cells

How oxygen enters the blood
Millions of minute air sacs in the lungs – the alveoli – contain blood vessels which exchange oxygen and carbon dioxide. The alveoli bring the blood into close contact with the breathed-in air, allowing oxygen to pass into the bloodstream and carbon dioxide to pass out of the body for expiration.

MAJOR DRUG GROUPS

Antibiotics	Decongestants
Bronchodilators	Drugs to treat coughs

BRONCHODILATORS

When air enters the lungs it passes through narrow tubes called bronchioles. In certain conditions the bronchioles become narrower, either as a result of contraction of the muscles in their walls, inflammation, or as a result of mucous congestion. This tightening of the bronchioles obstructs the flow of air into and out of the lungs and causes breathlessness.

Bronchodilators are prescribed to widen the bronchioles and improve breathing. There are three main groups of bronchodilators: *sympathomimetic* drugs, *anticholinergics*, and xanthine drugs, which are related to caffeine.

Why they are used

Bronchodilators are commonly used to relieve asthma and to compensate for narrowing of the bronchioles as a result of accumulation of mucus in chronic bronchitis. However, they are of little benefit when damage to the bronchioles is severe.

Bronchodilators together with anti-inflammatory agents are used in the management of asthma. Bronchodilators are generally taken as needed to relieve an attack of breathlessness that is in progress. Inhaled anti-inflammatory

INHALERS

Inhaling a bronchodilator drug directly into the lungs is usually the most effective method of ensuring maximum beneficial effect without excessive side effects.

Inhalers or **puffers** release a small dose when they are pressed, but require some skill to use effectively. Turbuhalers, Rotahalers, and Diskhalers are easier to use.

agents are used to prevent asthma attacks. Some people find it helpful to take an extra dose of their bronchodilator immediately before any activity likely to provoke an attack of breathlessness. Sympathomimetic drugs are mainly used for the rapid relief of breathlessness; inhaled anti-inflammatories, anti-cholinergic and xanthine drugs are more often used for the long-term prevention of breathless attacks.

How they work

Bronchodilator drugs act by relaxing the muscles surrounding the bronchioles. Sympathomimetic and anticholinergic drugs achieve this by interfering with nerve signals passed to the muscles

Insufflation cartridges deliver larger amounts of drug than inhalers and are easier to use because the drug is taken in as you breathe normally.

Nebulizers pump compressed air through a solution of drug to produce a fine mist which is inhaled through a face mask. They deliver large doses of the drug to the lungs, rapidly relieving breathing difficulty.

through the autonomic nervous system (see p.91). Xanthine drugs are thought to relax the muscles in the bronchioles by direct effect on the muscle fibers, but their precise action is not known. Corticosteroids decrease inflammation the lining of the lung.

How they affect you

When taken for the immediate relief of breathlessness, bronchodilators usually improve breathing within a few minutes. Taken to prevent attacks, anti-inflammatories usually start to increase one's capacity for exercise within a few days and most people find that the frequency of breathless attacks is reduced.

Bronchodilators can produce minor side effects, especially if taken too frequently or in too large a dose. Sympathomimetic drugs may sometimes cause palpitations and trembling. Typical side effects of anticholinergic drugs include dry mouth and blurred vision. Xanthine drugs may cause headaches and palpitations. Inhaled steroids may cause a sore, dry throat or oral thrush.

Risks and special precautions

Since bronchodilators are not often taken by mouth but inhaled (see Inhalers above), they do not commonly cause serious side effects. However, because of their possible effect on heart rate, sympathomimetic and xanthine drugs are prescribed with caution for those with heart problems, high blood pressure, or an overactive thyroid gland. Anticholinergic drugs may not be suitable for people with urinary retention or who have glaucoma.

ACTION OF BRONCHODILATORS

When bronchioles become narrow following contraction of the muscle layer and swelling of the mucous lining, the passage of air is impeded. Bronchodilators act on the nerve signals that govern muscle activity. Sympathomimetics enhance the action of neurotransmitters that encourage muscle relaxation. Anticholinergics block the neurotransmitters that trigger muscle contraction. Xanthines promote muscle relaxation by a direct effect on the muscles. Corticosteroids work to reduce inflammation of the lung lining.

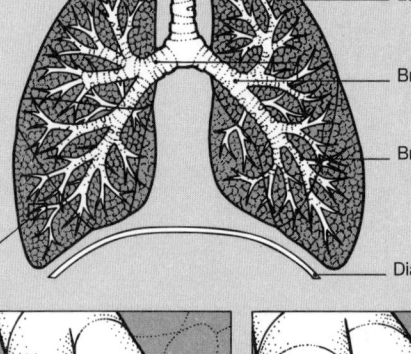

Trachea

Lung

Bronchi

Bronchioles

Diaphragm

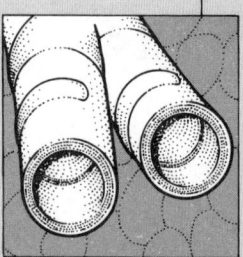

Normal bronchioles
The muscles surrounding the bronchioles are relaxed, leaving the airway open.

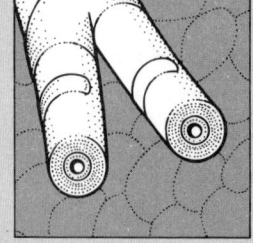

Asthmatic spasm
The muscles contract and the lining swells, narrowing the airway.

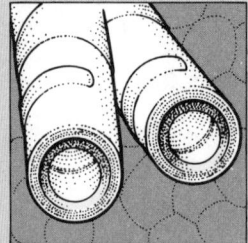

After drug treatment
The muscles relax, opening the airway, but the mucous lining remains swollen.

COMMON DRUGS

Sympathomimetics
Ephedrine
Epinephrine
Isoproterenol
Orciprenaline
Salbutamol
Salmeterol
Terbutaline

Anticholinergic
Ipratropium

Xanthines
Aminophylline
Oxtriphylline
Theophylline

Anti-inflammatories
Beclomethasone
Budesonide
Cromolyn sodium
Fluticasone
Nedocromil sodium

DECONGESTANTS

e usual cause of a blocked nose is
velling of the delicate mucous
embrane that lines the nasal passages
d excessive production of mucus as a
sult of inflammation. This may be
used by an infection (usually a
mmon cold) or it may be caused by an
ergy – for example, to pollen – a
indition known as allergic rhinitis or hay
ver. Congestion can also occur in the
uses (the air spaces in the skull),
sulting in sinusitis. Decongestants are
igs that reduce swelling of the mucous
embrane and suppress the production
mucus, therefore helping to clear
icked nasal passages and sinuses.
tihistamines, which counter the allergic
iponse in allergy-related conditions,
e discussed on p.136.

hy they are used

ist common colds do not need to be
ated with decongestants. Simple
me remedies such as steam
ialation, possibly with the addition of
aromatic oil – such as menthol or
calyptus – are often effective.
congestants are used when such
easures are ineffective or when there is
isk from untreated congestion – for
ample, in people who suffer from
current middle ear or sinus infections.
Decongestants can be taken by
uth. They also are available in the
m of drops or sprays that are applied
ectly into the nose (*topical* deconges-
its). Small quantities of decongestant
igs are often added to over-the-
inter cold remedies (see p.106).

ow they work

ien the mucous membrane lining the
ise is irritated by infection or allergy, the
od vessels supplying the membrane
come enlarged. This leads to fluid
cumulation in the surrounding tissue
d encourages the production of larger-
n-normal amounts of mucus.
Most decongestants belong to the
npathomimetic group of drugs which
nulate the sympathetic part of the
conomic nervous system (see p.91).
e effect of this action is to constrict
e blood vessels, so reducing swelling
the lining of the nose and sinuses.

ACTION OF DECONGESTANTS

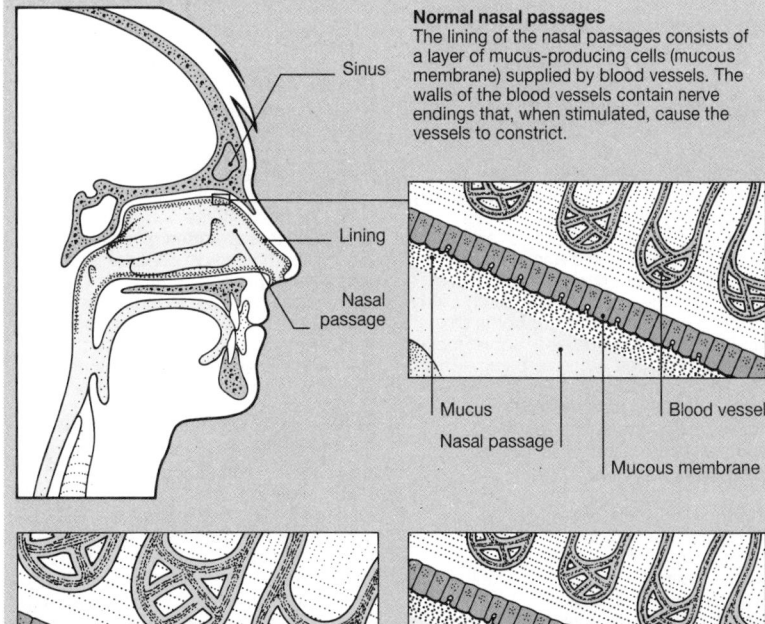

Normal nasal passages
The lining of the nasal passages consists of
a layer of mucus-producing cells (mucous
membrane) supplied by blood vessels. The
walls of the blood vessels contain nerve
endings that, when stimulated, cause the
vessels to constrict.

Sinus

Lining

Nasal
passage

Mucus

Nasal passage

Blood vessels

Mucous membrane

Congested nasal lining
When the blood vessels enlarge in response
to infection or irritation, increased amounts
of fluid pass into the mucous membrane,
which swells and produces more mucus.

Effect of decongestants
Decongestants enhance the action of
chemicals that stimulate constriction of the
blood vessels. Narrowing of the blood vessels
reduces swelling and mucus production.

How they affect you

When applied topically in drops or by
sprays, these drugs start to relieve
congestion within a few minutes. Decongestants by mouth take a little longer to
act, but their effect may last longer.
Topical decongestants used in
moderation have few adverse effects
because they are not absorbed by the
body in large amounts. Decongestants
taken by mouth are more likely to cause

symptoms related to their action on the
sympathetic nervous system, including
increased heart rate and trembling. For
these reasons they should be used with
caution by those with heart problems,
high blood pressure, or an overactive
thyroid gland.
Used for too long or in excess,
decongestants can, after giving initial
relief, do more harm than good, causing
a "rebound congestion" (see left). This
can be avoided by taking the minimum
effective dose and by using decongestant preparations only when absolutely
necessary for a very short period of time.

REBOUND CONGESTION

nis can happen when
econgestants are suddenly
ithdrawn after an extended
eriod of treatment, or when
econgestant nose drops or
prays are overused. The
sult is a sudden increase in
ongestion due to widening of
e blood vessels in the nasal
ning because blood vessels
e no longer constricted by
ie decongestant.

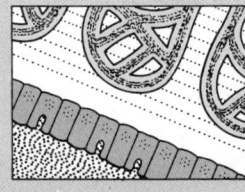

**Congestion before drug
treatment**

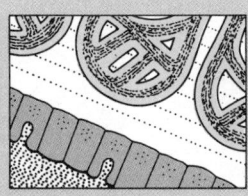

**Congestion after stopping
drug treatment**

COMMON DRUGS

Ephedrine
Oxymetazoline
Phenylephrine
Phenylpropanolamine
Pseudoephedrine
Xylometazoline

DRUGS TO TREAT COUGHS

Coughing is a natural response to irritation of the lungs and air passages, designed to expel harmful substances from the respiratory tract. Common causes of coughing include infection of the respiratory tract (for example, bronchitis or pneumonia), inflammation of the airways caused by asthma, or exposure to certain irritant substances such as smoke or chemical fumes. Depending on their cause, coughs may be productive – that is, phlegm producing – or they may be dry.

In most cases coughing is a helpful reaction that assists the body to get rid of excess phlegm or irritant substances; suppressing the cough may actually delay recovery. However, repeated bouts of coughing can be distressing, sometimes increasing irritation of the air passages. In such cases, medication to ease the cough may be recommended.

There are two main groups of cough remedies, according to whether the cough is productive or dry.

Productive coughs

Mucolytics and expectorants are the groups of drugs most commonly recommended for productive coughs when simple home remedies such as steam inhalation have failed to "loosen" the cough and make it easier to cough up phlegm. Mucolytics alter the consistency of the phlegm, making it less sticky and easier to cough up. These are often given by inhalation. Expectorants are drugs that are frequently included in over-the-counter cough and cold remedies. These are said to encourage the production of phlegm, but the overall benefits of such drugs are doubtful.

Dry coughs

In dry coughs there is no advantage to be gained from promoting the expulsion of phlegm. Drugs used for dry coughs are given to suppress the coughing mechanism by calming the part of the brain that governs the coughing reflex. Antihistamines are often given for mild coughs, particularly in children. For persistent coughs, mild narcotic drugs such as codeine are prescribed (see also Analgesics, p.92). All cough suppressants have a generally sedating effect on the brain and nervous system and commonly cause drowsiness and other side effects.

Selecting a cough medication

There is a bewildering variety of over-the-counter medications available for treating coughs. Most consist of a syrupy base to which active ingredients and flavorings are added. Many contain a number of different active ingredients, sometimes with contradictory effects: it is not uncommon to find an expectorant (for a productive cough) and a cough suppressant (for a dry cough) included in the same preparation.

It is important to select the correct type of medication for your cough to avoid the risk that you may make your condition

COLD REMEDIES

Many preparations are available over the counter to treat different symptoms of the common cold. The main ingredient is usually a mild analgesic such as acetaminophen, or ASA, and is often accompanied by a decongestant (p.105), an antihistamine (p.136), and sometimes caffeine. Often the dose of each added ingredient is too low to provide any benefit. Vitamin C (see p.528) is often included in cold relief products, but there is no evidence that it speeds recovery.

While some people find these preparations help to relieve symptoms, over-the-counter "cold cures" do not alter the course of the illness. Most physicians recommend preparations containing a single analgesic, as the best way of alleviating symptoms of the common cold. Additional decongestants or antihistamines may be taken as necessary if this does not provide adequate relief.

worse. For example, using a cough suppressant for a productive cough may prevent you from getting rid of excess phlegm and may thereby delay your recovery. It is best to choose a preparation with a single active ingredient that is appropriate for your type of cough. Diabetics may need to select a sugar-free product. If you are in any doubt ask your physician or pharmacist for advice. Because there is a danger that use of over-the-counter cough remedies to alleviate symptoms may delay the diagnosis of a more serious underlying disorder, it is important to seek medical advice for any cough that persists for longer than two days or if a cough is accompanied by additional symptoms such as fever or blood in the phlegm.

COMMON DRUGS

Expectorants
Ammonium chloride
Guaifenesin

Mucolytic
Acetylcysteine

Narcotic cough suppressants
Codeine
Hydrocodone

Non-narcotic cough suppressants
Antihistamines (see p.136)
Dextromethorphan

ACTION OF COUGH REMEDIES

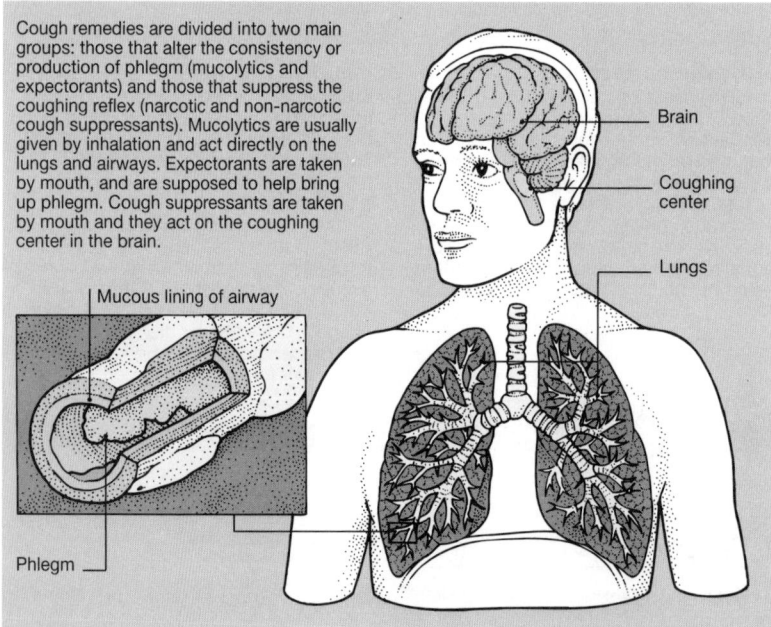

Cough remedies are divided into two main groups: those that alter the consistency or production of phlegm (mucolytics and expectorants) and those that suppress the coughing reflex (narcotic and non-narcotic cough suppressants). Mucolytics are usually given by inhalation and act directly on the lungs and airways. Expectorants are taken by mouth, and are supposed to help bring up phlegm. Cough suppressants are taken by mouth and they act on the coughing center in the brain.

Mucous lining of airway

Phlegm

Brain

Coughing center

Lungs

HEART AND CIRCULATION

The blood transports oxygen, nutrients, and heat, contains chemical messages in the form of drugs and hormones, and carries away waste products for excretion by the liver and kidneys. Pumped by the heart and carried in blood vessels (veins, arteries, and capillaries), blood circulates continuously around the body.

What can go wrong

Efficiency of the circulation may be impaired by a weakening of the heart's pumping action (heart failure) or irregularity of heartbeat (arrhythmia). In addition, the blood vessels may be narrowed and clogged by fatty deposits (atherosclerosis). This may reduce blood supply to the brain, the extremities (peripheral vascular disease), or to the heart muscle (coronary heart disease), causing angina. These last disorders can be complicated by the formation of clots which may block a blood vessel. In the arteries supplying the heart muscle, this is known as coronary thrombosis, and inside the brain it is the most frequent cause of stroke.

One common circulatory disorder is abnormally high blood pressure (hypertension), in which the pressure of the circulating blood on the vessel walls is increased for reasons not yet fully understood. One factor may be loss of elasticity of the blood vessel walls (arteriosclerosis).

A number of other conditions are caused by temporary alterations to blood vessel size. These include migraine and Raynaud's disease.

Why drugs are used

Because those suffering from heart disease often have more than one problem, several drugs may be prescribed at once. Many act directly on the heart to alter the rate and rhythm of the heartbeat. These are known as antiarrhythmics and include beta blockers and digitalis drugs.

Other drugs affect the diameter of blood vessels, either dilating them (vasodilators) to improve blood flow and reduce blood pressure and strain, or constricting them (vasoconstrictors).

Drugs may also reduce blood volume and fat levels, and alter clotting ability. Diuretics (used in the treatment of hypertension and heart failure) increase the body's excretion of water. Lipid-lowering drugs reduce blood fat levels, thereby lowering the risk of atherosclerosis. Drugs to reduce blood clotting are administered when there is a risk of abnormal blood clots forming in the veins or arteries. Drugs that increase clotting are given when the body's natural clotting mechanism is defective.

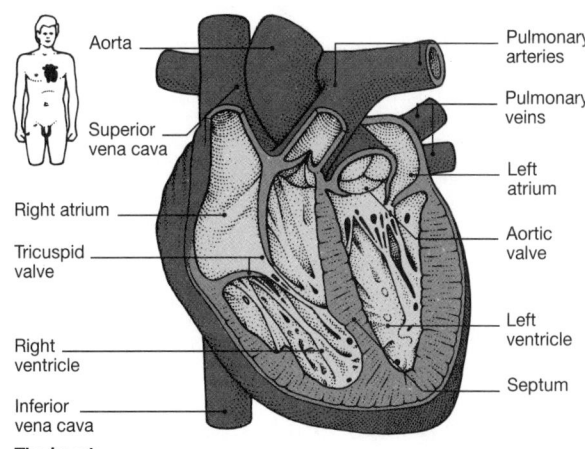

The heart
The heart is a pump containing four chambers. The atrium and ventricle on the left side pump oxygenated blood, while the corresponding chambers on the right pump deoxygenated blood. Backflow of blood is prevented by valves at the chamber exits.

How blood circulates
Deoxygenated blood is carried to the heart from all parts of the body. It is then pumped to the lungs where it becomes oxygenated. The oxygenated blood returns to the heart and from there is pumped throughout the body.

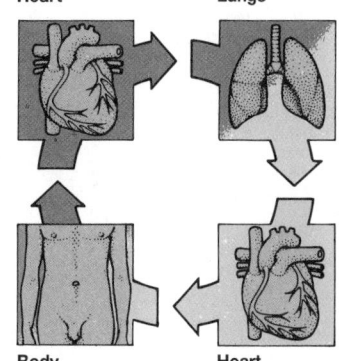

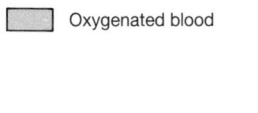

■ Deoxygenated blood

□ Oxygenated blood

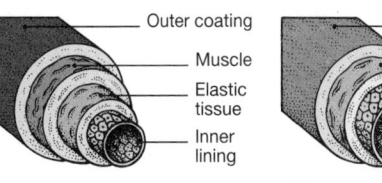

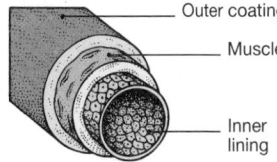

Arteries
Arteries carry blood away from the heart. Muscle walls contract and dilate in response to nerve signals.

Veins
Veins carry deoxygenated blood back to the heart. The walls are less elastic than artery walls.

MAJOR DRUG GROUPS

Digitalis drugs	Anti-angina drugs
Beta blockers	Antihypertensive drugs
Vasodilators	Lipid-lowering drugs
Diuretics	Drugs that affect blood
Anti-arrhythmic drugs	clotting

DIGITALIS DRUGS

Digitalis is the collective term for a number of naturally occurring substances (also called cardiac glycosides) found in the leaves of plants of the foxglove family and used for certain heart disorders. The principal drugs in this group are digoxin and digitoxin. Digoxin is more commonly used because it is shorter-acting and dosage is easier to adjust (see also Risks and special precautions, below).

Why they are used

Digitalis drugs do not cure heart disease but improve the heart's pumping action and so relieve many of the symptoms that result from poor heart function. They are useful for treating conditions in which the heart beats irregularly or too rapidly (notably in atrial fibrillation, see Anti-arrhythmic drugs, p.112), when it pumps too weakly (in congestive heart failure), or when the heart muscle is damaged and weakened following a heart attack.

Digitalis drugs can be used for a short period when the heart is working poorly, but in many cases they have to be taken indefinitely. Their effect may begin to wane after a time. In heart failure, digitalis drugs are often given together with a diuretic (see p.111).

How they work

The normal heartbeat results from electrical impulses generated in nerve tissue within the heart. These cause the heart muscle to contract and pump blood. By reducing the passage of electrical impulses in the heart, digitalis makes the heart beat more slowly.

The force with which the heart muscle contracts depends on chemical changes in the muscle. By promoting these chemical changes, digitalis increases the force of muscle contraction each time the heart is stimulated. This compensates for the loss of power that occurs when some of the muscle is damaged following a heart attack. The stronger heartbeat increases the flow of blood to the kidneys. This increases urine production and helps to remove the excess fluid that often accumulates as a result of heart failure.

How they affect you

Digitalis relieves symptoms of heart failure – fatigue, breathlessness, and swelling the legs – and increases your capacity for exercise. The frequency with which you need to pass urine is also increased initially.

Risks and special precautions

Digitalis drugs can be toxic and, if blood levels rise too high, may produce symptoms of digitalis poisoning. These include excessive tiredness, confusion, loss of appetite, nausea, vomiting, and diarrhea. If such symptoms occur, it is important to report them to your physician promptly.

Digoxin is normally removed from the body by the kidneys; if kidney function is impaired, the drug is more likely to accumulate in the body and cause toxic effects. Digitoxin, which is broken down in the liver, is sometimes preferred in such cases. Digitoxin can accumulate after repeated doses, especially if liver function is reduced.

Both digoxin and digitoxin are more toxic when blood potassium levels are low. Potassium deficiency is commonly caused by diuretic drugs, so that people taking these along with digitalis drugs need to have the effects of both drugs and blood potassium levels carefully monitored. Potassium supplements may be required.

ACTION OF DIGITALIS DRUGS

The heartbeat is triggered by electrical impulses that are generated by a small mass of nerve tissue in the right atrium called the pacemaker. Electrical signals pass from the pacemaker to the atrioventricular node. From here a wave of impulses spreads through the heart muscle, causing it to contract and pump blood to the body. The pumping action of the heart can become weak if the heart muscle is damaged or if the ventricles beat too fast, as in atrial fibrillation. In this condition (shown right), rapid signals from the pacemaker trigger fast and inefficient contractions of the ventricles.

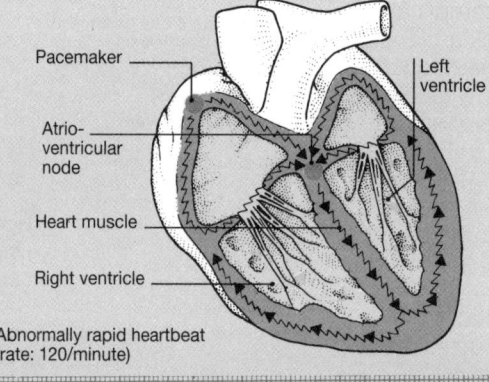

Pacemaker

Atrio-ventricular node

Heart muscle

Right ventricle

Left ventricle

Abnormally rapid heartbeat (rate: 120/minute)

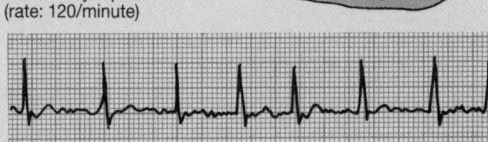

The effect of digitalis
Digitalis drugs reduce the flow of electrical impulses from the atrioventricular node so that the ventricles contract less often. In addition, by promoting the chemical changes in muscle cells necessary for muscular contraction, these drugs increase the force with which the heart muscle contracts and so improve the efficiency of each heartbeat.

Drug

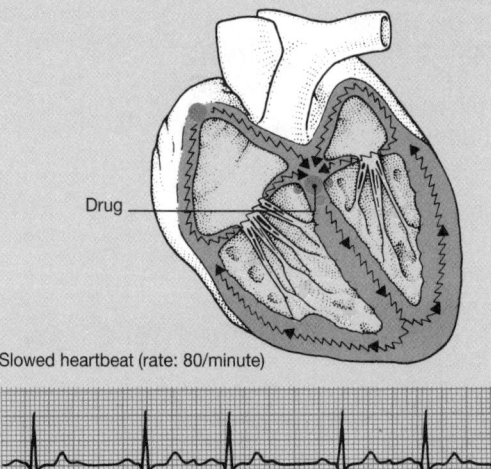

Slowed heartbeat (rate: 80/minute)

COMMON DRUGS

Digoxin
Digitoxin

BETA BLOCKERS

inephrine (from the adrenal gland) and milar substances act in part through eta *receptors* in the body. Beta blockers lso called beta adrenergic blocking gents) prevent the actions of inephrine-like substances on beta ceptors. Used mainly in heart disorders, ey are occasionally prescribed for other onditions.

Why they are used

eta blockers are used in the treatment of ngina (see p.113), hypertension (see 114), and irregular heart rhythms (see 112). They are sometimes given after a eart attack to reduce the likelihood of tal arrhythmia or further damage to the eart muscle. These drugs are also escribed to improve heart function in structive cardiomyopathy.

Beta blockers may also be given to event migraine headaches (see p.101) id to reduce some of the body mptoms associated with anxiety (see 95). They may be given to control mptoms of an overactive thyroid gland. beta blocker is sometimes given in the rm of eye drops in glaucoma to lower iid pressure inside the eye (see p.180).

low they work

/ occupying the beta receptors, beta ockers nullify the stimulating action of irepinephrine. Thus they reduce the rce and speed of the heartbeat, prevent e dilation of the airways to the lungs,

BETA RECEPTORS

Signals from the sympathetic nervous system are carried by norepinephrine, a *neurotransmitter* produced in the adrenal glands and it the ends of sympathetic nerve ibers. Beta blockers stop the signals from ne neurotransmitter.

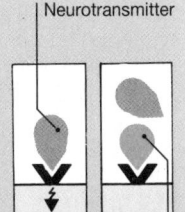

Neurotransmitter

Beta blocker

Types of beta receptor

There are two types of beta receptor: eta 1 and beta 2. Beta 1 receptors are ocated mainly in the eart muscle; beta 2 eceptors are found n the airways and lood vessels. Cardioselective drugs act mainly on eta 1 receptors; on-cardioselective drugs act on both ypes.

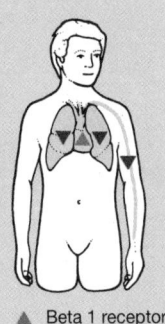

▲ Beta 1 receptors
▼ Beta 2 receptors

THE USES AND EFFECTS OF BETA BLOCKERS

The blockade of the transmission of signals through beta receptors in different parts of the body produces a wide variety of benefits and side effects according to the disease being treated. The illustration (right) shows the main areas and body systems affected by the action of beta blockers.

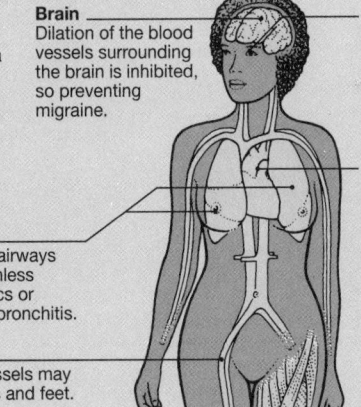

Brain
Dilation of the blood vessels surrounding the brain is inhibited, so preventing migraine.

Lungs
Constriction of the airways may provoke breathless attacks in asthmatics or those with chronic bronchitis.

Blood vessels
Constriction of the blood vessels may cause coldness of the hands and feet.

Blood pressure
This is lowered because the rate and force at which the heart pumps blood into the circulatory system is reduced.

Eyes
Beta blocker eye drops reduce fluid production and so lower pressure inside the eye.

Heart
Slowing of the heart rate and reduction of the force of the heartbeat reduce the work load of the heart, helping to prevent angina and abnormal heart rhythms. But this action may worsen heart failure.

Muscles
Muscle tremor in anxiety and overactivity of the thyroid gland is reduced.

and prevent the dilation of the blood vessels surrounding the brain and leading to the extremities. The effect of this "beta blockade" in a variety of disorders is shown in the box above.

How they affect you

Taken to treat angina, beta blockers reduce the frequency and severity of attacks. As part of the treatment for hypertension, they help to lower blood pressure and thus reduce the risks that are associated with this condition. Beta blockers help to prevent severe attacks of arrhythmia, marked by either irregular or rapid heartbeat.

Because beta blockers affect many parts of the body, they commonly produce minor side effects. By reducing heart rate and air flow to the lungs, they may reduce capacity for strenuous exercise, although this is unlikely to be noticed by somebody whose physical activity was previously limited by heart problems. Many people experience cold hands and feet while taking these drugs, due to the reduction in blood supply to the limbs. Reduced circulation can also lead to temporary impotence during beta blocker treatment.

Risks and special precautions

The main risk of beta blockers is that of provoking breathing difficulties as a result of their blocking effect on beta receptors in the lungs. Cardioselective beta blockers, which act principally on the heart, are thought to be less likely than non-cardioselective ones to cause such problems. But all beta blockers are

prescribed with caution for people with asthma, bronchitis, or other forms of respiratory disease.

Beta blockers are not usually prescribed for people who have poor circulation in the limbs, because they reduce the flow of blood and may aggravate such conditions. They are not normally given to people who are subject to heart failure because they may further reduce the force of the heartbeat. Diabetics who need to take beta blockers should be aware that they may notice a change in the warning signs of low blood sugar – in particular, symptoms such as palpitations and tremor may be suppressed.

Beta blockers should not be stopped suddenly after prolonged use; this may provoke a sudden and severe recurrence of symptoms of the original disorder, even a heart attack. Blood pressure may also rise markedly. When the treatment needs to be stopped, it should be withdrawn gradually under medical supervision.

COMMON DRUGS

Non-cardioselective
Labetalol
Nadolol
Oxprenolol
Pindolol
Propranolol
Sotalol
Timolol

Cardioselective
Acebutolol
Atenolol
Metoprolol

VASODILATORS

Vasodilators – drugs that dilate blood vessels – are commonly prescribed for disorders in which narrowing of the blood vessels leads to reduced blood flow and a consequent lower oxygen supply to parts of the body. Disorders of this type include angina, when a narrowing of the coronary arteries reduces the supply of blood, thereby causing painful spasm. They also include peripheral vascular disease, when blood vessels in the arms and legs cannot supply sufficient blood to the extremities. Vasodilators are also widely used in the treatment of high blood pressure (hypertension) and heart failure.

Several classes of vasodilator drugs are prescribed, including nitrates, *sympatholytics*, calcium channel blockers, and ACE (angiotensin-converting enzyme) inhibitors.

Why they are used

Vasodilators improve blood flow and oxygen supply to areas of the body where they are most needed. In angina, dilation of the blood vessels throughout the body reduces the force with which the heart needs to pump and therefore eases its work load (see also Anti-angina drugs, p.113). This effect is sometimes helpful in the treatment of congestive heart failure when other treatments are not effective. In peripheral vascular disease, vasodilators are usually taken on a continuing basis in order to improve blood circulation.

Vasodilator drugs have also been used for senile dementia, theoretically increasing the supply of oxygen needed by healthy brain cells. The benefits of this treatment have not been proved.

Because blood pressure depends partly on the diameter of the blood vessels, vasodilators are often helpful in treating hypertension (see Antihypertensive drugs, p.114).

ACTION OF VASODILATORS

The diameter of blood vessels is governed by the contraction of the surrounding muscle. The muscle contracts in response to signals from the sympathetic nervous system (p.91). Vasodilators encourage the muscles to relax, thus increasing the size of blood vessels.

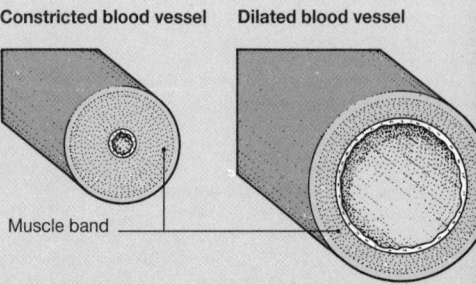

Constricted blood vessel   **Dilated blood vessel**

Muscle band

Where they act
Each type of vasodilator acts on a different part of the mechanism controlling blood vessel size to prevent contraction of the surrounding layer of muscles.

Nerves – Sympatholytics interfere with nerve signals to the muscles.

Muscle layer – Nitrates and calcium channel blockers act directly on the muscle to inhibit contraction.

Blood – ACE inhibitors block enzyme activity in the blood (see box below).

How they work

Vasodilators widen the blood vessels by relaxing the muscles that surround them. They achieve this either by affecting the action of the muscles directly (nitrates and calcium channel blockers) or by interfering with the nerve signals that govern contraction of the blood vessels (sympatholytics). ACE inhibitors act by blocking enzyme activity in the blood (see the box below).

How they affect you

In addition to relieving the symptoms of the disorders for which they are taken, vasodilators can have a number of minor adverse effects related to their action o the blood circulation. Flushing and headaches are common at the start of treatment. Dizziness and fainting may also occur as a result of lowered blood pressure. Dilation of the blood vessels can also cause a fluid buildup, leading swelling, particularly of the ankles.

Risks and special precautions

The major risk is that blood pressure m sometimes fall too low. For this reason these drugs are prescribed with cautio for those with unstable blood pressure may also be advisable to take the first dose of vasodilator drugs at a time wh you are able to sit or lie down afterwar

ACE INHIBITORS

ACE (angiotensin-converting enzyme) inhibitors are powerful vasodilators. They act by blocking the action of an enzyme in the blood-stream that is responsible for converting a chemical called angiotensin I into angiotensin II. Angiotensin II encourages constriction of the blood vessels and its absence permits them to dilate (see right).

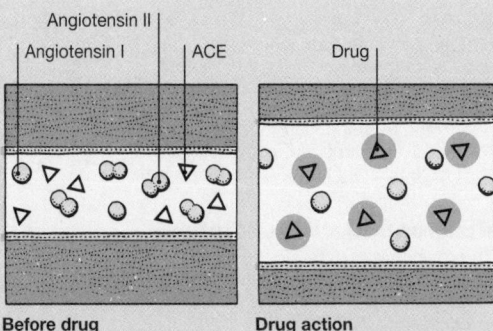

Before drug
Angiotensin I is converted by the enzyme into angiotensin II. The blood vessel constricts.

Drug action
ACE inhibitors block enzyme activity, thereby preventing the formation of angiotensin II. The blood vessel dilates.

COMMON DRUGS

Nitrates
Isosorbide dinitrate/mononitrate
Nitroglycerin

Calcium channel blockers
Amlodipine
Diltiazem
Felodipine
Nifedipine
Verapamil

ACE inhibitors
Captopril
Enalapril
Lisinopril
Quinapril

Sympatholytics
Hydralazine
Prazosin
Terazosin

IURETICS

retic drugs help to turn excess body
and water into urine. As more urine is
duced, two disorders are relieved:
ues become less water-swollen
ema) and heart action improves
ause a smaller volume of blood is
ulating. There are several classes of
etics, each of which has different
s, modes of action, and effects (see
es of diuretic, below). But all act on
kidneys, the organs that govern the
er content of the body.

y they are used

of the most common uses of
etics is in the treatment of high blood
ssure (hypertension). By removing
er-than-usual amounts of salt and
er from the bloodstream, the kidneys
uce the total volume of blood
ulating. This in turn reduces the
ssure within the blood vessels (see
hypertensive drugs, p.114).
iuretics are also widely used to treat
rt failure in which the heart's pumping
chanism has become weak. In this
rder they remove fluid that has
umulated in the tissues and lungs. The
lting drop in blood volume reduces
work of the heart.
ther conditions for which diuretics are
n prescribed include nephrotic
drome (a kidney disorder that causes
ma), cirrhosis of the liver (in which
may accumulate in the abdominal
ty), and rarely premenstrual fluid
ntion (when hormonal activity can
to swelling and bloating).
ess common uses for diuretics
ude treating glaucoma (see p.180)
Ménière's disease (see Vertigo and
ière's disease, p.102).

w they work

normal filtration process of the
eys takes water, salts (mainly
ssium and sodium), and waste
ucts out of the bloodstream. Most of
salts and water are returned to the
dstream, but certain amounts are
lled from the body together with the
te products in the urine. Diuretics
fere with this normal kidney action by

ACTION OF DIURETICS

As blood passes through the
kidney, water, sodium and
potassium salts, and waste
products are filtered out of the
bloodstream. Most of the water
and filtered salts are then
reabsorbed by the bloodstream
from the tubule, and the
remainder is excreted as urine.
By blocking the movement of
sodium back into the bloodstream, diuretics prevent the
reabsorption of water, so that
more is expelled from the body
as urine. Different diuretic drugs
act on different parts of the
tubule (see right).

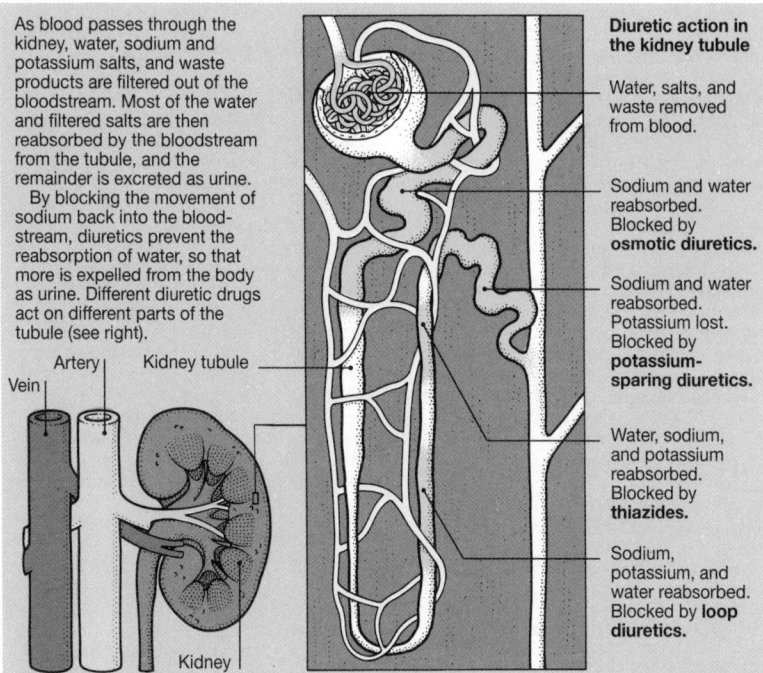

Artery   Kidney tubule

Vein

Kidney

**Diuretic action in
the kidney tubule**

Water, salts, and
waste removed
from blood.

Sodium and water
reabsorbed.
Blocked by
osmotic diuretics.

Sodium and water
reabsorbed.
Potassium lost.
Blocked by
**potassium-
sparing diuretics.**

Water, sodium,
and potassium
reabsorbed.
Blocked by
thiazides.

Sodium,
potassium, and
water reabsorbed.
Blocked by **loop
diuretics.**

reducing the amounts of sodium and
water taken back into the bloodstream,
thus increasing the volume of urine
produced. In this way the water content
of the blood is reduced and excess water
is drawn out of the tissues for elimination
in the urine.

How they affect you

All diuretics increase the frequency with
which you need to pass urine. This is
most noticeable at the start of treatment.
People who have suffered from edema
may notice that swelling – particularly of
the ankles – is reduced, and those with
heart failure may find that breathlessness
is relieved.

Risks and special precautions

Diuretics can cause chemical imbalances
in the blood. Most common of these is a
fall in potassium levels in the blood
(hypokalemia), which can cause
weakness, particularly in the elderly. Low
potassium can also trigger abnormal
heart rhythms, especially in those taking
digitalis drugs. The imbalance can usually
be corrected by potassium supplements
(see p.524) or by a potassium-sparing
diuretic. A diet that is rich in potassium
(containing plenty of fresh fruits and
vegetables) may be helpful.
Some diuretics may increase levels of
uric acid in the blood and thus the risk of
gout in susceptible people. They may also
raise blood sugar levels, which can cause
problems for diabetics.

YPES OF DIURETIC

azides The type most commonly
scribed, thiazides may lead to potassium
iciency and they are, therefore, sometimes
n together with a potassium supplement
n conjunction with a potassium-sparing
retic (see right).

op diuretics These fast-acting, powerful
gs increase the output of urine for a few
rs; they are sometimes used in
ergencies. They may cause excessive loss
otassium, which may need to be
untered as is done with thiazides. Large
ses may disturb hearing.

Potassium-sparing diuretics These mild
diuretics are usually used in conjunction with
a thiazide or a loop diuretic to prevent
excessive potassium loss.

Osmotic diuretics Prescribed only rarely,
these are used to maintain the flow of urine
through the kidneys after surgery or injury,
or sometimes during chemotherapy, and to
rapidly reduce pressure within fluid-filled
cavities.

Acetazolamide This mild diuretic drug is
used principally in the treatment of glaucoma
(see p.180).

COMMON DRUGS

Thiazides
Hydrochlorothiazide
Methyclothiazide

**Thiazide-like
diuretics**
Chlorthalidone
Indapamide
Metolazone

Osmotic diuretic
Mannitol

**Potassium-sparing
diuretics**
Amiloride
Spironolactone
Triamterene

Loop diuretics
Bumetanide
Ethacrynic acid
Furosemide

ANTI-ARRHYTHMIC DRUGS

The heart contains two upper and two lower chambers (see p.107). The pumping actions of these two sets of chambers are normally coordinated by electrical impulses so that the heart beats with a regular rhythm. If this coordination breaks down, the heart may beat abnormally, either irregularly or faster or slower than usual. The general term for abnormal heart rhythm is arrhythmia. There are several types of arrhythmia, depending on the part of the heart that is affected (see Types of arrhythmia, right).

The heart's rhythm can be disrupted in any disorder that affects the heart's mechanism for controlling its beat. Other conditions, including overactivity of the thyroid gland, and certain drugs – for example, *anticholinergic* drugs and caffeine – can also disturb heart rhythm.

A broad range of drugs is used to regulate heart rhythm, including digitalis drugs, beta blockers, and calcium channel blockers. Other drugs used are lidocaine, disopyramide, procainamide, and quinidine.

Why they are used

Minor disturbances of heart rhythm are common and do not usually require drug treatment. However, if the pumping action of the heart is seriously affected the circulation of blood throughout the body may become inefficient, and drug treatment may be necessary.

Drugs may be taken to treat individual attacks of arrhythmia, or they may be taken on a regular basis to prevent or control abnormal heart rhythms. The particular drug prescribed depends on the type of arrhythmia to be treated, but because people differ in their response, it may be necessary to try several in order to find the most effective one. When the arrhythmia is sudden and severe, it may be necessary to inject a drug immediately to restore normal heart function.

How they work

The heart's pumping action is governed by electrical impulses under the control of the sympathetic nervous system (see Autonomic nervous system, p.91). These signals pass through the heart muscle and cause each of the two pairs of heart chambers – the atria and the ventricles – to contract in turn (see Sites of drug action, left).

All anti-arrhythmic drugs alter the conduction of electrical signals in the heart, but each drug or drug group affects this sequence of events in a different way. Some block the transmission of signals to the heart (beta blockers); some affect the way signals are conducted within the heart (digitalis drugs); others affect the response of the heart muscle to the signals received (calcium channel blockers, disopyramide, procainamide, and quinidine).

How they affect you

These drugs usually prevent symptoms of arrhythmia and may restore a regular heart rhythm. Although they do not prevent all arrhythmias, they usually reduce the frequency and severity of any symptoms.

Unfortunately, as well as suppressing arrhythmias, many of these drugs tend to depress normal heart function, and may produce dizziness on standing up (postural hypotension), or increased breathlessness on exertion. Mild nausea and visual disturbances are also fairly frequent. Verapamil can cause constipation, especially in high doses. Disopyramide may interfere with the parasympathetic nervous system (see p.91), resulting in a number of anticholinergic effects.

SITES OF DRUG ACTION

Anti-arrhythmic drugs either impede the flow of electrical impulses to the heart muscle, or inhibit the ability of the muscle to contract. Beta blockers reduce the ability of the pacemaker to pass electrical signals to the atria. Digitalis drugs reduce the passage of signals from the atrioventricular node. Calcium channel blockers interfere with the ability of the heart muscle to contract by impeding the flow of calcium into muscle cells. Other drugs such as quinidine and disopyramide reduce the sensitivity of muscle cells to electrical impulses.

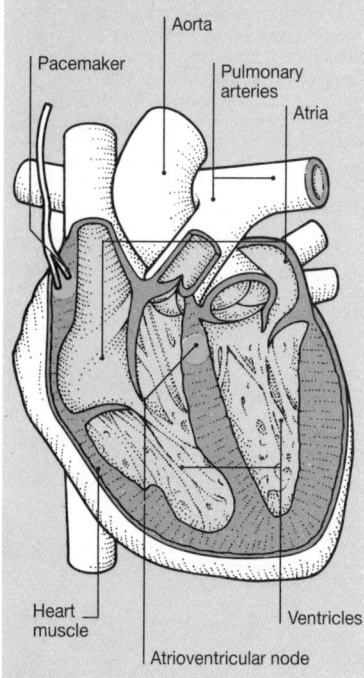

Aorta

Pacemaker

Pulmonary arteries

Atria

Heart muscle

Ventricles

Atrioventricular node

TYPES OF ARRHYTHMIA

Atrial fibrillation In this common arrhythmia, the atria contract irregularly at such a high rate that the ventricles cannot keep pace. It is treated with drugs such as digoxin, verapamil, diltiazem, a beta blocker or quinidine.

Ventricular tachycardia This arises from abnormal electrical activity in the ventricle that causes the ventricles to contract rapidly. Drugs such as disopyramide, procainamide, or quinidine may be used for long-term suppression.

Supraventricular tachycardia This occurs when extra electrical impulses arise in the atria or in the atrioventricular node. These extra impulses stimulate the ventricles to contract rapidly. Attacks may disappear on their own without treatment, but drugs such as adenosine, digoxin, verapamil, diltiazem or a beta blocker may be given.

Heart block When signals are not conducted from the atria to the ventricles, the ventricles start to beat at a slower rate. Some cases of heart block do not require treatment. For more severe heart block accompanied by dizziness and fainting, it usually necessary to fit an artificial pacemaker.

Risks and special precautions

These drugs may further disrupt heart rhythm under certain circumstances and therefore they are used only when the likely benefit outweighs the risks.

Quinidine can be toxic in overdose, resulting in a syndrome called cinchonism, which includes disturbed hearing, giddiness, and impaired vision (even blindness). Because some people are particularly sensitive to this drug, a test dose is usually given before regular treatment is started.

COMMON DRUGS

Beta blockers
(See p.109)

Calcium channel blockers
Diltiazem
Verapamil

Digitalis drugs
Digoxin
Digitoxin

Other drugs
Adenosine
Amiodarone
Bretylium
Disopyramide
Flecainide
Lidocaine
Mexiletine
Procainamide
Propafenone
Quinidine
Tocainide

ANTI-ANGINA DRUGS

ngina is chest pain produced when sufficient oxygen reaches the heart uscle. This is usually caused by a rrowing of the blood vessels (coronary teries) that carry blood and oxygen to e heart muscle. In the most common pe of angina (classic angina), pain pically occurs during exertion or notional stress. In variant angina, pain ay also occur at rest. In classic angina, rrowing of the coronary arteries results m deposits of fat – called atheroma – the walls of the arteries, whereas in riant angina it is caused by contraction pasm) of the muscle fibers in the artery lls.

Atheroma deposits build up in the teries, especially in smokers and in ople who eat a high-fat diet. This is iy, as a basic part of angina treatment, ysicians recommend that you stop noking and change your diet. verweight people are also advised to se weight in order to reduce the mands placed on their hearts. While ch changes in lifestyle often produce an provement in symptoms, drug atment to relieve angina is also quently necessary.

Three types of drugs are used to treat gina: beta blockers, nitrates, and lcium channel blockers.

hy they are used

equent episodes of angina can be sabling, and if left untreated can lead to increased risk of a heart attack. Drugs n be used both to relieve angina acks and to reduce their frequency. ople who suffer from only occasional isodes are usually prescribed a rapid-ting drug to take at the first signs of an ack, or prior to an activity that is known bring one on. A rapid-acting nitrate –

nitroglycerin – is usually prescribed for this purpose.

If attacks become more frequent or more severe, regular treatment to prevent them may be advised. Beta blockers, slow-acting nitrates, and calcium channel blockers are used as regular medication to prevent attacks. The introduction of adhesive patches for administering nitrates through the skin has extended the duration of action of nitroglycerin, making treatment easier on the individual.

Drug treatment can often control angina for many years, but it cannot cure the disorder. When severe angina cannot be controlled by drugs, heart surgery may be necessary.

How they work

Nitrates and calcium channel blockers dilate blood vessels by relaxing the muscle layer in the blood vessel wall (see also Vasodilators, p.110). This reduces strain on the heart by making it easier to pump blood.

Beta blockers interrupt the transmission of signals in the heart and so reduce stimulation of the heart muscle during exercise or stress. This also reduces the oxygen requirement of the heart muscle and makes angina attacks less likely to occur. For further information on beta blockers, see p.109.

How they affect you

Treatment with one or more of these drugs is usually effective in controlling angina. Drugs to prevent attacks allow sufferers to undertake more strenuous activities without provoking pain, and if an attack does occur, nitrates usually provide effective relief.

These drugs do not usually cause serious adverse effects, but they can

ACTION OF ANTI-ANGINA DRUGS

The pain of angina arises when the heart muscle cannot pump sufficient blood through the circulatory system. By dilating blood vessels, nitrates and calcium channel blockers make this easier. Beta blockers impede the stimulation of heart muscle, reducing its oxygen requirement, thus relieving or preventing angina pain.

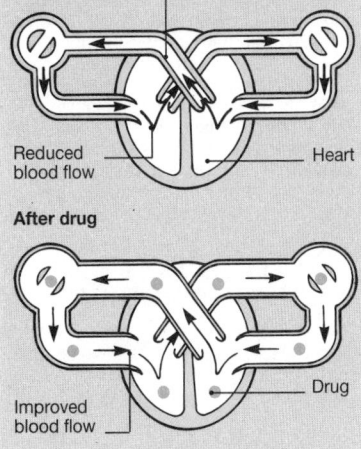

Before drug | Blood vessels of body
Reduced blood flow | Heart
After drug
Improved blood flow | Drug

produce a variety of minor symptoms. By dilating blood vessels throughout the body, nitrates and calcium channel blockers can cause dizziness and sometimes fainting (especially when standing). Other possible side effects are headaches at the start of treatment, flushing of the skin – especially of the face – and swelling of the ankles. Tolerance to nitrates can develop. A daily nitrate-free period of 10 to 12 hours is recommended with chronic use of these drugs. Beta blockers often cause cold hands and feet, and can produce tiredness and a feeling of heaviness in the legs.

COMMON DRUGS

Beta blockers
(see p.109)

Calcium channel blockers
Amlodipine
Diltiazem
Felodipine
Nifedipine
Verapamil

Nitrates
Isosorbide dinitrate/mononitrate
Nitroglycerin

CALCIUM CHANNEL BLOCKERS

he passage of calcium hrough special channels into muscle cells is an essential art of the mechanism of nuscle contraction (see ght). This relatively new lass of drugs prevents novement of calcium in the nuscles of the blood vessels nd so encourages them to ilate (see far right). The ction helps to reduce blood ressure and relieves the train on the heart muscle in ngina by making it easier or the heart to pump blood hroughout the body (see the ox above right). Calcium hannel blockers also slow e passage of nerve signals rough the heart muscle. his can be helpful for orrecting certain types of bnormal heart rhythm.

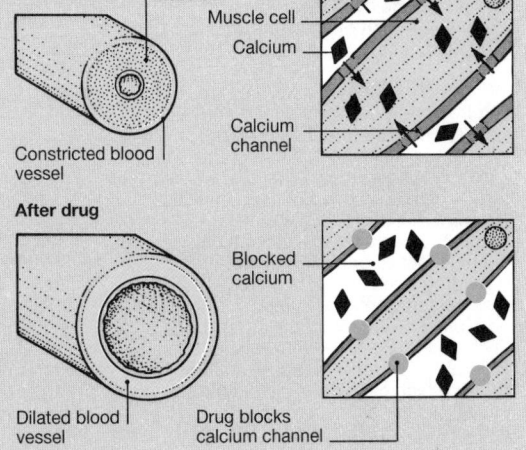

Before drug | Muscle
Muscle cell
Calcium
Calcium channel
Constricted blood vessel
After drug
Blocked calcium
Dilated blood vessel | Drug blocks calcium channel

ANTIHYPERTENSIVE DRUGS

Blood pressure is a measurement of the force exerted by the blood circulating in the arteries. Two readings are taken: one indicates force while the heart's ventricles are contracting (systolic pressure). It is a higher figure than the other reading, which measures the blood-flow push during ventricle relaxation (diastolic pressure). Blood pressure varies among individuals and normally increases with age. If a person's blood pressure is higher than normal on at least three separate occasions, a physician may diagnose hypertension.

Blood pressure may be raised as a result of an underlying disorder, which a physician will try to identify. Usually, however, it is not possible to find a cause. This condition is essential hypertension.

Although hypertension is usually without symptoms, severely raised pressure may produce headaches, palpitations, and general feelings of ill health. It is important to reduce high blood pressure, because it can have serious consequences, including stroke, heart attack, heart failure, and kidney damage. Certain groups are particularly at risk from high blood pressure. These include diabetics, smokers, people with preexisting heart damage, and those whose blood contains a high level of fat. High blood pressure is more common among black people than among whites.

A small reduction in blood pressure may be brought about by reducing weight, exercising regularly, and keeping to a low-salt diet. But for more severely raised blood pressure, one or more antihypertensive drugs may be prescribed. Several different classes of drugs have antihypertensive properties, including centrally acting antihypertensives, diuretics (p.111), beta blockers (p.109), calcium channel blockers (p.113), ACE (angiotensin converting enzyme) inhibitors (p.110), and sympatholytics. See also Vasodilators, p.110.

Why they are used

These drugs are prescribed when diet and exercise have not brought about an adequate reduction in blood pressure, and your physician sees a risk of serious consequences if the condition is not treated. Antihypertensive drugs do not cure hypertension and may have to be taken indefinitely. However, it is sometimes possible to taper off drug treatment when blood pressure has been reduced to a normal level for a year or more.

How they work

Blood pressure depends not only on the force with which the heart pumps blood, but also on the diameter of blood vessels and the volume of blood in circulation: blood pressure is increased if the vessels are narrow or the volume of blood is high.

Antihypertensive drugs lower blood pressure either by dilating the blood vessels or by reducing blood volume. Antihypertensive drugs work in different ways and some have more than one action (see Action of antihypertensive drugs, left).

Choice of drug

Drug treatment depends on the severity of hypertension. At the beginning of treatment for mild or moderately high blood pressure a single drug is used. A thiazide diuretic is often chosen for initial treatment, but it is also becoming common to use a beta blocker, a calcium channel blocker, or an ACE inhibitor. If a single drug does not reduce the blood pressure sufficiently, a diuretic in combination with one of the other drugs may be used. Some people with moderate hypertension require a third drug, in which case a sympatholytic or centrally acting antihypertensive may also be given. The choice of drug(s) may be influenced by the fact that some antihypertensive agents increase plasma lipids (fats).

Severe hypertension is usually controlled with a combination of several drugs, which may need to be given in high doses. A physician may need to try number of drugs before finding a combination that controls blood pressure without unacceptable side effects.

How they affect you

Since most people with hypertension have few, if any, symptoms, drug side effects may be more noticeable than an immediate beneficial effect. Some antihypertensive drugs may cause dizziness and fainting at the start of treatment because they can sometimes produce an excessive fall in blood pressure. It may take a while for the physician to determine a dosage that avoids such effects. For detailed information on the adverse effects of drugs used to treat hypertension, consult the individual drug profiles in Part 4.

Risks and special precautions

Since your physician needs to know exactly how treatment with a particular drug affects your hypertension – the benefits as well as side effects – it is important to keep using antihypertensive medication as prescribed, even though you may feel the problem is under control. Sudden withdrawal of some of these drugs may cause a dangerous rebound blood pressure: when treatment is stopped the dose needs to be reduced gradually under medical supervision.

COMMON DRUGS

Diuretics
(see p.111)

Beta blockers
(see p.109)

Calcium channel blockers
(see p.113)

ACE inhibitors
(see p.110)

Centrally acting antihypertensives
Clonidine
Methyldopa

Sympatholytics
Hydralazine
Prazosin
Terazosin

Other drugs
Minoxidil

ACTION OF ANTI-HYPERTENSIVE DRUGS

Each type of antihypertensive drug acts on a different part of the body to lower blood pressure.

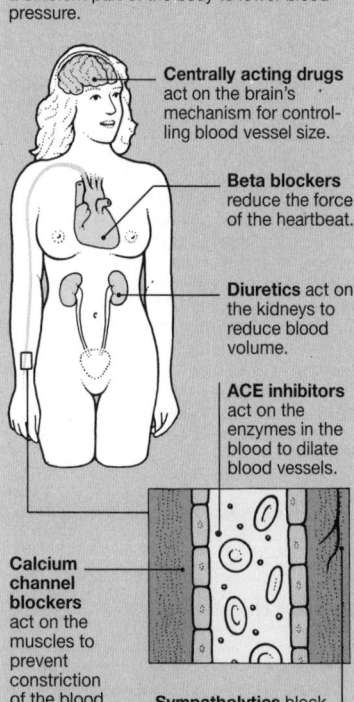

Centrally acting drugs act on the brain's mechanism for controlling blood vessel size.

Beta blockers reduce the force of the heartbeat.

Diuretics act on the kidneys to reduce blood volume.

ACE inhibitors act on the enzymes in the blood to dilate blood vessels.

Calcium channel blockers act on the muscles to prevent constriction of the blood vessels.

Sympatholytics block nerve signals that trigger constriction of blood vessels.

IPID-LOWERING DRUGS

e blood contains several types of fats
so known as lipids). Some of these are
eneficial but others – particularly
turated fats such as cholesterol found
meat and dairy products – can be
maging if present in excess. The main
k is atherosclerosis, in which fatty
eposits, called atheroma, build up in the
teries, restricting and disrupting the flow
blood. This can lead to a greater
elihood of the formation of abnormal
ood clots leading to potentially fatal
sorders such as stroke and heart attack.
For most people, cutting down the
mount of fat in the diet is sufficient to
duce the risk of atherosclerosis.
owever, for others, often those with an
herited tendency to high levels of fat in
e blood (hyperlipidemia), treatment with
id-lowering drugs may also be
commended.

hy they are used

id-lowering drugs are generally
escribed only when dietary measures
ve failed to control hyperlipidemia.
ey may also be given when an
dividual is considered to be at particular
k from atherosclerosis – for example,
abetics and people already suffering
m circulatory disorders. Research is
w being done to see if lowering
olesterol will remove existing atheroma
d prevent accumulation of new
posits.
For maximum benefit, these drugs
ed to be used in conjunction with a
v-fat diet, exercise, and a reduction in
er risk factors such as obesity and
oking. Because the choice of drug
pends to some extent on the particular
e of lipid that is causing problems, a
medical history and laboratory
alysis of blood samples are needed
fore drug treatment is prescribed.

ow they work

e salts, which contain large amounts of
olesterol, are normally released into the
wel to aid digestion and are then
absorbed into the bloodstream. By
cking the reabsorption of cholesterol-
rrying bile salts, some drugs, notably
olestyramine, colestipol, and neomycin,
rease the loss of cholesterol from the
dy and thus help to lower the level of
in the bloodstream. Other drugs –
fibrate, gemfibrozil, niacin, and
bucol – prevent conversion of fatty
ds to lipids in the liver (see Action of
d-lowering drugs, above right). Statin
gs inhibit an enzyme which produces
olesterol in the liver, so reducing
olesterol levels.
Lipid-lowering drugs do not correct the
derlying cause of raised levels of fat in
blood, therefore it is usually necessary
continue drug treatment indefinitely.
thdrawal of treatment almost always
ds to a return of high blood lipid levels.

ACTION OF LIPID-LOWERING DRUGS

Lipid-lowering drugs reduce the levels of fats
in the blood by interfering with the absorption
of bile salts in the bowel, or by altering the
way in which the liver converts fatty acids in
the blood into different types of lipids.

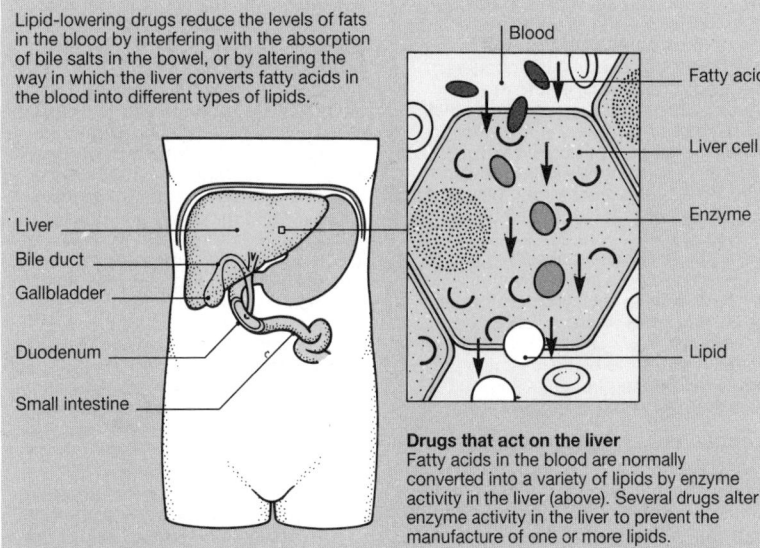

Liver
Bile duct
Gallbladder
Duodenum
Small intestine

Blood
Fatty acid
Liver cell
Enzyme
Lipid

Drugs that act on the liver
Fatty acids in the blood are normally
converted into a variety of lipids by enzyme
activity in the liver (above). Several drugs alter
enzyme activity in the liver to prevent the
manufacture of one or more lipids.

Drugs that act on bile salts
Bile is produced by the liver
and released into the small
intestine via the bile duct to
aid digestion. Salts in the
bile carry large amounts of
cholesterol and are normally
reabsorbed into the
bloodstream from the
intestine during digestion
(right). Some drugs combine
with bile salts in the intestine
and prevent their
reabsorption (far right). This
action reduces the levels of
bile salts in the blood, and
triggers the liver to convert
more cholesterol into bile
salts, thus reducing cholesterol levels in the blood.

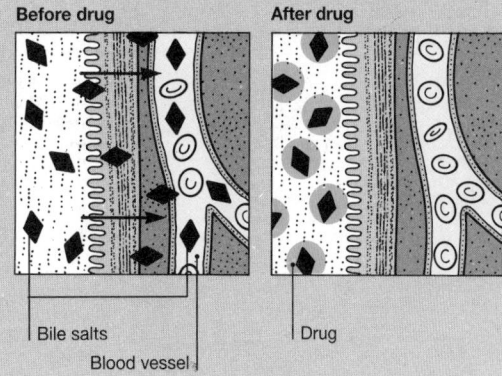

Before drug

After drug

Bile salts
Blood vessel
Drug

How they affect you

Because hyperlipidemia and atherosclerosis are without symptoms, you are unlikely
to notice any short-term benefits from
these drugs. By increasing the amount of
bile in the digestive tract, several of these
drugs can cause nausea and constipation
(colestipol and cholestyramine) or diarrhea
(clofibrate, niacin, and probucol).

Risks and special precautions

Cholestyramine, colestipol, and neomycin
are not absorbed from the bowel into the
bloodstream and therefore have few
adverse effects. They may, however, limit
absorption of certain fat-soluble vitamins;
supplements may be recommended (see
Vitamins, p.161). They may also interfere
with the absorption of other drugs. Other
lipid-lowering drugs that act in the liver, in
particular clofibrate, can increase suscep-

tibility to gallstones. They can occasionally upset the balance of different types of
lipids in the bloodstream. Regular monitoring of blood samples is often advised.
They are used with caution in those with
reduced liver function. Drugs that block
cholesterol formation, such as the statin
drugs, should be given with the evening
meal to achieve maximum benefit.

COMMON DRUGS

Drugs that act on the liver	Pravastatin
Bezafibrate	Probucol
Clofibrate	Simvastatin
Fenofibrate	
Gemfibrozil	**Drugs that act on bile salts**
Lovastatin	Cholestyramine
Niacin	Colestipol
	Neomycin

DRUGS THAT AFFECT BLOOD CLOTTING

When bleeding occurs from injury or surgery, the body normally acts swiftly to stem the flow by sealing the breaks in the blood vessels. This occurs in two stages – first when cells called platelets accumulate as a plug at the opening in the blood vessel wall, and then when these platelets produce chemicals that activate clotting factors in the blood to form a protein called fibrin. Vitamin K plays an important role in this process (see The clotting mechanism, below). An enzyme in the blood called plasmin ensures that clots are broken down when the injury has been repaired.

Some disorders interfere with this process, either preventing clot formation or creating clots uncontrollably. There is a danger that a lack of blood clotting will result in excessive blood loss; inappropriate development of clots can lead to blockage of the blood to a vital organ.

Drugs used to promote blood clotting

Fibrin formation depends on the presence in the blood of several clotting factor proteins. When Factor VIII is absent or at low levels, an inherited disease called hemophilia exists – the symptoms almost always appearing only in males. Factor IX deficiency causes another bleeding condition called Christmas disease, named after the person in whom it was first identified. Lack of these clotting factors can lead to uncontrolled bleeding or excessive bruising following injury.

Regular drug treatment for hemophilia is not normally required. But if severe bleeding or bruising occurs, a concentrated form of the missing factor, extracted from normal blood, may be injected in order to promote clotting and so halt bleeding. Injections may need to be repeated for several days after injury.

It is sometimes useful to promote blood clotting in non-hemophiliacs when bleeding is difficult to stop (for example, after surgery). In such cases, blood clots are sometimes stabilized by reducing the action of plasmin with an antifibrinolytic (or hemostatic) drug such as aminocaproic acid; this is also occasionally given to hemophiliacs prior to minor surgery such as tooth extraction.

A tendency to bleed may also occur as a consequence of vitamin K deficiency (see the box below).

Drugs used to prevent abnormal blood clotting

Blood clots normally form only in response to injury. In some people, however, there is a tendency for clots to form in the blood vessels without apparent cause. Disturbed blood flow as a result of the presence of fatty deposits – atheroma – inside the blood vessels increases the risk of the formation of this type of abnormal clot (or thrombus). In addition, a portion of a blood clot (known as an embolus) formed in response to injury or surgery may sometimes break off and be carried away in the bloodstream. The likelihood of this occurring is increased by long periods of little or no activity. When an abnormal clot forms, there is a risk that it may lodge in a blood vessel, thus blocking the blood supply to a vital organ such as the brain or heart.

Three main types of drugs are used to prevent and disperse clots: antiplatelet

THE CLOTTING MECHANISM

When a blood vessel wall is damaged, platelets accumulate at the site of damage and form a plug (1). Platelets clumped together release chemicals that activate blood clotting factors (2). These factors together with vitamin K act on a substance called fibrinogen and convert it to fibrin (3). Strands of fibrin become enmeshed in the platelet plug to form a blood clot (4).

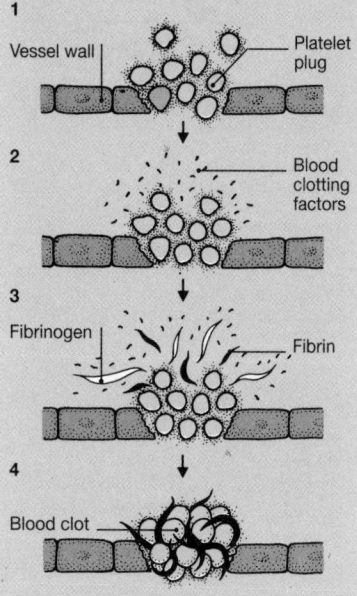

1

Vessel wall — Platelet plug

2

Blood clotting factors

3

Fibrinogen — Fibrin

4

Blood clot

VITAMIN K

Vitamin K is required for the production of several blood clotting factors. It is absorbed from the intestine in fats, but in some diseases of the small intestine or pancreas in which fat is poorly absorbed, the level of vitamin K in the circulation is low, resulting in impaired blood clotting. A similar problem sometimes occurs in newborn babies due to an absence of the vitamin. Injections of a vitamin K preparation called phytonadione are used to restore normal levels.

ACTION OF ANTIPLATELET DRUGS

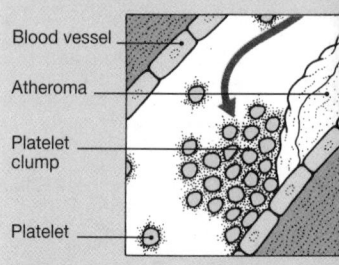

Blood vessel

Atheroma

Platelet clump

Platelet

Before drug
When blood flow is disrupted by atheroma in the blood vessels, platelets tend to clump together.

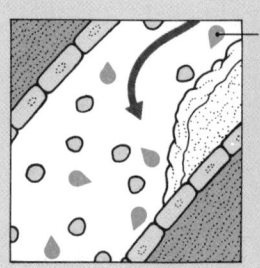

Antiplatelet drug

After drug
Antiplatelet drugs reduce the ability of platelets to stick together and so prevent clot formation.

drugs, anticoagulant drugs, and thrombolytic drugs.

Antiplatelet drugs

Taken regularly by people with a tendency to form clots in the fast-flowing blood of the heart and arteries, these are also given to prevent clots from forming after heart surgery. They reduce the tendency of platelets to stick together when blood flow is disrupted (see Action of antiplatelet drugs, above).

The most widely used antiplatelet drug is ASA (see also Analgesics, p.92). ASA has an antiplatelet action when given in much lower doses than would be necessary to reduce pain. In these low doses adverse effects that may occur when the drug is given in pain-relieving doses are unlikely. Other less common antiplatelet drugs include dipyridamole and sulfinpyrazone.

Anticoagulants

Anticoagulant drugs help to maintain normal blood flow in people who are at risk from clot formation. They can either prevent the formation of blood clots in veins or stabilize an existing clot so that does not break away and become a

rculation-stopping embolism. All anti-
oagulant drugs reduce the activity of
ertain blood-clotting factors, although
e precise mode of action of each drug
ffers (see Action of anticoagulant drugs,
ght). They do not, however, dissolve
ots that have already formed: these are
eated with thrombolytics (below).
Anticoagulants fall into two groups:
ose such as heparin and enoxaparin
at are given by injection and act
mmediately, and those that are given by
outh and take effect after a few days,
ch as warfarin.

jected anticoagulants

eparin is used mainly in the hospital
ring or after surgery. In addition, it is
so given during kidney dialysis to
event clots from forming in the dialysis
uipment. Heparin cannot be given by
outh; it is given intravenously or
bcutaneously. (Enoxaparin can only be
ven subcutaneously.)
Heparin is sometimes given prior to
arting regular treatment with an oral
ticoagulant.

ral anticoagulants

ese drugs are mainly used to prevent
e formation of clots in veins – they are
ss likely to prevent the formation of
ood clots in arteries. Oral
ticoagulants may be given following
ury or surgery (in particular, heart valve
placement) when there is a high risk of
bolism. They are also given as a
eventive treatment to people who are at
k from strokes.
A common problem with these drugs is
at overdosage may lead to bleeding
m the nose, gums, or in the urinary
ct, or easy bruising. For this reason the
sage needs to be carefully calculated;
gular blood tests are performed to

ACTION OF ANTICOAGULANT DRUGS

Anticoagulants block the
action of certain blood-clotting
factors which convert
fibrinogen into fibrin, the
protein that binds platelets
into blood clots.

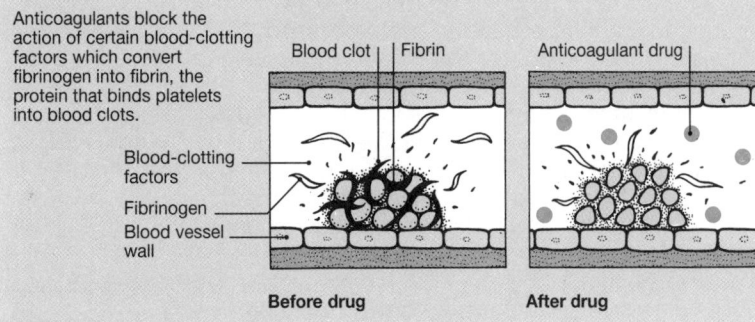

Blood clot | Fibrin | Anticoagulant drug
Blood-clotting factors
Fibrinogen
Blood vessel wall

Before drug   **After drug**

ensure that the clotting mechanism is
correctly adjusted. Warfarin is the most
widely used drug of this type.
The action of oral anticoagulant drugs
may be affected by many other drugs and
foods high in vitamin K such as green,
leafy vegetables. It may therefore be
necessary to alter the dosage of
anticoagulant when other drugs also are
needed. People who have been
prescribed anticoagulants should avoid
certain foods and carry a warning list of
drugs which should not be administered.
ASA, in particular, should not be taken
together with anticoagulants except on
the direction of a physician.

Thrombolytics

Also known as fibrinolytics, these drugs
are used to dissolve clots that have
already formed. They are usually
administered in the hospital by
intravenous injection to clear a blocked
blood vessel – for example, in coronary

thrombosis. As well as being given
intravenously, thrombolytic drugs may
also be administered directly into a
blocked blood vessel.
The main thrombolytic drugs are
streptokinase and tissue plasminogen
activator (tPA), both of which act by
increasing the blood level of plasmin, the
naturally occurring enzyme that normally
breaks down fibrin (see Action of
thrombolytic drugs, below).
The most common problems with the
use of these drugs are increased susceptibility to bleeding and bruising. Streptokinase can cause allergic reactions which
may take the form of hives (urticaria),
swelling, and breathing difficulty.

COMMON DRUGS

Normal blood extracts
Factor VIII (cryoprecipitated, concentrate)
Factor IX complex
Frozen plasma
Platelet concentrate

Antifibrinolytic drug
Aminocaproic acid
Tranexamic acid

Vitamin K
Phytonadione

Antiplatelet drugs
ASA
Dipyridamole
Sulfinpyrazone

Anticoagulant drugs
Enoxaparin
Heparin
Warfarin

Thrombolytic drugs
Streptokinase
Tissue plasminogen activator (tPA)
Urokinase

ACTION OF THROMBOLYTIC DRUGS

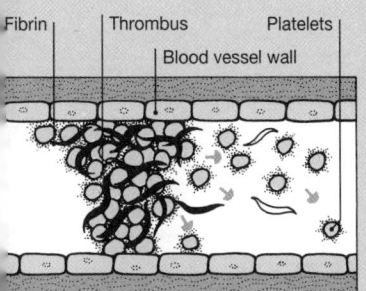

Fibrin | Thrombus | Platelets
Blood vessel wall

efore drug
Vhen platelets accumulate in a blood vessel
nd are reinforced by strands of fibrin, the
esultant blood clot, called a thrombus,
annot be dissolved either by antiplatelet
rugs or anticoagulant drugs.

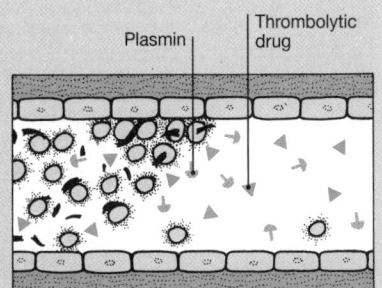

Plasmin | Thrombolytic drug

After drug
Thrombolytic drugs boost the action of
plasmin, an enzyme in the blood that breaks
up the strands of fibrin that bind the clot
together. This allows the accumulated
platelets to disperse and restores normal
blood flow.

GASTROINTESTINAL TRACT

The gastrointestinal tract (also known as the digestive or alimentary tract) is the pathway through which food passes as it is processed to enable the body to absorb the nutrients it contains. It consists of the mouth, esophagus, stomach, duodenum, small intestine, large intestine (including the colon and rectum), and anus. In addition, a number of other organs are involved in the digestion of food: the salivary glands in the mouth, the liver, pancreas, and gallbladder. These organs, together with the gastrointestinal tract, form the digestive system.

The digestive system breaks down large complex chemicals (proteins, fats, carbohydrates) present in the food we eat into simpler molecules that can be used by the body (see also Nutrition, p.160). Undigested or indigestible material, together with some of the body's waste products, pass to the large intestine. When a sufficient mass has reached the rectum, the contents are expelled from the body as feces.

What can go wrong

A common disorder is the inflammation of the lining of the stomach or intestine (gastroenteritis), usually the result of an infection or parasitic infestation. Damage can also be done by the inappropriate production of digestive juices, leading to minor complaints like acidity and major disorders like peptic ulcer. The lining of the intestines can be damaged by inflammation (inflammatory bowel disease). The rectum and anus can become painful and irritated by damage to the lining, tears in the skin at the opening of the anus (anal fissure), or enlarged veins (hemorrhoids).

The most frequent gastrointestinal disorders, constipation and diarrhea, usually occur when something disrupts the normal muscle contractions that propel food residue through the bowel.

Why drugs are used

Many drugs for gastrointestinal disorders are taken by mouth and act directly on the digestive tract without entering the bloodstream. Such drugs include certain antibiotics. Some antacids for peptic ulcers and excess stomach acidity, and bulk-forming agents for constipation and diarrhea, also pass through the system unabsorbed.

However, for many disorders, drugs with a systemic effect are required, including some anti-ulcer drugs, narcotic antidiarrheal drugs, and some of the drugs for inflammatory bowel disease.

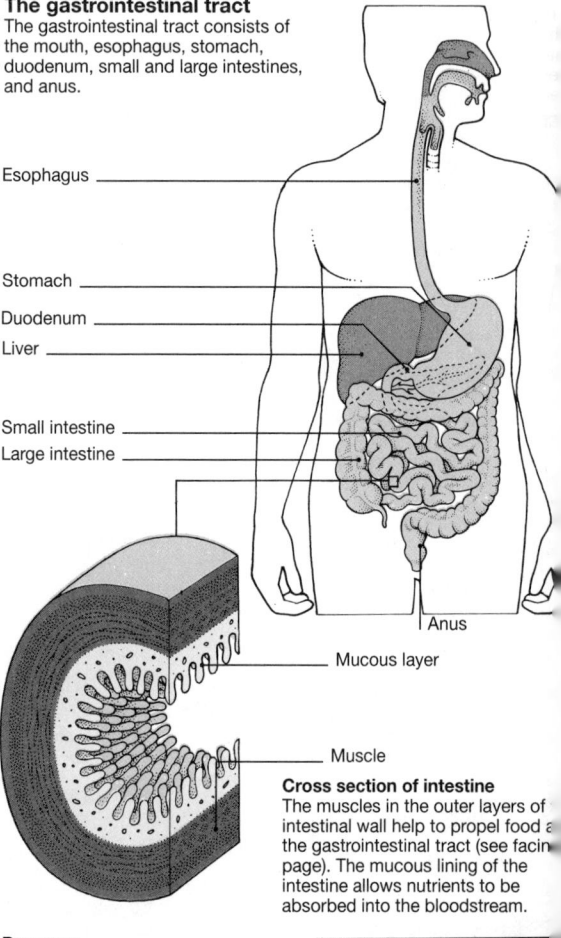

The gastrointestinal tract
The gastrointestinal tract consists of the mouth, esophagus, stomach, duodenum, small and large intestines, and anus.

Esophagus

Stomach

Duodenum

Liver

Small intestine

Large intestine

Anus

Mucous layer

Muscle

Cross section of intestine
The muscles in the outer layers of intestinal wall help to propel food a the gastrointestinal tract (see facin page). The mucous lining of the intestine allows nutrients to be absorbed into the bloodstream.

Pancreas
The pancreas produces *enzymes* that digest fats, proteins, and carbohydrates into simpler substances. Pancreatic juices neutralize acidity of the stomach contents.

Gallbladder
Bile produced by the liver is stored in the gallbladder and released into the small intestine. Bile improves the digestion of fats by reducing them to smaller units that are more easily acted upon by digestive enzymes.

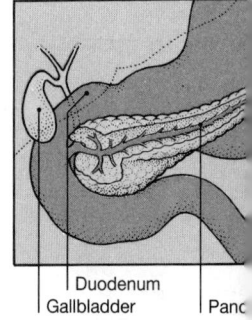

Duodenum

Gallbladder

Panc

MAJOR DRUG GROUPS

Antacids	Drugs for rectal and
Anti-ulcer drugs	anal disorders
Antidiarrheal drugs	Drug treatment
Laxatives	for gallstones
Drugs for inflammatory	
bowel disease	

The lining of the gastrointestinal tract

The internal lining of the different sections of the gastro-intestinal tract varies according to the function of that part, depending, for example, on whether its principal role is to secrete digestive juices or to absorb nutrients.

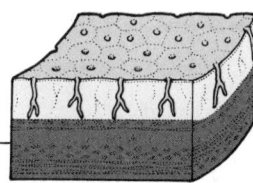

Stomach
Its main job is to store meals and pass food to the intestine. The lining of the stomach releases gastric juice that partly digests food. The stomach wall continuously produces thick mucus that forms a protective coating.

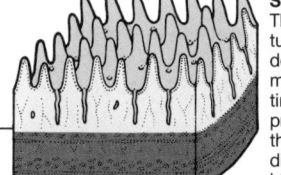

Duodenum
This is the tube that connects the stomach to the intestine. Its lining may be damaged by excess acid produced by the stomach.

Small intestine
The small intestine is a long tube in which food is broken down by digestive juices. The mucous lining is covered with tiny projections called villi that provide a large surface area through which the products of digestion are absorbed into the bloodstream.

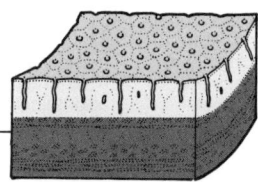

Large intestine
The large intestine receives undigested food and indigest-ible material from the small intestine. Water and mineral salts pass through the lining into the bloodstream.

MOVEMENT OF FOOD THROUGH THE GASTROINTESTINAL TRACT

Food is propelled through the gastrointestinal tract by rhythmic waves of muscular contraction known as peristalsis. The illustration (right) shows how peristaltic contractions of the bowel wall push food through the intestine.

Muscle contraction in the tract is controlled by the autonomic nervous system (p.91) and is therefore easily disrupted by drugs that either stimulate or inhibit the activity of the autonomic nervous system. Excessive peristaltic action may cause diarrhea; slowed peristalsis may cause constipation.

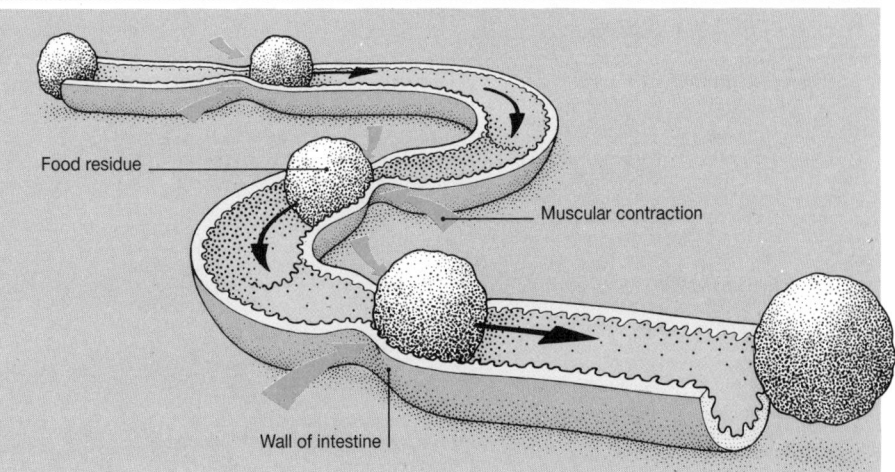

Food residue

Muscular contraction

Wall of intestine

ANTACIDS

Digestive juices in the stomach contain acid and enzymes that break down food before it passes into the intestine. The wall of the stomach is normally protected from the action of digestive acid by a layer of mucus that is constantly secreted by the stomach lining. Problems arise when the stomach lining is damaged or when too much acid is produced and eats away at the mucous layer. Excess acid leading to discomfort, commonly referred to as indigestion, may result from overeating, drinking coffee or alcohol, smoking, anxiety, or, in some people, from eating certain foods. Some drugs, notably ASA and non-steroidal anti-inflammatory drugs, can also irritate the stomach lining and even cause ulcers.

Antacids are used to neutralize acid and thus relieve pain. The types most regularly used are those that contain magnesium and aluminum. Some antacids contain calcium.

Why they are used

Antacids may be needed when simple remedies such as a change in diet or a glass of milk fail to relieve indigestion. They are especially useful one to three hours after meals to neutralize after-meal acid surge.

Physicians prescribe these drugs to relieve heartburn or acid indigestion (pain in the lower chest or upper abdomen caused by or aggravated by acid) in disorders such as inflammation or ulceration of the esophagus, stomach lining, and duodenum. Antacids usually relieve pain within a few minutes. Regular treatment with antacids reduces the acidity of the stomach and thereby encourages the healing of any ulcers that may have formed.

How they work

By neutralizing stomach acid, antacids prevent inflammation, relieve pain, and allow the mucous layer and lining to mend. When used in the treatment of ulcers, they prevent acid from attacking damaged stomach lining and so allow the ulcer to heal.

How they affect you

If antacids are taken according to instructions, they are usually effective in relieving abdominal discomfort caused by acid. The speed of action varies depending on the ability to neutralize acid. Their duration of action also varies; short-acting drugs may have to be taken quite frequently. Although most antacids have few serious side effects when used only occasionally, some may cause diarrhea, and others may cause constipation (see Types of antacids, below).

Risks and special precautions

Antacids should not be taken to prevent abdominal pain on a regular basis except under medical supervision, as they may suppress the symptoms of a serious disorder. Prolonged use of any antacid can cause an increase in the production of stomach acid when treatment is stopped suddenly.

All antacids can interfere with the absorption of other drugs. For this reason, if you are taking a prescription medicine, you should check with your physician before taking an antacid.

ACTION OF ANTACIDS

Excess acid in the stomach may eat away at the protective layer of mucus that lines the stomach. When this occurs, or when the mucous lining is damaged, for example, by an ulcer, stomach acid comes into contact with the underlying tissues, causing pain and inflammation (right). Antacids react with stomach acid to reduce the acidity of the digestive juices. This helps to prevent pain and inflammation, and allows the mucous layer to repair itself (far right).

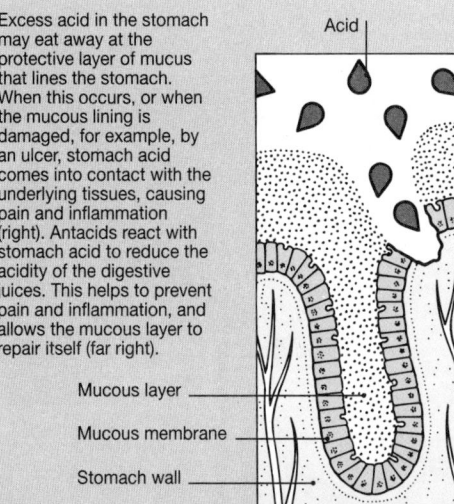

Acid | Drug

Mucous layer

Mucous membrane

Stomach wall

Before drug
Acid damages mucous layer and mucous membrane.

After drug
Acid is neutralized by antaci action.

COMMON DRUGS

Aluminum hydroxide
Calcium carbonate
Magnesium hydroxide
Sodium bicarbonate

TYPES OF ANTACIDS

Aluminum compounds These have a prolonged action and are widely used especially for the treatment of peptic ulcers. They may cause constipation, but this is often countered by combining this type of antacid with one that contains magnesium. Aluminum compounds can interfere with the absorption of phosphate from the diet, causing weakness and bone damage if taken in high doses over a long period.

Magnesium compounds Like the aluminum compounds, these have a prolonged action. In large doses they can cause diarrhea, and in people who have impaired kidney function, a high blood magnesium level may build up, causing weakness, lethargy, and drowsiness.

Sodium bicarbonate Sodium bicarbonate, the only sodium compound used as an antacid, acts quickly, but its effect soon passes. It reacts with stomach acids to produce gas, which may cause bloating and belching. This antacid is not advised for people with heart or kidney disease, as it can lead to the accumulation of water (edema) in the legs and lungs, or serious changes in the acid-base balance of the blood.

Combined preparations Antacids may be combined with other substances called alginates and antifoaming agents. Alginates are intended to float on the contents of the stomach and produce a neutralizing layer to subdue acid that can rise into the esophagus, causing heartburn.

Antifoaming agents, usually simethicone, are intended to relieve flatulence. In some preparations a local anesthetic is combined with the antacid to relieve discomfort in esophagitis. None of these additives is of primary benefit.

ANTI-ULCER DRUGS

ormally, the linings of the esophagus, tomach, and duodenum are protected om the irritant action of stomach acids y a layer of mucus. If this layer becomes amaged, stomach acid may erode the nderlying tissue, causing a peptic ulcer. his usually leads to abdominal pain, omiting, and loss of appetite. Duodenal cers, the most common peptic ulcers, e usually less of a problem than other pes.

The exact cause of peptic ulcers is not nderstood, but certain predisposing ctors have been identified; these clude heavy smoking, the regular use f ASA or similar drugs, the overuse of cohol and coffee, and a stressful estyle combined with irregular and shed meals. A bacterium called elicobacter pylori, found in the majority patients with duodenal ulcers, is now ought to be a causative agent. The sual first-line treatment is with either an 2 blocker (cimetidine, famotidine, zatidine, or ranitidine) or other anti-ulcer ug such as misoprostol, omeprazole, renzepine, or sucralfate.

SITES OF PEPTIC ULCERS

Peptic ulcers most commonly occur in the walls of the stomach or duodenum when damage to the mucous lining allows stomach acid to erode the underlying tissue. Ulcers may also form in the esophagus if acid backs up into the esophagus. Peptic ulcers also occur at the margin where the stomach has been sewn to the intestine after ulcer surgery. Similar drugs are prescribed for all three types of peptic ulcer.

Esophagus

Stomach

Duodenum

Why they are used

Drugs are prescribed both to relieve symptoms and to heal the ulcer. Until recently, drugs could heal but not cure ulcers. However, eradication of Helicobacter pylori by either "triple therapy" (bismuth subsalicylate and two antibiotics) or other combinations of an anti-ulcer drug with one or more antibiotics may provide a cure.

Surgical treatment is reserved for complications such as obstruction,

perforation, and hemorrhage and the possibility of malignancy in the case of stomach ulcers.

How they work

Drugs protect ulcers from the action of stomach acid, thereby allowing the underlying tissue to heal. H_2 blockers, misoprostol, omeprazole, and pirenzepine reduce the amount of acid released into the stomach, whereas sucralfate forms a protective coating over the ulcer (see Action of anti-ulcer drugs, left). Misoprostol and pirenzepine also have a protective action.

How they affect you

These drugs begin to reduce pain within a few hours, and in most cases allow the ulcer to heal in four to eight weeks. They produce few side effects, although one of the H_2 blockers, cimetidine, can cause confusion in the elderly, particularly if the stated dose is exceeded. Sucralfate may cause constipation, and misoprostol diarrhea. Because these drugs may mask symptoms of cancerous stomach ulcers, they are normally prescribed only when stomach cancer has been ruled out.

Risks and special precautions

The H_2 blockers are not usually prescribed for courses of more than six months because their safety over prolonged periods is not established. Long-term therapy with omeprazole is also not recommended. Sucralfate is prescribed for up to eight weeks at a time; it may interfere with absorption of fats and so reduce the absorption of vitamins A, D, E, and K, which are dissolved in fat. Prolonged use may require vitamin supplements.

ACTION OF ANTI-ULCER DRUGS

H_2 blockers
Histamine is a chemical released by mast cells (see Allergy, p.135). It can produce a number of effects, including dilation of the blood vessels in the nose and eyes, constriction of the airways, skin rashes hives), and increased secretion of stomach acid. Antihistamines (p.136), used medically for many years to block the effects of

histamine in allergic disorders, act only on receptors known as H_1 receptors. They do not block the effect of histamine on stomach acid production, which is triggered by the action of histamine on H_2 receptors. A new type of drug was therefore developed to block this action. Since their introduction in the 1970s, the H_2 blockers have been among the most widely prescribed drugs in Canada.

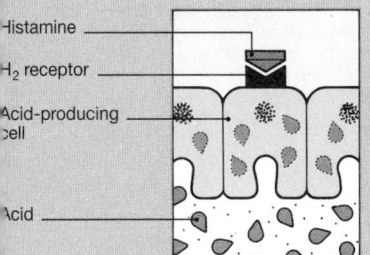

Histamine

H_2 receptor

Acid-producing Cell

Acid

The action of histamine on the stomach
Histamine binds to specialized H_2 receptors and stimulates acid-producing cells in the stomach wall to release acid.

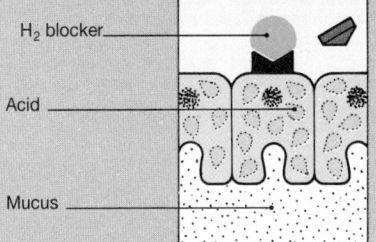

H_2 blocker

Acid

Mucus

The action of H_2 blockers
H_2 blockers occupy H_2 receptors, preventing histamine from triggering the production of acid. This allows the mucous lining to heal.

Sucralfate
This drug forms a coating over the ulcer, protecting it from the action of stomach acid and thus allowing it to heal.

Acid

Stomach wall

Ulcer

Sucralfate

COMMON DRUGS

H_2 blockers	Other drugs
Cimetidine	Antacids (see facing
Famotidine	page)
Nizatidine	Misoprostol
Ranitidine	Omeprazole
	Pirenzepine
	Sucralfate

ANTIDIARRHEAL DRUGS

Diarrhea is an increase in the fluidity and frequency of bowel movements. In some cases diarrhea protects the body from harmful substances in the intestine by hastening their removal. The most common causes of diarrhea are viral infection, food poisoning, and parasites. But diarrhea also occurs in other illnesses. It can be a side effect of some drugs and may follow radiation therapy for cancer. Diarrhea may also be caused by anxiety.

An attack of diarrhea usually clears up quickly without medical attention. The best treatment is to abstain from food and to drink plenty of clear fluids. Rehydration solutions containing sugar and potassium and sodium salts are recommended for preventing dehydration and chemical imbalances, particularly in children. You should consult your physician if: the condition does not improve within 48 hours; the diarrhea contains blood; there is severe abdominal pain and vomiting; you have just returned from a foreign country, or if the diarrhea occurs in a small child or an elderly person.

Severe diarrhea can impair absorption of drugs, and anyone taking a prescription medicine should call a physician. A woman taking oral contraceptives may need to take additional contraceptive measures (see p.175).

Nonspecific diarrhea may be relieved by drugs that act directly on the bowel (narcotics, loperamide), or by bulk-forming and adsorbent agents. Antispasmodic drugs may also be used to relieve pain (see Drugs for irritable bowel syndrome, below).

Why they are used

An antidiarrheal drug may be prescribed when simple remedies do not provide relief. They are generally prescribed to provide relief once it is certain that the diarrhea is neither infectious nor toxic. Narcotics are the most effective antidiarrheals. They are used when

ACTION OF ANTIDIARRHEAL DRUGS

Narcotic antidiarrheals
Narcotics reduce the propulsive muscle contraction of the intestine causing a delay in passage of the contents of the intestine. This allows more time for water to be absorbed from the food residue and therefore reduces the fluidity as well as the frequency of bowel movements.

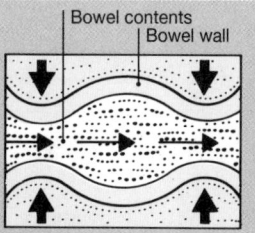
Bowel contents
Bowel wall

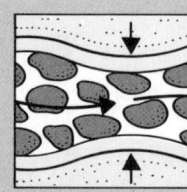

Before drug
Rapid bowel contraction prevents water from being absorbed.

After drug
Slowed bowel action allows more water to be absorbed.

Bulk-forming agents
These preparations contain particles that swell up as they absorb water from the large intestine. This makes bowel movements firmer and less fluid. It is thought that these agents may absorb irritants and harmful chemicals along with excess water.

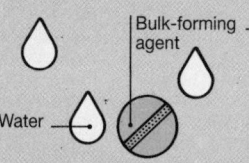
Bulk-forming agent
Water

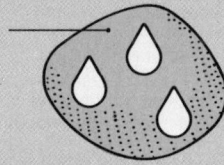

Water is attracted by bulk-forming agent.

Bulk-forming agent swells as water is absorbed.

diarrhea is severe and debilitating. Bulking and adsorbent agents have a milder effect and are often used when it is necessary to regulate bowel action over a prolonged period – for example, in those with colostomies or ileostomies.

How they work

Each type of antidiarrheal drug works differently. Narcotic drugs decrease the propulsive activity of the muscles so that fecal matter passes more slowly through the bowel.

Bulk-forming agents and adsorbents take on water and irritants present in the bowel, thus producing larger and firmer bowel movements less frequently.

How they affect you

Drugs used to treat diarrhea reduce the urge to move the bowels. Narcotic drugs and antispasmodics may relieve abdominal pain. All antidiarrheals may cause constipation if used in excess.

Risks and special precautions

Used in relatively low doses for a limited period of time, the narcotic drugs are unlikely to produce adverse effects. However, these drugs should be used with caution when diarrhea is caused by an infection, since they may slow the elimination of microorganisms from the intestine. All antidiarrheals should be taken with plenty of water. It is important not to take a bulk-forming agent together with a narcotic or antispasmodic drug, because a bulky mass could form and obstruct the bowel.

DRUGS FOR IRRITABLE BOWEL SYNDROME

Irritable bowel syndrome is a common stress-related condition in which the coordinated waves of muscular contraction responsible for moving the bowel contents smoothly through the intestines become strong and irregular, often causing pain. There may also be diarrhea or constipation.

Symptoms are often relieved by adjusting the amount of fiber in the diet, but medication may also be required. Bulk-forming agents may be given to regulate the consistency of the bowel contents. If pain is severe, an antispasmodic drug may be prescribed. These *anticholinergic* drugs reduce the transmission of nerve signals to the bowel wall, thus preventing spasm. Because irritable bowel is often made worse by anxiety, an anti-anxiety drug (p.95) may also be prescribed for short-term use.

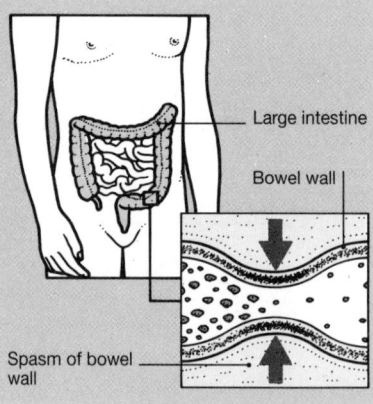
Large intestine
Bowel wall
Spasm of bowel wall

COMMON DRUGS

Antispasmodics
Belladonna
Dicyclomine

Bulk-forming and adsorbent agents
Kaolin
Methylcellulose
Psyllium

Narcotics
Codeine
Diphenoxylate

Others
Loperamide

LAXATIVES

hen your bowels do not move as equently as usual and the movements e hard and difficult to pass, you are uffering from constipation. The most ommon cause is the lack of sufficient ber in your diet; fiber supplies the bulk at makes the feces soft and easy to ass. The simple remedy is more fluid d a diet higher in fiber, i.e., more fruits, getables, and whole grain breads. onstipation is commonly relieved by xatives, although some physicians commend occasional small enemas.

Ignoring the urge to defecate can also use constipation, the feces becoming y (and hard to pass) and too small to mulate the muscles that propel them rough the intestine. Certain drugs may constipating such as narcotic algesics, tricyclic antidepressants, and tacids containing aluminum. Some seases, such as hypothyroidism, can d to constipation.

Because constipation may be a symp-m of something serious, consult your ysician about any change in bowel bits that lasts more than a week.

hy they are used

nce prolonged use is harmful, laxatives ould be used for very short periods ly. They may prevent pain and strain-j in people with aneurysms or hemor-oids (p.125). Physicians may prescribe atives for the same reason after ldbirth or abdominal surgery. Laxatives e also used to clear the bowel before ch investigative procedures as onoscopy. They may also be ministered to the elderly and dridden, because lack of exercise can d to constipation.

ow they work

xatives act on the large intestine – by reasing the speed with which fecal tter passes through the bowel or reasing its bulk and/or water content. mulants cause the bowel muscle to ntract, increasing the speed with which

ACTION OF LAXATIVES

Bulk-forming agents
Taken after a meal, these agents are not absorbed as they pass through the digestive tract. They contain particles that absorb many times their own volume of water. By doing so they increase the bulk of the bowel movements and thus encourage bowel action.

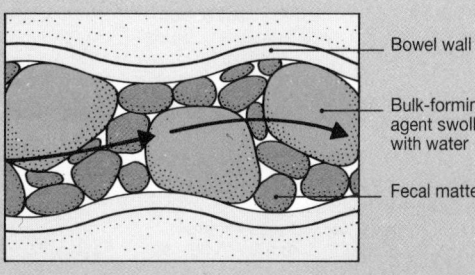

Bowel wall

Bulk-forming agent swollen with water

Fecal matter

Stimulant laxatives
These laxatives are thought to encourage bowel movement by acting on nerve endings in the wall of the intestines that trigger contraction of the intestinal muscles. This speeds the passage of fecal matter through the large intestine, allowing less time for water to be absorbed. Thus bowel movements become more frequent and more liquid.

Increased contractions speed passage of fecal matter

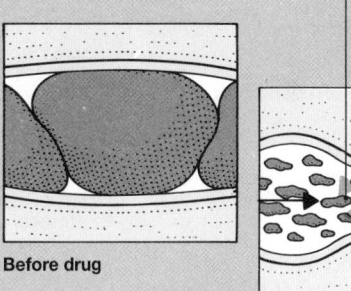

Before drug

After drug

fecal matter passes through the intestine. Bulk-forming laxatives absorb water in the bowel, thereby increasing the volume of fecal matter and making bowel movements softer and easier to pass. Lactulose also causes fluid to accumulate in the intestine. Saline laxatives prevent water from passing out of the large intestine by osmotic action without increasing the bulk of bowel movements. Lubricant mineral oil preparations and stool softeners make the bowel movements softer and easier to pass without increasing their bulk. But prolonged use of mineral oil leaves a

coating that can interfere with absorption of some essential vitamins.

Risks and special precautions

Laxatives can cause diarrhea if taken in overdose, and constipation if overused. The most serious risk of prolonged use of most laxatives is developing dependence on the laxative for normal bowel action. Use of a laxative should therefore be discontinued as soon as normal bowel movements have been reestablished. Children should not be given laxatives except in special circumstances on the advice of a physician.

TYPES OF LAXATIVES

ulk-forming agents These are relatively ow acting, but are less likely than other xatives to interfere with normal bowel ction. Only after consultation with your octor should they be taken for constipation ccompanied by abdominal pain, because of e risk of intestinal obstruction.

timulant (contact) laxatives These are uitable for occasional use when other eatments have failed or when a rapid onset f action is required. Stimulant laxatives nould not normally be used for longer than a eek, as they can cause abdominal cramps nd diarrhea.

ubricants Mineral oil (also called liquid etrolatum) is used as a fecal softener when

hard bowel movements cause pain on defecation – for example, if hemorrhoids are present. It is often recommended for the relief of fecal impaction (blockage of the bowel by fecal material).

Saline laxatives A variety of mineral salts are used to evacuate the bowel prior to surgery or investigative procedures. They are not used for the long-term relief of constipation because they can cause chemical imbalances in the blood.

Lactulose This is an alternative to bulk-forming laxatives for the long-term treatment of chronic constipation. It may cause stomach cramps and flatulence.

COMMON DRUGS

Stimulant laxatives
Bisacodyl
Phenolphthalein
Senna

Bulk-forming agents
Fiber tablets
Methylcellulose
Psyllium

Osmotic laxatives
Lactulose
Magnesium hydroxide
Sodium phosphate

Stool softeners
Docusate calcium
Docusate sodium

Lubricant laxatives
Mineral oil

DRUGS FOR INFLAMMATORY BOWEL DISEASE

"Inflammatory bowel disease" is the term used to describe certain disorders in which the wall of the intestine and other parts of the gastrointestinal tract become inflamed, causing symptoms that include periodic attacks of pain, general feelings of ill-health, and often diarrhea that is sometimes bloody. Loss of appetite and poor absorption of food often result in weight loss.

Although the exact cause of these disorders is unknown, the risks and severity of attacks are increased by some infections, antibiotics, and excessive stress.

Physicians identify two main types of inflammatory bowel disease: Crohn's disease and ulcerative colitis. In Crohn's disease (also called regional enteritis) any part of the digestive tract may be inflamed, although the small intestine and the colon are the most commonly affected sites. In ulcerative colitis the large intestine becomes inflamed and ulcerated, often producing blood-stained diarrhea (see the box, below).

Corticosteroids, mesalamine (5-aminosalicylic acid), sulfasalazine, and metronidazole are used to treat Crohn's disease and the first three agents are used in ulcerative colitis. Rarely, immunosuppressant drugs such as azathioprine are used in both conditions. Nutritional supplements are frequently given in Crohn's disease. Antidiarrheal agents are given with great caution. In severe cases, surgery may be necessary.

Why they are used

Drugs cannot cure inflammatory bowel disease. However, drug treatment can control symptoms and prevent compli-

SITES OF BOWEL INFLAMMATION

The two main types of bowel inflammation are called ulcerative colitis and Crohn's disease. The former occurs in the large intestine. Crohn's disease can occur anywhere along the gastrointestinal tract. It is typically found in the small intestine.

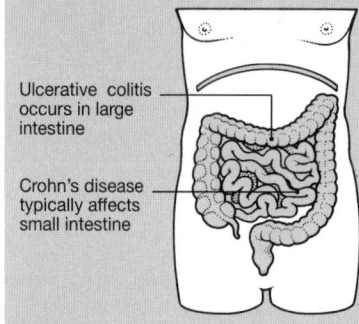

Ulcerative colitis occurs in large intestine

Crohn's disease typically affects small intestine

cations, especially severe anemia and perforation of the intestinal wall.

Corticosteroids are given in ulcerative colitis relapses and in Crohn's disease affecting either the small intestine (Crohn's ileitis) or colon (Crohn's colitis). Either sulfasalazine or mesalamine is used in Crohn's colitis and ulcerative colitis to treat attacks and prevent recurrences.

How they work

Corticosteroids, sulfasalazine, and mesalamine depress the inflammatory

process, thus allowing the damaged tissue to recover. They act in different ways to prevent migration of white blood cells into the bowel wall, which may be responsible in part for the inflammation of the bowel.

How they affect you

Taken to treat attacks, these drugs relieve symptoms within a few days, and general health improves gradually over a few weeks. Sulfasalazine and mesalamine are usually effective in providing longer-term relief from the symptoms of ulcerative colitis. Immunosuppressants are reserved for the treatment of severe disease that has not responded to other medications and are administered under strict medical supervision.

Risks and special precautions

Immunosuppressant and corticosteroid drugs can cause serious adverse effects and they are thus only prescribed when potential benefits outweigh the risks involved.

It is important to continue taking these drugs as instructed because stopping them abruptly may cause a sudden flare up of the disorder. Physicians usually supervise a gradual reduction in dosage when stopping the drug, even when given as a short course to treat an attack. Antidiarrheal drugs should not be taken on a routine basis because they may mask signs of deterioration or even aid sudden bowel dilation or rupture.

How they are administered

These drugs are usually taken in tablet form, although mild ulcerative colitis in the last part of the large intestine may be treated with suppositories or an enema containing a corticosteroid drug or mesalamine.

COMMON DRUGS

Corticosteroids
Betamethasone
Hydrocortisone
Prednisone

Immunosuppressants
Azathioprine
Mercaptopurine

Other drugs
Mesalamine
Metronidazole
Sulfasalazine

ACTION OF DRUGS IN ULCERATIVE COLITIS

Ulcerative colitis is the most common form of inflammatory bowel disease. It affects the large intestine, causing ulceration of the lining and producing pain and violent bloodstained diarrhea. It is often treated with corticosteroids, mesalamine, or sulfasalazine.

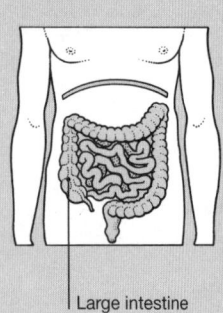

Large intestine

Bowel wall
Ulcerated area
Prostaglandins

White blood cells   Corticosteroid
Blood vessel   drug
                            Sulfasalazine
                            or mesalamine

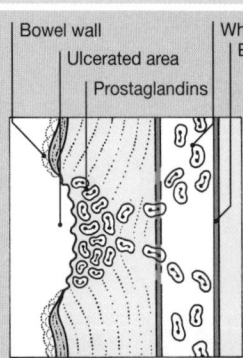

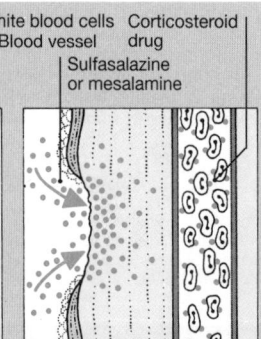

Before drug
Damage to the intestinal lining provokes the formation of chemicals known as prostaglandins which trigger the migration of white blood cells into the ulcerated area. The accumulation of white blood cells in the bowel wall causes inflammation.

Drug action
Sulfasalazine or mesalamine passes into the ulcerated area from inside the bowel. The drug prevents prostaglandins from forming in the damaged tissue. Corticosteroids reduce the ability of white blood cells to pass into the bowel wall.

DRUGS FOR RECTAL AND ANAL DISORDERS

he most common disorder affecting the
ectum (the last part of the large intestine)
nd anus (the opening from the rectum) is
emorrhoids, commonly called piles.
hey occur when hemorrhoidal veins
ecome swollen, irritated, or clotted,
ften the result of prolonged local back
ressure such as that caused by a
regnancy or a job requiring long hours of
tting. Hemorrhoids may cause irritation
nd pain, especially on defecation. The
ondition is aggravated by constipation
nd straining while passing a bowel
ovement. Sometimes hemorrhoids may
eed and occasionally clots may form in
e swollen veins, leading to severe pain,
condition called thrombosed
emorrhoids.

Other common disorders affecting the
nus include anal fissure (painful cracks in
e anus) and pruritus ani (itching around
e anus).

A number of over-the-counter and
rescription-only preparations are
vailable for the relief of such disorders.
arm sitz baths also help.

Why they are used

reparations for relief of hemorrhoids and
al discomfort fall into two main groups:
eams or suppositories that act locally to
lieve inflammation and irritation, and
easures that relieve constipation, which
ntributes to the formation of, and
scomfort from, hemorrhoids and anal
sure.

Preparations from the first group often
ntain a soothing agent with *antiseptic*,
tringent, or *vasoconstrictor* properties.
gredients of this type include zinc oxide,
smuth, hamamelis (witch hazel),
eruvian balsam, and ephedrine. Some
oducts also include a mild local
esthetic such as tetracaine (see p.92).

DISORDERS OF THE RECTUM AND ANUS

The rectum and anus form
the last part of the digestive
tract. Common conditions
affecting the area include
swelling of the veins around
the anus (hemorrhoids),
cracks in the anus (anal
fissure), and inflammation
and irritation of the anus
and surrounding area
(pruritus ani).

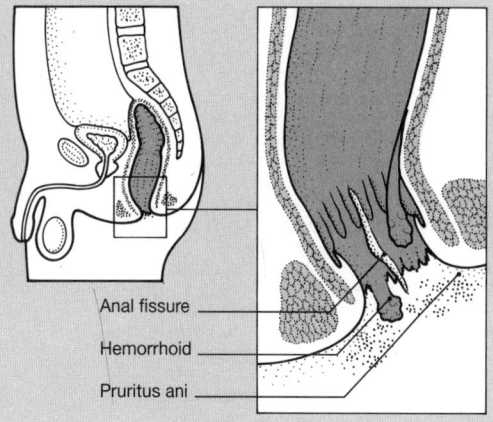

Anal fissure ⎯⎯

Hemorrhoid ⎯⎯

Pruritus ani ⎯⎯

In some cases a physician may prescribe
an ointment containing a corticosteroid to
relieve inflammation around the anus (see
Topical corticosteroids, p.186).

People who suffer from hemorrhoids or
anal fissure are generally advised to
include in their diets plenty of fluids and
fiber-rich foods (such as fresh fruits,
vegetables, and whole grain products) to
prevent constipation and to ease
defecation. A mild bulk-forming or
lubricant laxative may also be prescribed
(see p.123).

Neither type of treatment can shrink
large hemorrhoids, although they may
provide relief while healing occurs
naturally in anal fissure. Severe,
persistently painful hemorrhoids that
continue to be troublesome in spite of

these measures may need to be removed
surgically or, more commonly, by banding
with specially applied small rubber bands
(see below left).

How they affect you

The treatments described above usually
relieve discomfort, especially during
defecation. Most people experience no
adverse effects, although preparations
containing local anesthetics may cause
irritation or even a rash in the anal area. It
is rare for ingredients in locally acting
preparations to be absorbed into the
body in sufficient quantities to cause
generalized side effects.

The main risk is that self-treatment of
hemorrhoids may delay diagnosis of a
more serious bowel disorder. It is
therefore always wise to consult your
physician if you have symptoms of
hemorrhoids, especially if you have
noticed rectal bleeding.

SITES OF DRUG ACTION

he illustration below shows how and where
drugs for the treatment of rectal disorders
ct to relieve symptoms..

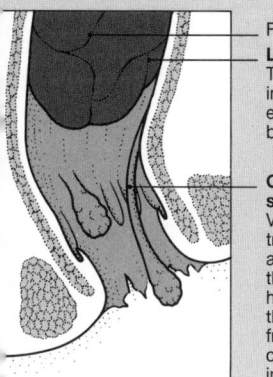

Fecal matter ⎯⎯

Laxatives
These act in the large
intestine to soften and
ease the passage of
bowel movements.

**Creams and
suppositories**
Vasoconstrictors and as-
tringents reduce swelling
and restrict blood supply,
thus helping to relieve
hemorrhoids. Local anes-
thetics numb pain signals
from the anus. Topical
corticosteroids relieve
inflammation.

Banding treatment
A small rubber band is applied
to a hemorrhoid, thereby
blocking off its blood supply.
The hemorrhoid will eventually
wither away.

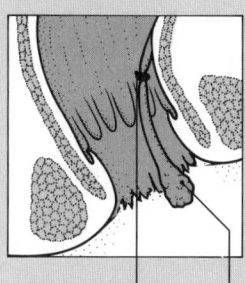

Rubber band ⎯⎯

Hemorrhoid ⎯⎯

COMMON DRUGS

Soothing and astringent agents
Bismuth
Hamamelis
Peruvian balsam
Zinc oxide
Zinc sulfate

Vasoconstrictors
Ephedrine

Topical corticosteroids
Fluocinolone
Hydrocortisone

Local anesthetics
(see p.92)

Laxatives
(see p.123)

DRUG TREATMENT FOR GALLSTONES

The formation of gallstones is the most common disorder of the gallbladder, which is the storage and concentrating unit for bile, a digestive juice produced by the liver. During digestion, bile passes from the gallbladder via the bile duct into the small intestine, where it aids the digestion of fats. Bile is made up of several ingredients, including bile acids, bile salts, and bile pigments. It also contains significant amounts of cholesterol dissolved in bile acid. If the amount of cholesterol in the bile increases or if that of bile acid is reduced, a proportion of the cholesterol cannot remain dissolved. This excess may accumulate in the gallbladder as gallstones.

Gallstones may be present in the gallbladder for years without causing symptoms. However, if they become lodged in the bile duct they cause pain and block the flow of bile, which could result in infection and inflammation.

Gallstones containing mostly cholesterol can be dissolved using drug therapy. However, when stones contain significant amounts of other material, such as calcium, or if a stone becomes lodged in the bile duct, surgical removal may be required. The most commonly used gallstone-dissolving drug is ursodiol.

Why they are used

Even if you do not have any symptoms, once gallstones have been diagnosed your physician may advise treatment because of the risk of blockage of the bile duct. Drug treatment is usually preferred to surgery when it is considered that surgery may be risky. Certain stones can also be treated by breaking them with shock waves (lithotripsy).

How they work

Ursodiol is a substance that is naturally present in bile. It acts on chemical processes in the liver to regulate the amount of cholesterol in the blood, by controlling the amount that passes into the bile. Once the level of cholesterol in the bile is reduced, the bile acids are able to start dissolving the stones in the gallbladder. For maximum effect, ursodiol treatment usually needs to be accompanied by adherence to a low-cholesterol, high-fiber diet.

DIGESTION OF FATS

The digestion of fats (or lipids) in the small intestine is assisted by the action of bile, a digestive juice produced by the liver and stored in the gallbladder. A complex sequence of chemical processes enables fats to be absorbed through the intestinal wall, broken down in the liver and converted for use in the body. Cholesterol, a lipid present in bile, plays an important part in this chain.

2 Bile salts act on fats to enable them to pass from the small intestine into the bloodstream, either directly or via the lymphatic system.

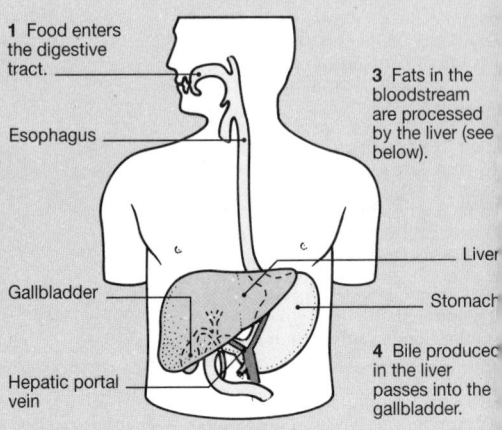

1 Food enters the digestive tract.

Esophagus

Gallbladder

Hepatic portal vein

3 Fats in the bloodstream are processed by the liver (see below).

Liver

Stomach

4 Bile produced in the liver passes into the gallbladder.

How fats are processed in the liver

Fat molecules are broken down in the liver into fatty acids and glycerol. Glycerol and some of the fatty acids pass back into the bloodstream. Other fatty acids are used to form cholesterol, some of which is then used to make bile salts. Unchanged cholesterol is dissolved in the bile, which then passes into the gallbladder.

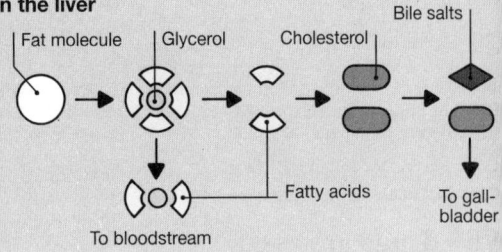

Fat molecule   Glycerol   Cholesterol   Bile salts

To bloodstream   Fatty acids   To gallbladder

How they affect you

Drug treatment may take up to two years, or longer, to dissolve gallstones completely. You will not, therefore, feel any immediate benefit from the drugs, but you may have some minor side effects, the most usual of which is diarrhea. If this occurs, your physician may adjust the dosage. The effect of drug treatment on the gallstones is usually monitored regularly by means of ultrasound or X-ray examinations.

Even after successful treatment with drugs, this condition can recur when ursodiol is stopped. In some cases drug treatment and dietary restrictions may be continued after the gallstones

have dissolved, in order to prevent a recurrence of the problem.

Ursodiol is not usually given to people with liver disorders because it can interfere with the normal liver function.

COMMON DRUGS

For gallstones
Ursodiol

Pancreatic enzymes
Pancreatin
Pancrelipase

AGENTS USED IN DISORDERS OF THE PANCREAS

The pancreas releases certain *enzymes* into the small intestine, which are necessary for digestion of a range of foods. If the release of pancreatic enzymes is impaired, for example by chronic pancreatitis or cystic fibrosis, enzyme replacement therapy may be necessary. Replacement of enzymes does not cure the underlying disorder, but restores normal digestion. Pancreatic enzymes should be taken just before or with meals, and

usually take effect immediately. Your physician will probably advise you to eat a diet that is high in protein and carbohydrates and low in fat.

The most frequently used replacements are pancreatin and pancrelipase, both of which are extracted from pig pancreas. Both must be taken indefinitely as long as the pancreatic disorder persists.

MUSCLES, BONES, AND JOINTS

The basic architecture of the human body relies on bones (206 of them), a variety of muscles, and a complex assortment of other tissues – ligaments, tendons, and cartilage – that enable them to function with remarkable efficiency.

What can go wrong

Though tough, these structures often suffer damage. Muscles, tendons, and ligaments can be strained or torn by violent movement. Such injury may cause inflammation, making the affected tissue swollen and painful. Joints, especially those that bear the body's weight – hips, knees, ankles, and vertebrae – are prone to wear and tear. The cartilage covering the bone ends may tear, causing pain and inflammation. Joint damage also occurs in rheumatoid arthritis, thought to be a form of autoimmune disorder. Gout, in which uric acid crystals form in some joints, may also cause inflammation, a condition known as gouty arthritis.

Other problems affecting the muscles, bones, and joints include those in which nerve control over muscle contraction is altered due to injury or a neurological disorder, or by poor nerve signals as in myasthenia gravis. The mineral composition of bone may be weakened by vitamin, mineral, or hormone deficiencies.

Why drugs are used

A simple analgesic drug or one that has an anti-inflammatory effect will provide pain relief in most of the above conditions. For more severe inflammation a physician may inject a drug with a more powerful anti-inflammatory effect – such as a corticosteroid – into the affected site. In cases of severe progressive rheumatoid arthritis, antirheumatic drugs may halt the disease process as well as relieving symptoms.

Drugs that help to eliminate excess uric acid from the body are often prescribed to treat gout. Muscle relaxants that inhibit transmission of nerve signals to the muscles are used to treat muscle spasm. Drugs that increase nervous stimulation of the muscle are prescribed for myasthenia gravis. Bone disorders in which the mineral content of the bone is reduced are treated with supplements of minerals, vitamins, and hormones.

MAJOR DRUG GROUPS

Non-steroidal anti-inflammatory drugs
Antirheumatic drugs
Locally acting corticosteroids
Drugs for gout

Muscle-relaxant drugs
Drugs used for myasthenia gravis
Drugs for bone disorders

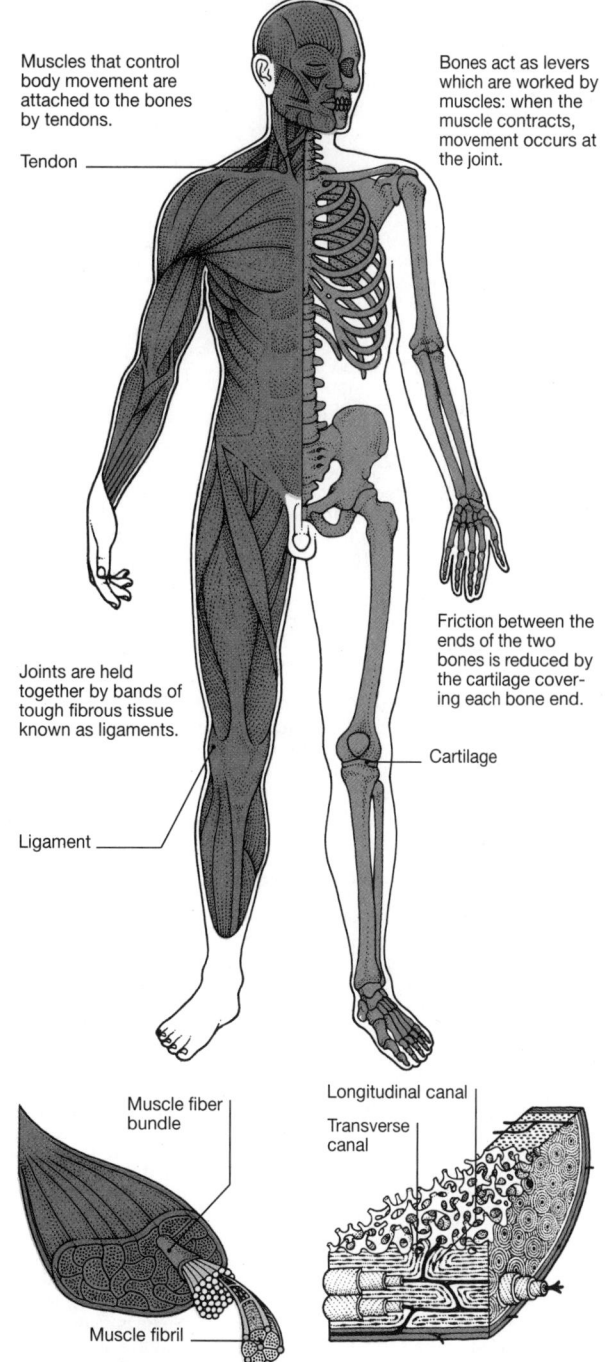

Muscles that control body movement are attached to the bones by tendons.

Tendon

Bones act as levers which are worked by muscles: when the muscle contracts, movement occurs at the joint.

Friction between the ends of the two bones is reduced by the cartilage covering each bone end.

Cartilage

Joints are held together by bands of tough fibrous tissue known as ligaments.

Ligament

Muscle fiber bundle

Muscle fibril

Longitudinal canal

Transverse canal

Muscle
Each muscle is made of thick bundles of fibers: each bundle in turn is made of fibrils. Tiny nerves and blood vessels enable the muscle to function.

Bone
Long bones, e.g., the femur, contain a network of longitudinal and transverse canals to carry blood, nerves, and lymph vessels through the bone.

NON-STEROIDAL ANTI-INFLAMMATORY DRUGS

Drugs in this group are used to relieve pain, stiffness, and inflammation associated with a wide variety of conditions, particularly those affecting the muscles, bones, and joints. NSAIDs are called non-steroidal to distinguish them from corticosteroid drugs (see p.153), which also have an anti-inflammatory effect.

Why they are used

NSAIDs are widely prescribed in the treatment of rheumatoid arthritis, osteoarthritis, and other rheumatic conditions. They do not alter the progress of those diseases, but reduce inflammation and thus relieve pain and swelling of joints.

An NSAID may be used as the first line of treatment, or may be given when an analgesic such as acetaminophen does not provide adequate relief or is unsuitable for other reasons. The response to the various drugs in this group varies among individuals, and the first drug chosen may not be effective. It is therefore sometimes necessary for the physician to prescribe a number of different NSAIDs before finding the one which best suits a particular individual.

Because NSAIDs do not alter the progress of the disease, additional treatment may be required, particularly in the case of rheumatoid arthritis (see facing page).

Some NSAIDs are also commonly prescribed to relieve back pain, gout (p.131), menstrual pain (p.172), headaches, mild pain following surgery, and pain from soft tissue injuries such as sprains and strains (see also Analgesics, p.92).

How they work

Prostaglandins are chemicals released at the site of an injury. They are believed to be the substances responsible for producing pain and inflammation following tissue damage and in immune reactions. All the NSAIDs block the production of prostaglandins and this may be how they reduce pain and inflammation (see p.93).

How they affect you

NSAIDs are usually effective in reducing joint pain and swelling. They are rapidly absorbed from the digestive system and most start to relieve symptoms within an hour. When used regularly for long-term treatment, they reduce stiffness and may restore or improve the function of a joint if this has been impaired. Common side effects include nausea, indigestion, and altered bowel action. But the potential of most NSAIDs to irritate the stomach is less than that of uncoated ASA.

Most NSAIDs are short-acting and need to be taken several times a day in order to provide optimal relief of pain. Some need to be taken only twice daily. Others such as piroxicam are very slowly eliminated from the body and are effective when taken once a day.

ACTION OF NSAIDs IN OSTEOARTHRITIS

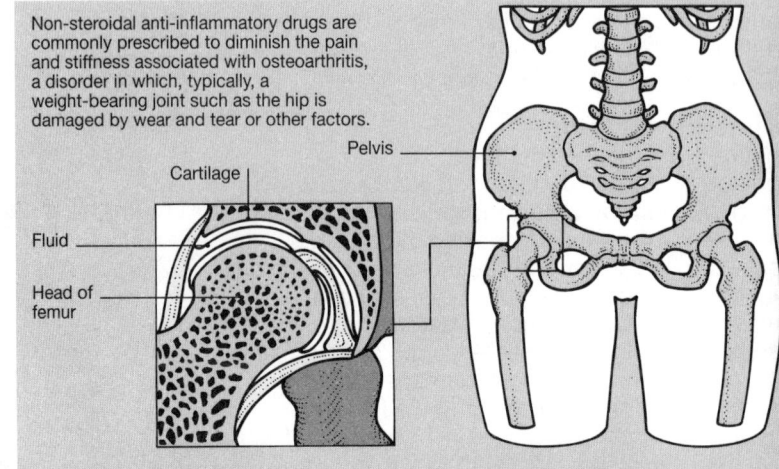

Non-steroidal anti-inflammatory drugs are commonly prescribed to diminish the pain and stiffness associated with osteoarthritis, a disorder in which, typically, a weight-bearing joint such as the hip is damaged by wear and tear or other factors.

Pelvis

Cartilage

Fluid

Head of femur

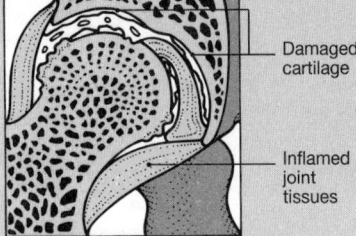

Damaged cartilage

Inflamed joint tissues

Before treatment
The protective layers of cartilage surrounding the joint are worn away and the joint becomes inflamed and painful.

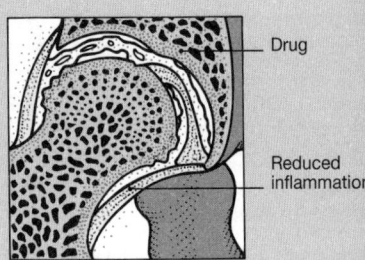

Drug

Reduced inflammation

Effect of NSAIDs
NSAIDs reduce inflammation and may thus relieve pain, but damage to the joint remains and symptoms may worsen or recur if the drug is stopped.

Risks and special precautions

With a few exceptions, most NSAIDs are free from serious adverse effects. The main danger is that they can occasionally cause bleeding in the stomach or duodenum. They should normally be avoided by people who have suffered from peptic ulcers. The NSAIDs' side effect of bleeding is due to their antiprostaglandin action. To protect against this, misoprostol, a prostaglandin-like drug, is sometimes prescribed with the NSAID.

Most NSAIDs are not recommended during pregnancy or for nursing mothers. Caution is also advised for those with kidney or liver abnormalities or with a history of hypersensitivity to other drugs. NSAIDs may also impair normal blood clotting and are, therefore, prescribed with caution for people with bleeding disorders or who are taking drugs that reduce blood clotting. One of the first NSAIDs, phenylbutazone, can impair the bone marrow's ability to produce blood cells. Early signs of this include sore throat or fever, and must be reported. Phenylbutazone is usually prescribed only for ankylosing spondylitis and acute attacks of gout with regular blood tests required.

COMMON DRUGS

Diclofenac	Nabumetone
Diflunisal	Naproxen
Fenoprofen	Phenylbutazone
Flurbiprofen	Piroxicam
Ibuprofen	Sulindac
Indomethacin	Tenoxicam
Ketoprofen	Tiaprofenic acid
Ketorolac	Tolmetin
Mefenamic acid	

ANTIRHEUMATIC DRUGS

These drugs are used in the treatment of various rheumatic disorders, the most crippling and deforming of which is rheumatoid arthritis. It is thought to be a form of autoimmune disease in which the body's mechanism for fighting infection contributes to the damage of its own joint tissue. The disease causes pain, stiffness, and swelling of the joints that over many months can lead to deformity. Flare-ups of rheumatoid arthritis also cause a generalized feeling of being unwell.

Treatments include drugs, rest, changes in diet, immobilization of joints, and physical therapy. Rheumatoid arthritis cannot yet be cured, although in many cases it does not progress far enough to cause permanent disability. The disease may subside spontaneously.

Why they are used

The aim of drug treatment is to relieve pain and stiffness, maintain mobility, and prevent deformity. There are two main approaches to drug treatment for rheumatoid arthritis: (1) to alleviate symptoms, and (2) to modify, halt, or slow the underlying disease process. Drugs in the first category include ASA (p.200) and the non-steroidal anti-inflammatory drugs (NSAIDs) (p.128). The second category of drugs may be given when rheumatoid arthritis is severe or when the initial drug treatment is inadequate. These can be of benefit where the disease is progressive because they may impede further joint damage and disability. They are not prescribed automatically because they have potentially severe adverse effects (see below) and because the disease may stop spontaneously.

Corticosteroids (p.153) are sometimes used in the treatment of rheumatoid arthritis, but only for limited periods.

How they work

It is not known precisely how most antirheumatic drugs stop or slow the disease process. Some may reduce the body's immune response, which is

THE EFFECTS OF ANTIRHEUMATIC DRUGS

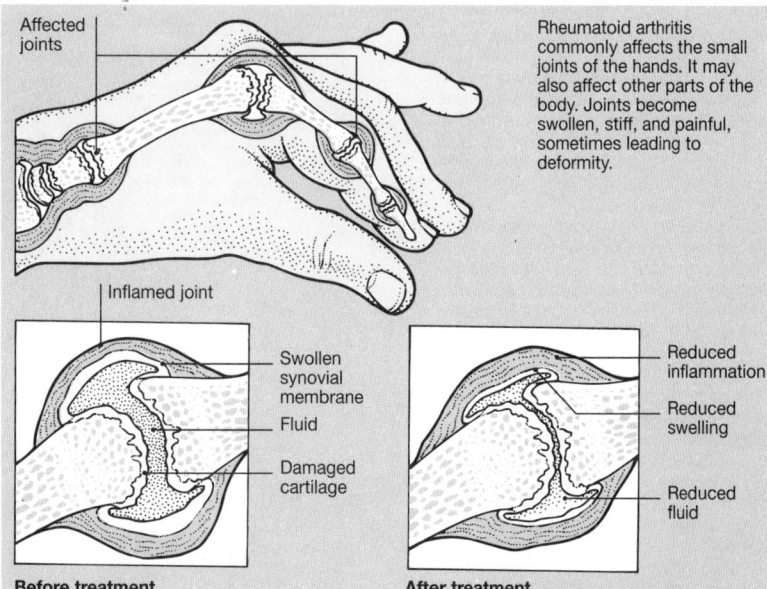

Affected joints

Rheumatoid arthritis commonly affects the small joints of the hands. It may also affect other parts of the body. Joints become swollen, stiff, and painful, sometimes leading to deformity.

Inflamed joint

Swollen synovial membrane
Fluid
Damaged cartilage

Reduced inflammation
Reduced swelling
Reduced fluid

Before treatment
The synovial membrane surrounding the joint is inflamed and thickened, producing increased fluid within the joint. The surrounding tissue is inflamed and joint cartilage damaged.

After treatment
Treatment with antirheumatic drugs relieves pain, swelling, and inflammation. Damage to cartilage and bone may be halted so that further deformity is minimized.

thought to be partly responsible for the disease (see also Immunosuppressant drugs, p.168). When effective, such drugs prevent damage to the cartilage and bone, thereby reducing progressive deformity and disability. The effectiveness of each drug varies depending on individual response.

How they affect you

These drugs are generally slow-acting; it may be weeks or even months before benefit is noticed. Treatment with NSAIDs

or ASA is usually continued. After this time, however, antirheumatic drugs can cause a marked improvement in symptoms. Pain is reduced, joint mobility increased, and generalized symptoms of ill health fade. Side effects, which vary among drugs, may be noticed before any beneficial effect, so patience is required. Severe adverse effects may necessitate abandoning the treatment.

COMMON DRUGS

Immunosuppressants
Azathioprine
Chlorambucil
Cyclophosphamide
Cyclosporine
Methotrexate

Gold-based drugs
Auranofin
Sodium aurothiomalate

Others
Chloroquine
Penicillamine
Sulfasalazine

TYPES OF ANTIRHEUMATIC DRUGS

Gold-based drugs These are believed to be the most effective and may be given by mouth or by injection for many years. Possible side effects include skin rash and digestive disturbances. Occasionally gold may cause kidney damage, so regular urine tests are usually carried out. Gold can also suppress production of blood cells in the bone marrow. For this reason, periodic blood tests are also carried out.

Penicillamine This drug may be used when rheumatoid arthritis is worsening, or when gold cannot be given. Improvement in symptoms may take three to six months. It has similar side effects to gold, and periodic blood and urine tests are usually performed.

Chloroquine Originally developed to treat malaria (see p.149), chloroquine and related drugs are less effective than penicillamine or gold. Since prolonged use may cause eye damage, regular eye checks are needed.

Immunosuppressants These may be prescribed if other drugs do not provide relief, and if rheumatoid arthritis is severe and disabling. Regular observation and blood tests are necessary to avoid severe complications.

Sulfasalazine Used mainly for ulcerative colitis, this drug is effective in treating some cases of rheumatoid arthritis that have not responded to first-line drugs.

LOCALLY ACTING CORTICOSTEROIDS

The adrenal glands, one atop each of the kidneys, produce a number of important hormones. Among them are the corticosteroids, so named because they are made in the outer part (cortex) of the glands. These hormones play an important role, influencing the immune system and regulating the carbohydrate and mineral *metabolism* of the body. A number of drugs that mimic the effects of natural corticosteroid hormones have been developed.

These drugs have many uses and are discussed in more detail under Corticosteroids (p.153). This section concentrates on corticosteroids given by injection into an affected site to treat various joint disorders.

Why they are used

Corticosteroids given by injection are particularly useful for treating joint disorders – notably rheumatoid arthritis and osteoarthritis – when one or only a few joints are involved and pain and inflammation have not been relieved. In such cases it is possible to relieve symptoms by injecting each of the affected joints individually. Cortico-steroids may also be injected to relieve pain and inflammation caused by strained or contracted muscles, ligaments, and/or tendons – for example, in frozen shoulder or tennis elbow. They may also be given for bursitis, tendinitis, or swelling that may be compressing a nerve.

Corticosteroid injections are sometimes used to relieve pain and stiffness sufficiently to allow physical therapy to be undertaken.

How they work

These drugs have two main actions that are thought to account for their effective-ness. They depress the activity of the

COMMON INJECTION SITES

Corticosteroids are often injected into joints affected by osteo- and rheumatoid arthritis. Joints commonly treated in this way are knee, shoulder, and finger joints.

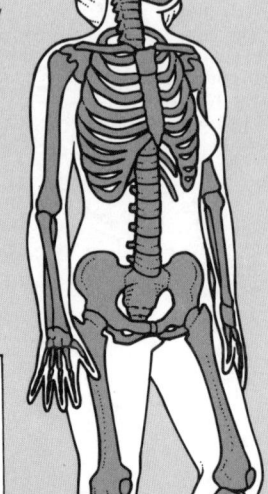

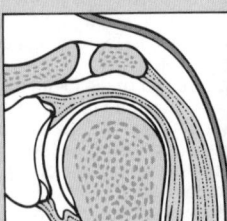
Shoulder joint

Finger joints

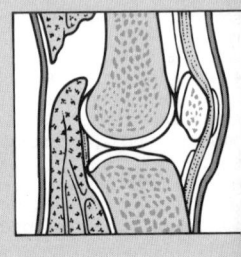
Knee joint

white blood cells, which are responsible for inflammation (below), and also block the production of chemicals called prostaglandins, which are responsible for triggering pain and inflammation. Administration by injection concentrates the effects of the corticosteroids at the site of the problem, producing maximum benefit where it is most needed with minimum side effects.

How they affect you

Corticosteroids usually produce dramat relief from symptoms when they are injected into a joint. Often a single injection is sufficient to relieve pain and swelling, and to improve mobility. When used to treat muscle or tendon pain the may not always be effective because it difficult to position the needle so that th drug reaches the right spot. In some cases repeated injections are necessar

Because these drugs are concentrate in the affected area, and are not dispersed in significant amounts in the body, the generalized adverse effects th may occur with corticosteroids taken b mouth are unlikely. Minor side effects such as loss of skin pigment at the injection site are uncommon. Occasionally, a temporary increase in pain (steroid flare) may occur. In such cases, local application of ice, rest, and analgesic medication may relieve the condition. Sterile injection technique is critically important.

COMMON DRUGS

Betamethasone
Methylprednisolone
Dexamethasone
Triamcinolone

ACTION OF CORTICOSTEROIDS ON INFLAMED JOINTS

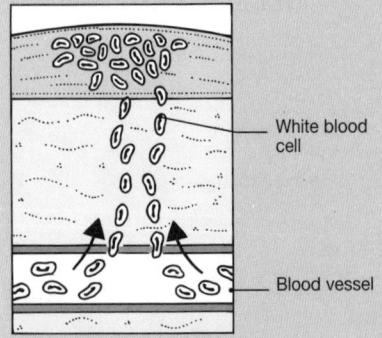

White blood cell

Blood vessel

Inflamed tissue
Inflammation occurs when disease or injury causes large numbers of white blood cells to accumulate in the affected area. In joints this leads to swelling and stiffness.

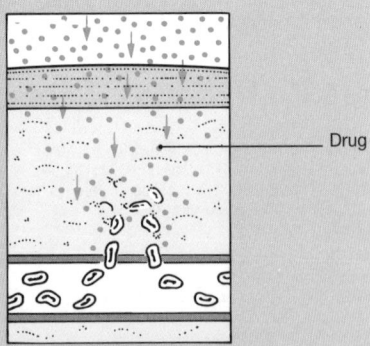

Drug

Action of corticosteroids
Corticosteroids injected into the area per-meate the joint lining (synovial membrane) and prevent accumulation of white blood cells.

DRUGS FOR GOUT

Gout is a disorder that arises when the blood contains increased levels of uric acid, a by-product of normal body metabolism. When its concentration in the blood is excessive, uric acid crystals may form in various parts of the body, especially in the joints of the foot (most often the big toe), the knee, and the hand, causing intense pain and inflammation known as gouty arthritis. Crystals may form as white masses, known as tophi, in soft tissue, and in the kidneys as stones. Attacks of gouty arthritis can recur, and may lead to damaged joints and deformity. Kidney stones can cause kidney damage.

An excess of uric acid can be caused either by increased production or by decreased elimination by the kidney which removes it from the body. The disorder tends to run in families and is far more common in men. The risk of attack is increased by high alcohol intake, obesity, and the consumption of certain foods (including red meat, sardines, anchovies, liver, and brains). An attack may be triggered by drugs such as thiazide diuretics (see p.111), anticancer drugs (see p.166), or excessive drinking. Changes in diet and a reduction in alcohol consumption may be an important part of treatment.

Drugs used to treat acute gout include non-steroidal anti-inflammatory drugs (see p.128), such as indomethacin, colchicine, and, less commonly today, corticosteroids and corticotropin (ACTH), which controls the production and release of adrenal corticosteroid hormones. Others which lower the blood level of uric acid are allopurinol and the uricosuric drugs, probenecid and sulfinpyrazone. ASA is not prescribed for pain relief because it slows the excretion of uric acid.

Why they are used

Drugs may be prescribed to treat an attack of gout or to prevent recurrent attacks that could lead to deformity of affected joints and kidney damage. Colchicine can halt an attack of gout; NSAIDs may also ease the symptoms. Either type of drug should be taken as soon as an attack begins. Because colchicine is relatively specific in relieving the pain and inflammation arising from gout, physicians sometimes administer it in order to confirm their diagnosis of the condition before prescribing an NSAID.

If symptoms recur, your physician may advise long-term treatment with allopurinol or uricosuric drugs.

These drugs usually have to be taken indefinitely. Since they can trigger attacks of gout at the beginning of treatment, colchicine is also given with these drugs for a few months.

How they work

Allopurinol reduces the level of uric acid in the blood by interfering with the activity of xanthine oxidase, an enzyme that is involved in the production of uric acid in the body. Probenecid and sulfinpyrazone increase the rate at which uric acid is excreted by the kidneys. Colchicine may decrease inflammation (and therefore pain) by interfering with the action of white blood cells in joints where uric acid crystals deposit.

How they affect you

Drugs used in the long-term treatment of gout are usually successful in preventing attacks and joint deformity. However, response may be slow.

Colchicine can disturb the digestive system, causing abdominal pain, which your physician can manage.

Risks and special precautions

Since they increase the output of uric acid through the kidneys, uricosuric drugs can cause uric acid crystals to form in the kidneys. They are not, therefore, usually prescribed for those who already have kidney problems. In such cases allopurinol may be preferred. It is always important to drink plenty of fluids while taking anti-gout drugs to prevent kidney crystals from forming. Regular blood tests to monitor levels of uric acid in the blood may be required.

ACTION OF URICOSURIC DRUGS

Uric acid is removed from the blood by the kidneys and excreted in the urine. Excess uric acid, caused by increased production or impaired kidney function, requires treatment with uricosuric drugs, which increase the rate at which uric acid is expelled.

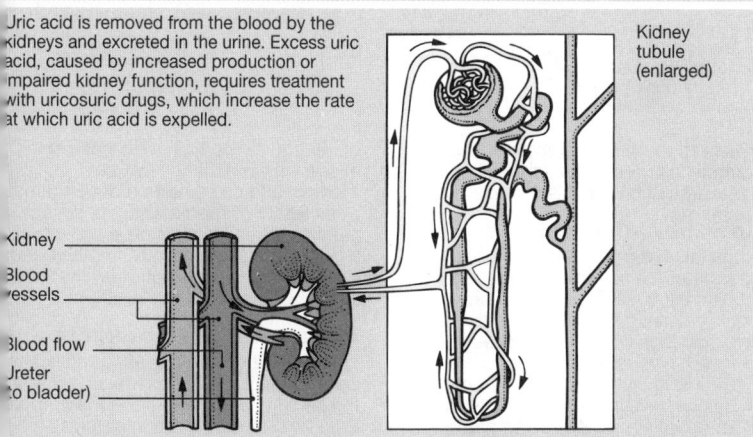

Kidney tubule (enlarged)

Kidney

Blood vessels

Blood flow

Ureter (to bladder)

Uric acid and gouty arthritis

Gouty arthritis occurs when uric acid crystals form in a joint, often in the toe, knee, or hand, causing inflammation and pain. This is the result of excessively high levels of uric acid in the blood. In some cases this is caused by over-production of uric acid, while in others it is the result of reduced excretion of uric acid by the kidneys.

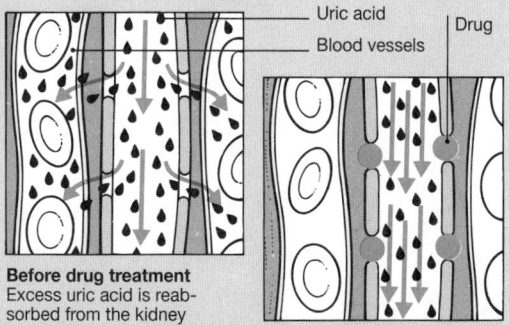

Uric acid

Blood vessels

Drug

Before drug treatment
Excess uric acid is reab-sorbed from the kidney tubule into the bloodstream which carries it to joints. Here uric acid precipitates out forming uric acid crystals, which can cause gouty arthritis.

After drug treatment
When the reabsorption of uric acid is blocked, excretion of uric acid is increased, lowering blood concentrations and reducing crystal formation.

COMMON DRUGS

Drugs to treat attacks
Colchicine
Corticosteroids (see p.153)
Some NSAIDs (see p.128)

Drugs to prevent attacks
Allopurinol
Probenecid
Sulfinpyrazone

MUSCLE-RELAXANT DRUGS

Several drugs are available to treat muscle spasm: the involuntary, painful contraction of a muscle or a group of muscles that can stiffen an arm or leg, or make it nearly impossible to straighten your back. There are various causes of muscle spasm. It can follow an injury, arise spontaneously, or be brought on by a disorder like osteoarthritis, the pain in the affected joint triggering abnormal tension in a nearby muscle.

Spasticity is another form of muscle tightness seen in some neurological disorders such as multiple sclerosis, stroke, or cerebral palsy. This can sometimes be helped by physical therapy but in severe cases drugs may be used to relieve symptoms.

Why they are used

Painful muscle spasm resulting from direct injury is usually and most effectively treated with an analgesic (see p.92) or non-steroidal anti-inflammatory drug (see p.128). However, if the spasm is severe, as it may be following a back injury, a muscle relaxant may be tried for a short period to relieve the symptoms. Muscle relaxants are sometimes added to analgesic preparations for the relief of spasm caused by painful conditions of this type.

In spasticity, the sufferer's legs may become so stiff and uncontrollable that it is impossible to walk unaided. In such cases a drug may be prescribed which relieves symptoms without taking all the strength away from the muscles. Relaxation of the muscles often permits physical therapy to be given for longer-term relief in certain spastic conditions.

How they work

Muscle-relaxant drugs work in one of two ways: the centrally acting drugs slow down the passage of the nerve signals from the brain and spinal cord that cause muscles to contract, thus reducing excessive stimulation of muscles and

SITES OF ACTION OF MUSCLE RELAXANTS

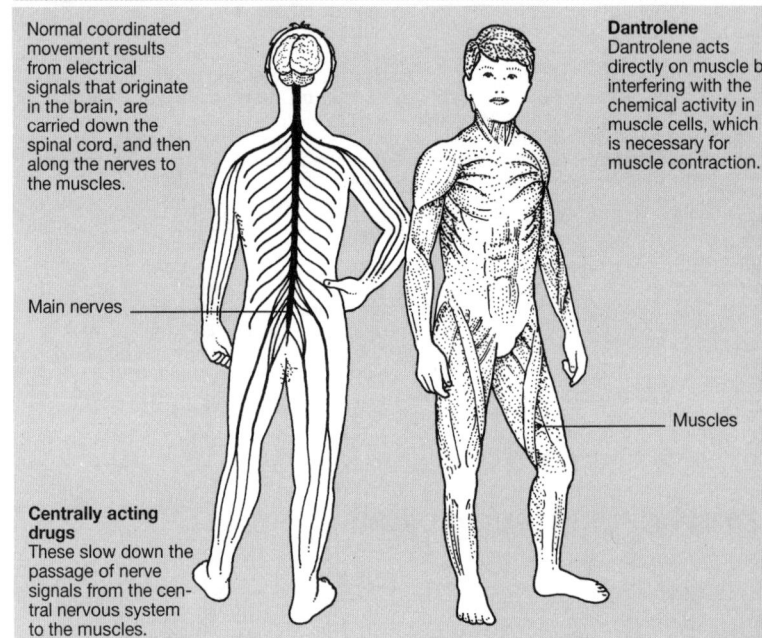

Normal coordinated movement results from electrical signals that originate in the brain, are carried down the spinal cord, and then along the nerves to the muscles.

Dantrolene
Dantrolene acts directly on muscle by interfering with the chemical activity in muscle cells, which is necessary for muscle contraction.

Main nerves

Muscles

Centrally acting drugs
These slow down the passage of nerve signals from the central nervous system to the muscles.

unwanted muscular contraction. Dantrolene reduces the sensitivity of the muscles to nerve signals.

How they affect you

Drugs taken regularly for a spastic disorder of the central nervous system usually reduce stiffness and improve mobility. They may restore the use of the arms and legs when this has been impaired by muscle spasm.

Unfortunately, most centrally acting drugs can have a generally depressant effect on nervous activity and produce drowsiness, particularly at the beginning

of treatment. Too high a dosage can excessively reduce the muscles' ability to contract and can therefore cause weakness. For this reason, the dosage must be carefully adjusted in order to find a level that controls symptoms and at the same time maintains sufficient muscular strength.

Risks and special precautions

The main long-term risk associated with centrally acting muscle relaxants is that the body may become dependent on the drug for depressing the excessive nervous activity responsible for muscle spasm. If the drug is withdrawn suddenly the stiffness may become worse than it was before drug treatment began.

Dantrolene can, in rare cases, cause serious liver damage, and for this reason those taking this drug should have their blood tested regularly to assess liver function.

ACTION OF CENTRALLY ACTING DRUGS

Centrally acting muscle relaxants restrict the passage of nerve signals to the muscles by occupying a proportion of the *receptors* in the central nervous system that are normally used by chemical *neurotransmitters* to transmit such impulses. Reduced nervous stimulation allows the muscles to relax: however, if the dose of the drug is too high, this action may give rise to excessive muscle weakness.

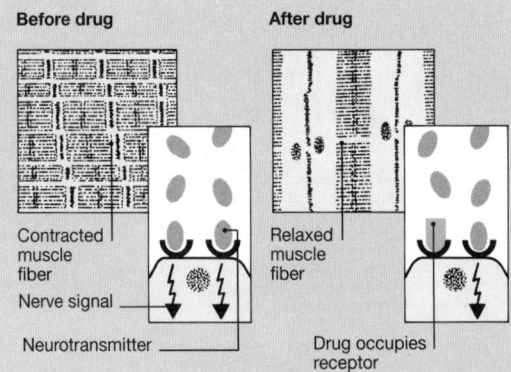

Before drug

After drug

Contracted muscle fiber

Relaxed muscle fiber

Nerve signal

Neurotransmitter

Drug occupies receptor

COMMON DRUGS

Centrally acting drugs
Baclofen
Carisoprodol
Chlorzoxazone
Cyclobenzaprine

Diazepam
Methocarbamol
Orphenadrine

Others
Dantrolene

DRUGS USED FOR MYASTHENIA GRAVIS

Myasthenia gravis is a disorder that occurs when the immune system (see p.164) becomes defective and produces antibodies that disrupt the signals being transmitted between the nervous system and the muscles under voluntary control. The result is a progressive weakening of muscular response. The muscles first affected are those controlling the eyes, eyelids, face, pharynx, and larynx, with muscles in the arms and legs becoming involved as the disease progresses. The disease is often linked to a disorder of the thymus gland, the source of the destructive antibodies concerned.

Treatment of myasthenia gravis can take several forms. It may involve the removal of the thymus gland (thymectomy). Temporary relief may be obtained by clearing the blood of antibodies, a procedure known as plasmapheresis. Drugs are available that improve muscle function, principally neostigmine and pyridostigmine. They may be used alone or together with other drugs that depress the immune system – usually corticosteroids (see p.153) or azathioprine (see immunosuppressant drugs, p.168).

Why they are used

Drugs may be given when it is not feasible to remove the thymus gland or when surgery does not provide adequate relief. Drugs may be taken in the long term to improve muscular strength, but these have no effect on the disease process itself. One of these, edrophonium, acts very rapidly and is used to confirm the diagnosis. When administered to a person suffering from myasthenia gravis, it brings about a dramatic improvement in symptoms, but as the benefits last for only a few minutes, it is not prescribed as a regular treatment for this disorder.

These drugs may also be given following surgery to counteract the effects of a muscle-relaxant drug given prior to certain surgical procedures.

THE EFFECTS OF MYASTHENIA GRAVIS

Myasthenia gravis initially causes weakness of the muscles in the face and throat, affecting the muscles around the eyes and the mouth. In the later stages, arms and legs may be affected.

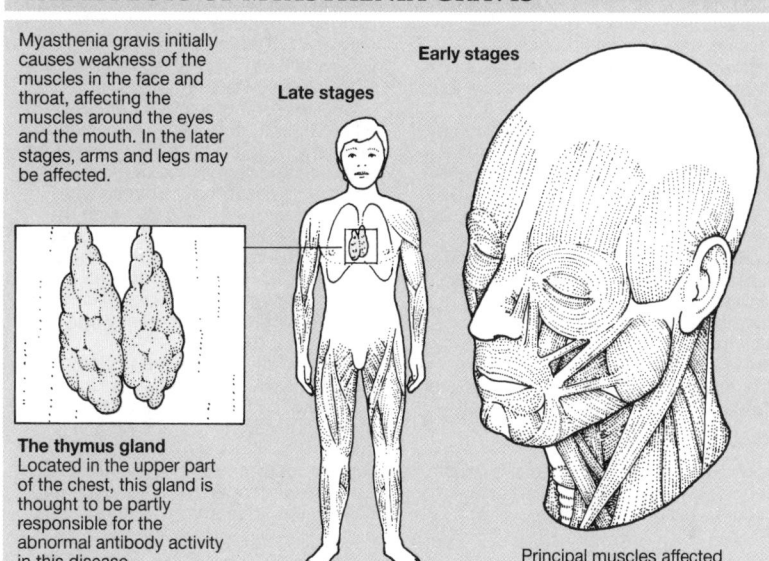

The thymus gland
Located in the upper part of the chest, this gland is thought to be partly responsible for the abnormal antibody activity in this disease.

Principal muscles affected

How they work

Normal muscle action occurs when a nerve impulse triggers a nerve ending to release a *neurotransmitter*, which combines with a specialized receptor on the muscle cells and causes the muscles to contract. In myasthenia gravis, the body's immune system destroys many of these receptors, so that the muscle is less responsive to nervous stimulation. Drugs used to treat the disorder, like neostigmine, increase the amount of neurotransmitter at the nerve ending by blocking the action of an *enzyme* which normally breaks it down. Increased levels of the neurotransmitter permit the remaining receptors to function more efficiently (see Action of drugs used for myasthenia gravis, below left).

How they affect you

These drugs usually restore muscle function to a normal or near normal level particularly when the disease takes a mild form. Unfortunately, they can produce unwanted muscular activity by enhancing the transmission of nerve impulses elsewhere in the body.

Common side effects include vomiting, nausea, diarrhea, and muscle cramps in the arms, legs, and abdomen.

Risks and special precautions

Muscle weakness can suddenly worsen even when it is being treated with drugs. Should this occur, it is important not to take larger doses of the drug in an attempt to relieve the symptoms, because excessive levels can interfere with the transmission of nerve impulses to muscles, causing further weakness. The administration of other drugs, including some antibiotics, can also markedly increase the symptoms of myasthenia gravis. If your symptoms become any worse, your physician should be consulted.

ACTION OF DRUGS USED FOR MYASTHENIA GRAVIS

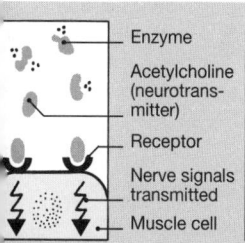

Enzyme
Acetylcholine (neurotransmitter)
Receptor
Nerve signals transmitted
Muscle cell

Normal nerve transmission
Muscles contract when a neurotransmitter (acetylcholine) binds to receptors on muscle cells. An enzyme breaks down acetylcholine.

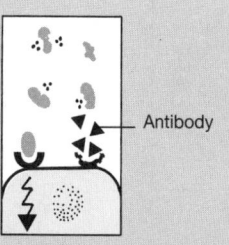

Antibody

In myasthenia gravis
Abnormal antibody activity destroys many receptors, reducing stimulation of muscle cells and weakening muscle action.

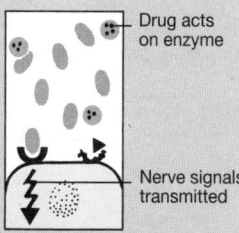

Drug acts on enzyme

Nerve signals transmitted

Drug action
Drugs block enzyme action, increasing acetylcholine and prolonging the muscle cell response to nervous stimulation.

COMMON DRUGS

Neostigmine
Pyridostigmine

DRUGS FOR BONE DISORDERS

Bone is a biologically active tissue of the body, its hard, mineralized quality created by the action of the bone cells. These continuously deposit and remove converted calcium and phosphorus stored in the pockets of a honeycombed protein framework called the matrix. Because the rates of deposit and removal (i.e., the bone *metabolism*) are about equal in adults, the bone mass remains fairly constant.

The bone metabolism is regulated by various hormones and influenced by many factors, notably the level of calcium in the blood. That, in turn, depends on the intake of calcium and vitamin D from the diet, the actions of various hormones, plus the movement and weight-bearing stress involved in everyday activities. When normal bone metabolism is altered, various bone disorders are the result.

Osteoporosis

In osteoporosis the strength and density of bone are reduced. Such wasting occurs when the rate of removal of

mineralized bone by the active cells exceeds the rate of renewal. In most people, bone density begins to decrease very gradually from the age of 30 onward. But bone loss can dramatically increase when a person is immobilized or bedridden for a prolonged period, and this is an important cause of osteoporosis in elderly people. Hormone deficiency is another important cause of osteoporosis, commonly occurring in women with lowered estrogen levels following the menopause or removal of the ovaries. Osteoporosis also occurs in disorders in which there is excess production of adrenal or thyroid hormones. It can be a result of long-term treatment with corticosteroid drugs.

People with osteoporosis often have no symptoms. But if the vertebrae become so weakened that they are unable to bear the body's weight, or if the person is injured in a fall, they may collapse. Subsequently, the individual suffers from back pain, reduced height and a round-shouldered appearance. Osteoporosis

also increases the likelihood of a fracture of the long bone in the arm or leg as a result of an injury or fall.

Most physicians emphasize the need to prevent the disorder by ensuring adequate intake of protein and calcium in the diet and regular exercise throughout adult life. If lack of calcium in the diet is a major cause, supplements are usually prescribed, possibly with vitamin D. Estrogen supplements during and after the menopause help to prevent osteoporosis in older women. For a discussion of such hormone replacement therapy, see p.159.

The condition of bones damaged by osteoporosis cannot usually be improved, although drug treatment can help prevent further deterioration and help fractures heal. The hormone calcitonin is involved with regulation of bone metabolism and calcium balance. Salmon calcitonin, a synthetic derivative, is more suitable for long-term use and is prescribed with dietary calcium and vitamin D. Etidronate, a biophosphate drug, reduces the rate of bone metabolism (p.307).

Osteomalacia and rickets

In osteomalacia – called rickets when it affects children – lack of vitamin D leads to loss of calcium, resulting in softening the bones. Sufferers experience pain and tenderness, and there is a risk of fracture and bone deformity. In children, growth is retarded.

The commonest cause of osteomalacia is lack of vitamin D. This can be caused by inadequate diet, inability to absorb the vitamin, or by insufficient exposure of the skin to sunlight (the action of the sun on the skin produces vitamin D inside the body). People at special risk include those whose absorption of vitamin D from the diet is impaired by an intestinal disorder such as Crohn's disease or celiac disease. Chronic kidney disease is an important cause of rickets in children and of osteomalacia in adults, since healthy kidneys play an essential role in the body's metabolism of vitamin D.

Long-term relief depends on treating the underlying disorder whenever possible. Treatment may in rare cases need to be lifelong.

BONE WASTING

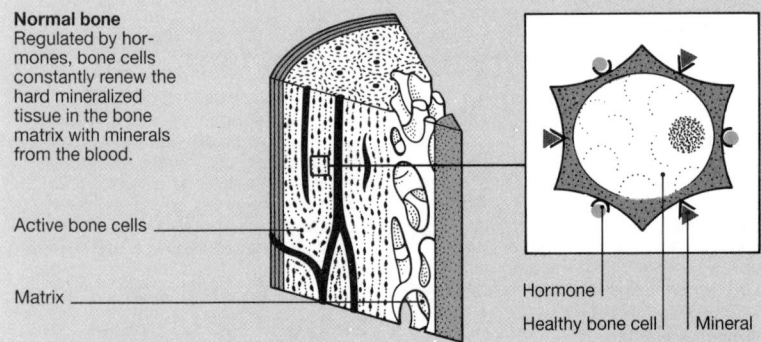

Normal bone
Regulated by hormones, bone cells constantly renew the hard mineralized tissue in the bone matrix with minerals from the blood.

Active bone cells

Matrix

Hormone

Healthy bone cell | Mineral

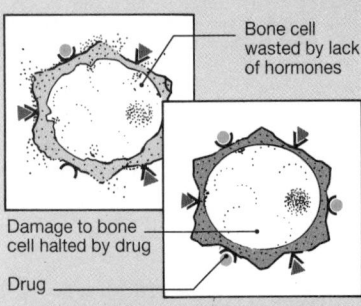

Bone cell wasted by lack of hormones

Damage to bone cell halted by drug

Drug

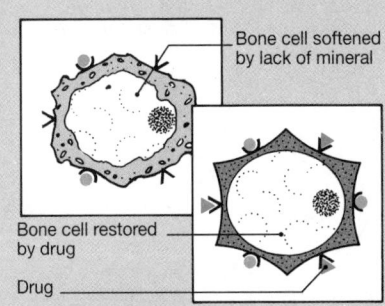

Bone cell softened by lack of mineral

Bone cell restored by drug

Drug

In osteoporosis
Hormonal disturbance leads to wasting of active bone cells. The bones become less dense and more fragile. Drug treatment with hormone and mineral supplements usually only prevents further bone loss.

In osteomalacia
Deficiency of calcium or vitamin D causes softening of the bone tissue. The bones become weaker and sometimes deformed. Drug treatment with specific vitamins and minerals usually restores bone strength.

COMMON DRUGS

Calcitonin
Calcium carbonate
Estrogens (see p.159)
Etidronate
Sodium fluoride
Vitamin D

ALLERGY

Allergy – a hypersensitivity to certain substances – reflects an excessive reaction of the body's immune system. Acting by means of a variety of mechanisms (see Malignant and immune disease, p.164), the immune system protects the body by trying to eliminate foreign substances that it does not recognize, such as invading bacteria or viruses.

One way in which it acts is through the production of *antibodies*. When a particular foreign substance (or allergen) is encountered for the first time, white blood cells known as lymphocytes produce antibodies that attach themselves to other white blood cells known as mast cells. If the same substance is encountered again, the allergen binds to the antibodies on the mast cells causing the release of chemicals called mediators, the most important of which is histamine. This chemical can produce rash, swelling, narrowing of the airways, and a drop in blood pressure.

What can go wrong

People differ widely in their response to allergens, and while some suffer severe allergic (hypersensitivity) reactions to insect bites or particular foods, others suffer no ill effects from exposure to the same substances.

One of the most common allergic disorders, however, is caused by an allergic reaction to inhaled grass pollen, leading to allergic rhinitis – swelling and irritation of the nasal passages and watering of the nose and eyes. Other substances, such as house-dust mites, animal fur, and feathers, may cause a similar reaction in susceptible people. Asthma, another allergic disorder, may result from the action of mediators other than histamine. Other allergic conditions include urticaria (hives) and other rashes (sometimes in response to a drug), some forms of eczema and dermatitis, and allergic alveolitis (farmer's lung).

Why drugs are used

Antihistamines and drugs that inhibit mast cell activity are used to prevent and treat allergic reactions. Other drugs are given for allergic symptoms, such as decongestants (p.105) to clear the nose in allergic rhinitis and bronchodilators (p.104) to widen the airways in asthma. Epinephrine may be used in severe allergic reactions.

MAJOR DRUG GROUPS

Antihistamines

Allergic response

Lymphocytes produce antibodies to allergens, which attach to mast cells. If the allergen enters the body again, it binds to the antibodies, and the mast cells release histamine.

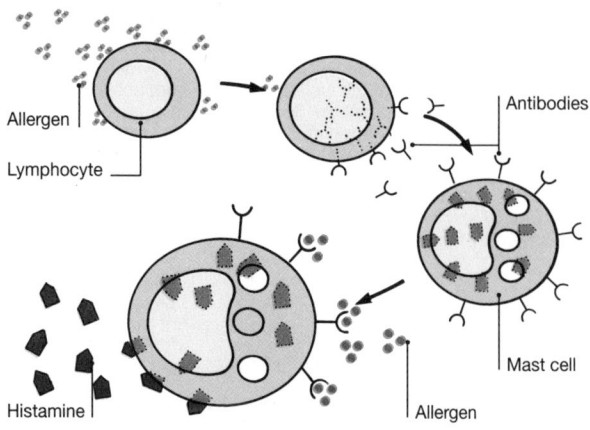

Histamine and histamine receptors

Histamine, released in response to injury or the presence of allergens, acts on H_1 *receptors* in the skin, blood vessels, nasal passages, and airways, and on H_2 receptors in the stomach lining, salivary and lacrimal (tear) glands. It provokes dilation of blood vessels, inflammation and swelling of tissues, and narrowing of the airways. Sometimes a reaction termed anaphylactic shock occurs caused by a dramatic fall in blood pressure and leading to collapse. Antihistamine drugs block H_1 receptors, and H_2 antagonists block H_2 receptors (see also Antihistamines, p.136, and Anti-ulcer drugs, p.121).

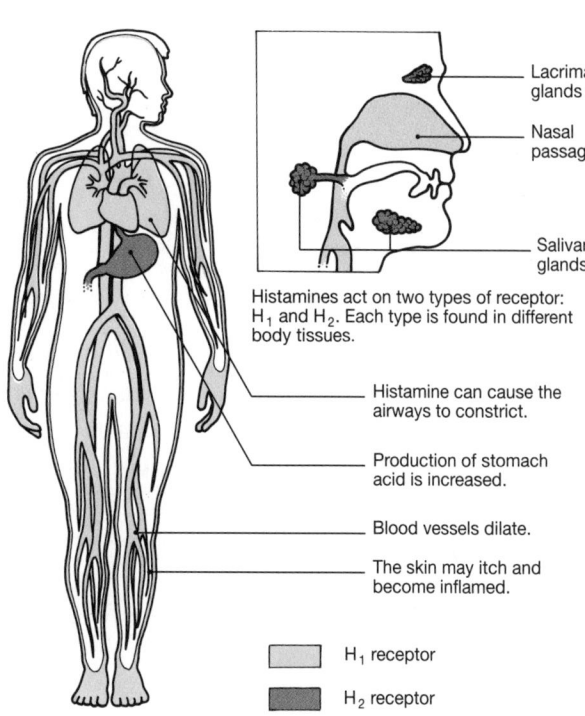

Histamines act on two types of receptor: H_1 and H_2. Each type is found in different body tissues.

Histamine can cause the airways to constrict.

Production of stomach acid is increased.

Blood vessels dilate.

The skin may itch and become inflamed.

H_1 receptor

H_2 receptor

ANTIHISTAMINES

Antihistamines are the most widely used drugs in the treatment of allergic reactions. They can be subdivided according to chemical structure, each subgrouping with slightly different actions and characteristics (see the table on the facing page). Their main action is to counter the effects of histamine, one of the chemicals released in the body when there is an allergic reaction. (For a full explanation of the allergy mechanism, see p.135.)

Histamine is also involved in a number of other body functions, including blood vessel dilation and constriction, the contraction of the muscles of the respiratory and gastrointestinal tracts, and the release of digestive juices in the stomach. The antihistamine drugs described here are also known as H_1 blockers because they only block the action of histamine on certain *receptors*, known as H_1 receptors. Another group of antihistamines, known as H_2 blockers, is used in the treatment of peptic ulcers (see Anti-ulcer drugs, p.121).

Most antihistamines have a significant *anticholinergic* action. Advantageous in a variety of conditions, this also accounts for certain undesired side effects.

Why they are used

Antihistamines relieve allergy-related symptoms when it is not possible or practical to prevent exposure to the substance that has provoked the reaction. Their most common use is in the prevention of allergic rhinitis, inflammation of the nose and upper airways resulting from an allergic reaction to a substance such as pollen, house dust, or animal fur. They are more effective when taken before the start of an attack. If they are taken only after an attack has already started, beneficial effects may not be observed or may be delayed.

Antihistamines are not generally effective in asthma caused by similar allergens because the symptoms of this allergic disorder are not solely caused by the action of histamine, but are likely to be the result of more complex mechanisms. When antihistamines fail to provide adequate relief, alternative treatments may be prescribed (see Other allergy treatments, below).

Antihistamines are also useful for relieving the itching, swelling, and redness characteristic of allergic reactions involving the skin – for example, urticaria (hives), infantile eczema, and other forms of dermatitis. Irritation from chickenpox may be reduced by these drugs. In addition, allergic reactions to insect sting may also be reduced by antihistamines. such cases the drug may be taken by mouth or applied *topically*. Applied as drops, antihistamines also reduce inflammation and irritation of the eyes a eyelids in allergic conjunctivitis.

An antihistamine is often included as an ingredient in cough and cold preparations (see p.106), when the anticholinergic effect of drying mucus secretions and the sedative effect on the coughing mechanism may be helpful.

Because most antihistamines have a depressant effect on the brain, they are sometimes used to promote sleep, especially when discomfort from itching is disturbing sleep (see also Sleeping drug p.94). However, newer antihistamines seem to cause less sedation. Because depressant effect on the brain also extends to the centers that control nausea and vomiting, antihistamines are therefore often effective for controlling these symptoms (see Anti-emetic drugs p.102).

Occasionally, antihistamines are used to treat fever, rash, and breathing difficulties that may occur in adverse reactions to blood transfusions and allergic reactions to drugs.

How they work

Antihistamines block the action of histamine on H_1 receptors. These are four on various body tissues, particularly the small blood vessels in the skin, nose, a eyes. This helps prevent the dilation of the vessels, thus reducing the redness and swelling.

Antihistamines pass from the blood into the brain, where their blocking acti on histamine activity produces general

SITES OF ACTION

Antihistamines act on a variety of sites and systems throughout the body. Their main action is on the muscles surrounding the small blood vessels that supply the skin and mucous membranes. They also act on the airways in the lungs and on the brain.

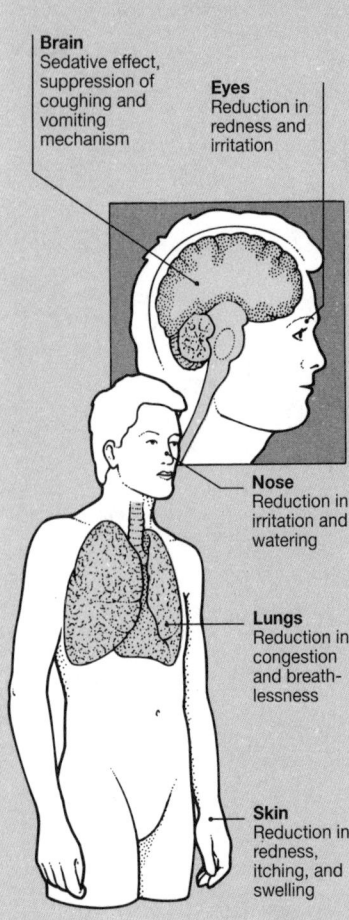

Brain
Sedative effect, suppression of coughing and vomiting mechanism

Eyes
Reduction in redness and irritation

Nose
Reduction in irritation and watering

Lungs
Reduction in congestion and breathlessness

Skin
Reduction in redness, itching, and swelling

OTHER ALLERGY TREATMENTS

Other drugs can replace antihistamines if they are unsuitable or may be added if the symptoms are not adequately controlled.

Anti-inflammatories
Cromolyn sodium curbs the release of histamine from mast cells (see p.135) in response to exposure to an allergen, thus preventing the physical symptoms of allergies. It is most commonly given by inhaler for the prevention of seasonal allergic rhinitis (hay fever) and allergy-induced asthma attacks. For further information on this drug, see p.274.

Corticosteroids are used to treat allergic rhinitis and asthma, usually by inhalers using doses much lower than given in tablet form.

Desensitization
This may be tried in such allergic conditions as allergic rhinitis due to pollen sensitivity, and insect venom hypersensitivity, when antihistamines and other treatments have not been effective and tests have shown one or two specific allergens to be responsible.

Desensitization is less likely to be effective when a large number of factors seem to provoke the allergic response. Also, because such treatment often provides only incomplete relief, it is usually attempted only when simpler measures such as avoidance the allergen have been tried unsuccessfully.

The treatment involves a series of injection containing gradually increasing doses of an extract of the allergen. How this prevents allergic reactions is not fully understood. On explanation is that such controlled exposure to the substance triggers the immune system to produce increasing levels of antibodies to the allergen, so that the body no longer responds dramatically when the allergen is encountered naturally.

Desensitization needs to be carried out under specialist medical supervision, becau it can occasionally provoke a severe allergic response. It is important to remain within close range of emergency medical facilities for at least 60 minutes after each injection.

COMPARISON OF ANTIHISTAMINES

Although antihistamines have broadly similar effects and uses, differences in their strength of anticholinergic action, the amount of drowsiness they produce, and also in their duration of action affect the uses for which each drug is commonly selected. The table at right indicates the main uses of each of the common antihistamines and gives an indication of the relative strengths of their anticholinergic and sedative effects and of their duration of action.

Legend:
- ■ Strong
- ◨ Medium
- □ Minimal
- ▲ Long (over 12 hours)
- ◮ Medium (6 – 12 hours)
- △ Short (4 – 6 hours)

Drug	Common uses					Actions and effects		
	Allergic rhinitis	Skin allergy	Sedation	Premedication	Nausea/vomiting	Drowsiness	Anticholinergic action	Duration of action
Astemizole	●	●				□	□	▲
Azatadine	●	●				■	◨	▲
Brompheniramine	●	●				◨	□	△
Cetirizine	●	●				◨	□	▲
Chlorpheniramine	●	●				◨	□	◮
Clemastine	●	●				◨	◨	◮
Cyproheptadine	●	●				◨	◨	△
Dimenhydrinate					●	◨	◨	△
Diphenhydramine			●		●	■	◨	△
Hydroxyzine		●	●			◨	□	△
Loratadine	●	●				□	□	▲
Meclizine					●	◨	◨	▲
Promethazine	●	●	●	●		■	◨	△
Terfenadine	●	●				□	□	▲
Trimeprazine		●	●			■	◨	◮
Triprolidine	●	●				◨	□	◮

...dation and depression of various brain ...ctions, including the vomiting and ...ughing mechanisms.

...ow they affect you

...tihistamines frequently cause drows-...ss and may adversely affect ...ordination, leading to clumsiness.

Some of the newer drugs have little or no sedative effect (see table above). Anticholinergic side effects, including dry mouth, blurred vision, and difficulty passing urine, are common. Most side effects diminish with continued use and can often be helped by an adjustment in dosage or a change to a different drug.

Risks and special precautions

Because older antihistamines may have a pronounced sedative effect, avoid driving or operating machinery until you know how they affect you.

Antihistamines can also increase the sedative effects of alcohol and anti-anxiety drugs.

In high doses, or in children, some antihistamines can cause excitement. Abnormal heart rhythms have occurred after high doses with some of the newer antihistamines, such as terfenadine, or when some antifungal agents or macrolide antibiotics have been taken at the same time or in people with liver disease, electrolyte disturbances, or heart abnormalities as detected by an electro-cardiogram. People with these conditions or with glaucoma or prostate trouble should seek medical advice before taking antihistamines because their various drug actions may make such conditions worse.

...ANTIHISTAMINES AND ALLERGIC RHINITIS

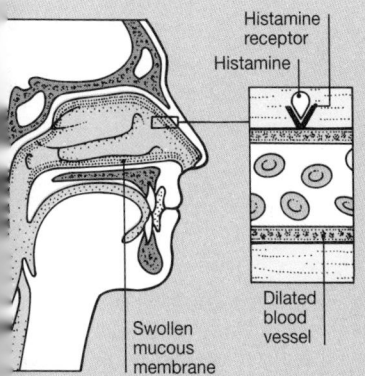

Histamine receptor
Histamine
Dilated blood vessel
Swollen mucous membrane

...efore drug treatment
...allergic rhinitis, histamine released in ...sponse to an allergen acts on histamine ...ceptors and produces dilation of the blood ...essels supplying the lining of the nose, ...ading to swelling and increased mucus ...roduction. There is also irritation that causes ...neezing, and often redness and watering of ...e eyes.

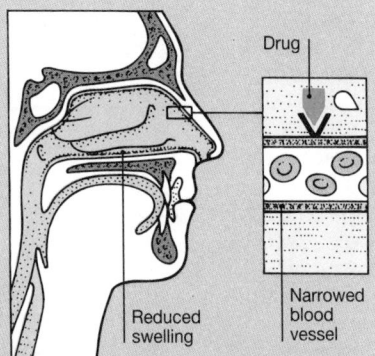

Drug
Narrowed blood vessel
Reduced swelling

After drug treatment
Antihistamine drugs prevent histamine from attaching to histamine receptors, thereby preventing the body from responding to allergens. Over a period of time, the blood vessels in the lining of the nose become narrower, and swelling, irritation, and watery discharge are reduced.

COMMON DRUGS

Astemizole	Diphenhydramine
Azatadine	Hydroxyzine
Brompheniramine	Loratadine
Cetirizine	Meclizine
Chlorpheniramine	Promethazine
Clemastine	Terfenadine
Cyproheptadine	Trimeprazine
Dimenhydrinate	Triprolidine

INFECTIONS AND INFESTATIONS

The human body is a suitable environment for many types of microorganisms, including bacteria, viruses, fungi, yeasts, and protozoa. It may also become the host for animal parasites such as insects, worms, and flukes.

Microorganisms (microbes) exist all around us and can be transmitted from person to person in many ways: direct contact, inhalation of infected air, and consumption of contaminated food or water (see Transmission of infection, facing page). Not all microorganisms cause disease; many types of bacteria exist on the skin surface or in the bowel without causing ill effects, while others cannot live either in or on the body.

Several systems exist to protect the body from infection. Invading microbes are killed before they can multiply in sufficient numbers to produce the symptoms of disease. (See also Malignant and immune disease, p.164.)

What can go wrong

Infectious diseases occur when the body is invaded by microbes against which its natural defenses are ineffective. This may be because the body has little or no natural immunity to the infection in question, or because the number of invading microbes is too great for the immune system to overcome. Serious infections can occur when the immune system does not function properly or when a disease weakens or destroys the immune system. That is what happens in AIDS (acquired immune deficiency syndrome).

Infections can be generalized (such as flu-like viruses and childhood infectious diseases) or they may affect one part of the body (as in wound infections). Some parts of the body are more susceptible to infection than others: respiratory tract infections are relatively common, whereas infections of the bones and muscles are rare.

Symptoms and consequences depend on the infecting organism and the parts of the body affected. Some are the result of damage to body tissues by the infection, others may be caused by *toxins* released by the microbes. In many cases, symptoms are the result of the activity of the body's defense mechanisms.

Most bacterial and viral infections cause fever. Infections may also cause inflammation and pus formation in the affected area.

Why drugs are used

Antibacterial and antibiotic drugs are frequently used to treat bacterial infections. They either kill the bacteria or prevent them from multiplying.

Types of infecting organisms
Bacteria
A typical bacterium (right) consists of a single cell with a protective wall. Some bacteria are aerobic – that is, they require oxygen – and therefore are more likely to infect surface areas such as the skin or respiratory tract. Others are anaerobic and multiply in oxygen-free surroundings such as the bowel or deep puncture wounds.

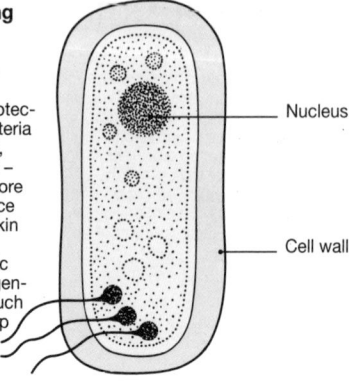

Nucleus

Cell wall

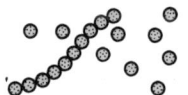

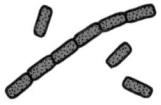

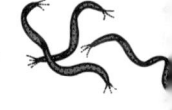

Cocci (spherical)
Streptococcus (above) can cause sore throats and pneumonia.

Bacilli (rod-shaped)
Mycobacterium tuberculosis (illustrated above) causes tuberculosis.

Spirochete (spiral shaped) This group includes those bac that cause syphilis infections of the g

Viruses
The smallest known infectious agents, viruses consist simply of a core of genetic material surrounded by a protein coat. A virus can multiply only in a living cell, using the host tissue's replicating material.

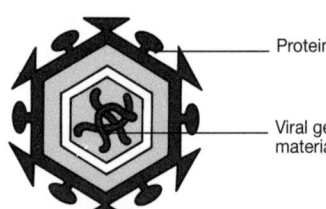

Protein c

Viral gen material

Protozoa
These single-celled parasites are slightly bigger than bacteria. Many live in the human intestine and are harmless. However, some types cause malaria, sleeping sickness, and dysentery.

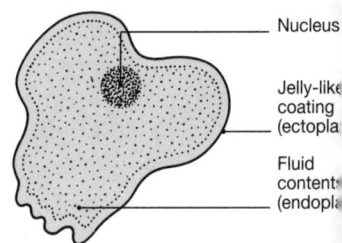

Nucleus

Jelly-like coating (ectopla

Fluid content (endopla

Treatment is necessary because the appearance symptoms shows that the body's defenses have failed to overcome the infection. Some antibiotic can be used against a broad range of bacteria w others have a specific effect against one particul type of bacterium.

There are fewer effective drugs available to tre viral infections. They are principally used in *topic* preparations for the treatment of viral infections the skin and eyes. Luckily, most viral infections a

▌low bacteria affect the body

▌acteria can cause symptoms of disease in two principal ways: first, by ▌leasing toxins that harm body cells; second, by provoking an ▌flammatory response in the infected tissues.

▌ffects of toxins

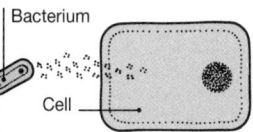
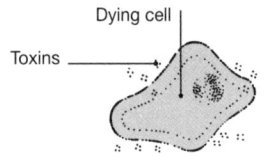

| Bacterium | Dying cell |
| Cell | Toxins |

▌e invading bacterium gives off ▌isons (toxins) which attack the ▌dy cell.

The toxins emanating from the bacterium break through the cell structure and destroy the cell.

▌flammatory response

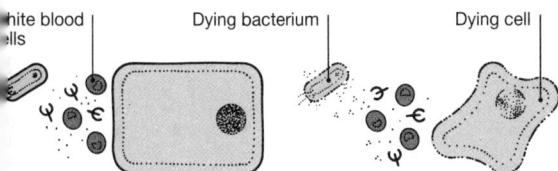

▌hite blood ▌lls — Dying bacterium — Dying cell

▌hite blood cells attack the ▌cterium by releasing inflam-▌atory substances and antibodies ▌owing the defending cells to kill ▌e bacterium.

A side effect of this attack on the bacterium is damage to the body's own cells, often resulting in swelling, redness, and sometimes pus formation.

▌ansmission of infection

▌ecting organisms can enter the human body through a variety of routes, ▌cluding direct contact between an infected person and someone else, ▌d eating or breathing in infected material.

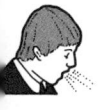

Droplet infection
Coughing and sneezing spread infected secretions.

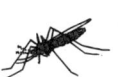

Insects
Insect bites may transmit infection.

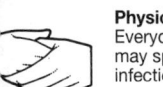

Physical contact
Everyday contact may spread infection.

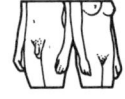

Sexual contact
Certain infections and infestations may be spread by genital contact.

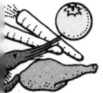

Food
Many infecting organisms can be ingested in food.

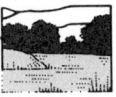

Water
Infections can be spread in polluted water.

▌ercome by the body's natural resistance ▌echanisms.

Other groups of drugs used in the fight against ▌fection include antiprotozoal drugs (including ▌timalarials) used for protozoal infections, ▌tifungal drugs used for infection by fungi and ▌asts, and anthelmintic drugs that eradicate worm ▌d fluke infestation. Infestation by skin parasites is ▌ually treated with topical application of ▌secticides (see p.188).

INFESTATIONS

Invasion by parasites that live on the body (such as lice) or in the body (such as tapeworm) is known as infestation. When infestations cause disease, use of antiparasitic drugs may be necessary. Infestations are often associated with tropical climates and poor hygiene; but head lice affect all of society.

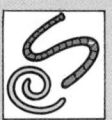

Tapeworms and roundworms live in the intestines and may cause diarrhea and anemia, as well as other problems. Roundworm eggs are spread by the fecal-oral route. Hookworm larvae in contaminated soil usually enter the body through the skin. Some worm infestations enter the body in undercooked meat.

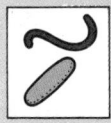

Flukes are of various types. The liver fluke (acquired from infected vegetation) lives in the bile duct in the liver and can lead to jaundice. Another more serious type (which lives in small blood vessels supplying the bladder or intestines) causes schistosomiasis, and is acquired from contact with infected water.

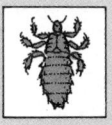

Lice and scabies spread by direct contact. Head, body, and crab lice need human blood to survive and die away from the body. The dried feces of lice spread typhus by being inhaled or infecting wounds. Scabies (caused by a tiny mite which does not carry disease) makes small, itchy tunnels in the skin.

Life cycle of a worm

Many worms have a complex life cycle. The life cycle of the worm that causes the group of diseases known as filariasis is illustrated below.

A mosquito ingests the filarial larvae and bites a human, thereby transmitting the larvae.

The mature larvae enter the lymph glands and vessels and reproduce there, often causing no ill effects.

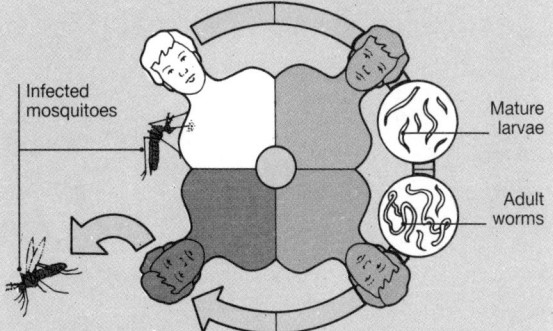

Infected mosquitoes

Mature larvae

Adult worms

The infestation is spread by mosquitoes biting infected people and restarting the cycle.

The larvae grow into adult worms. The severity of the infestation depends on the number of these in the body.

MAJOR DRUG GROUPS

Antibiotics
Antibacterial drugs
Antituberculous drugs
Antiviral drugs
Vaccines and immunization

Antiprotozoal drugs
Antimalarial drugs
Antifungal drugs
Anthelmintic drugs

ANTIBIOTICS

Of all the prescriptions that Canadian physicians write each year, some 15 percent call for the use of antibiotics. Usually safe and effective in the treatment of infections – ranging from minor problems like conjunctivitis to life-threatening diseases like pneumonia, meningitis, and septicemia – the antibiotics have played a major role in broadening the horizons of modern medical treatment.

Many different classes of antibiotics have been developed since 1941, when the first antibiotic – penicillin – was introduced. Each has a different chemical composition and is usually effective against a particular range of bacteria. Some have a broad spectrum of activity against a wide variety of bacteria. Others are used in the treatment of infection by only a few specific organisms. For a description of each common class of antibiotic, see the box on p.142.

Why they are used

A human being lives surrounded by bacteria – in the air he or she breathes, in the mucous membranes of the mouth and nose, on the skin, in the intestines. But we are protected, most of the time, by our defense mechanisms. When these break down, when bacteria already present migrate to a vulnerable new site, or when harmful bacteria not usually present invade the body, infectious disease sets in.

ANTIBIOTIC RESISTANCE

The increasing use of antibiotics in the treatment of infection over the past half century has led to the development of resistance in certain types of bacteria to the effects of particular antibiotics. This resistance to the drug usually occurs when bacteria develop mechanisms of growth and reproduction that are not disrupted by the effects of the antibiotics. In other cases, bacteria produce *enzymes* that neutralize the antibiotics.

Antibiotic resistance may develop in an individual during prolonged treatment when a drug has failed to eliminate the infection quickly, sometimes because the drug was not taken regularly. The resistant strain of bacteria is able to multiply, thereby prolonging the illness. It may also infect other people, causing the spread of resistant infection within a community.

Physicians try to prevent the development of antibiotic resistance by selecting the drug most likely to eliminate the bacteria present in each individual case as quickly and as thoroughly as possible. Failure to complete a course of antibiotics as prescribed by your physician increases the likelihood that the infection will recur in a resistant form.

The bacteria multiply uncontrollably, destroying tissue, releasing toxins, and in some cases threatening to spread via the bloodstream to such vital organs as the heart, brain, lungs, and kidneys. The symptoms of infectious disease vary widely, depending on the site of the infection and the type of bacteria.

Confronted with a sick person and suspecting a bacterial infection, the physician has an array of infection-destroying drugs that he can prescribe. Ideally, he should identify the organism causing the disease before prescribing any of them. But tests to analyze the blood, sputum, urine, stool, or pus usually take 24 hours or more. In the meantime, especially if the person is in discomfort or pain, the physician makes an initial drug choice, something of an educated guess. In starting this empiric treatment, as it is called, the physician is guided by the site of the infection, the severity of the symptoms, the likely source of infection, and the prevalence of similar illnesses in the community at that time.

In such circumstances, pending laboratory identification of the trouble-making bacteria, the physician may initially prescribe a broad-spectrum antibiotic – one effective against a wide variety of bacteria. As soon as tests provide more exact information, the physician may then choose an antibiotic that is the recommended treatment for the identified bacteria. Sometimes more than one antibiotic is prescribed, to be sure of eliminating all strains of bacteria.

In most cases, antibiotics can be given by mouth. However, in serious infection when high blood levels of the drug are needed rapidly, or when a type of antibiotic is needed that cannot be given by mouth, the drug may be given by injection or inhalation. Antibiotics are also included in *topical* preparations for localized skin, eye, and ear infections (see also Anti-infective skin preparations, p.187, and Drugs for ear disorders, p.183).

How they work

Depending on the type of drug and the dosage, antibiotics are either bactericidal, killing organisms directly, or bacteriostatic, halting the multiplication of bacteria and enabling the body's natural defenses to overcome the remaining infection.

There are two main mechanisms of action: penicillins and cephalosporins destroy bacteria by preventing them from making normal cell walls; most other antibiotics act inside the bacteria, interfering with the chemical activities essential to their life cycle.

How they affect you

Antibiotics stop most common types of infection within days. Because they do not relieve symptoms directly, your physician may advise additional

ACTION OF ANTIBIOTICS

Penicillins and cephalosporins
Drugs from these groups are bactericidal, that is, they kill bacteria. They interfere with the chemicals that bacteria need to form normal cell walls (right). The cell's outer lining disintegrates and the bacterium dies (far right).

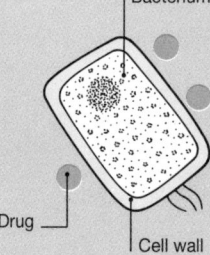
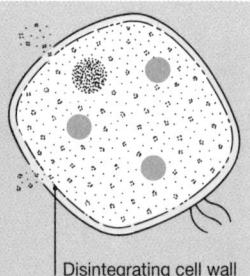

Drug

Bacterium

Cell wall

Disintegrating cell wall

Other antibiotics
These alter chemical activity inside the bacteria, thereby preventing the production of proteins that the bacteria need in order to multiply and survive (right). This may have a lethal effect in itself, or it may prevent reproduction (bacteriostatic action) (far right).

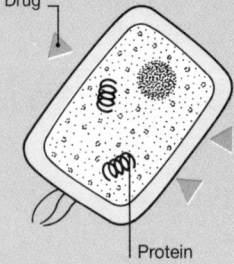
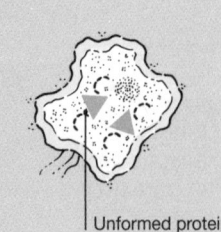

Drug

Protein

Unformed protein

THE USES OF ANTIBIOTICS

The table below shows which common drugs in each class of antibiotic are used for the treatment of infections in different parts of the body. For the purposes of comparison, the table also includes at the bottom some of the antibacterial drugs discussed on page 143.

This is not intended to be used as a guide to prescribing, but broadly to indicate the range of applications of each drug.

Some drugs have a wide range of theoretical applications, but this table concentrates on the most common uses of each drug. Selection of the most suitable agent for any individual is determined by the physician's assessment of the condition, the medical history of the person concerned, and also by the results of laboratory findings (see Why they are used, facing page).

Antibiotic	Ear, nose, throat, and mouth	Respiratory tract	Skin and soft tissue	Gastrointestinal tract	Eye	Kidney and urinary tract	Brain and nervous system	Heart	Bones and joints	Genital tract
Penicillins										
Amoxicillin	●	●		●		●		●	●	●
Ampicillin	●	●		●		●	●	●	●	●
Oxacillin		●	●						●	
Penicillin G	●	●	●				●	●	●	●
Penicillin V	●	●	●							
Cephalosporins										
Cefaclor	●	●				●				
Cefixime	●	●								●
Cefoxitin		●	●	●						●
Cefuroxime		●	●				●		●	●
Cephalexin		●	●							
Macrolides										
Azithromycin		●	●							●
Clarithromycin		●								
Erythromycin	●	●	●		●				●	●
Quinolones										
Ciprofloxacin		●	●	●		●			●	●
Norfloxacin					●	●				●
Ofloxacin		●	●							●
Aminoglycosides										
Gentamicin		●	●	●		●	●	●	●	
Neomycin			●	●						
Streptomycin		●						●		
Tobramycin		●	●	●		●	●		●	
Tetracyclines										
Doxycycline	●	●	●			●				●
Minocycline	●	●	●			●				●
Tetracycline	●	●			●	●				●
Sulfonamides										
Sulfacetamide					●					
Sulfamethoxazole						●				
Lincosamides										
Clindamycin		●	●	●					●	
Other drugs										
Chloramphenicol				●	●			●		
Imipenem/Cilastatin		●	●	●		●			●	●
Metronidazole	●		●	●			●	●	●	●
Nitrofurantoin						●				
Trimethoprim						●				
Trimethoprim/sulfamethoxazole	●	●		●		●				

ANTIBIOTICS continued

medication such as analgesics (see p.92) to relieve pain and fever until the antibiotics start to take effect. It is important to complete the course of medication as prescribed by your physician even if all symptoms seem to have disappeared. Failure to do this can lead to a resurgence of the infection in an antibiotic-resistant form (see Antibiotic resistance, p.140).

Most antibiotics used in the home do not cause side effects if taken in the recommended dosage. But digestive disturbances such as nausea and diarrhea, and yeast infections in women are among the more common reactions. Some people may be sensitive to particular types of antibiotics, and this can lead to serious adverse reactions.

Risks and special precautions

Most antibiotics prescribed for short periods outside a hospital setting are safe for the majority of people. The most common risk, particularly with penicillins and cephalosporins, is an allergic reaction, usually a rash or other skin eruption, but rarely a more serious reaction occurs. If this happens the drug should be stopped and immediate medical advice sought. A previous allergic reaction to an antibiotic means that all other drugs in that class and related classes should be avoided. It is therefore important to inform your physician if you have previously suffered an adverse reaction to treatment with an antibiotic drug.

Another risk of antibiotic treatment, especially if it is prolonged, is that the balance among microorganisms that normally inhabit the body may be disturbed. In particular, antibiotics may destroy the bacteria that normally limit the growth of candida, a yeast that is often present in the body in small amounts. This can lead to overgrowth of candida (also known as thrush) in the mouth, vagina, or bowel. In such cases an antifungal drug (p.150) may need to be prescribed. A rarer, but more serious, consequence of disruption of normal bacterial activity in the body is a disorder called pseudomembranous colitis, in which an antibiotic-resistant bacterium multiplies in the bowel, causing violent bloody diarrhea. Although this potentially fatal disorder can occur with any antibiotic, it is most common with the lincosamides.

Antibiotics taken by mouth or injection must be metabolized in the liver and excreted by the kidneys. Therefore, like many drugs, they should be prescribed with caution for those people who have reduced kidney or liver function (see also Kidney and liver disease, p.22). Specific risks associated with particular types of antibiotics are described under Classes of antibiotics, below.

COMMON DRUGS

Penicillins
Amoxicillin
Ampicillin
Cloxacillin
Penicillin G
Penicillin V
Pivampicillin

Cephalosporins
Cefaclor
Cefixime
Cefoxitin
Cefuroxime
Cephalexin

Aminoglycosides
Gentamicin
Neomycin
Streptomycin
Tobramycin

Tetracyclines
Doxycycline
Minocycline
Tetracycline

Macrolides
Azithromycin
Clarithromycin
Erythromycin

Lincosamides
Clindamycin

Other drugs
Chloramphenicol
Imipenem/cilastatin
Metronidazole
Nitrofurantoin
Trimethoprim
Trimethoprim/sulfa
  methoxazole

Quinolones
Ciprofloxacin
Norfloxacin
Ofloxacin

Sulfonamides
Sulfacetamide
Sulfamethoxazole

CLASSES OF ANTIBIOTICS

Penicillins The first antibiotic drugs to be developed, penicillins are still widely used to treat many common infections. Some penicillins are not effective when they are taken by mouth and therefore have to be given by injection in the hospital. Unfortunately, certain strains of bacteria are resistant to penicillin treatment, and other drugs may have to be substituted. Penicillins can cause allergic reactions.

Cephalosporins These are broad-spectrum antibiotics similar to the penicillins. Some cephalosporins can be given by mouth, but others are effective only when they are given by injection. Many people who are allergic to penicillins are also potentially allergic to cephalosporins. Allergic reactions are the most common adverse effect. Rarely, cephalosporins may cause interference with normal blood clotting and consequent bleeding, especially in the elderly.

Macrolides Erythromycin is the most common drug in this group. It is a broad-spectrum antibiotic that is often prescribed as an alternative to penicillins or cephalosporin antibiotics. Erythromycin is also effective for some diseases, such as Legionnaires' disease (a rare type of pneumonia), that cannot be treated with other antibiotics. Erythromycin is usually safe, although gastrointestinal upset is not uncommon and, occasionally, liver function may be disturbed.

Tetracyclines These have a broader spectrum of activity than any other class of antibiotic. However, increasing bacterial resistance to their effects (see Antibiotic resistance, p.140) has limited their use, although they remain widely prescribed. In addition to the treatment of infections, tetracyclines are also used in the long-term treatment of acne, although this application is probably not related to their antibacterial action. A major drawback to the use of tetracycline antibiotics in young children and in pregnant women is that they can discolor developing teeth.

Tetracyclines are adequately but incompletely absorbed from the intestine. The absorption of tetracyclines can be further reduced by interaction with calcium and other minerals. Drugs from this group therefore should not be taken with iron tablets or milk products. Tetracyclines deteriorate and may become poisonous with time. Leftover tablets or capsules should therefore always be discarded.

Aminoglycosides These potent drugs are effective against a broad range of bacteria, but they are not as widely used as some other antibiotics because, when given by injection they have potentially serious side effects. Aminoglycosides are also used in much smaller doses for eye and ear infections. They are often given in conjunction with other antibiotics.

Possible adverse effects include damage to the nerves in the ear, damage to the kidneys, and severe skin rashes.

Lincosamides These drugs are not commonly used because they are more likely to cause serious disruption of bacterial activity in the bowel than other antibiotics. They are mainly reserved for the treatment of bone, joint, abdominal, and pelvic infections that do not respond well to safer antibiotics.

ANTIBACTERIAL DRUGS

e use of prontosil and its metabolite
fanilamide to treat serious bacterial
ections in 1935 marked the beginning
the era of chemotherapy. Sulfanilamide
d the other "sulfa drugs" were known
antibacterials because they were
emical in origin and development.
nicillin and other later agents derived
m botanical sources, particularly molds
d fungi, were originally designated as
tibiotics. This distinction has become
s meaningful with time, and now
fonamides and other antibacterials are
nerally included within the broad
uping of antibiotics.

hy they are used

fonamides, the largest group of drugs
hin the antibacterial group, are today's
ccessors to the original sulfa drugs.
cause of the appearance of strains of
cteria resistant to their actions (see
tibiotic resistance, p.140), sulfon-
ides have in many cases been super-
ed by antibiotics that are more
ective and safe. Yet there are many
cumstances in which sulfonamides are
ticularly useful in treating infections.
Because they reach high concentra-
ns in the urine, sulfonamides are espe-
lly effective for treating many infections
the urinary tract. They are frequently
ed for chlamydial pneumonia and for
me middle ear infections; sulfacet-
ide is often included in *topical* prepara-
s for skin, eye, and outer ear infec-
ns. Sulfamethoxazole in combination
h trimethoprim is used for bladder
ections, certain types of bronchitis, and
me gastrointestinal infections. Not all
ibacterials are sulfonamides, of
urse. The antibacterials used for tuber-
osis are discussed on p.144. Other
ibacterials are used against protozoal
ctions (see Antiprotozoal drugs, p.148).

RUG TREATMENT FOR
EPROSY

prosy (also known as Hansen's disease)
a bacterial infection caused by an
ganism called *Mycobacterium leprae*. It is
re in Canada, but relatively common in
arts of Africa, Asia, and Latin America.
The disease progresses slowly, first
fecting the peripheral nerves and causing
ss of sensation in the hands and feet. This
ads to frequent unnoticed injuries and
nsequent scarring. Later, the nerves of
e face may also be affected.
Treatment with dapsone, an antibacterial
ug related to the sulfonamides, rapidly
lts infectivity and eventually eradicates
e disease (courses of treatment usually
st about two years). However, because
sistance to this drug is increasing, other
ugs, such as the antituberculous drugs
ampin and ethionamide, may also be
escribed.

ACTION OF SULFONAMIDES

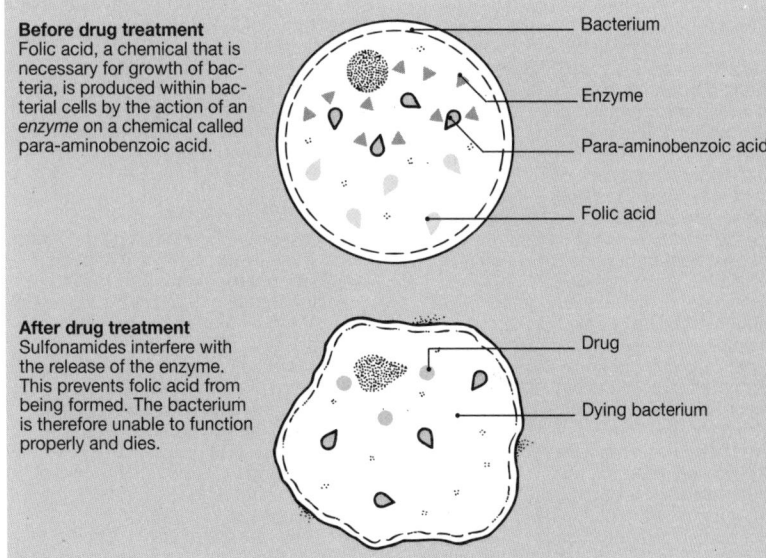

Before drug treatment
Folic acid, a chemical that is
necessary for growth of bacteria, is produced within bacterial cells by the action of an
enzyme on a chemical called
para-aminobenzoic acid.

- Bacterium
- Enzyme
- Para-aminobenzoic acid
- Folic acid

After drug treatment
Sulfonamides interfere with
the release of the enzyme.
This prevents folic acid from
being formed. The bacterium
is therefore unable to function
properly and dies.

- Drug
- Dying bacterium

Metronidazole is prescribed for a
variety of genital infections, and for some
serious infections of the abdomen, heart,
and central nervous system. Nalidixic
acid and nitrofurantoin are effective as
antiseptics for the urinary tract, and are
used to cure or prevent recurrent infections. Norfloxacin and ciprofloxacin are
two more potent derivatives of nalidixic
acid. Norfloxacin is primarily used in the
treatment of urinary tract infections, while
ciprofloxacin is used to treat a wide range
of serious bacterial infections.

How they work
Most antibacterials rid the body of
bacteria by preventing the growth and
multiplication of the organisms (see also
Action of antibiotics, p.140, and Action of
sulfonamides, above).

How they affect you
Antibacterials usually take several days to
eliminate bacteria. During this time your
physician may recommend additional
medication to alleviate pain and fever.
Sulfonamides can cause loss of appetite,
rash, nausea, and drowsiness.

Risks and special precautions
Like antibiotics, most antibacterials can
cause allergic reactions in susceptible
people. Possible symptoms that should
always be brought to your physician's
attention include rashes and fever. If such
a reaction occurs, a change to another
drug is likely to be necessary. Treatment
with sulfonamides carries a number of
risks, the most common being a variety of

rashes and other allergic reactions. Some
drugs in this group can cause crystals to
form in the kidneys, a risk that can be
reduced by drinking adequate amounts of
fluid during prolonged treatment. Because
sulfonamides may also occasionally
damage the liver, they are not usually
prescribed for people with impaired liver
function. There is also a slight risk of
damage to bone marrow, lowering the
production of white blood cells and
increasing the chances of infection.
Physicians therefore try to avoid
prescribing sulfonamides for prolonged
periods. Liver function and blood
composition are often monitored during
unavoidable long-term treatment.

COMMON DRUGS

Sulfonamides
Sulfacetamide
Sulfamethoxazole
Sulfisoxazole

Quinolones
Ciprofloxacin
Nalidixic acid
Norfloxacin
Ofloxacin

Other drugs
Dapsone
Metronidazole
Nitrofurantoin
Trimethoprim

ANTITUBERCULOUS DRUGS

Tuberculosis is a contagious bacterial disease acquired, often in childhood, by inhaling the tuberculosis bacilli (long, tube-shaped bacteria) present in the spray caused by a sneeze or cough from someone who is actively infected. Starting in a lung, tuberculosis takes one of two forms: primary infection or reactivation infection.

In 90 to 95 percent of those with primary infection, the body's immune system renders the bacilli quiescent. They remain alive, however, and they may spread via the lymphatic system and the bloodstream throughout the body (see Sites of infection, below).

Aside from some scarring and inflammation of the lungs, almost the only indication of infection is a reaction to an injection of tuberculin, a sterile extraction from the tuberculosis bacilli. When this is injected into the skin, only those people who have been previously infected show a reaction. Preventive measures are then undertaken (see box, right).

Reactivation tuberculosis (the gradual emergence of the destructive, progressive and sometimes fatal disease in adults) occurs in 5 to 10 percent of those with a primary infection when their bodily defensive mechanisms are reduced. A clinically identical form of the disease, called reinfection tuberculosis, occurs when someone with the dormant primary form of the disease is reinfected.

The symptoms of reactivation (or reinfection) tuberculosis can be deceiving,

SITES OF INFECTION

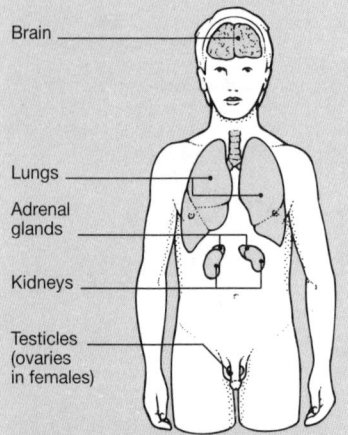

At first, tuberculosis usually affects only part of the lung. It may then spread to both lungs and may also affect the kidneys, leading to pyelonephritis; the adrenal glands, causing Addison's disease; and the membranes surrounding the brain, which may lead to meningitis. The testicles (in men) and the ovaries (in women) may also be affected.

for the disease may start in any part of the body originally seeded with bacilli. The disease is most often first seen in the upper lobes of the lung, and it is often diagnosed after a chest X ray. The early symptoms, which appear gradually, commonly include generally poor health, loss of appetite and weight, recurrent fever, and cough. Reactivation tuberculosis occurs in adults, most often in people over age 70.

Why they are used

Left untreated, tuberculosis continues to destroy tissue and spread. If it is not eventually treated death may result.

Antituberculous drugs can successfully eradicate the infection but they cannot restore destroyed tissue or scarring that has occurred as a result of the disease.

A person diagnosed as having tuberculosis is likely to be treated with three to four antituberculous drugs. This helps overcome the danger that the bacteria may develop resistance to one of the drugs (see Antibiotic resistance, p.140).

The drugs that are most likely to be prescribed first are rifampin, isoniazid, pyrazinamide, and ethambutol or streptomycin, but the choice of drug is determined by the areas of the body that are affected, and by the results of sensitivity tests. These tests may take up to two months to confirm whether the infection is sensitive or resistant to the drugs initially used. If the infection is found to be resistant, the initial treatment fails, or serious adverse effects are experienced, the treatment may be changed.

Drug treatment usually continues for months after the symptoms have subsided and laboratory investigations, such as sputum tests, have shown the person to be clear of infection. The usual length of therapy is nine months; however, in complicated cases, the duration of therapy can be extended to 18 months or longer.

How they work

Antituberculous drugs act either by directly killing the bacteria or by preventing them from multiplying (see Action of antibiotics, p.140).

How they affect you

Although the drugs start to combat the disease within days, benefits of drug treatment are not likely to be noticeable for a few weeks. As the infection is gradually eradicated, the body's healing processes repair the damage caused by the disease. Symptoms such as fever and coughing gradually subside, and weight is gained as appetite and general health improve.

Risks and special precautions

Some antituberculous drugs may cause adverse effects (nausea, vomiting, and abdominal pain), and they occasionally

TUBERCULOSIS PREVENTION

Uninfected people (mostly children) who are regularly exposed to someone with active pulmonary tuberculosis are at risk, and are given a year-long course of isoniazid and, except in children, pyridoxine. However, if the contact with the infected person ceases within that period, the therapy is stopped, provided that tuberculosis skin tests remain negative.

People with a primary tuberculosis infection are treated with the same drugs f a year. The preventive therapy is especially important for those taking certain drugs (especially corticosteroids or immunosuppressants) or those with other serious medical conditions (diabetes, leukemia, Hodgkin's disease, silicosis). The BCG (Bacille Calmette-Guérin) vaccine is sometimes given to people who are not infected but who are exposed frequently. However, many physicians question its effectiveness

lead to serious allergic reactions. These are most likely to occur during the sec month of treatment and may parallel the symptoms of the disease itself – fever general ill health, for instance. When th happens, another drug is substituted.

Some drugs may affect liver function (rifampin and isoniazid); others may adversely affect the nerves (isoniazid). Ethambutol can cause changes in visic and for this reason is not generally prescribed for young children because they are unable to report the warning symptoms. Isoniazid can cause pyridoxine deficiency, and this vitamin may be given with the drug.

Because the occurrence of adverse effects is usually related to levels of th drug in the bloodstream, dosage is carefully monitored. Special care is needed for children, the elderly, and th with reduced kidney function.

COMMON DRUGS

Ethambutol
Isoniazid
Pyrazinamide
Rifampin
Streptomycin

ANTIVIRAL DRUGS

simpler and smaller organism than the
cterium, the virus is less able to sustain
elf. It can survive and multiply only by
netrating body cells (see box, right).
cause the virus performs so few
nctions independently, medicines that
srupt or halt its life cycle without
rming human cells have been difficult
develop.

There are many different types of
uses, and viral infections cause
esses with various symptoms and
grees of severity. Common viral
esses include the cold, influenza and
-like illnesses, and the usual childhood
seases such as mumps and chicken
x. Throat infections, acute bronchitis,
eumonia, gastroenteritis, and
eningitis are often, but not always,
used by a virus.

Fortunately, the body's natural
fenses are usually strong enough to
ercome infections such as these, with
gs given to ease pain and lower fever.
wever, the more serious viral diseases,
ch as pneumonia and meningitis,
quire close medical supervision.

Another difficulty with viral infections is
e speed with which the virus multiplies.
the time symptoms appear, the viruses
e so numerous that drugs may have
e effect. Antiviral agents should be
en early in the course of an infection or
ey may be used prophylactically, i.e., as
reventive. Some viral infections can be
evented by vaccination (see p.146).

n recent years, a few drugs have been
roduced that are effective against
rtain viruses.

hy they are used

tiviral drugs are useful in the treatment
herpes virus infections. Some drugs
applied *topically* to treat herpes eye
ections; topical acyclovir may be used
treat the first outbreak of genital
rpes. An oral form of this drug is more
ective for genital herpes. Acyclovir also
be given by injection, and sometimes
mouth, to treat or prevent severe
rpes infections (e.g., cold sores,
cken pox, shingles) in people who
ve a weakened immune system.
hough antiviral drugs can reduce the
verity and duration of herpes virus
ections, they do not permanently
minate the virus from the body.

Another antiviral agent is amantadine,
ich is used to prevent, and in some
ople to treat, symptoms caused by the
uenza A virus. This drug is also used to
at parkinsonism.

AIDS (acquired immune deficiency
ndrome) is a viral infection that reduces
body's resistance to infection by
er viruses, bacteria, and protozoa, as
l as some types of cancer. Some anti-
l drugs may limit the progress of this
ease. Drug treatment for AIDS is
cussed on p.169.

ACTION OF ANTIVIRAL DRUGS

In order to reproduce, a virus requires a living
cell. The invaded cell eventually dies and the
new viruses are released, spreading and
infecting other cells. Most antiviral drugs act
to prevent the virus from using the cell's
genetic mechanisms to multiply. Unable to
divide, the virus dies and the spread of
infection is halted.

Before drug

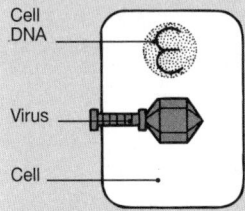

Cell
DNA

Virus

Cell

Virus attaches to and
penetrates body cell and
viral DNA is uncoated.

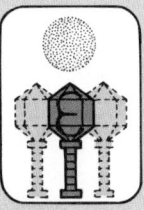

Viral DNA is replicated
in order to produce
new viruses.

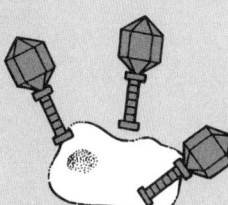

Cell dies and new
viruses are released.

After drug

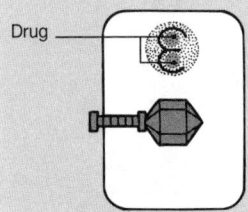

Drug

Virus enters cell that has
absorbed antiviral drug.

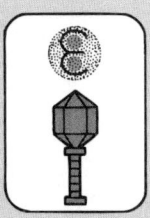

Drug prevents viral DNA
replication and new
viruses are not produced.

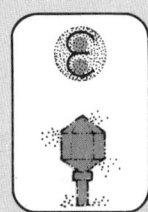

Virus dies and spread
of infection is halted.

How they work

Many antiviral drugs, such as acyclovir,
idoxuridine, trifluridine, and vidarabine,
act by preventing the formation of viral
genetic material (i.e., they inhibit viral
DNA replication). Thus, the virus cannot
multiply. Halting multiplication of the virus
prevents its spread to uninfected cells
and improves symptoms, but in the case
of herpes infections does not completely
eradicate the virus from the body.
Infection may therefore flare up on
another occasion.

Amantadine acts earlier in the influenza
virus life cycle to prevent it from
multiplying. This drug is most effective as
a *prophylactic*, given before the infection
has started.

How they affect you

Topical antiviral drugs do not begin to act
at once, but if the treatment is applied
early enough, an outbreak of herpes can
be cut short. Symptoms usually clear up
within two to four days. Antiviral
ointments may cause irritation and
redness. Antiviral drugs given by mouth
or injection can occasionally cause
nausea and dizziness.

Risks and special precautions

Because some of these drugs are
excreted by the kidneys, they are
prescribed with caution for people with
reduced kidney function. Some antiviral
drugs can adversely affect the activity of
normal body cells, particularly those in
the bone marrow. Idoxuridine is for this
reason available only for topical
application.

COMMON DRUGS

Acyclovir
Amantadine
Ganciclovir
Idoxuridine
Ribavirin
Trifluridine
Vidarabine

VACCINES AND IMMUNIZATION

Many infectious diseases, including most of the common viral infections, occur only once during a person's lifetime. The reason for this is that the antibodies produced in response to the disease remain afterward, prepared to repel any future invasion as soon as the first infectious germs appear. The duration of such immunity varies, but it can last a lifetime.

Protection from many infections can now be provided artificially by the use of vaccines derived from altered forms of the infecting organism. These vaccines stimulate the immune system in the same way as a real infection, and provide lasting, active immunity. A different vaccine is given for each disease because each type of microbe stimulates the production of a specific antibody.

Another type of immunization, called passive immunization, relies on the introduction of antibodies from someone who has recovered from a particular infectious disease. The transfer is made by means of serum (a part of the blood) containing antibodies (see Immune globulins, below).

Why they are used

Some infectious diseases cannot be treated effectively or are potentially so serious that prevention is the best treatment. The aim of routine immunization is not only to protect the individual, but gradually to eradicate the disease completely, as has been achieved with smallpox. Most children between the ages of 2 months and 15 years are routinely vaccinated against the common childhood infectious diseases. Newborn babies receive antibodies for many diseases from their mothers, but this protection lasts only for about three months. In addition, travelers to many underdeveloped countries are often urged to be vaccinated against the diseases common in those regions.

Effective lifelong immunization can sometimes be achieved by a single dose of the vaccine. However, in many cases reinforcing doses, commonly called booster shots, are needed later in order to maintain reliable immunity.

ACTIVE AND PASSIVE IMMUNIZATION

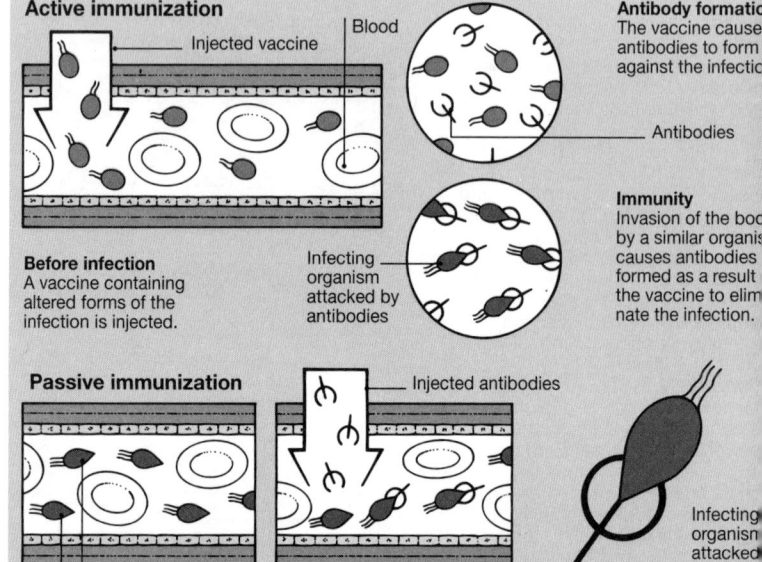

Active immunization

Injected vaccine

Blood

Antibody formatio
The vaccine cause antibodies to form against the infectio

Antibodies

Before infection
A vaccine containing altered forms of the infection is injected.

Infecting organism attacked by antibodies

Immunity
Invasion of the boc by a similar organis causes antibodies formed as a result the vaccine to elim nate the infection.

Passive immunization

Injected antibodies

Infecting organism attacked antibodi

Infecting organisms

After infection
Passive immunization is needed when the infection has entered the blood.

Immune globulin injection
A serum containing antibodies (immune globulin) extracte from donated blood is injected. This helps the body to figh the infection.

Vaccines do not provide immediate protection against infection, and it may be up to four weeks before full immunity develops. When immediate protection from a disease is needed – for example, following exposure to infection – it may be necessary to establish passive immunity with immune globulins.

How they work

Vaccines provoke the immune system into creating antibodies that help the body to resist specific infectious diseases. Many vaccines are made from

artificially weakened forms of the disease-causing germ (live vaccine). Bu these weak germs are nevertheless effective in stimulating sufficient growth antibodies. Other vaccines rely on inactive (or killed) disease-causing ger or inactive derivatives. But their effect the immune system remains the same. Effective antibodies are created; active immunity is established.

How they affect you

The degree of protection varies among different vaccines. Some provide reliab lifelong immunity; others may not give protection against a disease, and the effects may last for as little as six mon Any vaccine may cause side effects, b when these occur they are usually mild and soon disappear. The most commo reactions are a red, slightly raised tend area at the site of injection, and a sligh fever or a flu-like illness lasting for one two days.

Risks and special precautions

For most children, the risk of severe reactions with vaccines is far outweigh by the protection provided. Although there has been concern about a possi association of permanent neurologic disorder and pertussis (whooping coug vaccine, there is no scientific evidence

IMMUNE GLOBULINS

Antibodies, which can result from snake and insect venom as well as infectious disease, permeate the serum of the blood (the part remaining after the red cells and clotting agents are removed). The concentrated serum of people who have survived diseases or poisonous bites is called immune globulin, and given by injection, creates passive immunity. Immune globulin from blood donated by a wide cross section of donors is likely to contain antibodies to most common diseases. Specific immune globulins against rare diseases or toxins are derived from the blood of selected donors likely to have high levels of antibodies to that disease. These are called hyperimmune globulins. Some

immune globulins are extracted from horse blood.

Because immune globulins do not stimulate the body to produce its own antibodies their effect is not long lasting and diminishes progressively over three or four weeks. Continued protection requires repeated injections.

Adverse effects from immune globulins are uncommon. Some people are sensitive to horse globulins, and about a week after the injection may experience a reaction known as serum sickness, with fever, rash, joint swelling, and pain. This usually ends in a few days, but should be reported to your physician before any further immunization.

pport this concern. While the pertussis ccine – usually given in the combined m with diphtheria and tetanus as DPT – ay rarely cause a mild seizure, it is brief, uall ' associated with fever, and stops thout treatment. Children who have perienced such seizures recover com- tely without neurologic or develop-

mental problems. The risk of high fever following DPT can be reduced by giving acetaminophen at the time of vaccination. Children who have an infection more severe than a common cold will not be routinely vaccinated until they have recovered.

Live vaccines should not be given

during pregnancy, since they can affect the developing baby, nor should they be given to people whose immune systems are weakened by disease or drug therapy. It is also advisable for those taking corticosteroids (p.153) to delay their vaccination until the end of drug therapy.

COMMON VACCINATIONS

Disease	Age	How given	General information
Diphtheria	2 months, 4 months, 6 months, 18 months, 4 – 6 years.	Injection	Usually given routinely in infancy as a combined injection with tetanus and whooping cough vaccines. Immunity may diminish in later life.
Tetanus	2 months, 4 months, 6 months, 18 months, 4 – 6 years. Boosters every 5 years.	Injection	Given routinely in infancy, this gives protection for 5 to 10 years. Injury likely to result in tetanus infection in a person who has not been vaccinated within the last five years is usually treated immediately with immune globulin (see p.146), and at the same time the physician may start a course of booster injections of the active vaccine. Tetanus boosters in adulthood should not be given within five years of the previous booster, otherwise a hypersensitivity reaction may occur.
Whooping cough (pertussis)	2 months, 4 months, 6 months, 18 months, 4 – 6 years.	Injection	The pertussis vaccine may not give complete protection against whooping cough, but reduces the severity of symptoms that may develop following infection. Pertussis vaccine may cause mild fever, irritability, and, rarely, seizures.
Polio	2 months, 4 months, 18 months, 4 – 6 years. Boosters during adulthood as directed.	By mouth	Many physicians recommend a booster every 10 years, especially for people likely to be traveling to countries where polio is still prevalent.
Rubella (German measles)	12 – 15 months.	Injection	Given as a combined injection with measles and mumps vaccine in infancy, immunization against this disease is important because rubella can damage the developing baby if it affects a woman in early pregnancy. Women of childbearing age who have received the vaccine should be careful to avoid becoming pregnant for at least three months following the injection.
Measles	12 – 15 months.	Injection	Given together with mumps and rubella vaccine in infancy. It may cause a brief fever or rash, and there is a possibility of seizures.
Mumps	12 – 15 months.	Injection	Given in infancy together with measles and rubella vaccines.
Haemophilus influenzae type b	2 months, 4 months, 6 months, 18 months.	Injection	*Haemophilus influenzae* type b is the most common cause of bacterial meningitis and a leading cause of other severe infections in young children.
Influenza	People of any age who are at risk.	Injection	It is impossible to confer long-term immunity against all forms of this disease, but protection against some types may be given to people especially at risk from complications. Protection develops within four weeks and side effects are rare. Annual booster vaccinations are needed.
Hepatitis B	People of any age who are at risk.	Injection	Recommended for all children and adults at risk (health-care workers, children born to carrier mothers, male homosexuals, and intravenous drug users).

ANTIPROTOZOAL DRUGS

Protozoa, single-celled organisms that are often present in soil and may infect animals, can be transmitted to or between humans through contaminated food or water, sexual contact, or bites from insects. There are many types of protozoal infections, each causing a different disease, depending on the organism involved. Trichomoniasis, giardiasis, and pneumocystis pneumonia are probably the most common protozoal infections seen in Canada. The rarer infections are usually contracted as a result of exposure to infection in another part of the world.

Many types of protozoa infect the bowel, causing diarrhea and generalized symptoms of ill health. Others may infect the genital tract or skin. Some may penetrate vital organs such as the lungs, brain, and liver. Prompt diagnosis and treatment are important in order to limit the spread of the infection within the body and to other individuals. In many cases, increased attention to hygiene is an important factor in controlling the spread of the disease.

A variety of drugs are used in the treatment of these diseases. Some, such as metronidazole and tetracycline, are also used for their antibacterial action. Others, such as iodoquinol, are rarely used except in specific protozoal infections.

How they affect you

Protozoa are often difficult to eradicate from the body. Drug treatment may therefore need to be continued for months in order to eliminate the infecting organisms completely, and thus prevent recurrence of the disease. In addition, unpleasant side effects such as nausea, diarrhea, and abdominal cramps are often unavoidable because of the limited choice of drugs and the need to maintain dosage levels that will effectively cure the disease. For detailed information on the risks and adverse effects of individual antiprotozoal drugs, consult the appropriate drug profile in Part 4.

The table below describes the principal protozoal infections and some of the drugs used in their treatment. Malaria, probably the most common protozoal disease in the world today, is discussed on the facing page.

SUMMARY OF PROTOZOAL DISEASES

Disease	Protozoa	Description	Drugs
Amebiasis (amebic dysentery)	Entamoeba histolytica	Infection of the bowel and sometimes of the liver and other organs. Usually transmitted in contaminated food or water. Major symptom is violent, sometimes bloody diarrhea.	Iodoquinol Metronidazole Chloroquine Paromomycin
Balantidiasis	Balantidium coli	Infection of the bowel, specifically the colon, usually transmitted through contact with infected pigs. Possible symptoms include diarrhea and abdominal pain.	Tetracycline Iodoquinol Metronidazole
Dientamebiasis	Dientamoeba fragilis	Similar to amebiasis, but a milder disease. Possibly transmitted in the pinworm egg. Causes diarrhea and flu-like symptoms.	Tetracycline Iodoquinol Paromomycin
Giardiasis (lambliasis)	Giardia lamblia	Infection of the bowel, usually transmitted in contaminated food or water, but may also be spread by some types of sexual contact. Major symptoms are general ill health, diarrhea, flatulence, and abdominal pain.	Metronidazole Quinacrine Furazolidone Paromomycin
Leishmaniasis	Leishmania	A mainly tropical and subtropical disease spread through sand fly bites. It affects the mucous membranes of the mouth, nose, and throat, and may in its severe form invade organs such as the liver.	Antimony-based agents (stibogluconate) Amphotericin B Pentamidine
Pneumocystis pneumonia	Pneumocystis carinii	Potentially fatal lung infection that usually affects only those with reduced resistance to infection, such as AIDS victims. Symptoms include cough, breathlessness, fever, and chest pain.	Trimethoprim/sulfamethoxazole Pentamidine Trimethoprim/dapsone
Toxoplasmosis	Toxoplasma gondii	Infection usually spread through contacts with cat feces or by eating undercooked meat. It may also be transmitted from mother to baby during pregnancy. May be symptomless, but sometimes causes generalized ill health and low fever, and may affect vision.	Pyrimethamine/sulfadiazine Spiramycin
Trichomoniasis	Trichomonas vaginalis	Infection most commonly affects the vagina, causing irritation and an offensive discharge. In men infection may occur in the urethra. The disease is usually sexually transmitted.	Metronidazole
Trypanosomiasis	Trypanosoma	African trypanosomiasis (sleeping sickness) is spread by the tsetse fly and causes fever, swollen glands, and drowsiness. South American trypanosomiasis (Chagas' disease) is spread by cone-nosed bugs. It causes inflammation, enlargement of internal organs, and infection of the brain.	Pentamidine, suramin, melarsoprol, nifurtimox, benznidazole

ANTIMALARIAL DRUGS

all the infectious diseases that afflict ankind, the one that causes more illness d more deaths worldwide is malaria. evalent largely in the tropical zones (see ap below), malaria usually strikes only ose Canadians who travel there or ose who happen to receive a transfu- n of malaria-infected blood.

Malaria is caused by single-cell otozoa whose life cycle is far from nple. A parasite, the malaria plas- odium, as it is called, lives in and pends on the female anopheles osquito during one part of its life. It lives and depends on human beings during her parts of its life cycle.

Transferred to man in the saliva of the osquito as she penetrates ("bites") the n, the malaria parasite enters the oodstream and settles in the liver. hough no symptoms appear yet, the alaria parasite multiplies, asexually. Following its stay in the liver, the rasite enters another phase of its life cle, circulating in the bloodstream, netrating and destroying red blood ls and reproducing again, the results s time including male and female forms the parasite. If the sexual forms then nsfer back to a female anopheles osquito via another "bite," they breed ce more (bisexually), and are again dy to start a human infection.

It is after the emergence from the liver, when the plasmodia are entering and rupturing the red blood cells, that malaria appears in its classic, symptomatic form: high fever and profuse sweating, alternating with equally agonizing epi- sodes of shivering and chills. One strain of malaria (there are four) can produce a single severe attack, possibly fatal if untreated. The other forms of malaria cause recurrent attacks, sometimes extending over many years.

A number of drugs are available for malaria, the choice depending on many factors, such as the region in which the disease may have been contracted.

Why they are used

The medical response to malaria has three aims: suppression, the treatment of symptomatic attacks, and the complete eradication of the plasmodia.

For someone planning a trip to an area where malaria is prevalent, drugs are given that destroy the parasites before they can reach the liver. Treatment begins the week before arrival in the malarial area and will continue for four to eight weeks after return.

The same drugs are effective during the symptomatic period, relieving the episodes of fever and chills. However, these medicines do not destroy the

plasmodia remaining in the liver. Future malarial attacks are probable, sometimes occurring many years later.

The treatment of someone with malaria will depend on the chloroquine sensitivity of the infection. If it is known that the infection was definitely acquired in a chloroquine-sensitive area, the infection may be treated with chloroquine alone. Infections that are acquired in chloroquine- resistant zones should be treated with oral quinine in combination with either oral doxycycline, pyrimethamine/ sulfadoxine or clindamycin. A person who cannot tolerate oral medications or is suffering from a severe infection should be treated with intravenous quinidine or quinine. Halofantrine can be used if standard therapy fails.

How they work

Most antimalarial drugs act by rapidly killing plasmodia in the bloodstream. Taken as a suppressive, the drugs kill the plasmodia before they enter the liver, so stopping them from multiplying. Once the plasmodia have multiplied in the liver, the same drugs given in higher doses kill the parasites that reenter the bloodstream.

How they affect you

The low doses of antimalarial drugs taken to suppress the disease rarely cause noticeable effects. Drugs taken for an attack usually begin to relieve symptoms within a few hours. Most of them can cause nausea, vomiting, and diarrhea. More seriously, quinine can produce giddiness, noises in the ear, and disturbances in vision and hearing.

Risks and special precautions

When drugs are given to suppress or cure malaria the full course of treatment must be taken. No drugs give long-term protection: new treatment is needed for each journey. Because no drug is effective against every type of malaria, a change of antimalarial drug may be necessary when traveling from one malarial area to another where a differ- ent form of malaria may be prevalent.

Though most of these drugs do not produce severe adverse effects, prima- quine can cause the blood disorder hemolytic anemia, particularly in people with glucose-6-phosphate dehydro- genase (G6PD) deficiency. Hence, blood tests are taken before treatment to identify susceptible individuals.

CHOICE OF DRUGS

he parts of the world in hich malaria is prevalent lustrated on the map, ght), and travel to which ay make antimalarial drug eatment advisable, can be vided into two groups. he table below indicates e drug(s) currently commended for the evention and treatment of alaria for each group. It is, owever, advisable to take pecific medical advice efore traveling to these eas. Pregnant women and omen of childbearing age ay need alternative drug eatment.

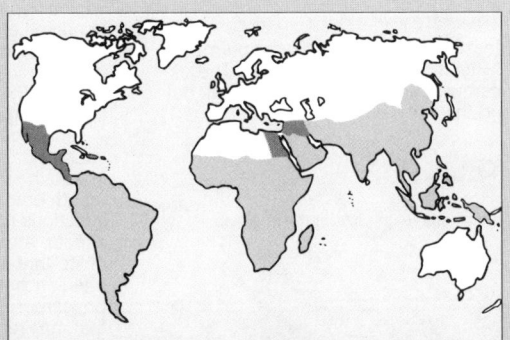

	Group 1 areas	Group 2 areas
	South America, Central and Southern Africa, China, Southeast Asia, and Oceania.	Central America west of the Panama Canal, Mexico, Haiti, the Dominican Republic, and parts of the Middle East including Egypt, Syria, and Iraq.

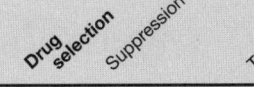

Drug selection	Suppression	Treatment
roup 1 areas	Mefloquine	Quinine with doxycyline, pyrimethamine/sulfadoxine or clindamycin
roup 2 areas	Chloroquine	Chloroquine only

COMMON DRUGS

Chloroquine	Primaquine
Clindamycin	Pyrimethamine/
Doxycycline	sulfadoxine
Halofantrine	Quinidine
(investigational)	Quinine
Mefloquine	

ANTIFUNGAL DRUGS

We are continually exposed to fungi – in the air we breathe, the food we eat, and the water we drink. Fortunately, most of them cannot live in the body, and few are harmful. But some can grow in the mouth, skin, hair, or nails, causing irritating or unsightly changes, and a few can cause serious and possibly fatal disease. The most common fungal infections are caused by the tinea group of infections. These include tinea pedis (athlete's foot), tinea cruris (jock itch), and tinea capitis (scalp ringworm). They are caused by a variety of organisms and may be spread by direct or indirect contact with infected humans or animals. Infection is encouraged by warm, moist conditions.

Problems may also result from the proliferation of a fungus normally present in the body; the most common example is excessive growth of candida, a yeast which causes thrush infection of the mouth, vagina, and bowel. It can also infect other organs if it spreads through the body via the bloodstream.

Overgrowth of candida may be provoked by diabetes, pregnancy, immune system disorders such as AIDS, treatment with antibiotics (p.140), or by taking oral contraceptives (p.173).

Superficial fungal infections – those that attack only the outer layer of the skin and mucous membranes – are relatively common and, although irritating, do not usually present a threat to general health. Internal fungal infections – for example, of the lungs, heart, or other organs – are rare, but may be serious and prolonged.

Because antibiotics and other anti-bacterial drugs have no effect on fungi and yeasts, a different type of drug is needed. Drugs for fungal infections are either applied *topically* to treat minor infections of the skin and mucous membranes or given by mouth or injection to eliminate serious fungal infections of the internal organs and nails.

Why they are used

Drug treatment is necessary for most fungal infections since they rarely improve alone. Measures such as careful washing and drying of affected areas may help, but are not a substitute for antifungal drugs. The use of over-the-counter preparations to increase the acidity of the vagina is not usually effective except when accompanied by drug treatment.

Fungal infections of the skin and scalp are usually treated with a cream or shampoo. Drugs for vaginal thrush may be applied in the form of vaginal suppositories or cream. A new oral tablet for vaginal thrush (fluconazole) is given as a single dose. It may be repeated once a month if necessary. Mouth infections are usually eliminated by lozenges dissolved in the mouth or an antifungal solution applied directly to the affected areas. When candida infects the bowel, an antifungal drug that is not absorbed into the bloodstream, nystatin for example, is given in tablet form.

In the rare cases in which fungal infections affect internal organs, or when the nails are severely affected by persistent tinea infection, drugs such as griseofulvin, amphotericin B, and ketoconazole, which pass into the bloodstream, are given by mouth or injection.

How they work

Most of these drugs alter the permeability of the fungal cell's walls. The chemicals essential for cell life leak out and the cell dies.

ACTIONS OF ANTIFUNGAL DRUGS

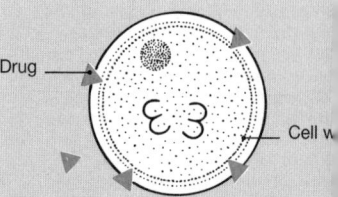

Drug — Cell w

Stage one
The drug acts on the wall of the fungal cell.

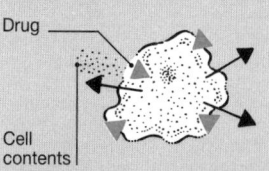

Drug — Cell contents

Stage two
The drug damages the cell wall and the ce contents leak out. The cell dies.

How they affect you

The speed with which antifungal drugs provide benefit varies with the type of infection. Thrush and most other funga yeast infections of the skin, mouth, anc vagina improve within a week. The condition of nails affected by fungal infections improves only when new nai growth occurs, and this takes many months. *Systemic* infections of the internal organs can take weeks to cure.

Antifungal drugs applied topically ra cause side effects, although they may irritate the skin. However, treatment by mouth or ingestion for systemic and na infections may produce more serious s effects. Amphotericin B, injected in cas of life-threatening systemic infections, often causes unpleasant and potentiall dangerous effects, notably a severe fev that may require other drugs. Because this drug may also cause kidney dama sufferers need regular blood tests. Griseofulvin, given for persistent nail infections, carries a risk of liver damag For this reason it is prescribed only wh topical treatments have failed and nail damage is severe.

CHOICE OF ANTIFUNGAL DRUG

The table below shows the range of uses for each antifungal drug. The particular drug chosen in each case depends on the precise nature and site of the infection.

Drug	Infection						Systemic candida	Administration		
	Skin ringworm	Scalp ringworm	Nail infection	Mouth thrush	Vaginal thrush	Candida of the skin	Systemic candida	Topical	Injection	Oral
Amphotericin B							●		●	
Ciclopirox	●				●			●		
Clotrimazole	●	●		●	●			●		
Econazole	●	●		●	●			●		
Fluconazole			●	●	●		●		●	●
Griseofulvin	●	●	●							●
Ketoconazole	●	●			●	●		●		●
Miconazole	●	●		●	●			●		
Nystatin			●					●		●
Terbinafine	●	●	●					●		●
Terconazole					●			●		
Tolnaftate	●	●						●		

COMMON DRUGS

Amphotericin B	Ketoconazole
Ciclopirox	Miconazole
Clotrimazole	Nystatin
Econazole	Terbinafine
Fluconazole	Terconazole
Griseofulvin	Tolnaftate

ANTHELMINTIC DRUGS

Anthelmintics are drugs that are used to eliminate the many types of worm (helminths) that can enter the body and live there as parasites, producing a general weakness in some cases, and serious harm in others. The body may be host to many different worms (see Choice of drug, below). Most species spend part of their life cycle in another animal, and the infestation is often passed on to humans in food contaminated with the eggs or larvae. Some larvae, such as those of hookworm, enter the body through the skin. Larvae or adults may attach themselves to the intestinal wall and feed on the bowel contents; others feed off the intestinal blood supply, causing *anemia*. Worms can also infest the bloodstream or lodge in the muscles or organs.

Many people have worms at some time during their life, especially during childhood; most can be effectively eliminated with anthelmintic drugs.

Why they are used

Most worms common in Canada cause only mild symptoms and generally do not pose any threat to general health. Anthelmintic drugs are usually necessary, however, because the body's natural

defenses against infection are not effective against most worm infestations. Certain types of worm infestation must always be treated since they can cause serious complications. Common roundworm (ascariasis) can block the intestine. In some cases, such as pinworm infestation, physicians may advise anthelmintic treatment for the whole family, to prevent reinfection. Laxatives are given with some anthelmintics to hasten expulsion of worms from the bowel. Other drugs may be prescribed to ease symptoms or to compensate for any blood loss or nutritional deficiency. If worms have invaded tissues and formed cysts, they may have to be removed surgically.

How they work

The anthelmintic drugs act in several ways. Many of them kill or paralyze the worms, and they pass out of the body in the feces. Others, that act *systemically*, are used to treat infection in the tissues. Many anthelmintics are specific for particular worms, and the physician must identify the worm before selecting the most appropriate treatment (see Choice of drug, below). Most common infestations of the intestine are easily

treated, often with only one or two doses of the drug. However, tissue infections may require more prolonged treatment.

How they affect you

Once the drug has eliminated the worms, symptoms caused by infestation rapidly disappear. Taken as a single dose, or a short course, anthelmintics do not usually produce side effects. However, treatment can disturb the digestive system, causing abdominal pain, nausea, and vomiting.

COMMON DRUGS

Diethylcarbamazine
Mebendazole
Praziquantel
Pyrantel
Thiabendazole

CHOICE OF DRUG

Pinworm (enterobiasis)
The most common worm infection in Canada. Commonly affects children. Eggs are usually swallowed in contaminated food or from sucking contaminated fingers or objects. Worms infect the intestines and lay eggs around the skin of the anus, often causing itching.
Drugs Mebendazole, pyrantel

Common roundworm (ascariasis)
The most common worm infection worldwide – transmitted in contaminated raw food or in soil. Infects the intestine. The worms are large and can block the intestine.
Drugs Mebendazole, pyrantel

Threadworm (strongyloidiasis)
Mainly occurs in the southern United States and southern Europe. Larvae penetrate skin in contact with contaminated soil, pass into the lungs and later are swallowed into the digestive tract.
Drugs Thiabendazole

Whipworm (trichuriasis)
Mainly occurs in tropical areas as a result of eating contaminated raw vegetables. Worms infest the intestines.
Drugs Mebendazole

Hookworm (uncinariasis)
Mainly found in tropical areas. Worm larvae penetrate skin and pass via the lymphatic system and bloodstream to the lungs. They then travel up the airways, are swallowed, and attach themselves to the intestinal wall.
Drugs Mebendazole, pyrantel

Pork roundworm (trichinosis)
Transmitted in infected undercooked pork. Initially worms lodge in the intestines, but larvae may invade muscle to form cysts that are often resistant to drug treatment.
Drugs Mebendazole, thiabendazole

Toxocariasis (visceral larva migrans)
Usually occurs as a result of eating soil contaminated by dog or cat feces. Eggs hatch in the intestine and may travel in the bloodstream to the lungs, liver, kidney, brain, and eyes.
Drugs Mebendazole, thiabendazole

Creeping eruption (cutaneous larva migrans)
Mainly occurs in tropical areas and coastal areas of southeastern United States as a result of skin contact with larvae from cat and dog feces. Infestation is usually confined to skin.
Drugs Thiabendazole

Filariasis (including onchocerciasis and loiasis)
Tropical areas only. Infection by this group of worms is spread by bites of insects that are carriers of worm larvae or eggs. May affect lymphatic system, blood, eyes, and skin.
Drugs Diethylcarbamazine

Flukes
Sheep liver fluke (fascioliasis) is indigenous to the United States. Infestation usually results from eating watercress grown in contaminated water. Mainly affects the liver and biliary tract. Other flukes found only abroad may infect the lungs, intestines, or blood.
Drugs Praziquantel

Tapeworms (including beef, pork, fish, and dwarf tapeworms)
Depending on type, may be carried by pigs, cattle, or fish and transmitted to humans in undercooked meat. Most types affect the intestines. Larvae of the pork tapeworm may form cysts in muscle and other tissues.
Drugs Mebendazole, praziquantel

Hydatid disease (echinococciasis)
Eggs are transmitted in dog feces. Larvae may form cysts over many years, commonly in the liver. Surgery is the usual treatment for cysts.
Drugs Mebendazole

HORMONES AND ENDOCRINE SYSTEM

The endocrine system is a collection of glands located throughout the body that produce *hormones* and release them into the bloodstream. Each endocrine gland produces one or more hormones, each of which governs a particular body function, including growth and repair of tissues, sexual development and reproductive function, and the body's response to stress.

Most hormones are released continuously from birth, but the amount produced fluctuates with the body's needs. Others are produced mainly at certain times: growth hormone is released principally during childhood and adolescence. Sex hormones are produced by the testicles and ovaries from puberty onward (see p.170).

Many endocrine glands release hormones in response to triggering hormones produced by the pituitary gland. The activity of the pituitary gland is partly controlled by the brain through the hypothalamus. This region of the brain produces "releasing" hormones that stimulate the release of a particular pituitary hormone that in turn stimulates hormone production by the appropriate endocrine gland. A "feedback" system usually regulates blood hormone levels: if the blood level rises too high, the pituitary decreases its release of stimulating hormones.

What can go wrong

Endocrine disorders, usually resulting in too much or too little of a particular hormone, have a variety of causes. Some are congenital in origin; others may be caused by cancer, autoimmune disease (including some forms of diabetes mellitus), injury, and certain drugs.

Why drugs are used

Natural hormone preparations or their synthetic versions are often prescribed to treat deficiency. Sometimes drugs are given to stimulate increased hormone production in the endocrine gland, such as oral antidiabetic drugs. When too much hormone is produced, drug treatment may reduce the activity of the gland.

Hormones or related drugs are also used to treat other conditions. Corticosteroids are related to adrenal hormones, and are used to relieve inflammation and to suppress immune system activity (see p.168). Several types of cancer are treated with sex hormones (see p.166). Female sex hormones are given as contraceptives (see p.173) and to treat menstrual disorders (p.172).

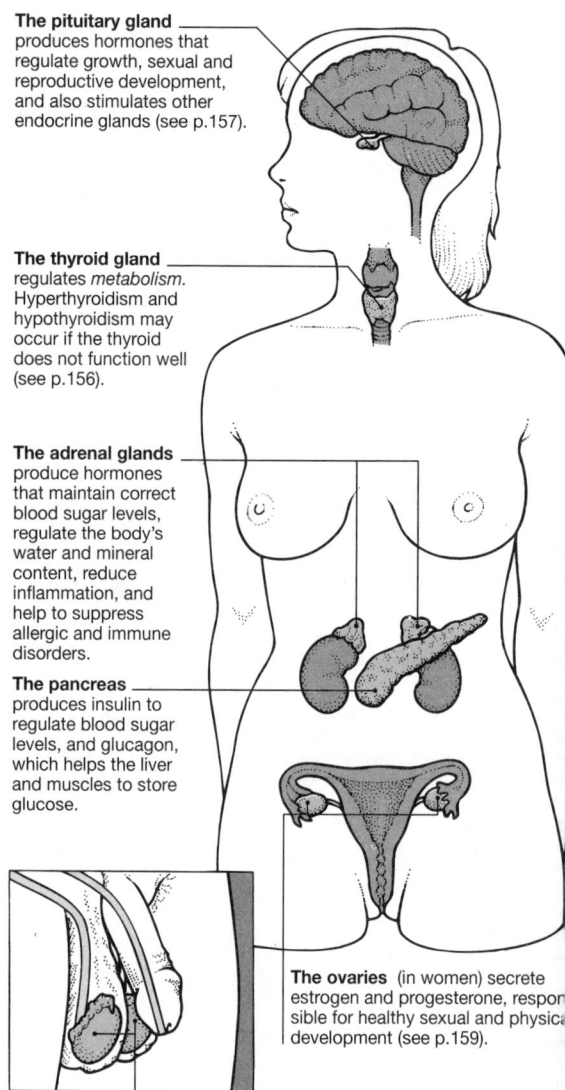

The pituitary gland produces hormones that regulate growth, sexual and reproductive development, and also stimulates other endocrine glands (see p.157).

The thyroid gland regulates *metabolism*. Hyperthyroidism and hypothyroidism may occur if the thyroid does not function well (see p.156).

The adrenal glands produce hormones that maintain correct blood sugar levels, regulate the body's water and mineral content, reduce inflammation, and help to suppress allergic and immune disorders.

The pancreas produces insulin to regulate blood sugar levels, and glucagon, which helps the liver and muscles to store glucose.

The ovaries (in women) secrete estrogen and progesterone, responsible for healthy sexual and physical development (see p.159).

The testicles (in men) produce testosterone, which controls the development of male sexual and physical characteristics (see p.158).

MAJOR DRUG GROUPS

Corticosteroids
Drugs used in diabetes
Drugs for thyroid disorders
Drugs for pituitary disorders
Male sex hormones
Female sex hormones

CORTICOSTEROIDS

The adrenal glands, atop each kidney, produce *hormones* that regulate a variety of body functions. One important group of hormones produced in the outer part of each adrenal gland (cortex) is the corticosteroids. Release of these hormones is governed by the pituitary gland (see p.157). Corticosteroids have two types of effect: glucocorticoid and mineralocorticoid. The glucocorticoid effects include the maintenance of normal levels of sugar in the blood and the promotion of recovery from injury and stress. The main mineralocorticoid effect is the regulation of the balance of mineral salts and the water content of the body. When present in large amounts, corticosteroids reduce inflammation and suppress allergic reactions and immune system activity.

Corticosteroid drugs – often referred to simply as steroids – are derived from or are synthetic variants of the natural corticosteroid hormones. They are distinct from another group of hormones, the anabolic steroids (see p.158).

ADVERSE EFFECTS OF CORTICOSTEROIDS

Corticosteroids are effective and useful drugs that often provide benefit when other drugs are ineffective. However, long-term use of high doses can lead to a variety of unwanted effects on the body as shown below.

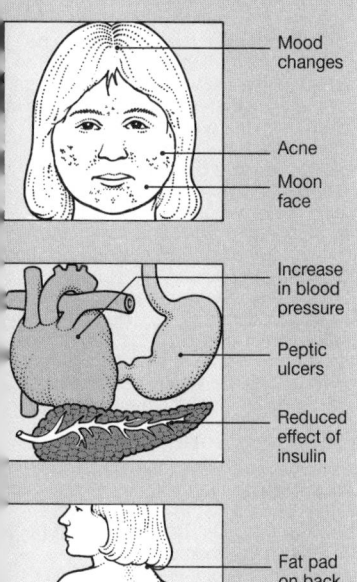

Mood changes

Acne

Moon face

Increase in blood pressure

Peptic ulcers

Reduced effect of insulin

Fat pad on back

Osteoporosis (p.134)

Although corticosteroids have broadly similar actions, they vary in their relative strength and duration of action. The strength of mineralocorticoid effects also varies.

Why they are used

Corticosteroid drugs are used primarily for their anti-inflammatory effect. *Topical* preparations containing corticosteroids are frequently used for the treatment of many inflammatory skin disorders (see p.186). These drugs may also be injected directly into a joint or around a tendon to relieve inflammation caused by injury or disease (see p.130). However, when local administration of the drug is not possible or effective, corticosteroids may be given *systemically*, by mouth or intravenous injection.

An important use of oral corticosteroids is to replace the natural hormones that are deficient when adrenal gland function is reduced, as in Addison's disease. In these cases, drugs that most closely resemble the actions of the natural hormones are selected and a combination of these may be used.

Corticosteroids are an important part of the treatment of many disorders in which inflammation is thought to be caused by excessive or inappropriate activity of the immune system. Such disorders include rheumatoid arthritis (p.129), inflammatory bowel disease (p.124), glomerulonephritis (a kidney disease), and some rare connective tissue disorders such as systemic lupus erythematosus. In these conditions they relieve symptoms and may temporarily halt the disease.

Corticosteroids may be given regularly by mouth or inhaler to treat asthma, although they are not effective for the relief of asthma attacks in progress.

Some cancers of the blood (leukemias) and lymphatic system (lymphomas) may also respond to corticosteroid treatment. These drugs are also widely used to prevent or treat rejection of organ transplants, usually in conjunction with other drugs (see Immunosuppressant drugs, p.168).

How they work

Given in high doses, corticosteroid drugs reduce inflammation by blocking the action of chemicals called prostaglandins that are responsible for triggering the inflammatory response. They also temporarily depress the immune system by reducing the activity of certain types of white blood cells.

How they affect you

Corticosteroid drugs often produce a dramatic improvement in symptoms. Given systemically, corticosteroids may also act on the brain to produce a heightened sense of well-being and, in some people, a sense of euphoria.

Troublesome day-to-day side effects are rare. However, long-term, high-dose corticosteroid treatment carries a number of serious risks.

Risks and special precautions

Few risks are associated with these drugs when they are given in low doses by mouth for the treatment of Addison's disease. Expected adverse effects from higher doses depend on the drug used and the duration of treatment.

Drugs with strong mineralocorticoid effects such as hydrocortisone may cause water retention, swelling (particularly of the ankles), and an increase in blood pressure. Because corticosteroids reduce the effect of insulin they create problems in diabetics. They may even give rise to diabetes in susceptible individuals. They can also contribute to peptic ulcers.

Since corticosteroids suppress the immune system, they increase susceptibility to infection. They also suppress symptoms of infectious disease. With long-term use, corticosteroids may cause a variety of adverse effects as described in the box on the left. Physicians try to avoid long-term prescription of corticosteroids to children because prolonged use may retard growth.

Long-term use of corticosteroids suppresses the production of the body's own corticosteroid hormones. For this reason, treatment lasting for more than a few weeks should be withdrawn gradually to give the body time to adjust. If the drug is stopped abruptly, the lack of corticosteroid hormones may lead to sudden collapse. People taking corticosteroids by mouth for longer than one month are advised to carry a warning card for two years. In the case of an accident, their defenses against shock may need to be quickly strengthened with extra hydrocortisone.

COMMON DRUGS

Beclomethasone
Betamethasone
Budesonide
Clobetasol
Cortisone
Dexamethasone
Flunisolide
Fluocinolone
Fluticasone
Hydrocortisone
Methylprednisolone
Prednisolone
Prednisone
Triamcinolone

DRUGS USED IN DIABETES

The body obtains most of its energy from glucose, a simple form of sugar broken down in the intestine from starch and other sugars and absorbed into the bloodstream. The hormone insulin, produced by the pancreas, enables body tissues to take up glucose from the blood, either to use it for energy or store it. In diabetes mellitus (also called sugar diabetes) not enough insulin is produced by the pancreas, so that little glucose is taken up by the tissues and glucose in the blood rises to abnormal levels, a condition known as hyperglycemia.

There are two main types of diabetes mellitus. Insulin-dependent, or type 1, diabetes, the most severe form, usually first appears in people under 35 and commonly between the ages of 10 and 16. It develops rapidly when insulin-secreting cells in the pancreas are destroyed, probably as a result of antibodies attacking the pancreas, possibly triggered by a virus. Insulin production ceases, often rapidly, leading to symptoms of hyperglycemia: lethargy, general ill health, weight loss, thirst, and increased urination. If treatment is not given, coma and death may result.

The other main form of the disorder, non-insulin-dependent, maturity-onset, or type 2 diabetes, is usually of gradual onset and occurs mainly in people over 40. Insulin is produced, but not in sufficient amounts to meet the body's needs. It is especially common among overweight people who eat large amounts of sugary foods. This form of diabetes may also be caused by chronic pancreatitis and may occasionally be triggered by drugs such as oral contraceptives (p.173) or cortico-steroids (p.153).

In both types of diabetes it is necessary to change the diet to reduce consumption of sugary foods. For many obese type 2 diabetics, control of sugar intake and loss of excess weight reduce the body's insulin requirements to a sufficiently low level without the need for further treatment. However, many type 2 diabetics and all type 1 diabetics require

ADMINISTRATION OF INSULIN

Insulin is given in a way that attempts to mimic the body's production of insulin, which is at a constant overall level with increased production as food is eaten. In practice, a common method of administration is injections twice a day with a mixture of short- and long-acting insulin preparations. The long-acting insulin produces an overall level, while the short-acting one produces the higher level that is needed to cope with the increase in blood sugar following a meal.

Older diabetics may be advised to have injections once a day, which may be necessary if they need someone else to give the injection. Unstable diabetics or those with irregular mealtimes may need to inject short-acting insulin before each meal or snack as well as using a long-acting preparation once or twice a day. In difficult cases a device that continuously delivers insulin into the bloodstream may be needed in order to maintain a finer control over the body's insulin needs.

Duration of action of types of insulin

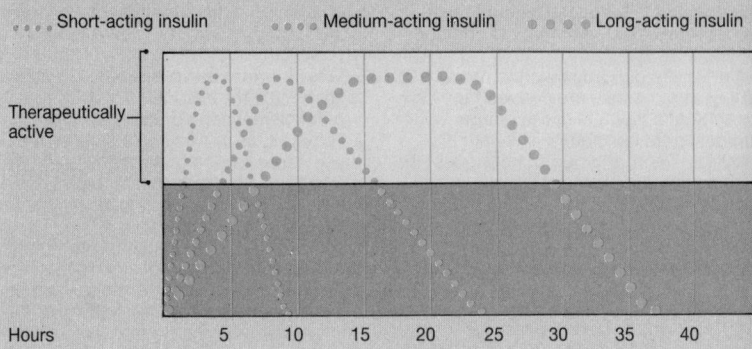

some form of drug treatment in addition to those simpler measures. Two types of drug can be used – insulin and oral antidiabetic drugs, the sulfonylureas and metformin.

Why they are used

Treatment of diabetes is essential to prevent hyperglycemia and to avoid some serious long-term risks. These include an increased likelihood of heart and circulatory problems, and kidney and eye damage.

Oral antidiabetic drugs are prescribed for people with type 2 diabetes who still produce some insulin but whose blood glucose level cannot be adequately

controlled by diet alone. Insulin is prescribed for all sufferers from type 1 diabetes, and treatment must be continued for life. Insulin may also be given to type 2 diabetics to provide control of hyperglycemia before treatme with oral antidiabetic drugs. Insulin is als used if the oral drugs fail to provide adequate control over the condition. Insulin may also be substituted for other treatments for shorter periods of time when these become temporarily unsuitable or insufficient, for example, during pregnancy, severe illness, or pric to undergoing surgery.

A variety of types of insulin are available. Some have a long duration of action; others are short-acting. Sometimes more than one type of insulin is given to provide steady diabetic control (see Administration of insulin, above).

How they work

Sulfonylurea oral antidiabetic drugs encourage the pancreas to release insulin and allow the insulin to work better in the cells. They are therefore effective only when some insulin-secreting cells remain active. Insulin injection directly replaces the natural hormone that is deficient in diabetes mellitus.

By increasing insulin levels in the blood, both types of drug promote the uptake of glucose into body tissues and

ACTION OF ORAL ANTIDIABETIC DRUGS

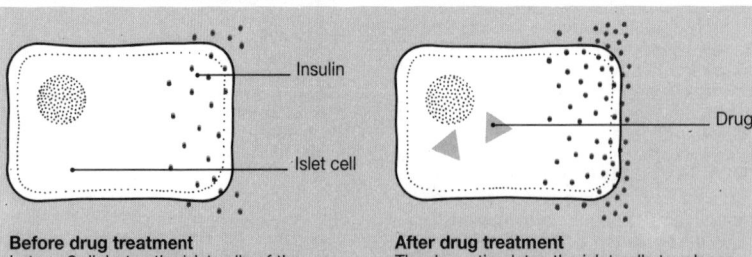

Before drug treatment
In type 2 diabetes the islet cells of the pancreas secrete insufficient insulin to meet the body's needs.

After drug treatment
The drug stimulates the islet cells to release increased amounts of insulin.

elp to prevent an excessive rise in the evel of glucose in the blood.

Insulin cannot be given by mouth ecause it is broken down in the digesve tract before it reaches the bloodream. Regular injections are therefore ecessary (see Administration of insulin, icing page).

low they affect you

ntidiabetic drugs rapidly relieve sympoms of diabetes and, in combination ith dietary measures, usually permit a abetic to lead a full and healthy life. uccessful control of blood glucose levels elps to reduce the long-term risks of abetes mellitus.

Because the body's requirement for ucose and therefore for insulin varies ccording to the level of activity and the te at which the body burns up energy, e main day-to-day problems arise out of e difficulty in establishing a dosage and chedule to meet individual variations. ymptoms of hyperglycemia may develop the dose is too low, and those of hypoycemia (low blood glucose) may arise if e dose is too high. The warning sympms of hypoglycemia include sweating, zziness, and faintness.

Insulin regimens are tailored to each dividual's particular needs. Dosage is tablished for a particular calorie intake d exercise level, making it important to aintain regular eating habits and levels activity.

Insulin was traditionally extracted from e pancreases of pigs and cattle. Animal insulin may, however, cause allergic reactions in some people. A skin rash at the injection site develops, along with reduced effectiveness of the drug. A human insulin, produced by genetic engineering or by modifying pork insulin, is now available and is prescribed instead. Repeated injection at the same site may disturb the fat layer beneath the skin, producing a swelling or dimpling. This can usually be avoided by regularly changing the injection site.

Risks and special precautions

The most serious risk of treatment with drugs for diabetics is an excessive reduction in the blood glucose level. This is usually caused by insufficient food intake, particularly if a person taking insulin misses a meal or snack, or takes unaccustomed exercise. Unless compensating action is taken, the diabetic may lose consciousness; in rare circumstances prolonged hypoglycemia may result in seizures or brain damage. Diabetics should always carry glucose tablets or candy to take if warning symptoms of hypoglycemia occur. People who take insulin may also be advised to carry glucagon, a drug which rapidly increases the blood glucose level by blocking the effects of insulin, together with instructions for its use in the event of loss of consciousness. As a precaution, family and colleagues should be told about the symptoms of hypoglycemia and what treatment to give. If attacks of hypoglycemia occur frequently, a

SITES OF INJECTION

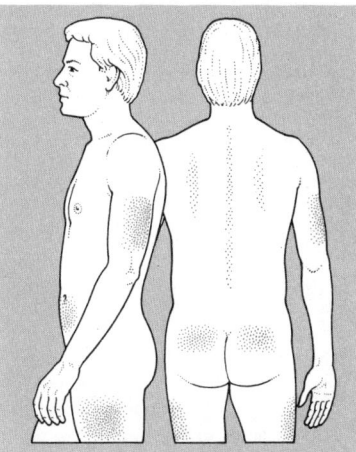

The shaded areas indicate suitable sites for the injection of insulin.

reduction in insulin dosage may be advised. Diabetics should carry a "Medic-Alert" or similar identification in case of severe hypoglycemia.

Because exercise increases the body's glucose requirement, extra glucose may be needed before undertaking unaccustomed physical activity. Serious illness often increases the need for insulin, and dosage may need to be increased until after recovery. A woman taking sulfonylurea drugs who wishes to become pregnant should discuss her drug treatment with a physician before conceiving because these drugs can cross the placenta and affect the developing baby; a temporary change to insulin treatment until after the baby is born is advised.

There are many types of insulin preparations, each available in different strengths. It is important that you receive exactly the same one each time you renew your prescription, since the dosage is tailored for your needs. You will be given an identification card stating type of drug and dosage.

COMMON DRUGS

Sulfonylurea drugs
Acetohexamide
Chlorpropamide
Gliclazide
Glyburide
Tolbutamide

Other drugs
Glucagon
Insulin
Metformin

MONITORING BLOOD GLUCOSE

Diabetics need to check either heir blood or urine glucose evel at home. Blood tests are he most accurate. The kit hown here consists of a rogrammable meter that eads the glucose levels of lood samples applied to a pecial testing strip. Carefully ollow the instructions for your it to ensure accuracy.

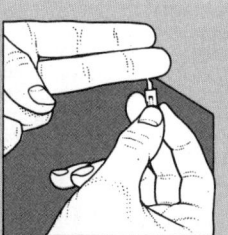

1 Prick your finger to produce a large drop of blood.

2 Touch the blood onto the test pads of the testing strip.

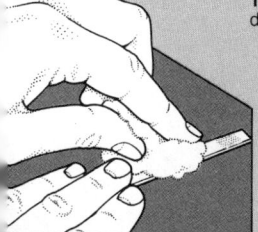

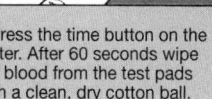

Press the time button on the eter. After 60 seconds wipe e blood from the test pads ith a clean, dry cotton ball.

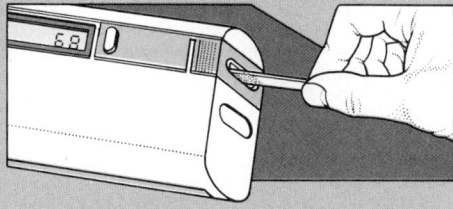

4 Within 120 seconds insert the test strip into the meter as shown. Your reading will appear after 120 seconds.

DRUGS FOR THYROID DISORDERS

The thyroid gland, located in the neck, produces *hormones* that regulate *metabolism*. During childhood, thyroid hormones are essential for normal mental and physical development. The thyroid also produces calcitonin, a hormone involved with normal calcium balance.

The thyroid gland can become overactive, producing excess amounts of hormones, causing a condition known as hyperthyroidism or thyrotoxicosis. The gland can also become underactive, producing insufficient hormones, a condition called hypothyroidism.

ACTION OF DRUGS FOR THYROID DISORDERS

Thyroid hormone production
Iodine combines with other chemicals (precursors) in the thyroid gland to make thyroid hormones.

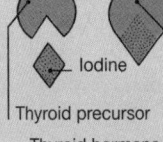

Iodine

Thyroid precursor

Thyroid hormone

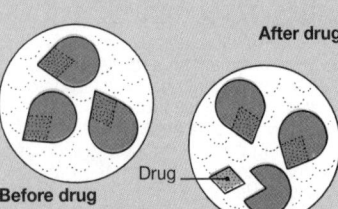

Thyroid hormone

Normal output of thyroid hormones
Thyroid output is normally regulated according to the body's needs.

After drug

Drug

Before drug

Action of antithyroid drugs
In thyrotoxicosis, antithyroid drugs partly reduce the production of thyroid hormones by preventing iodine from combining with thyroid precursors in the thyroid gland.

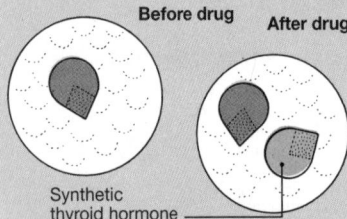

Before drug

After drug

Synthetic thyroid hormone

Action of thyroid hormones
In hypothyroidism, when the thyroid gland is underactive, supplements of synthetic or (rarely) natural thyroid hormones restore hormone levels to normal.

Thyrotoxicosis
Overactivity of the thyroid causes thyrotoxicosis. Symptoms include anxiety, trembling, sweating, palpitations, an increased appetite, weight loss, and intolerance to heat. Diarrhea and menstrual disturbances may occur. Thyrotoxicosis can also cause abnormal protrusion of the eyes, exophthalmos.

Drugs for thyrotoxicosis
Antithyroid drugs reduce production of thyroid hormones to near normal levels. These drugs may take about four to six weeks to produce any effect, because the thyroid gland contains a store of hormones that is only gradually depleted. Therefore, a beta blocker (p.109) may be prescribed to control symptoms at the beginning of treatment.

A course of antithyroid drug treatment is usually started with a high dose to give a rapid improvement in symptoms; the dosage is gradually reduced, depending on the individual response. Some people recover completely after one course of treatment, but symptoms may return, especially in children, making further treatment necessary. Antithyroid drugs may not improve exophthalmos, although they may prevent it from worsening. To relieve this condition a corticosteroid (p.153) may be given. Surgery may be necessary.

The initial high dose of an antithyroid drug may occasionally produce nausea, vomiting, headache, or skin rashes. More seriously, these drugs may reduce the white blood cell count, thus increasing susceptibility to infection, and causing recurrent fevers and sore throats. Such symptoms need prompt medical advice.

Radioactive iodine may also be used for the treatment of hyperthyroidism; occasionally, surgery is advised.

Hypothyroidism
In an adult, a low thyroid hormone level may result in a condition called hypothyroidism. It may be caused by an autoimmune disorder, in which the body's immune system attacks the thyroid gland. Reduced thyroid output may also arise after surgery or radioactive iodine treatment for hyperthyroidism. In newborn babies, hypothyroidism may be the result of an inborn *enzyme* disorder.

Symptoms of adult hypothyroidism usually develop slowly and include tiredness, slowing of mental processes, puffy facial appearance with dry skin and some hair loss, and increased sensitivity to cold. Women may develop heavy or prolonged menstrual periods.

Drugs for hypothyroidism
Hypothyroidism is usually permanent, necessitating lifelong treatment with synthetic thyroid hormone preparations. These are usually given by mouth, but

TREATMENT FOR GOITER

A goiter is a swelling of the thyroid gland. It may occur temporarily during puberty or pregnancy, or may be due to an abnormal growth of thyroid tissue that may require surgical removal. It may rarely be brought about by an iodine deficiency. This last cause is treated with iodine supplements (see also p.522).

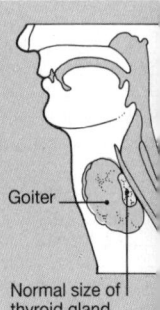

Goiter

Normal size of thyroid gland

may be given by injection or by using a nasogastric tube if an individual's level of thyroid hormone falls so low that consciousness is lost.

Babies are routinely checked after birth for thyroid deficiency because low level may cause cretinism – permanent mental and physical retardation. If the level is low, a thyroid drug is injected immediately and administered at regular intervals thereafter. Prompt treatment should establish normal development.

Thyroid drugs do not usually produce adverse effects, since they are simply supplying a substance that the body would normally produce. However, if the dose is too high, symptoms of thyrotoxicosis may arise. Regular blood tests are usually performed to check that the correct dose is being given. It is common practice to start with a low dose of the drug and to increase it gradually. A sudden rise in hormone levels can put a strain on the heart. For this reason, thyroid drugs are prescribed with caution to the elderly and those with heart disease or high blood pressure. A beta blocker may also be given to reduce adverse effects on the heart.

COMMON DRUGS

Drugs for thyrotoxicosis
Methimazole
Propylthiouracil

Drugs for hypothyroidism
Levothyroxine
Liothyronine
Thyroid

Other drug
Iodine

DRUGS FOR PITUITARY DISORDERS

The pituitary gland, which lies at the base of the brain, produces a number of hormones that regulate physical growth, metabolism, sexual development, and reproductive function. Many of these hormones act indirectly by stimulating other glands, such as the thyroid, adrenal glands, ovaries, and testicles, to release their own hormones. A summary of the actions and effects of each pituitary hormone is given below.

An excess or a lack of a pituitary hormone may produce serious effects, the nature of which depends on the hormone involved. Abnormal levels of a particular hormone may be caused by a pituitary tumor sometimes treated surgically. In other cases, drugs may be used to correct the hormonal imbalance.

The more common pituitary disorders that can be treated with drugs are those involving growth hormone, antidiuretic hormone, prolactin, adrenal hormones, and the gonadotropins. The first three are discussed below. For information on the use of drugs to treat infertility arising from inadequate levels of gonadotropins, see p.176. Lack of corticotropin, leading to inadequate production of adrenal hormones, is usually treated with corticosteroid drugs (see p.153).

Drugs for growth hormone disorders

Growth hormone (somatropin) is the principal hormone required for normal growth in childhood and adolescence. Lack of growth hormone impairs normal physical growth, a condition known as pituitary dwarfism. Physicians administer growth hormone only after tests have shown that a lack of this hormone is the cause of the disorder. If treatment begins early, regular injections of hormone until the end of adolescence usually allow normal growth and development to take place.

Less often, the pituitary produces an excess of growth hormone. In children this can result in pituitary gigantism; in adults, it can produce a deformity known as acromegaly. Acromegaly is usually the result of a pituitary tumor and is characterized by thickening of the skull, face, hands, and feet, and the enlargement of some internal organs.

Although these conditions cannot be cured, gigantism may be halted and some of the deformities of acromegaly reversed by reducing the output of growth hormone. This is usually achieved by destroying part of the pituitary gland, either by surgery or radiation treatment. The drug bromocriptine, which reduces growth hormone levels, is also used.

Drugs for diabetes insipidus

Antidiuretic hormone (also known as ADH or vasopressin) acts on the kidneys, controlling the amount of water retained in the body and returned to the blood. A lack of ADH is usually caused by damage to the pituitary, and this in turn causes diabetes insipidus. In this rare condition, the kidneys cannot retain water, and large quantities pass into the urine. The chief symptoms of diabetes insipidus are constant thirst and the production of large volumes of urine.

Diabetes insipidus is treated with vasopressin or desmopressin. Vasopressin has to be given by injection. Desmopressin, an artificial form of vasopressin, is inhaled from a nasal spray. Mild cases of this disease may be treated either with clofibrate (see also Lipid-lowering drugs, p.115), which increases the amount of ADH released by the pituitary, or chlorpropamide, which also increases ADH release. In addition the drug makes the kidneys more sensitive to the hormone. Alternatively, a thiazide-like diuretic (such as chlorthalidone) may be prescribed for mild cases (see Diuretics, p.111). The usual effect of such drugs is to increase urine production, but in diabetes insipidus they have the opposite effect, reducing water loss from the body.

Drugs used to reduce prolactin levels

Prolactin, or lactogenic hormone, is produced in both men and women. In women, prolactin controls the secretion of breast milk following childbirth; its function in men is not understood, although it appears to be necessary for normal sperm production. The disorders associated with prolactin are all concerned with overproduction. High levels of prolactin in women can cause lactation unassociated with pregnancy and birth (galactorrhea), lack of menstruation (amenorrhea), and infertility. If excessive amounts are produced in men, the result may be galactorrhea and/or infertility. Some drugs, notably phenothiazine antipsychotics, estrogen, and methyldopa, can all raise the level of prolactin in the blood. More often, however, increased prolactin results from a pituitary tumor that is sometimes treated surgically. Bromocriptine inhibits the production of prolactin and is also used in the treatment of prolactin tumors.

THE EFFECTS OF PITUITARY HORMONES

The pituitary gland produces a large number of hormones, many of which control the activities of other glands. The illustration shows the principal sites of action of the major pituitary hormones.

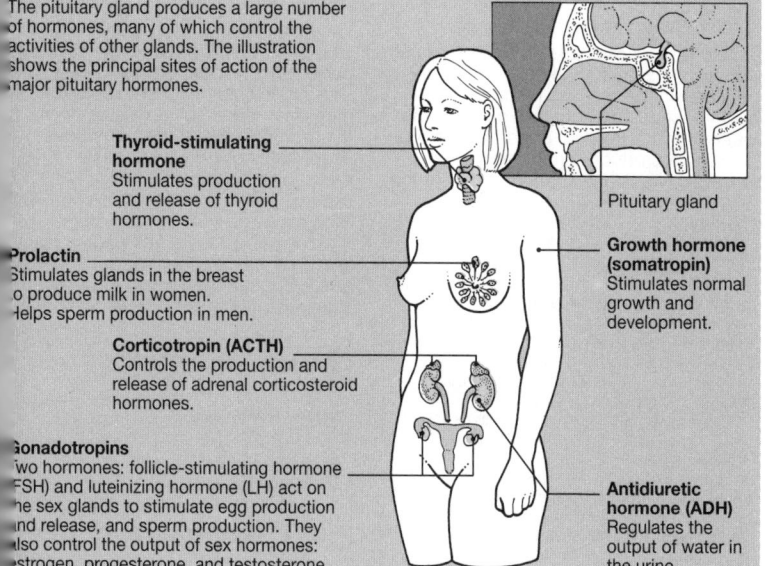

Thyroid-stimulating hormone
Stimulates production and release of thyroid hormones.

Prolactin
Stimulates glands in the breast to produce milk in women. Helps sperm production in men.

Corticotropin (ACTH)
Controls the production and release of adrenal corticosteroid hormones.

Gonadotropins
Two hormones: follicle-stimulating hormone (FSH) and luteinizing hormone (LH) act on the sex glands to stimulate egg production and release, and sperm production. They also control the output of sex hormones: estrogen, progesterone, and testosterone.

Pituitary gland

Growth hormone (somatropin)
Stimulates normal growth and development.

Antidiuretic hormone (ADH)
Regulates the output of water in the urine.

COMMON DRUGS

Drugs for growth hormone disorders
Bromocriptine
Growth hormone

Drugs for diabetes insipidus
Chlorpropamide
Chlorthalidone
Clofibrate
Desmopressin
Vasopressin

Drugs to reduce prolactin levels
Bromocriptine

MALE SEX HORMONES

Male sex hormones – androgens – are responsible for the development of male sexual characteristics. The principal androgen is testosterone, which in men is produced by the testicles from puberty onward. Women also produce testosterone in small amounts in the adrenal glands, but its exact function in the female body is not known.

Testosterone has two major effects: an androgenic effect and an anabolic effect. Its androgenic effect is to stimulate the appearance of secondary sexual characteristics at puberty, such as the growth of body hair, deepening of the voice, and an increase in the size of the genitals. Its anabolic effect is to increase muscle bulk and accelerate rate of growth.

There are a number of synthetically produced derivatives of testosterone that produce varying degrees of the androgenic and anabolic effects mentioned above. Those having a mainly anabolic effect are known as anabolic steroids (see box below), although all anabolic drugs have some androgenic activity.

Testosterone and its derivatives have been used in both men and women to treat a number of conditions.

Why they are used

Male sex hormones are mainly given to men to promote the development of male sexual characteristics when hormone production is deficient. This may be the result of an abnormality of the testicles or of inadequate production of the pituitary hormones that stimulate the testicles to release testosterone.

A course of treatment with male sex hormones is sometimes prescribed for adolescent boys in whom the onset of puberty is delayed by pituitary problems. This treatment may also help to stimulate the development of secondary male sexual characteristics and to increase sex drive (libido) in adult men who are producing inadequate levels of testosterone. However, such hormone treatment is unlikely to promote the production of sperm. (For information

EFFECTS OF MALE SEX HORMONES

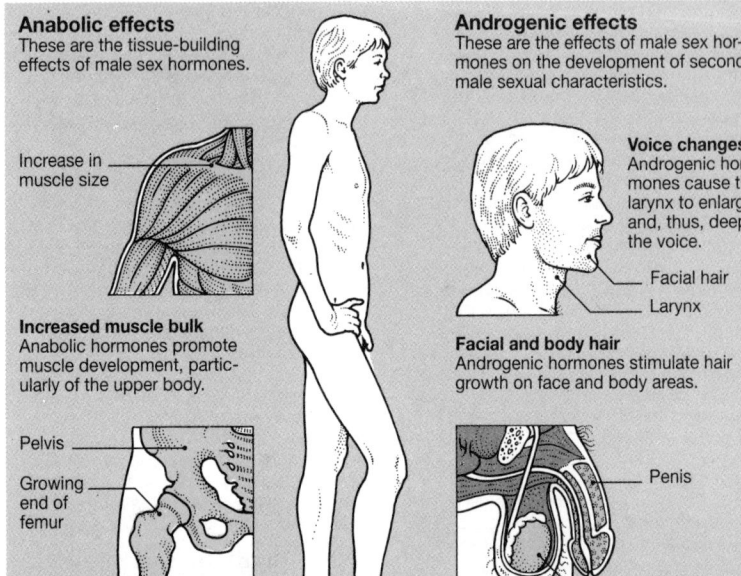

Anabolic effects
These are the tissue-building effects of male sex hormones.

Increase in muscle size

Increased muscle bulk
Anabolic hormones promote muscle development, particularly of the upper body.

Pelvis

Growing end of femur

Bone growth
Anabolic hormones increase bone density. They also halt growth of the bone ends.

Androgenic effects
These are the effects of male sex hormones on the development of secondary male sexual characteristics.

Voice changes
Androgenic hormones cause the larynx to enlarge and, thus, deepen the voice.

Facial hair

Larynx

Facial and body hair
Androgenic hormones stimulate hair growth on face and body areas.

Penis

Testicles

Genital development
Androgenic hormones stimulate enlargement of the testicles and penis.

on the drug treatment of male infertility, see p.176.)

Male sex hormones and mainly some of their synthetic variants may also be prescribed for women to treat certain types of cancer of the breast and uterus (see Anticancer drugs, p.166).

How they work

Taken in low doses as part of replacement therapy when natural production is low, male sex hormones act in the same way as the natural hormones. In adolescents suffering from delayed puberty, hormone treatment produces androgenic and anabolic effects (see above), initiating the

development of secondary sexual characteristics over a few months; full sexual development usually takes place over three to four years. In adult men, the effects of hormone treatment may begin to be felt within a few weeks.

Risks and special precautions

The main risks with these drugs occur when they are given to boys with delayed puberty and to women with breast cancer. Given to initiate the onset of puberty, they may stunt growth by prematurely sealing the growing ends of the long bones. Physicians normally try to avoid prescribing hormones in these circumstances until growth is complete. High doses given to women have masculinizing effects – increased facial and body hair, deeper voice. They may also produce enlargement of the clitoris, acne, and changes in libido.

COMMON DRUGS

Primarily androgenic
Testosterone

Primarily anabolic
Nandrolone

ANABOLIC STEROIDS

Anabolic steroids are synthetically produced variants that mimic the anabolic effects of the natural hormones. They increase muscle bulk and body growth.

Physicians occasionally prescribe anabolic steroids and a high protein diet to promote recovery after serious illness or major surgery. The steroids may also help to increase the production of blood cells in some forms of anemia. They have also been used in the treatment of the bone-wasting disorder osteoporosis in postmenopausal women, but because of the risk of serious side effects alternative forms of treatment are usually given (see p.134).

Anabolic steroids have been widely abused by athletes because they speed up the recovery of muscles after a session of intense exercise. This enables the athlete to go through a more demanding daily exercise program, resulting in a significant improvement in muscle power. The use of anabolic steroids by athletes to improve their performance is condemned by physicians and athletic organizations because of the risks to health, particularly for women. Adverse effects range from acne and baldness to fluid retention, reduced fertility in men and women, hardening of the arteries, a long-term risk of liver disease, and certain forms of cancer.

FEMALE SEX HORMONES

There are two types of female sex hormones, estrogens and progesterone. In women these are secreted by the ovaries from puberty until after the menopause. Additional estrogens and progesterone are produced by the placenta during pregnancy. Small amounts of estrogens are also produced in the adrenal glands.

Estrogens are responsible for the development of female sexual characteristics including breast development, growth of pubic hair, and widening of the pelvis. Progesterone acts on the lining of the uterus and prepares it for implantation of a fertilized egg. It is also important for the maintenance of pregnancy. On a monthly basis, levels of estrogens and progesterone fluctuate, producing the menstrual cycle (see p.171).

The production of these hormones is regulated by the action of two gonadotropin hormones produced by the pituitary gland (see p.157).

Estrogens and progesterone and synthetic variants of these hormones synthetic progesterone drugs are known as progestins) are used medically to treat number of conditions.

Why they are used

The best-known use of these drugs is in oral contraceptive preparations. These are discussed on p.173. Other uses include the treatment of menstrual disorders (p.172) and certain hormone-sensitive cancers (p.166). This page focuses on the use of hormones in conditions in which the levels of natural hormones are deficient.

Hormone deficiency

Deficiency of female sex hormones may occur as a result of deficiency of gonadotropins (caused by a pituitary disorder) or of abnormal development of the ovaries (ovarian failure). This may lead to the absence of menstruation and sexual development. If tests show a deficiency of gonadotropins, preparations of these hormones may be prescribed if fertility is desired. These trigger the release of estrogens and progesterone from the ovaries. If pituitary function is normal and ovarian failure is diagnosed as the cause of hormone deficiency, estrogen and progesterone supplements may be given. In this situation, hormone supplements ensure development of normal female sexual characteristics, but cannot stimulate ovulation.

Menopause

A fall in levels of estrogens and progesterone occurs naturally after the menopause, when the menstrual cycle ceases. The sudden reduction in estrogen levels often causes distressing symptoms including sweating, hot flashes, dryness of the vagina, and mood changes. Many physicians advocate the use of hormone supplements following the menopause. Such hormone replacement therapy helps to reduce the symptoms of the menopause and also helps to delay some of the long-term consequences of reduced estrogen levels in old age, including osteoporosis (p.134) and deposition of fat in the arteries (atherosclerosis). When dryness of the vagina is a particular problem, estrogen cream may be prescribed. The duration of hormonal treatment after menopause is controversial, but may be continued for many years.

Hormone replacement therapy may also be prescribed for women who have undergone a premature menopause as a result of surgical removal of the ovaries or following radiation treatment for ovarian cancer.

How they affect you

Hormones given to treat ovarian failure or delayed puberty may take three to six months to produce a noticeable effect on sexual development. Taken for menopausal symptoms, they can dramatically lessen the number of hot flashes within a week.

Both estrogens and progestins can cause fluid retention, and estrogens may cause nausea, vomiting, breast tenderness, headache, dizziness, and depression. Progestins may cause "breakthrough" bleeding between menstrual periods. In the comparatively low doses used to treat these disorders, however, side effects are unlikely.

Risks and special precautions

Treatment with estrogens and progestins for ovarian failure carries few risks for otherwise healthy young women. However, there are risks linked to long-term estrogen treatment in older women. The hormone increases the risk of abnormal blood clotting (thrombosis) and raised blood pressure (hypertension). For these reasons, estrogen treatment is used with caution in women with heart or circulatory disorders, or who are overweight or smoke. Estrogens may also trigger diabetes mellitus in susceptible people. The risks of estrogen hormones are reduced by prescribing them with progestins, which oppose some of the harmful effects. However, the danger of adverse effects increases with age. Postmenopausal women on hormonal therapy should have regular gynecological examinations.

COMPARATIVE HORMONE LEVELS DURING THE MENSTRUAL CYCLE AND PREGNANCY

In an adult woman of child-bearing years the production of female sex hormones fluctuates during a monthly cycle. During pregnancy the levels of both estrogen and progesterone rise dramatically. After the menopause hormone production falls to a level similar to that which occurs during menstruation.

The large graph (right) shows the rise in hormone levels during the 40 weeks of pregnancy. The smaller graph (inset) illustrates hormone levels in a typical 28-day menstrual cycle. Because the hormone levels in pregnancy are so much greater, each unit of measurement on the pregnancy graph represents 100 units in the menstrual cycle graph.

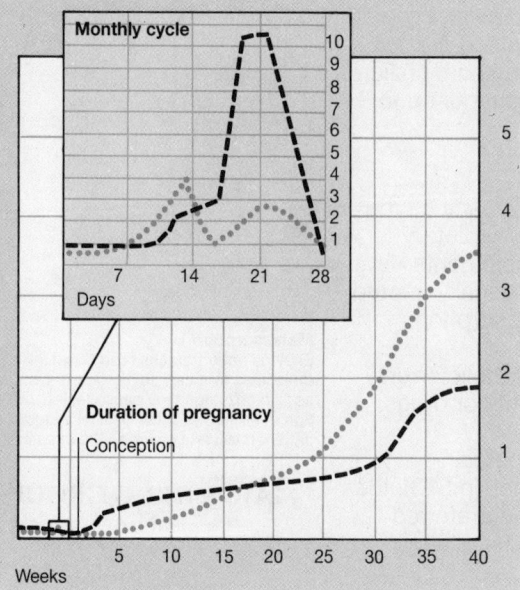

Monthly cycle

Days

Duration of pregnancy

Conception

Weeks

..... Estrogen

---- Progesterone

COMMON DRUGS

Estrogens
Conjugated estrogens
Estradiol
Ethinyl estradiol

Progestins
Medroxyprogesterone
Megestrol
Norgestrel
Progesterone

NUTRITION

Food provides energy (as calories) and materials called nutrients needed for growth and renewal of tissues. Protein, carbohydrate, and fat are the three major nutrient components of food. Vitamins and minerals are found in small amounts in food but are just as important for normal function of the body. Fiber, found only in foods from plants, is needed for a healthy digestive system.

During digestion, large molecules of food are broken down into smaller molecules, releasing nutrients that can be absorbed into the bloodstream. Carbohydrate and fat are then *metabolized* by body cells to produce energy. They may also be incorporated with protein into cell structure. Each metabolic process inside cells is promoted by a specific *enzyme* and often requires the presence of a particular vitamin or mineral.

What can go wrong

Dietary deficiency of essential nutrients can lead to illness. In poorer countries where there is a shortage of food, marasmus (resulting from lack of food energy) and kwashiorkor (from lack of protein) are common. In the developed world, however, excessive food intake leading to obesity is more common. Nutritional deficiencies in developed countries result from poor food choices and usually stem from a lack of a specific vitamin or mineral as in iron-deficiency anemia.

Some nutritional deficiencies may be caused by an inability of the body to absorb a nutrient from food (malabsorption) or to utilize it once it has been absorbed. Malabsorption may be caused by lack of an enzyme or an abnormality of the digestive tract. Errors of metabolism are often inborn and are not yet fully understood. They may be caused by failure of the body to produce the chemicals required to process nutrients for use.

Why supplements are used

Deficiencies of the kwashiorkor or marasmus type are not usually treated by drugs, but by dietary improvement, and perhaps food supplements. Vitamin and mineral deficiencies are usually treated with appropriate supplements. Malabsorption disorders may require continued use of supplements or changes in diet. Metabolic errors are not easily treated with supplements or drugs. Dietary changes may be tried.

Obesity has been treated with appetite suppressants related to amphetamines (p.533), the use of which is now discouraged. The preferred treatment includes reduced food intake, altered eating patterns, and increased exercise.

Major food components

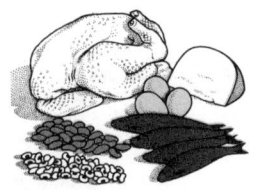

Proteins
Vital for growth and repair of tissue. In meat, fish, dairy products, cereals, and legumes.

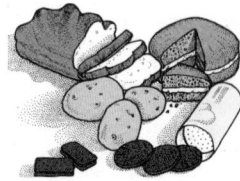

Carbohydrates
A major energy source, stored as fat when taken in excess. In cereals, sugar, and vegetables.

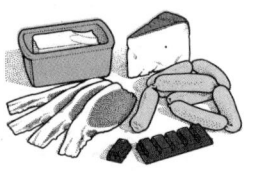

Fats
A concentrated energy form but needed only in small quantities. In animal products and oils.

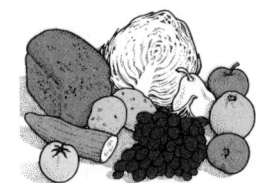

Fiber
The indigestible part of any plant product which, though it contains no nutrients, adds bulk to feces.

Absorption of nutrients

Food passes through mouth, esophagus, and stomach to the small intestine. The lining of the small intestine secretes many enzymes and is covered by tiny projections (villi) which enable nutrients to pass into the blood.

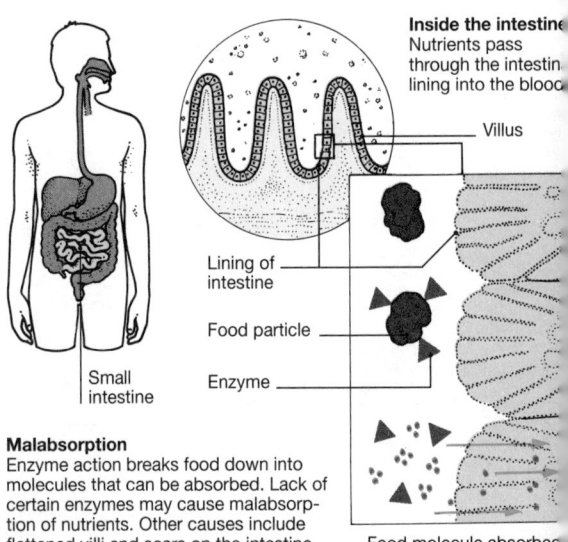

Inside the intestine
Nutrients pass through the intestinal lining into the blood

Villus

Lining of intestine

Food particle

Enzyme

Small intestine

Malabsorption
Enzyme action breaks food down into molecules that can be absorbed. Lack of certain enzymes may cause malabsorption of nutrients. Other causes include flattened villi and scars on the intestine.

Food molecule absorbed

MAJOR DRUG GROUPS

Vitamins

VITAMINS

Vitamins are complex chemicals that are essential for a variety of body functions. The body is unable to manufacture these substances itself and therefore we need to take them in in the diet. There are 13 major vitamins: A, C, D, E, K, and the eight B complex vitamins – thiamine (B_1), riboflavin (B_2), niacin (B_3), folic acid, biotin (vitamin H), pantothenic acid (B_5), pyridoxine (B_6), and cobalamin (B_{12}). Most are required in extremely small amounts, and each vitamin is present in one or more foods (see Main food sources of vitamins and minerals, p.162). Vitamin D is also produced in the body when the skin is exposed to sunlight. Vitamins fall into two groups: those that dissolve in fat and those that dissolve in water (see Fat-soluble and water-soluble vitamins, p.163).

A balanced diet that includes a variety of different types of foods is likely to contain adequate amounts of all the vitamins. Inadequate intake of any vitamin over an extended period can lead to symptoms of deficiency. The nature of these symptoms depends on the vitamin concerned.

A physician may recommend supplements of one or more vitamins in a variety of circumstances: to prevent vitamin deficiency from occurring in people considered at special risk, to treat symptoms of deficiency, and to treat certain medical conditions.

Why they are used
Preventing deficiency
Most people in Canada obtain sufficient quantities of vitamins in their diet, and it is therefore unnecessary in most cases to take additional vitamins in the form of supplements. People who are unsure as to whether their present diet is adequate are advised to look at the table on p.162 to check that foods that are rich in vitamins are eaten regularly. Vitamin intake can often be boosted simply by increasing the quantities of fresh foods and raw fruit and vegetables in the diet.

Certain groups in the population are, however, at increased risk of vitamin deficiency. These include those who have an increased need for certain vitamins that may not be met from dietary sources – in particular, women who are pregnant or nursing, infants, and young children. The elderly who may not be eating a varied diet may also be at risk. Strict vegetarians and others on restricted diets may not receive adequate amounts of all vitamins.

In addition, people being fed intravenously or by stomach tube on artificial nutrients for prolonged periods, those suffering from disorders in which absorption of nutrients from the bowel is impaired, and those who need to take drugs (for example, lipid-lowering drugs) which reduce vitamin absorption, are usually given additional vitamins.

In these cases, a physician is likely to advise supplements of one or more vitamins. Although most vitamin preparations are available without a prescription, it is important to seek medical advice before starting a course of vitamin supplements, so that a proper assessment can be made of your individual requirements.

Vitamin supplements should not be used as a general tonic to improve well-being – they do not do so – nor should they be used as a substitute for a balanced diet.

Vitamin deficiency
It is rare for a diet to be completely lacking in a particular vitamin. But if intake of a particular vitamin is regularly

PRIMARY FUNCTIONS OF VITAMINS

The role of vitamins in the body is not yet fully understood; most of our knowledge is based on the evidence provided by symptoms that occur as a result of deficiency of a particular vitamin. Most vitamins have been found to have a number of important actions on one or more body systems or functions. Many are involved in the activity of *enzymes* (substances that promote biochemical reactions in the body). The illustration indicates the organs and body systems on which each vitamin has its principal effect.

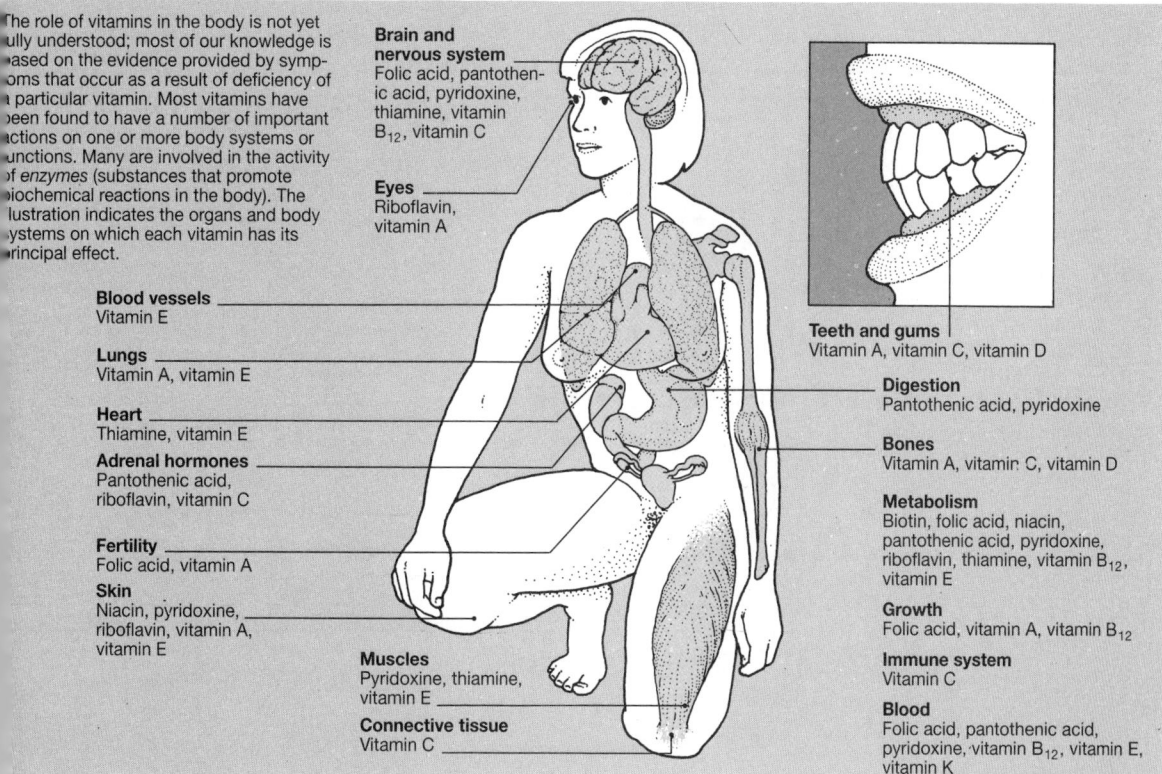

Brain and nervous system
Folic acid, pantothenic acid, pyridoxine, thiamine, vitamin B_{12}, vitamin C

Eyes
Riboflavin, vitamin A

Blood vessels
Vitamin E

Lungs
Vitamin A, vitamin E

Heart
Thiamine, vitamin E

Adrenal hormones
Pantothenic acid, riboflavin, vitamin C

Fertility
Folic acid, vitamin A

Skin
Niacin, pyridoxine, riboflavin, vitamin A, vitamin E

Muscles
Pyridoxine, thiamine, vitamin E

Connective tissue
Vitamin C

Teeth and gums
Vitamin A, vitamin C, vitamin D

Digestion
Pantothenic acid, pyridoxine

Bones
Vitamin A, vitamin C, vitamin D

Metabolism
Biotin, folic acid, niacin, pantothenic acid, pyridoxine, riboflavin, thiamine, vitamin B_{12}, vitamin E

Growth
Folic acid, vitamin A, vitamin B_{12}

Immune system
Vitamin C

Blood
Folic acid, pantothenic acid, pyridoxine, vitamin B_{12}, vitamin E, vitamin K

VITAMINS continued

MAIN FOOD SOURCES OF VITAMINS AND MINERALS

The table below indicates which foods are especially good sources of particular vitamins and minerals. Regularly selecting foods from a variety of categories helps to maintain adequate intake for most people, without a need for supplements. It is important to remember that processed and overcooked foods are likely to contain fewer vitamins than fresh, raw, or lightly cooked foods.

	Red meat	Poultry	Liver	Milk	Cheese	Butter/margarine	Eggs	Fish	Cereals and bread	Green vegetables	Root vegetables	Legumes	Nuts	Fruit	Other	
Vitamins																
Biotin			●				●					●	●			Especially peanut butter. Cauliflower is good vegetable source.
Folic acid			●				●			●				●		Wheat germ and mushrooms are rich sources.
Niacin	●	●	●				●	●	●			●	●			Protein-rich foods such as milk and eggs contain tryptophan, which can be converted to niacin in the body.
Pantothenic acid			●				●	●								Each food group contributes some pantothenic acid.
Pyridoxine	●	●	●				●	●	●							Especially white meat (chicken, fish) and whole grain cereals.
Riboflavin			●	●	●		●		●			●	●	●		Found in most foods.
Thiamine	●		●					●		●	●					Brewer's yeast, wheat germ, and bran are also good sources.
Vitamin A			●	●	●	●	●			●				●		Fish liver oil, dark green leafy vegetables such as spinach, and orange or yellow-orange vegetables and fruits such as carrots, apricots, and peaches, are especially good sources of vitamin A.
Vitamin B$_{12}$	●		●	●	●		●	●								Obtained only from animal products.
Vitamin C										●				●		Especially citrus fruits, tomatoes, potatoes, broccoli, strawberries, and cantaloupe.
Vitamin D				●			●									Fortified milk is the only good source. Other dietary sources are unreliable. Also obtained by the body when the skin is exposed to sunlight.
Vitamin E			●				●	●	●	●				●		Vegetable oils, whole grain cereals, and wheat germ are the best sources.
Vitamin K										●						Found in small amounts in fruits, seeds, tubers, dairy and meat products.
Minerals																
Calcium				●	●				●	●	●					Dark green leafy vegetables, soybean products, and nuts are good non-dairy alternatives. Also present in hard, or alkaline, water supplies.
Chromium	●				●		●	●								Especially unrefined whole grain cereals.
Copper	●	●	●				●	●	●	●		●				Especially shellfish, whole grain cereals, and mushrooms.
Fluoride								●								Primarily obtained from fluoridated water supplies. Also in seafood and tea.
Iodine				●	●			●	●							Provided by iodized table salt, but adequate amounts can be obtained from dairy products, saltwater fish, and bread made without table salt.
Iron	●	●	●				●	●	●	●						Especially liver, red meat, and enriched or whole grains.
Magnesium				●			●	●	●			●	●			Dark green leafy vegetables such as spinach are rich sources. Also present in alkaline water supplies.
Phosphorus	●	●	●	●	●		●	●	●	●	●	●	●	●		Common food additive. Large amounts found in some carbonated beverages.
Potassium								●	●		●			●		Best sources are fruits and vegetables, especially oranges, bananas, and potatoes.
Selenium	●		●	●			●	●								Seafood is the richest source. Amounts in most foods are variable depending on soil where plants were grown and animals grazed.
Sodium	●	●	●	●	●	●	●	●	●	●	●	●	●	●		Sodium is present in all foods, especially table salt, processed foods, potato chips, crackers, and pickled, cured, or smoked meats, seafood, and vegetables. Also present in softened water.
Zinc	●						●	●		●						Sufficient amounts only in whole grain breads and cereals.

ower than the body's requirements, over a period of time the body's stores of the vitamin may become depleted and symptoms of deficiency may gradually begin to appear.

In Canada vitamin deficiency disorders are found mostly among vagrants and alcoholics and those on low incomes who fail to eat an adequate diet. Deficiencies of water-soluble vitamins are the most common since most of these are not stored in large quantities in the body. For descriptions of individual deficiency disorders, see the appropriate vitamin profile in Part 4.

Dosages of vitamins prescribed to treat vitamin deficiency are likely to be larger than those used to prevent deficiency. Medical supervision is required in these cases.

Other medical uses of vitamins

A number of claims have been made for the value of vitamins in the treatment of a range of medical disorders other than vitamin deficiency.

The "antioxidant" vitamins beta-carotene, vitamin C, and vitamin E are believed to be important in preventing cancer and heart disease by countering the damaging effects of free radicals and other highly reactive chemical entities produced by oxidation.

Vitamin D has long been used in the treatment of bone-wasting disorders (p.134). Niacin, a B vitamin, is sometimes used as a lipid-lowering drug (p.115). Derivatives of vitamin A (retinoids) are an established part of the treatment of severe acne (p.189).

Many sufferers from premenstrual syndrome take supplements of pyridoxine (vitamin B6) (see also Drugs used to treat menstrual disorders, p.172).

MINERALS

Minerals are elements – the simplest form of matter – many of which are essential in trace amounts for normal bodily processes. A balanced diet usually contains all of the minerals that the body requires; mineral deficiency diseases, except iron-deficiency anemia, are uncommon.

Dietary supplements are necessary only as part of the treatment for a medical disorder or when a physician has diagnosed a specific deficiency. Physicians commonly prescribe minerals for people with intestinal diseases that reduce the absorption of minerals from the diet. Iron supplements are advised for women who are pregnant or nursing, and iron-enriched cereals are recommended for infants over 6 months.

Much of the general advice given for vitamins also applies to minerals: taking supplements unless under medical direction is not advisable, exceeding the body's daily requirements is not beneficial, and large doses may be harmful.

CALCULATING DAILY VITAMIN REQUIREMENTS

Guidelines for assessing the nutritional value of diets are called Recommended Nutrient Intakes (RNIs) and are based on the estimated requirement of individuals with the highest needs. For most people, the RNI is several times their requirement.

RNIs do not cover individual variation due to acquired or inherited disease, but are designed to cover the needs of about 97 per cent of the population. Those consuming much less than the RNIs may not be consuming less than their needs but the risk of doing so is increased.

The current RNIs (see table below) were set by the Scientific Review Committee of Health and Welfare Canada in 1990 as part of a general review of national nutritional guidelines initiated in 1987.

Daily recommended nutrient intakes of vitamins for adults (aged 25-49)

Vitamin (unit)	RNI		
	Men	Women	Pregnancy and breast feeding
Biotin (mcg)	10 – 200*	10 – 200*	Not established
Folic acid (mcg)	230	185	285 – 385
Niacin as nicotinic acid (mg)	19	14	15 – 17
Pantothenic acid (mg)	3 – 7*	3 – 7*	3 – 7*
Pyridoxine (mg)	1.8	1.5	1.5
Riboflavin (mg)	1.4	1	1.1 – 1.3
Thiamine (mg)	1.1	0.8	0.9 – 1
Vitamin A (mcg)	1,000	800	800 – 1,200
(IU)	5,000	4,000	4,000 – 6,000
Vitamin B12 (mcg)	1	1	1.2
Vitamin C (mg)	40	30	40 – 55
Vitamin D (mcg)	2.5	2.5	5
(IU)	100	100	200
Vitamin E (mg)	9	6	8 – 9

*Estimated requirement

Risks and special precautions

Vitamins are natural substances, and supplements can be taken without risk by most people. It is, however, important to be careful not to exceed the recommended dosage, particularly in the case of fat-soluble vitamins, which may accumulate in the body. Dosage needs to be carefully calculated, taking account of the degree of deficiency, dietary intake, and duration of treatment. Overdosage has at best no therapeutic value and at worst may incur the risk of serious harmful effects. Preparations containing several times the recommended daily intake are best avoided except on medical advice. Multivitamin preparations containing a large number of different vitamins are widely available. Fortunately, the amounts of each vitamin contained in each tablet are not usually large and are not likely to be harmful unless the dose is greatly exceeded. Single vitamin supplements can be harmful because an excess of one vitamin may increase requirements for others. For specific information on each vitamin, see Part 4, pp.518–530.

FAT-SOLUBLE AND WATER-SOLUBLE VITAMINS

Fat-soluble vitamins
Vitamins A, D, E, and K are absorbed from the small intestine into the bloodstream together with fat (see also How drugs pass through the body, p.17). Deficiency of these fat-soluble vitamins may occur as a result of any disorder (for example, sprue) that affects the absorption of fat. These vitamins are stored in the liver and reserves of some of them may last for several years. But taking an excess of a fat-soluble vitamin for a long time may cause it to build up to a harmful level in the body. Ensuring that foods rich in these vitamins are regularly consumed usually provides a sufficient supply to meet dietary requirements without the risk of overdosage.

Water-soluble vitamins
Vitamin C and the B vitamins dissolve in water. Most are stored in the body for only a short period and are rapidly excreted by the kidneys if taken in higher amounts than the body requires. Vitamin B12 is the exception; it is stored in the liver, which may hold up to four years' supply. For these reasons foods containing water-soluble vitamins need to be eaten daily. These vitamins are easily lost in cooking, so raw foods containing them should be eaten regularly. An overdose of water-soluble vitamins does not usually cause toxic effects, but adverse reactions to large dosages of vitamin C and pyridoxine (vitamin B6) have been reported.

MALIGNANT AND IMMUNE DISEASE

The creation and growth of new cells are continuously needed by the body – to replace cells that wear out and die naturally, and to repair injured tissue. Under normal circumstances the rate at which cell reproduction takes place is carefully regulated.

But sometimes abnormal cells are formed, and sometimes they multiply uncontrollably. They may form lumps of abnormal tissue (tumors), which are considered benign if they merely occupy space in a tissue, malignant when they invade and destroy body tissues or spread to other parts of the body. Growth, invasion, destruction, and spread of abnormal cells define cancer.

The workings of a healthy immune system can oppose the development of cancer as well as deal effectively with bacteria, viruses, and other microbes. Abnormal cells can be recognized, rendered harmless or killed. The immune system employs a variety of types of white blood cells for this purpose (facing page). An immune system that malfunctions can provoke allergic reactions of several varieties (see p.135).

What can go wrong

There are many different types of cancer. Some are more deadly than others. Cancer can originate in any tissue or organ of the body. Although medical science cannot identify a single "cause" of cancer, it is known that many noxious outside influences, collectively known as "carcinogens," can provoke the formation of abnormal cells. Tobacco smoke is such a factor in lung cancer. Long-term over-exposure to sunlight induces skin cancer. Some forms of cancer are provoked by the malfunctioning of certain genes inherited from parents. In old age, cancer is a common disease.

Failure of the immune system can lead to increased susceptibility to infections and the development of some kinds of cancer. Such failure can result from infection by human immuno-deficiency virus (HIV), the virus that causes AIDS. The functions of the immune system may be deliberately decreased in order to treat certain disorders, while in other instances decreased immune system function may occur as an unfortunate side effect or consequence of a necessary drug treatment.

In some cases, the immune system can trigger an inappropriate attack on the body's own tissues, leading to what are known collectively as auto-immune disorders. Some common disorders of this type are rheumatoid arthritis, inflammatory skin conditions (lupus erythematosus), inflammation of

Types of cancer

Uncontrolled multiplication of cells leads to the formation of tumors that may be benign or malignant. Benign tumors do not spread to other tissues: malignant (cancerous) tumors do. Some of the main types of cancer are defined below.

Type of cancer	Tissues affected
Carcinoma	Skin and glandular tissue lining cells of internal organs
Sarcoma	Muscles, bones, and fibrous tissues and lining cells of vessels
Leukemia	White blood cells
Lymphoma	Lymph glands

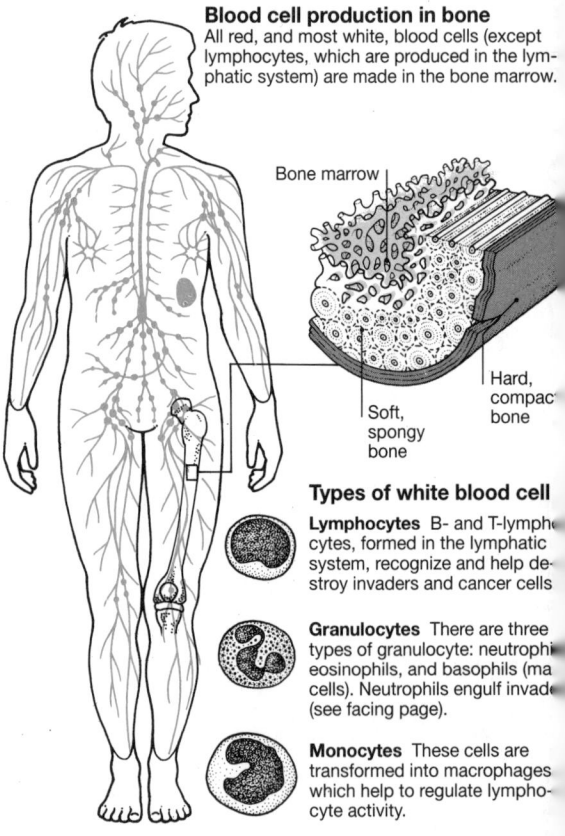

Blood cell production in bone
All red, and most white, blood cells (except lymphocytes, which are produced in the lymphatic system) are made in the bone marrow.

Bone marrow

Hard, compact bone

Soft, spongy bone

Types of white blood cell

Lymphocytes B- and T-lymphocytes, formed in the lymphatic system, recognize and help destroy invaders and cancer cells

Granulocytes There are three types of granulocyte: neutrophil, eosinophils, and basophils (mast cells). Neutrophils engulf invader (see facing page).

Monocytes These cells are transformed into macrophages which help to regulate lymphocyte activity.

blood vessels, and some forms of hypothyroidism. The immune system is responsible for the rejection of organ transplants (kidney, heart, liver, etc.), and because of this may have to be partially "turned off" by special medications.

Why drugs are used

Various kinds of drugs can affect the viability of cancer cells as well as influence the mechanisms work within the cells of the immune system. Cytotoxic (cell-killing) drugs are used to eliminate

Types of immune response

A specific response occurs when the immune system recognizes an invader. Two types of specific response, humoral and cellular, are described below. Phagocytosis, a non-specific response that does not depend on recognition of the invader, is also described.

Humoral response

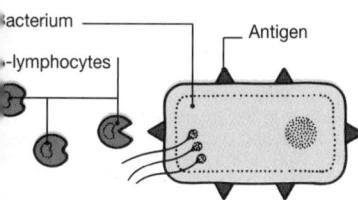

Bacterium — Antigen
B-lymphocytes

B-lymphocytes are activated by unfamiliar proteins (antigens) on the surface of the invading bacterium.

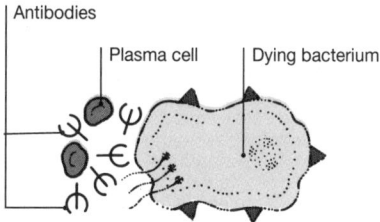

Antibodies
Plasma cell — Dying bacterium

The activated B-lymphocytes form plasma cells, which release antibodies that bind to the invader and kill it.

Cellular response

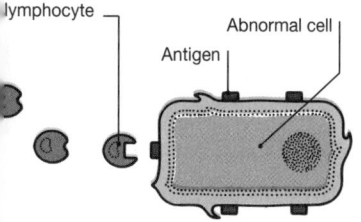

T-lymphocyte
Abnormal cell
Antigen

T-lymphocytes recognize the antigens on abnormal or invading cells.

Dying cell
T-lymphocyte

The T-lymphocytes bind to the abnormal cell and destroy it by altering chemical activity within the cell.

Engulfing invaders (phagocytosis)

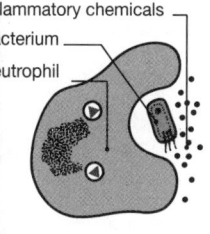

Inflammatory chemicals
Bacterium
Neutrophil

Certain cells, such as neutrophils, are attracted by inflammatory chemicals to the area of bacterial infection.

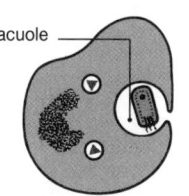

Vacuole

The neutrophil flows around the bacterium, enclosing it within a fluid-filled space called a vacuole.

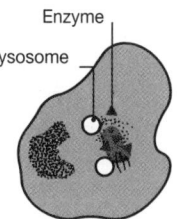

Enzyme
Lysosome

When the vacuole is formed, enzymes from areas called lysosomes within the neutrophil destroy the bacterium.

INTERFERONS

Interferons are natural proteins that limit viral infection by inhibiting viral replication within body cells. These substances also assist in the destruction of cancer cells.

Effect on viral infection

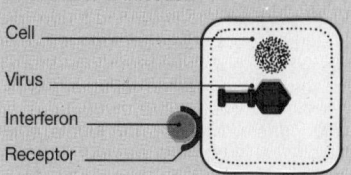

Cell
Virus
Interferon
Receptor

Interferon binds to receptors on a virus-infected cell.

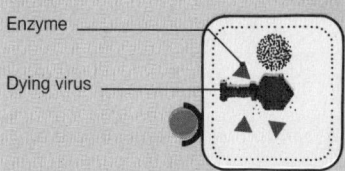

Enzyme
Dying virus

The presence of interferon triggers the release of enzymes that block viral replication. The virus is thus destroyed.

Effect on cancer cells

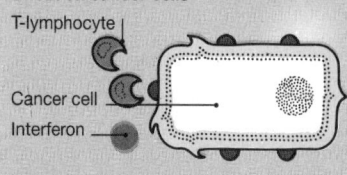

T-lymphocyte
Cancer cell
Interferon

Interferon produced in response to a cancer cell activates T-lymphocytes.

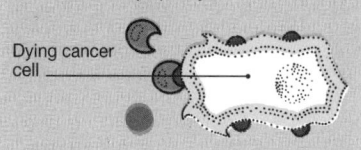

Dying cancer cell

T-lymphocytes attack and destroy the cancer cell.

---

abnormally dividing cells in cancer. These drugs act against all rapidly dividing cells. They also reduce the numbers of blood cells being produced by the bone marrow. While this can induce low white cell counts or *anemia* in cancer patients, this side effect can be beneficial in limiting white cell activity in autoimmune disorders. Other drugs that have immunosuppressant effects include corticosteroids, such as prednisone and cyclosporine, both of which are used after transplant surgery. No drugs are yet available that directly stimulate immune system activity for use in the treatment of immune deficiency diseases. Deficient plasma factors may be replaced, however, and drugs may also be used to treat the infections and other consequences of immune deficiency.

MAJOR DRUG GROUPS

Anticancer drugs
Immunosuppressant drugs
Drugs for AIDS and immune deficiency

ANTICANCER DRUGS

The body's cells normally grow and divide in an organized way; cells that are old or damaged are regularly replaced by new, healthy cells. Sometimes, however, a single cell becomes free from the controls that regulate cell division, and it multiplies at an unchecked rate. Such excessive growth usually leads to the production of a tumor, which may be either benign or malignant (cancerous).

A benign tumor grows slowly and is restricted to a particular area; it produces harmful effects only when it causes pressure on surrounding tissues. A malignant tumor tends to spread to other parts of the body; this occurs when the original tumor invades neighboring tissues or when cells break off and are carried to other parts of the body, where they start to grow. The secondary growths that result are known as metastases. Cancerous cells are frequently unable to perform their usual functions, and this leads to progressively impaired function of the organ or area concerned.

There are many different factors that can provoke cancerous changes in cells. A combination of factors may be involved, notably an individual's genetic background, immune system failure, and over-exposure to cancer-causing substances (carcinogens). Known carcinogens include strong sunlight (for those who are fair-skinned), viruses, dietary factors, certain chemicals, radiation, and tobacco smoke.

Treating cancer is a complicated process that depends on the type of cancer, its stage of development, and the patient's condition and wishes. Any of the following treatments may be used on its own or in combination: surgical removal of the cancer, radiation treatment, and chemotherapy (that is, the use of anti-cancer drugs).

Anticancer drugs that kill cancer cells are sometimes referred to as cytotoxic drugs. They fall into several classes, according to their chemical composition and principal mode of action: alkylating

agents, antimetabolites, and cytotoxic antibiotics are among the most widely used classes. In addition to these drugs, sex hormones and related substances are also used to treat some types of cancer.

Why they are used

Anticancer drugs are the treatment of choice for leukemias, lymphatic cancers, and certain forms of cancer of the testicles. They are particularly useful for rapidly spreading cancers, but are less effective in the treatment of solid tumors. A fuller listing of cancers in which treatment with drugs may be of benefit is included in the box below. Hormone treatment is offered in most cases of hormone-sensitive cancer, including some forms of breast cancer, cancer of the uterus, and cancer of the prostate.

Since all anticancer drugs may produce severe adverse effects (see facing page), they are used only when there is a reasonable chance of achieving a complete cure, significantly prolonging

SUCCESSFUL CHEMOTHERAPY

Not all cancers respond to treatment with anticancer drugs. Some cancers can be cured by drug treatment. In others, drug treatment can slow or temporarily halt the progress of the disease. In a certain number of cases, drug treatment has no beneficial effect, although in some of these cases other treatments, such as surgery, often produce significant benefits. The table at right summarizes the main cancers that fall into each of the three groups described.

Successful drug treatment of cancer normally requires repeated courses of

anticancer drugs, because treatment needs to be halted periodically to allow the blood-producing cells in the bone marrow to recover. The diagram below shows the number of cancer cells and normal blood cells before and after each course of treatment with cytotoxic anticancer drugs during successful chemotherapy. Both cancer cells and blood cells are reduced, but the blood cells recover quickly between courses of drug treatment. When treatment is effective, the number of cancer cells is reduced, so that they no longer cause symptoms.

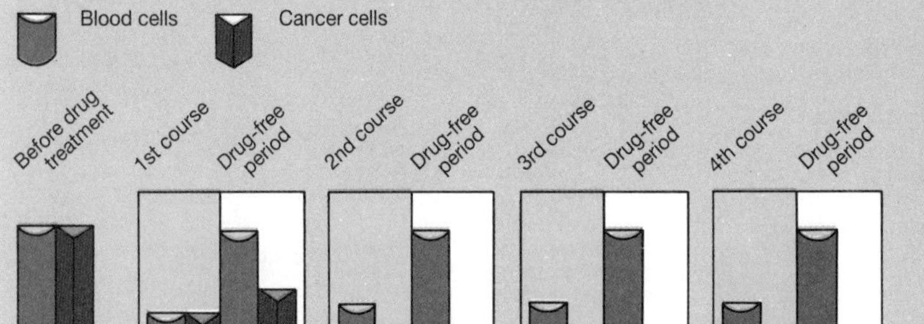

Response to chemotherapy

Cancers that can be cured by drugs
Some cancers of the lymphatic system (including Hodgkin's disease)
Acute lymphoblastic leukemia (a form of blood cancer)
Choriocarcinoma (cancer of the placenta)
Germ cell tumors (cancers affecting sperm and egg cells)
Wilms' tumor (a rare form of kidney cancer that affects children)
Cancer of the testicles

Cancers in which drugs produce worthwhile benefits
Breast cancer
Ovarian cancer
Some leukemias
Multiple myeloma (a bone marrow cancer)
Many types of lung cancer
Head and neck cancers
Cancer of the stomach
Cancer of the prostate
Some cancers of the lymphatic system
Bladder cancer
Cancer of the islet cells of the pancreas
Endometrial cancer (cancer affecting the lining of the uterus)
Cancer of the large intestine
Cancer of the esophagus

Cancers in which drugs are unlikely to be of benefit
Thyroid cancer
Brain cancer in adults
Malignant melanoma (a form of skin cancer)
Cancer of the soft tissues
Liver cancer
Cancer of the pancreas
Cancer of the cervix
Kidney cell cancer

Blood cells   Cancer cells

Before drug treatment · 1st course · Drug-free period · 2nd course · Drug-free period · 3rd course · Drug-free period · 4th course · Drug-free period

e, or relieving distressing symptoms.
ieir effectiveness varies a great deal,
epending primarily on the type of cancer
id the extent of its spread.

Chemotherapy can also be useful after
irgical removal of a tumor, or following
diation treatment, to kill any cancer
ells that remain.

The choice of anticancer drug depends
i the type of cancer and the condition of
e person being treated. No class of
iticancer drugs is used specifically for a
irticular cancer; individual drugs have
parate properties and uses. Often
veral drugs are used, either simulta-
ously or successively.

Certain anticancer drugs are also used
r their effect in suppressing immune
stem activity (see p.168).

ow they work

cytotoxic anticancer drugs kill cancer
lls by preventing them from growing or
viding. Cells grow and divide in several
iges. Most anticancer drugs act on one
ecific stage. During treatment, several
igs may be given in sequence in order
eliminate abnormal cells at all stages
development.

Hormone treatments work by opposing
effects of the hormone that encour-
es the growth of the cancer. For
ample, some breast cancers are
mulated by the female sex hormone
trogen. Spread of the cancer may thus
limited by a drug, such as tamoxifen
it opposes the effects of estrogen.
ier hormone-sensitive cancers are
maged by high doses of a particular
< hormone. Medroxyprogesterone, a
igesterone, often halts the spread of
dometrial cancer.

ow they affect you

the start of treatment adverse effects
cytotoxic anticancer drugs are likely
be more noticeable than benefits. The
st common side effect is nausea and
niting, for which an anti-emetic drug
e p.102) may be prescribed. Diarrhea
lso a common side effect. Many anti-
icer drugs cause hair loss because
he effect of their activity on the cells
he hair follicles, but the hair usually
rts to regrow after chemotherapy has
en completed. Individual drugs may
duce other side effects which
sicians monitor.

Anticancer drugs are usually
ninistered in the highest doses that
be tolerated in order to kill as many
cer cells as quickly as possible, and
refore to reduce the risk of the cancer
eading to other parts of the body and
ning metastases.

Beneficial effects on the underlying
ease may not be apparent for several
eks. The unpleasant side effects of
nsive cancer chemotherapy, combined
a the lack of immediate response to the

ACTION OF CYTOTOXIC ANTICANCER DRUGS

Each type of cytotoxic drug affects a separate stage of the cancer cell's development, and each type of drug kills the cell by a different mechanism of action. The action of some of the principal classes of cytotoxic drugs is described below.

Alkylating agents and cytotoxic antibiotics
These act within the cell's nucleus to damage the cell's genetic material, DNA. This prevents the cell from growing and dividing.

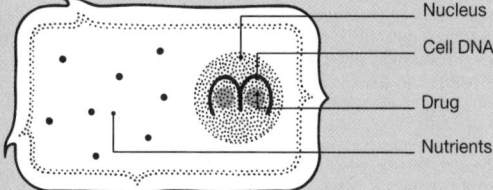

Nucleus
Cell DNA
Drug
Nutrients

Antimetabolites
These drugs prevent the cell from *metabolizing* (processing) nutrients and other substances that are necessary for normal activity in the cell.

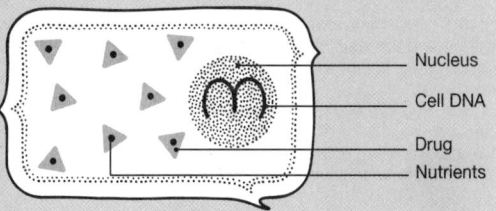

Nucleus
Cell DNA
Drug
Nutrients

treatment, often lead to depression among those receiving anticancer drugs. Specialist counseling may be helpful.

Risks and special precautions

All cytotoxic anticancer drugs interfere with the activity of non-cancerous cells and for this reason they often produce serious adverse effects during long-term treatment. In particular, these drugs often adversely affect the blood-producing cells in the bone marrow. The number of both red and white cells and the number of platelets (particles in the blood which are responsible for clotting) may all be reduced. In some cases, symptoms of *anemia* (weakness and fatigue) and an increased risk of abnormal or excessive bleeding may develop as a result of treatment. In addition, wounds may take longer to heal, and susceptible people can develop gout as a result of increased release of uric acid (a by-product of cell destruction). Reduction in the number of white blood cells may result in an increased susceptibility to infection.

Because of these problems, anticancer chemotherapy is often given in a hospital, where the effects can be closely monitored. Several short courses of drug treatment are often given, thus allowing the bone marrow time to recover in the intervening period (see Successful chemotherapy, facing page). Blood tests are performed regularly. Where necessary, blood transfusions, antibiotics, or other forms of treatment are used to overcome the adverse effects. Where relevant, contraceptive advice is given early in

treatment, because most anticancer drugs can damage a developing baby.

In addition to these general effects, individual drugs may have adverse effects on particular organs. These are described in the drug profiles in Part 4.

COMMON DRUGS

Alkylating agents
Carboplatin
Chlorambucil
Cisplatin
Cyclophosphamide
Melphalan

Antimetabolites
Cytarabine
Fluorouracil
Mercaptopurine
Methotrexate

Cytotoxic antibiotics
Doxorubicin
Epirubicin
Idarubicin

Hormone treatments
Aminoglutethimide
Flutamide
Goserelin
Leuprolide
Medroxyprogesterone
Megestrol
Tamoxifen

Other drugs
Amsacrine
Asparaginase
Etoposide
Fludarabine
Paclitaxel
Procarbazine
Vincristine

IMMUNOSUPPRESSANT DRUGS

The body is protected against attack from bacteria and viruses by the specialized cells and proteins in the blood and tissues that make up the immune system (see p.164). White blood cells known as lymphocytes either kill these invading organisms directly or produce special proteins (*antibodies*) to destroy them. These mechanisms are also responsible for eliminating abnormal or unhealthy cells that could otherwise multiply and develop into a cancer.

In certain conditions, it is medically necessary to dampen the activity of the immune system. These include a number of autoimmune disorders in which the immune system attacks normal body tissue. Autoimmune disorders may affect a single organ – for example, the kidneys in Goodpasture's syndrome or the thyroid gland in Hashimoto's disease – or may cause widespread damage, as in rheumatoid arthritis or systemic lupus erythematosus.

Immune system activity may also need to be reduced following an organ transplant, when the body's defenses would otherwise attack and reject the transplanted tissue.

Several types of drugs are used as immunosuppressants: anticancer drugs (p.166), corticosteroids (p.153), and cyclosporine.

Why they are used

Immunosuppressant drugs are given in autoimmune disorders such as rheumatoid arthritis when symptoms are severe and other treatments have not provided adequate relief. Corticosteroids are usually prescribed initially. The pronounced anti-inflammatory effect of these drugs, in addition to their immunosuppressant action, helps to promote healing of tissue damaged by abnormal immune system activity. Anticancer drugs such as azathioprine may be used in addition to corticosteroids if these do not produce sufficient improvement or if their effect wanes (see also Antirheumatic drugs, p.129).

Immunosuppressant drugs are given before and after organ and other tissue transplants. Treatment may have to continue permanently following the transplant to prevent rejection. A number of drugs and drug combinations are used, depending on the organ or tissue being transplanted and the underlying condition of the recipient. Corticosteroids in conjunction with azathioprine were, until recently, the most widely used therapy. However, cyclosporine and muromonab-CD3 are now being used for preventing organ rejection. Cyclosporine is currently being studied to evaluate its possible usefulness in the treatment of autoimmune disorders.

How they work

Immunosuppressant drugs reduce the effectiveness of the immune system either by depressing the production of lymphocytes or by altering their activity.

How they affect you

When immunosuppressants are given to treat an autoimmune disorder they reduce the severity of the symptoms and in many cases temporarily halt the progress of the disease. However, they cannot restore major tissue damage, such as damage to the joints in rheumatoid arthritis.

Corticosteroids often promote a general feeling of well-being, but given in doses high enough to produce an immunosuppressant effect, they may also produce unwanted effects. These are described in more detail on p.153. Anticancer drugs, when prescribed as immunosuppressants, are given in low doses that produce only mild side effec[t]. They may cause nausea and vomiting, [for] which an anti-emetic drug (p.102) may [be] prescribed. Hair loss may occur, but ha[ir] growth usually resumes when the drug [is] discontinued. Cyclosporine may cause increased growth of facial hair, swelling the gums, and tingling in the hands.

Risks and special precautions

All of these drugs may produce potentially serious adverse effects. By reducin[g] immune system activity, immunosuppre[s]sant drugs can affect the body's ability t[o] fight invading microorganisms, thereby increasing the risk of serious infections, such as those described on the facing page. Because lymphocyte activity is al[so] important for preventing the multiplicatio[n] of abnormal cells, there is an increased [risk] of certain types of cancer. A major drawback of anticancer drugs is that, in addition to their effect on the productio[n] of lymphocytes, they interfere with the growth and division of other blood cells [in] the bone marrow. Reduced production [of] red blood cells can cause *anemia*; when the production of blood platelets is suppressed, blood clotting may be less efficient.

Because cyclosporine is more specif[ic] in its action than corticosteroids or anti[-] cancer drugs, it produces fewer trouble[some] side effects. However, it may cau[se] kidney damage, and in too high a dose may affect the brain, causing hallucinations or seizures. Cyclosporine also tends to raise blood pressure, and anot[her] drug may be required to counteract thi[s] effect (see Antihypertensive drugs, p.1[...]).

ACTION OF IMMUNOSUPPRESSANTS

Before treatment
Many types of blood cell, each with a distinct role, form in the bone marrow. Lymphocytes respond to infection and foreign tissue. B-lymphocytes produce antibodies to attack invading organisms, whereas T-lymphocytes directly attack invading cells. Others help the action of the B- and T-cells.

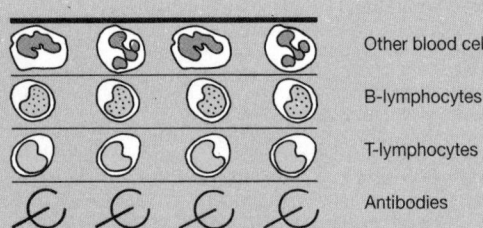

Other blood cells

B-lymphocytes

T-lymphocytes

Antibodies

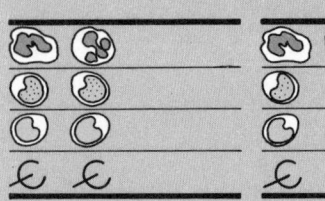

Anticancer drugs
Anticancer drugs slow the production of all cells in the bone marrow.

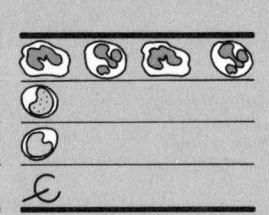

Corticosteroids
These reduce both B- and T-lymphocyte activity.

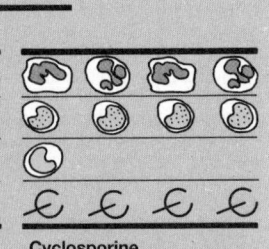

Cyclosporine
This inhibits the activity of T-lymphocytes only, and not the activity of B-lymphocytes.

COMMON DRUGS

Anticancer drugs
Azathioprine
Chlorambucil
Cyclophosphamide
Methotrexate

Corticosteroids
(see p.153)

Other drugs
Anti-thymocyte globulin
Cyclosporine
Muromonab-CD3

DRUGS FOR AIDS AND IMMUNE DEFICIENCY

Immune deficiency occurs when the body's immune system, which normally protects the body against infecting organisms and the development of cancer, fails. Immune deficiency may be present from birth because the body's immune system has not developed normally, or it may occur during drug treatment (for example, with cortico-steroids or anticancer drugs), or as a result of cancer or infection.

AIDS (acquired immune deficiency syndrome) is a disorder caused by infection with HIV (human immuno-deficiency virus). The virus invades certain types of cells, particularly the white blood cells known as T-helper lymphocytes. T-helper lymphocytes normally activate other cells in the immune system to produce antibodies to fight infection. Because the AIDS virus attacks T-helper lymphocytes, the body is unable to fight the AIDS virus or any subsequent infection.

There may be a long interval between infection with the HIV virus and the development of AIDS. Not everybody who is HIV positive progresses to AIDS. Illnesses that commonly affect people with AIDS include candidiasis (thrush), herpes simplex infections, tuberculosis, cryptococcal meningitis, lymphomas, Kaposi's sarcoma (a rare form of skin cancer), pneumocystis carinii pneumonia (PCP), and dementia.

Why they are used

Various infections are the most common consequence of all immune-deficiency disorders. These are treated with a variety of antibiotics (p.140), antiviral drugs (p.145), and antifungal drugs (p.150). The antiprotozoal pentamidine may be used to treat PCP.

Kaposi's sarcoma and other cancers are not consistently treated with anti-cancer drugs, since there is an added risk of depressing the immune system. Radiation therapy may be given instead. When serious AIDS-related infections have occurred, the antiviral drugs zidovudine (AZT), didanosine, or zalcitabine may be prescribed. They do not provide a cure but may prolong life expectancy. HIV patients may be given treatment to prevent some of these conditions, especially PCP and tuberculosis.

New drugs

Current research into new drug treatment of AIDS is proceeding along two principal lines. Scientists are searching for a vaccine that will provide immunity against the AIDS virus, and they are also trying to develop drugs to eradicate the HIV virus from the body once infection has occurred (see box, right).

AIDS INFECTION AND POSSIBLE TREATMENTS

The illustrations below show how the AIDS virus enters body cells and, once inside, replicates itself to produce new viruses. The stages at which drugs might in the future be used to block the action of AIDS viruses, or destroy them, are also indicated.

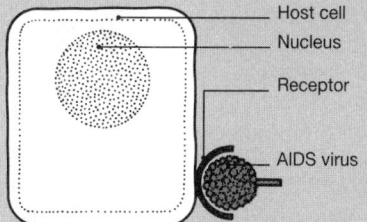
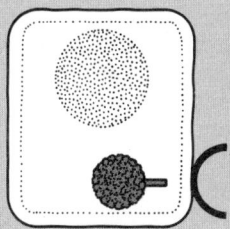

Stage 1
The virus binds to a specialized site (receptor) on a body cell.

Possible drug intervention
Binding could be blocked by the production of antibodies to destroy the virus or the cell's receptor.

Stage 2
The virus enters the cell.

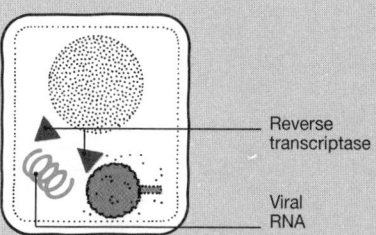
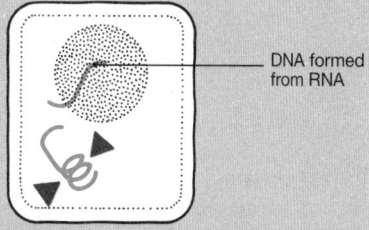

Stage 3
The virus loses its protective coat and releases RNA, its genetic material, and an enzyme known as reverse transcriptase.

Possible drug intervention
Drugs may be developed to prevent the virus from losing its protective coat. Amantadine has this effect on the influenza A virus but not on HIV.

Stage 4
The enzyme reverse transcriptase converts the viral RNA into DNA that can then enter the host cell's nucleus and may become integrated with the cell's genetic material.

Possible drug intervention
Zidovudine blocks the action of reverse transcriptase.

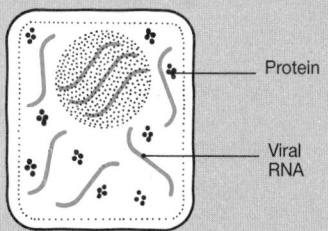
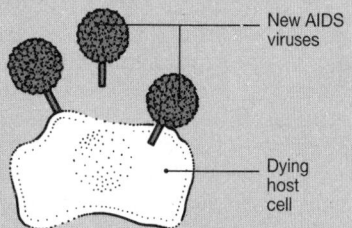

Stage 5
The host cell starts to produce new viral RNA and protein from the viral material that has been incorporated into its nucleus.

Possible drug intervention
There is a possibility that in the future drugs may be available to inhibit the production of new viral RNA and proteins by altering genes on the viral material.

Stage 6
The new viral RNA and proteins are assembled to produce new viruses. These leave the host cell (which then dies) and are free to attack other cells in the body.

Possible drug intervention
The drug alpha interferon prevents the new viruses from leaving the cell. It is under investigation for limiting the spread of AIDS infection within the body.

REPRODUCTIVE & URINARY TRACTS

The reproductive systems of men and women consist of those organs which produce and release sperm (male), store and release eggs (female), and then nurture a fertilized egg until it becomes a baby (female).

The urinary system filters wastes and water from the blood, producing urine, which is then expelled from the body. The reproductive and urinary systems of men are partially linked, but those of women form two physically close but functionally separate systems.

The female reproductive organs comprise the ovaries, fallopian tubes, and uterus (womb). The uterus opens via the cervix (neck of the uterus) into the vagina. The principal male reproductive organs are the two sperm-producing glands – the testicles (testes) contained in the scrotum – and the penis. Other parts of the male reproductive tract include the prostate gland and several tubular structures: the epididymis, the vas deferens, the seminal vesicles, and the urethra (see right).

The urinary organs in both sexes comprise the kidneys, which filter blood and excrete urine (see also p.111), the ureters down which urine passes, and the bladder, where urine is stored until it is released from the body via the urethra.

What can go wrong
The reproductive and urinary tracts are both subject to infection. Such infections (apart from those transmitted by sexual activity) are relatively uncommon in men because the long male urethra prevents bacteria and other organisms from passing easily to the bladder and upper urinary tract and to the male sex organs. The shorter female urethra allows infection of the urinary tract, especially of the bladder (cystitis) and of the urethra (urethritis), to occur commonly. The female reproductive tract is also vulnerable to infection, sometimes sexually transmitted.

Reproductive function may also be disrupted by hormonal disturbances that lead to reduced fertility. Women may be troubled by symptoms arising from normal activity of the reproductive organs, including menstrual disorders and problems associated with childbirth.

The most common urinary problems apart from infection are those related to bladder function. Urine may be released involuntarily (incontinence) or it may be retained in the bladder. Such disorders are usually the result of abnormal nerve signals to the bladder or sphincter muscle. The filtering action of the kidneys may be disrupted by alteration of the composition of the blood or the hormones that

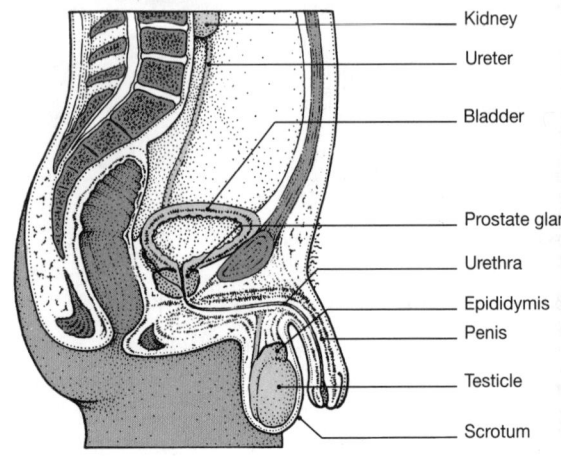

Kidney

Ureter

Bladder

Prostate glan

Urethra

Epididymis

Penis

Testicle

Scrotum

Male reproductive system
Sperm produced in each of the testicles pass into the epididymis, a tightly coiled tube in which the sperm mature before passing along the vas deferens to the seminal vesicles. Sperm are stored in the seminal vesicles u they are ejaculated from the pe via the urethra together with seminal fluid and secretions fro the prostate gland.

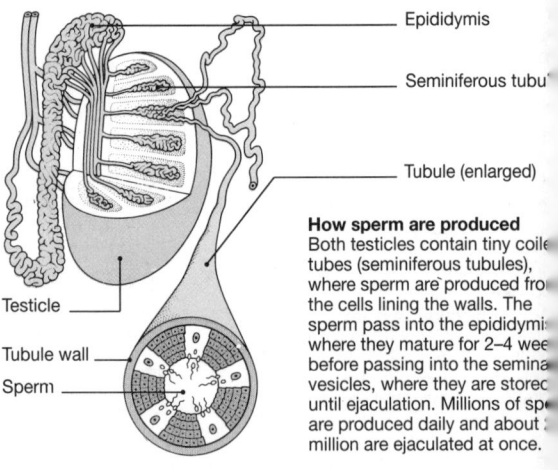

Epididymis

Seminiferous tubu

Tubule (enlarged)

Testicle

Tubule wall

Sperm

How sperm are produced
Both testicles contain tiny coile tubes (seminiferous tubules), where sperm are produced fro the cells lining the walls. The sperm pass into the epididymi where they mature for 2–4 wee before passing into the semina vesicles, where they are storec until ejaculation. Millions of sp are produced daily and about million are ejaculated at once.

regulate urine production, or by damage (from infection or inflammation) to the filtering units themselves.

Why drugs are used
Antibiotic drugs (p.140) are used to eliminate bot urinary and reproductive tract infections (includin sexually transmitted infections). Certain infection of the vagina are caused by fungi or yeasts and require antifungal drugs (p.150).

Hormone drugs are used both to reduce fertili deliberately (oral contraceptives) and to increase fertility in certain conditions that make it impossi for a couple to conceive. Hormones may also be

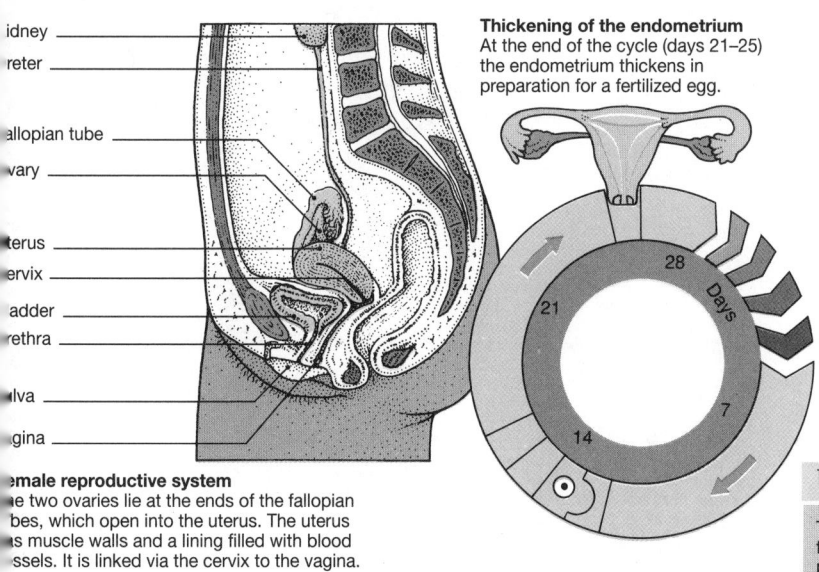

idney
reter
allopian tube
vary
terus
ervix
adder
rethra
ilva
agina

emale reproductive system
ie two ovaries lie at the ends of the fallopian
bes, which open into the uterus. The uterus
is muscle walls and a lining filled with blood
ssels. It is linked via the cervix to the vagina.

Thickening of the endometrium
At the end of the cycle (days 21–25) the endometrium thickens in preparation for a fertilized egg.

28
Days
21
14
7

Menstrual cycle
A monthly cycle of hormone interactions allows an egg to be released and, if it is fertilized, creates the correct environment for it to implant in the uterus. Major body changes occur, most obviously, monthly vaginal bleeding (menstruation). The cycle usually starts between 11 and 14 years, and continues until the menopause, which occurs at around 50. After the menopause, childbearing is no longer possible. The cycle is usually 28 days, but this varies with individuals.

Menstruation
If no egg is fertilized, the endometrium is shed (days 1–5).

Fertile period
Conception may take place in the two days after ovulation (days 14–16).

Endometrium

The fertilized egg divides continually on the way down the fallopian tube.

One sperm fuses with the egg in the fallopian tube.

Fallopian tube

Ovarian follicle

A fluid-filled cell cluster (follicle) nourishes the maturing egg. When the egg is ripe, it is released from the follicle.

Ovary

The fertilized egg implants in the uterine wall and develops into an embryo.

Journey of the egg
Every month, hormone activity causes an egg within an ovarian follicle in one of the ovaries to ripen. It is then released (ovulation) and travels down the fallopian tube to the womb.

URINARY SYSTEM

The kidneys extract waste and excess water from the blood. The waste liquid (urine) passes into the bladder, from where it is expelled via the urethra.

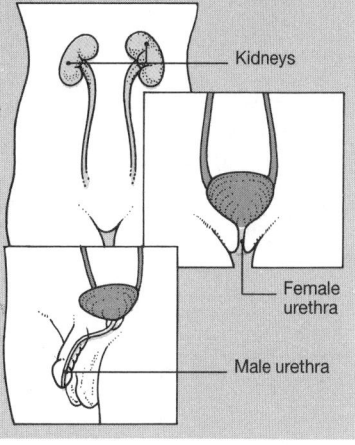

Kidneys

Female urethra

Male urethra

---

ed to regulate menstruation when this is irregular
excessively painful or heavy. Analgesic drugs
92) are used to treat menstrual period pain and
e also used for pain relief in labor. Other drugs
ed in labor include those that increase contrac-
n of the muscles of the uterus and those that
iit blood loss after the birth. Drugs may also be
iployed to halt premature labor (see Drugs used
labor, p.177).
Drugs that alter the transmission of nerve signals
the bladder muscles have an important role in
e treatment of urinary incontinence and retention.
ugs that increase the filtering action of the
Ineys are commonly used to reduce blood

pressure and fluid retention (see Diuretics, p.111). Other drugs may alter the composition of the urine, such as the uricosuric drugs used in the treatment of gout (p.131).

MAJOR DRUG GROUPS

Drugs used to treat menstrual disorders
Oral contraceptives
Drugs for infertility
Drugs used in labor
Drugs used for urinary disorders

DRUGS USED TO TREAT MENSTRUAL DISORDERS

The menstrual cycle results from the actions of female sex hormones that each month cause ovulation (release of an egg) and thickening of the endometrium (lining of the uterus) in preparation for pregnancy. Unless the egg is fertilized, the endometrium is shed about two weeks later during menstruation (see also p.171).

The main problems associated with menstruation that may require medical treatment are excessive blood loss (menorrhagia), pain during menstruation (dysmenorrhea), and distressing symptoms prior to menstruation (premenstrual syndrome). Absence of periods (amenorrhea) is discussed under Female sex hormones (p.159).

The drugs most commonly used to treat the menstrual disorders described above include estrogens and progesterone (or synthetic progesterone drugs known as progestins), danazol, and analgesics.

Why they are used

Drug treatment for menstrual disorders is undertaken only when the physician has ruled out the possibility of an underlying gynecological disorder such as pelvic infection or fibroids. In some cases, especially in women over the age of 35, a D and C (dilatation and curettage) may be recommended. When no underlying reason for the problem has been found, drug treatment aimed primarily at the relief of symptoms is usually prescribed.

Dysmenorrhea

Painful menstrual periods are usually treated initially with a simple analgesic (see also p.92). ASA and non-steroidal anti-inflammatory drugs (such as ibuprofen, naproxen, mefenamic acid and others) are often effective because they counter the effects of chemicals called prostaglandins, which are considered to be partly responsible for transmission of pain. When these drugs fail to provide sufficient relief of pain, hormonal drug treatment may be advised. If contraception is also required, treatment may take the form of an oral contraceptive tablet containing an estrogen and a progestin, or a progestin alone. However, non-contraceptive progestin preparations are also used. These may be taken for only a few days during each month. Treatment of dysmenorrhea caused by endometriosis is described in the box above right.

Menorrhagia

Excessive blood loss during menstruation can sometimes be reduced by the use of non-steroidal anti-inflammatory drugs. However, in many cases, hormone treatment, as described under dysmenorrhea (above), is advised. Alternatively, danazol, a drug that reduces production of the hormone estrogen, may be prescribed.

ENDOMETRIOSIS

Endometriosis is a condition in which fragments of endometrial tissue (uterine lining) occur outside the uterus in the pelvic cavity. This disorder causes severe pain during menstruation and often pain during intercourse; it may sometimes lead to infertility.

Drugs used for this disorder are similar to those prescribed for heavy periods (menorrhagia). However, in this case the intention is to suppress endometrial development for an extended period so that the abnormal tissue eventually withers away. Progesterone supplements that suppress thickening of endometrium may be prescribed throughout the menstrual cycle. Alternatively, danazol, a drug that suppresses endometrial development by reducing estrogen production, may be prescribed. Any drug treatment usually needs to be continued for a minimum of six months.

When drug treatment is unsuccessful, surgical removal of the abnormal tissue is usually necessary.

Sites of endometriosis

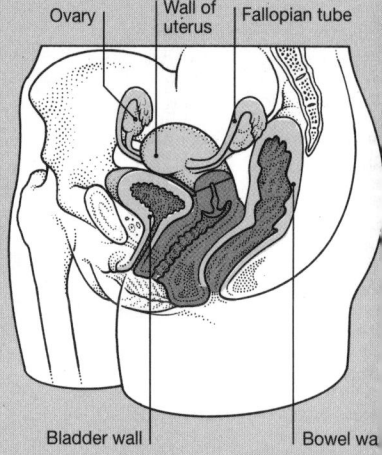

Ovary | Wall of uterus | Fallopian tube

Bladder wall | Bowel wa[ll]

☐ Endometrial tissue

Premenstrual syndrome

This is a collection of emotional and physical symptoms that affect many women to some degree in the days prior to menstruation. Psychological symptoms include mood changes such as increased irritability, depression, and anxiety. Principal physical symptoms are bloating, headache, and breast tenderness. Non-drug treatment includes ensuring optimal nutrition, rest, and exercise as well as reduction of excessive stress. Because premenstrual syndrome may be the result of a drop in progesterone levels in the last half of the menstrual cycle, supplements of this hormone may be given in the week or so prior to menstruation. Other drugs sometimes used include pyridoxine (vitamin B_6) for depression, diuretics (p.111) if bloating is a problem, and bromocriptine when breast tenderness is the major symptom. Anti-anxiety drugs (p.95) may be prescribed in rare cases where severe premenstrual psychological disturbance is experienced.

How they work

Drugs used in menstrual disorders act in a variety of ways. Hormonal treatments are aimed at suppressing the pattern of hormonal changes that is causing troublesome symptoms. Contraceptive preparations override the normal menstrual cycle. Ovulation does not occur and the endometrium does not thicken normally. Bleeding that occurs at the end of a cycle is less likely to be abnormally heavy, to be preceded by

distressing symptoms, or to be accompanied by severe discomfort. For further information on oral contraceptive see p.173.

Non-contraceptive progesterone preparations taken in the days prior to menstruation do not suppress ovulation. Increased progesterone during this time reduces premenstrual symptoms and prevents excessive thickening of the endometrium.

Danazol, a potent and expensive drug prevents the thickening of the endometrium, thereby correcting excessively heavy periods. Blood loss is reduced; in some cases menstruation ceases altogether during treatment.

COMMON DRUGS

Estrogens and progestins
(see p.159)

Analgesics
ASA
Ibuprofen
Mefenamic acid
Naproxen

Diuretics
(see p.111)

Others
Bromocriptine
Danazol
Nafarelin
Pyridoxine

ORAL CONTRACEPTIVES

here are many different means of nsuring that conception and pregnancy o not follow sexual intercourse. For many women the oral contraceptive is a ghly effective method (see Comparison f reliability of different methods of ontraception, right). In addition to its ontraceptive qualities, it is well tolerated, onvenient, and unobtrusive during vemaking. About 25 per cent of women eking contraceptive protection in anada choose a form of oral ontraceptive.

There are two main types of oral ontraceptive: the combined pill and the hased pill. Both types contain a natural synthetic estrogen and a progestin (a nthetic form of the female sex hormone ogesterone). (See also Female sex ormones, p.159.) Both types are taken a cyclic basis.

Another type of oral contraceptive, the ogestin-only pill, which was introduced the 1970s, is rarely used in Canada day because of its relatively high failure te and the frequent occurrence of ublesome side effects.

hy they are used

e combined pill
ese contain a fixed amount of an trogen and a progestin drug. The west formulations are a further inement of the original combined pills roduced in the 1960s. These eparations are effective, safe, and do t usually cause significant adverse ects. They may be especially beneficial some women who experience painful, avy, or prolonged periods (see Drugs ed to treat menstrual disorders, p.172).

ased pills
ch pack of phased pills, the newest m of oral contraceptive, contains pills vided into three groups, or phases. ch phase of the pills contains a ferent proportion of an estrogen and a

VAILABLE ORMULATIONS

ealth Canada recommends that oral ontraceptives contain not more than 5mcg of estrogen and a progestin of low ological activity. Occasionally, depending individual circumstances, it may be ecessary to select a formulation with a gher dose of estrogen or progestin.

Most formulations can be divided into ose that contain 35mcg or less of strogen and those that contain more than 5mcg of estrogen. In considering the oice of formulation, the risks as well as e benefits are considered.

COMPARISON OF RELIABILITY OF DIFFERENT METHODS OF CONTRACEPTION

The table (right) indicates the number of pregnancies that occur with each method of contraception among 100 women using that method in a year. The wide variation that occurs with some methods takes into account pregnancies that occur as a result of incorrect use of the method.

Method	Pregnancies*
Combined and phased pills	Less than 1 – 2
Progestin-only pill	3 – 6
IUCD**	Less than 1 – 6
Condom/diaphragm	2 – 18
Rhythm	2 – 20
Contraceptive sponge	3 – 28
Vaginal spermicide alone	3 – 21
No contraception	60 – 85

*Per 100 users per year
** Intra-uterine contraceptive device

ORAL CONTRACEPTIVE PRODUCTS AVAILABLE IN CANADA

Brand Name	Estrogen	Progestin
Combined pills – 35mcg or less of estrogen		
Minestrin 1/20	Ethinyl estradiol 20mcg	Norethindrone acetate 1mg
Demulen 30	Ethinyl estradiol 30mcg	Ethynodiol diacetate 2mg
Loestrin 1.5/30	Ethinyl estradiol 30mcg	Norethindrone acetate 1.5mg
Marvelon	Ethinyl estradiol 30mcg	Desogestrel 0.15mg
Min-Oval	Ethinyl estradiol 30mcg	Levonorgestrel 0.15mg
Ortho-Cept	Ethinyl estradiol 30mcg	Desogestrel 0.15mg
Brevicon 0.5/35	Ethinyl estradiol 35mcg	Norethindrone acetate 0.5mg
Brevicon 1/35	Ethinyl estradiol 35mcg	Norethindrone 1mg
Cyclen	Ethinyl estradiol 35mcg	Norgestimate 0.25mg
Ortho 0.5/35	Ethinyl estradiol 35mcg	Norethindrone 0.5mg
Ortho 1/35	Ethinyl estradiol 35mcg	Norethindrone 1mg
Tri-Cyclen (days in brackets for each component)	Ethinyl estradiol 35mcg (21)	Norgestimate 0.18mg (7) Norgestimate 0.215mg (7) Norgestimate 0.25mg (7)
Combined pills – 50mcg of estrogen		
Demulen 50	Ethinyl estradiol 50mcg	Ethynodiol diacetate 1mg
Ortho Novum 1/50	Mestranol 50mcg	Norethindrone 1mg
Ovral	Ethinyl estradiol 50mcg	Norgestrel 0.25mg
Norinyl 1 + 50	Mestranol 50mcg	Norethindrone 1mg
Phased pills (days in brackets for each component)		
Ortho 10/11	Ethinyl estradiol 35mcg (21)	Norethindrone 0.5mg (10) Norethindrone 1mg (11)
Ortho 7/7/7	Ethinyl estradiol 35mcg (21)	Norethindrone 0.5mg (7) Norethindrone 0.75mg (7) Norethindrone 1mg (7)
Synphasic	Ethinyl estradiol 35mcg (21)	Norethindrone 0.5mg (7) Norethindrone 1mg (9) Norethindrone 0.5mg (5)
Triphasil	Ethinyl estradiol 30mcg (6) Ethinyl estradiol 40mcg (5) Ethinyl estradiol 30mcg (10)	Levonorgestrel 0.05mg (6) Levonorgestrel 0.075mg (5) Levonorgestrel 0.125mg (10)
Triquilar	Ethinyl estradiol 30mcg (6) Ethinyl estradiol 40mcg (5) Ethinyl estradiol 30mcg (10)	Levonorgestrel 0.05mg (6) Levonorgestrel 0.075mg (5) Levenorgestrel 0.125mg (10)
Progestin-only pill		
Micronor		Norethindrone 0.35mg

ORAL CONTRACEPTIVES continued

progestin. The aim is to reduce the total amount of progestin taken during the cycle. Phased pills, taken in the same way as the combined pill, provide effective contraceptive protection. They are especially beneficial for many women who suffer side effects from the combined pill.

How they work

In a normal menstrual cycle, the ripening and release of an egg, and the preparation of the uterus for implantation of the fertilized egg, are the result of a complex interplay between the natural female sex hormones, estrogen and progesterone, and the pituitary hormones, follicle-stimulating hormone (FSH) and luteinizing hormone (LH) (see also p.159). Estrogens and progestins contained in oral contraceptives act in a variety of ways to disrupt the normal cycle in such a way as to make conception less likely.

In combined and phased pills, levels of estrogen and progestin inhibit the production of FSH and LH, and thereby prevent the egg from ripening in the ovary and from being released.

All pills (combined, phased, and progestin-only) change cervical mucus and the lining of the uterus to interfere with the ability of sperm to fertilize the egg.

How they affect you

Each course of combined and phased pills lasts for 21 days, followed by a pill-free seven days during which menstruation occurs. Some brands contain seven additional inactive pills. This means that the new course directly follows the last, so that the habit of taking the pill daily is not broken. Progestin-only pills are taken for 28 days each month. Menstruation usually occurs during the last few days of the cycle.

HOW TO MINIMIZE YOUR HEALTH RISKS WHILE TAKING THE PILL

▼ Give up smoking.

▼ Maintain a healthy weight.

▼ Have a regular blood pressure and blood fat checks.

▼ Have regular cervical smear tests.

▼ Remind your physician that you are taking oral contraceptives before taking any other medications, such as antibiotics.

▼ Stop taking estrogen-containing oral contraceptives four weeks before planned major surgery (use alternative contraception).

BALANCING THE RISKS AND BENEFITS OF ORAL CONTRACEPTIVES

Oral contraceptives are safe for the vast majority of women. However every woman considering using this method of contraception should see her physician to discuss the risks involved, possible adverse effects, the particular advantages of these drugs, and other factors involved before deciding that a hormonal method is the most suitable in her case. A variety of factors must be taken into account, including the woman's age, her own medical history and that of her close relatives, and factors such as whether or not she is overweight or a smoker. Many risks have been reduced with the introduction of the lower-dose hormonal pills. The table below summarizes the main advantages and disadvantages of currently available oral contraceptives.

Advantages	● Very reliable
	● Convenient/unobtrusive
	● Regularizes menstruation
	● Reduced menstrual pain and blood loss
	● Reduced risk of:
	▼ benign breast disease
	▼ endometriosis
	▼ ectopic pregnancy
	▼ ovarian cysts
	▼ pelvic infection
	▼ ovarian and endometrial cancer
Side effects	● Weight gain
	● Depression
	● Breast swelling
	● Reduced sex drive
	● Headaches
	● Increased vaginal discharge
	● Nausea
Risks	● Thrombosis/embolism
	● Heart disease
	● High blood pressure
	● Jaundice
	● Cancer of the liver (rare)
	● Gallstones
Factors that may prohibit use	● Previous thrombosis
	● Heart disease
	● High levels of fat in blood
	● Liver disease
	● Blood disorders
	● High blood pressure
	● Unexplained vaginal bleeding
	● Migraine
	● Otosclerosis
	● Presence of several risk factors (below)
Factors that increase risks	● Smoking
	● Obesity
	● Increasing age
	● Diabetes mellitus
	● Family history of heart or circulatory disease
	● Current treatment with other drugs

Most women notice little change in
r overall feeling of well-being with the
ver types of oral contraceptive. Ten to
per cent of women may experience
al breakthrough bleeding, missed
ods, mood changes, headaches,
ast tenderness, weight gain, and/or
sea. Many of these troublesome side
cts disappear after three months, and
majority of women can continue
ng the pill. In some cases it may be
essary to switch to another
nulation in order to reduce side
cts. Many women find relief from
nful, heavy, or prolonged menstrual
ods while taking the pill.

ks and special precautions

ral contraceptives need to be taken
larly for maximum protection against
gnancy. Contraceptive protection can
educed by missing a pill (see What to
f you miss a pill, right). It may also be
ced by vomiting or diarrhea. If you
er from either of these symptoms, it is
isable to act as if you had missed your
pill. Many drugs may also affect the
on of oral contraceptives, so it is
ential to inform your physician that
are taking oral contraceptives before
take any additional medications.
ral contraceptives have been found to
y a number of risks. These are
marized on the facing page. Almost
of the serious potential adverse effects
ral contraceptive therapy have been
ced to minimal levels as a result of
following factors: the introduction of
nulations containing less than 50mcg
strogen; the low progestin content of
sed pills; a greater awareness of the
eased risks for women over 35 years
smoke and take the oral
traceptive pill.
woman considering using the
traceptive pill is encouraged to
uss with her physician the specific
s and benefits as they apply to the
icular formulation selected. Each pill
kage contains an insert which can
e as a framework for this discussion.
here are some common myths and
conceptions associated with the use
ral contraceptives, that it alters
lity, increases cancer potential, and
ses fetal damage. There is no evi-
ce to support such myths.
number of benefits have been dem-
trated conclusively in women who
e been using oral contraceptives.
se include a reduced risk of ovarian
ts, pelvic infections, anemia, and
ine and ovarian cancers.

IF YOU DECIDE TO TAKE THE PILL

Should you and your physician decide that,
for you, the benefits of the birth control pill
outweigh its risks, you should be aware that
periodic medical supervision is necessary.

Cigarette smoking increases the risk of
serious adverse effects on the heart and
blood vessels in women who use oral
contraceptives. This risk increases with age
and heavy smoking (15 or more cigarettes a
day) and is more marked in women over 35
years of age.

▼ Take the tablets only on the advice of
your physician and carefully follow all
directions given to you. It is important to
take the tablets exactly as prescribed,
otherwise you may become pregnant.

▼ After the age of 35 years, your physician
should be consulted regarding the special
risks of using the pill.

▼ See your physician at least once a year
after the initial visits.

▼ Common, troublesome side effects of
the pill such as nausea, unusual tiredness,
mood changes, abnormal menstruation,
breast swelling and/or tenderness, acne,
weight gain, and increase or decrease in
appetite may occur. See your physician
three months after starting the pill and be
sure to report any side effects experienced
that persist or are bothersome.

Serious side effects experienced while
using the pill are rare. However, if you
develop chest pain, sudden shortness of
breath, visual changes, severe headaches,
vomiting, pain or swelling of a leg,
unexplained weakness or numbness in an
arm or leg, or jaundice call your physician
immediately.

▼ Never take an oral contraceptive if you
think you are pregnant. It will not prevent
the pregnancy from continuing.

▼ It is not recommended that the pill be
discontinued periodically for "rest periods."
However, many physicians suggest that you
wait for at least one normal spontaneous
menstrual cycle after stopping the pill
before becoming pregnant.

▼ Recent studies suggest that women who
are breast-feeding may take the pill safely.
However, consult your physician.

▼ Discuss with your physician the benefits
of stopping the pill before major surgery.

▼ Because some laboratory tests,
medications, and physical signs may be
influenced by the pill, any physician that you
see should be made aware that you are
taking oral contraceptives.

WHAT TO DO IF YOU MISS A PILL

Contraceptive protection may be reduced if
blood levels of the hormones in the body fall
as a result of missing a pill. It is particularly
important to ensure that the progestin-only
pills are taken punctually. If you miss a pill,
however, take it as soon as you remember.
This may mean that you might take two pills
in one day. It is always wise to use a backup
form of contraception for the remainder of
the cycle.

POSTCOITAL CONTRACEPTION

Pregnancy following intercourse without
contraception may be avoided by taking a
short course of postcoital ("morning after")
contraceptive pills. This entails taking two
doses of a contraceptive pill within 72 hours
following intercourse. These drugs postpone ovulation and act on the lining of the
uterus to prevent implantation of the egg.
However, the high doses required make
them unsuitable for regular use, and they
are used only in special circumstances.

COMMON DRUGS

Estrogens
Ethinyl estradiol
Mestranol

Progestins
Desogestrel
Ethynodiol diacetate
Levonorgestrel
Norethindrone
Norethindrone acetate
Norgestimate
Norgestrel

DRUGS FOR INFERTILITY

Conception and establishment of pregnancy require a healthy reproductive tract in both partners. The man must produce sufficient numbers of healthy sperm; the woman must be able to produce a healthy egg that is able to pass freely down the fallopian tube to the uterus. The lining of the uterus must be in a condition that allows the implantation of the fertilized egg.

Although the cause of infertility sometimes remains undiscovered, in the majority of cases it is found to be due to one of the following factors: intercourse taking place at the wrong time during the menstrual cycle; the man producing too few or unhealthy sperm; the woman failing to ovulate (release an egg), or having blocked fallopian tubes as a result of previous pelvic infection. The production of female hormones necessary for ovulation and implantation of the egg in the uterus may be disturbed by physical illness or psychological stress.

Physicians do not usually begin to investigate the cause of failure to conceive until normal sexual intercourse without contraception has been taking place regularly for over a year. The first step is usually a thorough medical examination of both partners. If no simple explanation can be found, the man's semen will be analyzed to find out if he is producing healthy sperm in sufficient quantity. If these tests show abnormally low numbers of sperm or if a large proportion of the sperm produced are unhealthy, some of the treatments described in the box below may be tried.

At the same time, the female partner will be investigated. Ovulation is monitored and blood tests may be performed to assess hormone levels throughout the menstrual cycle. If ovulation does not occur, the woman may be offered treatment with a fertility drug.

Why they are used

Drugs are useful in helping to achieve pregnancy only when a hormone defect that inhibits ovulation has been diag-

MALE INFERTILITY

When the quality of the sperm is normal but the numbers produced are insufficient, the cause may be excessively low production of FSH and LH by the pituitary gland. In such cases, regular treatment with a pituitary-stimulating drug such as clomiphene, or with menotropins or human chorionic gonadotropin (which mimic the actions of FSH and LH), may be prescribed. Such drug treatment may need to be continued for many months before any increase in sperm production can be detected.

If, however, abnormal sperm production is due to an abnormality of the testicles or another part of the genitourinary tract, drug treatment is unlikely to be helpful.

ACTION OF FERTILITY DRUGS

Menotropins and HCG Menotropins contains FSH and LH. It acts on the ovary to initiate the development of an egg and stimulates the cells surrounding the developing egg (the follicle) to ripen.

HCG mimics the action of the hormone LH, causing the ripened follicle to release the egg into the fallopian tube. It also ensures that, after ovulation, progesterone is produced to prepare the uterus for the implantation of a fertilized egg.

Clomiphene Normally, estrogen acts on part of the brain (the hypothalamus) to suppress the output of FSH and LH by the pituitary gland. Clomiphene opposes the action of estrogen, so that FSH and LH continue to be produced.

Comparison of normal hormone fluctuation and timing of drug treatment

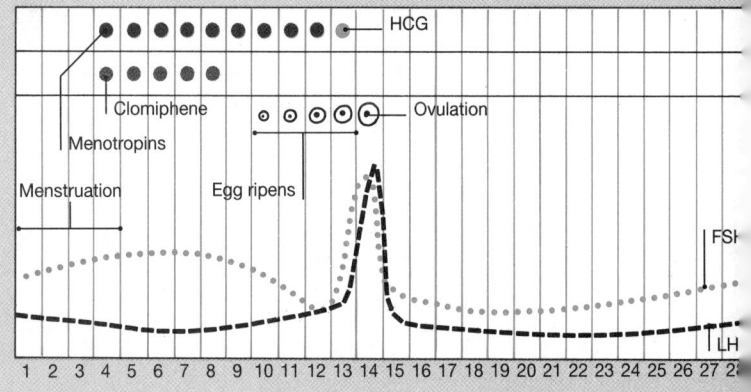

nosed. Fertility drug treatment may need to be continued for many months and does not always produce a pregnancy.

Women in whom the pituitary gland does not produce enough of the gonadotropin hormones – follicle-stimulating hormone (FSH) and luteinizing hormone (LH) – may be given courses of clomiphene for several days during each month. An effective dose produces ovulation 5 to 10 days after the last tablet is taken. Couples are advised to have intercourse during this phase.

Clomiphene occasionally thickens the cervical mucus, thereby impeding the passage of sperm. If this happens, an estrogen drug that counteracts this effect may be given prior to the course of clomiphene.

If treatment with clomiphene fails to produce ovulation, or if a disorder of the pituitary gland prevents the production of FSH and LH, treatment with menotropins and human chorionic gonadotropin (HCG) may be given.

Menotropins is given during the second week of the menstrual cycle, followed by an injection of HCG. Courses of these drugs may have to be repeated several times before pregnancy occurs.

How they work

Fertility drugs increase the chance of ovulation by boosting the levels of LH and FSH, the pituitary hormones that govern

ovulation. Clomiphene stimulates the pituitary gland to increase its output of these hormones. Menotropins acts to stimulate the ripening of the egg in the same way as natural FSH. HCG has an action similar to that of LH; it triggers the release of the egg and promotes the production of progesterone after ovula has taken place.

How they affect you

Each of these drugs may produce min adverse effects. Clomiphene may caus hot flushes, nausea, and headache, wh HCG can cause tiredness, headache, and mood changes. Menotropins can make the ovaries enlarge, producing abdominal discomfort that may contin for several days.

All these drugs increase the likeliho of multiple births (usually twins). A less common adverse effect is an increase risk of ovarian cysts with clomiphene.

COMMON DRUGS

Clomiphene
HCG (human chorionic gonadotropin)
Menotropins
Urofollitropin

RUGS USED IN LABOR

mal labor has three stages. In the first ge the uterus begins to contract, first gularly and then gradually more ularly and powerfully, while the cervix tes until it is fully stretched. During the ond stage, powerful contractions of uterus push the baby down the birth al and out of the body. The third stage he delivery of the placenta.

rugs may be required during one or e stages of labor for any of the owing reasons: to induce or augment or; to delay premature labor (see rine muscle relaxants, below right); to relieve pain. While the admin- ation of some drugs may be viewed as of routine obstetric care, most drugs administered only when the condition he mother or baby requires inter- tion. The possible adverse effects of drug on both parties are always efully balanced against the benefits.

ugs to induce or augment or

action of labor may be advised when a sician considers it risky for the health he mother or baby for the pregnancy continue – for example, if natural labor s not occur within two weeks of the date or when a woman has pre- ampsia. Other common reasons for acing labor include premature rupture he membrane surrounding the baby aking of the waters), delayed growth he baby due to poor nourishment by placenta, or death of the fetus in the us.

When labor needs to be induced, oxy- n, a uterine stimulant, is usually inistered intravenously. A prosta- ndin hormone and laminaria are being estigated for initiation of labor and tion of the cervix. If these methods are fective or cannot be used because of erse effects (see Risks and special cautions, above right), a cesarean de- ry may have to be performed.

Oxytocin may also be used to ngthen the force of contractions in or that has started spontaneously but ot progressing. This drug is also given

RUGS USED TO ERMINATE PREGNANCY

rugs may be used in a hospital or clinic to rminate pregnancy up to 20 weeks, or to npty the uterus after the death of the aby. Before the 14th week of pregnancy, e fetus is usually removed under general esthetic.

After the 14th week, labor is induced with e injection of saline or a prostaglandin ug into the uterus. These methods may all e supplemented by oxytocin given by travenous drip (see Drugs to induce or gment labor, above).

to most women as the baby is being born or immediately following birth to prevent excessive bleeding following the delivery of the placenta. This medication encourages the uterus to contract after delivery, thereby restricting the flow of blood. Ergonovine (ergometrine) is also sometimes used to decrease excessive postpartum bleeding.

Risks and special precautions
When oxytocin is used to induce labor, the dosage is carefully monitored throughout to prevent the possibility of excessively violent contractions. It is administered to women who have had surgery of the uterus only with careful monitoring. The drug is not known to affect the baby adversely. Ergonovine is not given to women who have suffered from high blood pressure during the course of pregnancy.

Drugs used for pain relief
Narcotics
Narcotic drugs such as meperidine may be given once active labor has been established (see Analgesics, p.92). Possible side effects for the mother include drowsiness, nausea, and vomiting. Narcotics may cause respiratory problems for the new baby and are usually not administered within one to two hours of delivery.

Epidural anesthesia
This provides pain relief during labor and birth by numbing the nerves leading to the uterus and pelvic area. It is often used during a planned cesarean delivery thus enabling the mother to be fully conscious for the birth.

An epidural involves the injection of a local anesthetic drug (see p.92) into the epidural space between the spinal cord and the vertebrae. An epidural may block the mother's urge to push during the second stage, and a forceps delivery may be necessary. Headaches may occasionally occur following epidural anesthesia.

Oxygen and nitrous oxide
These gases are combined to produce a mixture that reduces the pain of contrac- tions. During the first and second stages of labor it is self-administered by inhalation through a mask or mouthpiece. If it is used over too long a period it may produce nausea, confusion, and dehydration in the mother.

Local anesthetics
These drugs are injected inside the vagina or near the vaginal opening and are used to numb sensation during forceps delivery, before an episiotomy (an incision made to enlarge the vaginal opening), and whenever stitches are necessary. Side effects are rare.

WHEN DRUGS ARE USED IN LABOR

The drugs used in each stage of labor are described below.

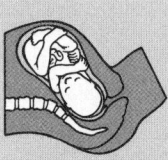
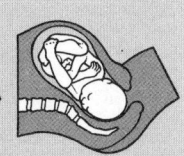

Before labor
Oxytocin
Prostaglandins

First stage
Epidural anesthetics
Meperidine
Oxytocin

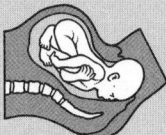
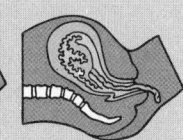

Second stage
Local anesthetics
Nitrous oxide
Oxytocin

Third stage
Ergonovine
Oxytocin

Uterine muscle relaxants
When contractions of the uterus start before the 34th week of pregnancy, physicians usually advise bed rest and may also administer a drug to relax the muscles of the uterus and thus halt labor. Initially the drug is given by injection in the hospital but may be continued orally at home. These drugs stimulate the sympathetic nervous system (see Autonomic nervous system, p.91) and may cause palpitations and anxiety in the mother. They have not been shown to have adverse effects on the baby.

COMMON DRUGS

Uterine stimulants
Ergonovine
Oxytocin

Prostaglandins
Dinoprostone

Uterine muscle relaxants
Ritodrine

Narcotics
Meperidine

DRUGS USED FOR URINARY DISORDERS

Urine is produced by the kidneys and stored in the bladder. As urine accumulates, the bladder walls stretch, and pressure within the bladder increases. Eventually, the stretching stimulates nerve endings that produce the urge to urinate. The ring of muscle (sphincter) around the bladder neck normally keeps the bladder closed until it is consciously relaxed, allowing urine to pass via the urethra out of the body.

A number of disorders can affect the urinary tract. The most common are infection in the bladder (cystitis) and urethra (urethritis), benign prostatic hyperplasia (BPH), and loss of reliable control over urination (urinary incontinence). A less common problem is inability to expel urine (urinary retention). Drugs used to treat these problems include antibiotics, analgesics, and drugs that act on nerve control over the muscles of the bladder and sphincter.

Drugs for urinary infection

Bladder infections – generally due to bacteria – may cause the following symptoms: burning on urination, urge to urinate small amounts frequently, and sometimes lower abdominal pain.

Antibiotic drugs are used to eradicate infection. Co-trimoxazole and amoxicillin, sometimes given in a single large dose or in longer courses, are among the most common treatments. Other antibiotics include the cephalosporins, the quinolones, and nitrofurantoin (see also Antibiotics, p.140).

Symptoms may be relieved by a urinary analgesic, phenazopyridine, which concentrates in the urine and has a soothing effect on the lining of the bladder and

urethra. It is often combined with an antibacterial drug.

BPH is a non-cancerous enlargement of the prostate gland that commonly occurs in older men. Symptoms include weak or interrupted urinary stream, dribbling, inability to empty the bladder completely, delay or hesitation on starting urination and the need to urinate frequently. Whereas severe forms of BPH with blockage must be treated surgically, drugs may help milder cases. Finasteride, a drug that blocks the effect of androgen, works to reduce prostate size. Alpha-adrenergic blocking agents work by decreasing the tone of the muscles surrounding the prostate and bladder.

Drugs for urinary incontinence

Urinary incontinence can occur for a number of reasons. A weak sphincter muscle allows the involuntary passage of urine when abdominal pressure is raised by coughing or physical exertion. This is known as stress incontinence and commonly affects women who have had children. Urgency – the sudden need to urinate – stems from increased sensitivity of the bladder muscle; small quantities of urine stimulate the urge to urinate frequently.

Incontinence can also occur due to loss of nerve control in neurological disorders such as multiple sclerosis. In children, inability to control urination at night (nocturnal enuresis) is also a form of urinary incontinence.

Drug treatment is not necessary or appropriate for all forms of incontinence. In stress incontinence, exercises to strengthen the pelvic floor muscles or surgery to tighten stretched ligaments

may be effective. In urgency, regular emptying of the bladder can often avo the need for medical intervention. Incontinence caused by loss of nerve control can sometimes be helped by c therapy. Frequency of urination in urge may be reduced by *anticholinergic* an antispasmodic drugs. These reduce n signals from the muscles in the bladde allowing greater volumes of urine to accumulate without stimulating the ur to pass urine. When a decision is mad treat childhood enuresis, desmopress nasal spray – a synthetic derivative of antidiuretic hormone – is the preferred drug. Tricyclic antidepressants are nov rarely used for bedwetting, due to the of adverse effects.

Drugs for urinary retention

Urinary retention is the inability to emp the bladder. This usually results from t failure of the bladder muscle to contra sufficiently to expel accumulated urine Possible causes include an enlarged prostate gland or tumor or a longstanc neurological disorder.

Most cases of urinary retention nee be relieved by inserting a tube (cathet into the urethra, and surgery may be needed to prevent a recurrence of the problem. Bethanechol, a *parasympath mimetic* drug which increases the strength of contraction of the bladder muscle, may relieve urinary retention following surgery. This drug is not suit for long-term therapy.

COMMON DRUGS

Antibiotics
(see pp.140 – 143)

Urinary analgesic
Phenazopyridine

Anticholinergic drugs
Hyoscine butylbromide
Flavoxate
Oxybutynin

Parasympathomimetic
Bethanechol

Alpha-adrenergic blockers
Prazosin
Terazosin
Doxazosin

Anti-androgen drug
Finasteride

ACTION OF DRUGS ON URINATION

Normal bladder action
Urination occurs when the sphincter that keeps the exit from the bladder into the urethra closed is consciously relaxed in response to signals from the bladder indicating that it is full. As the sphincter opens, the bladder wall contracts and urine is expelled.

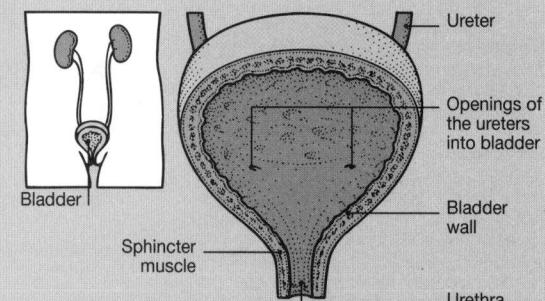

Ureter

Openings of the ureters into bladder

Bladder wall

Urethra

Sphincter muscle

Bladder

How drugs act to improve bladder control
Anticholinergics relax the bladder muscle by interfering with the passage of nerve impulses to the muscle.

Sympathomimetics act directly on the sphincter muscle, causing it to contract.

How drugs act to relieve urinary retention
Parasympathomimetics (cholinergics) stimulate contraction of the bladder wall.

EYES AND EARS

The eyes and ears are the two sense organs that provide us with most information about the world around us. The eye is the organ of vision that converts light images into nerve signals, which are transmitted to the brain for interpretation.

The ear not only provides the means by which sound is detected and communicated to the brain but it also contains the organ of balance that tells the brain about the position and movement of the body. It is divided into three parts – outer, middle, and inner ear.

What can go wrong

The most common eye and ear disorders are infection and inflammation (sometimes caused by allergy). Many parts of the eye may be affected, notably the conjunctiva (membrane that covers the front of the eye and lines the eyelids) and the iris. The middle and outer ear are more commonly affected by infection than the inner ear.

The eye is subject to a disorder known as glaucoma, in which pressure of fluid within the eye builds up and may eventually threaten vision. An eye disorder such as retinopathy (disease of the retina) may occur as a result of diabetes or hypertension and is controlled by treatment of the primary problem. Disorders for which no drug treatment is appropriate are beyond the scope of this book.

Other disorders affecting the ear include buildup of wax (cerumen) in the outer ear canal and disturbances to the balance mechanism (see Vertigo and Ménière's disease, p.102).

Why drugs are used

Physicians usually prescribe antibiotics (see p.140) to clear ear and eye infections. These may be given by mouth or *topically*. Topical eye and ear preparations may contain a corticosteroid (p.153) to reduce inflammation. When inflammation has been caused by allergy, antihistamines (p.136) may also be taken. Decongestant drugs (p.105) are often prescribed to help clear the eustachian tube in middle ear infections.

A variety of drugs are used to reduce fluid pressure in glaucoma. These include diuretics (p.111), beta blockers (p.109), and *miotics* to narrow the pupil. In other cases, the pupil may need to be widened by *mydriatic* drugs.

MAJOR DRUG GROUPS

Drugs for glaucoma
Drugs affecting the pupil

Drugs for ear disorders

How the eye works
Light enters the eye through the cornea. The muscles of the iris control pupil size and thus the amount of light passing into the eye. The optic nerve carries signals received by the retina to be interpreted in the brain.

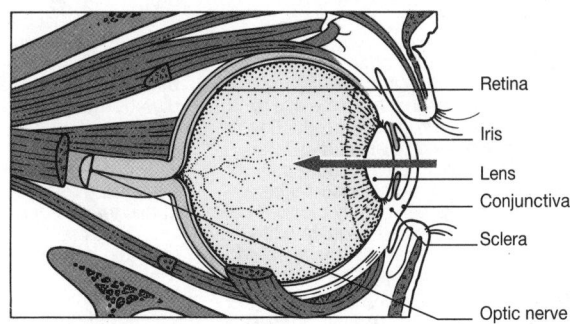

Retina
Iris
Lens
Conjunctiva
Sclera
Optic nerve

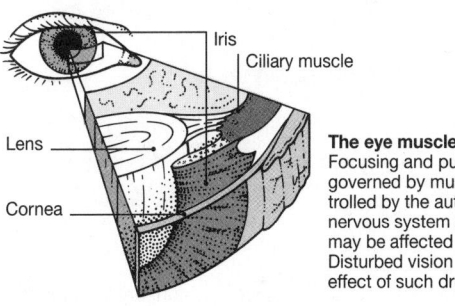

Iris
Ciliary muscle
Lens
Cornea

The eye muscles
Focusing and pupil size are governed by muscles controlled by the autonomic nervous system (p.91), which may be affected by many drugs. Disturbed vision is often a side effect of such drugs.

The ear
The outer ear canal is separated from the middle ear by the eardrum. Three bones in the middle ear connect it to the inner ear. This contains the cochlea (organ of hearing) and the labyrinth (organ of balance).

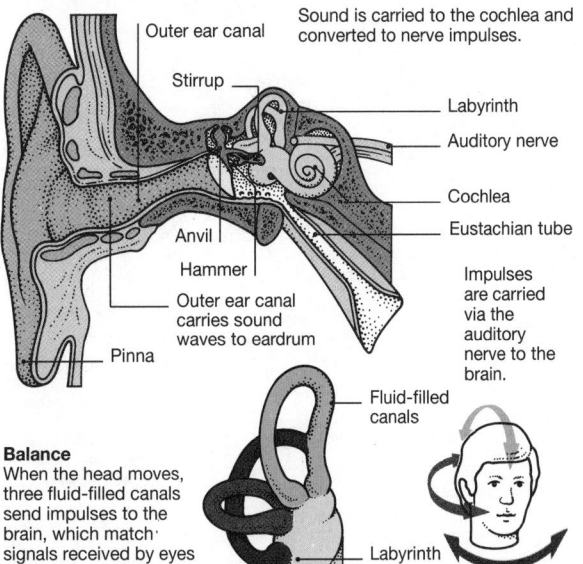

Outer ear canal
Sound is carried to the cochlea and converted to nerve impulses.
Stirrup
Labyrinth
Auditory nerve
Cochlea
Eustachian tube
Anvil
Hammer
Outer ear canal carries sound waves to eardrum
Pinna
Impulses are carried via the auditory nerve to the brain.
Fluid-filled canals
Labyrinth

Balance
When the head moves, three fluid-filled canals send impulses to the brain, which match signals received by eyes and limb muscles.

DRUGS FOR GLAUCOMA

Glaucoma is the name given to a group of conditions in which the pressure in the eye builds up to an abnormally high level. This compresses the blood vessels supplying the nerve that connects the eye to the brain (optic nerve) and may lead to irreversible nerve damage and permanent loss of vision.

In the most common type of glaucoma known as chronic (or open-angle) glaucoma, reduced drainage of fluid from the eye causes pressure inside the eye to build up slowly. Progressive reduction in the peripheral field of vision may take months or years to be noticed. Acute (or closed-angle) glaucoma occurs when drainage of fluid is suddenly blocked by the iris. Fluid pressure builds up quite suddenly, blurring vision in the affected eye (see the box below). The eye becomes red and painful, accompanied by a headache and sometimes vomiting. The main attack is often preceded by milder warning attacks such as seeing halos

around lights in the previous weeks or months. Elderly, farsighted people are particularly at risk of developing acute glaucoma. The angle may also narrow suddenly following injury or after taking certain drugs, for example, *anticholinergic* drugs.

Drugs are used in the treatment of both types of glaucoma. These include miotics (see also Drugs affecting the pupil, p.182), beta blockers (p.109), and certain diuretics (carbonic anhydrase inhibitors and osmotics).

Why they are used

Chronic glaucoma

In this form of glaucoma, drugs are used to reduce pressure inside the eye and to maintain normal pressure thereafter (lifelong treatment is often necessary). This prevents further deterioration of vision, but cannot restore any damage that has already been sustained.

Initially, drops containing a beta blocker

(such as timolol or levobunolol) are giv to reduce secretion of fluid within the A miotic drug such as pilocarpine may also have to be given, which improves drainage of fluid from the eye. Epinephrine or dipivefrin drops may al be helpful. If these measures fail to br about the necessary reduction of pressure within the eye, acetazolamid carbonic anhydrase inhibitor, may be given by mouth to further reduce fluid production. Treatment with acetazolar is usually continued only until laser treatment or surgery can be arranged.

Acute glaucoma

People who have acute glaucoma nee immediate medical treatment in order prevent total loss of vision. Drugs are used initially to bring down blood pres sure within the eye. Laser treatment o eye surgery is then carried out to prev a recurrence of the problem. It is rare drug treatment to be continued long t

WHAT HAPPENS IN GLAUCOMA

Normal eye

The ciliary body, situated at the root of the iris, continuously produces aqueous humor – a watery fluid that helps maintain the normal shape of the eyeball. Aqueous humor continuously drains via the angle between the cornea and iris through a mesh of fibers (the trabecular meshwork) into a channel in the sclera (white of the eye).

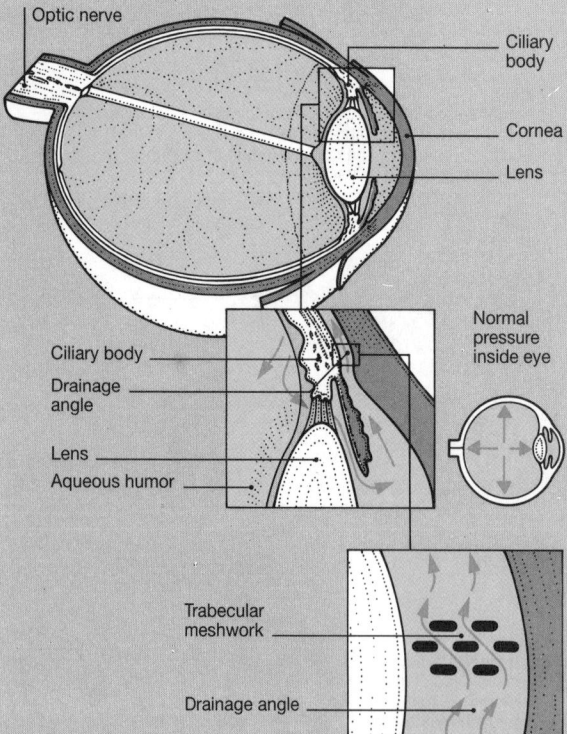

Optic nerve
Ciliary body
Cornea
Lens
Ciliary body
Drainage angle
Lens
Aqueous humor
Trabecular meshwork
Drainage angle
Normal pressure inside eye

How vision is lost

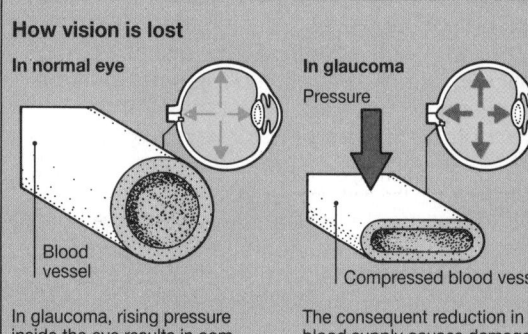

In normal eye
In glaucoma
Pressure
Blood vessel
Compressed blood vess

In glaucoma, rising pressure inside the eye results in compression of the blood vessels that supply the optic nerve.

The consequent reduction in blood supply causes damage to the nerve fibers and permanent loss of vision.

Acute glaucoma

In acute glaucoma, the drainage angle between the cornea and the iris becomes completely closed – so that the pressure inside the eye rises rapidly. This may lead to permanent damage to the nerve fibers.

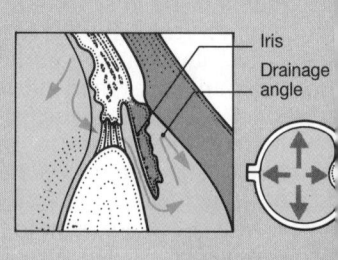

Iris
Drainage angle

Chronic glaucoma

In chronic glaucoma, the trabecular meshwork through which the aqueous humor normally drains gradually closes off, so that fluid pressure builds up slowly, gradually damaging the optic nerve.

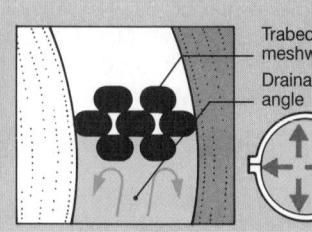

Trabecula meshwork
Drainage angle

etazolamide is usually the first drug ministered when the condition is ignosed. This is initially injected for id effect and thereafter administered mouth. Frequent applications of eye ops containing pilocarpine or another otic drug are given. Occasionally an motic diuretic is administered. This aws fluid out of all body tissues, luding the eye, and reduces pressure hin the eye.

ow they work
e drugs used to treat glaucoma act in ious ways to reduce the pressure of d in the eye. Miotics improve the inage of the fluid out of the eye. In onic glaucoma this is achieved by reasing the outflow of aqueous humor ough the drainage channel called the becular meshwork. In acute glaucoma pupil-constricting effect of miotics s the iris away from the drainage nnel, allowing the aqueous humor to v out normally. Beta blockers and bonic anhydrase inhibitors act on the d-producing cells inside the eye to uce the output of aqueous humor.

w they affect you
gs for acute glaucoma act quickly, eving pain and other symptoms within w hours. The benefits of drug tment in chronic glaucoma may not immediately apparent since treatment y halts a further deterioration of vision. People receiving miotic eye drops are y to notice darkening of vision and culty seeing in the dark. Increased rtsightedness may be noticeable. ne miotics also cause irritation and ness of the eyes.
eta blocker eye drops have few day-lay side effects but carry risks for a people (see right). Acetazolamide

---

ACTION OF DRUGS FOR GLAUCOMA

Miotics
These act on the circular muscle in the iris to reduce the size of the pupil. In acute glaucoma this relieves any obstruction to the flow of aqueous humor by pulling the iris away from the cornea (right). In chronic glaucoma, miotic drugs act directly to increase the outflow of aqueous humor.

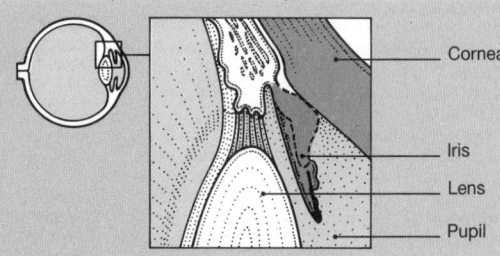

Cornea
Iris
Lens
Pupil

Beta blockers
The fluid-producing cells in the ciliary body are stimulated by signals passed through beta receptors. Beta blocking drugs prevent the transmission of signals through these receptors, thereby reducing the stimulus to produce fluid.

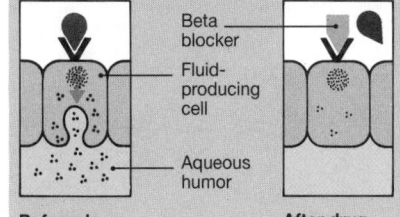

Beta blocker
Fluid-producing cell
Aqueous humor

Before drug

After drug

Fluid-producing cell
Carbonic anhydrase
Drug

Carbonic anhydrase inhibitors
These block carbonic anhydrase, an *enzyme* involved in the production of aqueous humor in the ciliary body.

---

usually causes an increase in frequency of urination and thirst. Nausea and general malaise are also common.

Risks and special precautions
Miotics are generally risk-free. If beta blockers are absorbed into the body they can affect the lungs, heart, and circulation. For this reason, they are prescribed with caution to people with

asthma or certain circulatory disorders and in some cases they are withheld altogether. The amount of the drug absorbed into the body can be reduced by applying the eye drops carefully, as described in the box (left). Acetazolamide is not normally prescribed for prolonged treatment because of its troublesome adverse effects, including painful tingling of the hands and feet. It may encourage the formation of kidney stones and may in rare cases cause kidney damage. People with existing kidney problems are not usually given this drug.

COMMON DRUGS

Miotics
Carbachol
Pilocarpine

Beta blockers
Betaxolol
Levobunolol
Timolol

Carbonic anhydrase inhibitor
Acetazolamide

Other drugs
Dipivefrin
Epinephrine

PPLYING EYE DROPS IN GLAUCOMA

reduce the amount of drug absorbed into e blood via the lacrimal (tear) duct, apply e drops as described. This also improves e effectiveness of the drug.

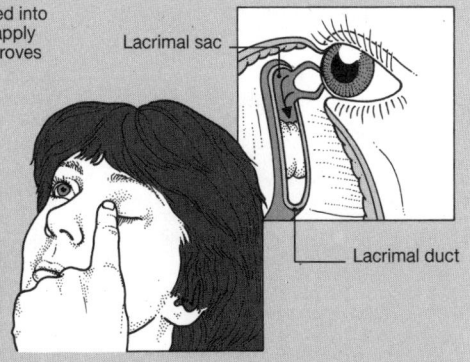

Lacrimal sac

Lacrimal duct

Press firmly on the lacrimal c in the corner of the eye and oly the number of drops scribed by your physician.

2 Maintain pressure on the lacrimal sac for a few moments after applying the drops.

DRUGS AFFECTING THE PUPIL

The pupil of the eye is the circular opening in the center of the iris (the colored part of the eye) through which light enters. It continually changes in size to adjust to variations in the intensity of light; in bright light it becomes quite small (constricts), but in dim light the pupil enlarges (dilates).

Eye drops containing drugs that act on the pupil are widely used by specialist eye physicians. They are of two types: those that dilate the pupil, known as *mydriatics*; and those that constrict the pupil, known as *miotics*.

Why they are used

Mydriatics are most often used to allow the physician to view the inside of the eye – particularly the retina, the optic nerve head, and the blood vessels that supply the retina. Many of these drugs cause a temporary paralysis of the eye's focusing mechanism, a state known as cycloplegia.

Cycloplegia is sometimes induced to help determine the presence of any focusing errors, especially in babies and young children. By producing cycloplegia, physicians can determine the precise optical prescription required for a small child, especially in the case of a squint.

Dilation of the pupil is part of the treatment for uveitis, an inflammatory disease of the iris and focusing muscle. In uveitis, the inflamed iris may stick to the lens, and thus cause severe damage to the eye. This complication can be prevented by early dilation of the pupil so that the iris is no longer in contact with the lens.

Constriction of the pupil with miotic drugs is often required in the treatment of glaucoma (see p.180). Miotics can also be used to restore the pupil to a normal size after dilation has been induced artificially by drugs.

How they work

The size of the pupil of the eye is con-trolled by two separate sets of muscles in the iris, the circular muscle and the radial muscle (see the box above). Each set of

ACTION OF DRUGS AFFECTING THE PUPIL

The muscles of the iris
The pupil is made smaller and larger by the coordi-nated action of the circular and radial muscles in the iris. The circular muscle forms a ring around the pupil; when it contracts, the pupil becomes smaller. The radial muscle is composed of fibers that run from the pupil to the base of the iris like the spokes of a wheel. Contraction of these fibers causes the pupil to become larger.

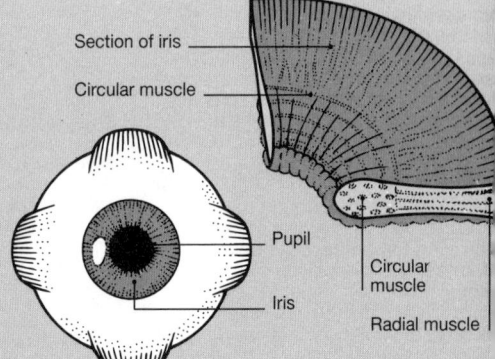

Section of iris
Circular muscle
Pupil
Iris
Circular muscle
Radial muscle

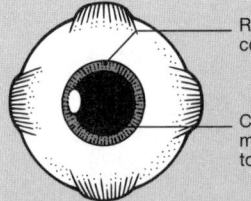

Radial muscle contracts
Circular muscle unable to contract

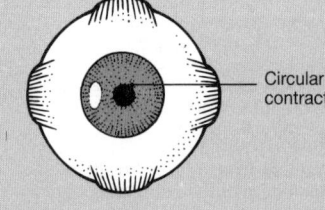

Circular muscle contracts

Mydriatics
Mydriatics enlarge the pupil in one of two ways. The *sympathomimetics* stimulate the radial muscle to contract. The *anticholinergics* prevent the circular muscle from contracting.

Miotics
Most miotics reduce the size of the pupil by stimulating the activity of the parasympathe[tic] nervous system, which causes the circular muscle to contract.

muscles is governed by a separate branch of the autonomic nervous system (see p.91): the sympathetic nervous system controls the radial muscle, and the parasympathetic nervous system controls the circular muscle.

Individual mydriatic and miotic drugs act on different branches of the autonomic nervous system, and cause the pupil of the eye either to dilate or to contract, depending on the type of drug being used.

How they affect you

Mydriatic drugs – especially the long-acting types – impair the ability to focu[s] the eye(s) for several hours after use. [It] interferes particularly with close activit[y] such as reading. Bright light may caus[e] discomfort. Miotics often interfere wit[h] night vision and may cause temporary short sight (myopia).

Normally, these eye drops produce [no] serious adverse effects. *Sympatho-mimetic* mydriatics may raise blood pressure and are used with caution in people with heart disease or hyper-tension. Miotics may irritate the eye, b[ut] rarely cause generalized effects.

ARTIFICIAL TEAR PREPARATIONS

Tears are continually produced to keep the front of the eye covered with a thin moist film. This is essential for clear vision and for keeping the front of the eye free from dirt and other irritants. In some conditions, known collectively as dry eye syndromes (for example, Sjögren's syndrome), inadequate tear production may make the eyes feel dry and sore. Sore eyes can also occur in disorders where the eyelids do not close properly, causing the eye to become dry.

Why they are used
Since prolonged deficiency of natural tears can damage the cornea, regular application of

artificial tears in the form of eye drops is recommended in all of the conditions described. Artificial tears may also be used to provide temporary relief from any feeling of discomfort and dryness in the eye caused by irritants, exposure to wind or sun, or the initial wearing of contact lenses.

Although artificial tears are non-irritating, the preparations containing them often in-clude a preservative (for example, thimerosal or benzalkonium chloride) that may cause irritation. This risk is increased for wearers of soft contact lenses, who should ask their physician for advice before using any type of eye drops.

COMMON DRUGS

Sympathomimetic mydriatics
Epinephrine
Phenylephrine

Anticholinergic mydriatics
Atropine
Cyclopentolate
Homatropine
Tropicamide

Miotics
Carbachol
Pilocarpine

DRUGS FOR EAR DISORDERS

Inflammation and infection of the outer and the middle ear are the most common disorders affecting the ear that are treated with drugs. Drug treatment of Ménière's disease, which affects the inner ear, is described under Vertigo and Ménière's disease, p.102.

The type of drug treatment given for ear inflammation depends on the cause of the trouble and the site affected.

Inflammation of the outer ear

Inflammation of the external ear canal (otitis externa) can be caused by eczema, or by a bacterial or fungal infection. The risk of inflammation is increased by swimming in dirty water, the accumulation of wax in the ear, or by too frequent poking or scratching at the ear.

Symptoms vary, but often there is itching, pain (which may be severe if there is a boil in the ear canal), tenderness, and possibly some loss of hearing. If the ear is infected as well there will probably be a discharge.

Drug treatment

A weak corticosteroid (see p.153), in the form of ear drops, may be used to treat inflammation of the outer ear when there is no infection. Aluminum acetate solution, as drops or applied on a piece of gauze, may also be used. Relief is usually obtained within a day or two. Prolonged use of corticosteroids is not advisable because they may reduce the ear's resistance to infection.

If there is both inflammation and infection, the physician may prescribe ear drops containing an antibiotic (see p.140) combined with a weak corticosteroid to relieve the inflammation. Usually, a combination of antibiotics is prescribed, commonly neomycin, polymyxin B, or chloromycetin – to make the treatment effective against a wide range of bacteria. These antibiotics are not usually applied for long periods, since prolonged appli-

cation can irritate the skin that lines the ear canal. Sometimes an antibiotic given in the form of drops is not effective, and another type of antibiotic may also have to be taken by mouth.

Infection of the middle ear

Infection of the middle ear (otitis media) often causes severe pain and hearing loss. It is particularly common in young children in whom infecting organisms are able to spread easily into the middle ear from the nose or throat via the eustachian tube.

Viral infections of the middle ear usually cure themselves and are less serious than those caused by bacteria. Bacterial infections often cause the eustachian tube to swell and become blocked. When a blockage occurs, pus builds up in the

middle ear and puts pressure on the eardrum, which may then perforate.

Drug treatment

Physicians sometimes prescribe a decongestant (see p.105) or antihistamine (see p.136) to reduce swelling in the eustachian tube, thus allowing the pus to drain out of the middle ear. Usually, an antibiotic is then given by mouth to clear the infection.

Antibiotics are not effective against viral infections, but as it is often difficult to distinguish between a viral and a bacterial infection of the middle ear, your physician may prescribe an antibiotic as a precautionary measure. Acetaminophen, an analgesic (see p.92), may be given to relieve pain. When infection is recurrent, antibiotic treatment lasting several weeks may be prescribed.

EAR WAX REMOVAL

Ear wax (or cerumen) is a natural secretion from the outer ear canal that keeps it free from dust and skin debris. Occasionally, wax may build up in the outer ear canal and become hard, leading to irritation and/or hearing loss.

A number of over-the-counter products are available to soften ear wax and hasten its expulsion. Such products may contain irritating substances that can cause inflammation. Physicians advise instead application of mineral oil or glycerin. A cotton plug should be inserted to retain the oil in the outer ear. When ear wax is not dislodged by such home treatment, a physician may syringe the ear with warm water.

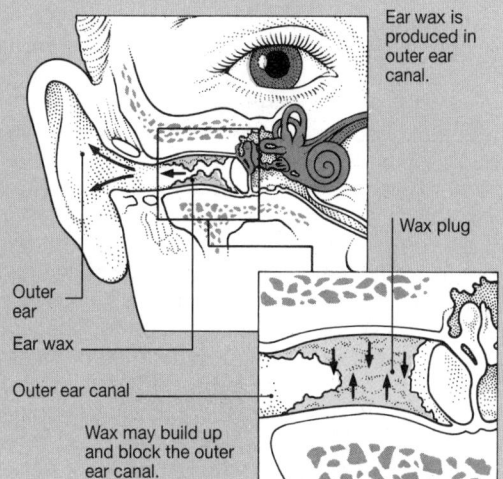

Ear wax is produced in outer ear canal.

Wax plug

Outer ear

Ear wax

Outer ear canal

Wax may build up and block the outer ear canal.

HOW TO USE EAR DROPS

Ear drops for outer ear disorders are more easily and efficiently administered if you have someone to help you. Lie on your side while the other person drops the medication into the ear cavity, ensuring that the dropper does not touch the ear. If possible, it is advisable to remain lying in that position for a few minutes in order to allow the drops to bathe the ear canal. Ear drops should be discarded when the course of treatment has been completed.

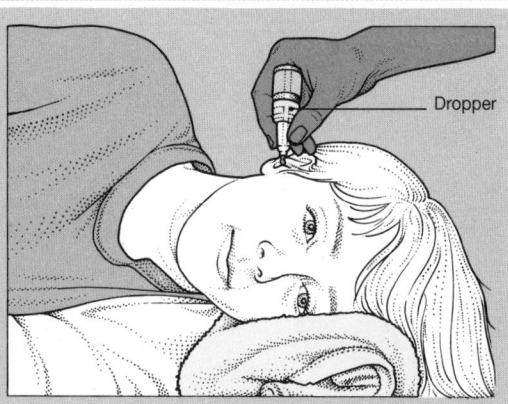

Dropper

COMMON DRUGS

Antibiotic and antibacterial ear drops
Chloramphenicol
Clioquinol
Colistin
Framycetin
Gentamicin
Neomycin
Polymyxin B

Oral antibiotics
See p.140

Other drugs
Aluminum acetate
Antihistamines (see p.136)
Corticosteroids (see p.153)
Decongestants (see p.105)

SKIN

The largest organ of the human body, the skin performs a variety of essential tasks. It provides a barrier against innumerable infections and infestations; it helps the body retain its vital fluids; it plays a major role in temperature control; and it houses the sensory nerves of touch.

The skin consists of two main layers: a thin, tough top layer, the epidermis, and below it a thicker layer, the dermis. The epidermis divides into two: the skin surface, or stratum corneum (horny layer) consisting of dead skin cells, and below, a layer of active cells. The active layer cells divide and eventually die, maintaining the horny layer. Living cells produce keratin, which toughens the epidermis and is the basic substance of hair and nails. Some living cells in the epidermis contain melanin, a pigment released following exposure to sunlight, which protects the dermis.

The dermis contains different types of nerve endings for sensing pain, pressure, and temperature; sweat glands to cool the body; sebaceous glands that release an oil (sebum) that lubricates and waterproofs the skin; and white blood cells that help keep the skin clear of infection.

What can go wrong

Most skin complaints are not serious, but they may be distressing if visible. They include infection, inflammation and irritation, infestation by skin parasites, and changes in skin structure and texture (psoriasis and acne).

Why drugs are used

Skin problems often resolve themselves without drug treatment. Over-the-counter preparations containing active ingredients are available, but physicians generally advise against their use without medical supervision because they can aggravate some skin conditions if used inappropriately. Drugs prescribed by physicians are often highly effective: antibiotics (p.140) for bacterial infections; antifungal drugs (p.150) for fungal infections; anti-infestation agents for skin parasites (p.188); and corticosteroids (p.186) for inflammatory conditions. Specialized drugs are available for conditions like psoriasis and acne.

Although many drugs are *topical* medications, you must use them as carefully as drugs taken by mouth, since they too can cause adverse effects.

Structure of the skin
The epidermis contains keratin and melanin, while the dermis contains sweat glands, sebaceous glands, and nerve endings that sense pain, temperature, and pressure.

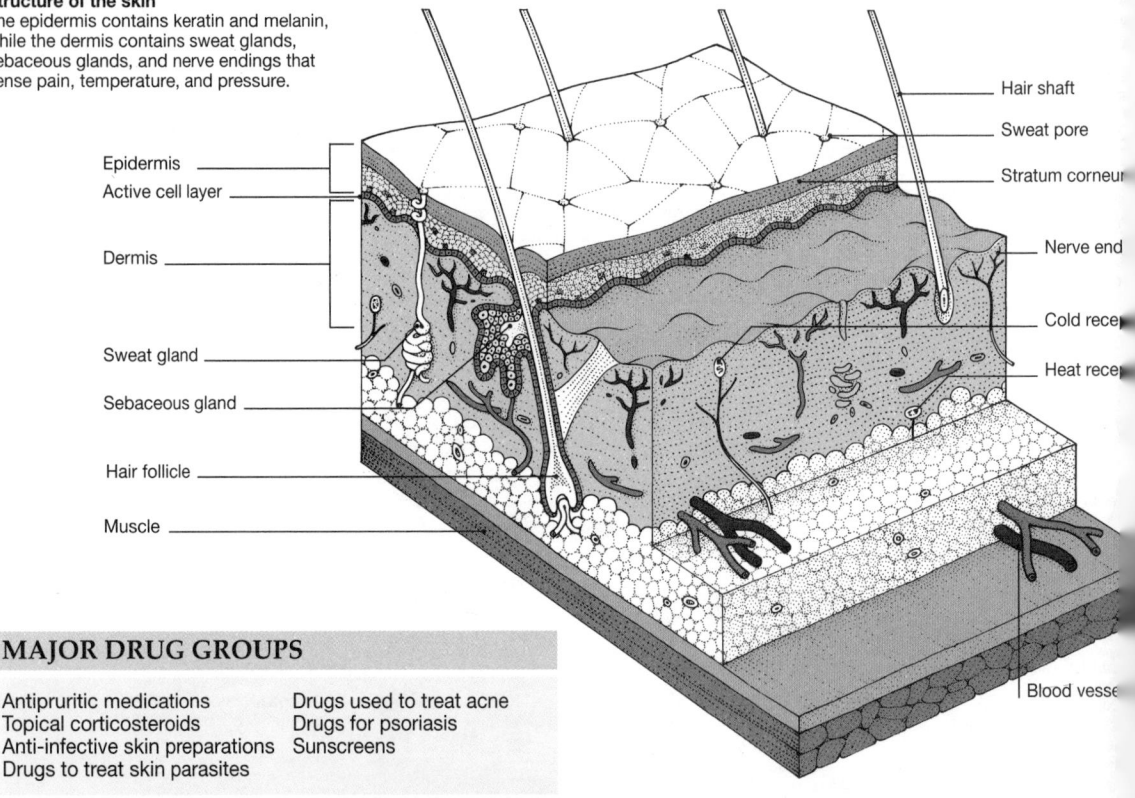

Epidermis
Active cell layer
Dermis
Sweat gland
Sebaceous gland
Hair follicle
Muscle

Hair shaft
Sweat pore
Stratum corneum
Nerve end
Cold recep
Heat recep
Blood vesse

MAJOR DRUG GROUPS

Antipruritic medications
Topical corticosteroids
Anti-infective skin preparations
Drugs to treat skin parasites

Drugs used to treat acne
Drugs for psoriasis
Sunscreens

ANTIPRURITIC MEDICATIONS

ching (irritation of the skin that creates he urge to scratch), also known as pruritus, probably occurs as a result of chemical changes in the skin caused by disease, allergy, inflammation, or exposure to irritant substances. People differ in their tolerance of itching, and an individual's threshold can be altered by stress and other psychological factors.

Itching is a common symptom of many skin disorders, including eczema and allergic conditions such as urticaria (hives). It may also be caused by localized fungal infection or parasitic infestation. Diseases such as chicken pox and psoriasis may also cause itching. Itching may also occur in diabetes mellitus, jaundice, and kidney failure.

In many cases, generalized itching is caused by dry skin. Itching in particular parts of the body often has special causes: itching around the anus (pruritus ani) may result from hemorrhoids or worm infestation, genital itching in women (pruritus vulvae) may be caused by vaginal infection or, in older women, hormone deficiency.

Although scratching provides temporary relief, it often increases skin inflammation and thus may make the condition worse. In some cases, continued scratching of an area of irritated skin can lead to a vicious circle of scratching and itching that continues long after the original cause of the trouble has been removed.

A number of different types of medication are used for the relief of skin irritation. These include soothing preparations that are applied to the affected skin and drugs that are taken by mouth. The principal drugs used in antipruritic medications include corticosteroids (see Topical corticosteroids, p.186), local anesthetics (p.92), and antihistamines (p.136). Plain *emollient* or cooling creams and ointments containing no active ingredients are often recommended.

Why they are used

For mild itching arising from sunburn, urticaria, or insect bites, a cooling lotion such as calamine, perhaps containing menthol, phenol, or camphor, may be the most appropriate treatment. Local anesthetic creams are sometimes helpful for small areas of irritation such as insect bites, but are unsuitable for widespread itching. Itching from dry skin is often soothed by a simple emollient. Avoidance of excessive bathing and use of moisturizing bath oils may also help.

Severe itching from eczema or other inflammatory skin conditions may be treated with a topical corticosteroid preparation. Where the irritation prevents sleep, a physician may prescribe an antihistamine drug to be taken at night to promote sleep as well as relieve itching (see also Sleeping drugs, p.94). Antihistamines are sometimes included in topical preparations for the relief of skin irritation but their effectiveness when administered in this way is doubtful. For the treatment of pruritus ani, see Drugs for rectal and anal disorders (p.125). Post-menopausal pruritus vulvae may be helped by vaginal creams containing estrogen. For further information, see Female sex hormones (p.159). Itching that is caused by an underlying illness cannot be helped by skin creams and requires treatment for the principal disorder.

Risks and special precautions

The main risk with any of these preparations other than simple emollient and soothing preparations is that prolonged or heavy use may cause skin irritation, thereby aggravating itching. Antihistamine and local anesthetic creams are especially likely to irritate or cause allergic reactions. If this occurs, stop therapy. Antihistamines taken by mouth to relieve itching are likely to cause drowsiness. The special risks of topical corticosteroids are discussed on p.186.

Because itching can be a symptom of many underlying conditions, self-treatment should be continued for no longer than a week before seeking medical advice.

ACTION OF ANTIPRURITICS

Irritation of the skin causes the release of substances from the blood that cause blood vessels to dilate and fluid to accumulate under the skin. This causes itching and inflammation. Antipruritic drugs act either by reducing inflammation and therefore irritation, or by numbing the nerve impulses that transmit sensation to the brain.

Corticosteroids applied to the skin surface reduce itching caused by allergy within a few days, although the soothing effect of the cream may produce an immediate improvement. They pass into the underlying tissues and blood vessels and reduce the release of histamine, the chemical that causes itching and inflammation.

Antihistamines act within a few hours to reduce allergy-related skin inflammation. Applied to the skin, they pass into the underlying tissue and block the effects of histamine on the blood vessels beneath the skin. Taken by mouth they also act on the brain to reduce the perception of irritation.

Local anesthetics absorbed through the skin numb the transmission of signals from the nerves in the skin to the brain.

Soothing and emollient creams Calamine lotion and similar preparations applied to the skin surface reduce inflammation and itching by cooling the skin. Emollient creams lubricate the skin surface and prevent dryness.

COMMON DRUGS

Corticosteroids
(see p.153)

Local anesthetics
Benzocaine
Lidocaine
Tetracaine

Antihistamines
(see p.136)

Emollient and cooling preparations
Cold cream
Calamine lotion
Hydrophilic ointment USP

Other drugs
Crotamiton

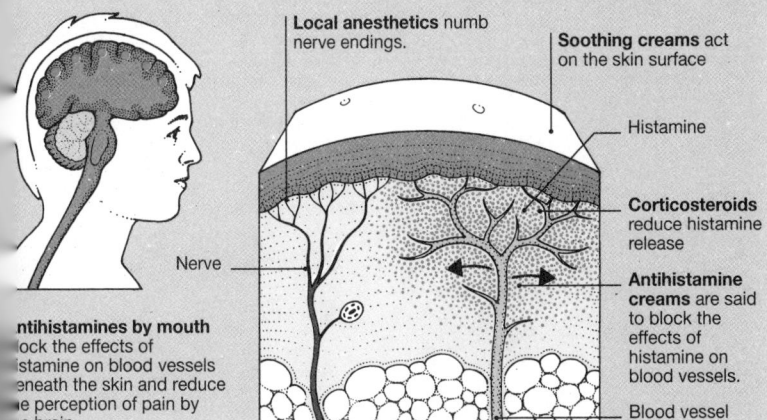

Local anesthetics numb nerve endings.

Soothing creams act on the skin surface

Histamine

Corticosteroids reduce histamine release

Antihistamine creams are said to block the effects of histamine on blood vessels.

Nerve

Blood vessel

Antihistamines by mouth block the effects of histamine on blood vessels beneath the skin and reduce the perception of pain by the brain.

TOPICAL CORTICOSTEROIDS

Corticosteroid drugs (often simply called steroids) are related to hormones produced by the adrenal glands. For a full description of these drugs, see p.153. *Topical* preparations containing a corticosteroid drug are often used to treat skin conditions in which inflammation is a prominent symptom.

Why they are used

Corticosteroid creams and ointments are most commonly given to relieve itching and inflammation associated with skin diseases such as eczema and dermatitis. These preparations may also be prescribed for psoriasis (see p.190). Corticosteroids do not affect the underlying cause of skin irritation, and the condition is therefore likely to recur unless the substance (allergen or irritant) that has provoked the irritation is itself removed, or the underlying condition treated.

A physician may not prescribe a corticosteroid as the initial treatment, preferring to try a topical medicine that has fewer adverse effects (see Antipruritic medications, p.185).

In most cases treatment is started with a preparation containing a low concentration of a mild corticosteroid drug. A stronger preparation may be prescribed subsequently if the first product is ineffective.

How they affect you

Corticosteroids prevent the release of chemicals that trigger the symptoms of inflammation (see Action of corticosteroids on the skin, above right). Conditions for which topical corticosteroids are prescribed improve within a few days of starting treatment. Applied topically, corticosteroids rarely cause adverse effects, but the stronger drugs carry certain risks when used in high concentrations.

ACTION OF CORTICOSTEROIDS ON THE SKIN

Skin inflammation
Irritation of the skin caused by allergens or irritant substances provokes the release by white blood cells of substances that dilate the blood vessels. This makes the skin hot, red and swollen.

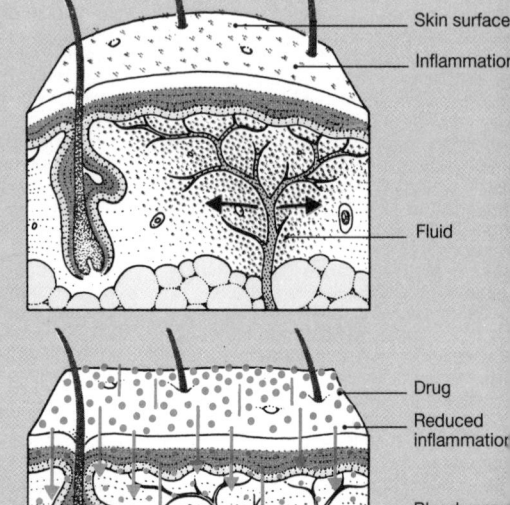

Skin surface

Inflammation

Fluid

Drug action
Applied to the skin surface, corticosteroids are absorbed into the underlying tissue. There they inhibit the action of the substances that cause inflammation, thereby allowing the blood vessels to return to normal and reducing the swelling.

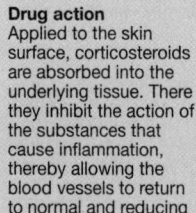

Drug

Reduced inflammation

Blood vessel

Swelling reduced

Risks and special precautions

Prolonged use of potent corticosteroids in high concentrations can lead to permanent changes in the skin. The most common effect is thinning of the skin, sometimes resulting in stretch marks that may be permanent. Fine blood vessels under the surface of the skin may become prominent (a condition known as telangiectasia). The vessels may become damaged, resulting in a red rash beneath the skin. Because the skin on the face is especially vulnerable to such damage, only weak corticosteroids are sometimes prescribed for use on the face. Dark-skinned people sometimes suffer a temporary reduction in pigmentation at the site of application.

When powerful corticosteroid preparations have been used for a prolonged period, abrupt discontinuation of the treatment can result in a general reddening of the skin called "rebound erythroderma." This may be avoided by gradual reduction in dosage. Corticosteroids suppress the body's immune system (see p.168), thus increasing the risk of infection. For this reason, they are not used alone to treat skin inflammation caused by bacterial or fungal infection. However, they may sometimes be included in a topical preparation that also contains an antibiotic drug or antifungal agent (see Anti-infective skin preparations, facing page).

LONG-TERM EFFECTS OF TOPICAL CORTICOSTEROIDS

Prolonged use of topical corticosteroids causes drying and thinning of the epidermis, so that tiny blood vessels close to the skin surface become visible. In addition, long-term use of these drugs weakens the underlying connective tissue of the dermis, leading to an increased susceptibility to stretch marks.

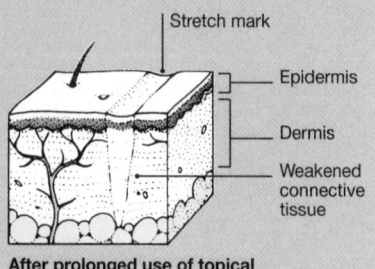

Epidermis

Dermis

Normal skin

Stretch mark

Epidermis

Dermis

Weakened connective tissue

After prolonged use of topical corticosteroids

COMMON DRUGS

Betamethasone
Clobetasol propionate
Fluocinolone
Hydrocortisone
Mometasone
Triamcinolone

NTI-INFECTIVE SKIN PREPARATIONS

skin is the body's first line of defense
inst infection. Yet it can also become
cted itself, especially if the outer layer
dermis) is damaged by a burn, cut,
pe, insect bite, or an inflammatory
condition such as eczema or
natitis.

everal different types of organism may
ct the skin, including bacteria, viruses,
ji, and yeasts. This page concentrates
Jrugs applied *topically* to treat bac-
al skin infections. These include anti-
tics, antibiotics, and other antibac-
al agents. Infection by other organisms
overed elsewhere (see Antiviral drugs,
45, Antifungal drugs, p.150, and Drugs
eat skin parasites, p.188).

ny they are used

terial infections of the skin can usually
prevented by thorough cleansing of an
a of skin damage and the application
ntiseptic creams and lotions as
cribed in the box (right). Once
ction has occurred (causing redness,
lling, and sometimes formation of
), treatment with an antibiotic prepara-
may be necessary. An antibiotic or
bacterial skin cream may be used to
vent infection when a physician con-
rs this to be a particular risk – for
mple, in the case of severe burns.
ther skin disorders in which topical
biotic treatment may be prescribed
ude impetigo and infected eczema,
ulcers, bedsores, and diaper rash.
sually, a preparation containing two or
e antibiotics is used in order to ensure
all bacteria are eradicated. The
piotics selected for inclusion in topical
parations are usually drugs that are
rly absorbed through the skin. Thus
drug remains concentrated on the
ace and in the skin's upper layers
re it is intended that it should have its
ct. However, if the infection is deep
er the skin, or is causing fever and

ANTISEPTICS

Antiseptics (sometimes called germicides or
skin disinfectants) are chemicals that kill or
prevent the growth of microorganisms. They
are weaker than household disinfectants,
which are irritating to the skin.

Antiseptic lotions, creams, and solutions
may be effective for preventing infection
following surface wounds to the skin. Solutions
can be added to water while bathing wounds

Soaps, shampoos,
throat lozenges and
mouthwashes, skin
lotions, creams, and
ointments may
contain antiseptic
ingredients.

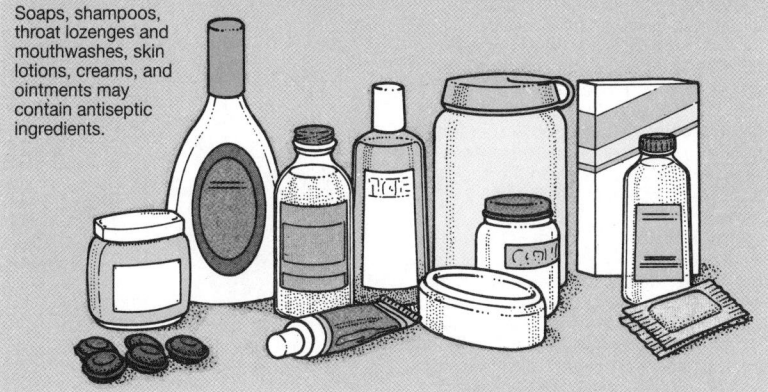

(used undiluted they may cause inflammation
and increase the risk of infection). Creams
may be applied to wounds after cleansing.

Antiseptics are also included in some soaps
and shampoos for the prevention of acne and
dandruff, but their benefits in these disorders
are doubtful. They are also included as
ingredients of some throat lozenges, but their
effectiveness in curing infections is unproven.

malaise, antibiotics may need to be
administered by mouth or injection.

Risks and special precautions

Some ointments containing antibiotics are
available without prescription, but
physicians do not encourage the use of
these preparations for self-medication
because of the risk of encouraging the
formation of drug-resistant strains of
bacteria if an inappropriate medication is
used (see Antibiotic resistance, p.140).
Seek medical advice if you suspect that
a wound or other skin condition has

become infected, and follow your
physician's instructions concerning the
duration of treatment even though the
infection may appear to have cleared.

Any topical antibiotic product can
irritate the skin or cause an allergic
reaction. Irritation is sometimes caused
by another ingredient of the preparation
rather than the active drug, for example, a
preservative contained in the preparation.
Allergic reactions causing swelling and
reddening of the skin are more likely to be
caused by the antibiotic itself. Any
adverse reaction of this kind should be
reported to your physician, who may
substitute another drug, or prescribe a
different preparation.

ASES FOR SKIN PREPARATIONS

ugs that are applied to the skin are usually
a preparation known as a base (or vehicle),
ch as cream, lotion, ointment, or paste.
ny bases are beneficial on their own.

eams These have an *emollient* effect. They
usually composed of an oil-in-water base
d are used in the treatment of dry skin
orders, such as psoriasis and dry eczema.
ey may contain other ingredients such as
mphor, or menthol. Barrier creams protect
skin against water and irritating
stances. They may be used in the
atment of diaper rash and to protect the
n around an open sore. They may contain
wders and water-repellent substances,
ch as silicones.

tions Thin, semi-liquid preparations often
d to cool and soothe inflamed skin. They
most suitable for use on large, hairy areas.
ake lotions contain fine powder which

remains on the surface of the skin when the
liquid has evaporated. They are used to
encourage scabs to form.

Ointments These are usually greasy and are
suitable for treating wet (weeping) eczema.
Most ointments contain mineral oil or wax and
are insoluble in water.

Pastes Containing large amounts of finely
powdered solids such as starch or zinc oxide,
pastes protect the skin as well as absorb
unwanted moisture and are used for skin
conditions that affect clearly defined areas,
such as psoriasis.

Collodions These are preparations that,
when applied to damaged areas of the skin
such as ulcers and minor wounds, dry to form
a protective film. They are sometimes used to
keep a dissolved drug in contact with the
skin.

COMMON DRUGS

Antibiotics
Bacitracin
Clindamycin
Framycetin
Fusidic acid
Gentamicin
Gramicidin
Mupirocin
Neomycin

Antiseptics and other antibacterials
Cetrimide
Chlorhexidine
Potassium permanganate
Povidone-iodine
Silver sulfadiazine

DRUGS TO TREAT SKIN PARASITES

Mites and lice are the most common parasites that live on the skin. Mites cause the skin disease known as scabies; they burrow into the skin and lay eggs, causing an intense itching. Scratching the affected area results in bleeding and the formation of scabs, and increases the risk of infection.

There are three types of lice, each of which infests a different part of the body: the head louse, the body (or clothes) louse, and the crab louse, which often infests the pubic areas but is also sometimes found on other hairy areas such as the eyebrows. All lice cause itching and lay eggs (nits) that look like white grains attached to hairs.

Both mites and lice are passed on by direct contact with an infected person (during sexual intercourse in the case of pubic lice) or, particularly in the case of body lice, by contact with infected bedding or clothing.

The drugs most commonly used to eliminate skin parasites are insecticides that kill both the adult insects and their eggs. The principal drugs are permethrin and lindane (both scabies and louse infestations), crotamiton (scabies only), and a combination of pyrethrins and piperonyl butoxide (louse infestations only).

Why they are used

Skin parasites do not represent a serious threat to health, but require prompt treatment because they can cause severe irritation and spread rapidly if untreated. Drugs are used to eradicate the parasites from the body, but it may also be necessary to disinfect bedding and clothing to avoid the possibility of reinfestation.

How they are used

Scabies infestations are usually treated by applying a preparation containing permethrin, lindane, or crotamiton as instructed by the leaflet with the preparation.

SITES AFFECTED BY SKIN PARASITES

Scabies
The female scabies mite burrows into the skin and lays its eggs under the skin surface. After hatching, the larvae travel to the skin surface, where they mature for 10 – 17 days before starting the cycle again.

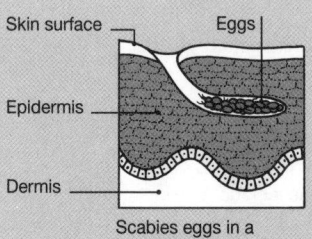

Skin surface · Epidermis · Dermis · Eggs

Scabies eggs in a burrow under the skin

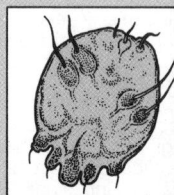

Scabies mite

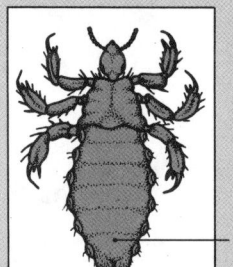

Head louse

Head lice
These tiny brown insects are transmitted from person to person (commonly among children). Their bites often cause itching.

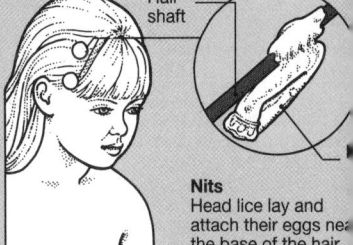

Hair shaft

Nits
Head lice lay and attach their eggs nea the base of the hair shaft, especially around the ears.

One or two treatments are normally sufficient to remove the scabies mites. However, the itch associated with scabies may persist after the mite has been removed, so it may be necessary to use a soothing cream or medication containing an antipruritic drug (see p.185) to ease this. People who have skin-to-skin contact with a sufferer from scabies – family members and sexual partners – should also undergo treatment with antiparasitic preparations at the same time.

Head and pubic lice infestations are usually treated by applying a preparation of one of the products, and washing it off with water as instructed by the leaflet with the preparation. If the skin has become infected as a result of scratching, a *topical* antibiotic (see Anti-infective ski preparations, p.187) may also be prescribed.

Risks and special precautions

Preparations prescribed to control parasites can cause irritation and sting that may be intense if the medication i allowed to come into contact with the eyes, mouth, or other moist membran Care is therefore needed when applyin these preparations. Because they are applied *topically*, antiparasitic drugs seldom have generalized effects. Nevertheless, it is important not to app these preparations more often than directed and to keep them well out of reach of children at all times.

COMMON DRUGS

Crotamiton
Lindane
Permethrin
Pyrethrins/piperonyl butoxide

ELIMINATING PARASITES FROM BEDDING AND CLOTHING

Most skin parasites may also infest bedding and clothing that has been next to the skin of an infected person. Therefore, to avoid reinfestation following removal of the parasites from the body, it is essential to eradicate insects and eggs that may be lodged in them.

Washing
Since all skin parasites are killed by heat, washing affected items of clothing and bedding in hot water and drying them in a hot dryer is an effective and convenient method of dealing with the problem.

Non-washable items
Items that cannot be washed should be isolated in plastic bags. The insects and their eggs cannot survive long without their human

hosts and die within days. The length of time they can survive, and therefore the period of isolation, varies depending on the type of parasite (see the table below).

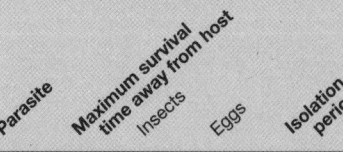

Parasite	Maximum survival time away from host		Isolation period
	Insects	Eggs	
Scabies	2 days	0 days	2 days
Head lice	2 days	10 days	10 days
Crab lice	1 day	10 days	10 days
Body lice	10 days	30 days	30 days

DRUGS USED TO TREAT ACNE

Acne, known medically as acne vulgaris, is a common condition caused by an excess production of the skin's natural oil (sebum), which leads to blockage of hair follicles (see What happens in acne, right). Though it chiefly affects adolescents, acne may occur at any age as a result of taking certain drugs, exposure to industrial chemicals, oily cosmetics, or hot and humid conditions.

Acne primarily affects the skin on the face, neck, back, and chest. The principal skin symptoms are blackheads, papules (inflamed spots), and pustules (raised pus-filled spots with a white center). Mild acne may produce only blackheads and an occasional papule or pustule. Moderate cases are characterized by larger numbers of pustules and papules. In severe cases of acne, painful, inflamed cysts also develop. These can sometimes cause permanent pitting and scarring of the skin.

Medication for acne can be divided into two groups: *topical* preparations applied directly to the skin and *systemic* treatments taken by mouth.

Why they are used

Mild acne does not normally require medical intervention. It can be controlled by regular washing and moderate exposure to sunlight or ultraviolet light. Over-the-counter antibacterial soaps and lotions have only a limited usefulness and may cause irritation. When a physician

CLEARING BLOCKED HAIR FOLLICLES

The most common treatment for acne is the application of keratolytic skin ointments. These encourage the layer of dead and hardened skin cells that form the skin surface to peel off. This action simultaneously clears blocked hair follicles that give rise to the formation of acne spots.

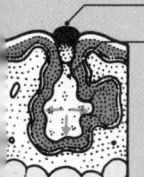

Blackhead
Trapped sebum

Blocked hair follicle
A hair follicle blocked by a plug of skin debris and sebum is ideal for acne spot formation.

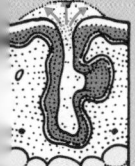

Freed sebum

Cleared hair follicle
Once the follicle is unblocked, sebum can escape and air can enter, thereby limiting bacterial activity.

WHAT HAPPENS IN ACNE

In normal skin, sebum produced by a sebaceous gland attached to a hair follicle is able to flow out of the follicle along the hair. An acne spot forms when the flow of the sebum from the sebaceous gland is blocked by a plug of skin debris and hardened sebum, leading to an accumulation of sebum.

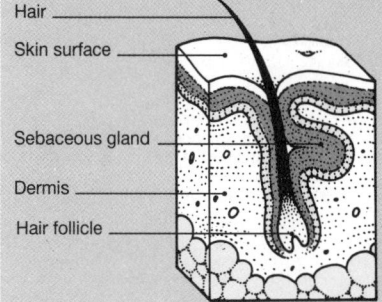

Hair
Skin surface
Sebaceous gland
Dermis
Hair follicle

Acne papules and pustules
Bacterial activity leads to the formation of pustules and papules. Irritant substances may leak into the surrounding skin, causing inflammation.

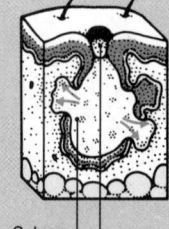

Sebum
Blackhead
Cyst

Cystic acne
When acne is severe, cysts may form in the inflamed dermis. These are pockets of pus enclosed within scar tissue.

considers acne is severe enough to warrant medical treatment, he or she is likely initially to recommend a topical preparation containing benzoyl peroxide, sulfur, or salicylic acid. If this treatment is inadequate, a cream containing tretinoin, a drug related to vitamin A, may be prescribed. Antibiotics such as erythromycin or clindamycin may also be used topically.

If acne is severe or does not respond to topical treatments, a physician may prescribe a course of antibiotics (a tetracycline or erythromycin) by mouth. If all these measures are unsuccessful, the more powerful vitamin A-like drug isotretinoin may be prescribed by mouth.

Estrogen drugs may have a beneficial effect on acne. A woman who suffers from troublesome acne and who also requires contraceptive protection may therefore be advised to try an estrogen-containing oral contraceptive (p.173).

How they work

Drugs used to treat acne act in different ways. Some have a keratolytic effect, that is, they loosen the dead cells on the skin surface (see Clearing blocked hair follicles, left). Other drugs counter bacterial activity in the skin or reduce sebum production.

Topical anti-acne preparations containing drugs such as benzoyl peroxide, salicylic acid, tretinoin, and sulfur, have a keratolytic effect. Benzoyl peroxide and sulfur also have an antibacterial effect. Antibiotics applied topically or taken systemically reduce bacterial activity, but may also have a direct anti-inflammatory effect on the skin. Isotretinoin reduces the production of sebum, soothes inflammation, and also helps to unblock hair follicles.

How they affect you

Keratolytic preparations often cause soreness of the skin, especially at the start of treatment. If this persists, a change to a milder preparation may be recommended. Day-to-day side effects are rare with antibiotics.

Isotretinoin treatment often causes dryness and scaling of the skin, particularly on the lips. The skin may become itchy and some hair loss may occur.

Risks and special precautions

Antibiotics applied topically may, in rare cases, provoke an allergic reaction requiring discontinuation of treatment. The tetracyclines, some of the most commonly used antibiotics for acne, are not suitable for use by mouth in pregnancy since they can discolor the teeth of the developing baby. Isotretinoin can increase levels of fat in the blood. More seriously, the drug may cause major abnormalities of the developing baby if taken during pregnancy. Women taking this drug must be certain to use effective contraception.

COMMON DRUGS

Oral drugs
Clindamycin
Isotretinoin
Erythromycin
Minocycline
Tetracycline

Topical treatments
Benzoyl peroxide
Clindamycin
Erythromycin
Isotretinoin
Salicylic acid
Sulfur
Tretinoin

DRUGS FOR PSORIASIS

The skin is constantly being renewed; as fast as dead cells in the outermost layer (epidermis) are shed, they are replaced by cells from the base of the epidermis. Psoriasis occurs when the production of new cells increases while the shedding of old cells remains normal. As a result, the live skin cells accumulate and produce patches of inflamed, thickened skin covered by silvery scales. In some cases, the area of skin affected is extensive and causes severe embarrassment and physical discomfort. Psoriasis may occasionally be accompanied by arthritis in which the joints become swollen and painful.

The underlying cause of psoriasis is unknown. It usually first occurs between the ages of 10 and 30, and recurs throughout life. Outbreaks may be triggered by emotional stress, skin damage, and physical illnesses. Psoriasis can also be a consequence of the withdrawal of corticosteroid drugs.

There is no complete cure for psoriasis. Simple measures such as careful sunbathing or using an ultraviolet lamp may help to clear mild psoriasis. An *emollient* cream (see p.185) often soothes the irritation. When such measures fail to provide adequate relief, additional drug therapy is needed.

Why they are used

Drugs are used to reduce the size of areas of affected skin and to reduce inflammation and scaling. Mild or moderate psoriasis is usually treated with a *topical* preparation. Coal tar preparations in the form of creams, pastes, and bath additives are often helpful, although some people dislike the smell. Anthralin is also widely used. Applied to the affected areas, it is then left for a few minutes or overnight (depending on the preparation), after which it is washed off. Both anthralin and coal tar can stain clothes and bed linen.

If these agents alone do not produce adequate benefit, ultraviolet light therapy in the form of regulated exposure to natural sunlight or to ultraviolet lamps may be advised. Salicylic acid may be applied to help remove thick scale and crusts, especially from the scalp.

Topical corticosteroids (see p.186) may be used in difficult cases that do not respond to those treatments. They are particularly useful for the skinfold areas and may be given to counter irritation caused by anthralin.

For more severe psoriasis not improved by any of these treatments, your physician may recommend special treatment with more powerful drugs. These include acitretin and etretinate, vitamin A derivatives that are taken by mouth in courses lasting about 6 months, and methotrexate, an anticancer drug. Another form of treatment, using the psoralen drug meth-

PUVA

PUVA is the combined use of a psoralen drug and ultraviolet A light (UVA). The drug is applied *topically* or taken by mouth some hours before exposure to UVA, which enhances the effect of the drug on skin cells.

This therapy is given two to three times a week, producing an improvement in skin condition within about four to six weeks.

Possible adverse effects include nausea, itching, and painful reddening of the normal areas of skin. More seriously, there is a risk of the skin aging prematurely and a long-term risk of skin cancer, particularly in fair-skinned people. For these reasons, PUVA therapy is generally recommended only for severe psoriasis after other treatments have failed.

In psoriasis
Skin cells form at the base of the epidermis faster than they can be shed from the skin surface. This causes the formation of patches of thickened, inflamed skin covered by a layer of flaking dead skin.

Normal skin   **Skin in psoriasis**

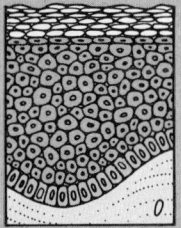
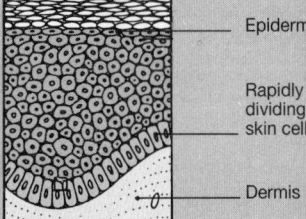

- Epiderm
- Rapidly dividing skin cell
- Dermis

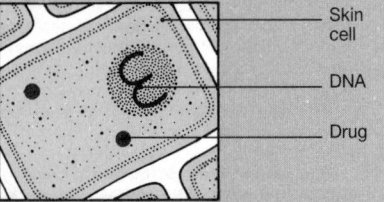

- Skin cell
- DNA
- Drug
- UVA rays
- Drug
- DNA restricte

Psoralen drugs
In PUVA, psoralen drugs administered by mouth or as ointment penetrate the skin cells.

Ultraviolet light
The drug is activated by exposure of the skin to ultraviolet light. It acts on the cell's genetic material (DNA) to regulate its rate of division.

oxsalen in conjunction with ultraviolet light therapy (PUVA), is described above.

How they work

Anthralin, etretinate, and methotrexate slow down the rapid rate of cell division that is responsible for skin thickening. Acitretin and etretinate also reduce production of keratin, the hard protein that forms in the outer layer of skin. Salicylic acid and coal tar remove the layers of dead skin cells. Corticosteroids reduce inflammation of the underlying skin.

How they affect you

Appropriate treatment usually improves the appearance of the skin. However, because drugs cannot cure the underlying cause of the disorder, psoriasis tends to recur even after successful treatment.

Individual drugs may cause side effects. Topical preparations can cause stinging and inflammation, especially if applied to normal skin. Coal tar and methoxsalen increase the skin's sensitivity to sunlight; excessive sunbathing

or over exposure to artificial ultraviolet light may damage skin and worsen the condition.

Acitretin and etretinate may damage the developing baby if taken during pregnancy. Women taking these drugs must use effective contraception. Both agents can also damage the liver. Methotrexate can cause gastrointestina upsets and bone marrow damage. Topi corticosteroids may also cause reboun worsening of psoriasis when stopped.

COMMON DRUGS

Acitretin
Anthralin
Calcipotriol
Coal tar
Cyclosporine
Etretinate
Methotrexate
Methoxsalen
Salicylic acid
Topical corticosteroids (see p.186)

SUNSCREENS

Sunscreens are chemicals usually formulated as creams, lotions, or oils, that protect the skin from the damaging effects of ultraviolet radiation from the sun.

People vary widely in their sensitivity to sunlight. Fair-skinned people generally have the least tolerance to direct sunlight and tend to burn easily, while people with darker skin can usually withstand exposure to the sun for much longer periods without suffering noticeable harm.

In a few cases the skin is made more sensitive to sunlight by a disease such as pellagra (a form of malnutrition primarily due to a deficiency of niacin; see p.523) or herpes simplex infection. Certain drugs - such as the thiazide diuretics, phenothiazine antipsychotics, sulfonamide antibacterials, quinolone and tetracycline antibiotics, psoralens, and coal tar - can also increase the skin's sensitivity to sunlight.

Why they are used

Sunscreens are usually applied before and during sunbathing to prevent burning while allowing the skin to tan. Prolonged exposure of unprotected skin to strong sunlight increases the risk of skin cancer, especially among fair-skinned people, and can cause premature aging of the skin. A sunscreen is particularly advisable for people traveling to tropical and semitropical countries who are unaccustomed to strong sunlight.

Sunscreens are graded according to the degree of protection they offer – the sun protection factor (SPF). This is a measure of the amount of ultraviolet radiation that the sunscreen absorbs; the higher the number, the greater the protection afforded. Thus people of various skin types can choose the most suitable sunscreen. Sunscreens should have an SPF factor of at least 15. Waterproof sunscreens maintain their effectiveness after 80 minutes of water immersion; water-resistant sunscreens after 40 minutes of water immersion.

ACTION OF SUNSCREENS

Fair skin unprotected by a sunscreen suffers damage as ultraviolet rays pass through to the layers beneath, causing pain and inflammation. Sunscreens block out some of these ultraviolet rays, while allowing a proportion of them to pass through the skin surface to the epidermis to stimulate the activity of melanin, the pigment that gives the skin a tan and helps to protect it during further exposure to the sun.

Skin unprotected

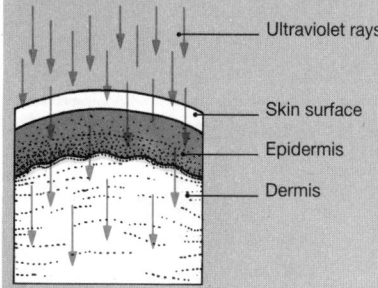

- Ultraviolet rays
- Skin surface
- Epidermis
- Dermis

Skin protected by sunscreen

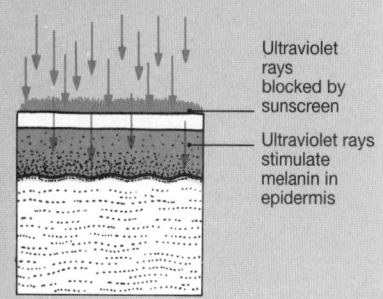

- Ultraviolet rays blocked by sunscreen
- Ultraviolet rays stimulate melanin in epidermis

How they work

Sunlight is composed of different wavelengths of electromagnetic radiation. Of these, ultraviolet radiation can be particularly harmful to the skin. The chemicals in sunscreens absorb ultraviolet radiation, ensuring that a smaller proportion of it reaches the skin.

Risks and special precautions

Sunscreens only form a physical barrier to the passage of ultraviolet radiation. They do not alter the skin to make it more resistant to sunlight. Therefore a sunscreen lotion must be applied frequently to maintain protection.

Even sunscreens with the highest blocking effect do not completely exclude radiation from the sun. Accordingly, people who are fair-skinned or very sensitive to sunlight should never expose themselves to direct sun, even if they are using a sunscreen.

Sunscreens can irritate the skin and some may cause an allergic rash. People who are sensitive to drugs such as procaine and benzocaine, certain hair dyes, and sulfonamides, may develop a rash following application of a preparation containing para-aminobenzoic acid (PABA) or benzophenones such as oxybenzone.

TREATMENT FOR DANDRUFF AND HAIR LOSS

Dandruff treatments

The condition in which dead cells accumulate on the scalp and form white flaky scales is commonly referred to as dandruff. It is not a sign of ill health, but most people find it unsightly and want to get rid of it. In some cases frequent washing (four to six times a week) with a mild shampoo keeps the scalp free of dandruff. Many people, however, find that a medicated shampoo is more effective.

Medicated shampoos usually contain active ingredients such as tar, sulfur, or salicylic acid that soften the dead scales and make them easier to remove.

Shampoos that contain zinc pyrithione or selenium sulfide are often effective for more severe cases. These reduce the formation of dandruff by slowing down the growth of skin cells. They also have a mild antifungal action. Ketoconazole shampoo has a more potent antifungal action. (Some physicians believe that yeast infection is a cause of dandruff.)

If the dandruff is severe and does not respond to any of those treatments, a physician may prescribe a weak corticosteroid lotion or gel (see also Topical corticosteroids, p.186).

Drugs used for hair loss

One of the most common causes of hair loss is male pattern baldness, in which hair lost from the temples and crown is initially replaced by fine downy hair, and finally lost permanently. It is probably caused by hormonal changes and most commonly affects men, although women can also suffer this type of hair loss.

Traditionally, response to male pattern baldness has included the use of wigs and toupees, and hair transplants. However, minoxidil, a vasodilator and antihypertensive drug, has been found to stimulate hair growth in some people. A topical preparation of the drug is being prescribed by some physicians as a possible treatment for hair loss. It is thought to act by increasing blood flow in the skin, and elongating the hair follicles, as well as reducing the number of white cells around hair follicles. However, minoxidil may be absorbed through the scalp and in excessive concentrations can produce harmful effects. Temporary thinning of the hair may be caused by fungal infection, stress, serious illness, childbirth, or treatment with anticancer drugs (see p.166). In these cases drug treatment is not effective and hair growth returns to normal once the cause has been removed.

COMMON DRUGS

2-Ethylhexylsalicylate
Avobenzone (Parsol 1789)
Benzophenone
Homosalate
Octyl methoxycinnamate
Oxybenzone
Padimate O
Para-aminobenzoic acid (PABA)
Titanium dioxide

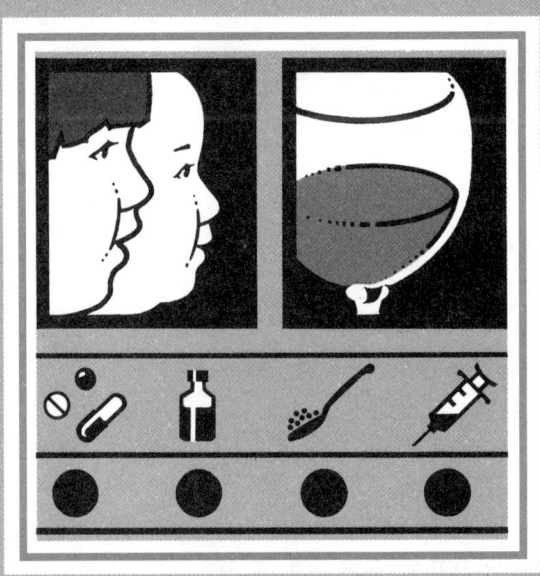

PART

4

A - Z
OF DRUGS

A - Z OF MEDICAL DRUGS
A - Z OF VITAMINS AND MINERALS
DRUGS OF ABUSE
FOOD ADDITIVES

A – Z OF MEDICAL DRUGS

The drug profiles in this section provide information and practical advice on 320 individual drugs. It is intended that these profiles should provide reference and guidance for non-medical reader on drug therapy. However, it is impossible for a book of this kind to take into account every variation in individual circumstances, and readers should always follow their physician's instructions where these differ from the advice in this section.

The drugs have been selected to provide representative coverage of the principal classes of medications in use today. For disorders where a number of different drugs are available for treatment, the ones which are used most commonly have been selected. Emphasis has also been

placed on those drugs which are likely to be used in the home, although in a few cases those that are administered only in the hospital have been included when it has been judged a drug is of sufficient interest.

Each drug profile is organized in the same way, using standard headings (see sample page, below). To help you make the most of the information provided, the terms used and the instructions given under each heading are discussed and explained on the following pages.

Supplementary profiles on vitamins and mineral (pp.518 – 530), drugs of abuse (pp.531 – 538), and food additives (pp.539 – 543) are provided at the end of this section.

HOW TO UNDERSTAND THE PROFILES

For ease of reference, the information on each drug is arranged in a consistent format under standard headings.

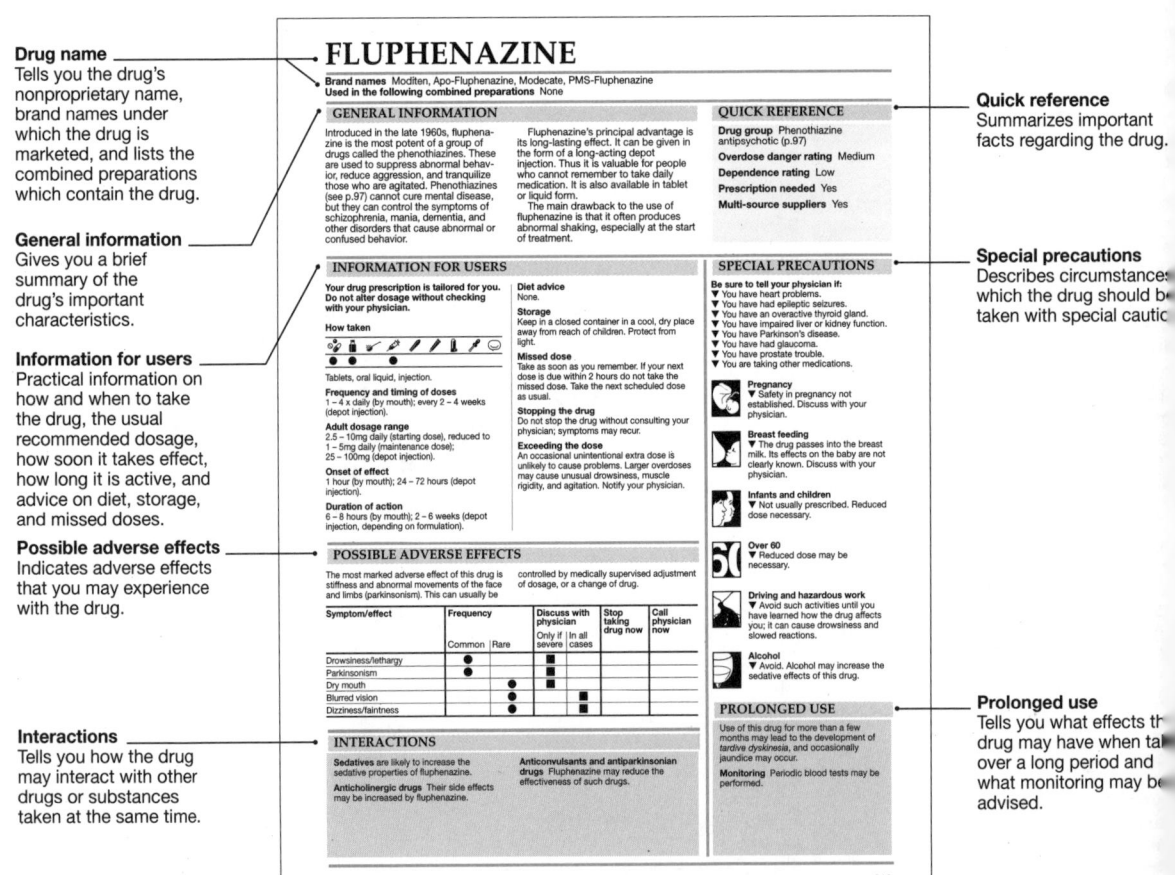

Drug name
Tells you the drug's nonproprietary name, brand names under which the drug is marketed, and lists the combined preparations which contain the drug.

General information
Gives you a brief summary of the drug's important characteristics.

Information for users
Practical information on how and when to take the drug, the usual recommended dosage, how soon it takes effect, how long it is active, and advice on diet, storage, and missed doses.

Possible adverse effects
Indicates adverse effects that you may experience with the drug.

Interactions
Tells you how the drug may interact with other drugs or substances taken at the same time.

Quick reference
Summarizes important facts regarding the drug.

Special precautions
Describes circumstances which the drug should be taken with special caution

Prolonged use
Tells you what effects the drug may have when taken over a long period and what monitoring may be advised.

DRUG NAME

Nonproprietary name

The main heading on the page is the shortest form of the drug's nonproprietary name, unless the short form causes confusion with another drug, in which case the full nonproprietary name is given. For example, neomycin sulfate, an antibiotic, is listed as neomycin, as there is no other nonproprietary drug of this name. However, magnesium hydroxide, an antacid, is listed under its full name to avoid confusing it with the mineral magnesium, or other compounds of the mineral, such as magnesium sulfate.

Brand names

Under the nonproprietary name are the brand names of products in which the drug is the major single active ingredient;

if there are many different brand-named forms of the drug, several of the most commonly used ones are given. Wherever possible, the innovator's brand is listed first. The names of the principal preparations, if any, in which the drug is combined with other drugs, are also listed. For more information about brand and nonproprietary names, see page 13.

HALOPERID

Brand names Haldol, Apo-Haloperidol, N
Used in the following combined prepara

GENERAL INFORMATION

GENERAL INFORMATION

The information here provides an overall picture of the drug. It may include notes on the drug's history (for example, when it was first introduced), and the principal disorders for which it is prescribed. This section also discusses the drug's major advantages and disadvantages.

GENERAL INFORMATION

Introduced in the early 1960s, haloperidol is the most widely used of a group of drugs known as butyrophenones. It is effective in reducing the violent, aggressive manifestations of mental illness such as schizophrenia, mania

QUICK REFERENCE

The text in this box summarizes the important facts regarding your drug and is organized under five headings, which are explained in detail below.

Drug group

This tells you which of the major groups the drug belongs to, and the page on which you can find out more about the drugs in the group and the various disorders or conditions they are used to treat. Where a drug belongs to more than one group, each group in the book is listed. For example, dimenhydrinate is listed as an antihistamine drug (p.136) and an anti-emetic drug (p.102).

Overdose danger rating

Gives a general indication of the seriousness of the drug's effects if the dosage prescribed by your physician, or that recommended on the label of an over-the-counter drug, is exceeded. The ratings – low, medium and high – are

QUICK REFERENCE

Drug group Antihistamine (p.136) and anti-emetic drug (p.102)

Overdose danger rating Medium

Dependence rating Low

Prescription needed No

Multi-source suppliers Yes

explained below. The rating also determines the advice given under Exceeding the dose.

- **Low** Symptoms unlikely. Death unknown.
- **Medium** Medical advice needed. Death rare.
- **High** Medical attention needed urgently. Potentially fatal.

If you do exceed the dose, advice is given under Exceeding the dose.

Dependence rating

Drugs are classified on the basis of the risk of dependence, and are given a rating of low, medium, or high.

- **Low** Dependence unknown.
- **Medium** Rare possibility of dependence.
- **High** Dependence is likely in long-term use.

Prescription needed

This tells you if a prescription is required to obtain the drug. The sale of certain drugs, however, may be subject to special provincial regulations and conditions. See How drugs are classified, page 13.

Multi-source suppliers

Tells you if a drug is marketed by more than one manufacturer.

INFORMATION FOR USERS (for common forms of each medication)

Information on the following: administration, dosage frequency and amount, effects and actions, and advice on diet, storage, missed doses, overdose and stopping drug treatment. **All information is generalized and is in no way a recommendation for an individual dosing schedule. Always follow your physician's instructions in the case of prescription drugs, and those of the manufacturer or pharmacist for over-the-counter medications.**

How taken

The symbols in the box represent the ways in which drugs can be administered. The dot that appears below the

symbol indicates the form in which the drug is available. This acts as a visual backup to the written information which follows immediately below the box.

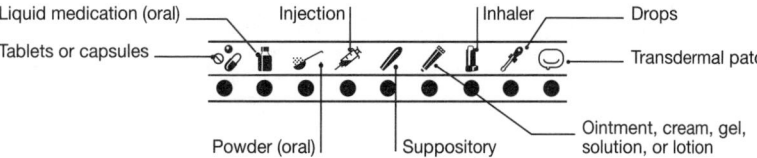

Liquid medication (oral)　　Injection　　Inhaler　　Drops

Tablets or capsules　　Transdermal patch

Powder (oral)　　Suppository　　Ointment, cream, gel, solution, or lotion

A – Z OF MEDICAL DRUGS continued

INFORMATION FOR USERS continued

Frequency and timing of doses

This refers to the standard number of times each day that the drug should be taken and, where relevant, whether it should be taken with liquid, with meals, or on an empty stomach.

> **Frequency and timing of doses**
> *Relief of pain and fever* Every 4 hours as necessary, with food or milk. (Slow-release capsules or tablets every 8 – 12 hours.)
> *Prevention of blood clots* Once daily.

> **Frequency and timing of doses**
> 1 – 3 x daily with meals.

Dosage range

This is generally given as the normal oral dosage range for an adult; dosages for injection are not usually given. In cases where the dosages for specific age groups vary significantly from the normal adult dosage, these will also be given. Where dosage varies according to use, the dosage for each use is included. Most drug dosages are expressed in Système International (SI) units, usually milligrams (mg) or micrograms (mcg). In a few, dosage is given in units (u) or international units (IU). See also Weights and measures, facing page.

> **Adult dosage range**
> *Prevention of gout attacks* 0.6 – 1.2mg daily. *Relief of gout attacks* 1.0 – 1.2mg per dose initially, then 0.6mg every 2 hours, up to a maximum of 4 – 8mg daily until joint is better or gastrointestinal problems arise.

> **Dosage range**
> *Adults* 60 – 180mL daily (liquid); 1.5 – 9.5g daily (tablets).
> *Children over 6 years* Reduced dose according to age and weight.

Onset of effect

The onset of effect is the time it takes for the drug to become active in the body. This sometimes coincides with the onset of beneficial effects, but there may sometimes be an interval between the time when a drug is pharmacologically active and when you start to notice improvement in your symptoms or your underlying condition.

> **Onset of effect**
> In Parkinson's disease some benefits may be noticed within 1 hour, but full effect may not be felt for up to 2 weeks. In viral infections the severity and duration of symptoms is likely to be reduced during a 2-week course of treatment if the drug is begun within 48 hours

> **Onset of effect**
> 15 – 60 minutes.

Duration of action

The information given here refers to the length of time that one dose of the drug remains active in the body.

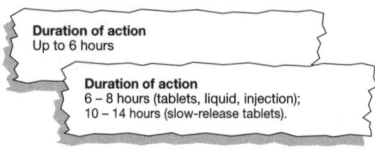

> **Duration of action**
> Up to 6 hours

> **Duration of action**
> 6 – 8 hours (tablets, liquid, injection); 10 – 14 hours (slow-release tablets).

Diet advice

With some drugs, it is important to avoid certain foods, either because they reduce the effect of the drug or because they interact adversely. This section of the profile tells you what, if any, dietary changes are necessary.

> **Diet advice**
> It is necessary to drink plenty of water during the 24 hours following treatment to reduce the risk of kidney damage.

Storage

Drugs will deteriorate and may become inactive if they are not stored under suitable conditions. The advice given in the profiles is usually to store in a cool, dry place out of the reach of children. Some drugs must also be protected from light. Others, especially liquid medications, need to be kept in a refrigerator, but should not be frozen. For further advice on storing drugs, see page 29.

> **Storage**
> Keep in a closed container in a cool, dry place away from reach of children. Protect from light.

Missed dose

This section gives advice on what to do if you forget a dose of your drug, so that the effectiveness and safety of your treatment is maintained as far as possible. If you forget to take several doses in succession, consult your physician. You can read more about missed doses on page 28.

> **Missed dose**
> Take as soon as your remember. If your next dose is due within 2 hours, take a single dose now and skip the next

> **Missed dose**
> No cause for concern, but make up the missed dose or application as soon as you remember.

Stopping the drug

If you are taking a drug regularly you should know how and when you can safely stop taking it. Some drugs can be safely stopped as soon as you feel better or as soon as your symptoms have disappeared. Others must not be stopped until the full course of treatment has been completed, or they must be gradually withdrawn under the supervision of a physician. Failure to comply with instructions for stopping a drug may lead to adverse effects. It may also cause your condition to worsen or your symptoms to reappear. See also Ending drug therapy, page 28.

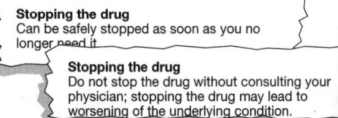

> **Stopping the drug**
> Can be safely stopped as soon as you no longer need it

> **Stopping the drug**
> Do not stop the drug without consulting your physician; stopping the drug may lead to worsening of the underlying condition.

Exceeding the dose

The information in this section expands on that in the quick reference box on the drug's overdose danger rating. It explains the possible consequences of exceeding the dose and what to do if an overdose is taken. Examples of wording used for low, medium, and high overdose ratings are as follows:

Low
An occasional unintentional extra dose is unlikely to be a cause for concern. But if you notice unusual symptoms, or if a large overdose has been taken, notify your physician.

Medium
An occasional unintentional extra dose is unlikely to cause problems. Large overdoses may cause [relevant symptoms]. Notify your physician.

High
Seek immediate medical advice in all cases. Take emergency action if [relevant symptoms] occur.

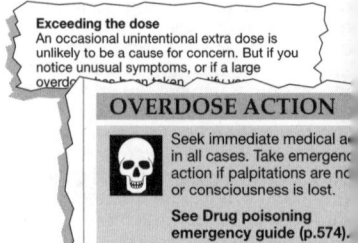

> **Exceeding the dose**
> An occasional unintentional extra dose is unlikely to be a cause for concern. But if you notice unusual symptoms, or if a large overdose has been taken, notify your...

> **OVERDOSE ACTION**
> Seek immediate medical advice in all cases. Take emergency action if palpitations are not or consciousness is lost.
>
> See Drug poisoning emergency guide (p.574).

SPECIAL PRECAUTIONS

Many drugs need to be taken with care by people with a history of particular conditions. The profile lists conditions you should tell your physician about when a drug is prescribed for you, and conditions you should discuss with your physician or pharmacist before taking an over-the-counter drug. Certain groups of people (pregnant women, nursing mothers, children, and those over 60) may also be at special risk from drug therapy. Advice for these groups is given in every profile. Information is also included about drinking alcohol, driving, and undertaking hazardous work.

SPECIAL PRECAUTIONS

Be sure to tell your physician if:
▼ You have impaired liver or kidney function.
▼ You have heart or circulation problems.
▼ You have had epileptic seizures.
▼ You have an overactive thyroid gland.
▼ You have Parkinson's disease.
▼ You have had glaucoma.

Pregnancy
▼ Safety in pregnancy not established. Discuss with your physician.

Breast feeding
▼ The drug passes into the breast milk. Its effects on the baby are not known. Discuss with your physician.

Infants and children
▼ Rarely required. Reduced dose necessary.

Over 60
▼ Reduced dose may be necessary.

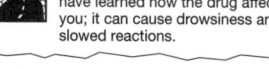

Driving and hazardous work
▼ Avoid such activities until you have learned how the drug affects you; it can cause drowsiness and slowed reactions.

Alcohol
▼ Avoid. Alcohol may increase the sedative effect of this drug.

WEIGHTS AND MEASURES

Système International (SI) equivalents of measurements used in this book:

1,000mcg (microgram) = 1mg (milligram)
1,000mg = 1g (gram)
1,000mL (millilitre) = 1L (litre)

POSSIBLE ADVERSE EFFECTS

The adverse effects discussed in the drug profile are symptoms or reactions that may arise when you take the drug. The emphasis is on symptoms that you, the patient, are likely to notice, rather than on the findings of laboratory tests that your physician may order. The bulk of the section is in the form of a table that lists the adverse effects and indicates how commonly they occur, when to tell your physician about them, and when to stop the drug. The headings in the table are explained below.

Frequency
Tells you whether the adverse effect is common or rare. Common effects are listed first.

Discuss with physician
The marker in this section indicates under what circumstances you need to inform your physician about an adverse effect you are experiencing.

Only if severe A marker in this column means that the symptom is unlikely to be serious, but that you should seek your physician's advice if it troubles you. *In all cases* Adverse effects marked in this column require prompt, but not necessarily emergency, medical attention. (See also Call physician now, below.)

Stop taking drug now
In cases where certain unpleasant or dangerous adverse effects of a drug may override its beneficial effects, you are advised to stop taking the drug immediately, if necessary before seeing your physician.

Call physician now
Effects marked in this column require immediate medical help. They indicate a potentially dangerous response to the drug treatment, for which you should seek emergency medical attention.

Symptom/effect	Frequency		Discuss with physician		Stop taking drug now	Call physician now
	Common	Rare	Only if severe	In all cases		
Nausea	●		■			
Diarrhea/abdominal pain	●		■			
Headache/dizziness		●	■			
Rash		●		■	▲	‖
Blurred vision		●		■	▲	‖

INTERACTIONS

The interactions discussed here are those that may occur between the drug under discussion and other drugs. Information includes the name of the interacting drug or drug groups and the effect of the interaction.

INTERACTIONS

Sedatives All drugs, including alcohol, that have sedative effects are likely to increase the sedative properties of haloperidol.

PROLONGED USE

The information given here concerns the adverse, and sometimes beneficial, effects of the drug which may occur during long-term use. These may differ from those listed under Possible Adverse Effects. This section of the profile also includes information on monitoring the effects of the drug during long-term treatment, explaining the tests you may be given if your physician thinks they are necessary.

PROLONGED USE

Sudden onset of abnormal heart rhythms or abnormalities of the blood may occur.

Monitoring Periodic checks on blood levels of the drug may be required.

Units or international units
Units (u) and international units (IU) are also used to express drug dosages. They represent the biological activity of a drug (its effect on the body). This ability cannot be measured in terms of weight or volume, but must be calculated in a laboratory.

ACEBUTOLOL

Brand names Monitan, Rhotral, Sectral
Used in the following combined preparations None

GENERAL INFORMATION

Acebutolol, introduced in 1986, is a beta blocker that is most commonly prescribed to treat hypertension and angina.

Unlike some similar drugs that act on both the heart and lungs, acebutolol is cardioselective – that is, it acts mainly on the heart. It is less dangerous than other beta blockers in people with asthma, bronchitis, or other lung problems, although special caution is still required. In common with other beta blockers, acebutolol affects the body's response to low blood sugar, which can cause problems for diabetics. It can sometimes cause cold hands and feet by reducing circulation to the limbs.

INFORMATION FOR USERS

Your drug prescription is tailored for you. Do not alter dosage without checking with your physician.

How taken

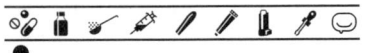

Tablets.

Frequency and timing of doses
2 x daily.

Adult dosage range
Hypertension 200 – 800mg daily.
Angina 200 – 600mg daily.

Onset of effect
1 – 4 hours. Full beneficial effect on blood pressure may take some weeks.

Duration of action
Up to 24 hours.

Diet advice
None.

Storage
Keep in a closed container in a cool, dry place away from reach of children.

Missed dose
Take as soon as you remember. If your next dose is due within 2 hours, take a single dose now and skip the next.

Stopping the drug
Do not stop the drug without consulting your physician; stopping the drug may lead to dangerous worsening of the underlying condition or precipitation of a heart attack.

OVERDOSE ACTION

 Seek immediate medical advice in all cases. Take emergency action if collapse or loss of consciousness occurs.

See Drug poisoning emergency guide (p.574).

SPECIAL PRECAUTIONS

Be sure to tell your physician if:
▼ You have impaired liver or kidney function.
▼ You have heart failure.
▼ You have a lung disorder such as asthma, emphysema, or bronchitis.
▼ You have allergies.
▼ You have diabetes.
▼ You have circulatory disease.
▼ You are taking other medications.

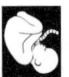 **Pregnancy**
▼ Safety in pregnancy not established. Discuss with your physician.

 Breast feeding
▼ The drug passes into the breast milk. Discuss with your physician.

 Infants and children
▼ Not prescribed.

 Over 60
▼ Increased likelihood of adverse effects.

 Driving and hazardous work
▼ Avoid such activities until you have learned how the drug affects you; it can cause dizziness.

 Alcohol
▼ No known problems with moderate intake.

Surgery and general anesthetics
▼ Acebutolol may need to be stopped before you have a general anesthetic. Discuss this with your physician or dentist before any surgery.

POSSIBLE ADVERSE EFFECTS

Acebutolol has adverse effects that are common to most beta blockers. Symptoms such as fatigue and nausea are usually temporary and diminish with long-term use. Acebutolol can occasionally provoke or worsen asthma and heart problems. Fainting may be a sign that the drug has slowed the heartbeat excessively.

Symptom/effect	Frequency		Discuss with physician		Stop taking drug now	Call physician now
	Common	Rare	Only if severe	In all cases		
Lethargy/fatigue	●		■			
Cold hands and feet		●	■			
Nausea/vomiting		●	■			
Nightmares/vivid dreams		●	■			
Rash		●		■	▲	
Breathlessness/fainting		●		■	▲	▮

INTERACTIONS

Calcium channel blockers Taken with acebutolol, some of these drugs may further decrease blood pressure and/or heart rate and may also reduce the force of the heart's pumping action.

Non-steroidal anti-inflammatory drugs (NSAIDs) may reduce the antihypertensive effect of acebutolol.

Cimetidine may increase the levels of acebutolol in the blood.

Sympathomimetic decongestants used with acebutolol may increase blood pressure and/or heart rate.

PROLONGED USE

No special problems expected.

ACETAMINOPHEN

Brand names Tylenol, Abenol, Apo-Acetaminophen, Atasol, Tempra, 222 AF
Used in the following combined preparations Contac Sinus Pain, Oxycocet, Parafon Forte, Percocet, Tylenol w/codeine

GENERAL INFORMATION

Although acetaminophen has been known since the early 1900s, it has been widely used as an analgesic only since the 1950s. One of a group of drugs known as the non-narcotic analgesics, it is kept in the home to relieve occasional bouts of mild pain and to reduce fever. It is suitable for children as well as adults.

One of the advantages of taking acetaminophen is that it does not cause stomach upset or bleeding problems. That makes it a particularly useful alternative for people who suffer from peptic ulcers or who cannot tolerate ASA. Occasional doses can also be safely taken if you are receiving treatment with anticoagulants.

An overdose of acetaminophen is dangerous, capable of causing serious damage to the liver and kidneys. Large dosages of acetaminophen may be toxic if you are a regular consumer of even moderate amounts of alcohol.

QUICK REFERENCE

Drug group Non-narcotic analgesic (p.92)

Overdose danger rating High

Dependence rating Low

Prescription needed No

Multi-source suppliers Yes

INFORMATION FOR USERS

Follow instructions on the label. Call your physician if symptoms worsen.

How taken

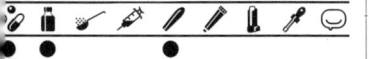

Tablets, capsules, oral liquid, rectal suppositories.

Frequency and timing of doses
Every 4 – 6 hours as necessary.

Dosage range
Adults 500mg – 1g per dose up to a maximum of 4g daily.
Children 10mg per kg body weight.

Onset of effect
Within 10 – 60 minutes.

Duration of action
Up to 6 hours.

Diet advice
None.

Storage
Keep in a closed container in a cool, dry place, away from reach of children.

Missed dose
Take as soon as you remember if required to relieve pain. Otherwise do not take the missed dose, and take a further dose only when you are in pain.

Stopping the drug
Can be safely stopped as soon as you no longer need it.

OVERDOSE ACTION

 Seek immediate medical advice in all cases. Take emergency action if nausea, vomiting, or stomach pain occurs.

See Drug poisoning emergency guide (p.574).

POSSIBLE ADVERSE EFFECTS

Acetaminophen has rarely been found to produce any side effects if you take the drug as recommended.

Symptom/effect	Frequency		Discuss with physician		Stop taking drug now	Call physician now
	Common	Rare	Only if severe	In all cases		
Nausea		●		■		
Rash		●		■	■	▲

INTERACTIONS

Cholestyramine inhibits absorption of acetaminophen.

Anticoagulant drugs such as warfarin may need dosage adjustment if acetaminophen is taken regularly in high doses.

SPECIAL PRECAUTIONS

Be sure to consult your physician or pharmacist before using this drug if:
▼ You have impaired liver or kidney function.
▼ You are taking other medications.

 **Pregnancy**
▼ Safety in pregnancy not established. Discuss with your physician.

 Breast feeding
▼ In normal doses the drug does not significantly affect the breast milk or baby. Discuss with your physician.

 Infants and children
▼ Reduced dose necessary.

 Over 60
▼ No special problems.

 Driving and hazardous work
▼ No special problems.

 Alcohol
▼ Prolonged heavy intake of alcohol in combination with acetaminophen may substantially increase the risk of injury to the liver.

PROLONGED USE

You should not normally take this drug for a period longer than 5 days except on the advice of your physician.

ACETYLSALICYLIC ACID (ASA)

Brand names Aspirin, Apo-ASA, Entrophen, Novasen
Used in the following combined preparations Anacin, Asasantine, Oxycodan, Percodan, Robaxisal

GENERAL INFORMATION

Commonly used since 1919, ASA is a non-narcotic analgesic that relieves pain, reduces fever, and alleviates the symptoms of arthritis. In small doses, it helps prevent blood clots from forming.

It is present in numerous combination medicines for colds, menstrual period pains, headaches, and joint or muscular aches.

One disadvantage of ASA is its tendency to irritate the stomach and even cause bleeding. Another is the possibility that it may be a causative factor in Reye's syndrome, a rare brain and liver disorder usually occurring in children. Only under close medical supervision should it be given to children with fever caused by viral illness.

QUICK REFERENCE

Drug group Non-narcotic analgesic (p.92) and antiplatelet drug (p.116)

Overdose danger rating High

Dependence rating Low

Prescription needed No

Multi-source suppliers Yes

INFORMATION FOR USERS

Follow instructions on the label. Call your physician if symptoms worsen.

How taken

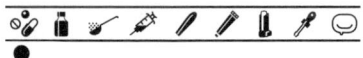

Tablets, enteric-coated tablets.

Frequency and timing of doses
Relief of pain and fever Every 4 – 6 hours as necessary, with food or milk.
Prevention of blood clots Once daily.

Adult dosage range
Relief of pain and fever 325 – 650mg per dose. Larger doses may be required in arthritis.
Prevention of blood clots Dose uncertain: 80 – 325mg daily or higher as prescribed.

Onset of effect
30 – 60 minutes (regular tablets);
1¹/₂ – 8 hours (enteric-coated tablets).

Duration of action
Up to 12 hours. The antiplatelet effect which helps prevent blood clots persists for several days.

Diet advice
None.

Storage
Keep in a closed container in a cool, dry place away from reach of children.

Missed dose
Do not make up the dose you missed. Take your next dose on your original schedule. If you are taking the medicine long term, take the missed dose as soon as you remember.

Stopping the drug
If you have been prescribed ASA by your physician for a long-term condition, you should seek medical advice before stopping the drug. Otherwise it can be safely stopped as soon as you no longer need it.

OVERDOSE ACTION

Seek immediate medical advice in all cases. Take emergency action if there is restlessness, stomach pain, ringing noises in the ears, blurred vision, or vomiting.

See Drug poisoning emergency guide (p.574).

SPECIAL PRECAUTIONS

Be sure to consult your physician or pharmacist before taking this drug if:
▼ You have impaired liver or kidney function.
▼ You have asthma.
▼ You have nasal polyps.
▼ You have a blood clotting disorder.
▼ You have a peptic ulcer.
▼ You are taking other medications.

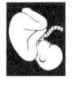

Pregnancy
▼ Not usually recommended. ASA may prolong labor and may cause bleeding in the newborn baby. An alternative drug may be safer. Discuss with your physician.

Breast feeding
▼ Not usually recommended. The drug passes into the breast milk. An alternative drug may be safer. Discuss with your physician.

Infants and children
▼ Not recommended.

Over 60
▼ No special problems.

Driving and hazardous work
▼ No special problems.

Alcohol
▼ Avoid. Alcohol increases the likelihood of stomach irritation with this drug.

Surgery and general anesthetics
▼ Treatment with ASA may need to be stopped about one week before surgery. Discuss with your physician or dentist before any operation.

POSSIBLE ADVERSE EFFECTS

Adverse effects are more likely to occur with high dosage of ASA, but may be reduced by taking the drug with food or in enteric-coated forms.

Symptom/effect	Frequency		Discuss with physician		Stop taking drug now	Call physician now
	Common	Rare	Only if severe	In all cases		
Indigestion/nausea/vomiting	●			■		
Ringing in ears (tinnitus)		●		■		■
Rash		●		■	▲	
Breathlessness/wheezing		●		■	▲	■
Black/bloodstained feces		●		■	▲	■

INTERACTIONS

Anticoagulants ASA may add to the anticoagulant effect of such drugs, leading to an increased risk of abnormal bleeding.

NSAIDs and corticosteroids These drugs may increase the likelihood of stomach irritation when taken with ASA.

Drugs for gout ASA may reduce the effect of these drugs, especially probenecid and sulfinpyrazone.

Oral antidiabetic drugs ASA may increase the effect of these drugs.

PROLONGED USE

ASA should not be taken for longer than 5 days except on your physician's advice. Prolonged use of ASA may lead to bleeding in the stomach and to stomach ulcers.

ACYCLOVIR

Brand names Zovirax, Avirax
Used in the following combined preparations None

GENERAL INFORMATION

Acyclovir is an antiviral drug used in the treatment of herpes infections of all types. Originally, acyclovir ointment was used to treat primary (first case) genital herpes. However, oral acyclovir is now used to treat both primary herpes infections and unusually frequent recurrences. Treatment reduces the severity of the episodes by decreasing discomfort, but it does not prevent infection from recurring. Oral acyclovir is also used to treat acute herpes zoster (shingles) and acute varicella (chickenpox) infections.

Acyclovir may also be administered as an ointment for herpes infections of the cornea, almost always under the care of a specialist.

Intravenous acyclovir is used to treat herpes infections in people with reduced immunity. This injected form is prescribed with caution to those with impaired kidney function.

INFORMATION FOR USERS

Your drug prescription is tailored for you. Do not alter dosage without checking with your physician.

How taken

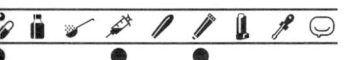

Tablets, capsules, injection, ointment, cream.

Frequency and timing of doses
4 – 5 x daily (oral forms); 4 – 6 x daily (topical forms).

Adult dosage range
Capsules, tablets Established individually on basis of condition under treatment.
Ointment, cream Using a finger cot or rubber glove, apply a sufficient quantity to adequately cover all affected areas.

Onset of effect
Within 24 hours.

Duration of action
Up to 8 hours.

Diet advice
Increase intake of fluids.

Storage
Keep in a closed container in a cool, dry place away from reach of children. Protect from light.

Missed dose
Ointment, cream Do not apply the missed dose. Apply your next dose as usual.
Capsules, tablets Take as soon as you remember.

Stopping the drug
Complete the full course as directed.

Exceeding the dose
An occasional unintentional extra dose is unlikely to be a cause for concern. But if you notice unusual symptoms, or if a large overdose has been taken, notify your physician.

POSSIBLE ADVERSE EFFECTS

Serious adverse effects are rare. *Topical* forms commonly cause discomfort at the site of application. Confusion, hallucinations, and blood in urine occur rarely with injections.

Symptom/effect	Frequency		Discuss with physician		Stop taking drug now	Call physician now
	Common	Rare	Only if severe	In all cases		
Ointment, cream						
Burning/stinging/itching	●		■			
Rash	●			■	▲	
Capsules, tablets						
Nausea/vomiting	●		■			
Headache/dizziness	●		■			
Injection						
Blood in urine		●		■	▲	
Confusion/hallucinations		●		■	▲	

INTERACTIONS (by mouth and injection only)

General note Any drug that affects the kidneys increases the risk of side effects with acyclovir.

Probenecid may increase the level of acyclovir in the blood.

Interferon and methotrexate Taken with acyclovir, these may increase the risk of adverse effects on the nervous system.

SPECIAL PRECAUTIONS

Be sure to tell your physician if:
▼ You have impaired kidney function.
▼ You are taking other medications.

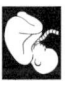

Pregnancy
▼ Topical preparations carry no known risk, but oral and injectable forms are not usually prescribed, as the effects on the developing baby are unknown. Discuss with your physician.

Breast feeding
▼ No evidence of risk with topical forms. The drug passes into the breast milk following injection or oral administration. Discuss with your physician.

Infants and children
▼ Reduced dose necessary.

Over 60
▼ Reduced dose may be necessary.

Driving and hazardous work
▼ Avoid such activities after oral or injected acyclovir until you have learned how the drug affects you; it can cause dizziness.

Alcohol
▼ No known problems.

PROLONGED USE

There is a rare risk of resistance to acyclovir with prolonged use.

ALLOPURINOL

Brand names Zyloprim, Apo-Allopurinol, Purinol
Used in the following combined preparations None

GENERAL INFORMATION

Allopurinol is prescribed as a long-term preventive of recurrent attacks of gout. By decreasing the formation of uric acid, it lowers blood concentrations and thus prevents the formation in the joints of uric acid crystals, which cause the inflammation characteristic of gout. Allopurinol is also employed to lower high uric acid levels (hyperuricemia) caused by other drugs, especially anticancer drugs.

Its effects tend to be long-term, so allopurinol is not effective in relieving the pain of an acute flare-up. In fact, gout attacks may increase during the first months of allopurinol treatment, so colchicine is often given as well initially.

Unlike the gout drugs that reduce uric acid levels by increasing the quantity excreted in the urine, allopurinol does not raise the risk of kidney stones. This makes it particularly suitable for those with poor kidney function or a tendency to form kidney stones.

QUICK REFERENCE

Drug group Drug for gout (p.131)
Overdose danger rating Medium
Dependence rating Low
Prescription needed Yes
Multi-source suppliers Yes

INFORMATION FOR USERS

Your drug prescription is tailored for you. Do not alter dosage without checking with your physician.

How taken

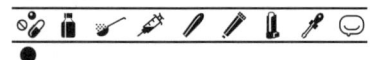

Tablets.

Frequency and timing of doses
1 – 3 x daily with meals.

Adult dosage range
Gout 200 – 600mg daily, usually 300mg.
With anticancer drugs 600 – 800mg daily.

Onset of effect
Within 24 – 48 hours. Full effect may not be felt for several weeks.

Duration of action
Up to 30 hours. Some effect may last for 1 – 2 weeks after the drug has been stopped.

Diet advice
A high fluid intake (2 litres of fluid daily) is recommended.

Storage
Keep in a closed container in a cool, dry place away from reach of children.

Missed dose
Take as soon as you remember. If your next dose is due within 12 hours, take a dose now and take the next one on time. Otherwise skip the missed dose, and take your next dose on schedule.

Stopping the drug
Do not stop the drug without consulting your physician; symptoms may recur.

Exceeding the dose
An occasional unintentional extra dose is unlikely to cause problems. Large overdoses may cause nausea, vomiting, abdominal pain, and diarrhea. Notify your physician.

SPECIAL PRECAUTIONS

Be sure to tell your physician if:
▼ You have impaired liver or kidney function
▼ You are taking other medications.

Pregnancy
▼ Safety in pregnancy not established. Discuss with your physician.

Breast feeding
▼ The drug passes into the breast milk and may affect the baby. Discuss with your physician.

Infants and children
▼ Not usually prescribed. Reduced dose necessary.

Over 60
▼ Reduced dose may be necessary.

Driving and hazardous work
▼ Avoid such activities until you have learned how the drug affects you; it can cause drowsiness.

Alcohol
▼ Avoid. Alcohol increases the adverse effects of this drug and increases the risk of an attack of gout.

POSSIBLE ADVERSE EFFECTS

Adverse effects of allopurinol are not very common. The most serious is an allergic rash that may require the drug to be stopped and an alternative treatment substituted.

Symptom/effect	Frequency		Discuss with physician		Stop taking drug now	Call physician now
	Common	Rare	Only if severe	In all cases		
Nausea	●		■			
Rash/itching	●			■	▲	▮
Drowsiness		●	■			
Headache		●		■		
Tingling hands/feet		●		■		
Metallic taste		●		■		
Fever and chills		●		■		

PROLONGED USE

Apart from an increased risk of gout in the first weeks or months, no problems are expected.

Monitoring Periodic checks on uric acid levels in the blood are usually performed.

INTERACTIONS

Thiazide diuretics may increase the risk of adverse effects from allopurinol.

Chlorpropamide Allopurinol may prolong or increase the blood sugar lowering effect of chlorpropamide.

Anticoagulant drugs Allopurinol may increase the effects of these drugs.

Mercaptopurine and azathioprine Allopurinol blocks the breakdown of these drugs; they are given in reduced doses.

Amoxicillin- and ampicillin-related skin rashes may be increased in patients taking allopurinol.

ALPRAZOLAM

Brand names Xanax, Apo-Alpraz, Novo-Alprazol, Nu-Alpraz
Used in the following combined preparations None

GENERAL INFORMATION

Alprazolam, introduced in 1981, belongs to a group of drugs known as benzodiazepines. See page 95 for a fuller description of the actions and adverse effects of this category of drugs.

Alprazolam is indicated for the short-term symptomatic relief of excessive anxiety. It is also used in the treatment of panic disorders and anxiety that accompanies agitated depression. Physicians may also prescribe it for agoraphobia (fear of open spaces), other phobias, and anxiety disorders of a general nature.

In common with other benzodiazepines, alprazolam can be addictive if taken regularly over a long period. Its effects may also become weaker over time. For those reasons, treatment with alprazolam is reviewed at regular intervals.

QUICK REFERENCE

Drug group Benzodiazepine anti-anxiety drug (p.95)

Overdose danger rating Medium

Dependence rating High

Prescription needed Yes

Multi-source suppliers Yes

INFORMATION FOR USERS

Your drug prescription is tailored for you. Do not alter dosage without checking with your physician.

How taken

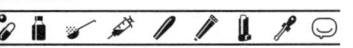

Tablets.

Frequency and timing of doses
1 – 3 x daily.

Adult dosage range
0.75 – 1.5mg daily. Occasionally, larger doses may be prescribed.

Onset of effect
1 – 2 hours.

Duration of action
Up to 24 hours.

Diet advice
None.

Storage
Keep in a tightly closed container in a cool, dry place away from reach of children. Protect from light.

Missed dose
No cause for concern, but take when you remember. If your next dose is due within 2 hours, take a single dose now and skip the next.

Stopping the drug
If you have been taking the drug continuously for less than 2 weeks, it can be safely stopped as soon as you feel you no longer need it. However, if you have been taking it for longer, consult your physician, who may advise a gradual reduction in dosage. Stopping abruptly may lead to withdrawal symptoms (see p.95).

Exceeding the dose
An occasional unintentional extra dose is unlikely to cause problems. Larger overdoses may cause unusual drowsiness, unsteadiness, or coma. Notify your physician.

SPECIAL PRECAUTIONS

Be sure to tell your physician if:
▼ You have impaired liver or kidney function.
▼ You have myasthenia gravis.
▼ You have glaucoma.
▼ You have had problems with alcohol or drug abuse.
▼ You are taking other medications.

Pregnancy
▼ Safety in pregnancy not established. Discuss with your physician.

Breast feeding
▼ The drug passes into the breast milk. Its effects on the baby are not clearly known. Discuss with your physician.

Infants and children
▼ Not recommended in patients under 18 years.

Over 60
▼ Increased likelihood of adverse effects. Reduced dose may therefore be necessary.

Driving and hazardous work
▼ Avoid such activities until you have learned how the drug affects you: it can cause reduced alertness, blurred vision, and slowed reactions.

Alcohol
▼ Avoid. Alcohol may increase the sedative effects of this drug.

POSSIBLE ADVERSE EFFECTS

The principal adverse effects of this drug are related to its sedative and tranquilizing properties. These effects normally diminish after the first few days of treatment. If adverse effects persist, they can often be reduced by adjustment of dosage.

Symptom/effect	Frequency		Discuss with physician		Stop taking drug now	Call physician now
	Common	Rare	Only if severe	In all cases		
Drowsiness	●			■		
Dizziness/unsteadiness	●			■		
Blurred vision		●		■		
Forgetfulness/confusion		●		■		
Headache		●		■		
Rash		●		■	▲	
Jaundice		●		■	▲	■

PROLONGED USE

Regular use of this drug over several weeks can lead to a reduction in its effect as the body adapts. It may also be habit-forming when taken for extended periods, especially if larger-than-average doses are taken.

INTERACTIONS

Sedatives All drugs that have a sedative effect on the central nervous system are likely to increase the sedative properties of alprazolam. Such drugs include alcohol, sleeping drugs, antihistamines, antidepressants, narcotic analgesics, and antipsychotics.

ALUMINUM HYDROXIDE

Brand names Amphojel, Alu-Tab, Basaljel
Used in the following combined preparations Amphojel 500, Diovol Ex, Gaviscon, Maalox, Neutralca-S

GENERAL INFORMATION

Commonly used for more than 50 years to neutralize stomach acid, aluminum hydroxide is the ingredient basic to most of the over-the-counter remedies for indigestion and heartburn. Because it is constipating (it is sometimes used for diarrhea), aluminum hydroxide is usually combined with a magnesium-containing antacid with a balancing laxative effect.

The action of aluminum hydroxide is prolonged, making it useful in preventing the pain caused by stomach and duodenal ulcers or reflux esophagitis. Aluminum hydroxide can also promote the healing of ulcers.

In the intestine, aluminum hydroxide inactivates phosphate. This makes it helpful in the treatment of high blood phosphate (hyperphosphatemia), a condition of some people suffering impaired kidney function. But prolonged use of aluminum hydroxide can lead to phosphate deficiency and a consequent weakening of the bones.

Some preparations include large amounts of sodium and should be used with caution by those on low-sodium diets. Liquid preparations of the drug may be more effective than tablets.

QUICK REFERENCE

Drug group Antacid (p.120)
Overdose danger rating Low
Dependence rating Low
Prescription needed No
Multi-source suppliers Yes

INFORMATION FOR USERS

Follow instructions on the label. Call your physician if symptoms worsen.

How taken

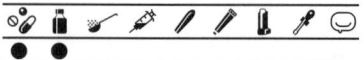

Tablets, capsules, oral liquid (gel suspension).

Frequency and timing of doses
As antacid 4 – 6 x daily as needed, or 1 hour before and after meals.
Peptic ulcer Every 1 – 2 hours while awake.
Hyperphosphatemia 3 – 4 x daily with meals.
Diarrhea 3 – 6 x daily.

Dosage range
Adults 60 – 180mL daily (liquid), 1.5 – 9.5g daily (tablets); as directed by physician (capsules).
Children over 6 years Reduced dose according to age and weight.

Onset of effect
Within 15 minutes.

Duration of action
2 – 4 hours.

Diet advice
For hyperphosphatemia, aluminum hydroxide may be given with a low-phosphate diet.

Storage
Keep in a closed container in a cool, dry place away from reach of children.

Missed dose
Do not take the missed dose. Take your next dose as usual.

Stopping the drug
Can be safely stopped as soon as you no longer need it (indigestion). When given as ulcer treatment or for hyperphosphatemia resulting from kidney failure, do not stop without consulting your physician.

Exceeding the dose
An occasional unintentional extra dose is unlikely to be a cause for concern. But if you notice unusual symptoms, or if a large overdose has been taken, notify your physician.

POSSIBLE ADVERSE EFFECTS

Constipation is common with aluminum hydroxide; nausea and vomiting may occur due to the granular, powdery nature of the drug. Bone pain and muscle weakness occur only when large doses have been taken regularly for months or years.

Symptom/effect	Frequency		Discuss with physician		Stop taking drug now	Call physician now
	Common	Rare	Only if severe	In all cases		
Constipation	●		■			
Nausea		●	■			
Vomiting		●			■	
Bone pain		●			■	
Muscle weakness		●			■	

INTERACTIONS

General note Aluminum hydroxide interferes with the absorption or excretion of a wide range of drugs taken by mouth, including tetracyclines, warfarin, digoxin, iron supplements, penicillamine, phenytoin, and corticosteroids.

Enteric-coated tablets This drug may break up the enteric coating of tablets such as bisacodyl, sometimes leading to stomach irritation.

SPECIAL PRECAUTIONS

Be sure to consult your physician or pharmacist before taking this drug if:
▼ You have impaired kidney function.
▼ You have heart problems.
▼ You have high blood pressure.
▼ You suffer from constipation.
▼ You have a bone disease.
▼ You are taking other medications.

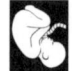

Pregnancy
▼ No evidence of risk with occasional use. Discuss with your physician.

Breast feeding
▼ No evidence of risk.

Infants and children
▼ Not recommended in children under 6 years except on the advice of a physician.

Over 60
▼ Increased likelihood of adverse effects. Reduced dose may therefore be necessary.

Driving and hazardous work
▼ No known problems.

Alcohol
▼ No known problems.

PROLONGED USE

Aluminum hydroxide should not be used for longer than 4 weeks without consulting your physician. Prolonged use in high doses may deplete blood phosphate and calcium levels, leading to weakening of the bones and fractures.

AMANTADINE

rand names Symmetrel, Endantadine, PMS-Amantadine
sed in the following combined preparations None

GENERAL INFORMATION

mantadine was introduced in the
960s as an antiviral drug used for the
revention and treatment of influenza A.
urrently it is used in conjunction with
accination to prevent and control
utbreaks of influenza A. Amantadine
an also be used alone in high-risk
dividuals who have not been
accinated.
　Amantadine has been found to be
oderately useful in *parkinsonism* and
this is now its main use. Though
amantadine usually produces symptomatic improvement during the first
few weeks, its effectiveness wears off in
a period of months, and replacement by
another drug is required. It is sometimes
given with levodopa (see p.358), another
antiparkinsonism drug.
　Marked adverse effects with the use
of amantadine are unusual.

(see p.358)

QUICK REFERENCE

Drug group Antiparkinsonism drug
(p.99) and antiviral drug (p.145)

Overdose danger rating Medium

Dependence rating Low

Prescription needed Yes

Multi-source suppliers Yes

(p.99) ... (p.145)

INFORMATION FOR USERS

ur drug prescription is tailored for you.
 not alter dosage without checking
th your physician.

ow taken

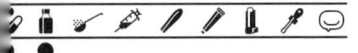

psules, oral liquid.

equency and timing of doses
 2 x daily.

ult dosage range
 – 200mg daily.

set of effect
Parkinson's disease some benefits may be
ticed within 1 hour, but full effect may not
 felt for up to 2 weeks. In viral infections the
verity and duration of symptoms is likely to
 reduced during a 2-week course of
atment if the drug is begun within 48 hours
onset of symptoms.

Duration of action
Up to 24 hours.

Diet advice
None.

Storage
Keep in a closed container in a cool, dry place
away from reach of children.

Missed dose
Take as soon as you remember. If your next
dose is due within 2 hours, take a single dose
now and skip the next.

Stopping the drug
Do not stop taking the drug without consulting
your physician; symptoms may recur.

Exceeding the dose
An occasional unintentional extra dose is
unlikely to cause problems. But if you notice
unusual symptoms, or if a large overdose has
been taken, notify your physician.

SPECIAL PRECAUTIONS

Be sure to tell your physician if:
▼ You have impaired liver or kidney function.
▼ You suffer from eczema.
▼ You have had a peptic ulcer.
▼ You have had epileptic seizures.
▼ You are taking other medications.

Pregnancy
▼ Safety in pregnancy not
established. Discuss with your
physician.

Breast feeding
▼ The drug passes into the breast
milk and may affect the baby.
Discuss with your physician.

Infants and children
▼ Not usually prescribed. Reduced
dose necessary.

Over 60
▼ Increased likelihood of adverse
effects. Reduced dose may
therefore be necessary.

Driving and hazardous work
▼ Avoid such activities until you
have learned how the drug affects
you because of the possibility of
blurred vision, confusion, and
agitation.

Alcohol
▼ Avoid in the first few days of
treatment; thereafter keep
consumption low.

POSSIBLE ADVERSE EFFECTS

verse effects are uncommon and often
ar off during continued treatment. They are
rarely serious enough to require treatment to
be stopped.

mptom/effect	Frequency		Discuss with physician		Stop taking drug now	Call physician now
	Common	Rare	Only if severe	In all cases		
rvousness/agitation		●	■			
omnia	●		■			
nfusion		●		■		
ziness	●			■		
rred vision		●		■		
estive disturbances	●			■		
kle swelling		●		■		
sh		●		■	▲	

NTERACTIONS

nticholinergic drugs Amantadine may
 ld to the effects of *anticholinergic* drugs.
In that event your physician will probably
reduce the dosage of the anticholinergic
drugs.

AMILORIDE

Brand name Midamor
Used in the following combined preparations Moduret, Apo-Amilzide, Novamilor, Nu-Amilzide

GENERAL INFORMATION

Amiloride belongs to the class of drugs known as potassium-sparing diuretics. Combined with thiazide or loop diuretics, amiloride is used in the treatment of hypertension, and for edema (fluid retention) resulting from heart failure or liver disease.

Amiloride's effect on urine flow is apparent within two to four hours. For this reason, avoid taking it after about 4 p.m.; otherwise you may need to pass urine during the night.

As with other potassium-sparing diuretics, amiloride can contribute to dangerously high levels of potassium in the blood, especially in the presence of diabetes or diseases of the kidneys. The drug is therefore prescribed with caution for people with kidney disorders.

INFORMATION FOR USERS

Your drug prescription is tailored for you. Do not alter dosage without checking with your physician.

How taken

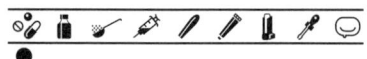

Tablets.

Frequency and timing of doses
1 – 2 x daily with food or milk.

Adult dosage range
5 – 20mg daily.

Onset of effect
Within 2 – 4 hours.

Duration of action
12 – 24 hours.

Diet advice
Avoid salt substitutes unless advised by your physician.

Storage
Keep in a closed container in a cool, dry place away from reach of children.

Missed dose
Take as soon as you remember. However, if it is late in the day, do not take the missed dose, or you may need to get up at night to pass urine. Take the next scheduled dose as usual.

Stopping the drug
Do not stop the drug without consulting your physician; symptoms may recur.

Exceeding the dose
An occasional unintentional extra dose is unlikely to be a cause for concern. But if you notice unusual symptoms, or if a large overdose has been taken, notify your physician.

POSSIBLE ADVERSE EFFECTS

Amiloride has few adverse effects; the main problem is the possibility that potassium may be retained by the body. This can only be detected by blood tests.

Symptom/effect	Frequency		Discuss with physician		Stop taking drug now	Call physician now
	Common	Rare	Only if severe	In all cases		
Headache	●		■			
Digestive disturbances	●		■			
Confusion	●			■		
Muscle weakness	●			■		
Rash	●			■	▲	

INTERACTIONS

Lithium Amiloride may increase the blood levels of lithium, leading to an increased risk of lithium poisoning.

ACE inhibitors may increase the risk of potassium retention with amiloride.

SPECIAL PRECAUTIONS

Be sure to tell your physician if:
▼ You have impaired kidney function.
▼ You have diabetes.
▼ You are taking other medications.

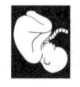

Pregnancy
▼ Not usually prescribed. May cause a reduction in the blood supply to the developing baby. Discuss with your physician.

Breast feeding
▼ It is not known whether the drug passes into breast milk. Discuss with your physician.

Infants and children
▼ Safety in children not established.

Over 60
▼ Increased likelihood of adverse effects. Reduced dose may therefore be necessary.

Driving and hazardous work
▼ Avoid such activities until you have learned how the drug affects you; it may cause confusion.

Alcohol
▼ No special problems.

PROLONGED USE

Serious problems are unlikely.

Monitoring Blood tests may be performed to check on kidney function and levels of body salts.

AMIODARONE

...and name Cordarone
...sed in the following combined preparations None

GENERAL INFORMATION

...miodarone was introduced in 1986 ...treat a variety of abnormal heart ...ythms (arrhythmias). It works by ...owing nerve impulses in the heart ...uscle.
Currently, amiodarone is reserved for ...e treatment of abnormal heart ...ythms, notably atrial fibrillation and ...ntricular tachycardia.
Amiodarone is generally used only ...en other drugs have proved ineffec-tive. However, there are serious adverse effects associated with amiodarone and patients receiving the drug must be carefully monitored. These effects include liver damage, thyroid problems, and eye and lung damage.

Treatment with amiodarone should be started under specialist supervision and the dosage carefully controlled so as to achieve the desired effect with the lowest effective dose.

INFORMATION FOR USERS

...ur drug prescription is tailored for you. ...not alter dosage without checking ...h your physician.

...w taken

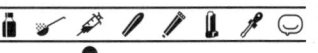

...lets, injection.

...quency and timing of doses
...ally 3 x daily with meals, then once or ...e daily with meals (maintenance dose).

...ult dosage range
...– 1,600mg daily (starting dose), reduced ...00 – 400mg daily (maintenance dose).

...set of effect
...me effects may be noticed within 72 hours, ...full benefits may not be felt for up to ...eeks.

...ration of action
...to 1 month.

Diet advice
None.

Storage
Keep in a closed container in a cool, dry place away from reach of children. Protect from light.

Missed dose
Take as soon as you remember. If your next dose is due within 12 hours, do not take the missed dose. Take your next scheduled dose as usual.

Stopping the drug
Do not stop the drug without consulting your physician; symptoms may recur.

Exceeding the dose
An occasional unintentional extra dose is unlikely to cause problems. Large overdoses may cause nausea, vomiting, dizziness, and abnormal heartbeat. Notify your physician.

POSSIBLE ADVERSE EFFECTS

...odarone has a number of unusual *side ...cts*, including a metallic taste in the mouth, increased sensitivity of the skin to sunlight, and a grayish skin color.

...mptom/effect	Frequency		Discuss with physician		Stop taking drug now	Call physician now
	Common	Rare	Only if severe	In all cases		
...sea/vomiting	●		■			
...allic taste		●	■			
...dache		●		■		
...red vision		●		■		
...t-sensitive rash	●			■		
...akness/fatigue		●		■		
...ful breathing		●		■		
...y skin color		●		■		

INTERACTIONS

...arfarin Amiodarone may increase the ...ticoagulant effect of warfarin.

...uretics The potassium loss caused by ...ese drugs may increase toxic effects of ...niodarone.

Other anti-arrhythmic drugs Amiodarone is likely to increase the effects of drugs such as beta blockers, disopyramide, digoxin, procainamide, and quinidine, causing abnormal heart rhythms.

SPECIAL PRECAUTIONS

Be sure to tell your physician if:
▼ You have impaired liver function.
▼ You have heart disease.
▼ You have eye disease.
▼ You have a lung disorder such as asthma or bronchitis.
▼ You have a thyroid disorder.
▼ You are taking other medications.

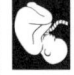

Pregnancy
▼ Not usually prescribed. May cause thyroid disease and slow heartbeat in newborn infants. Discuss with your physician.

Breast feeding
▼ The drug passes into the breast milk and may affect the baby. Discuss with your physician.

Infants and children
▼ Not recommended.

Over 60
▼ Increased likelihood of adverse effects. Reduced dose may therefore be necessary.

Driving and hazardous work
▼ No known problems.

Alcohol
▼ No known problems.

Surgery and general anesthetics
▼ Amiodarone treatment may need to be stopped before you have a general anesthetic. Discuss with your physician or dentist before any surgery.

PROLONGED USE

Prolonged use of this drug may cause a number of adverse effects on the eyes, lungs, thyroid gland, and liver.

Monitoring Blood may be taken periodically to measure levels of the drug and to check hormone levels and liver function. Regular ophthalmic examination is recommended.

AMITRIPTYLINE

Brand names Elavil, Apo-Amitriptyline, Novo-Tryptin
Used in the following combined preparations Elavil Plus, Etrafon, PMS-Levazine, Triavil

GENERAL INFORMATION

Amitriptyline belongs to a class of antidepressant drugs known as the tricyclics. It is used mainly in the long-term treatment of depression. It elevates mood, increases physical activity, improves appetite, and restores interest in everyday activities.

More sedating than some of the other tricyclic antidepressants, amitriptyline is useful when depression is accompanied by anxiety and insomnia. Taken at night, it encourages sleep and helps to eliminate the need for additional sleeping drugs. It is sometimes used for treating bedwetting in children.

In overdose amitriptyline may cause coma and dangerously abnormal heart rhythms.

QUICK REFERENCE

Drug group Tricyclic antidepressant drug (p.96)

Overdose danger rating High

Dependence rating Low

Prescription needed Yes

Multi-source suppliers Yes

INFORMATION FOR USERS

Your drug prescription is tailored for you. Do not alter dosage without checking with your physician.

How taken

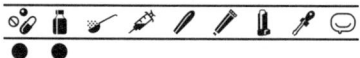

Tablets, oral liquid.

Frequency and timing of doses
1 – 4 x daily.

Dosage range
Adults 25 – 300mg daily.
Children (for bedwetting) 10 – 25mg, according to age, at bedtime.

Onset of effect
Can appear within hours, though full antidepressant effect may not be felt for 2 – 4 weeks.

Duration of action
Antidepressant effect may last for 6 weeks; adverse effects, only a few days.

Diet advice
None.

Storage
Keep in a closed container in a cool, dry place away from reach of children. Protect from light.

Missed dose
Take as soon as you remember. If your next dose is due within 3 hours, take a single dose now and skip the next.

Stopping the drug
Consult your physician, who may supervise a gradual reduction in dosage.

OVERDOSE ACTION

 Seek immediate medical advice in all cases. Take emergency action if palpitations are noted or consciousness is lost.

See Drug poisoning emergency guide (p.574).

SPECIAL PRECAUTIONS

Be sure to tell your physician if:
▼ You have heart problems.
▼ You have had epileptic seizures.
▼ You have impaired liver or kidney function
▼ You have had glaucoma.
▼ You have urinary difficulties.
▼ You have thyroid disease.
▼ You are taking other medications.

 **Pregnancy**
▼ Safety in pregnancy not established. Discuss with your physician.

 Breast feeding
▼ The drug passes into the breast milk. Discuss with your physician.

 Infants and children
▼ Not recommended for the treatment of depression in children under 12 years. Reduced dose necessary in older children.

 Over 60
▼ Increased likelihood of adverse effects. Reduced dose may therefore be necessary initially.

 Driving and hazardous work
▼ Avoid such activities until you have learned how the drug affects you; it can cause blurred vision and reduced alertness.

 Alcohol
▼ Avoid. Alcohol may increase the sedative effects of this drug.

Surgery and general anesthetics
▼ Amitriptyline treatment may need to be stopped before you have a general anesthetic. Discuss this with your physician or dentist before any operation.

POSSIBLE ADVERSE EFFECTS

The possible adverse effects of this drug are mainly the result of its *anticholinergic* action and its blocking action on the transmission of signals through the heart.

Symptom/effect	Frequency		Discuss with physician		Stop taking drug now	Call physician now
	Common	Rare	Only if severe	In all cases		
Drowsiness	●		■			
Sweating/flushing	●		■			
Dry mouth	●		■			
Blurred vision	●			■		
Dizziness/fainting	●			■		
Difficulty passing urine		●		■	▲	
Palpitations		●		■	▲	■

INTERACTIONS

Sedatives All drugs, including alcohol, that have sedative effects intensify those of amitriptyline.

Antihypertensive drugs Amitriptyline may reduce the effectiveness of some of these drugs.

Monoamine oxidase inhibitors (MAOIs) Usually, amitriptyline should not be given during or within 14 days of treatment with an MAOI. Serious reaction may occur. Such drugs are prescribed together only under strict medical supervision.

PROLONGED USE

No problems expected.

Monitoring Periodic blood tests may be performed.

AMLODIPINE

rand name Norvasc
sed in the following combined preparations None

GENERAL INFORMATION

mlodipine belongs to a group of drugs
nown as calcium channel blockers,
hich interfere with the conduction of
gnals in the muscles of the heart and
ood vessels.
Amlodipine is used in the treatment
angina to help prevent attacks of
nest pain. Unlike some other anti-
ngina drugs (i.e., beta blockers), it can
used safely by asthmatics and non-
sulin-dependent diabetics. It is often
successful when other treatments have
failed. Amlodipine is also used to reduce
raised blood pressure.

In common with other drugs of its
class, amlodipine may cause blood
pressure to fall too low. In rare cases,
angina may become worse at the start
of amlodipine therapy. This drug may
cause mild to moderate leg and ankle
swelling.

INFORMATION FOR USERS

ur drug prescription is tailored for you.
not alter dosage without checking
th your physician.

w taken

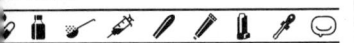

lets.

equency and timing of doses
gina – once daily.
pertension – once daily.

ult dosage range
gina 5 – 10mg daily.
pertension 5 – 10mg daily.

set of effect
12 hours.

ration of action
hours.

t advice
ne.

Storage
Keep in a closed container in a cool, dry place
away from reach of children. Protect from
light.

Missed dose
If you miss a dose and you remember it within
12 hours, take it as soon as you remember.
However, if you do not remember until later,
do not take the missed dose at all and do not
double up the next one. Instead, go back to
your regular schedule.

Stopping the drug
Do not stop taking the drug without consulting
your physician; symptoms may recur.

Exceeding the dose
An occasional unintentional extra dose is
unlikely to cause problems. Large overdoses
may cause a marked lowering of blood
pressure. Notify your physician immediately.

SPECIAL PRECAUTIONS

Be sure to tell your physician if:
▼ You have impaired kidney or liver function.
▼ You have heart failure.
▼ You have diabetes.
▼ You are taking other medications.

Pregnancy
▼ Safety in pregnancy not
established. Discuss with your
physician.

Breast feeding
▼ It is not known if the drug passes
into the breast milk. Discuss with
your physician.

Infants and children
▼ Not recommended.

Over 60
▼ Increased likelihood of adverse
effects. Reduced dose may
therefore be necessary.

Driving and hazardous work
▼ Avoid such activities until you
have learned how the drug affects
you; it can cause dizziness owing to
lowered blood pressure.

Alcohol
▼ Avoid. Alcohol may further
reduce blood pressure, causing
dizziness or other symptoms.

POSSIBLE ADVERSE EFFECTS

lodipine can cause a variety of minor
erse effects, including leg and ankle
elling, headache, dizziness, fatigue, and
sea. Dizziness, especially on rising, may be
sed by an excessive reduction in blood
pressure. The most serious effect is the rare
possibility of angina becoming worse after
starting amlodipine treatment. This should be
reported to your physician.

mptom/effect	Frequency		Discuss with physician		Stop taking drug now	Call physician now
	Common	Rare	Only if severe	In all cases		
and ankle swelling	●		■			
adache	●		■			
ziness/fatigue	●		■			
shing	●		■			
sea/abdominal pain		●		■		
cramps		●	■			
wsiness		●	■			
itations		●				■

INTERACTIONS

eta blockers Amlodipine may increase
e effect of these drugs.

AMOXICILLIN

Brand names Amoxil, Apo-Amoxi, Novamoxin, Nu-Amoxi
Used in the following combined preparation Clavulin

GENERAL INFORMATION

Amoxicillin is a penicillin antibiotic. It is prescribed to treat a variety of infections but is particularly useful for the treatment of ear, nose, and throat infections, cystitis, uncomplicated gonorrhea, and certain skin and soft tissue infections.

When taken by mouth, amoxicillin is absorbed well by the body, and it works quickly and effectively.

As with other penicillin antibiotics, the most common *side effect* of amoxicillin is a blotchy skin rash. It can also provoke a more severe allergic reaction, causing symptoms of fever, swelling of the mouth and tongue, itching, and breathing difficulties.

INFORMATION FOR USERS

Your drug prescription is tailored for you. Do not alter dosage without checking with your physician.

How taken

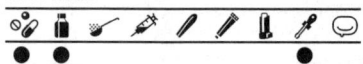

Capsules, chewable tablets, oral liquid, pediatric drops.

Frequency and timing of doses
3 x daily.

Dosage range
Adults 750mg – 1.5g daily.
Children Reduced dose according to age and weight.

Onset of effect
Symptoms usually improve within 1 – 2 days, depending on the condition.

Duration of action
Up to 8 hours.

Diet advice
None.

Storage
Keep tablets and capsules in a closed container in a cool, dry place away from reach of children. Refrigerate liquid and pediatric drops, but do not freeze and keep for no longer than 14 days.

Missed dose
Take as soon as you remember. If your next dose is due at this time, double the usual dose to make up the missed dose.

Stopping the drug
Take the full course. Even if you feel better, the original infection may still be present and symptoms may recur if treatment is stopped too soon.

Exceeding the dose
An occasional unintentional extra dose is unlikely to be a cause for concern. But if you notice any unusual symptoms, or if a large overdose has been taken, notify your physician.

SPECIAL PRECAUTIONS

Be sure to tell your physician if:
▼ You have impaired kidney function.
▼ You have an allergy (for example, asthma, hay fever, or eczema).
▼ You have had a rash after being given a penicillin or cephalosporin antibiotic.
▼ You have ulcerative colitis.
▼ You have infectious mononucleosis.
▼ You are taking other medications.

Pregnancy
▼ Is prescribed during pregnancy, but risks to baby have not been fully established. Discuss with your physician.

Breast feeding
▼ The drug passes into the milk and may affect the baby. Discuss with your physician.

Infants and children
▼ Reduced dose necessary.

Over 60
▼ No known problems.

Driving and hazardous work
▼ No known problems.

Alcohol
▼ No known problems.

POSSIBLE ADVERSE EFFECTS

If you develop a rash, wheezing, itching, fever, or joint swelling, this may indicate an allergy. Call your physician, who may prescribe a different antibiotic.

Symptom/effect	Frequency		Discuss with physician		Stop taking drug now	Call physician now
	Common	Rare	Only if severe	In all cases		
Diarrhea	●			■		
Rash	●			■	▲	▮
Nausea/vomiting		●	■			
Unusual thirst		●	■			
Tiredness/weakness		●	■			
Wheezing		●		■	▲	▮
Itching		●		■	▲	▮
Swollen mouth/tongue		●		■	▲	▮

INTERACTIONS

Oral contraceptives Amoxicillin may reduce the effectiveness of oral contraceptive tablets and also increase the risk of breakthrough bleeding. Discuss with your physician.

PROLONGED USE

Amoxicillin is usually given only for short courses of treatment.

AMPHOTERICIN B

Brand name Fungizone
Used in the following combined preparations None

GENERAL INFORMATION

Amphotericin B is a highly effective and powerful antifungal drug. Usually administered by intravenous injection, it is used in cases of serious *systemic* fungal infections.
Treatment by injection is carefully supervised, usually in the hospital, because of adverse effects.

INFORMATION FOR USERS

The drug is given only under medical supervision and is not for self-administration.

How taken

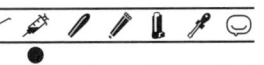

Action.

Frequency and timing of doses
Daily over a period of approximately 6 hours.

Adult dosage range
The dosage for injection is determined individually. Total daily dosage should not exceed 50mg/day.

Onset of effect
Several weeks of amphotericin B therapy may be required to clear an infection.

Duration of action
The effect may persist for several weeks after treatment has been stopped.

Diet advice
Amphotericin B may reduce the levels of potassium and magnesium in the blood. Mineral supplements may be recommended.

Storage
Not applicable. This drug is not normally kept at home.

Missed dose
Not applicable. This drug is given only in a hospital under close medical supervision.

Stopping the drug
This drug is stopped under medical supervision.

Exceeding the dose
Overdosage is unlikely, since treatment is carefully monitored.

POSSIBLE ADVERSE EFFECTS

Amphotericin B is given under close medical supervision only. Adverse effects are thus carefully monitored and promptly treated.

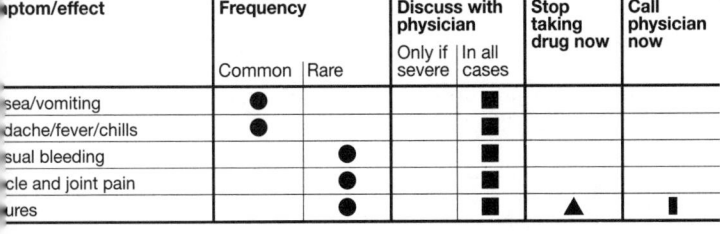

Symptom/effect	Frequency		Discuss with physician		Stop taking drug now	Call physician now
	Common	Rare	Only if severe	In all cases		
Nausea/vomiting	●			■		
Headache/fever/chills	●			■		
Unusual bleeding		●		■		
Muscle and joint pain		●		■		
Seizures		●		■	▲	∎

INTERACTIONS

Digoxin Amphotericin B increases the toxicity of digoxin.

Diuretics Amphotericin B increases the risk of low potassium levels with diuretics.

Aminoglycoside antibiotics Taken with amphotericin B, these drugs increase the likelihood of kidney damage.

SPECIAL PRECAUTIONS

Be sure to tell your physician if:
▼ You have impaired kidney function.
▼ You have previously had an allergic reaction to amphotericin.
▼ You are taking other medications.

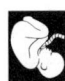 **Pregnancy**
▼ Injections are given only when the infection is life-threatening.

 Breast feeding
▼ Given by injection, the drug passes into the breast milk. Discuss with your physician.

 Infants and children
▼ The drug is given by injection only in life-threatening conditions.

 Over 60
▼ No special problems.

 Driving and hazardous work
▼ No known problems.

 Alcohol
▼ No known problems.

PROLONGED USE

Amphotericin B injection may cause a reduction in blood levels of potassium and magnesium. It may also damage the kidneys and cause blood disorders.

Monitoring Regular blood tests to monitor kidney function are advised during treatment.

AMPICILLIN

Brand names Penbritin, Ampicin, Apo-Ampi, Novo-Ampicillin, Nu-Ampi
Used in the following combined preparations None

GENERAL INFORMATION

Ampicillin, a penicillin antibiotic available since 1962, is prescribed to treat a variety of infections.

In common with other penicillin antibiotics, it is particularly useful for treating ear, nose, and throat infections, infections in the respiratory tract, cystitis, uncomplicated gonorrhea, and certain skin and soft tissue infections.

When given in large doses by injection, ampicillin is effective in the treatment of more serious infections, such as meningitis and pyelonephritis. It may also be prescribed to treat biliary tract infections and typhoid fever.

Gastrointestinal infections caused by salmonella and shigella bacteria may sometimes by treated with ampicillin. As with other penicillin antibiotics, rashes are not uncommon. More severe allergic reactions are also possible.

QUICK REFERENCE

Drug group Penicillin antibiotic (p.140)

Overdose danger rating Low

Dependence rating Low

Prescription needed Yes

Multi-source suppliers Yes

INFORMATION FOR USERS

Your drug prescription is tailored for you. Do not alter dosage without checking with your physician.

How taken

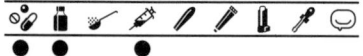

Capsules, oral liquid, injection.

Frequency and timing of doses
4 x daily on an empty stomach.

Dosage range
Adults 1 – 2g daily (by mouth).
Children Reduced dose according to age and weight.

Onset of effect
Symptoms usually improve within 1 – 2 days, depending on the condition.

Duration of action
6 – 8 hours.

Diet advice
None.

Storage
Keep capsules in a closed container in a cool, dry place away from reach of children. Refrigerate liquid, but do not freeze and do not keep for longer than 14 days.

Missed dose
Take as soon as you remember. If your next dose is due at this time, double the usual dose to make up the missed dose.

Stopping the drug
Take the full course. Even if you feel better, the original infection may still be present and symptoms may recur if treatment is stopped too soon.

Exceeding the dose
An occasional unintentional extra dose is unlikely to be a cause for concern. But if you notice unusual symptoms, or if a large overdose has been taken, notify your physician.

SPECIAL PRECAUTIONS

Be sure to tell your physician if:
▼ You have impaired kidney function.
▼ You have an allergy (for example, asthma, hay fever, eczema, or hives).
▼ You have had a rash after taking a penicillin or cephalosporin antibiotic.
▼ You have had ulcerative colitis.
▼ You have recently had infectious mononucleosis.
▼ You are taking other medications.

Pregnancy
▼ Is prescribed during pregnancy, but risks to baby have not been fully established. Discuss with your physician.

Breast feeding
▼ The drug passes into the breast milk and may affect the baby. Discuss with your physician.

Infants and children
▼ Reduced dose necessary.

Over 60
▼ No known problems.

Driving and hazardous work
▼ No known problems.

Alcohol
▼ No known problems.

POSSIBLE ADVERSE EFFECTS

If you develop a rash, wheezing, itching, fever, or joint swelling, this may indicate an allergy.

Call your physician, who may prescribe a different antibiotic.

Symptom/effect	Frequency		Discuss with physician		Stop taking drug now	Call physician now
	Common	Rare	Only if severe	In all cases		
Diarrhea	●			■		
Rash	●			■	▲	∎
Nausea/vomiting		●	■			
Unusual thirst		●	■			
Tiredness/weakness		●	■			
Wheezing		●		■	▲	∎
Itching		●		■	▲	∎
Swollen mouth/tongue		●		■	▲	∎

PROLONGED USE

Ampicillin is usually only given for short courses of treatment.

INTERACTIONS

Oral contraceptives Ampicillin may reduce the effectiveness of oral contraceptive tablets and also increase the risk of breakthrough bleeding. Discuss with your physician.

ANTHRALIN

and names Anthraforte, Anthranol, Anthrascalp
ed in the following combined preparations None

GENERAL INFORMATION

thralin, introduced in 1936, is an
ective *topical* non-steroidal agent for
derately severe psoriasis. Applied as
tion, cream, or ointment, it restores
cessive skin growth to normal. It is
metimes accompanied by periodic
aviolet (UVA) treatments to boost its
ect.
f psoriasis is particularly severe,
atment at a specialized outpatient
ter may be recommended.
wever, most people can use the drug
home, leaving it on either overnight or
up to 30 minutes each day. Since the

drug may stain clothes and bed linen,
these should be protected.
Anthralin frequently causes irritation
or redness of normal skin around the
treated areas, especially at high
concentrations. A protective coat of
petrolatum applied to normal skin
before using the drug helps to minimize
such effects; plastic gloves should be
worn during application. Raw, blistered,
or oozing areas should never be treated,
and the drug should not be used on the
face, genital area, or skin folds such as
those of the neck or groin.

INFORMATION FOR USERS

d the product information carefully
ore using anthralin. Do not use more
n recommended amounts without
sulting your physician.

w taken

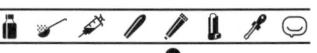

ment, cream, lotion.

quency and timing of doses
e daily, either low concentration (0.1 –
per cent) at bedtime for 8 – 12 hours
rnight treatment) or high concentration
r cent) during the day for 10 – 30 minutes
irected (short-contact treatment).
ove the medicine by washing as directed
each application.

lt dosage range
ly thinly to the affected area as directed.
strength of the preparation is increased, if
ired, as treatment continues.

et of effect
days. Full beneficial effect of the drug
not be felt for several days.

Duration of action
Up to 72 hours.

Diet advice
None.

Storage
Keep in a closed container in a cool, dry place
away from reach of children. Protect from
light.

Missed dose
Apply as soon as you remember. If not
remembered until the next morning (overnight
treatment), skip the missed application and
apply your next dose as usual. If your next
dose is due within 4 hours (short-contact
treatment), apply a single dose now and skip
the next dose.

Stopping the drug
For best results, apply the full course of
treatment.

Exceeding the dose
An occasional unintentional extra application
is unlikely to cause problems. If the cream is
left on the skin longer than recommended,
irritation and redness may result. If this occurs,
notify your physician.

SPECIAL PRECAUTIONS

**Be sure to consult your physician or
pharmacist before using this drug if:**
▼ You have impaired kidney function.
▼ You are taking other medications.

Pregnancy
▼ Safety in pregnancy not
established. Discuss with your
physician.

Breast feeding
▼ The drug passes into the breast
milk, and may affect the baby
adversely. Discuss with your
physician.

Infants and children
▼ Not recommended under
12 years.

Over 60
▼ No special problems.

Driving and hazardous work
▼ No known problems.

Alcohol
▼ No known problems.

PROLONGED USE

No special problems.

POSSIBLE ADVERSE EFFECTS

tion or redness of the skin around the
ed areas is fairly common and is usually

helped by reducing the amount or frequency
of application. Allergic skin rashes are rare.

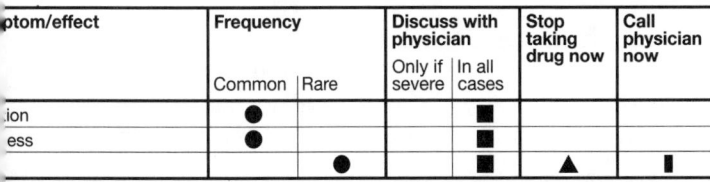

ptom/effect	Frequency		Discuss with physician		Stop taking drug now	Call physician now
	Common	Rare	Only if severe	In all cases		
ion	●			■		
ess	●			■		
		●		■	▲	∎

INTERACTIONS

neral note Any drug that increases the
sitivity of the skin to light may increase
risk of redness or irritation with
hralin. Such drugs include coal tar or

coal tar derivatives, thiazide diuretics,
griseofulvin, nalidixic acid, phenothiazine
antipsychotic drugs, sulfonamides, and
tetracycline antibiotics.

ASTEMIZOLE

Brand name Hismanal
Used in the following combined preparations None

GENERAL INFORMATION

Astemizole is an antihistamine with a prolonged duration of action. Its main use is in the treatment of allergic rhinitis, particularly hay fever. Taken as tablets or liquid, it reduces sneezing and irritation of the eyes and nose. Allergic skin conditions such as chronic urticaria (hives) may also be helped by astemizole.

The main difference between this drug and the older, traditional antihistamines is that it has little or no sedative effect on the central nervous system. It is therefore useful for people who need to avoid drowsiness – for example, at work. It also has fewer *anticholinergic* effects than older antihistamines.

Astemizole's slow onset of full thera-peutic effect makes it unsuitable for treating allergic conditions such as re-actions to food and the intense itching of skin reactions. Moreover, because of the drug's extended action in the body, it should be discontinued for at least 4 weeks prior to skin testing for allergy.

QUICK REFERENCE

Drug group Antihistamine (p.136)
Overdose danger rating Low
Dependence rating Low
Prescription needed No
Multi-source suppliers No

INFORMATION FOR USERS

Follow instructions on the label. Call your physician if symptoms worsen.

How taken

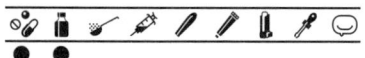

Tablets, oral liquid.

Frequency and timing of doses
Once daily on an empty stomach.

Adult dosage range
10mg daily.

Onset of effect
1 – 3 hours.

Duration of action
Up to 24 hours.

Diet advice
None.

Storage
Keep in a closed container in a cool, dry place away from reach of children.

Missed dose
If it is almost time for your next dose, take a single dose now and skip the next.

Stopping the drug
Can be safely stopped as soon as you no longer need it.

Exceeding the dose
An occasional unintentional extra dose is unlikely to be a cause for concern. But if you notice unusual symptoms, or if a large overdose has been taken, notify your physician.

SPECIAL PRECAUTIONS

Be sure to consult your physician or pharmacist before taking this drug if:
▼ You have impaired liver or kidney functio
▼ You have chronic lung disease or asthm
▼ You have had heart problems.
▼ You are taking other medications.

Pregnancy
▼ Safety in pregnancy not established. Discuss with your physician.

Breast feeding
▼ Effect on breast feeding uncertain. Discuss with your physician.

Infants and children
▼ Patients under 12 years shoul be given the drug only on a physician's advice.

Over 60
▼ Reduced dose may be necessary.

Driving and hazardous work
▼ No known problems. Unlike th older antihistamines, drowsiness does not appear to be a problem

Alcohol
▼ No known problems.

POSSIBLE ADVERSE EFFECTS

Weight gain, perhaps due to an increase in appetite, occurs occasionally with astemizole; other *side effects* are very rare. A rash may be a sign of an unusual allergic reaction.

Symptom/effect	Frequency		Discuss with physician		Stop taking drug now	Call physician now
	Common	Rare	Only if severe	In all cases		
Weight gain/increased appetite	●		■			
Headache		●	■			
Nausea/vomiting		●	■			
Rash		●		■	▲	
Confusion		●		■	▲	∎

INTERACTIONS

Antifungal drugs Ketoconazole, fluconazole, itraconazole, and possibly other antifungal drugs increase levels of astemizole, and may lead to adverse effects on the heart.

Antidepressants/antipsychotics These drugs increase the possibility of abnormal heart rhythms.

Anticholinergic drugs The anticholinergic effects of astemizole may be increased by all drugs that have anticholinergic effects, including antipsychotics and tricyclic antidepressants.

Erythromycin This drug may increase levels of astemizole and lead to adverse effects on the heart.

PROLONGED USE

Astemizole should be discontinued at least 4 weeks prior to allergy skin testing

ATENOLOL

Brand names Tenormin, Apo-Atenol, Novo-Atenol, Nu-Atenol
Used in the following combined preparation Tenoretic

GENERAL INFORMATION

Atenolol belongs to the class of drugs known as beta blockers (see p.109). It prevents the heart from beating too quickly and is mainly used to treat angina and high blood pressure.

Atenolol is sometimes given to people with lung problems because unlike some other beta blockers, it acts mainly on the heart rather than other parts of the body. It may also be given just after a heart attack to protect the heart from further damage.

Because atenolol does not cure heart disease, but only controls the symptoms, it may have to be taken continuously over a long period, even for the rest of a person's life. Atenolol stays in the body for a long time, so it only needs to be taken once a day.

INFORMATION FOR USERS

Your drug prescription is tailored for you. Do not alter dosage without checking with your physician.

How taken

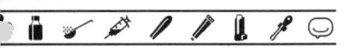

Tablets.

Frequency and timing of doses
Once daily.

Adult dosage range
Hypertension 50 – 100mg daily.
Angina 50 – 200mg daily.

Onset of effect
2 – 4 hours.

Duration of action
20 – 30 hours. Some effects may last for 2 – 3 days in people with impaired kidney function.

Diet advice
None.

Storage
Keep in a tightly closed container in a cool, dry place away from reach of children. Protect from light.

Missed dose
Take as soon as you remember. If your next dose is due within 6 hours, do not take the missed dose but take the next scheduled dose as usual.

Stopping the drug
Do not stop taking the drug without consulting your physician; withdrawal of the drug may lead to dangerous worsening of the underlying condition or precipitation of a heart attack.

OVERDOSE ACTION

Seek immediate medical advice in all cases. Take emergency action if consciousness is lost.

See Drug poisoning emergency guide (p.574).

POSSIBLE ADVERSE EFFECTS

Atenolol has adverse effects that are common to most beta blockers. Symptoms are usually temporary and diminish with long-term use.

Symptom/effect	Frequency		Discuss with physician		Stop taking drug now	Call physician now
	Common	Rare	Only if severe	In all cases		
Muscle ache	●		■			
Dizziness/lightheadedness		●	■			
Cold hands and feet		●	■			
Nightmares/sleeplessness		●	■			
Rash		●		■		
Digestive disturbances		●		■		
Breathing difficulties		●		■		■
Fatigue/depression		●		■		

SPECIAL PRECAUTIONS

Be sure to tell your physician if:
▼ You have impaired kidney function.
▼ You have poor circulation.
▼ You have allergies.
▼ You have diabetes.
▼ You have heart failure.
▼ You have a lung disorder such as emphysema, asthma, or bronchitis.
▼ You are taking other medications.

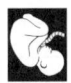

Pregnancy
▼ Safety in pregnancy not established. Discuss with your physician.

Breast feeding
▼ The drug passes into the breast milk. Discuss with your physician.

Infants and children
▼ Not recommended.

Over 60
▼ Reduced dose may be necessary if there is impaired kidney function.

Driving and hazardous work
▼ Avoid such activities until you have learned how the drug affects you; it can cause dizziness.

Alcohol
▼ No special problems with moderate intake.

Surgery and general anesthetics
▼ Atenolol may need to be stopped before you have a general anesthetic. Discuss this with your physician or dentist before any surgery.

PROLONGED USE

No special problems expected.

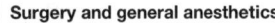

INTERACTIONS

General note Atenolol may interact with many drugs, most notably non-steroidal anti-inflammatory drugs (NSAIDs), calcium channel blockers, clonidine, and sympathomimetic decongestants.

Anti-arrhythmic drugs When used together with atenolol they may increase the risk of adverse effects on the heart.

Antidiabetic drugs used with atenolol may increase the risk and/or mask many symptoms of low blood sugar.

AURANOFIN

Brand name Ridaura
Used in the following combined preparations None

GENERAL INFORMATION

Introduced in 1985, auranofin is the only gold-based drug for rheumatoid arthritis that can be taken by mouth. The other gold drugs have to be injected, usually in a physician's office or a hospital.

Most of the drugs for rheumatoid arthritis ease the pain and soothe the inflammation (ASA and non-steroidal anti-inflammatory drugs). They do not change the course of the disease. But, auranofin and the other gold drugs are able to arrest or slow the progression of the disease. The gold drugs are toxic, however, and so long as an arthritic condition remains stable, most physicians prefer to keep a person on other treatment. But when early signs of deformity appear, signaling an increase in the pace of the disease, treatment by auranofin is appropriate. Since it can take 3 to 6 months to work, the use of analgesics and anti-inflammatory drugs is continued for that period.

Diarrhea commonly occurs and may be severe enough for treatment to be stopped. More serious effects, such as blood disorders, rashes, and impaired kidney function, occur only rarely.

INFORMATION FOR USERS

Your drug prescription is tailored for you. Do not alter dosage without checking with your physician.

How taken

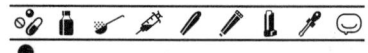

Capsules.

Frequency and timing of doses
1 – 2 x daily with food.

Adult dosage range
6mg daily. This may be increased up to a maximum of 9mg daily in some people.

Onset of effect
Adverse effects may be felt within 2 weeks. Beneficial effects may not be felt for 3 – 6 months.

Duration of action
Effects may last for several months after stopping the drug.

Diet advice
None.

Storage
Keep in a closed container in a cool, dry place away from reach of children.

Missed dose
Take as soon as you remember. If your next dose is due within 2 hours, take a single dose now and skip the next.

Stopping the drug
Do not stop the drug without consulting your physician; stopping suddenly could lead to a flare-up of rheumatoid arthritis.

Exceeding the dose
An occasional unintentional extra dose is unlikely to cause problems. Large overdoses may cause vomiting. Notify your physician.

SPECIAL PRECAUTIONS

Be sure to tell your physician if:
▼ You have impaired liver or kidney function.
▼ You have previously had an allergic reaction to gold treatment.
▼ You have inflammatory bowel disease.
▼ You have severe eczema.
▼ You have had a blood disorder.
▼ You are taking other medications.

 **Pregnancy**
▼ Safety in pregnancy not established. Discuss with your physician.

 Breast feeding
▼ The drug may pass into the breast milk and may affect the baby. Discuss with your physician.

 Infants and children
▼ Not recommended.

 Over 60
▼ No special problems.

 Driving and hazardous work
▼ No known problems.

 Alcohol
▼ No known problems.

Sunlight
▼ Direct sunlight may increase the risk of skin reactions.

POSSIBLE ADVERSE EFFECTS

The most common adverse effects of this drug include rashes that may sometimes be serious, nausea, and diarrhea. Cloudy urine may be a sign of kidney problems.

Symptom/effect	Frequency		Discuss with physician		Stop taking drug now	Call physician now
	Common	Rare	Only if severe	In all cases		
Diarrhea/nausea	●		■			
Indigestion/abdominal pain	●			■		
Conjunctivitis	●			■		
Mouth ulcers/soreness	●			■		
Rash/itching	●			■	▲	∎
Blood-tinged urine		●		■		
Easy bruising or bleeding		●		■		∎

INTERACTIONS

Penicillamine may increase the risk of impaired kidney function with auranofin and may also increase the risk of blood disorders.

PROLONGED USE

Prolonged use may rarely lead to kidney damage and blood disorders.

Monitoring Periodic blood counts, urine examination, and tests of kidney function are required.

AZATADINE

Brand name Optimine
Used in the following combined preparation Trinalin

GENERAL INFORMATION

Azatadine is an antihistamine used for treating allergic conditions. It relieves the itching, swelling, and redness of the skin caused by allergy, insect bites, or contact with irritant chemicals. Because of its relatively strong sedative effect, it is especially useful for the relief of itching at night.

Azatadine is also effective for treating allergic rhinitis because its *anticholinergic* action helps to dry up runny eyes and nose.

Longer acting than many similar drugs, azatadine retains its effect for about 12 hours. Its main disadvantage is that it frequently causes drowsiness.

INFORMATION FOR USERS

Your drug prescription is tailored for you. **Do not alter dosage without checking with your physician.**

How taken

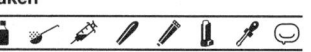

Tablets.

Frequency and timing of doses
daily.

Dosage range
Adults 2 – 4mg daily.
Children 6 – 12 years 1 – 2mg daily.

Onset of effect
60 minutes.

Duration of action
to 12 hours.

Diet advice
None.

Storage
Keep in a closed container in a cool, dry place away from reach of children.

Missed dose
Take as soon as you remember. If your next dose is due within 2 hours, take a single dose now and skip the next.

Stopping the drug
Can be safely stopped as soon as you no longer need it.

Exceeding the dose
An occasional unintentional extra dose is unlikely to cause problems. Large overdoses may cause unusual drowsiness. Notify your physician.

SPECIAL PRECAUTIONS

Be sure to tell your physician if:
▼ You have impaired liver function.
▼ You have chronic lung disease.
▼ You have had epileptic seizures.
▼ You have glaucoma.
▼ You have difficulty passing urine.
▼ You are taking other medications.

Pregnancy
▼ Safety in pregnancy not established. Discuss with your physician.

Breast feeding
▼ The drug passes into the breast milk and may affect the baby adversely. Discuss with your physician.

Infants and children
▼ Not recommended for children under 6 years.

Over 60
▼ Reduced dose may be necessary.

Driving and hazardous work
▼ Avoid such activities until you have learned how the drug affects you; it may cause drowsiness.

Alcohol
▼ Avoid. Alcohol may increase the sedative effects of this drug.

POSSIBLE ADVERSE EFFECTS

Drowsiness is the most significant adverse effect of this drug. Certain other side effects such as dry mouth and blurred vision are due to its *anticholinergic* action. Nausea and other digestive disturbances can be avoided by taking the drug with food or milk.

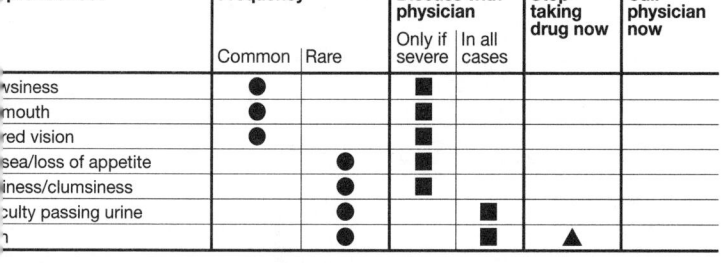

Symptom/effect	Frequency		Discuss with physician		Stop taking drug now	Call physician now
	Common	Rare	Only if severe	In all cases		
Drowsiness	●		■			
Dry mouth	●		■			
Blurred vision	●		■			
Nausea/loss of appetite		●	■			
Dizziness/clumsiness		●	■			
Difficulty passing urine		●		■		
Rash		●		■	▲	

INTERACTIONS

Sedatives All drugs, including alcohol, that have a sedative effect on the central nervous system are likely to enhance the sedative effect of azatadine.

Anticholinergic drugs The anticholinergic effects of azatadine are likely to be increased by all drugs that have anticholinergic effects, including some antiparkinsonism drugs, antipsychotic and tricyclic antidepressant drugs.

Monoamine oxidase inhibitors (MAOIs)
There is a risk of a dangerous rise in blood pressure if azatadine is taken within 14 days of MAOIs.

PROLONGED USE

The effect of the drug may become weaker over a period of weeks or months as the body adapts. Transfer to a different antihistamine may be recommended.

Antihistamines should be discontinued approximately 48 hours before allergy skin testing.

AZATHIOPRINE

Brand name Imuran
Used in the following combined preparations None

GENERAL INFORMATION

Azathioprine is an immunosuppressant drug used to prevent immune system rejection of transplanted organs. The drug is also given for severe rheumatoid arthritis that has failed to respond to conventional drug therapy.

Autoimmune and collagen diseases (including systemic lupus erythematosus, polymyositis, dermatomyositis, myasthenia gravis, and chronic inflammatory bowel disease) may also be treated with azathioprine. Often prescribed when corticosteroids have proved insufficient, azathioprine boosts the effects of these drugs, thus allowing a reduction in the dose of corticosteroids in some cases.

Azathioprine is given only under close supervision because of the risk of serious adverse effects. These include suppression of the production of white blood cells, thereby increasing the risk of infection, and the risk of excessive or prolonged bleeding.

QUICK REFERENCE

Drug group Antirheumatic drug (p.129) and immunosuppressant drug (p.168)

Overdose danger rating Medium

Dependence rating Low

Prescription needed Yes

Multi-source suppliers No

INFORMATION FOR USERS

Your drug prescription is tailored for you. Do not alter dosage without checking with your physician.

How taken

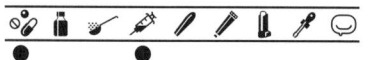

Tablets, injection.

Frequency and timing of doses
Usually once daily with food.

Dosage range
Initially according to body weight and the condition being treated and then adjusted according to response.

Onset of effect
2 – 4 weeks. Antirheumatic effect may not be felt for 8 weeks or more.

Duration of action
Immunosuppressant effects may last for several weeks after the drug is stopped.

Diet advice
None.

Storage
Keep in a closed container in a cool, dry place away from reach of children. Protect from light.

Missed dose
Take as soon as you remember, then return to your normal schedule. If more than 2 doses are missed, consult your physician.

Stopping the drug
Do not stop the drug without consulting your physician. If taken to prevent graft transplant rejection, stopping treatment could provoke rejection of the transplant.

Exceeding the dose
An occasional unintentional extra dose is unlikely to cause problems. Large overdoses may cause nausea, vomiting, abdominal pains, and diarrhea. Notify your physician.

SPECIAL PRECAUTIONS

Be sure to tell your physician if:
- ▼ You have impaired kidney or liver function.
- ▼ You have recently had shingles or chicken pox.
- ▼ You have an infection.
- ▼ You have pancreatitis.
- ▼ You have a blood disorder.
- ▼ You are taking other medications.

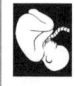

Pregnancy
▼ Not usually prescribed. But azathioprine has been taken in pregnancy without problems. Discuss with your physician.

Breast feeding
▼ The drug passes into the breast milk and may affect the baby. Discuss with your physician.

Infants and children
▼ No special problems.

Over 60
▼ Increased likelihood of adverse effects.

Driving and hazardous work
▼ No known problems.

Alcohol
▼ No known problems.

POSSIBLE ADVERSE EFFECTS

Digestive disturbances and adverse effects on the blood which could lead to sore throat, fever, and weakness are common with azathioprine. Unusual bleeding or bruising while taking this drug may be a sign of reduced levels of platelets in the blood.

Symptom/effect	Frequency		Discuss with physician		Stop taking drug now	Call physician now
	Common	Rare	Only if severe	In all cases		
Nausea/vomiting	●		■			
Weakness/fatigue	●			■		
Sore throat	●			■		▮
Fever/chills	●			■		▮
Unusual bleeding/bruising		●		■	▲	▮
Jaundice		●		■	▲	▮
Rash		●		■	▲	▮

INTERACTIONS

General note Any drug that affects the breakdown of other drugs in the liver or kidneys may alter the blood levels of azathioprine. These include phenytoin, phenobarbital, rifampin, allopurinol, and certain antibiotics. Dosage adjustments may be necessary.

PROLONGED USE

There may be an increased risk of some cancers with long-term use of azathioprine. Blood changes may also occur, but may be corrected by adjusting the dosage.

Monitoring Checks on blood composition should be carried out at regular intervals.

AZITHROMYCIN

rand name Zithromax
sed in the following combined preparations None

GENERAL INFORMATION

zithromycin is a macrolide antibiotic
fective against a wide range
f bacteria. It is a useful alternative to
enicillins and tetracyclines for people
ho are allergic to those drugs.
Azithromycin is commonly prescribed
r sinus, throat, middle ear, and chest
fections, including some rare types of
eumonia such as walking (myco-
asma) pneumonia, and in sexually
ansmitted diseases caused by

chlamydia. It can also be used to treat
infection of the skin and skin structures.
Azithromycin shows promise in the
treatment of uncommon, difficult-to-
treat infections associated with AIDS
and other states of weakened immunity.
Azithromycin may sometimes cause
abdominal cramping and discomfort or
nausea and vomiting. Other possible
adverse effects include rash and a rare
risk of liver disorders.

QUICK REFERENCE

Drug group Macrolide antibiotic
(p.138)

Overdose danger rating Low

Dependence rating Low

Prescription needed Yes

Multi-source suppliers No

INFORMATION FOR USERS

ur drug prescription is tailored for you.
 not alter dosage without consulting
ur physician.

w taken

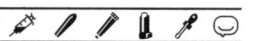

psules.

quency and timing of doses
ce daily at least 1 hour before or 2 hours
er food.

sage range
 – 500mg daily.
amydia: 1g as a single dose.

set of effect
 3 days.

ration of action
hours.

Diet advice
None.

Storage
Keep in a closed container in a cool, dry place
away from reach of children.

Missed dose
Take as soon as you remember. If your next
dose is within 6 hours, take a single dose now
and skip the next.

Stopping the drug
Take the full course. Even if you feel better, the
original infection may still be present and
symptoms may recur if treatment is stopped
too soon.

Exceeding the dose
An occasional unintentional extra dose is
unlikely to be a cause for concern. But if you
notice unusual symptoms, or if a large overdose has been taken, notify your physician.

SPECIAL PRECAUTIONS

Be sure to tell your physician if:
▼ You have a liver disease or impaired liver
function.
▼ You have had a previous allergic reaction
to a macrolide antibiotic.
▼ You are taking other medications.

Pregnancy
▼ Safety in pregnancy not
established. Discuss with your
physician.

Breast feeding
▼ It is not known if azithromycin
passes into the breast milk. Discuss
with your physician.

Infants and children
▼ Not recommended for children
under 16 years.

Over 60
▼ No special problems.

Driving and hazardous work
▼ No known problems.

Alcohol
▼ No known problems.

POSSIBLE ADVERSE EFFECTS

sea and vomiting are the most common
erse effects and are most likely to occur
large doses. Symptoms such as fever,

rash, and jaundice may be a sign of a liver
disorder and should always be reported to
your physician.

mptom/effect	Frequency		Discuss with physician		Stop taking drug now	Call physician now
	Common	Rare	Only if severe	In all cases		
sea/vomiting	●		■			
rhea	●		■			
ominal discomfort	●		■			
h/itching		●		■	▲	
ndice		●		■	▲	▌
lling/breathing difficulties		●		■	▲	▌

PROLONGED USE

Prolonged use may increase the risk of
liver damage in patients with impaired
liver function.

INTERACTIONS

me of the following interactions have
en reported with another macrolide
tibiotic, erythromycin, and may occur
th azithromycin.

closporine, digoxin, triazolam, and
eophylline Erythromycin may increase
 risk of *side effects* with these drugs.

rfenadine and astemizole Erythro-
ycin increases the risk of adverse effects
these antihistamines on the heart.

Warfarin Erythromycin increases the risk
of bleeding with warfarin.

Ergotamine Erythromycin may increase
the risk of side effects with this drug.

Antacids may reduce the absorption of
azithromycin and should not be taken
simultaneously with the antibiotic.

BACITRACIN

Brand names Baciguent, Bacitin
Used in the following combined preparations Bioderm, Cortisporin, Neosporin, Polysporin (ointments), Polytopic

GENERAL INFORMATION

Introduced in 1948, bacitracin is a *topical* antibiotic used mainly for staphylococcal and streptococcal infections of the skin, outer ear, and eyelids. It is combined with other drugs into ointments that have a wide spectrum of bacteria-killing action. Some bacitracin preparations contain a corticosteroid to help in the relief of skin inflammation.

When applied to the skin, bacitracin rarely causes adverse effects. What harmful reactions do occur usually result from the other drugs in a combined preparation.

Not readily absorbed in the digestive tract, bacitracin has been used on an investigational basis to treat certain inflammatory infections of the large intestine. Other newer drugs are just as effective, however, and less risky. Bacitracin can cause kidney damage, especially in the rare cases when it is given by injection.

INFORMATION FOR USERS

Follow instructions on the label. Call your physician if symptoms worsen.

How taken

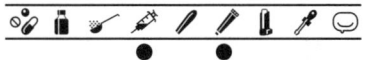

Injection, ointment.

Frequency and timing of doses
1 – 4 x daily.

Dosage range
Enough to cover the affected area at each application (ointment).

Onset of effect
1 – 2 hours (ointment).

Duration of action
Up to 24 hours.

Diet advice
None.

Storage
Keep ointment in a closed container in a cool, dry place away from reach of children.

Missed dose
Apply ointment as soon as you remember.

Stopping the drug
Apply the full course. Even if you feel better, the original infection may still be present and may recur if treatment is stopped too soon.

Exceeding the dose
An occasional unintentional extra dose is unlikely to be a cause for concern. But if you notice unusual symptoms, or if the drug has been swallowed, notify your physician.

SPECIAL PRECAUTIONS

Be sure to consult your physician or pharmacist before using this drug if:
▼ You have impaired kidney function.
▼ You are allergic to bacitracin.
▼ You are taking other medications.

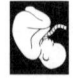
Pregnancy
▼ No evidence of risk with topical preparations. Doses by injection may adversely affect the developing baby. Discuss with your physician.

Breast feeding
▼ No evidence of risk with topical preparations. Injected, this drug passes into the breast milk and may affect the baby adversely. Discuss with your physician.

Infants and children
▼ No special problems with topical preparations.

Over 60
▼ Use by injection is avoided because of the risk of kidney damage.

Driving and hazardous work
▼ No known problems.

Alcohol
▼ No known problems.

POSSIBLE ADVERSE EFFECTS

Used topically, bacitracin rarely causes adverse effects. Injection treatment is only undertaken in the hospital, where any side effects can be closely monitored.

Symptom/effect	Frequency		Discuss with physician		Stop taking drug now	Call physician now
	Common	Rare	Only if severe	In all cases		
Topical preparations						
Skin irritation/rash		●		■	▲	
Injection						
Rash		●		■		▮
Dark/cloudy urine		●		■		▮

INTERACTIONS

General note Any drug that has adverse effects on kidney function increases the risk of such effects with bacitracin injection. Such drugs include streptomycin, polymyxin B, and neomycin.

PROLONGED USE

Prolonged use of this drug by injection may lead to kidney damage.

Monitoring Periodic kidney function tests are recommended when the drug is taken by injection.

BACLOFEN

Brand names Lioresal, Alpha-Baclofen, PMS-Baclofen
Used in the following combined preparations None

GENERAL INFORMATION

Baclofen is a muscle-relaxant drug that acts on the central nervous system, including the spinal cord. It relieves the spasms, cramping, and rigidity of muscles caused by such disorders as multiple sclerosis and spinal cord injury. It is also used to treat spasticity due to brain injury, cerebral palsy, and some other spinal cord disorders.

Although this drug does not cure these disorders, it increases mobility, allowing other treatment, such as physiotherapy, to be carried out.

Baclofen is less likely to cause muscle weakness than similar drugs, and its *side effects*, such as dizziness and drowsiness, are usually temporary. Elderly people in particular may experience unusual excitement, and confusion or hallucinations.

INFORMATION FOR USERS

Your drug prescription is tailored for you. Do not alter dosage without checking with your physician.

How taken

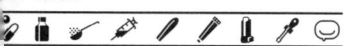

Tablets.

Frequency and timing of doses
1 x daily with food or milk.

Adult dosage range
5mg daily (starting dose) for 3 days, increased by 5mg every 3 days as required up to 80mg daily.

Onset of effect
Some benefits may appear after 2 – 3 hours, but full beneficial effects may not be felt for several weeks.

Duration of action
Up to 8 hours.

Diet advice
None.

Storage
Keep in a closed container in a cool, dry place away from reach of children. Protect from light.

Missed dose
Take as soon as you remember. If your next dose is due within 2 hours, take a single dose now and skip the next.

Stopping the drug
Do not stop taking the drug without consulting your physician. Abrupt cessation may cause hallucinations and seizures.

Exceeding the dose
An occasional unintentional extra dose is unlikely to cause problems. Large overdoses may cause weakness, vomiting, and severe drowsiness. Notify your physician.

SPECIAL PRECAUTIONS

Be sure to tell your physician if:
▼ You have impaired liver or kidney function.
▼ You have had a peptic ulcer.
▼ You have had epileptic seizures.
▼ You have diabetes.
▼ You have breathing problems.
▼ You are taking other medications.

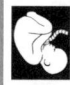

Pregnancy
▼ Safety in pregnancy not established. Discuss with your physician.

Breast feeding
▼ The drug passes into the breast milk and may affect the baby adversely. Discuss with your physician.

Infants and children
▼ Not recommended in patients under 12 years.

Over 60
▼ Increased likelihood of adverse effects. Reduced dose necessary.

Driving and hazardous work
▼ Avoid such activities until you have learned how the drug affects you, because the drug can cause dizziness and drowsiness.

Alcohol
▼ Avoid. Alcohol may increase the sedative effects of this drug.

Surgery and general anesthetics
▼ Be sure to inform your physician or dentist that you are taking baclofen before you have a general anesthetic.

POSSIBLE ADVERSE EFFECTS

The common adverse effects are related to the sedative effects of the drug. Such effects can be minimized by starting with a low dose that is gradually increased.

Symptom/effect	Frequency		Discuss with physician		Stop taking drug now	Call physician now
	Common	Rare	Only if severe	In all cases		
Dizziness	●		■			
Drowsiness	●		■			
Nausea	●		■			
Muscle fatigue/weakness	●			■		
Constipation/diarrhea		●	■			
Headache		●	■			
Confusion		●		■		

INTERACTIONS

Antidiabetic drugs Baclofen may increase blood sugar levels, so the dosage may need to be adjusted accordingly.

Antihypertensive drugs Baclofen may increase the blood pressure-lowering effect of such drugs.

Sedatives and monoamine oxidase inhibitors (MAOIs) All such drugs with central nervous system depressant effects may increase the sedative properties of baclofen.

Antiparkinsonian drugs Some drugs used to treat Parkinson's disease may cause confusion and hallucinations if taken with baclofen.

Tricyclic antidepressants may increase the effects of baclofen leading to muscle weakness.

PROLONGED USE

No problems expected.

BECLOMETHASONE

Brand names Beclodisk, Becloforte, Beclovent, Beconase, Propaderm, Vancenase, Vanceril
Used in the following combined preparations Propaderm C

GENERAL INFORMATION

Beclomethasone is a corticosteroid drug prescribed to relieve the symptoms of allergic rhinitis (as a nasal spray) and to control asthma (as an inhalant). It controls nasal symptoms by reducing inflammation and mucus production in the nose. It also helps to reduce chest symptoms, such as wheezing and coughing, by reducing inflammation in the bronchi. People who suffer from asthma may take beclomethasone to reduce the severity and frequency of attacks. However, once an attack has started, this drug does not relieve symptoms.

Beclomethasone is given primarily to people with asthma who require regular use of *bronchodilators* (p.104). Fungal infection causing irritation of the mouth and throat is a possible *side effect* of beclomethasone treatment that can, to a certain degree, be avoided by thoroughly rinsing the mouth and gargling with water after each inhalation.

Creams, lotions, and ointments are available for relief of inflammatory skin conditions. As beclomethasone is given *topically* it is not absorbed by the body to any great extent. Instructions must be followed carefully for the drug to be fully effective.

QUICK REFERENCE

Drug group Corticosteroid (p.153)

Overdose danger rating Low

Dependence rating Low

Prescription needed Yes

Multi-source suppliers Yes

INFORMATION FOR USERS

Your drug prescription is tailored for you. Do not alter dosage without checking with your physician.

How taken

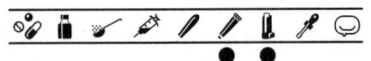

Topical lotion, cream, ointment, inhaler, nasal spray.

Frequency and timing of doses
2 – 4 x daily (inhaler, nasal spray);
1 – 2 x daily (lotion, cream, ointment).

Dosage range
Adults 1 – 2 puffs 2 – 4 x daily (asthma);
1 – 2 sprays in each nostril 2 – 4 x daily (allergic rhinitis); as directed (skin conditions).
Children Reduced dose according to age and weight.

Onset of effect
Within 1 week (asthma); 1 – 3 days (allergic rhinitis). Full benefit may not be felt for up to 4 weeks.

Duration of action
Several days after stopping the drug.

Diet advice
None.

Storage
Keep in a closed container in a cool, dry place away from reach of children. Protect from light.

Missed dose
Take as soon as you remember. If your next dose is due within 2 hours, take a single dose now and skip the next.

Stopping the drug
Do not stop the drug without consulting your physician; symptoms may recur. A gradual reduction in dosage may be recommended.

Exceeding the dose
An occasional unintentional extra dose is unlikely to be a cause for concern. But if you notice unusual symptoms, or if a large overdose has been taken, notify your physician. Adverse effects may occur if the recommended dose is regularly exceeded over a prolonged period.

SPECIAL PRECAUTIONS

Be sure to tell your physician if:
▼ You have had tuberculosis or another respiratory infection.
▼ You are taking other medications.

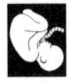

Pregnancy
▼ No evidence of risk. Discuss wit your physician.

Breast feeding
▼ The drug passes into the breast milk, but at normal doses adverse effects on the baby are unlikely. Discuss with your physician.

Infants and children
▼ Not recommended in patients under 3 years. Reduced dose necessary in older children.

Over 60
▼ No known problems.

Driving and hazardous work
▼ No known problems.

Alcohol
▼ No known problems.

POSSIBLE ADVERSE EFFECTS

Adverse effects are unlikely as the dose used is low. The main *side effects* are irritation of the nasal passages and fungal infection of the throat and mouth.

Symptom/effect	Frequency		Discuss with physician		Stop taking drug now	Call physician now
	Common	Rare	Only if severe	In all cases		
Nasal discomfort/irritation	●		■			
Cough	●		■			
Sore/dry throat	●			■		
Nosebleed		●		■		

PROLONGED USE

Long-term topical application may cause permanent thinning of the skin.

Monitoring Periodic checks to make sure that the adrenal glands are functioning healthily may be required if large doses are being used.

INTERACTIONS

None.

BENZOCAINE

Brand names Orajel, Topicaine
Used in the following combined preparations Anbesol Gel, Auralgan, Bionet, Dermoplast, Slim Mint

GENERAL INFORMATION

Benzocaine, introduced in 1905, is one of the earliest local anesthetics. A gel formulation is available for short-term relief of toothache in adults and teething pains in infants. The pain of minor burns, sunburn, abrasions, and anal discomfort may be relieved by benzocaine in spray form.

Benzocaine is also given to relieve pain and prevent gagging prior to dental treatment, oral surgery, and medical examination of the mouth, throat, trachea, or esophagus. Occasionally, it is used in ear drops

to relieve pain caused by ear inflammation. It can also be taken as a lozenge either for the relief of sore throat or for suppressing appetite, although there is no proof of its effectiveness as a diet aid.

Poorly absorbed through the skin and mucous membranes, the drug rarely causes adverse effects, though allergic reactions may occur occasionally. It should not be used for more than a few days except under medical supervision, since it could mask the symptoms of a more serious disease.

QUICK REFERENCE

Drug group Local anesthetic (p.92)
Overdose danger rating Low
Dependence rating Low
Prescription needed No
Multi-source suppliers Yes

INFORMATION FOR USERS

Follow instructions on the label. Call your physician if symptoms worsen.

How taken

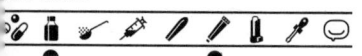

Oral liquid, gel, lozenges, spray.

Frequency and timing of doses
As needed.

Dosage range
Apply gel or liquid thinly to the affected area. Apply spray for 1 second, and repeat the application if necessary.

Onset of effect
About 1 minute.

Duration of action
0 – 30 minutes.

Diet advice
Benzocaine by mouth causes numbness of the mouth and throat and may interfere with

swallowing. To avoid choking and injury to the inside of your mouth from hot food or drink, do not eat or drink anything for 1 hour afterwards.

Storage
Keep in a closed container in a cool, dry place away from reach of children.

Missed dose
Use as soon as you remember if still required.

Stopping the drug
Can be safely stopped as soon as you no longer need it.

Exceeding the dose
An occasional unintentional extra application is unlikely to be a cause for concern. But if you notice unusual symptoms, or if a large overdose has been taken, notify your physician.

SPECIAL PRECAUTIONS

Be sure to consult your physician or pharmacist before using this drug if:
▼ You have ever had an allergic reaction to a local anesthetic.
▼ You are taking other medications.

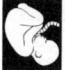
Pregnancy
▼ No evidence of risk to the developing baby.

Breast feeding
▼ No evidence of risk. Avoid use on or around nipples.

Infants and children
▼ Use with caution.

Over 60
▼ No special problems.

Driving and hazardous work
▼ No known problems.

Alcohol
▼ No known problems.

POSSIBLE ADVERSE EFFECTS

Adverse effects are rare with short-term use of benzocaine. Allergic reactions such as

burning, stinging, redness, itching, and swelling may occasionally occur.

Symptom/effect	Frequency		Discuss with physician		Stop taking drug now	Call physician now
	Common	Rare	Only if severe	In all cases		
Burning/stinging		●		■	▲	
Itching/redness		●		■	▲	
Swelling		●		■	▲	
Rash		●		■	▲	

INTERACTIONS

None.

PROLONGED USE

This drug should not be used for prolonged periods. If your symptoms do not improve within a few days, consult your physician.

BENZOYL PEROXIDE

Brand names Acnomel B.P.5, Benzac W, Benzagel, Dermoxyl, Loroxide, Solugel
Used in the following combined preparations Persol, Persol Forte, Sulfoxyl

GENERAL INFORMATION

Benzoyl peroxide, introduced for medical use in 1931, is used in *topical* preparations for the treatment of acne. Available over the counter and by prescription, it comes in concentrations of varying strengths. It is often added to tinted preparations that camouflage as well as treat the condition.

Benzoyl peroxide works by removing the top layer of skin and unblocking the sebaceous glands. It also reduces inflammation of blocked hair follicles by killing bacteria that infect them.

It may cause irritation due to its drying effect on the skin, but this generally diminishes with time. The drug should be left on the skin for about 15 minutes initially and then washed off. The length of exposure can then be increased as the body adapts. *Side effects* are less likely if treatment is started with a preparation containing a low concentration of benzoyl peroxide and changed to a stronger preparation only if necessary. Marked dryness and peeling of the skin, which may occur with overuse, can usually be controlled by reducing the frequency of application. Avoid contact with eyes, nose, and mouth.

INFORMATION FOR USERS

Follow instructions on the label. Call your physician if symptoms worsen.

How taken

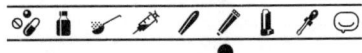

Cream, lotion, gel, cleansing bar.

Frequency and timing of doses
1 – 2 x daily (cream, gel, lotion); 2 – 3 x daily (cleansing bar).

Adult dosage range
Apply to affected skin sparingly.

Onset of effect
Reduces oiliness of skin immediately. Acne usually improves within 4 – 6 weeks.

Duration of action
24 – 48 hours.

Diet advice
None.

Storage
Keep in a closed container in a cool, dry place away from reach of children.

Missed dose
Apply as soon as you remember.

Stopping the drug
Can be safely stopped as soon as you no longer need it.

Exceeding the dose
A single extra application is unlikely to cause problems. Regular overuse may cause irritation, peeling, redness, and swelling.

POSSIBLE ADVERSE EFFECTS

Application of benzoyl peroxide may cause temporary burning or stinging of the skin. Redness, peeling, and swelling may result from excessive drying of the skin with overuse and usually clear up if treatment is stopped or used less frequently. If severe burning, blistering, or crusting occurs, stop using the product, and consult a physician.

Symptom/effect	Frequency		Discuss with physician		Stop taking drug now	Call physician now
	Common	Rare	Only if severe	In all cases		
Irritation	●		■			
Dryness/peeling	●		■			
Stinging/redness		●	■			
Blistering/crusting/swelling		●		■	▲	▌
Rash		●		■	▲	▌

INTERACTIONS

Skin-drying preparations Medicated cosmetics, soaps, toiletries, and anti-acne preparations increase the likelihood of dryness and irritation of the skin with benzoyl peroxide.

SPECIAL PRECAUTIONS

Be sure to consult your physician or pharmacist before using this drug if:
▼ You have eczema.
▼ You have sunburn.
▼ Your skin is highly sensitive to sunlight.
▼ You are taking other preparations.

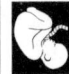

Pregnancy
▼ Not usually prescribed. Safety in pregnancy not established. Discuss with your physician.

Breast feeding
▼ No evidence of risk.

Infants and children
▼ Not recommended in patients under 12 years.

Over 60
▼ Not usually required.

Driving and hazardous work
▼ No known problems.

Alcohol
▼ No known problems.

PROLONGED USE

Benzoyl peroxide should not be used for longer than 6 weeks except on the advice of your physician.

BENZTROPINE

Brand names Cogentin, Apo-Benztropine, PMS Benztropine
Used in the following combined preparations None

GENERAL INFORMATION

Benztropine was introduced for the treatment of Parkinson's disease in the 1940s. It is still used for relieving early symptoms of the disease, and is also used in conjunction with the stronger, levodopa-based drugs for treatment of more advanced cases of Parkinson's disease. It is particularly helpful in treating the rigidity and tremor of Parkinson's disease and in the reduction of excess salivation. However, it does

little to improve the slow physical movements that also characterize the disease.

Benztropine is also used for the treatment of drug-induced dystonia (acute muscular rigidity and cramping).

Dosage has to be determined individually in order to find the best balance between relief of symptoms and the occurrence of adverse effects.

QUICK REFERENCE

Drug group Anticholinergic antiparkinsonism drug (p.99)

Overdose danger rating Medium

Dependence rating Low

Prescription needed Yes

Multi-source suppliers Yes

INFORMATION FOR USERS

Your drug prescription is tailored for you. Do not alter dosage without checking with your physician.

How taken

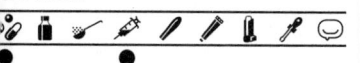

Tablets, injection.

Frequency and timing of doses
1 – 4 x daily.

Adult dosage range
0.5 – 6mg daily.

Onset of effect
Within 30 minutes.

Duration of action
6 – 24 hours.

Diet advice
None.

Storage
Keep in a closed container in a cool, dry place away from reach of children.

Missed dose
Take as soon as you remember. If your next dose is due within 2 hours, take a single dose now and skip the next.

Stopping the drug
Do not stop the drug without consulting your physician; symptoms may recur.

Exceeding the dose
An occasional unintentional extra dose is unlikely to cause problems. Larger overdoses may cause agitation and/or an increase in heart rate. Notify your physician.

SPECIAL PRECAUTIONS

Be sure to tell your physician if:
▼ You have impaired liver or kidney function.
▼ You have had glaucoma.
▼ You have urinary difficulties.
▼ You have high blood pressure.
▼ You suffer from depression.
▼ You have peptic ulcers.
▼ You are taking other medications.

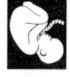

Pregnancy
▼ Unlikely to be required. Safety in pregnancy not established.

Breast feeding
▼ Unlikely to be required.

Infants and children
▼ Not for use in patients under 3 years of age. Reduced dose necessary in older children.

Over 60
▼ Increased likelihood of adverse effects. Reduced dose may therefore be necessary.

Driving and hazardous work
▼ Avoid such activities until you have learned how the drug affects you, because the drug can cause blurred vision and drowsiness.

Alcohol
▼ Avoid. Alcohol may increase the sedative effects of this drug.

POSSIBLE ADVERSE EFFECTS

The possible adverse effects of benztropine are mainly the result of its *anticholinergic* action. Some of the more common symptoms, such as dry eyes and mouth, drowsiness, and blurred vision, can be overcome by an adjustment in dosage.

Symptom/effect	Frequency		Discuss with physician		Stop taking drug now	Call physician now
	Common	Rare	Only if severe	In all cases		
Dry mouth/eyes	●		■			
Difficulty in passing urine	●		■			
Constipation	●		■			
Nervousness	●		■			
Blurred vision	●			■		
Confusion		●		■		
Nausea/vomiting		●		■		
Rash		●		■	▲	
Palpitations		●		■	▲	■

INTERACTIONS

Anticholinergic drugs and antihistamines Benztropine adds to the actions of such drugs, so increasing the likelihood of adverse effects.

PROLONGED USE

Prolonged use of this drug may contribute to the onset of glaucoma.

Monitoring Periodic eye examinations are usually required.

BENZYDAMINE

Brand name Tantum
Used in the following combined preparations None

GENERAL INFORMATION

Benzydamine is a *topical* non-steroidal anti-inflammatory drug (NSAID) that is available in the form of an oral rinse. This means that this drug is swished or gargled and then spat out: it is not meant to be swallowed. It is used for the relief of pain of bacterial and viral sore throat.

It is also used for the relief of pain and inflammation of the mouth and throat caused by radiation therapy. Benzydamine use should begin the day prior to the start of radiation therapy and continue daily. After radiation is completed, it can still be used until the mouth and throat are comfortable.

The most common adverse effects are local numbness, burning, and stinging.

QUICK REFERENCE

Drug group Non-steroidal anti-inflammatory drug (p.128)

Overdose danger rating Low

Dependence rating Low

Prescription needed Yes

Multi-source suppliers No

INFORMATION FOR USERS

Your drug prescription is tailored for you. Do not alter dosage without checking with your physician.

How taken

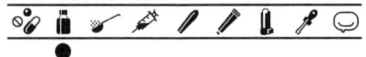

Oral rinse.

Frequency and timing of doses
3 – 4 x daily (general pain relief); every 1½ – 3 hours (acute sore throat).

Adult dosage range
15mL of liquid held in the mouth for at least 30 seconds (gargle, then spit out: do not swallow).

Onset of effect
Within 15 minutes.

Duration of action
4 – 6 hours.

Diet advice
None.

Storage
Keep in a closed container in a cool place away from children.

Missed dose
Take as needed. Allow at least 1½ hours between doses.

Stopping the drug
Can be safely stopped as soon as you no longer need it.

Exceeding the dose
An occasional unintentional extra dose is unlikely to be a cause for concern. But if you notice unusual symptoms, or if a large overdose has been taken, notify your physician.

SPECIAL PRECAUTIONS

Be sure to tell your physician if:
▼ You have impaired kidney function.
▼ You are allergic to ASA.
▼ You have asthma.
▼ You are taking other medications.

Pregnancy
▼ Safety in pregnancy not established. Discuss with your physician.

Breast feeding
▼ Effects on breast feeding uncertain. Discuss with your physician.

Infants and children
▼ Not recommended for children under 5 years.

Over 60
▼ No special problems.

Driving and hazardous work
▼ Avoid such activities until you have learned how the drug affects you; it can cause drowsiness.

Alcohol
▼ Avoid. Alcohol may increase the risk of local irritation and/or dryness

POSSIBLE ADVERSE EFFECTS

The most common adverse effect is local numbness. Burning and stinging can be reduced by diluting benzydamine oral rinse with an equal volume of water.

Symptom/effect	Frequency		Discuss with physician		Stop taking drug now	Call physician now
	Common	Rare	Only if severe	In all cases		
Local numbness	●			■		
Local burning/stinging	●			■		
Nausea/vomiting		●		■		
Dry mouth/thirst		●		■		
Drowsiness		●		■		
Headache		●		■		

PROLONGED USE

Not usually given for prolonged treatment.

INTERACTIONS

None.

BETAMETHASONE

Brand names Betnesol, Betnovate, Celestoderm, Celestone, Diprosone, Occlucort
Used in the following combined preparations Diprogen, Diprosalic, Garasone, Lotriderm, Valisone-G

GENERAL INFORMATION

Betamethasone is a corticosteroid prescribed to treat a variety of conditions. *Topical* preparations are available for skin complaints such as eczema and psoriasis. It can be injected directly into the joints to relieve the pain and stiffness of rheumatoid arthritis and other forms of joint inflammation. Given as an enema, it provides relief of inflammatory bowel disease. The drug is also given by mouth or injection to treat certain endocrine conditions affecting the pituitary and adrenal glands.

Low or moderate doses of betamethasone taken for short periods rarely cause serious *side effects*. Prolonged use or high dosages can lead to peptic ulcers, fragile bones, muscle weakness, and thin skin, and may retard growth in children.

INFORMATION FOR USERS

Your drug prescription is tailored for you. Do not alter dosage without checking with your physician.

How taken

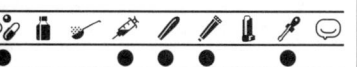

Tablets, slow-release tablets, injection, enema, cream, ointment, lotion, eye/ear drops.

Frequency and timing of doses
According to disorder being treated and method of administration.

Adult dosage range
Considerable variation according to the method of administration and condition. Follow your physician's instructions.

Onset of effect
2 – 48 hours.

Duration of action
Up to 24 hours.

Diet advice
A low-sodium, high-potassium diet may be recommended when the oral form of the drug is prescribed for extended periods. Follow the advice of your physician.

Storage
Keep in a closed container in a cool, dry place away from reach of children. Protect from light.

Missed dose
Take as soon as you remember. If your next dose is due within 2 hours, take a single dose now and skip the next.

Stopping the drug
Do not stop tablets without consulting your physician, who may supervise a gradual reduction in dosage. Abrupt cessation after long-term treatment may cause adrenal collapse.

Exceeding the dose
An occasional unintentional extra dose is unlikely to be a cause for concern. But if you notice unusual symptoms, or if a large overdose has been taken, notify your physician.

SPECIAL PRECAUTIONS

Be sure to tell your physician if:
▼ You suffer from a mental disorder.
▼ You have had glaucoma.
▼ You have high blood pressure.
▼ You have had a peptic ulcer.
▼ You have had tuberculosis.
▼ You have an infection.
▼ You have diabetes.
▼ You are taking other medications.

Pregnancy
▼ No evidence of risk with topical preparations or joint injections. Prescribed in tablet form in low doses, harm to baby is unlikely. Discuss with your physician.

Breast feeding
▼ No evidence of risk with topical preparations or joint injections. Taken by mouth, the drug passes into the breast milk and may adversely affect the baby's growth. Discuss with your physician.

Infants and children
▼ Reduced dose may be necessary.

Over 60
▼ Reduced dose may be necessary.

Driving and hazardous work
▼ No known problems.

Alcohol
▼ Avoid. Alcohol may increase the risk of peptic ulcers with betamethasone tablets. No special problems with other dosage forms.

POSSIBLE ADVERSE EFFECTS

Serious adverse effects only occur when high doses are taken by mouth for long periods.

Topical preparations may cause serious skin damage if used inappropriately.

Symptom/effect	Frequency		Discuss with physician		Stop taking drug now	Call physician now
	Common	Rare	Only if severe	In all cases		
Indigestion	●			■		
Weight gain	●			■		
Acne		●		■		
Muscle weakness		●		■		
Mood changes		●		■		
Bloody/black feces		●		■	▲	▌

INTERACTIONS (by mouth or injection only)

Insulin and oral hypoglycemic agents Betamethasone reduces the action of these drugs.

Antihypertensive drugs Betamethasone can cause fluid retention, which may reduce the effect of these drugs.

Vaccines Serious reactions can occur when certain vaccinations are given during betamethasone treatment. Discuss with your physician.

Phenytoin may reduce the effectiveness of betamethasone.

PROLONGED USE

Prolonged use of high doses of betamethasone by mouth can lead to peptic ulcers, thin skin, fragile bones, and muscle weakness, and can retard growth in children.

BEZAFIBRATE

Brand name Bezalip
Used in the following combined preparations None

GENERAL INFORMATION

Bezafibrate belongs to a group of drugs that lower lipid levels in the blood. Other drugs in the same chemical group (usually called fibrates) include clofibrate, fenofibrate, and gemfibrozil. These drugs are particularly effective in decreasing blood levels of triglycerides. They also reduce levels of cholesterol. Raised levels of lipids (fats) in the blood are associated with atherosclerosis (deposition of fat in blood vessel walls). This can lead to coronary heart disease (e.g. angina and heart attacks) and cerebrovascular disease (e.g. stroke). There is growing evidence that maintaining normal levels of blood lipids helps prevent heart attacks and strokes.

QUICK REFERENCE

Drug group Lipid-lowering drug (p.115)

Overdose danger rating Low

Dependence rating Low

Prescription needed Yes

Multi-source suppliers No

INFORMATION FOR USERS

Your drug prescription is tailored for you. Do not alter dosage without checking with your physician.

How taken

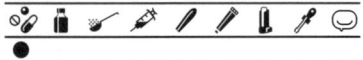

Tablets, slow-release tablets.

Frequency and timing of doses
2 – 3 x daily with or after meals (tablets); 1 x daily in the morning or evening with or after meals (slow-release tablets).

Adult dosage range
400 – 600mg daily.

Onset of effect
A beneficial effect on blood fat levels may not occur for weeks.

Duration of action
About 6 – 24 hours. This may vary according to the individual.

Diet advice
A low-fat diet may be recommended. Follow the advice of your physician.

Storage
Keep in a closed container in a cool, dry place away from reach of children.

Missed dose
Take as soon as your remember. If your next dose is due within 4 hours (and you take once daily), take a single dose now and skip the next. If you take 2 – 3 times daily, take the next dose as normal.

Stopping the drug
Do not stop the drug without consulting your physician.

Exceeding the dose
An occasional unintentional extra dose is unlikely to be a cause for concern. But if you notice unusual symptoms, notify your physician.

SPECIAL PRECAUTIONS

Be sure to tell your physician if:
▼ You have impaired liver or kidney function.
▼ You have a history of gallbladder disease.
▼ You are taking other medications.

Pregnancy
▼ Not recommended. If pregnancy occurs despite contraceptive measures, discontinue bezafibrate and inform your physician.

Breast feeding
▼ Not recommended. Discuss with your physician.

Infants and children
▼ Not usually prescribed.

Over 60
▼ Reduced dose may be necessary.

Driving and hazardous work
▼ Avoid such activities until you have learned how the drug affects you; it can cause dizziness.

Alcohol
▼ No special problems.

POSSIBLE ADVERSE EFFECTS

The most common adverse effects are those on the gastrointestinal tract, such as diarrhea, constipation, and nausea. These effects normally improve as treatment continues.

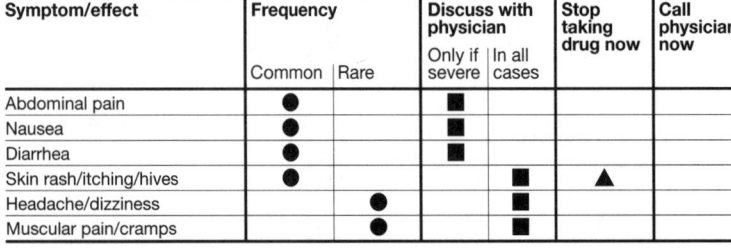

Symptom/effect	Frequency		Discuss with physician		Stop taking drug now	Call physician now
	Common	Rare	Only if severe	In all cases		
Abdominal pain	●		■			
Nausea	●		■			
Diarrhea	●		■			
Skin rash/itching/hives	●			■	▲	
Headache/dizziness		●		■		
Muscular pain/cramps		●		■		

PROLONGED USE

No problems expected.

Monitoring Blood tests will be undertaken to monitor the effect of the drug on lipids in the blood.

INTERACTIONS

Anticoagulants Bezafibrate may increase the effect of anticoagulants such as warfarin.

Lovastatin (and other "statins") as well as cyclosporine are not usually prescribed with bezafibrate because of the risk of severe muscle inflammation.

Monoamine oxidase inhibitors (MAOIs) with a potential for producing liver damage should not be taken with bezafibrate.

Cholestyramine An interval of 2 hours should be maintained between doses of cholestyramine and bezafibrate.

BISACODYL

Brand names Dulcolax, Apo-Bisacodyl
Used in the following combined preparations None

GENERAL INFORMATION

Bisacodyl is a powerful stimulant laxative. It encourages bowel activity by keeping the stool moist and soft and by stimulating the muscle contractions that propel feces through the bowel.

Available without a prescription, it is widely used for relief of constipation. It is also sometimes given after abdominal surgery or a heart attack so that strained efforts for bowel movement are unnecessary. It may also be used to evacuate the bowel prior to surgery or labor or before medical or X-ray examinations of the colon or rectum.

Since bisacodyl can irritate the stomach, tablets are covered with a protective coating to prevent their breakdown before reaching the intestine; they should be swallowed whole and not crushed or chewed. Taken at bedtime with a snack, they stimulate a bowel action in the morning. Rectal suppositories are faster-acting, but sometimes cause stinging and inflammation.

Regular long-term use of this drug may seriously upset normal bowel action, leading to severe, prolonged diarrhea. This may disrupt the balance of potassium in the body and affect nerve and muscle activity, causing weakness and debility.

QUICK REFERENCE

Drug group Laxative (p.123)
Overdose danger rating Medium
Dependence rating Medium
Prescription needed No
Multi-source suppliers Yes

INFORMATION FOR USERS

Follow instructions on the label. Call your physician if symptoms worsen.

How taken

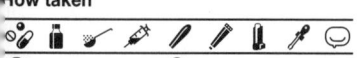

Tablets, rectal suppositories, enema.

Frequency and timing of doses
Tablets Once daily in the evening or before breakfast. Do not chew.
Rectal suppositories Once daily, usually in the morning.
Enema 1 – 2 hours prior to diagnostic or surgical procedure.

Adult dosage range
5 – 15mg daily (tablets); 10mg daily (suppositories); 5mL (enema).

Onset of effect
6 – 8 hours (tablets); 15 – 60 minutes (suppositories, enema).

Duration of action
Several days.

Diet advice
None.

Storage
Keep in a closed container in a cool, dry place away from reach of children.

Missed dose
Do not take the missed dose. Take your next dose only if relief of severe constipation is required.

Stopping the drug
Can be safely stopped as soon as you no longer need it.

Exceeding the dose
An occasional unintentional extra dose is unlikely to cause problems. Large overdoses may cause colicky lower abdominal pain. Notify your physician.

POSSIBLE ADVERSE EFFECTS

Side effects are rarely serious. Tablets may cause irritation of the stomach or bowel, leading to abdominal cramps. Soreness and itching around the anus and rectum are the most common adverse effects of bisacodyl suppositories.

Symptom/effect	Frequency		Discuss with physician		Stop taking drug now	Call physician now
	Common	Rare	Only if severe	In all cases		
Abdominal pain	●		■			
Rectal irritation	●		■			
Belching		●	■			
Nausea		●	■			
Diarrhea		●		■	▲	

INTERACTIONS

Antacids and milk If taken within one hour of bisacodyl tablets, these may cause premature disintegration of the enteric coating, leading to stomach irritation.

SPECIAL PRECAUTIONS

Be sure to consult your physician or pharmacist before taking this drug if:
▼ You have severe abdominal pain.
▼ You have severe constipation and/or hard stools.
▼ You have unexplained rectal bleeding.
▼ You are taking other medications.

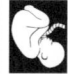

Pregnancy
▼ Not usually prescribed. Other laxatives are more widely used and regarded as safer in pregnancy.

Breast feeding
▼ No evidence of risk.

Infants and children
▼ Not recommended except on the advice of a physician.

Over 60
▼ Increased likelihood of adverse effects.

Driving and hazardous work
▼ No known problems.

Alcohol
▼ No known problems.

PROLONGED USE

Not recommended. Bisacodyl should not be taken regularly for longer than one week except on the advice of your physician. Overuse of laxatives – the laxative habit – reduces spontaneous, normal bowel activity and leads to dependence on the drug for bowel movement.

BROMAZEPAM

Brand name Lectopam
Used in the following combined preparations None

GENERAL INFORMATION

Bromazepam, introduced in 1981, belongs to a group of drugs known as the benzodiazepines, which are effective for the short-term relief of anxiety and tension and also insomnia. See page 95 for a full description of the actions and adverse effects of this category of drugs.

Bromazepam is used in the short-term symptomatic relief of anxiety.

In common with other benzodiazepines, bromazepam can be habit-forming if taken regularly over a long period. Its effects may also become weaker with time. For these reasons, treatment with bromazepam should be limited to a few weeks and then reviewed.

QUICK REFERENCE

Drug group Benzodiazepine anti-anxiety drug (p.95)

Overdose danger rating Medium

Dependence rating Medium

Prescription needed Yes

Multi-source suppliers No

INFORMATION FOR USERS

Your drug prescription is tailored for you. Do not alter dosage without checking with your physician.

How taken

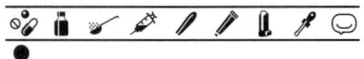

Tablets.

Frequency and timing of doses
2 – 3 x daily.

Adult dosage range
6 – 30mg daily.

Onset of effect
1 – 2 hours.

Duration of action
Up to 19 hours.

Diet advice
None.

Storage
Keep in a closed container in a cool, dry place away from reach of children.

Missed dose
No cause for concern, but take the missed dose when you remember. If your next dose is due within 2 hours, take a single dose now and skip the next.

Stopping the drug
If you have been taking the drug continuously for less than 2 weeks, it can be safely stopped as soon as you feel you no longer need it. However, if you have been taking it for longer, consult your physician who may advise a gradual reduction in dosage. Stopping abruptly may lead to withdrawal symptoms (see p.95).

Exceeding the dose
An occasional unintentional extra dose is unlikely to cause problems. Larger overdoses may cause unusual drowsiness. Notify your physician.

SPECIAL PRECAUTIONS

Be sure to tell your physician if:
▼ You have impaired liver or kidney function.
▼ You have myasthenia gravis.
▼ You have had problems with alcohol or drug abuse.
▼ You are taking other medications.

Pregnancy
▼ Safety in pregnancy not established. Discuss with your physician.

Breast feeding
▼ This drug probably passes into the breast milk. Its effects on the baby are uncertain. Discuss with your physician.

Infants and children
▼ Not recommended.

Over 60
▼ Increased likelihood of adverse effects. Reduced dose may therefore be necessary.

Driving and hazardous work
▼ Avoid such activities until you have learned how the drug affects you; it can cause blurred vision, reduced alertness, and slowed reactions.

Alcohol
▼ Avoid. Alcohol may increase the sedative effects of this drug.

POSSIBLE ADVERSE EFFECTS

The principal adverse effects of this drug are related to its sedative properties. These effects, including drowsiness and dizziness, normally diminish after the first few days and, if troublesome, can often be reduced by adjustment of dosage.

Symptom/effect	Frequency		Discuss with physician		Stop taking drug now	Call physician now
	Common	Rare	Only if severe	In all cases		
Daytime drowsiness	●			■		
Dizziness/unsteadiness	●			■		
Forgetfulness/confusion		●		■		
Blurred vision/headache		●		■		
Rash		●			■	▲	▮

INTERACTIONS

Sedatives All drugs, including alcohol, that have a sedative effect on the central nervous system are likely to increase the sedative properties of bromazepam. Such drugs include other anti-anxiety and sleeping drugs, antihistamines, antidepressants, antipsychotics, anticonvulsants, and narcotic analgesics.

PROLONGED USE

Regular use of this drug over several weeks can lead to a reduction in its effect as the body adapts. It may also be habit-forming when taken for extended periods, especially if larger-than-average doses are taken.

BROMOCRIPTINE

Brand names Parlodel, Apo-Bromocriptine
Used in the following combined preparations None

GENERAL INFORMATION

By inhibiting the secretion of the hormone prolactin from the pituitary gland, bromocriptine is helpful in treating conditions associated with excessive prolactin production. Such conditions include some types of female infertility and occasionally male infertility and impotence. Bromocriptine is effective in treating some benign breast conditions and other symptoms of menstrual disorders.

Bromocriptine reduces the release of growth hormone, and it is useful in the treatment of acromegaly (see p.157).

Bromocriptine may be used with the combination agent levodopa-carbidopa to treat those in advanced stages of Parkinson's disease when other drugs have failed or are unsuitable.

Although bromocriptine is generally well tolerated, adverse reactions may occur. The most common of these is dizziness, sometimes accompanied by fainting. Less common but much more serious are hypertension, heart attack, seizures, and stroke in the postpartum period. Higher doses may cause gastrointestinal ulceration with bleeding as well as mental disturbances including agitation, nightmares, and hallucinations.

QUICK REFERENCE

Drug group Antiparkinsonism drug (p.99) and pituitary agent (p.157)

Overdose danger rating Low

Dependence rating Low

Prescription needed Yes

Multi-source suppliers Yes

INFORMATION FOR USERS

Your drug prescription is tailored for you. Do not alter dosage without checking with your physician.

How taken

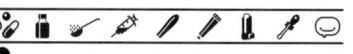

Tablets, capsules.

Frequency and timing of doses
1 – 3 x daily with food or milk.

Adult dosage range
The dose given depends on the condition being treated and your response. In most cases treatment starts with a daily dose of 1.25mg. This is gradually increased until a satisfactory response is achieved.

Onset of effect
Within 1 hour.

Duration of action
About 8 hours.

Diet advice
None.

Storage
Keep in a closed container in a cool, dry place away from reach of children. Protect from light.

Missed dose
Take as soon as you remember. If your next dose is due within 2 hours, take a single dose now and skip the next.

Stopping the drug
Do not stop the drug without consulting your physician; symptoms may recur.

Exceeding the dose
An occasional unintentional extra dose is unlikely to be a cause for concern. But if you notice unusual symptoms, or if a large overdose has been taken, notify your physician.

SPECIAL PRECAUTIONS

Be sure to tell your physician if:
▼ You have impaired liver or kidney function.
▼ You have poor circulation in hands or feet.
▼ You have a stomach ulcer.
▼ You are taking other medications.

Pregnancy
▼ Safety in pregnancy not established. Discuss with your physician.

Breast feeding
▼ The drug suppresses lactation and prevents it completely if given within 12 hours of delivery. Consult your physician if you wish to breast feed.

Infants and children
▼ Not usually prescribed. Reduced dose necessary.

Over 60
▼ Reduced dose may be necessary.

Driving and hazardous work
▼ Avoid such activities until you have learned how the drug affects you; it can reduce alertness.

Alcohol
▼ Avoid. Alcohol increases the likelihood of confusion while taking this drug.

POSSIBLE ADVERSE EFFECTS

Nausea and vomiting, the most common problems, can be minimized by taking bromocriptine with food. When taken for Parkinson's disease, bromocriptine may cause abnormal movements of the face and limbs, and hallucinations. Ulceration of the stomach is rare.

Symptom/effect	Frequency		Discuss with physician		Stop taking drug now	Call physician now
	Common	Rare	Only if severe	In all cases		
Nausea/vomiting	●		■			
Confusion/dizziness	●			■		
Headache/constipation		●	■			
Abnormal movements		●		■		
Hallucinations		●		■		
Collapse		●		■	▲	▮

INTERACTIONS

Antipsychotic drugs oppose the action of bromocriptine and increase the risk of parkinsonism.

Domperidone and metoclopramide may reduce some of the effects of bromocriptine.

PROLONGED USE

Long-term use may rarely lead to abnormal growth of fibrous tissue in the lungs, chest, urinary tract, or blood vessels, causing chest pain, loin pain, urinary difficulties, and reduced blood supply to the limbs.

Monitoring Periodic blood tests may be performed to check hormone levels.

BROMPHENIRAMINE

Brand name Dimetane
Used in the following combined preparations Dimetane Expectorant, Dimetapp, Dimetapp-A Sinus

GENERAL INFORMATION

Brompheniramine, an antihistamine introduced in 1957, is used for treating allergies such as hay fever, allergic conjunctivitis, urticaria (hives), and angioedema (allergic swellings). It is also a common ingredient of over-the-counter cold remedies (see p.106).

Like other antihistamines, it relieves allergic skin symptoms such as itching, swelling, and redness. It also reduces sneezing and runny nose and the itching eyes in hay fever. It has a mild *anticholinergic* action, which enhances its drying effect on the nose.

Brompheniramine may also be used to prevent or treat allergic reactions to blood transfusions or X-ray contrast material, and to supplement epinephrine injections for people with acute allergic shock (anaphylaxis).

QUICK REFERENCE

Drug group Antihistamine (p.136)
Overdose danger rating Medium
Dependence rating Low
Prescription needed No
Multi-source suppliers No

INFORMATION FOR USERS

Follow instructions on the label. Call your physician if symptoms worsen.

How taken

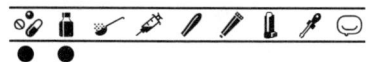

Tablets, slow-release tablets, oral liquid.

Frequency and timing of doses
3 – 4 x daily (tablets, oral liquid); 2 – 3 x daily (slow-release tablets).

Dosage range
Adults 12 – 32mg daily (tablets, liquid).
Children 6 – 8mg daily (3 – 6 years, liquid); 12 – 16mg daily (6 – 12 years, tablets, liquid).

Onset of effect
Within 60 minutes.

Duration of action
4 – 6 hours (tablets, liquid); 10 – 14 hours (slow-release tablets).

Diet advice
None.

Storage
Keep in a closed container in a cool, dry place away from reach of children. Protect from light.

Missed dose
Take as soon as you remember. If your next dose is due within 2 hours, take a single dose now and skip the next.

Stopping the drug
Can be safely stopped as soon as you no longer need it.

Exceeding the dose
An occasional unintentional extra dose is unlikely to cause problems. Large overdoses may cause unusual drowsiness or agitation. Notify your physician.

SPECIAL PRECAUTIONS

Be sure to consult your physician or pharmacist before taking this drug if:
▼ You have impaired liver function.
▼ You have chronic lung disease.
▼ You have had epileptic seizures.
▼ You have had glaucoma.
▼ You have urinary difficulties.
▼ You are taking other medications.

Pregnancy
▼ Safety in pregnancy not established. Discuss with your physician.

Breast feeding
▼ The drug passes into breast milk and may affect the baby adversely. Discuss with your physician.

Infants and children
▼ Not recommended for newborn or premature infants. Reduced dose necessary for older children.

Over 60
▼ Reduced dose may be necessary. Increased likelihood of adverse effects.

Driving and hazardous work
▼ Avoid such activities until you have learned how the drug affects you; it can cause drowsiness.

Alcohol
▼ Avoid. Alcohol may increase the sedative effects of this drug.

POSSIBLE ADVERSE EFFECTS

Brompheniramine has few adverse effects. The most common is drowsiness. Other symptoms, such as dryness of the mouth, blurred vision, and difficulty passing urine, are due to the *anticholinergic* effects of brompheniramine. Gastrointestinal irritation may be reduced by taking tablets or liquid with food or drink.

Symptom/effect	Frequency		Discuss with physician		Stop taking drug now	Call physician now
	Common	Rare	Only if severe	In all cases		
Drowsiness	●		■			
Blurred vision		●	■			
Dizziness/incoordination		●	■			
Digestive disturbances		●		■		
Urinary difficulties		●		■		
Dry mouth		●		■		
Excitation (in children)		◐		■	▲	

INTERACTIONS

Alcohol and other sedatives All drugs that have a sedative effect are likely to enhance the sedative effect of brompheniramine.

Anticholinergic drugs are likely to increase the anticholinergic effects of brompheniramine.

Monoamine oxidase inhibitors (MAOIs)
There is a risk of a dangerous rise in blood pressure if brompheniramine is taken with MAOIs.

PROLONGED USE

The effect of the drug may become weaker with prolonged use over a period of weeks or months as the body adapts. Transfer to a different antihistamine may be recommended.

Antihistamines should be discontinued approximately 48 hours prior to allergy skin testing.

BUDESONIDE

Brand names Entocort, Pulmicort, Rhinocort
Used in the following combined preparations None

GENERAL INFORMATION

Budesonide is a corticosteroid drug prescribed to relieve the symptoms of allergic rhinitis (as a nasal inhaler or spray), to control asthma (as an inhaler or nebulizer solution), and to control ulcerative colitis (as an enema). It controls nasal symptoms by reducing inflammation and mucus production in the nose. It also helps to reduce chest symptoms, such as wheezing and coughing, by reducing inflammation in the bronchi. People who suffer from asthma may take budesonide to reduce the severity and frequency of attacks. However, once an attack has started, this drug does not relieve symptoms.

Fungal infection (thrush) causing irritation of the mouth and throat is a possible adverse effect of budesonide asthma treatment. It can be minimized by thoroughly rinsing the mouth and gargling with water after each inhalation.

INFORMATION FOR USERS

Your drug prescription is tailored for you. **Do not alter dosage without checking with your physician.**

How taken

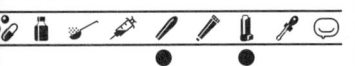

Enema, inhaler, nasal inhaler, nasal spray, nebulizer.

Frequency and timing of doses
Once nightly (enema). 2 – 4 x daily (nasal spray, inhaler)

Dosage range
Adults 1 – 2 sprays 2 – 4 x daily (asthma); 1 spray in each nostril 2 – 4 x daily (allergic rhinitis); 1 enema nightly (ulcerative colitis). *Children* Reduced dose according to age and weight.

Onset of effect
Within 1 week (asthma); 1 – 3 days (allergic rhinitis); within a week (ulcerative colitis).

Duration of action
Several days after stopping the drug.

Diet advice
None.

Storage
Store away from heat and direct light, away from reach of children. Keep the medicine from getting too cold or freezing. This medicine may be less effective if the container is cold when you use it. Do not puncture, break, or burn the aerosol container, even after it is empty.

Missed dose
Take as soon as you remember. However, if it is almost time for your next dose, skip the missed dose and go back to your regular schedule. Do not double doses.

Stopping the drug
Do not stop the drug without consulting your physician; symptoms may recur.

Exceeding the dose
An occasional unintentional extra dose is unlikely to be a cause for concern. But if you do notice unusual symptoms, or if a large overdose has been taken, notify your physician. Adverse effects may occur if the recommended dose is regularly exceeded over a prolonged period.

SPECIAL PRECAUTIONS

Be sure to tell your physician if:
▼ You have had any nasal ulcers or surgery.
▼ You have had tuberculosis or another respiratory infection.
▼ You are taking other medications.

Pregnancy
▼ Safety in pregnancy not established. Discuss with your physician.

Breast feeding
▼ The drug passes into the breast milk, but at normal doses adverse effects on the baby are unlikely. Discuss with your physician.

Infants and children
▼ Not recommended for children under 6 years. Reduced dose necessary in older children.

Over 60
▼ No known problems.

Driving and hazardous work
▼ No known problems.

Alcohol
▼ No known problems.

PROLONGED USE

Monitoring Periodic checks to make sure that the adrenal glands are functioning properly may be required if large doses are being used.

POSSIBLE ADVERSE EFFECTS

Adverse effects are unlikely as the dose used is low. The main *side effects* are irritation of the nasal passages and fungal infection of the throat and mouth with the nasal spray or inhaler; and gastrointestinal disturbances (e.g., flatulence, diarrhea) with the enema.

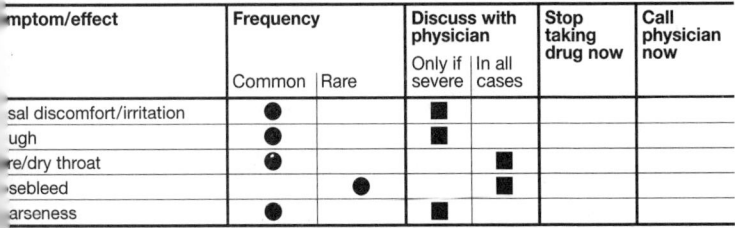

Symptom/effect	Frequency		Discuss with physician		Stop taking drug now	Call physician now
	Common	Rare	Only if severe	In all cases		
Nasal discomfort/irritation	●		■			
Cough	●		■			
Sore/dry throat	●			■		
Nosebleed		●		■		
Hoarseness	●		■			

INTERACTIONS

None.

BUMETANIDE

Brand name Burinex
Used in the following combined preparations None

GENERAL INFORMATION

Bumetanide is a powerful, short-acting loop diuretic. Like other diuretics, it is used to treat edema (fluid retention) resulting from heart failure, nephrotic syndrome, and cirrhosis of the liver. Bumetanide is particularly useful in the treatment of people with impaired kidney function who do not respond well to thiazide diuretics.

Bumetanide increases the loss of potassium in the urine, which can result in a wide variety of symptoms (see p.111). For this reason, potassium supplements or a diuretic that conserves potassium are often given with the drug.

QUICK REFERENCE

Drug group Loop diuretic (p.111)
Overdose danger rating Low
Dependence rating Low
Prescription needed Yes
Multi-source suppliers No

INFORMATION FOR USERS

Your drug prescription is tailored for you. Do not alter dosage without checking with your physician.

How taken

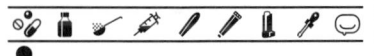

Tablets.

Frequency and timing of doses
Usually once daily in the morning. In some cases, twice daily.

Dosage range
0.5 – 5mg daily.

Onset of effect
Within 30 minutes.

Duration of action
3 – 4 hours.

Diet advice
Use of this drug may reduce potassium in the body. Eat plenty of potassium-rich fruit and vegetables.

Storage
Keep in a closed container in a dry place at room temperature away from reach of children. Protect from light.

Missed dose
No cause for concern, but take as soon as you remember. However, if it is late in the day do not take the missed dose, or you may need to get up during the night to pass urine. Take the next scheduled dose as usual.

Stopping the drug
Do not stop the drug without consulting your physician; symptoms may recur.

Exceeding the dose
An occasional unintentional extra dose is unlikely to be cause for concern. But if you notice unusual symptoms, or if a large overdose has been taken, notify your physician.

SPECIAL PRECAUTIONS

Be sure to tell your physician if:
▼ You have impaired liver or kidney function.
▼ You have diabetes.
▼ You have prostate trouble.
▼ You have gout.
▼ You have hearing problems.
▼ You are allergic to sulfonamides.
▼ You are taking other medications.

Pregnancy
▼ Not usually prescribed. Discuss with your physician.

Breast feeding
▼ Not recommended. Discuss with your physician.

Infants and children
▼ Safety and effectiveness in patients under 18 years not established.

Over 60
▼ Dosage is often reduced.

Driving and hazardous work
▼ Avoid such activities until you have learned how the drug affects you because of the possibility of dizziness and faintness.

Alcohol
▼ Keep consumption low. Bumetanide increases the likelihood of dehydration and hangovers after drinking alcohol.

POSSIBLE ADVERSE EFFECTS

Adverse effects are caused mainly by the rapid fluid loss produced by bumetanide. These diminish as the body adjusts to the drug.

Symptom/effect	Frequency		Discuss with physician		Stop taking drug now	Call physician now
	Common	Rare	Only if severe	In all cases		
Dizziness/faintness		●	■			
Lethargy/fatigue		●	■			
Cramps		●	■			
Rash		●		■		
Nausea/vomiting		●		■		
Joint pain		●		■		▲

PROLONGED USE

Serious problems are unlikely, but levels of certain salts such as potassium, sodium, and calcium may occasionally become depleted during prolonged use.

Monitoring Periodic checks may be performed to check on kidney function and levels of body salts.

INTERACTIONS

Non-steroidal anti-inflammatory drugs (NSAIDs) Some of these drugs may reduce the diuretic effect of bumetanide.

Aminoglycoside antibiotics may increase the risk of hearing problems when taken with high doses of bumetanide.

Lithium Bumetanide may increase the blood levels of lithium, leading to an increased risk of lithium poisoning.

Digoxin The adverse effects of digoxin may be increased if excessive potassium is lost.

BUSPIRONE

Brand name Buspar
Used in the following combined preparations None

GENERAL INFORMATION

Buspirone is a new anti-anxiety drug which shares some of the properties of the benzodiazepines (see p.95), but generally has fewer and less severe side effects.

In conjunction with counseling, buspirone is used for the treatment of anxiety disorders marked by persistent, unrealistic, and excessive worry and anxiety. One such disorder is general-ized anxiety disorder. Buspirone is not used to treat the tension and stress of everyday life.

Although some studies have shown little potential for it to be habit-forming, only more extensive studies and experience will provide conclusive evidence.

QUICK REFERENCE

Drug group Anti-anxiety drug (p.95.)

Overdose danger rating Medium

Dependence rating Low to medium

Prescription needed Yes

Multi-source suppliers No

INFORMATION FOR USERS

Your drug prescription is tailored for you. Do not alter dosage without checking with your physician.

How taken

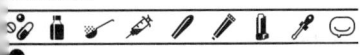

Tablets.

Frequency and timing of doses
1 – 3 x daily.

Adult dosage range
15 – 30mg daily.

Onset of effect
30 – 90 minutes.

Duration of action
Up to 11 hours.

Diet advice
None.

Storage
Keep in a closed container in a cool, dry place away from the reach of children.

Missed dose
No cause for concern, but take when you next feel you need the drug. If your next dose is due within 2 hours, take a single dose now and skip the next dose.

Stopping the drug
If you have been taking the drug continuously for less than 2 weeks, it can be safely stopped if you no longer need it. However, if you have been taking it for a longer period of time, consult your physician. Stopping abruptly may lead to *withdrawal symptoms*.

Exceeding the dose
An occasional unintentional extra dose is unlikely to cause problems. Larger overdoses may cause unusual drowsiness. Notify your physician.

SPECIAL PRECAUTIONS

Be sure to tell your physician if:
▼ You have impaired kidney or liver function.
▼ You have any form of epilepsy or any other convulsive disorder.
▼ You have a problem with alcohol or drug abuse.
▼ You are taking other medications.

Pregnancy
▼ Safety in pregnancy not established. Discuss with your physician.

Breast feeding
▼ Safety in breast feeding not established. Discuss with your physician.

Infants and children
▼ Not recommended for patients under 18 years of age.

Over 60
▼ Increased chance of adverse effects. Reduced dosage, therefore, may be necessary.

Driving and hazardous work
▼ Avoid such activities until you have learned how the drug affects you; it can cause reduced alertness and slowed reactions.

Alcohol
▼ Avoid. Alcohol may increase the sedative effects of this drug.

POSSIBLE ADVERSE EFFECTS

The most common adverse reactions encountered with buspirone are dizziness, headache, drowsiness, and nausea. They normally diminish after the first few days and if troublesome, they can usually be reduced by adjustment of dosage.

Symptom/effect	Frequency		Discuss with physician		Stop taking drug now	Call physician now
	Common	Rare	Only if severe	In all cases		
Dizziness/lightheadedness	●		■			
Headache	●			■		
Daytime drowsiness	●		■			
Numbness	●		■			
Nausea	●		■			
Skin rash		●		■	▲	▮
Sore throat		●		■	▲	▮

PROLONGED USE

If buspirone is taken for longer than 3 – 4 weeks, the need for continued therapy should be reassessed regularly.

INTERACTIONS

Sedatives All drugs, including alcohol, that have a sedative effect on the central nervous system are likely to increase the sedative effects of buspirone.

Haloperidol Buspirone may increase blood levels of haloperidol.

Monoamine oxidase inhibitors (MAOIs) Phenelzine, tranylcypromine, and moclobemide taken with buspirone may cause increased blood pressure; therefore, they should not be used together.

BUTORPHANOL

Brand name Stadol NS
Used in the following combined preparations None

GENERAL INFORMATION

Butorphanol is an analgesic agent similar in action to narcotic analgesics. It is available in a nasal spray formulation to provide rapid relief of moderate to severe pain following surgery and in situations such as acute migraine.

Patients who use narcotic medications regularly may experience *withdrawal symptoms* when butorphanol is given. Such patients should have an adequate period of withdrawal from narcotic drugs prior to starting butorphanol.

Although butorphanol has a lower abuse and/or *dependence* potential than morphine or other narcotics, patients with a history of severe emotional problems or drug abuse may be at higher risk of developing dependency problems.

INFORMATION FOR USERS

Your drug prescription is tailored for you. Do not alter dosage without checking with your physician.

How taken

Nasal spray.

Frequency and timing of doses
Usual dose is 1 spray (1mg) into one nostril only with an additional spray into 1 nostril after 60 to 90 minutes if adequate pain relief has not been achieved. In post-surgical pain, this may be increased to 1 spray in each nostril (total of 2 sprays). Timing of dose: every 3 to 4 hours, when necessary.

Dosage range
4 – 16mg daily. Doses may vary considerably for each individual.

Onset of effect
Within 15 – 30 minutes.

Duration of action
3 – 6 hours.

Diet advice
For relief of constipation, increase intake of fluids and high fiber foods.

Storage
Keep the drug in its original closed container in a cool, dry place away from the reach of children.

Missed dose
As it is used on an as needed basis, use only when required for pain control.

Stopping the drug
If you have been taking butorphanol for less than one week, it can be safely stopped as soon as you feel that you no longer need it. However, if you have been taking the drug for longer than one week, consult your physician, who may supervise a gradual reduction in dosage.

OVERDOSE ACTION

 Seek immediate medical advice in all cases. Take emergency action if there are symptoms such as slow or irregular breathing, severe drowsiness, or loss of consciousness.

See Drug poisoning emergency guide (p.574).

SPECIAL PRECAUTIONS

Be sure to tell your physician if:
▼ You have a history of drug and/or alcohol misuse or abuse.
▼ You have impaired liver or kidney function.
▼ You have a central nervous system disease.
▼ You have a heart, circulatory, or high blood pressure problem.
▼ You have a lung disorder such as asthma or bronchitis.
▼ You are taking other medications.

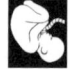 **Pregnancy**
▼ Not recommended. Discuss with your physician.

 Breast feeding
▼ Not recommended. Discuss with your physician.

 Infants and children
▼ Not recommended in patients under 18 years.

 Over 60
▼ Increased likelihood of adverse effects. Reduced dose may therefore be necessary.

 Driving and hazardous work
▼ Avoid such activities until you have learned how the drug affects you; it can cause dizziness and drowsiness.

 Alcohol
▼ Avoid. Alcohol may increase the side effects of drowsiness and dizziness.

PROLONGED USE

Butorphanol is not used for prolonged periods.

POSSIBLE ADVERSE EFFECTS

Adverse effects may occur more frequently in migraine sufferers. Drowsiness, dizziness, nausea, and vomiting are common and appear related to the dosage given.

Symptom/effect	Frequency		Discuss with physician		Stop taking drug now	Call physician now
	Common	Rare	Only if severe	In all cases		
Drowsiness/dizziness	●		■			
Nausea/vomiting	●		■			
Confusion		●		■	▲	▮
Breathing difficulties		●		■	▲	▮
Slow heart rate/palpitations		●		■	▲	▮
Rash/hives/itching		●		■	▲	▮

INTERACTIONS

Sedatives Butorphanol increases the sedative properties of all drugs that have a sedative effect. Such drugs include alcohol, barbiturates, antipsychotics, sleeping drugs, and antihistamines.

Monoamine oxidase inhibitors (MAOIs) These drugs may produce a severe rise in blood pressure when taken with butorphanol.

CALCIPOTRIOL

Brand name Dovonex
Used in the following combined preparations None

GENERAL INFORMATION

Calcipotriol is a new drug used in the treatment of mild to moderate psoriasis. It is effective in plaque psoriasis affecting up to 40 per cent of the patient's skin area.

Calcipotriol is a derivative of vitamin D and is thought to work by reducing the production of certain skin cells that cause skin thickening and scaling, which are the most common symptom of psoriasis. Because calcipotriol is related to vitamin D,

excessive widespread use can lead to a rise in calcium levels in the body; otherwise calcipotriol is unlikely to cause any serious adverse effects.

The drug is applied to the affected areas in cream or ointment form. It should not be used on the face. Hands should be washed afterward to avoid accidental transfer to unaffected areas. Local irritation may occur during the early stages of treatment.

QUICK REFERENCE

Drug group Psoriasis drugs (p.190)
Overdose danger rating Low
Dependence rating Low
Prescription needed Yes
Multi-source suppliers No

INFORMATION FOR USERS

Your drug prescription is tailored for you. Do not alter dosage without checking with your physician.

How taken

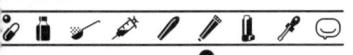

Cream, ointment.

Frequency and timing of doses
2 x daily, in the morning and in the evening.

Adult dosage range
Applied twice daily; maximum of 100g each week.

Onset of effect
Improvement is usually seen within 2 weeks.

Duration of action
One application lasts up to 12 hours. Beneficial effects are longer lasting.

Diet advice
None.

Storage
Store at room temperature away from reach of children.

Missed dose
Apply the next dose at the scheduled time.

Stopping the drug
Do not stop taking the drug without consulting your physician; symptoms may recur.

Exceeding the dose
Excessive prolonged use may lead to an increase in blood calcium levels, causing nausea, constipation, thirst, and frequent urination. Notify your physician.

POSSIBLE ADVERSE EFFECTS

Adverse effects are rarely a problem. A temporary local irritation may occur during the early phases of treatment.

Symptom/effect	Frequency		Discuss with physician		Stop taking drug now	Call physician now
	Common	Rare	Only if severe	In all cases		
Local irritation	●		■			
Rash on face/mouth		●		■		
Thirst/frequent urination		●		■		
Nausea/constipation		●		■		

INTERACTIONS

None known.

SPECIAL PRECAUTIONS

Be sure to tell your physician if:
▼ You have a metabolic disorder.
▼ You are taking other medications.

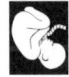 **Pregnancy**
▼ Safety in pregnancy not established. Discuss with your physician.

 Breast feeding
▼ It is not known whether the drug passes into the breast milk. Discuss with your physician.

 Infants and children
▼ Not recommended.

 Over 60
▼ No problems expected.

 Driving and hazardous work
▼ No problems expected.

 Alcohol
▼ No problems expected.

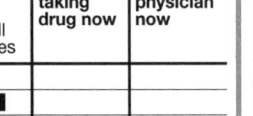

PROLONGED USE

The drug is not normally used for longer than 6 weeks.

Monitoring Regular checks on calcium levels in the blood are required.

CAPSAICIN

Brand names Zostrix, Zostrix H.P.
Used in the following combined preparations None

GENERAL INFORMATION

Capsaicin is an analgesic cream used for the temporary relief of neuralgia (severe throbbing or burning pain that comes from nerves near the surface of the skin). The regular strength cream is used to treat the pain associated with and also following episodes of herpes zoster (shingles), once the sores have healed. Both the regular and high strength (H.P.) creams may also be used for the temporary relief of pain in rheumatoid arthritis and osteoarthritis. High strength capsaicin is used for the more severe types of neuralgia associated with diabetes, and for pain following surgery.

It is very important to avoid contact with eyes. Do not apply the cream to open wounds or damaged skin and do not apply a bandage over the cream.

QUICK REFERENCE

Drug group Analgesic (p.92)

Overdose danger rating Low

Dependence rating Low

Prescription needed No

Multi-source suppliers No

INFORMATION FOR USERS

Follow instructions on the label. Call your physician if symptoms worsen.

How taken

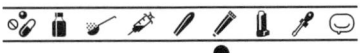

Cream.

Frequency and timing of doses
Not less than 3 or 4 x daily.

Adult dosage range
Apply to affected areas 3 – 4 x daily.

Onset of effect
Within a few minutes.

Duration of action
4 – 6 hours.

Diet advice
None.

Storage
Keep in a closed container in a cool, dry place away from the reach of children.

Missed dose
No cause for concern, but make up the missed application as soon as you remember.

Stopping the drug
Can be safely stopped when no longer required.

Exceeding the dose
Exceeding the dose may cause a burning sensation on the skin.

SPECIAL PRECAUTIONS

Be sure to consult your physician or pharmacist before using this drug if:
▼ You have broken, damaged, or irritated skin.
▼ You have other skin problems or conditions.
▼ You are taking any other medications.

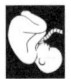

Pregnancy
▼ Safety in pregnancy not established. Discuss with your physician.

Breast feeding
▼ It is not known if capsaicin passes into breast milk. Discuss with your physician.

Infants and children
▼ Not recommended for children under 2 years.

Over 60
▼ No known problems.

Driving and hazardous work
▼ No known problems.

Alcohol
▼ No known problems.

POSSIBLE ADVERSE EFFECTS

A transient burning sensation may occur on application. This burning is observed more frequently when application schedules of less than 3 or 4 times a day are used. Do not apply to open wounds or damaged skin. Avoid contact with eyes. Wash hands immediately after application.

Symptom/effect	Frequency		Discuss with physician		Stop taking drug now	Call physician now
	Common	Rare	Only if severe	In all cases		
Skin irritation	●		■			
Transient burning	●		■			
Rash		●		■	▲	∎

INTERACTIONS

None.

PROLONGED USE

No problems expected unless skin becomes irritated or rash-like symptoms develop. However, if condition worsens or does not improve after 28 days, discontinue use and consult your physician.

CAPTOPRIL

Brand names Capoten, Apo-Capto, Novo-Captoril, Nu-Capto, Syn-Captopril
Used in the following combined preparations None

GENERAL INFORMATION

Captopril belongs to the class of drugs called ACE inhibitors and it is used to treat high blood pressure and heart failure. It works by dilating the blood vessels and easing blood flow. Captopril lowers blood pressure rapidly but may require several weeks to achieve maximum effect. People with heart failure may be given captopril in addition to diuretics. It can achieve dramatic improvement, relieving blood vessel muscle spasm and reducing the work load of the heart.

The first dose is usually very small and should be taken while lying down as there is a risk of a sudden fall in blood pressure. Diuretics are often prescribed with captopril.

A variety of minor *side effects* may occur. Some people experience upset in their sense of taste, others develop a persistent dry cough. A reduction in dose may help minimize these effects.

INFORMATION FOR USERS

Your drug prescription is tailored for you. Do not alter dosage without checking with your physician.

How taken

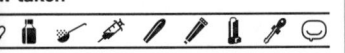

Tablets.

Frequency and timing of doses
3 x daily one hour before food.

Adult dosage range
12.5 – 37.5mg daily (starting dose), gradually increased to 75 – 150mg daily (maintenance dose).

Onset of effect
30 – 60 minutes.

Duration of action
6 – 8 hours.

Diet advice
None.

Storage
Keep in a closed container in a cool, dry place away from reach of children. Protect from light.

Missed dose
Take as soon as you remember. If your next dose is due within 2 hours, take a single dose now and skip the next.

Stopping the drug
Do not stop the drug without consulting your physician; stopping the drug may lead to worsening of the underlying condition.

Exceeding the dose
An occasional unintentional extra dose is unlikely to cause problems. Large overdoses may cause dizziness or fainting. Notify your physician.

POSSIBLE ADVERSE EFFECTS

Captopril may cause a variety of minor adverse effects on the gastrointestinal system.

Rashes, which may occur, usually disappear soon after treatment is begun.

Symptom/effect	Frequency		Discuss with physician		Stop taking drug now	Call physician now
	Common	Rare	Only if severe	In all cases		
Dizziness/fainting		●		■		
Loss of taste	●		■			
Rash/itching	●			■		
Persistent dry cough	●			■		
Nausea/vomiting		●		■		
Swelling of tongue or face		●		■	▲	■

INTERACTIONS

Non-steroidal anti-inflammatory drugs (NSAIDs) Some of these drugs may reduce the effectiveness of captopril.

Potassium supplements, potassium-sparing diuretics, and cyclosporine Captopril may increase the risk of high blood levels of potassium with these drugs.

Antihypertensive drugs are likely to add to the blood pressure-lowering effect of captopril.

SPECIAL PRECAUTIONS

Be sure to tell your physician if:
▼ You have impaired liver or kidney function.
▼ You have coronary artery disease.
▼ You have an autoimmune disease.
▼ You are taking other medications.

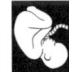

Pregnancy
▼ Can cause abnormalities in the unborn baby. Discuss with your physician if planning a pregnancy or immediately upon becoming pregnant.

Breast feeding
▼ The drug passes into the breast milk, but at normal doses adverse effects on the baby are unlikely. Discuss with your physician.

Infants and children
▼ Not usually prescribed. Reduced dose necessary.

Over 60
▼ Reduced dose may be necessary.

Driving and hazardous work
▼ Avoid such activities until you have learned how the drug affects you; it can cause dizziness and ·fainting.

Alcohol
▼ Avoid. Alcohol may increase the likelihood of an excessive drop in blood pressure.

Surgery and general anesthetic
▼ Captopril treatment may need to be stopped before you have a general anesthetic. Discuss with your physician or dentist before any operation.

PROLONGED USE

No problems expected.

Monitoring Periodic checks required on the white blood cell count and the urine during the first three months of treatment.

CARBAMAZEPINE

Brand names Tegretol, Apo-Carbamazepine, Novo-Carbamaz
Used in the following combined preparations None

GENERAL INFORMATION

Chemically related to the tricyclic antidepressants (see p.96), carbamazepine reduces the likelihood of seizures caused by abnormal nerve signals in the brain. Physicians have used it in the long-term treatment of epilepsy since 1969, and it is considered particularly suitable for treating children because side effects are less of a problem compared to some other drugs for epilepsy. Carbamazepine is also prescribed to relieve the intermittent severe pain caused by damage to the cranial nerves – for example, in trigeminal neuralgia (tic douloureux).

Carbamazepine may also be prescribed to treat mania or to stabilize mood in bipolar affective disorder (manic-depressive disorder).

(see p.96)

QUICK REFERENCE

Drug group Anticonvulsant drug (p.98) and antipsychotic drug (p.97)

Overdose danger rating Medium

Dependence rating Low

Prescription needed Yes

Multi-source suppliers Yes

INFORMATION FOR USERS

Your drug prescription is tailored for you. Do not alter dosage without checking with your physician.

How taken

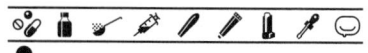

Tablets, slow-release tablets, chewable tablets.

Frequency and timing of doses
1 – 4 x daily with food or milk.

Adult dosage range
Epilepsy 100 – 1,200mg daily.
Pain relief 200 – 1,200mg daily.
Mania 400 – 1,600mg daily.

Onset of effect
Within 4 hours.

Duration of action
12 – 24 hours.

Diet advice
None.

Storage
Keep in a closed container in a cool, dry place away from reach of children. Protect from light.

Missed dose
Take as soon as you remember. If your next dose is due within 2 hours, take a single dose now and skip the next.

Stopping the drug
Do not stop the drug without consulting your physician; symptoms may recur.

Exceeding the dose
An occasional unintentional extra dose is unlikely to cause problems. Large overdoses may cause dizziness or drowsiness. Notify your physician.

SPECIAL PRECAUTIONS

Be sure to tell your physician if:
▼ You have impaired liver or kidney function
▼ You have heart problems.
▼ You have poor circulation.
▼ You have prostate trouble.
▼ You have a blood disease.
▼ You have glaucoma.
▼ You are hypersensitive to tricyclic antidepressants.
▼ You are taking other medications.

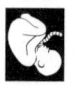 **Pregnancy**
▼ Safety in pregnancy not established. Discuss with your physician.

 Breast feeding
▼ The drug passes into the breast milk and may affect the baby. Discuss with your physician.

 Infants and children
▼ Reduced dose necessary.

 Over 60
▼ May cause confused or agitated behavior in the elderly. Reduced dose may be necessary.

 Driving and hazardous work
▼ Discuss with your physician. Your underlying condition, as well as the possibility of reduced alertness while taking this drug, may make such activities inadvisable.

 Alcohol
▼ Avoid. Alcohol may increase the sedative effects of this drug.

POSSIBLE ADVERSE EFFECTS

Most people experience very few adverse effects with this drug, but when blood levels get too high, adverse effects are common and the dose may need to be reduced.

Symptom/effect	Frequency		Discuss with physician		Stop taking drug now	Call physician now
	Common	Rare	Only if severe	In all cases		
Dizziness/unsteadiness	●		■			
Drowsiness	●		■			
Nausea/vomiting	●		■			
Blurred vision	●			■		
Ankle swelling		●		■		
Rash		●		■	▲	▌

INTERACTIONS

General note Carbamazepine may reduce the effect of many other drugs, including oral anticoagulants, theophylline, anticonvulsants, haloperidol, doxycycline, and oral corticosteroids.

Monoamine oxidase inhibitors (MAOIs) Carbamazepine should not be given within 14 days of treatment with an MAOI.

Diuretics Taken with diuretics, carbamazepine may increase loss of sodium.

Lithium, verapamil, diltiazem, erythromycin, isoniazid, cimetidine, danazol, propoxyphene, and tricyclic antidepressants may increase the risk of adverse effects from carbamazepine.

Oral contraceptives Carbamazepine may reduce the effectiveness of oral contraceptives. An alternative form of contraceptive may need to be used.

PROLONGED USE

There is a slight risk of blood abnormalities occurring during prolonged use.

Monitoring Periodic blood tests may be performed to monitor levels of the drug in the body and the composition of the blood.

CEFACLOR

Brand name Ceclor
Used in the following combined preparations None

GENERAL INFORMATION

Cefaclor, introduced in 1979, is an antibiotic given by mouth to treat a variety of bacterial infections, mainly those affecting the respiratory tract, sinuses, skin, soft tissue, urinary tract, and middle ear. It may be active against some types of bacteria that are resistant to penicillin.

The main use for cefaclor is in the treatment of childhood ear infections that are resistant to ampicillin. Sometimes it is prescribed as follow-up treatment for more severe infections after a different cephalosporin has been given by injection.

Unlike many similar drugs, cefaclor is not affected by the action of digestive juices. Because food may delay its absorption, it is best taken on an empty stomach.

Diarrhea is the most common *side effect* of cefaclor. Some people may suffer from nausea or vomiting, itching, skin rash, and fever especially if they are sensitive to penicillin. In such cases another drug is substituted.

INFORMATION FOR USERS

Your drug prescription is tailored for you. Do not alter dosage without checking with your physician.

How taken

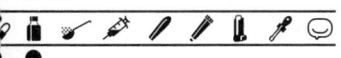

Capsules, oral liquid.

Frequency and timing of doses
2 daily on an empty stomach.

Dosage range
Adults 750mg – 2g daily.
Children Reduced dose according to age and weight up to a maximum of 1g/day.

Onset of effect
1 - 2 days.

Duration of action
8 hours.

Diet advice
None.

Storage
Keep capsules in a closed container in a cool, dry place away from children. Refrigerate liquid, but do not freeze, and keep for no longer than 14 days.

Missed dose
Take as soon as you remember. If your next dose is due at this time, take both doses now.

Stopping the drug
Take the full course. Even if you feel better, the original infection may still be present and may recur if treatment is stopped too soon.

Exceeding the dose
An occasional unintentional extra dose is unlikely to be a cause for concern. But if you notice unusual symptoms, or if a large overdose has been taken, notify your physician.

POSSIBLE ADVERSE EFFECTS

Most people do not suffer any adverse effects while taking cefaclor. Diarrhea occurs fairly commonly but tends not to be severe. Most other adverse effects are due to an allergic reaction that may necessitate stopping the drug.

Symptom/effect	Frequency		Discuss with physician		Stop taking drug now	Call physician now
	Common	Rare	Only if severe	In all cases		
Diarrhea	●		■			
Nausea/vomiting		●	■			
Itching		●		■		
Fever		●		■		▮
Rash		●		■	▲	▮
Joint pain/swelling		●		■	▲	▮

INTERACTIONS

None.

SPECIAL PRECAUTIONS

Be sure to tell your physician if:
▼ You have impaired kidney function.
▼ You have had a previous allergic reaction to penicillin or cephalosporin antibiotics.
▼ You have a history of bleeding disorders.
▼ You are taking other medications.

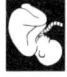
Pregnancy
▼ While there is no evidence of risk to developing baby, absolute safety in pregnancy has not been established. Discuss with your physician.

Breast feeding
▼ The drug passes into the breast milk and may affect the baby. Discuss with your physician.

Infants and children
▼ Reduced dose necessary.

Over 60
▼ No special problems.

Driving and hazardous work
▼ No special problems.

Alcohol
▼ No special problems.

PROLONGED USE

Cefaclor is usually given only for short courses of treatment.

CEFIXIME

Brand name Suprax
Used in the following combined preparations None

GENERAL INFORMATION

Cefixime is a cephalosporin antibiotic given by mouth to treat a variety of mild to moderate bacterial infections. Cefixime does not have as wide a range of effectiveness as some other cephalosporins, but it is helpful in treating infections affecting the middle ear, the respiratory tract, sinuses, and the urinary tract. It is also used to treat uncomplicated gonorrhea.

Sometimes cefixime is prescribed as follow-up treatment for severe infections after a more powerful cephalosporin has been given by injection.

Diarrhea is the most common adverse effect of cefixime. Some people may suffer from nausea or vomiting, itching, skin rash, and fever especially if they are sensitive to penicillin. In such cases, another antibiotic is substituted.

QUICK REFERENCE

Drug group Cephalosporin antibiotic (p.156)

Overdose danger rating Low

Dependence rating Low

Prescription needed Yes

Multi-source suppliers No

INFORMATION FOR USERS

Your drug prescription is tailored for you. Do not alter dosage without checking with your physician.

How taken

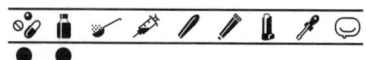

Tablets, oral liquid.

Frequency and timing of doses
Once daily on an empty stomach.

Dosage range
Adults 400mg daily.
Children over 6 months 8mg/kg/day.

Onset of effect
4 hours.

Duration of action
24 hours.

Diet advice
None.

Storage
Keep in a closed container in a cool, dry place away from reach of children. Protect from light. Refrigerate liquid, but do not freeze, and keep for no longer than 14 days.

Missed dose
Take as soon as you remember. If your next dose is due within 6 hours, take a single dose now and skip the next, then follow your regular schedule.

Stopping the drug
Take the full course. Even if you feel better, the original infection may still be present and may recur if treatment is stopped too soon.

Exceeding the dose
An occasional unintentional extra dose is unlikely to be a cause for concern. But if you notice unusual symptoms, or if a large overdose has been taken, notify your physician.

SPECIAL PRECAUTIONS

Be sure to tell your physician if:
▼ You have impaired kidney function.
▼ You have had a previous allergic reaction to penicillin or cephalosporin antibiotics.
▼ You are taking other medications.

Pregnancy
▼ Safety in pregnancy not established. Discuss with your physician.

Breast feeding
▼ It is not known if the drug passes into the breast milk. Discuss with your physician.

Infants and children
▼ Not recommended for children under 6 months. Reduced dose is necessary for older children.

Over 60
▼ Reduced dose may be necessary especially if kidney function is severely impaired.

Driving and hazardous work
▼ Avoid such activities until you have learned how the drug affects you; it may cause dizziness.

Alcohol
▼ No known problems.

POSSIBLE ADVERSE EFFECTS

Most people do not suffer serious adverse effects while taking cefixime. Diarrhea is common but it tends not to be severe. The rarer adverse effects are usually due to an allergic reaction and may necessitate stopping the drug.

Symptom/effect	Frequency		Discuss with physician		Stop taking drug now	Call physician now
	Common	Rare	Only if severe	In all cases		
Diarrhea	●		■			
Headache	●		■			
Nausea/vomiting	●		■			
Abdominal pain		●	■			
Skin rash		●		■	▲	▌
Itching/swelling/wheezing		●		■	▲	▌

INTERACTIONS

None.

PROLONGED USE

Cefixime is usually given only for short courses of treatment.

CEFOXITIN

Brand name Mefoxin
Used in the following combined preparations None

GENERAL INFORMATION

Cefoxitin is a cephalosporin antibiotic. Available in injection form only, it is given in the hospital to prevent infection in surgery of the bowel or female genital tract. It is also used to treat serious conditions such as blood poisoning (septicemia), infections of the abdominal cavity (peritonitis), pelvic infections (salpingitis, endometritis), and certain pneumonias. Cefoxitin is also effective against gonorrhea, but drugs that are less expensive or that can be taken orally are usually preferred. Possible *side effects* include nausea, vomiting, and diarrhea, as well as allergic reactions.

QUICK REFERENCE

Drug group Cephalosporin antibiotic (p.140)

Overdose danger rating Low

Dependence rating Low

Prescription needed Yes

Multi-source suppliers No

INFORMATION FOR USERS

This drug is given only under medical supervision and is not for self-administration.

How taken

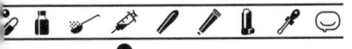

Injection.

Frequency and timing of doses
Every 6 – 8 hours.

Adult dosage range
6 to 12g daily.

Onset of effect
Symptoms usually improve within 1 – 2 days, depending on the condition.

Duration of action
6 – 12 hours

Diet advice
None.

Storage
Not applicable. This drug is not normally kept in the home.

Missed dose
A missed dose is unlikely, since treatment is given by a physician or nurse.

Stopping the drug
The course of treatment should be completed as prescribed. Even if you feel better, the original infection may still be present and may recur if treatment is stopped too soon.

Exceeding the dose
Overdose is unlikely, since treatment is administered by a physician or nurse.

SPECIAL PRECAUTIONS

Be sure to tell your physician if:
▼ You have impaired liver or kidney function.
▼ You have previously suffered an allergic reaction to penicillin or cephalosporin antibiotics.
▼ You are taking other medications.

Pregnancy
▼ Safety in pregnancy not established. Discuss with your physician.

Breast feeding
▼ The drug passes into the breast milk, but at normal doses adverse effects on the baby are unlikely. Discuss with your physician.

Infants and children
▼ Not usually prescribed for babies under 1 month. Reduced dose necessary for older children.

Over 60
▼ Reduced dose may be necessary.

Driving and hazardous work
▼ No known problems.

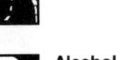
Alcohol
▼ No known problems.

POSSIBLE ADVERSE EFFECTS

Cefoxitin rarely causes serious adverse effects. Development of a rash or fever may be due to an allergic reaction that makes stopping the drug necessary.

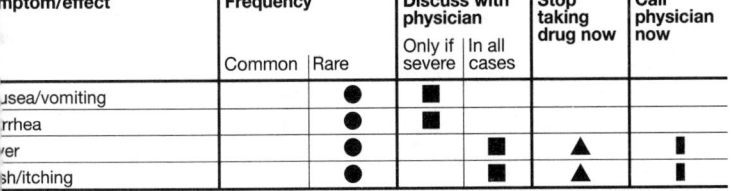

Symptom/effect	Frequency		Discuss with physician		Stop taking drug now	Call physician now
	Common	Rare	Only if severe	In all cases		
Nausea/vomiting		●	■			
Diarrhea		●	■			
Fever		●		■	▲	▮
Rash/itching		●		■	▲	▮

INTERACTIONS

None.

PROLONGED USE

Cefoxitin is usually only given for short courses of treatment.

CEFUROXIME

Brand names Ceftin, Kefurox, Zinacef
Used in the following combined preparations None

GENERAL INFORMATION

Cefuroxime is a cephalosporin antibiotic given by mouth to treat a variety of mild to moderate bacterial infections. Cefuroxime does not have as wide a range of effectiveness as some other cephalosporins, but it is helpful in treating infections affecting the middle ear, the respiratory tract, sinuses, the skin, and the urinary tract. It is also used to treat uncomplicated gonorrhea.

Cefuroxime injection is given in hospital for susceptible infections.
   Diarrhea is the most common adverse effect of cefuroxime. Some patients may suffer from nausea or vomiting, itching, skin rash, and fever, especially if they are sensitive to penicillin. In such cases, another antibiotic is substituted.

QUICK REFERENCE

Drug group Cephalosporin antibiotic (p.156)

Overdose danger rating Low

Dependence rating Low

Prescription needed Yes

Multi-source suppliers Yes

INFORMATION FOR USERS

Your drug prescription is tailored for you. Do not alter dosage without checking with your physician.

How taken

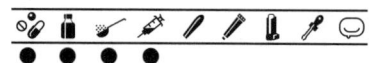

Tablets, oral liquid, granules, injection.

Frequency and timing of doses
2 x daily (by mouth); 3 – 4 x daily (injection).

Dosage range
Adults 250 – 1,000mg daily (by mouth); higher doses according to severity of infection (injection).
Children over 6 months Reduced dosage according to age and weight.

Onset of effect
Within 4 hours (by mouth); within 30 minutes (injection).

Duration of action
12 hours (oral forms); 4 hours (injection).

Diet advice
None.

Storage
Keep tablets in a closed container in a cool, dry place away from reach of children. Protect from light. Refrigerate liquid, but do not freeze, and keep no longer than 14 days.

Missed dose
Take oral forms as soon as you remember. If your next dose is due within 3 hours, take a single dose now and skip the next, then follow your regular schedule.

Stopping the drug
Take the full course. Even if you feel better, the original infection may still be present and may recur if treatment is stopped too soon.

Exceeding the dose
An occasional unintentional extra dose is unlikely to be a cause for concern. But if you notice unusual symptoms, or if a large overdose has been taken, notify your physician.

SPECIAL PRECAUTIONS

Be sure to tell your physician if:
▼ You have impaired kidney function.
▼ You have had a previous allergic reaction to penicillin or cephalosporin antibiotics.
▼ You are taking other medications.

Pregnancy
▼ Safety in pregnancy not established. Discuss with your physician.

Breast feeding
▼ The drug passes into the breast milk and may affect the baby. Discuss with your physician.

Infants and children
▼ Not recommended for children under 6 months. Reduced dose is necessary for older children.

Over 60
▼ Reduced dose may be necessary, especially if kidney function is severely impaired.

Driving and hazardous work
▼ Avoid such activities until you have learned how the drug affects you; it may cause dizziness.

Alcohol
▼ No known problems.

POSSIBLE ADVERSE EFFECTS

Most people do not suffer adverse effects while taking cefuroxime tablets. Diarrhea is common but it tends not to be severe. The rarer adverse effects are usually due to an allergic reaction and may necessitate stopping the drug.

Symptom/effect	Frequency		Discuss with physician		Stop taking drug now	Call physician now
	Common	Rare	Only if severe	In all cases		
Diarrhea	●		■			
Headache/dizziness		●	■			
Nausea/vomiting		●	■			
Skin rash		●		■	▲	▌
Itching/swelling/wheezing		●		■	▲	▌

INTERACTIONS

Antacids Drugs that lower gastric acidity may decrease absorption of cefuroxime given by mouth and should be taken 2 hours before or after cefuroxime.

PROLONGED USE

Cefuroxime is usually given orally for short courses of treatment (7 – 10 days).

CEPHALEXIN

Brand names Keflex, Apo-Cephalex, Novo-Lexin, Nu-Cephalex
Used in the following combined preparations None

GENERAL INFORMATION

Cephalexin, introduced in 1971, is a cephalosporin antibiotic prescribed for a variety of mild to moderate infections. Cephalexin does not have such a wide range of use as some other cephalosporins, but it is helpful in treating bronchitis, cystitis, and certain skin and soft tissue infections. Sometimes it is prescribed as follow-up treatment for severe infections after a more powerful cephalosporin has been given by injection.

Diarrhea is the most common *side effect* of cephalexin. Some people may find that they are allergic to this drug, especially if they are sensitive to penicillin.

INFORMATION FOR USERS

Your drug prescription is tailored for you. Do not alter dosage without checking with your physician.

How taken

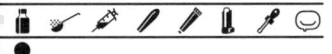

Tablets, capsules, oral liquid.

Frequency and timing of doses
2 – 4 x daily.

Dosage range
Adults 1 – 4g daily.
Children Reduced dose according to age and weight.

Onset of effect
Symptoms usually improve within 1 – 2 days, depending on the condition.

Duration of action
6 hours.

Diet advice
None.

Storage
Keep in a closed container in a cool, dry place away from reach of children. Refrigerate liquid, but do not freeze, and keep no longer than 14 days.

Missed dose
Take as soon as you remember. If your next dose is due at this time, take both doses now.

Stopping the drug
Take the full course. Even if you feel better, the original infection may still be present and may recur if treatment is stopped too soon.

Exceeding the dose
An occasional unintentional extra dose is unlikely to be a cause for concern. But if you notice unusual symptoms, or if a large overdose has been taken, notify your physician.

SPECIAL PRECAUTIONS

Be sure to tell your physician if:
▼ You have impaired kidney function.
▼ You have had a previous allergic reaction to penicillin or cephalosporin antibiotics.
▼ You are taking other medications.

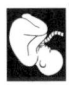 **Pregnancy**
▼ While there is no evidence of risk to developing baby, absolute safety in pregnancy has not been established. Discuss with your physician.

 Breast feeding
▼ The drug passes into the breast milk but at normal doses adverse effects on the baby are unlikely. Discuss with your physician.

 Infants and children
▼ Reduced dose necessary.

 Over 60
▼ No special problems.

 Driving and hazardous work
▼ No known problems.

 Alcohol
▼ No known problems.

POSSIBLE ADVERSE EFFECTS

Most people do not suffer serious adverse effects while taking cephalexin. Diarrhea is common but it tends not to be severe. The rarer adverse effects are usually due to an allergic reaction and may necessitate stopping the drug.

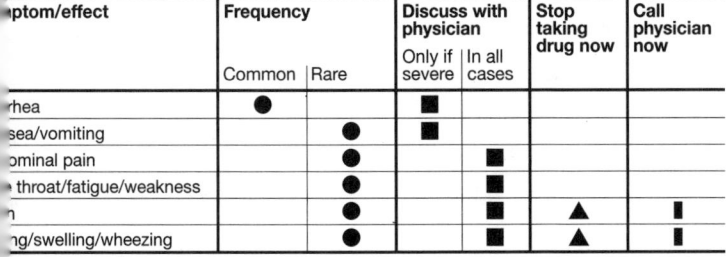

Symptom/effect	Frequency		Discuss with physician		Stop taking drug now	Call physician now
	Common	Rare	Only if severe	In all cases		
Diarrhea	●		■			
Nausea/vomiting		●	■			
Abdominal pain		●		■		
Sore throat/fatigue/weakness		●		■		
Rash		●		■	▲	▍
Itching/swelling/wheezing		●		■	▲	▍

INTERACTIONS

Probenecid This drug increases the level of cephalexin in the blood. The dosage of cephalexin may need to be adjusted accordingly.

PROLONGED USE

Cephalexin is usually given only for short courses of treatment.

CETIRIZINE

Brand name Reactine
Used in the following combined preparations None

GENERAL INFORMATION

Cetirizine is a long-acting antihistamine. Its main use is in the treatment of allergic rhinitis, particularly hay fever.

Cetirizine is also used to treat allergic skin conditions such as urticaria (hives).

The main difference between this drug and older, traditional antihistamines is that it has less *sedative* effect on the central nervous system. It may therefore be suitable for people who need to avoid sleepiness – for example, at work. However, because cetirizine can cause drowsiness in some people, learn how the drug affects you before undertaking activities requiring concentration.

INFORMATION FOR USERS

Follow instructions on the label. Call your physician if symptoms worsen.

How taken

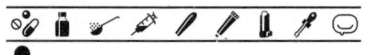

Tablets.

Frequency and timing of doses
Once daily.

Adult dosage range
5 – 20mg daily.

Onset of effect
1 – 3 hours. Some effects may not be felt for 1 – 2 days.

Duration of action
Up to 24 hours.

Diet advice
None.

Storage
Keep in a closed container in a cool, dry place away from reach of children.

Missed dose
No cause for concern, but take as soon as you remember. If your next dose is due within 8 hours, take a single dose now and skip the next.

Stopping the drug
Can be safely stopped as soon as you no longer need it.

Exceeding the dose
An occasional unintentional extra dose is unlikely to cause problems. Large overdoses may cause nausea or drowsiness and have adverse effects on the heart. Notify your physician.

SPECIAL PRECAUTIONS

Be sure to consult your physician or pharmacist before taking this drug if:
▼ You have liver or kidney problems.
▼ You have glaucoma.
▼ You are taking other medications.

 **Pregnancy**
▼ Safety in pregnancy not established. Discuss with your physician.

 Breast feeding
▼ The drug passes into the breast milk. Discuss with your physician.

 Infants and children
▼ Not recommended for children under 12 years of age.

 Over 60
▼ No problems expected.

 Driving and hazardous work
▼ Problems are unlikely. However, avoid such activities until you have learned how the drug affects you because the drug can cause drowsiness in some people.

 Alcohol
▼ Avoid. Alcohol may increase the sedative effects of this drug.

POSSIBLE ADVERSE EFFECTS

The most common adverse effects are somnolence, dry mouth, and fatigue.

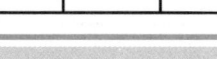

Symptom/effect	Frequency		Discuss with physician		Stop taking drug now	Call physician now
	Common	Rare	Only if severe	In all cases		
Drowsiness/fatigue	●		■			
Dry mouth	●		■			

INTERACTIONS

Anticholinergic drugs The *anticholinergic* effects of cetirizine may be increased by all drugs that have anticholinergic effects, including antipsychotics and tricyclic antidepressants.

Sedatives Cetirizine may increase the sedative effects of anti-anxiety drugs, sleeping drugs, antidepressants, and antipsychotics.

PROLONGED USE

Antihistamines should be discontinued approximately 48 hours before allergy skin testing.

CHLORAL HYDRATE

Brand names None
Used in the following combined preparations None

GENERAL INFORMATION

Chloral hydrate is one of the oldest sleeping drugs in use. Although it has largely been superseded by the benzodiazepines, it is still prescribed for the short-term treatment of insomnia or for relief of anxiety before a surgical or diagnostic procedure. Unlike many sleeping drugs, chloral hydrate is suitable for occasional use in the treatment of sleeplessness in children. The liquid form of the drug has an unpleasant taste; it is also available in capsule form. *Tolerance* can develop to this drug.

QUICK REFERENCE

Drug group Non-barbiturate, non-benzodiazepine sleeping drug (p.94)

Overdose danger rating High

Dependence rating Medium

Prescription needed Yes

Multi-source suppliers Yes

INFORMATION FOR USERS

Your drug prescription is tailored for you. **Do not alter dosage without checking with your physician.**

How taken

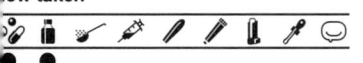

Capsules, syrup.

Frequency and timing of doses
Once daily 15 – 30 minutes before bedtime. Capsules should be taken with a full glass of water. Syrup should be well diluted with fruit juice, ginger ale, or water.

Dosage range
Adults 500mg – 1g daily or 30 minutes before surgery.
Children Reduced dose according to age and weight.

Onset of effect
30 – 60 minutes.

Duration of action
6 – 9 hours.

Diet advice
None.

Storage
Keep in a closed container in a cool, dry place away from reach of children.

Missed dose
If you fall asleep without having taken a dose and wake some hours later, do not take the missed dose. If necessary, return to your normal dose schedule the following night.

Stopping the drug
If you have been taking the drug for less than 4 weeks, it can be safely stopped as soon as you feel that you no longer need it. However, if you have been taking the drug for longer than a few weeks, consult your physician, who may supervise a gradual reduction in dosage. Stopping abruptly may lead to withdrawal symptoms (see p.94).

OVERDOSE ACTION

 Seek immediate medical advice in all cases. Take emergency action if severe confusion, vomiting, or loss of consciousness occur.

See Drug poisoning emergency guide (p.574).

SPECIAL PRECAUTIONS

Be sure to tell your physician if:
▼ You have impaired liver or kidney function.
▼ You have heart problems.
▼ You suffer from porphyria.
▼ You have had problems with alcohol or drug abuse.
▼ You have a stomach ulcer.
▼ You are taking other medications.

 **Pregnancy**
▼ Safety in pregnancy not established. Discuss with your physician.

 Breast feeding
▼ The drug passes into the breast milk. Its effects on the baby are not clearly known. Discuss with your physician.

 Infants and children
▼ Reduced dose necessary.

 Over 60
▼ Reduced dose may be necessary.

 Driving and hazardous work
▼ Avoid such activities until you have learned how the drug affects you; it can cause drowsiness.

 Alcohol
▼ Avoid. Alcohol may increase the sedative effects of this drug.

PROLONGED USE

Regular use of this drug over several weeks can lead to a reduction in its effect as the body adapts. It may also be habit-forming when taken for extended periods, especially if larger-than-average doses are taken.

POSSIBLE ADVERSE EFFECTS

The principal adverse effects of this drug are related to its sedative properties. These effects normally diminish after the first few days of treatment.

Symptom/effect	Frequency		Discuss with physician		Stop taking drug now	Call physician now
	Common	Rare	Only if severe	In all cases		
Nausea/vomiting	●		■			
Clumsiness/unsteadiness		●	■			
Daytime drowsiness		●	■			
Unusual excitement		●		■		
Headache		●		■		
Rash		●		■	▲	

INTERACTIONS

Sedatives All drugs, including alcohol, that have a sedative effect on the central nervous system are likely to increase the sedative properties of chloral hydrate.

Anticoagulants Increased anticoagulant effects may occur when chloral hydrate is taken with anticoagulants such as warfarin.

CHLORAMBUCIL

Brand name Leukeran
Used in the following combined preparations None

GENERAL INFORMATION

Introduced in 1957, this anticancer drug interferes with the growth of cancer cells, thereby helping the immune system overcome the disease. Taken in tablet form, chlorambucil is mainly used to treat certain types of leukemia (cancer of the blood cells) and lymphoma (cancer of the lymph glands), but can affect some cancers of the ovaries and testicles.

Because chlorambucil has an immunosuppressant action, it is sometimes prescribed for such disorders of the immune system as certain types of kidney disease and severe rheumatoid arthritis.

As with other anticancer drugs, chlorambucil may reduce blood cell production by the bone marrow, thereby increasing the risk of abnormal bleeding, anemia, and infection. Long-term use of the drug can also lead to sterility in men and to cessation of periods in women; both these problems may improve after the treatment is stopped. Unlike other anticancer drugs, chlorambucil rarely causes nausea and vomiting.

INFORMATION FOR USERS

Your drug prescription is tailored for you. Do not alter dosage without checking with your physician.

How taken

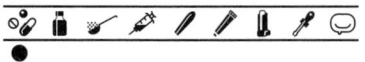

Tablets.

Frequency and timing of doses
Once daily.

Dosage range
Dosage is determined individually according to body height, weight, and response.

Onset of effect
Active in the body within 2 hours. Beneficial effects may not be noticed for 3 – 4 weeks.

Duration of action
24 hours.

Diet advice
None.

Storage
Keep in a closed container in a cool, dry place away from the reach of children.

Missed dose
Take as soon as you remember. If your next dose is due within 6 hours, take a single dose now and skip the next. Tell your physician that you missed a dose.

Stopping the drug
Do not stop the drug without consulting your physician; stopping the drug may lead to worsening of the underlying condition.

Exceeding the dose
An occasional unintentional extra dose is unlikely to cause problems. Large overdoses may cause nausea and vomiting. Notify your physician.

SPECIAL PRECAUTIONS

Chlorambucil is prescribed only under close medical supervision, taking account of your present condition and medical history.

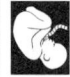

Pregnancy
▼ Not usually prescribed. May cause abnormalities in the unborn baby. Discuss with your physician.

Breast feeding
▼ Discontinue breast feeding. The drug passes into the breast milk and may affect the baby adversely.

Infants and children
▼ Reduced dose necessary.

Over 60
▼ No special problems.

Driving and hazardous work
▼ No known problems.

Alcohol
▼ No known problems.

Surgery and general anesthetics
▼ Before any surgery advise your physician, dentist, or anesthetist that you are taking chlorambucil.

POSSIBLE ADVERSE EFFECTS

Noticeable adverse effects are uncommon with chlorambucil, but always require medical attention. Irregular menstruation in women and sterility in men are usually temporary and disappear when treatment is stopped.

Symptom/effect	Frequency		Discuss with physician		Stop taking drug now	Call physician now
	Common	Rare	Only if severe	In all cases		
Nausea/vomiting		●		■		
Seizures		●		■		
Difficult breathing		●		■	▲	▌
Rash		●		■	▲	▌
Jaundice		●		■	▲	▌

INTERACTIONS

Allopurinol This drug may increase blood levels of chlorambucil, leading to an increased risk of adverse effects.

Radiation treatment Usually there is a short period of delay after radiation before chlorambucil is started.

PROLONGED USE

Prolonged use of this drug may reduce production of blood cells, and may cause temporary sterility in men and disrupted periods in women.

Monitoring Frequent checks on blood composition are required.

CHLORAMPHENICOL

Brand names Chloromycetin, Chloroptic, Ophtho-Chloram, Pentamycetin
Used in the following combined preparations Actinac, Ophthocort, Pentamycetin-HC, Sopamycetin-HC

GENERAL INFORMATION

Chloramphenicol is an antibiotic that is commonly included in *topical* preparations for eye and ear infections. Given by mouth or injection, it is widely distributed in the body and penetrates the brain effectively, making it useful in the treatment of meningitis and brain abscesses. It is also prescribed for typhoid fever and abdominal infections. It is particularly useful for combating epiglottitis, pneumonia, or meningitis caused by Hemophilus bacteria that have acquired resistance to other antibiotics. Q fever, Rocky Mountain spotted fever, and similar infections may also be treated with the drug.

Although most people experience few adverse effects, chloramphenicol occasionally causes serious or even fatal blood disorders. For this reason, chloramphenicol is reserved for serious or life-threatening infections that do not respond to safer drugs.

QUICK REFERENCE

Drug group Antibiotic (p.140)
Overdose danger rating Low
Dependence rating Low
Prescription needed Yes
Multi-source suppliers Yes

INFORMATION FOR USERS

Your drug prescription is tailored for you. Do not alter dosage without checking with your physician.

How taken

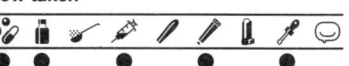

Capsules, oral liquid, injection, cream, eye ointment, eye and ear drops.

Frequency and timing of doses
Every 6 – 8 hours (by mouth, injection); every 2 hours (eye preparations); 3 – 4 x daily (ear drops, cream).

Adult dosage range
Varies according to preparation and condition. Follow your physician's instructions.

Onset of effect
1 – 3 days, depending on the condition and preparation.

Duration of action
6 – 8 hours.

Diet advice
None.

Storage
Keep in a closed container in a cool, dry place away from reach of children.

Missed dose
Take as soon as you remember (capsules, liquid). If your next dose is due, double the dose to make up the missed dose. For skin, eye, and ear preparations, apply as soon as you remember.

Stopping the drug
Take the full course. Even if you feel better, the infection may still be present and may recur if treatment is stopped too soon.

Exceeding the dose
An occasional unintentional extra dose is unlikely to be a cause for concern. But if you notice unusual symptoms, or if a large overdose has been taken, notify your physician.

SPECIAL PRECAUTIONS

Be sure to tell your physician if:
▼ You have impaired liver or kidney function.
▼ You have a blood disorder.
▼ You are taking other medications.

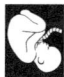

Pregnancy
▼ Taken by mouth or injection in late pregnancy, chloramphenicol may cause vomiting, breathing difficulties, and poor circulation in the newborn infant. Discuss with your physician.

Breast feeding
▼ No evidence of risk with skin, eye or ear preparations. Taken by mouth, the drug passes into the breast milk and may increase the risk of blood disorders in the baby. Discuss with your physician.

Infants and children
▼ Reduced dose necessary.

Over 60
▼ Reduced dose may be necessary.

Driving and hazardous work
▼ No known problems.

Alcohol
▼ No known problems.

POSSIBLE ADVERSE EFFECTS

Transient irritation may occur with eye or ear drops. Sore throat, fever, and unusual redness with any form of chloramphenicol may be signs of blood abnormalities and should be reported to your physician without delay even after treatment has been stopped.

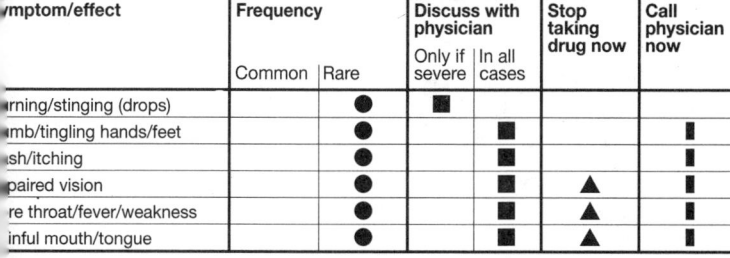

Symptom/effect	Frequency		Discuss with physician		Stop taking drug now	Call physician now
	Common	Rare	Only if severe	In all cases		
Burning/stinging (drops)		●	■			
Numb/tingling hands/feet		●		■		▮
Rash/itching		●		■		▮
Impaired vision		●		■	▲	▮
Sore throat/fever/weakness		●		■	▲	▮
Painful mouth/tongue		●		■	▲	▮

INTERACTIONS

General note Chloramphenicol may increase the effect of certain other drugs, including phenytoin, oral antidiabetics, and oral anticoagulants. Phenobarbital, phenytoin, and rifampin may reduce the effect of chloramphenicol.

Other antibiotics Chloramphenicol may inhibit the antibacterial effects of penicillin and erythromycin antibiotics.

PROLONGED USE

Prolonged use of this drug may increase the risk of serious blood disorders and eye damage.

Monitoring Periodic blood cell counts and eye tests may be performed. Blood levels of the drug are usually monitored in young children given chloramphenicol by mouth or injection.

CHLORDIAZEPOXIDE

Brand names Librium, Apo-Chlordiazepoxide, Solium
Used in the following combined preparations Apo-Chlorax, Librax

GENERAL INFORMATION

Introduced in the mid-1960s, chlordiazepoxide belongs to a group of drugs known as benzodiazepines. These are used to help relieve nervousness and tension and encourage sleep. The actions and adverse effects of this group of drugs are described more fully on page 95.

Prescribed primarily to treat anxiety, chlordiazepoxide is also administered to relieve the symptoms of alcohol withdrawal.

Chlordiazepoxide is combined with clidinium bromide for the treatment of some gastrointestinal disorders associated with anxiety.

Addictive if taken regularly over a long period, chlordiazepoxide may also lose effectiveness with time. For these reasons, treatment is regularly reviewed.

(p.95)

QUICK REFERENCE

Drug group Benzodiazepine anti-anxiety drug (p.95)

Overdose danger rating Medium

Dependence rating Medium

Prescription needed Yes

Multi-source suppliers Yes

INFORMATION FOR USERS

Your drug prescription is tailored for you. Do not alter dosage without checking with your physician.

How taken

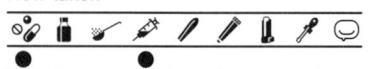

Capsules, injection.

Frequency and timing of doses
1 – 4 x daily with food or milk.

Adult dosage range
10 – 100mg daily (by mouth). The dosage varies considerably from person to person.

Onset of effect
1 – 3 hours.

Duration of action
12 – 24 hours.

Diet advice
None.

Storage
Keep in a closed container in a cool, dry place away from reach of children. Protect from light.

Missed dose
No cause for concern, but take when you remember. If your next dose is due within 2 hours, take a single dose now and skip the next.

Stopping the drug
If you have been taking the drug for less than 2 weeks, it can be safely stopped as soon as you feel you no longer need it. However, if you have been taking the drug for longer, consult your physician, who may supervise a gradual reduction in dosage. Stopping abruptly may lead to withdrawal symptoms (see p.95).

Exceeding the dose
An occasional unintentional extra dose is unlikely to cause problems. Large overdoses may cause unusual drowsiness. Notify your physician.

SPECIAL PRECAUTIONS

Be sure to tell your physician if:
▼ You have impaired liver or kidney function.
▼ You have had problems with alcohol or drug abuse.
▼ You have myasthenia gravis.
▼ You are taking other medications.

Pregnancy
▼ Safety in pregnancy not established. Discuss with your physician.

Breast feeding
▼ The drug passes into the breast milk and may affect the baby. Discuss with your physician.

Infants and children
▼ Not usually prescribed. Reduced dose necessary.

Over 60
▼ Increased likelihood of adverse effects. Reduced dose may therefore be necessary.

Driving and hazardous work
▼ Avoid such activities until you have learned how the drug affects you; it can cause reduced alertness and slowed reactions.

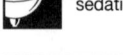

Alcohol
▼ Avoid. Alcohol may increase the sedative effects of this drug.

POSSIBLE ADVERSE EFFECTS

The principal adverse effects of this drug are related to its sedative and tranquilizing properties. These effects normally diminish after the first few days of treatment.

Symptom/effect	Frequency		Discuss with physician		Stop taking drug now	Call physician now
	Common	Rare	Only if severe	In all cases		
Daytime drowsiness	●		■			
Dizziness/unsteadiness	●		■			
Forgetfulness/confusion		●	■			
Headache		●	■			
Blurred vision		●		■		
Rash		●		■	▲	
Hallucinations		●		■	▲	■

PROLONGED USE

Regular use of this drug over several weeks can lead to a reduction in its effect as the body adapts. It may also be habit-forming when taken for extended periods, especially if larger-than-average doses are taken.

INTERACTIONS

Sedatives All drugs, including alcohol, that have a sedative effect on the central nervous system are likely to increase the sedative properties of chlordiazepoxide.

Cimetidine may cause a buildup of chlordiazepoxide levels in the blood, which increases the likelihood of adverse effects.

CHLORPHENIRAMINE

Brand names Chlor-Tripolon, Novo-Pheniram
Used in the following combined preparations Chlor-Tripolon Decongestant, Contac C, Corsym, Ornade

GENERAL INFORMATION

Chlorpheniramine, an antihistamine used for over 35 years, is given to treat allergies such as hay fever, allergic conjunctivitis, urticaria (hives), and angioedema (allergic swellings). It is included in several over-the-counter cold remedies (see p.106).

Like other antihistamines, it relieves allergic skin symptoms such as itching, swelling, and redness. It also reduces sneezing and runny nose and itching eyes in hay fever. Chlorpheniramine also has a mild *anticholinergic* action, which suppresses mucus secretion.

Chlorpheniramine may also be used to prevent or treat allergic reactions to blood transfusions or X-ray contrast material, and as a supplement to epinephrine injections for acute allergic shock (anaphylaxis).

INFORMATION FOR USERS

Follow instructions on the label. Call your physician if symptoms worsen.

How taken

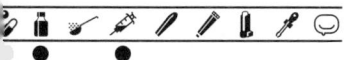

Tablets, slow-release tablets, oral liquid, injection.

Frequency and timing of doses
1 – 4 x daily (tablets, oral liquid); every 8 – 12 hours (slow-release tablets); single dose as needed (injection).

Dosage range
Adults 8 – 24mg daily (orally); up to 40mg daily (injection).
Children over 6 years Reduced dose according to age and weight.

Onset of effect
Within 60 minutes (orally); within 20 minutes (injection).

Duration of action
6 – 8 hours (tablets, oral liquid, injection); 10 – 14 hours (slow-release tablets).

Diet advice
None.

Storage
Keep in a closed container in a cool, dry place away from reach of children.

Missed dose
Take as soon as you remember. If your next dose is due within 2 hours, take a single dose now and skip the next.

Stopping the drug
Can be safely stopped as soon as you no longer need it.

Exceeding the dose
An occasional unintentional extra dose is unlikely to cause problems. Large overdoses may cause drowsiness or agitation. Notify your physician.

SPECIAL PRECAUTIONS

Be sure to consult your physician or pharmacist before taking this drug if:
▼ You have impaired liver function.
▼ You have chronic lung disease.
▼ You have had epileptic seizures.
▼ You have had glaucoma.
▼ You have urinary difficulties.
▼ You are taking other medications.

Pregnancy
▼ Safety in pregnancy not established. Discuss with your physician.

Breast feeding
▼ The drug passes into breast milk, but at normal doses adverse effects on the baby are unlikely. Discuss with your physician.

Infants and children
▼ Not recommended in children under 6 years old. Reduced dose necessary in older children.

Over 60
▼ Reduced dose may be necessary. Increased likelihood of adverse effects.

Driving and hazardous work
▼ Avoid such activities until you have learned how the drug affects you; it can cause drowsiness.

Alcohol
▼ Avoid. Alcohol may increase the sedative effects of this drug.

POSSIBLE ADVERSE EFFECTS

Drowsiness is the most common adverse effect of chlorpheniramine. Other side effects are rare. Some of these, such as dryness of the mouth, blurred vision, and difficulty passing urine, are due to its *anticholinergic* effects. Gastrointestinal irritation may be reduced by taking tablets or liquid with food or drink.

Symptom/effect	Frequency		Discuss with physician		Stop taking drug now	Call physician now
	Common	Rare	Only if severe	In all cases		
Drowsiness	●			■		
Digestive disturbances		●		■		
Urinary difficulties		●		■		
Dry mouth		●		■		
Shaking/tremor		●		■		
Excitation (children)		●			■	▲
Rash		●			■	▲

INTERACTIONS

Alcohol and other sedatives All drugs that have a sedative effect are likely to enhance the sedative effect of chlorpheniramine.

Anticholinergic drugs The anticholinergic effects of chlorpheniramine are likely to be increased by all drugs that have anticholinergic effects, including trihexyphenidyl, antipsychotic drugs, and tricyclic antidepressants.

PROLONGED USE

The effect of the drug may become weaker with prolonged use over a period of weeks or months as the body adapts. Transfer to a different antihistamine may be recommended.

Antihistamines should be discontinued approximately 48 hours prior to allergy skin testing.

CHLORPROMAZINE

Brand name Largactil
Used in the following combined preparations None

GENERAL INFORMATION

Chlorpromazine, introduced in the early 1950s, was the first antipsychotic drug to be marketed. It remains one of the most widely used of this group of drugs, effective in suppressing abnormal behavior, reducing aggression, and inducing a generally tranquilizing effect. For further information, see page 97.

Chlorpromazine is used in the treatment of schizophrenia, mania, dementia, and other disorders where confused, aggressive, or abnormal behavior may occur and a degree of sedation is required. It does not cure the underlying disorder, but it does relieve the distressing symptoms. Another use of chlorpromazine is in the treatment of nausea and vomiting, especially when caused by drug or radiation treatment, or anesthetics.

The main drawback to the use of chlorpromazine is that it can produce serious side effects (see below).

INFORMATION FOR USERS

Your drug prescription is tailored for you. Do not alter dosage without checking with your physician.

How taken

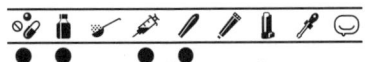

Tablets, oral liquid, injection, rectal suppositories.

Frequency and timing of doses
1 – 4 x daily.

Adult dosage range
30 – 300mg daily. Dose may be increased in severe illness.

Onset of effect
30 – 60 minutes (by mouth); 15 – 20 minutes (injection); up to 30 minutes (rectal suppository).

Duration of action
10 – 12 hours (by mouth or injection); 3 – 4 hours (rectal suppository). Some effect may persist for up to 3 weeks when stopping the drug after regular use.

Diet advice
None.

Storage
Keep in a closed container in a cool, dry place away from reach of children. Protect from light.

Missed dose
Take as soon as you remember. If your next dose is due within 2 hours, do not take the missed dose. Take your next scheduled dose as usual.

Stopping the drug
Do not stop the drug without consulting your physician; symptoms may recur.

Exceeding the dose
An occasional unintentional extra dose is unlikely to cause problems. Larger overdoses may cause unusual drowsiness, fainting, muscle rigidity, and agitation. Notify your physician.

SPECIAL PRECAUTIONS

Be sure to tell your physician if:
▼ You have impaired liver or kidney function
▼ You have had heart problems.
▼ You have prostate trouble.
▼ You have had epileptic seizures.
▼ You have Parkinson's disease.
▼ You have glaucoma.
▼ You are taking other medications.

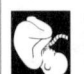

Pregnancy
▼ Not usually prescribed. Taken near the time of delivery it can prolong labor and may cause drowsiness in the newborn baby.

Breast feeding
▼ The drug passes into the breast milk and may affect the baby. Discuss with your physician.

Infants and children
▼ Not recommended for children under one year. Reduced dose is necessary for older children.

Over 60
▼ Initial dosage is low; it may be increased if there are no adverse reactions, such as abnormal limb movements or low blood pressure on arising.

Driving and hazardous work
▼ Avoid such activities until you have learned how the drug affects you; it can cause drowsiness and slowed reactions.

Alcohol
▼ Avoid. Alcohol may increase the sedative effects of this drug.

Surgery and general anesthetics
▼ Chlorpromazine treatment may need to stopped before you have a general anesthetic. Discuss this with your physician or dentist before any operation.

POSSIBLE ADVERSE EFFECTS

Chlorpromazine has a strong *anticholinergic* effect, which can cause serious symptoms. The most significant adverse effect is abnormal movements of the face and limbs (*parkinsonism*).

Symptom/effect	Frequency		Discuss with physician		Stop taking drug now	Call physician now
	Common	Rare	Only if severe	In all cases		
Drowsiness/lethargy	●		■			
Weight gain	●		■			
Blurred vision	●			■		
Dizziness/fainting	●			■		
Parkinsonism	●			■		
Infrequent periods		●		■		
Rash		●		■		▲

INTERACTIONS

Anticonvulsants and antiparkinsonian drugs Chlorpromazine may reduce the effect of these drugs.

Sedatives All drugs, including alcohol, that have a sedative effect on the central nervous system are likely to increase the sedative properties of chlorpromazine.

Anticholinergic drugs may intensify the anticholinergic properties of chlorpromazine.

PROLONGED USE

If used for more than a few months, chlorpromazine may cause *tardive dyskinesia*, a movement disorder. Occasionally, jaundice may occur.

CHLORPROPAMIDE

Brand names Diabinese, Apo-Chlorpropamide, Novo-Propamide
Used in the following combined preparations None

GENERAL INFORMATION

Chlorpropamide is an oral antidiabetic drug. Given in conjunction with a diet that limits carbohydrates and fats, it is used in the treatment of adult (maturity-onset) diabetes mellitus. It lowers blood sugar by stimulating insulin secretion from the pancreas and by promoting the uptake of sugar into body cells.

Chlorpropamide is also prescribed for mild forms of diabetes insipidus, in which it reduces the volume of urine produced by increasing water reabsorption in the kidneys.

The longest acting of the oral antidiabetic drugs, chlorpropamide needs to be taken only once daily. It is not given to people with kidney failure and it is used with caution in the elderly and in children with diabetes insipidus, since it may build up in the body and cause excessive lowering of blood sugar.

QUICK REFERENCE

Drug group Oral antidiabetic drug (p.154)

Overdose danger rating High

Dependence rating Low

Prescription needed Yes

Multi-source suppliers Yes

INFORMATION FOR USERS

Your drug prescription is tailored for you. Do not alter dosage without checking with your physician.

How taken

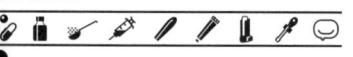

Tablets.

Frequency and timing of doses
Once daily with breakfast.

Dosage range
Adults 100 – 500mg daily.
Children Reduced dose necessary.

Onset of effect
Within 1 hour.

Duration of action
– 3 days.

Diet advice
For treatment of diabetes mellitus, a low-carbohydrate, low-fat diet must be maintained. Follow your physician's advice.

Storage
Keep in a closed container in a cool, dry place away from reach of children.

Missed dose
Take before your next meal.

Stopping the drug
Do not stop the drug without consulting your physician; stopping the drug may lead to worsening of your diabetes.

OVERDOSE ACTION

Seek immediate medical advice in all cases. If symptoms of low blood sugar such as faintness, confusion, sweating, or shaking occur, eat or drink something sugary. Take emergency action if seizures or loss of consciousness occurs.

See Drug poisoning emergency guide (p.574).

SPECIAL PRECAUTIONS

Be sure to tell your physician if:
▼ You have impaired liver or kidney function.
▼ You have thyroid problems.
▼ You are allergic to sulfonamide drugs.
▼ You are taking other medications.

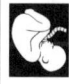

Pregnancy
▼ Not recommended. Insulin is generally used in pregnancy because it gives better diabetic control.

Breast feeding
▼ The drug passes into the breast milk and may cause low blood sugar in the baby. Discuss with your physician.

Infants and children
▼ Not prescribed for diabetes mellitus. Reduced dose necessary for diabetes insipidus.

Over 60
▼ Signs of low blood sugar may be more difficult to recognize. Reduced dose may be necessary.

Driving and hazardous work
▼ Usually no problem. Avoid these activities if you have warning signs of low blood sugar.

Alcohol
▼ Avoid. Alcoholic drinks upset diabetic control and chlorpropamide may cause intolerance to alcohol.

Surgery and general anesthetics
▼ Surgery may reduce the response to this drug. Notify your physician that you are diabetic before any surgery; insulin treatment may need to be substituted.

POSSIBLE ADVERSE EFFECTS

Serious adverse effects are rare. Faintness, sweating, tremor, weakness, and confusion may be signs of low blood sugar due to lack of food or too high a dose.

Symptom/effect	Frequency		Discuss with physician		Stop taking drug now	Call physician now
	Common	Rare	Only if severe	In all cases		
Faintness/confusion	●			■		
Weakness/tremor	●			■		
Sweating	●			■		
Nausea/vomiting	●			■		
Heartburn/indigestion		●	■			
Thirst		●		■		
Rash/itching		●		■		

PROLONGED USE

No problems expected.

Monitoring If the drug is taken for diabetes mellitus, regular monitoring of urine or blood sugar is required.

INTERACTIONS

General note A variety of drugs may reduce the effect of chlorpropamide and so raise blood sugar levels. Such drugs include corticosteroids, estrogens, diuretics, and niacin. Other drugs increase the risk of low blood sugar. These include warfarin, sulfonamides, clofibrate, beta blockers and probenecid.

Barbiturates Chlorpropamide may prolong the action of barbiturates.

CHLORTHALIDONE

Brand names Hygroton, Apo-Chlorthalidone, Uridon
Used in the following combined preparations Combipres, Hygroton-Reserpine, Tenoretic

GENERAL INFORMATION

Chlorthalidone is similar to drugs in the thiazide group of diuretics (p.111). It is longer-acting than many thiazides. These drugs remove excess salt and water from the body and reduce edema (fluid retention) in people with congestive heart failure, and cirrhosis of the liver.

Chlorthalidone is frequently used to treat high blood pressure (see Antihypertensive drugs, p.114), and because it reduces the amount of calcium in the urine, it is sometimes used to prevent the recurrence of certain types of kidney stones.

It increases the loss of potassium and other body salts in the urine, which can result in a variety of symptoms (see p.524), increasing the likelihood of irregular heart rhythms, particularly in those taking drugs such as digoxin for heart failure. For this reason, potassium supplements may be prescribed along with chlorthalidone.

QUICK REFERENCE

Drug group Thiazide-like diuretic (p.111)

Overdose danger rating Low

Dependence rating Low

Prescription needed Yes

Multi-source suppliers Yes

INFORMATION FOR USERS

Your drug prescription is tailored for you. Do not alter dosage without checking with your physician.

How taken

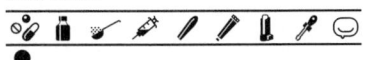

Tablets.

Frequency and timing of doses
Once daily, early in the day, with food.

Adult dosage range
25 – 200mg daily, or three times a week.

Onset of effect
Within 2 hours.

Duration of action
60 hours.

Diet advice
Use of this drug may reduce potassium in the body. Eat plenty of fresh fruit and vegetables.

Discuss the advisability of reducing your salt intake with your physician.

Storage
Keep in a closed container in a cool, dry place away from reach of children.

Missed dose
No cause for concern, but take as soon as you remember.

Stopping the drug
Do not stop taking the drug without consulting your physician; symptoms may recur.

Exceeding the dose
An occasional unintentional extra dose is unlikely to be a cause for concern. But if you do notice unusual symptoms, or if a large overdose has been taken, notify your physician.

SPECIAL PRECAUTIONS

Be sure to tell your physician if:
▼ You have impaired liver or kidney function.
▼ You have had gout.
▼ You have diabetes.
▼ You have had lupus erythematosus.
▼ You have a high level of fat in your blood.
▼ You are allergic to sulfonamide drugs.
▼ You are taking other medications.

Pregnancy
▼ Not usually prescribed. May cause jaundice in the newborn baby. Discuss with your physician.

Breast feeding
▼ The drug passes into the breast milk, but at normal doses adverse effects on the baby are unlikely. Discuss with your physician.

Infants and children
▼ Not usually prescribed. Reduced dose necessary.

Over 60
▼ Increased likelihood of adverse effects.

Driving and hazardous work
▼ No special problems.

Alcohol
▼ Keep consumption low. Chlorthalidone increases the likelihood of dehydration and hangovers after consumption of alcohol.

POSSIBLE ADVERSE EFFECTS

Most adverse effects are caused by the excessive loss of potassium from the body. This can usually be put right by taking a potassium supplement.

Symptom/effect	Frequency		Discuss with physician		Stop taking drug now	Call physician now
	Common	Rare	Only if severe	In all cases		
Lethargy	●		■			
Dizziness	●		■			
Digestive disturbance	●		■			
Temporary impotence	●		■			
Rash	●			■		▲

INTERACTIONS

Non-steroidal anti-inflammatory drugs (NSAIDs) Some of these drugs may reduce the diuretic effect of chlorthalidone. The dosage of chlorthalidone may need to be adjusted accordingly.

Digoxin The effects of digoxin may be increased if excessive amounts of potassium are lost.

Corticosteroids further increase the loss of potassium from the body when taken with chlorthalidone.

Lithium Chlorthalidone may increase lithium levels in the blood, leading to a risk of serious adverse effects.

PROLONGED USE

Prolonged use of this drug can lead to excessive loss of potassium and imbalances of other salts.

Monitoring Blood tests may be performed periodically to check kidney function and levels of blood sugar, potassium, and other salts.

CHOLESTYRAMINE

Brand names Questran, PMS-Cholestyramine
Used in the following combined preparations None

GENERAL INFORMATION

Cholestyramine is a resin which binds bile acids in the intestine, preventing their reabsorption. Cholesterol in the liver is normally converted to bile acids. Therefore, the use of cholestyramine results in a reduction of cholesterol levels in the blood. This action on the bile acids makes bowel movements bulkier, thus creating an antidiarrheal effect. The action on cholesterol helps people with hyperlipidemia (high levels of fat in the blood) who have not responded to dietary measures, and who are at particular risk from heart disease.

If bile salts accumulate in the bloodstream, as sometimes happens in liver disorders such as primary biliary cirrhosis, cholestyramine may be prescribed to alleviate any accompanying itching that might occur.

In large doses, cholestyramine often causes bloating, mild nausea, and constipation. Cholestyramine may also interfere with the body's ability to absorb fat, and certain vitamins dissolved in fat, causing pale, bulky, foul-smelling feces (steatorrhea).

QUICK REFERENCE

Drug group Lipid-lowering drug (p.115)

Overdose danger rating Low

Dependence rating Low

Prescription needed Yes

Multi-source suppliers Yes

INFORMATION FOR USERS

Your drug prescription is tailored for you. Do not alter dosage without checking with your physician.

How taken

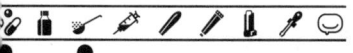

Tablets, powder mixed with water or other fluids before ingesting.

Frequency and timing of doses
1 – 3 x daily with meals.

Adult dosage range
4 – 24g daily.

Onset of effect
Some effect may be noticed within one week, but full beneficial effects may not be felt for several weeks.

Duration of action
12 – 24 hours.

Diet advice
A low-fat, low-calorie diet may be recommended for those overweight. Use of this drug may deplete levels of certain vitamins. Supplements may be advised.

Storage
Keep in a closed container in a cool, dry place away from reach of children.

Missed dose
Take as soon as you remember.

Stopping the drug
Do not stop taking the drug without consulting your physician.

Exceeding the dose
An occasional unintentional extra dose is unlikely to cause problems. But if you notice unusual symptoms, or if a large overdose has been taken, notify your physician.

SPECIAL PRECAUTIONS

Be sure to tell your physician if:
▼ You suffer from constipation.
▼ You have jaundice.
▼ You have a kidney disorder.
▼ You have a peptic ulcer.
▼ You suffer from hemorrhoids.
▼ You are taking other medications.

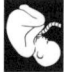

Pregnancy
▼ Safety in pregnancy not established. Discuss with your physician.

Breast feeding
▼ Possible lack of proper vitamin absorption may affect the baby. Discuss with your physician.

Infants and children
▼ Dosage for infants and children not established.

Over 60
▼ Increased likelihood of adverse effects.

Driving and hazardous work
▼ No special problems.

Alcohol
▼ Although this drug does not interact with alcohol, your underlying condition may make it inadvisable to take alcohol.

POSSIBLE ADVERSE EFFECTS

Adverse effects are more likely if large doses are taken by people over 60. Minor side effects such as indigestion and abdominal pain are uncomfortable but rarely cause for concern. More serious adverse effects are usually the result of vitamin deficiency.

Symptom/effect	Frequency		Discuss with physician		Stop taking drug now	Call physician now
	Common	Rare	Only if severe	In all cases		
Indigestion	●		■			
Abdominal pain	●		■			
Nausea/vomiting	●		■			
Constipation	●		■			
Steatorrhea		●		■		
Diarrhea		●		■		

INTERACTIONS

General note Cholestyramine considerably reduces the body's ability to absorb other drugs. It may be necessary to organize a schedule in consultation with your physician whereby you take other medications at a fixed time before you take cholestyramine. Usually, taking other medications at least 1 hour before or 4 to 6 hours after cholestyramine solves the problem. The dosage of other drugs may need to be adjusted.

PROLONGED USE

As this drug reduces vitamin absorption, supplements of vitamins A, D, and K and folic acid may be advised.

Monitoring Periodic blood checks are usually required to monitor the level of cholesterol in the blood.

CICLOPIROX

Brand name Loprox
Used in the following combined preparations None

GENERAL INFORMATION

This relatively new antifungal drug is prescribed as a *topical* treatment for fungal and yeast infections of the skin, such as athlete's foot and jock itch. It may also be prescribed to treat the less common skin disease known as tinea versicolor, characterized by fine scales over the skin, usually on the chest.

Ciclopirox has two clear advantages over most other topical antifungal preparations: it has a more rapid onset of effect; and its adverse reactions are rare, and tend to be minor.

INFORMATION FOR USERS

Your drug prescription is tailored for you. Do not alter dosage without checking with your physician.

How taken

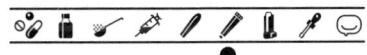

Cream, lotion.

Frequency and timing of doses
2 x daily.

Adult dosage range
Gently massage sufficient cream or lotion on the affected and surrounding skin areas twice daily, in the morning and evening, for a minimum of 4 weeks.

Onset of effect
1 – 2 days.

Duration of action
12 hours.

Diet advice
None.

Storage
Keep in a closed container in a cool, dry place away from reach of children.

Missed dose
No cause for concern, but apply as soon as you remember.

Stopping the drug
Apply the full course. Even if symptoms disappear, the original infection may still be present and may recur if treatment is stopped too soon.

Exceeding the dose
An occasional unintentional extra application is unlikely to be a cause for concern.

POSSIBLE ADVERSE EFFECTS

Ciclopirox rarely causes adverse effects. It may occasionally cause local irritation, and this may mean that a different antifungal may need to be substituted.

Symptom/effect	Frequency		Discuss with physician		Stop taking drug now	Call physician now
	Common	Rare	Only if severe	In all cases		
Irritation/burning	●			■	▲	
Itching	●			■	▲	

INTERACTIONS

None.

SPECIAL PRECAUTIONS

Be sure to tell your physician if:
▼ You are taking other medications.

Pregnancy
▼ Safety in pregnancy not established. Discuss with your physician.

Breast feeding
▼ No evidence of risk.

Infants and children
▼ Safety for children under 10 years not established.

Over 60
▼ No special problems.

Driving and hazardous work
▼ No known problems.

Alcohol
▼ No known problems.

PROLONGED USE

No problems expected.

CIMETIDINE

Brand names Tagamet, Apo-Cimetidine, Novo-Cimetine, Nu-Cimet, Peptol
Used in the following combined preparations None

GENERAL INFORMATION

Introduced in 1977, cimetidine reduces the secretion of gastric acid and of pepsin, an enzyme which helps the digestion of protein. By reducing levels of acid and pepsin, it promotes healing of ulcers in the stomach and duodenum (see p.121). Cimetidine is also used in reflux esophagitis, a condition that may cause acid stomach contents to flow partway up the esophagus. Treatment is usually given in courses of 4 to 8 weeks, followed by maintenance therapy.

Cimetidine also affects the actions of certain enzymes in the liver, where many drugs are broken down. It is therefore prescribed with caution if you are receiving drugs, particularly anticoagulants and anticonvulsants, whose levels need to be carefully controlled. As cimetidine promotes healing of the stomach lining, it may mask the symptoms of stomach cancer, delaying diagnosis. It is therefore prescribed with due caution.

INFORMATION FOR USERS

Your prescription is tailored for you. Do not alter dosage without checking with your physician.

How taken

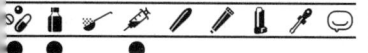

Tablets, oral liquid, injection.

Frequency and timing of doses
4 x daily (after meals and at bedtime).

Adult dosage range
800 – 2,400mg daily.

Onset of effect
15 – 90 minutes.

Duration of action
4 hours.

Diet advice
None.

Storage
Keep in a closed container in a cool, dry place away from reach of children. Protect from light.

Missed dose
Do not take the missed dose. Take your next dose as usual.

Stopping the drug
Do not stop taking the drug without consulting your physician; symptoms may recur.

Exceeding the dose
An occasional unintentional extra dose is unlikely to be a cause for concern. But if you notice unusual symptoms, or if a large overdose has been taken, notify your physician.

SPECIAL PRECAUTIONS

Be sure to tell your physician if:
▼ You have impaired liver or kidney function.
▼ You are taking other medications.

Pregnancy
▼ Safety in pregnancy not established. Discuss with your physician.

Breast feeding
▼ The drug passes into the breast milk and may affect the baby adversely. Discuss with your physician.

Infants and children
▼ Reduced dose necessary.

Over 60
▼ No special problems unless kidney function is impaired and/or the patient is taking other medications. Reduced dose may therefore be necessary.

Driving and hazardous work
▼ Avoid such activities until you have learned how the drug affects you, because the drug can cause dizziness and confusion.

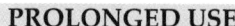

Alcohol
▼ Avoid. Alcohol may aggravate the underlying condition and counter the beneficial effects of cimetidine.

POSSIBLE ADVERSE EFFECTS

Adverse effects of cimetidine are uncommon. They are usually related to dosage level and almost always disappear when the drug is stopped.

Symptom/effect	Frequency		Discuss with physician		Stop taking drug now	Call physician now
	Common	Rare	Only if severe	In all cases		
Diarrhea		●		■		
Dizziness/unsteadiness		●		■		
Confusion		●		■		
Breast enlargement (men)		●		■		
Impotence		●		■		
Rash		●		■		

PROLONGED USE

Courses of longer than 12 months are not usually necessary.

INTERACTIONS

Anticonvulsant drugs Cimetidine may increase the blood levels of such drugs, and the dose may need to be reduced.

Anticoagulant drugs Cimetidine may increase the effect of these drugs. The dosage of anticoagulants may need to be reduced.

Beta blockers Cimetidine may increase blood levels of these drugs.

Benzodiazepine drugs Cimetidine may cause an increase in blood levels of some of these drugs, leading to an increased risk of adverse effects.

CIPROFLOXACIN

Brand name Cipro
Used in the following combined preparations None

GENERAL INFORMATION

Ciprofloxacin, a quinolone antibiotic, is effective against several types of bacteria that tend to be resistant to other commonly used antibiotics. It is prescribed to treat a wide range of infections, and is particularly useful for infections of the chest, intestine, and urinary tract. It is also used as a single dose in treating uncomplicated gonorrhea.

When taken in the form of tablets, ciprofloxacin is well absorbed by the body and works quickly and effectively. In more severe systemic bacterial infections, however, it may need to be given by injection.

Ciprofloxacin has a long duration of action and needs to be taken only once or twice daily depending on the condition being treated. The drug causes few *side effects*, of which gastrointestinal disturbance is the most common.

INFORMATION FOR USERS

Your drug prescription is tailored for you. Do not alter dosage without checking with your physician.

How taken

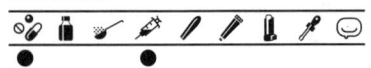

Tablets, injection.

Frequency and timing of doses
1 – 2 x daily.

Adult dosage range
0.2 – 1.5g daily (tablets); 400 – 800mg daily (injection).

Onset of effect
The drug begins to work within a few hours, although full beneficial effect may not be felt for several days.

Duration of action
About 12 hours.

Diet advice
Do not get dehydrated. Ensure that you drink fluids regularly. Avoid excessive caffeine.

Storage
Keep in a closed container in a cool, dry place away from reach of children. The injection must be protected from light.

Missed dose
Take as soon as you remember, and take your next dose as usual.

Stopping the drug
Take the full course. Even if you feel better the original infection may still be present, and symptoms may recur if treatment is stopped too soon.

Exceeding the dose
An occasional unintentional extra dose is unlikely to cause problems. Large overdoses may cause mental disturbance and convulsions. Notify your physician.

SPECIAL PRECAUTIONS

Be sure to tell your physician if:
▼ You have impaired liver or kidney function.
▼ You have had epileptic seizures.
▼ You are taking other medications.

Pregnancy
▼ Safety in pregnancy not established. Discuss with your physician.

Breast feeding
▼ The drug passes into the breast milk and may affect the baby. Discuss with your physician.

Infants and children
▼ Not recommended.

Over 60
▼ No special problems.

Driving and hazardous work
▼ Avoid such activities until you have learned how the drug affects you because it can cause dizziness

Alcohol
▼ Avoid. Alcohol may increase the sedative effects of this drug.

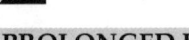

POSSIBLE ADVERSE EFFECTS

Although ciprofloxacin may cause nausea and vomiting, other side effects are less common, except when very high doses are given for severe infections.

Symptom/effect	Frequency		Discuss with physician		Stop taking drug now	Call physician now
	Common	Rare	Only if severe	In all cases		
Nausea/vomiting	●		■			
Diarrhea	●		■			
Abdominal pain	●		■			
Dizziness		●	■			
Joint pain		●	■			
Headache		●	■			
Rash		●		■		

INTERACTIONS

Antacids containing magnesium or aluminum hydroxide interfere with the absorption of ciprofloxacin. Do not take antacids within 2 hours of taking ciprofloxacin tablets.

Iron Oral iron preparations will reduce the absorption of ciprofloxacin.

Theophylline Ciprofloxacin may increase the blood levels of theophylline. Dose adjustment may be necessary, and blood levels of theophylline may need monitoring.

Oral anticoagulants Ciprofloxacin may increase the anticoagulant effect of these drugs.

PROLONGED USE

No problems expected. Blood tests may be necessary to monitor kidney and liver function.

CISAPRIDE

Brand name Prepulsid
Used in the following combined preparations None

GENERAL INFORMATION

Cisapride is a new drug that stimulates forward movement in the esophagus and intestines. It is useful in a number of gastrointestinal disorders including gastroesophageal reflux, which gives symptoms such as dyspepsia, heartburn, and regurgitation. Cisapride may be useful when stomach emptying is delayed. This happens in some diabetics and patients suffering from systemic sclerosis (scleroderma) and autonomic neuropathy.

Cisapride produces its effect by increasing the release of acetylcholine in the gut wall; this in turn increases the contractions of the muscles in the gut wall. Adverse effects on the gastrointestinal tract rarely require discontinuing the drug and tend to diminish as treatment continues.

QUICK REFERENCE

Drug group Motility stimulant
Overdose danger rating Medium
Dependence rating Low
Prescription needed Yes
Multi-source suppliers No

INFORMATION FOR USERS

Your drug prescription is tailored for you. Do not alter dosage without checking with your physician.

How taken

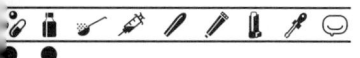

Tablets, oral liquid.

Frequency and timing of doses
3 – 4 x daily, 15 minutes before meals and/or at bedtime (for symptoms during the night).

Adult dosage range
15 – 40mg daily in divided doses.

Onset of effect
5 – 30 minutes.

Duration of action
5 to 10 hours.

Diet advice
None, unless your physician has advised according to the condition you have.

Storage
Keep in a closed container in a cool, dry place away from reach of children. Protect from light.

Missed dose
Do not take unless you have symptoms. Take the next dose as usual unless you took the last dose less than 2 hours ago.

Stopping the drug
Do not stop the drug without consulting your physician; symptoms may recur.

Exceeding the dose
An occasional unintentional extra dose is unlikely to be a cause for concern. But if you notice unusual symptoms, or if a large overdose has been taken, notify your physician.

SPECIAL PRECAUTIONS

Be sure to tell your physician if:
▼ You have impaired liver or kidney function.
▼ You have a history of gastrointestinal illness.
▼ You are taking other medications.

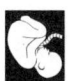
Pregnancy
▼ Safety in pregnancy not established. Discuss with your physician.

Breast feeding
▼ The drug passes into the breast milk and breast feeding is not recommended. Discuss with your physician.

Infants and children
▼ Not usually prescribed.

Over 60
▼ Reduced dose may be necessary.

Driving and hazardous work
▼ Avoid such activities until you have learned how the drug affects you because the drug can cause dizziness.

Alcohol
▼ Avoid. Alcohol's sedative effects may be increased by cisapride.

POSSIBLE ADVERSE EFFECTS

The most common adverse effects are those of the gastrointestinal system. These are usually transient and rarely require discontinuing the drug.

Symptom/effect	Frequency		Discuss with physician		Stop taking drug now	Call physician now
	Common	Rare	Only if severe	In all cases		
Abdominal pain/cramps	●		■			
Diarrhea	●		■			
Dizziness		●		■		
Headaches		●		■		
Tremor		●		■		

PROLONGED USE

Cisapride is normally given for a course of treatment lasting between 4 and 12 weeks depending on the condition being treated.

INTERACTIONS

General note Cisapride may decrease the absorption of some drugs from the stomach (e.g. digoxin) whereas absorption of other drugs from the small bowel may be accelerated (e.g. acetaminophen, tetracycline antibiotics, levodopa).

Anticholinergic drugs may reduce the beneficial effects of cisapride.

Anticoagulants The effect of anticoagulants such as warfarin may be increased by cisapride.

Cimetidine, ranitidine The effects of cisapride may be increased by these drugs.

259

CLARITHROMYCIN

Brand name Biaxin
Used in the following combined preparations None

GENERAL INFORMATION

Clarithromycin is a macrolide antibiotic effective against a wide range of bacteria. It is a useful alternative to penicillins and tetracyclines for people who are allergic to those drugs.

Clarithromycin is commonly prescribed for sinus, throat, middle ear, and chest infections, including some rare types of pneumonia such as walking (mycoplasma) pneumonia. It can also be used to treat infections of the skin and skin structures.

Clarithromycin shows promise in the treatment of uncommon, difficult-to-treat infections associated with AIDS and other states of weakened immunity.

Clarithromycin may sometimes cause abdominal cramping and discomfort, or nausea and vomiting. Other possible adverse effects include headache, altered taste, and a rare risk of liver disorders.

INFORMATION FOR USERS

Your drug prescription is tailored for you. Do not alter dosage without consulting your physician.

How taken

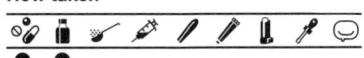

Tablets, oral liquid.

Frequency and timing of doses
2 x daily. May be taken with or without meals.

Dosage range
Adults 500 – 1,000mg daily.
Children Reduced dose according to weight.

Onset of effect
Symptoms usually improve within 1 – 3 days, depending on the condition.

Duration of action
12 hours.

Diet advice
None.

Storage
Keep in a closed container in a cool, dry place away from reach of children.

Missed dose
Take as soon as you remember. If your next dose is within 4 hours, take a single dose now and skip the next.

Stopping the drug
Take the full course. Even if you feel better, the original infection may still be present and symptoms may recur if treatment is stopped too soon.

Exceeding the dose
An occasional unintentional extra dose is unlikely to be a cause for concern. But if you notice unusual symptoms, or if a large overdose has been taken, notify your physician.

SPECIAL PRECAUTIONS

Be sure to tell your physician if:
▼ You have a liver disease or impaired liver function.
▼ You have had a previous allergic reaction to a macrolide antibiotic.
▼ You are taking other medications.

Pregnancy
▼ Safety in pregnancy not established. Discuss with your physician.

Breast feeding
▼ The drug passes into the breast milk. Discuss with your physician.

Infants and children
▼ Reduced dose necessary.

Over 60
▼ No special problems.

Driving and hazardous work
▼ No known problems.

Alcohol
▼ No known problems.

POSSIBLE ADVERSE EFFECTS

Nausea and vomiting are the most common adverse effects and are most likely to occur with large doses. Symptoms such as fever, rash, and jaundice may be a sign of a liver disorder and should always be reported to your physician.

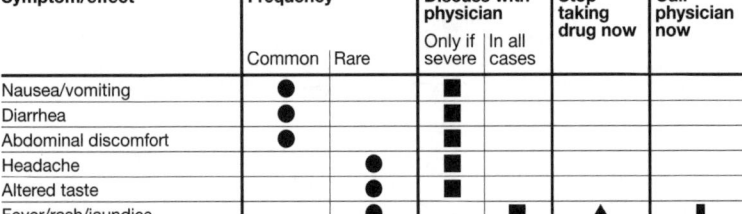

Symptom/effect	Frequency		Discuss with physician		Stop taking drug now	Call physician now
	Common	Rare	Only if severe	In all cases		
Nausea/vomiting	●		■			
Diarrhea	●		■			
Abdominal discomfort	●		■			
Headache		●	■			
Altered taste		●	■			
Fever/rash/jaundice		●		■	▲	■

PROLONGED USE

Prolonged use may increase the risk of liver damage.

INTERACTIONS

The following interactions have been reported with another macrolide antibiotic, erythromycin, and may occur with clarithromycin.

Carbamazepine, cyclosporine, digoxin, triazolam, and theophylline Erythromycin may increase the risk of *side effects* with these drugs.

Terfenadine and astemizole Erythromycin increases the risk of adverse effects of these antihistamines on the heart.

Warfarin Erythromycin increases the risk of bleeding with warfarin.

Ergotamine Erythromycin may increase the risk of side effects with this drug.

CLINDAMYCIN

Brand names Dalacin C, Dalacin T
Used in the following combined preparations None

GENERAL INFORMATION

Clindamycin is a powerful antibiotic that can be taken by mouth and is absorbed into the bloodstream in high concentrations. It is used in the treatment of serious infections, particularly those that commonly involve penicillin-resistant bacteria. These include gynecological and pelvic infections in women, peritonitis, serious lung infections, and skin infections such as abscesses and infected bedsores.

Since clindamycin penetrates bone and joints well, it is sometimes prescribed for bone and joint infections, including osteomyelitis and septic arthritis. It may be given to prevent infection in people undergoing surgery of the mouth, throat, or bowel. *Topical* solution is used to treat acne, and vaginal cream is used to treat bacterial vaginosis.

Although clindamycin can be safely used in most people, it may occasionally cause a potentially fatal disorder called pseudomembranous colitis. This disorder is caused by an overgrowth of clindamycin-resistant bacteria in the bowel, leading to severe bloody diarrhea with cramping abdominal pain and fever.

QUICK REFERENCE

Drug group Lincosamide antibiotic (p.142)

Overdose danger rating Low

Dependence rating Low

Prescription needed Yes

Multi-source suppliers No

INFORMATION FOR USERS

Your drug prescription is tailored for you. Do not alter dosage without checking with your physician.

How taken

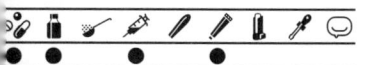

Capsules, oral liquid, injection, vaginal cream, topical solution.

Frequency and timing of doses
By mouth 3 – 4 x daily with food or water.
Injection 2 – 4 x daily or continuously by infusion.

Dosage range
Adults 600 – 1,800mg daily (by mouth).
Children Reduced dose according to age and weight.

Onset of effect
1 – 3 days.

Duration of action
8 – 12 hours.

Diet advice
None.

Storage
Keep in a closed container in a cool, dry place away from reach of children.

Missed dose
Take as soon as you remember. If your next dose is due within 2 hours, take a single dose now and skip the next.

Stopping the drug
Take the full course. Even if you feel better the original infection may still be present and may recur if treatment is stopped too soon.

Exceeding the dose
An occasional unintentional extra dose is unlikely to be a cause for concern. But if you notice unusual symptoms, or if a large overdose has been taken, notify your physician.

POSSIBLE ADVERSE EFFECTS

The most common *side effect* of clindamycin is mild diarrhea. More severe diarrhea, especially if bloodstained or accompanied by abdominal pain or fever, may be a sign of pseudomembranous colitis and requires immediate medical attention.

Symptom/effect	Frequency		Discuss with physician		Stop taking drug now	Call physician now
	Common	Rare	Only if severe	In all cases		
Diarrhea	●			■	▲	▮
Nausea/vomiting		●	■			
Fever		●		■		▮
Rash/itching		●		■	▲	
Abdominal cramps		●		■	▲	▮
Blood/mucus in stools		●		■	▲	▮

INTERACTIONS

Drugs for myasthenia gravis Clindamycin may oppose the beneficial effects of these drugs on myasthenia gravis.

SPECIAL PRECAUTIONS

Be sure to tell your physician if:
▼ You have impaired liver function.
▼ You have myasthenia gravis.
▼ You have had a bowel disorder.
▼ You are taking other medications.

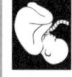

Pregnancy
▼ Not usually prescribed. Safety in pregnancy not established. Discuss with your physician.

Breast feeding
▼ The drug passes into the breast milk, but at normal doses adverse effects on the baby are unlikely. Discuss with your physician.

Infants and children
▼ Reduced dose necessary.

Over 60
▼ Reduced dose may be necessary. Increased likelihood of adverse effects.

Driving and hazardous work
▼ No known problems.

Alcohol
▼ No known problems.

PROLONGED USE

Monitoring Continued monitoring is essential where there are signs of pseudomembranous colitis.

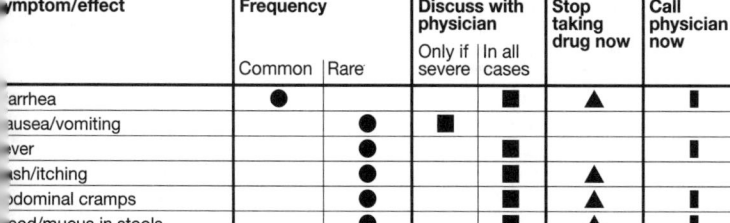

CLOBETASOL PROPIONATE

Brand names Dermasone, Dermovate
Used in the following combined preparations None

GENERAL INFORMATION

Clobetasol propionate is a powerful corticosteroid applied *topically* to treat skin conditions that have failed to improve after treatment with milder corticosteroids. Such conditions include severe psoriasis and eczematous dermatitis.

Clobetasol is for short-term treatment only because, if applied to large areas for prolonged periods, it may be absorbed in amounts great enough to cause systemic effects.

Adverse effects that may occur with any topically applied corticosteroid are more likely to occur with this drug because of its powerful action, especially if applied to the skin folds or face. The effects include local burning, irritation, itching, thinning of the skin, streaks or lines, change in pigmentation, secondary infection, excessive hair growth, and adrenal suppression.

INFORMATION FOR USERS

Your drug prescription is tailored for you. Do not alter dosage without checking with your physician.

How taken

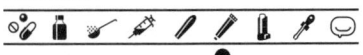

Ointment, cream, scalp lotion.

Frequency and timing of doses
2 – 3 x daily.

Dosage range
Apply thinly to the affected area and rub gently into the skin. The total dose applied weekly should not exceed 50g (cream, ointment) or 50mL (lotion).

Onset of effect
Within a few days.

Duration of action
24 hours.

Diet advice
None.

Storage
Keep in a closed container in a cool, dry place away from reach of children.

Missed dose
No cause for concern, but apply as soon as you remember.

Stopping the drug
Use as directed by your physician. When symptoms improve, discuss stopping the drug with your physician.

Exceeding the dose
An occasional unintentional extra dose is unlikely to be a cause for concern. But if you notice unusual symptoms, notify your physician.

SPECIAL PRECAUTIONS

Be sure to tell your physician if:
▼ You are taking other medications.

Pregnancy
▼ No evidence of risk to developing baby.

Breast feeding
▼ No evidence of risk.

Infants and children
▼ Not recommended.

Over 60
▼ No special problems.

Driving and hazardous work
▼ No known problems.

Alcohol
▼ No known problems.

POSSIBLE ADVERSE EFFECTS

Clobetasol propionate is a highly potent topical corticosteroid. All suspected adverse effects should be promptly reported to your physician.

Symptom/effect	Frequency		Discuss with physician		Stop taking drug now	Call physician now
	Common	Rare	Only if severe	In all cases		
Thinning of the skin		●		■	▲	
Local irritation		●		■	▲	
Reddening of the skin		●		■	▲	

INTERACTIONS

None.

PROLONGED USE

The drug is not prescribed for prolonged periods because long-term treatment can cause permanent damage to the skin.

CLOMIPHENE

Brand names Clomid, Serophene
Used in the following combined preparations None

GENERAL INFORMATION

Clomiphene increases the output of hormones by the pituitary gland, stimulating ovulation (release of egg) in women.

For female infertility, tablets are taken for five consecutive days each month early in the menstrual cycle. This stimulates ovulation. If clomiphene fails to stimulate ovulation after several months, other drugs may be prescribed.

Multiple pregnancies (usually twins) occur more commonly in women treated with clomiphene. Birth defects have occasionally been reported in association with clomiphene therapy. Other adverse effects include an increased risk of ovarian cysts. In rare cases, the ovaries become greatly enlarged, leading to abdominal pain and swelling.

INFORMATION FOR USERS

Your drug prescription is tailored for you. Do not alter dosage without checking with your physician.

How taken

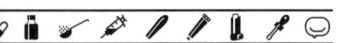

Tablets.

Frequency and timing of doses
Once daily for 5 days during each menstrual cycle.

Dosage range
50mg daily initially; dose may be increased up to 100mg daily.

Onset of effect
Ovulation occurs 4 – 10 days after the last dose in any cycle. However, it may be several months before this occurs.

Duration of action
5 days.

Diet advice
None.

Storage
Keep in a closed container in a cool, dry place away from reach of children. Protect from light.

Missed dose
Take as soon as you remember. If your next dose is due at this time, take the missed dose and the next scheduled dose together.

Stopping the drug
Take as directed by your physician. Stopping the drug will reduce chances of conception.

Exceeding the dose
An occasional unintentional extra dose is unlikely to be a cause for concern. But if you notice unusual symptoms, or if a large overdose has been taken, notify your physician.

SPECIAL PRECAUTIONS

Be sure to tell your physician if:
▼ You have impaired liver function.
▼ You are taking other medications.

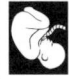

Pregnancy
▼ Not prescribed. The drug is stopped as soon as pregnancy occurs. Ensure that you are not pregnant before starting a new course of clomiphene.

Breast feeding
▼ Not prescribed.

Infants and children
▼ Not prescribed.

Over 60
▼ Not prescribed.

Driving and hazardous work
▼ Avoid such activities until you have learned how the drug affects you; it can cause blurred vision.

Alcohol
▼ Keep consumption low. Alcohol does not interact directly with clomiphene but taken in excess may reduce the chance of conception.

POSSIBLE ADVERSE EFFECTS

Abdominal pain and swelling, due to enlargement of the ovaries or the formation of cysts, are fairly common. In rare cases, massive enlargement of the ovaries may occur about a week after ovulation, but usually disappears over several weeks.

Symptom/effect	Frequency		Discuss with physician		Stop taking drug now	Call physician now
	Common	Rare	Only if severe	In all cases		
Hot flushes	●		■			
Abdominal pain/swelling	●			■		
Nausea/vomiting		●		■		
Breast tenderness		●		■		
Dry skin/hair loss/rash		●		■		
Jaundice		●		■	▲	∎
Impaired vision		●		■	▲	∎

INTERACTIONS

None.

PROLONGED USE

Prolonged use may cause visual impairment.

Monitoring Eye tests are recommended if symptoms of visual impairment are noted. Monitoring of body temperature and blood or urine hormone levels is performed to detect signs of ovulation and pregnancy.

CLOMIPRAMINE

Brand names Anafranil, Apo-Clomipramine
Used in the following combined preparations None

GENERAL INFORMATION

Clomipramine belongs to a class of antidepressant drugs known as the tricyclics. It is mainly used in the long-term treatment for depression.

Clomipramine elevates mood, increases physical activity, improves appetite, and restores interest in every-day activities. The drug seems to have a mild sedative effect which may alleviate the anxiety often accompanying depression.

Clomipramine is particularly useful in the treatment of irrational fears and obsessive-compulsive disorders. In overdose it may cause coma and dangerously abnormal heart rhythms, but in normal use serious *side effects* are rare.

INFORMATION FOR USERS

Your drug prescription is tailored for you. Do not alter dosage without checking with your physician.

How taken

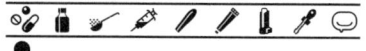

Tablets.

Frequency and timing of doses
Single dose at bedtime or 2 – 3 x daily.

Adult dosage range
20 – 300mg daily.

Onset of effect
Some effects may be felt within a few days, but full antidepressant effect may not be felt for up to 4 weeks.

Duration of action
Following prolonged treatment antidepressant effect may last up to 2 weeks.

Diet advice
None.

Storage
Keep in a closed container in a cool, dry place away from reach of children. Protect from light.

Missed dose
If taken once at bedtime, take the next dose as usual. If taken 2 – 3 times daily, take as soon as you remember. If your dose is due within 3 hours, take a single dose now and skip the next.

Stopping the drug
Consult your physician, who may supervise a gradual reduction in dosage.

OVERDOSE ACTION

 Seek immediate medical advice in all cases. Take emergency action if palpitations are noted or consciousness is lost.

See Drug poisoning emergency guide (p.574).

SPECIAL PRECAUTIONS

Be sure to tell your physician if:
▼ You have heart problems.
▼ You have had epileptic seizures.
▼ You have impaired liver or kidney function.
▼ You have had glaucoma.
▼ You have had prostate trouble.
▼ You have a blood disease.
▼ You have a thyroid disorder.
▼ You are taking other medications.

 **Pregnancy**
▼ Safety in pregnancy not established. Discuss with your physician.

 Breast feeding
▼ The drug passes into the breast milk and may affect the baby. Discuss with your physician.

 Infants and children
▼ Reduced dose necessary.

 Over 60
▼ Increased likelihood of adverse effects. Reduced dose may therefore be necessary.

 Driving and hazardous work
▼ Avoid such activities until you have learned how the drug affects you; it can cause blurred vision and reduced alertness.

 Alcohol
▼ Avoid. Alcohol may increase the sedative effects of this drug.

Surgery and general anesthetics
▼ Clomipramine treatment may need to be stopped before you have a general anesthetic. Discuss this with your physician or dentist before any operation.

POSSIBLE ADVERSE EFFECTS

The possible adverse effects of this drug are mainly the result of its *anticholinergic* action and its blocking action on the transmission of signals through the heart. Some problems can be overcome by medically supervised adjustment of dosage.

Symptom/effect	Frequency		Discuss with physician		Stop taking drug now	Call physician now
	Common	Rare	Only if severe	In all cases		
Sweating/dry mouth	●		■			
Weight gain	●		■			
Trembling/shaking	●		■			
Dry mouth/constipation	●		■			
Drowsiness/dizziness/fainting	●		■			
Blurred vision	●			■		
Rash		●		■	▲	
Urinary or ejaculation difficulties		●		■	▲	
Palpitations		●		■	▲	■

SPECIAL PRECAUTIONS (cont.)

PROLONGED USE

No problems expected.

INTERACTIONS

Sedatives All drugs that have sedative effects may intensify those of clomipramine.

Antihypertensive drugs Clomipramine may reduce the effectiveness of some of these drugs.

Monoamine oxidase inhibitors (MAOIs) Usually clomipramine should not be given during or within 2 weeks of treatment with an MAOI. Serious reactions may occur.

CLONAZEPAM

Brand names Rivotril, PMS-Clonazepam
Used in the following combined preparations None

GENERAL INFORMATION

Clonazepam belongs to a group of drugs known as the benzodiazepines, which are mainly used in the treatment of anxiety and insomnia (see p.95). Clonazepam, however, is used principally as an anticonvulsant to prevent and treat epileptic seizures. It is particularly useful for the prevention of brief muscle spasms and absence seizures (petit mal) in children, but other forms of epilepsy, such as sudden flaccidity or seizures induced by bright lights, also respond to clonazepam treatment.

Clonazepam is used either alone or together with other anticonvulsant drugs. Its anticonvulsant effect may begin to wear off after a few months. Being a benzodiazepine, clonazepam has tranquilizing and sedating effects. It is sometimes used to treat anxiety.

QUICK REFERENCE

Drug group Benzodiazepine anticonvulsant drug (p.98)

Overdose danger rating Medium

Dependence rating High

Prescription needed Yes

Multi-source suppliers Yes

INFORMATION FOR USERS

Your drug prescription is tailored for you. Do not alter dosage without checking with your physician.

How taken

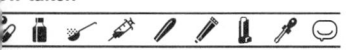

Tablets.

Frequency and timing of doses
1 – 3 x daily.

Dosage range
Adults 1.5 – 20mg daily.
Children Reduced dose according to age and weight.

Onset of effect
Within 1 hour.

Duration of action
Approximately 30 hours.

Diet advice
None.

Storage
Keep in a closed container in a cool, dry place away from reach of children.

Missed dose
No cause for concern, but take as soon as you remember. If your next dose is due within 2 hours, take both doses now.

Stopping the drug
Do not stop the drug without consulting your physician; symptoms may recur.

Exceeding the dose
An occasional unintentional extra dose is unlikely to cause problems. Larger overdoses may cause unusual drowsiness and confusion. Notify your physician.

SPECIAL PRECAUTIONS

Be sure to tell your physician if:
▼ You have severe respiratory disease.
▼ You have impaired liver or kidney function.
▼ You have had glaucoma.
▼ You have had problems with alcohol or drug abuse.
▼ You are taking other medications.

Pregnancy
▼ Safety in pregnancy not established. Discuss with your physician.

Breast feeding
▼ The drug passes into the breast milk and may affect the baby adversely. Discuss with your physician.

Infants and children
▼ Reduced dose necessary.

Over 60
▼ Reduced dose may be necessary.

Driving and hazardous work
▼ Your underlying condition as well as the possibility of drowsiness while taking this drug may make such activities inadvisable. Discuss with your physician.

Alcohol
▼ Avoid. Alcohol may increase the sedative effects of this drug.

POSSIBLE ADVERSE EFFECTS

The principal adverse effects of this drug are related to its sedative and tranquilizing properties. These effects normally diminish after the first few days of treatment and can often be reduced by medically supervised adjustment of dosage.

Symptom/effect	Frequency		Discuss with physician		Stop taking drug now	Call physician now
	Common	Rare	Only if severe	In all cases		
Daytime drowsiness	●		■			
Dizziness/unsteadiness	●		■			
Increased salivation	●		■			
Altered behavior	●			■		
Forgetfulness/confusion		●		■		
Headache		●		■		❙
Rash		●		■	▲	❙

INTERACTIONS

Sedatives All drugs, including alcohol, that have a sedative effect on the central nervous system are likely to increase the sedative properties of clonazepam. Such drugs include anti-anxiety and sleeping drugs, antihistamines, antidepressants, narcotic analgesics, and antipsychotics.

Other anticonvulsants Clonazepam may alter the effects of other anticonvulsants you are taking, and adjustment of dosage or change of drug may be necessary.

PROLONGED USE

Both beneficial and adverse effects of clonazepam may become less marked during prolonged treatment as the body adapts.

CLONIDINE

Brand names Catapres, Dixarit, Apo-Clonidine, Novo-Clonidine, Nu-Clonidine
Used in the following combined preparation Combipres

GENERAL INFORMATION

Clonidine, a centrally acting antihypertensive, is principally used to treat high blood pressure. By reducing the stimulatory nerve impulses from the brain to the heart and circulatory system, clonidine lowers the blood pressure to a safe level. It is sometimes prescribed together with a diuretic to enhance its effect.

Clonidine has also been used for other conditions such as menopausal flushing, migraine, and *withdrawal symptoms* during drug detoxification.

Its main drawback is that when used in the doses required to control blood pressure, there may be a severe rise in blood pressure if doses are missed or if the drug is stopped suddenly.

INFORMATION FOR USERS

Your drug prescription is tailored for you. Do not alter dosage without checking with your physician.

How taken

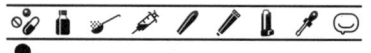

Tablets.

Frequency and timing of doses
2 – 4 x daily.

Adult dosage range
High blood pressure 0.2mg – 1.2mg daily. Doses of up to 5mg daily have been used in some resistant cases.
Menopausal flushing 0.1mg daily.

Onset of effect
2 – 5 hours.

Duration of action
6 – 20 hours.

Diet advice
None.

Storage
Keep in a closed container in a cool, dry place away from reach of children.

Missed dose
Take as soon as you remember, then resume your normal schedule. Discuss with your physician if you miss two or more doses.

Stopping the drug
Do not stop the drug without consulting your physician, who will supervise a gradual reduction in dosage. Abrupt withdrawal may cause a dangerous rise in blood pressure.

Exceeding the dose
An occasional unintentional extra dose is unlikely to cause problems. You may experience vomiting or drowsiness. Notify your physician.

SPECIAL PRECAUTIONS

Be sure to tell your physician if:
▼ You have impaired liver or kidney function.
▼ You have poor circulation.
▼ You have coronary artery disease.
▼ You have had depression.
▼ You are taking other medications.

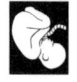

Pregnancy
▼ Not usually prescribed. Safety in pregnancy not established. Discuss with your physician.

Breast feeding
▼ The drug passes into the breast milk. Discuss with your physician.

Infants and children
▼ Not recommended.

Over 60
▼ Reduced dose may be necessary.

Driving and hazardous work
▼ Avoid such activities until you have learned how the drug affects you; it can cause drowsiness and dizziness.

Alcohol
▼ Avoid. Alcohol may increase the sedative effects of this drug.

POSSIBLE ADVERSE EFFECTS

Clonidine may cause drowsiness, dry mouth, and constipation. These effects usually decrease after long-term therapy. An adjustment in dosage may help.

Symptom/effect	Frequency		Discuss with physician		Stop taking drug now	Call physician now
	Common	Rare	Only if severe	In all cases		
Drowsiness	●		■			
Constipation	●		■			
Dry mouth	●		■			
Dizziness/weakness		●		■		
Rash		●		■		
Depression		●		■		
Ankle swelling		●		■		
Cold hands		●		■		
Impotence		●		■		

PROLONGED USE

The more common adverse effects, such as drowsiness, constipation, and dry mouth, may decrease with long-term use.

INTERACTIONS

Tricyclic antidepressant drugs may reduce the effect of clonidine.

Sedatives Clonidine increases the effect of these drugs.

Beta blockers may reverse the effects of clonidine, producing a rise in blood pressure.

CLORAZEPATE

Brand names Tranxene, Apo-Clorazepate, Novo-Clopate
Used in the following combined preparations None

GENERAL INFORMATION

Clorazepate is a member of the drug group known as the benzodiazepines. These drugs help relieve nervousness and tension and encourage sleep. The actions and adverse effects of this group of drugs are described more fully on page 95.

Clorazepate is principally used in the treatment of anxiety and anxiety-related insomnia. It can also be prescribed in the treatment of alcohol withdrawal.

Clorazepate can be habit-forming if taken regularly over a long period. Its effects may also diminish with time. Treatment with clorazepate is usually reviewed frequently.

QUICK REFERENCE

Drug group Benzodiazepine anti-anxiety drug (p.95)

Overdose danger rating Medium

Dependence rating Medium

Prescription needed Yes

Multi-source suppliers Yes

INFORMATION FOR USERS

Your drug prescription is tailored for you. Do not alter dosage without checking with your physician.

How taken

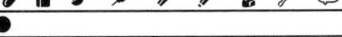

Capsules.

Frequency and timing of doses
1 – 4 x daily.

Adult dosage range
7.5 – 60mg daily.

Onset of effect
Within 2 hours.

Duration of action
Up to 24 hours. Some effect may last up to 4 days.

Diet advice
None.

Storage
Keep in a closed container in a cool, dry place away from reach of children.

Missed dose
No cause for concern, but take when you next feel you need the drug. If your next dose is due within 2 hours, take a single dose now and skip the next.

Stopping the drug
If you have been taking the drug continuously for less than 2 weeks, it can be safely stopped as soon as you feel you no longer need it. However, if you have been taking it for longer, consult your physician, who will supervise a gradual reduction in dosage. Stopping abruptly may lead to withdrawal symptoms (see p.95).

Exceeding the dose
An occasional unintentional extra dose is unlikely to cause problems. Larger overdoses may cause unusual drowsiness. Notify your physician.

POSSIBLE ADVERSE EFFECTS

The principal adverse effects of this drug are related to its sedative properties. These effects, including drowsiness and dizziness, normally diminish after the first few days and, if troublesome, can often be reduced by adjustment of dosage.

Symptom/effect	Frequency		Discuss with physician		Stop taking drug now	Call physician now
	Common	Rare	Only if severe	In all cases		
Daytime drowsiness	●		■			
Dizziness/unsteadiness	●			■		
Headache		●	■			
Blurred vision/dry mouth		●		■		
Forgetfulness/confusion		●		■		
Rash		●		■	▲	

INTERACTIONS

Sedatives All drugs, including alcohol, that have a sedative effect on the central nervous system are likely to increase the sedative properties of clorazepate.

Antacids The onset of action of clorazepate may be slowed by antacids; take these drugs as far apart as possible.

SPECIAL PRECAUTIONS

Be sure to tell your physician if:
▼ You have severe respiratory disease.
▼ You have impaired liver or kidney function.
▼ You have had problems with alcohol or drug abuse.
▼ You have myasthenia gravis.
▼ You have glaucoma.
▼ You are taking other medications.

Pregnancy
▼ Safety in pregnancy not established. Discuss with your physician.

Breast feeding
▼ The drug passes into the breast milk and may affect the baby. Discuss with your physician.

Infants and children
▼ Not recommended in patients under 18 years.

Over 60
▼ Increased likelihood of adverse effects. Reduced dose may therefore be necessary.

Driving and hazardous work
▼ Avoid such activities until you have learned how the drug affects you; it can cause reduced alertness and slowed reactions.

Alcohol
▼ Avoid. Alcohol may increase the sedative effects of this drug.

PROLONGED USE

Regular use of this drug over several weeks can lead to a reduction in its effect as the body adapts. It may also be habit-forming when taken for extended periods. Severe withdrawal reactions have occurred.

CLOTRIMAZOLE

Brand names Canesten, Clotrimaderm, Myclo
Used in the following combined preparations None

GENERAL INFORMATION

Clotrimazole is prescribed for yeast and fungal infections. It is effective for treating tinea (ringworm) infections of the skin and candida infections of the vagina. The drug is applied in the form of cream or solution to the affected area and inserted as vaginal tablets or cream for vaginal conditions.

Adverse effects from clotrimazole are very rare, although some people may experience burning and irritation on the skin surface where the cream has been applied.

QUICK REFERENCE

Drug group Antifungal drug (p.150)
Overdose danger rating Low
Dependence rating Low
Prescription needed No
Multi-source suppliers Yes

INFORMATION FOR USERS

Follow instructions on the label. Call your physician if symptoms worsen.

How taken

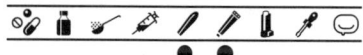

Vaginal tablets, skin cream, skin solution, vaginal cream.

Frequency and timing of doses
Skin infections 2 x daily (cream or solution).
Vaginal infections Once daily at bedtime (vaginal cream or vaginal tablet).

Adult dosage range
Skin infections Sufficient cream or solution to cover the infected and surrounding area at each application.
Vaginal infections 100 – 500mg per dose (vaginal tablets); 1 applicatorful per dose (vaginal cream).

Onset of effect
Within 3 – 7 days (skin conditions); within 24 hours (vaginal conditions).

Duration of action
Over 25 hours (cream); over 72 hours (500mg vaginal tablets).

Diet advice
None.

Storage
Keep in a closed container in a cool, dry place away from reach of children.

Missed dose
No cause for concern, but make up the missed dose or application as soon as you remember.

Stopping the drug
Apply the full course. Even if symptoms disappear, the original infection may still be present and symptoms may recur if treatment is stopped too soon.

Exceeding the dose
An occasional unintentional extra dose is unlikely to be a cause for concern. But if you notice unusual symptoms or if a large amount has been swallowed, notify your physician.

POSSIBLE ADVERSE EFFECTS

Clotrimazole rarely causes adverse effects. Skin creams and vaginal applications may occasionally cause localized burning and irritation.

Symptom/effect	Frequency		Discuss with physician		Stop taking drug now	Call physician now
	Common	Rare	Only if severe	In all cases		
Local burning or stinging		●	■			
Skin irritation		●		■		
Rash		●		■	▲	
Hives		●		■	▲	

INTERACTIONS

None.

SPECIAL PRECAUTIONS

Be sure to consult your physician or pharmacist before using this drug if:
▼ You have impaired liver function.
▼ You are taking other medications.

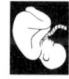

Pregnancy
▼ No evidence of risk with skin preparations. Vaginal preparations are prescribed with caution in the first 3 months of pregnancy. Use of the vaginal applicator may be undesirable. Discuss with your physician.

Breast feeding
▼ No evidence of risk.

Infants and children
▼ No special problems.

Over 60
▼ No special problems.

Driving and hazardous work
▼ No known problems.

Alcohol
▼ No known problems.

PROLONGED USE

No problems expected from the drug. However, recurrent or intractable candidiasis may require further assessment by your physician.

CLOXACILLIN

Brand names Orbenin, Apo-Cloxi, Novo-Cloxin, Nu-Cloxin, Tegopen
Used in the following combined preparations None

GENERAL INFORMATION

Cloxacillin, a penicillin antibiotic first available in 1963, is prescribed to treat staphylococcal infections. These are usually resistant to treatment with other forms of penicillin because the bacteria produce an enzyme that breaks down the antibiotic. Cloxacillin, however, is not affected by the enzyme. Common sites where staphylococcal infection may occur include the skin and soft tissues.

For maximum effect, cloxacillin needs to be taken on an empty stomach, because food interferes with absorption of the drug from the digestive tract.

Diarrhea is the most common side effect. As with other penicillin antibiotics, there is a risk of an allergic reaction – rash and possibly fever, itching, swelling of the mouth and tongue, and breathing difficulty.

QUICK REFERENCE

Drug group Penicillin antibiotic (p.140)

Overdose danger rating Low

Dependence rating Low

Prescription needed Yes

Multi-source suppliers Yes

INFORMATION FOR USERS

Your drug prescription is tailored for you. Do not alter dosage without checking with your physician.

How taken

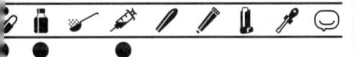

Capsules, oral liquid, injection.

Frequency and timing of doses
4 daily at least 1 hour before, or 2 hours after eating.

Dosage range
Adults 1 – 4g daily (by mouth).
Children Reduced dose according to age and weight.

Onset of effect
Symptoms usually improve within 1 – 3 days, depending on the condition.

Duration of action
4 to 6 hours.

Diet advice
None.

Storage
Keep capsules in a closed container in a cool, dry place away from reach of children. Refrigerate liquid, but do not freeze and do not keep for longer than 14 days.

Missed dose
Take as soon as you remember. If your next dose is due at this time, take both doses now.

Stopping the drug
Take the full course. Even if you feel better, the original infection may still be present and symptoms may recur if treatment is stopped too soon.

Exceeding the dose
An occasional unintentional extra dose is unlikely to be a cause for concern. But if you notice unusual symptoms, or if a large overdose has been taken, notify your physician.

SPECIAL PRECAUTIONS

Be sure to tell your physician if:
▼ You have an allergy (for example, asthma, hay fever, eczema, or hives).
▼ You have ulcerative colitis.
▼ You have had a rash after taking a penicillin or cephalosporin antibiotic.
▼ You are taking other medications.

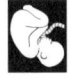
Pregnancy
▼ Is prescribed during pregnancy, but risks to baby have not been fully established. Discuss with your physician.

Breast feeding
▼ The drug passes into the breast milk and may affect the baby adversely. Discuss with your physician.

Infants and children
▼ Safety in premature and newborn infants not established. Reduced dose necessary for older children.

Over 60
▼ Reduced dose necessary.

Driving and hazardous work
▼ No known problems.

Alcohol
▼ No known problems.

POSSIBLE ADVERSE EFFECTS

If you develop a rash, wheezing, itching, fever, or joint swelling, this may indicate an allergy to cloxacillin, making it necessary to take a different antibiotic.

Symptom/effect	Frequency		Discuss with physician		Stop taking drug now	Call physician now
	Common	Rare	Only if severe	In all cases		
Rash	●			■	▲	■
Nausea/vomiting		●		■		
Unusual thirst		●		■		
Tiredness/weakness		●		■		
Diarrhea		●		■		
Wheezing/breathlessness		●		■	▲	■
Itching		●		■	▲	■
Swollen mouth/tongue		●		■	▲	■

INTERACTIONS

None.

PROLONGED USE

Cloxacillin is usually given only for short courses of treatment.

CODEINE

Brand names None
Used in the following combined preparations Empracet, Novahistex C, Penntuss, 222 Tablets, Tylenol with codeine

GENERAL INFORMATION

In common medical use since the beginning of the century, codeine is a mild narcotic analgesic, similar to, but weaker than, morphine.

It is primarily used to relieve mild to moderate pain, often in combination with a non-narcotic analgesic, but it is also an effective cough suppressant. It is an ingredient in many cough and cold preparations and analgesic compounds. Like other narcotic drugs,

codeine is constipating.

Codeine is habit-forming, but addiction seldom occurs if the drug is used for a limited period of time and the recommended dosage is followed.

QUICK REFERENCE

Drug group Narcotic analgesic (p.92), and cough suppressant (p.106)

Overdose danger rating High

Dependence rating Medium

Prescription needed Yes (most preparations)

Multi-source suppliers Yes

INFORMATION FOR USERS

Your drug prescription is tailored for you. Do not alter dosage without consulting your physician.

How taken

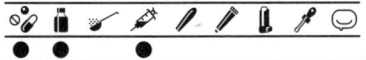

Tablets, oral liquid, injection.

Frequency and timing of doses
4 – 6 x daily (pain); every 4 – 6 hours when necessary (cough).

Adult dosage range
120 – 240mg daily (pain); 40 – 120mg daily (cough).

Onset of effect
30 – 60 minutes.

Duration of action
4 – 6 hours.

Diet advice
Due to the likelihood of constipation, plenty of fluids and fiber-rich foods should be taken.

Storage
Keep in a closed container in a cool, dry place away from reach of children. Protect from light.

Missed dose
Take as soon as you remember if needed for relief of symptoms. If not needed, do not take the missed dose, and return to your normal dose schedule when necessary.

Stopping the drug
Can be safely stopped as soon as you no longer need it.

OVERDOSE ACTION

 Seek immediate medical advice in all cases. Take emergency action if there are symptoms such as slow or irregular breathing, severe drowsiness, or loss of consciousness.

See Drug poisoning emergency guide (p.574).

POSSIBLE ADVERSE EFFECTS

Serious adverse effects are rare with codeine. Constipation occurs frequently, but other side effects, such as nausea, vomiting, and drowsiness, are not usually troublesome at recommended doses, and usually disappear if the dose is reduced.

Symptom/effect	Frequency		Discuss with physician		Stop taking drug now	Call physician now
	Common	Rare	Only if severe	In all cases		
Constipation	●		■			
Nausea/vomiting		●		■		
Drowsiness		●		■		
Dizziness		●		■		
Agitation/restlessness		●		■	▲	
Rash/hives		●		■	▲	▎
Wheezing/breathlessness		●		■	▲	▎

INTERACTIONS

Sedatives All drugs, including alcohol, that have a sedative effect on the central nervous system are likely to increase sedation with codeine. Such drugs include antidepressant drugs, sleeping drugs, and antihistamines.

Monoamine oxidase inhibitors (MAOIs) Codeine may interact with these drugs to cause a dangerous rise in blood pressure.

SPECIAL PRECAUTIONS

Be sure to tell your physician if:
▼ You have impaired liver or kidney function
▼ You have a lung disorder such as asthma or bronchitis.
▼ You have inflammatory bowel disease.
▼ You are taking other medications.

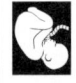 **Pregnancy**
▼ No evidence of risk, but may adversely affect the baby's breathing if taken during labor. Discuss with your physician.

 Breast feeding
▼ The drug passes into the breast milk and may affect the baby. Discuss with your physician.

 Infants and children
▼ Reduced dose necessary.

 Over 60
▼ Reduced dose may be necessary.

 Driving and hazardous work
▼ Avoid such activities until you have learned how the drug affects you; it may cause dizziness and drowsiness.

Alcohol
▼ Avoid. Alcohol may increase the sedative effects of this drug.

PROLONGED USE

Codeine is normally used only for short-term relief of symptoms. It can be habit-forming if taken for extended periods, especially if higher-than-average doses are taken.

COLCHICINE

Brand names None
Used in the following combined preparations None

GENERAL INFORMATION

Colchicine, a drug originally extracted from the autumn crocus flower and later synthesized, has been used since the 18th century for gout. It is still often used to relieve joint pain and inflammation in flare-ups of gout. It is most effective when taken at the first sign of symptoms, and it almost always produces an improvement. Colchicine is also often given in the first few months of treatment with allopurinol or probenecid (other drugs used for treating gout), because these may at first increase the frequency of gout attacks.

Colchicine is also occasionally prescribed for the relief of symptoms of familial Mediterranean fever (a rare congenital condition).

INFORMATION FOR USERS

Your drug prescription is tailored for you. Do not alter dosage without checking with your physician.

How taken

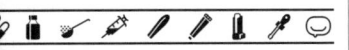

Tablets.

Frequency and timing of doses
Prevention of gout attacks 1 – 2 x daily.
Relief of gout attacks Every 2 hours.

Adult dosage range
Prevention of gout attacks 0.6 – 1.2mg daily.
Relief of gout attacks 1.0 or 1.2mg initially, then 0.6mg every 2 hours, up to a maximum of 4 – 8mg daily until joint is better or gastrointestinal problems arise.

Onset of effect
Relief of symptoms in an acute attack of gout may be felt in 6 – 24 hours. Full effect in gout prevention may not be felt for several days.

Duration of action
1 to 2 hours. Some effect may last longer.

Diet advice
Certain foods are known to make gout worse. Discuss with your physician.

Storage
Keep in a closed container in a cool, dry place away from reach of children. Protect from light.

Missed dose
Take as soon as you remember. If your next dose is due within 30 minutes, take a single dose now and skip the next.

Stopping the drug
When taking colchicine frequently during an acute attack, stop if diarrhea or abdominal pain develops. In other cases do not stop without consulting your physician.

OVERDOSE ACTION

Seek immediate medical advice in all cases; some reactions can be fatal. Take emergency action if severe nausea, vomiting, bloody diarrhea, severe abdominal pain, or loss of consciousness occurs.

See Drug poisoning emergency guide (p.574).

SPECIAL PRECAUTIONS

Be sure to tell your physician if:
▼ You have impaired liver or kidney function.
▼ You have heart problems.
▼ You have a blood disorder.
▼ You have stomach ulcers.
▼ You have chronic inflammation of the bowel.
▼ You are taking other medications.

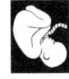

Pregnancy
▼ Not usually prescribed. May cause defects in the unborn baby. Discuss with your physician.

Breast feeding
▼ The drug passes into the breast milk and may affect the baby. Discuss with your physician.

Infants and children
▼ Not recommended.

Over 60
▼ Increased likelihood of adverse effects.

Driving and hazardous work
▼ No special problems.

Alcohol
▼ Avoid. Alcohol may increase stomach irritation caused by colchicine. It may also worsen gout.

PROLONGED USE

Prolonged use of this drug may lead to hair loss, rashes, tingling in the hands and feet, muscle pain and weakness, and blood disorders.

Monitoring Periodic blood checks are usually required.

POSSIBLE ADVERSE EFFECTS

The appearance of any symptom that may be an adverse effect of the drug is a sign that you should stop the drug until you have received further medical advice. Drugs are sometimes prescribed to relieve adverse effects.

Symptom/effect	Frequency		Discuss with physician		Stop taking drug now	Call physician now
	Common	Rare	Only if severe	In all cases		
Nausea/vomiting	●			■	▲	❘
Diarrhea/abdominal pain	●			■	▲	❘
Numbness and tingling		●		■	▲	
Unusual bleeding/bruising		●		■	▲	❘
Rash		●		■		❘

INTERACTIONS

Vitamin B$_{12}$ Colchicine may interfere with vitamin B$_{12}$ absorption.

CONJUGATED ESTROGENS

Brand names Premarin, C.E.S., Congest
Used in the following combined preparations None

GENERAL INFORMATION

Conjugated estrogen preparations consist of naturally occurring estrogens similar to those found in the urine of pregnant mares.

Given by mouth, they are used to relieve menopausal symptoms such as hot flushes and sweating, to treat hypogonadism (underdeveloped ovaries), and to control abnormal bleeding from the womb due to hormone imbalance. They are also used to treat and prevent osteoporosis (brittle bones), which may occur after the menopause, and to treat certain cases of cancer of the prostate or female breast cancer.

As replacement therapy, conjugated estrogens are usually taken on a cyclic dosing schedule, often in conjunction with a progestin, to simulate the hormonal changes of a normal menstrual cycle. They are also prescribed in the form of vaginal cream to relieve pain and dryness of the vagina or vulva after the menopause.

INFORMATION FOR USERS

Your drug prescription is tailored for you. Do not alter dosage without checking with your physician.

How taken

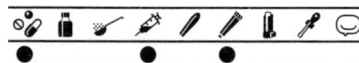

Tablets, injection, vaginal cream.

Frequency and timing of doses
Tablets 1 – 3 x daily, with food.
Cream Once daily.

Adult dosage range
Replacement therapy 0.625 – 1.25mg daily (tablets), generally in cycles of 21 – 25 days; 2 – 4g daily (cream).
Prostate cancer 3.75 – 7.5mg daily.
Breast cancer 30mg daily.

Onset of effect
5 – 20 days.

Duration of action
1 – 2 days.

Diet advice
None.

Storage
Keep in a closed container in a cool, dry place away from reach of children.

Missed dose
Take as soon as you remember.

Stopping the drug
Do not stop the drug without consulting your physician; symptoms may recur.

Exceeding the dose
An occasional unintentional extra dose is unlikely to be a cause for concern. But if you notice unusual symptoms, or if a large overdose has been taken, notify your physician.

POSSIBLE ADVERSE EFFECTS

The most common adverse effects of conjugated estrogens are similar to symptoms that occur in the early stages of pregnancy, and generally diminish or disappear after 2 – 3 months of treatment. Sudden, sharp pain in the chest, groin, or legs may indicate an abnormal blood clot and requires urgent medical attention.

Symptom/effect	Frequency		Discuss with physician		Stop taking drug now	Call physician now
	Common	Rare	Only if severe	In all cases		
Nausea/vomiting	●		■			
Breast swelling/tenderness	●		■			
Increase in weight	●		■			
Reduced sex drive		●	■			
Depression		●		■		
Vaginal bleeding		●		■		
Pain in chest/groin/legs		●		■	▲	▮

INTERACTIONS

Tobacco smoking Smoking increases the risk of serious adverse effects on the heart and circulation with conjugated estrogens.

Oral anticoagulant drugs Conjugated estrogens reduce the anticoagulant effect of these drugs.

SPECIAL PRECAUTIONS

Be sure to tell your physician if:
▼ You have heart failure or high blood pressure.
▼ You have had blood clots or a stroke.
▼ You have impaired liver or kidney function.
▼ You have diabetes or asthma.
▼ You have serious eye disease.
▼ You suffer from migraine or epilepsy.
▼ You are taking other medications.

Pregnancy
▼ Not prescribed. May adversely affect the baby. Discuss with your physician.

Breast feeding
▼ Not prescribed. The drug may inhibit the flow of milk. Discuss with your physician.

Infants and children
▼ Not usually prescribed.

Over 60
▼ Reduced dose may be necessary. Discuss with your physician.

Driving and hazardous work
▼ No known problems.

Alcohol
▼ No known problems.

Surgery and general anesthetics
▼ Conjugated estrogens may need to be stopped several weeks before you have surgery. Discuss with your physician.

PROLONGED USE

There is a slightly higher risk of cancer of the uterus after the menopause when used without a progestin. The risk of gallstones is also increased.

Monitoring Physical examinations and blood pressure checks may be needed.

CO-TRIMOXAZOLE

rand names Bactrim, Apo-Sulfatrim, Novo-Trimel, Nu-Cotrimox, Roubac, Septra
sed in the following combined preparations (Co-trimoxazole is a combination of trimethoprim and sulfamethoxazole)

GENERAL INFORMATION

o-trimoxazole is an antibacterial drug at is a combination of one part methoprim and five parts sulfa-ethoxazole. It is prescribed for the evention and treatment of urinary tract ections and the treatment of ections of the respiratory tract, astrointestinal tract, skin, and ear. o-trimoxazole is also used to treat ostatitis and pneumocystis

pneumonia. Treatment is usually continued for at least five days and should not be stopped sooner, otherwise the infection is likely to recur.

The *side effects* of co-trimoxazole are a combination of those caused by the two antibacterial drugs it contains. These can be nausea, vomiting, sore tongue, rash, and rarely blood disorders and jaundice.

INFORMATION FOR USERS

ur drug prescription is tailored for you. not alter dosage without checking th your physician.

w taken

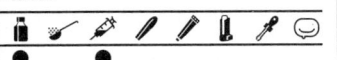

lets (standard and double strength [DS]), l liquid, injection.

equency and timing of doses
rmally 2 x daily, preferably with food.

ult dosage range
ually 4 – 6 standard tablets daily. Higher ses are required for the treatment of eumocystis pneumonia.

set of effect
4 hours.

ration of action
hours.

t advice
nk plenty of fluids, particularly in warm ather.

Storage
Keep in a closed container in a cool, dry place away from reach of children. Protect from light.

Missed dose
Take as soon as you remember. If your next dose is due at this time, double the usual dose to make up the missed dose.

Stopping the drug
Take the full course. Even if you feel better the original infection may still be present and symptoms may recur if treatment is stopped too soon.

Exceeding the dose
An occasional unintentional extra dose is unlikely to be a cause for concern. Large overdoses may cause nausea, vomiting, dizziness, and confusion. Notify your physician.

SPECIAL PRECAUTIONS

Be sure to tell your physician if:
▼ You have long-term liver or kidney problems.
▼ You have a blood disorder.
▼ You have glucose-6-phosphate dehydrogenase (G6PD) deficiency.
▼ You are allergic to sulfonamide drugs.
▼ You suffer from porphyria.
▼ You are taking other medications.

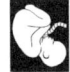

Pregnancy
▼ Not usually prescribed. May cause defects in the baby. Discuss with your physician.

Breast feeding
▼ The drug passes into the breast milk and may affect the baby adversely. Discuss with your physician.

Infants and children
▼ Not recommended in infants under 6 weeks old. Reduced dose necessary in older children.

Over 60
▼ Side effects are more likely. Used only when necessary.

Driving and hazardous work
▼ No known problems.

Alcohol
▼ No known problems.

POSSIBLE ADVERSE EFFECTS

e effects can be caused by either the ethoprim or the sulfamethoxazole

ingredient of this preparation. The most common problems are nausea and rash.

nptom/effect	Frequency		Discuss with physician		Stop taking drug now	Call physician now
	Common	Rare	Only if severe	In all cases		
rhea		●	■			
sea/vomiting	●			■		
h/itching	●			■	▲	▮
e tongue		●		■		
dache		●		■		
ndice		●		■		▮

INTERACTIONS

arfarin Co-trimoxazole may increase its ticoagulant effect; the dose of warfarin ay have to be reduced.

enytoin Co-trimoxazole may cause a ildup of phenytoin in the body; the dose phenytoin may have to be reduced.

Oral antidiabetic drugs Co-trimoxazole may increase the blood sugar lowering effect of these drugs.

Cyclosporine Taking cyclosporine with co-trimoxazole can impair kidney function.

PROLONGED USE

Long-term use of this drug may lead to folic acid deficiency which, in turn, can cause a blood abnormality. Folic acid supplements may be prescribed.

Monitoring Periodic blood tests to monitor blood composition are usually carried out.

CROMOLYN SODIUM

Brand names Intal, Nalcrom, Novo-Cromolyn, Opticrom, Rynacrom, Vistacrom
Used in the following combined preparations None

GENERAL INFORMATION

Cromolyn sodium, introduced in the 1970s, is used primarily as a preventive for asthma and allergic conditions.

Taken by inhaler as a powder (Spinhaler) or a spray, it is commonly prescribed to prevent mild to moderate asthma. It also reduces the frequency and severity of asthmatic attacks induced by exercise or cold air. Cromolyn sodium has a slow onset of action, taking from a few days to up to 6 weeks of regular dosage to produce its anti-asthmatic effect. It is not effective for the relief of an asthmatic attack in progress.

Aside from its use in asthma, cromolyn sodium eye preparations may be used to prevent allergic conjunctivitis. When taken as a nasal spray, it is helpful in preventing allergic rhinitis (hay fever). It is also given in the form of capsules for gastrointestinal food allergy.

Side effects are mild. Coughing and wheezing on inhalation may be prevented by using a *sympathomimetic* bronchodilator (p.104) first. Hoarseness and throat irritation can be avoided by rinsing the mouth with water after inhalation.

INFORMATION FOR USERS

Your drug prescription is tailored for you. Do not alter dosage without checking with your physician.

How taken

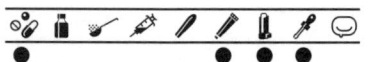

Capsules, eye ointment, inhaler (various types), eye drops, and nasal spray.

Frequency and timing of doses
4 x daily before meals. Allow contents of capsules to dissolve in warm water and take as solution (by mouth); 4 – 8 x daily (inhaler, nasal preparations); 4 x daily (eye drops); 2 – 3 x daily (eye ointment).

Dosage range
800mg daily (by mouth); as directed (inhaler, nasal preparations); 1 – 2 drops per application (eye drops); 0.5 – 1cm per application (eye ointment).

Onset of effect
Varies with dosage form and condition treated. Eye conditions and allergic rhinitis may respond after several days' treatment, while asthma and chronic allergic rhinitis may take 2 – 6 weeks to show improvement.

Duration of action
4 – 6 hours. Some effect persists for several days after treatment is stopped.

Diet advice
None.

Storage
Keep in a closed container in a cool, dry place away from reach of children. Protect from light.

Missed dose
Take as soon as you remember. If your next dose is due within 2 hours, take a single dose now and skip the next.

Stopping the drug
Do not stop the drug without consulting your physician; symptoms may recur.

Exceeding the dose
An occasional unintentional extra dose is unlikely to be a cause for concern. But if you notice unusual symptoms, or if a large overdose has been taken, notify your physician.

SPECIAL PRECAUTIONS

Be sure to tell your physician if:
▼ You have impaired liver or kidney function.
▼ You are taking other medications.

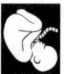

Pregnancy
▼ No evidence of risk to developing baby.

Breast feeding
▼ No evidence of risk.

Infants and children
▼ Reduced dose necessary.

Over 60
▼ No known problems.

Driving and hazardous work
▼ Exercise caution if dizziness occurs.

Alcohol
▼ No known problems.

POSSIBLE ADVERSE EFFECTS

Coughing and hoarseness are common with inhalation of cromolyn sodium, and burning and stinging may occur with all topical dosage forms. Nasal spray may cause sneezing. All these symptoms diminish with continued use.

Symptom/effect	Frequency		Discuss with physician		Stop taking drug now	Call physician now
	Common	Rare	Only if severe	In all cases		
Coughing/hoarseness	●		■			
Local irritation	●		■			
Nausea/vomiting (by mouth)		●		■		
Dizziness/headache		●		■		
Wheezing/breathlessness		●		■		
Rash/itching (by mouth)		●		■	▲	

INTERACTIONS

None.

PROLONGED USE

No problems expected.

CYCLOBENZAPRINE

Brand names Flexeril, Novo-Cycloprine
Used in the following combined preparations None

GENERAL INFORMATION

Chemically similar to the tricyclic antidepressant drugs (p.96), cyclobenzaprine acts on nerve cells in the central nervous system to relieve spasm and rigidity of the muscles. It may also help to relieve pain. Cyclobenzaprine is mainly used in the short term to treat painful symptoms caused by injury. Such treatment is usually accompanied by rest and physical therapy.

Because cyclobenzaprine is not recommended for prolonged treatment, it is not useful for neurological disorders, such as multiple sclerosis, or after injury to the spinal cord. As with all muscle relaxants, drowsiness is one of the most common side effects of cyclobenzaprine.

QUICK REFERENCE

Drug group Muscle-relaxant drug (p.132)

Overdose danger rating High

Dependence rating Low

Prescription needed Yes

Multi-source suppliers Yes

INFORMATION FOR USERS

Your drug prescription is tailored for you. Do not alter dosage without checking with your physician.

How taken

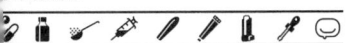

Tablets.

Frequency and timing of doses
× daily.

Adult dosage range
– 40mg daily. Larger doses may be given in some cases.

Onset of effect
Within 1 hour.

Duration of action
up to 24 hours.

Diet advice
None.

Storage
Keep in a closed container in a cool, dry place away from reach of children.

Missed dose
Take as soon as you remember. If your next dose is due within 2 hours, take a single dose now and skip the next.

Stopping the drug
Do not stop the drug without consulting your physician; symptoms may recur.

OVERDOSE ACTION

 Seek immediate medical advice in all cases. Take emergency action if abnormal heart rhythm, breathing difficulties, loss of consciousness, or coma occurs.

See Drug poisoning emergency guide (p.574).

POSSIBLE ADVERSE EFFECTS

Most adverse effects of cyclobenzaprine are due to its sedative and *anticholinergic* properties and disappear when a course of treatment with the drug is stopped.

Symptom/effect	Frequency		Discuss with physician		Stop taking drug now	Call physician now
	Common	Rare	Only if severe	In all cases		
Drowsiness	●		■			
Dizziness	●		■			
Dry mouth	●		■			
Blurred vision		●		■		
Nausea/indigestion		●		■		
Weakness		●		■	▲	
Palpitations		●		■	▲	■

INTERACTIONS

Sedatives All drugs, including alcohol, that have a sedative effect on the central nervous system are likely to increase the sedative properties of cyclobenzaprine.

Anticholinergic drugs There is an increased risk of *side effects* if these drugs are taken with cyclobenzaprine.

Monoamine oxidase inhibitors (MAOIs) There is a risk of severe high blood pressure if cyclobenzaprine is taken during or within 14 days of treatment with an MAOI.

Guanethidine Cyclobenzaprine interferes with the blood pressure-lowering effect of guanethidine.

SPECIAL PRECAUTIONS

Be sure to tell your physician if:
▼ You have had a recent heart attack or heart problems.
▼ You have had glaucoma.
▼ You have an overactive thyroid gland.
▼ You have urinary difficulties.
▼ You are taking other medications.

 **Pregnancy**
▼ Safety in pregnancy not established. Discuss with your physician.

 Breast feeding
▼ The drug passes into the breast milk. Discuss with your physician.

 Infants and children
▼ Not recommended.

 Over 60
▼ Reduced dose may be necessary.

 **Driving and hazardous work**
▼ Avoid such activities until you have learned how the drug affects you, because the drug can cause drowsiness and dizziness.

 Alcohol
▼ Avoid. Alcohol may increase the adverse effects of this drug.

Surgery and general anesthetics
▼ Cyclobenzaprine may need to be stopped before you have a general anesthetic. Discuss this with your physician or dentist before any surgery.

PROLONGED USE

Cyclobenzaprine is not prescribed for prolonged periods and should not be taken for longer than 2 or 3 weeks.

CYCLOPHOSPHAMIDE

Brand names Cytoxan, Procytox
Used in the following combined preparations None

GENERAL INFORMATION

Cyclophosphamide is a widely used anticancer drug. It interferes with the growth of cancer cells, which are later destroyed by the immune system.

It is used for a wide range of cancers including leukemias, lymphomas (lymph gland cancers), and solid tumors, particularly of the lung and breast. Cyclophosphamide is also used in certain malignant conditions occurring in childhood. It is commonly given with other drugs to treat cancer or with radiotherapy.

Cyclophosphamide causes nausea, vomiting, and loss of hair; it can affect the heart, lungs, liver, and bladder. The drug often reduces blood cell production, resulting in abnormal bleeding and increased risk of infection, and reduced fertility in men.

Effective contraception should be used during cyclophosphamide therapy.

INFORMATION FOR USERS

Your drug prescription is tailored for you. Do not alter dosage without checking with your physician.

How taken

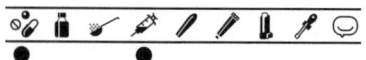

Tablets, injection.

Frequency and timing of doses
Varies from once daily to every 7 – 10 days or 2 x weekly, depending on the condition being treated.

Dosage range
Dosage is determined individually according to the nature of the condition, body weight, and response.

Onset of effect
Some effects may appear within hours of starting treatment. Full beneficial effects may not be felt for up to 6 weeks.

Duration of action
Several weeks.

Diet advice
High fluid intake with frequent bladder emptying is advised. This will usually prevent the drug causing bladder irritation.

Storage
Keep in a closed container in a cool, dry place away from reach of children. Protect from light.

Missed dose
Injections are given only in the hospital. If you are taking tablets, take the missed dose as soon as you remember. If your next dose is due within 6 hours, take a single dose now and skip the next. Tell your physician that you missed a dose.

Stopping the drug
The drug will be stopped under medical supervision (injection). Do not stop taking the drug without consulting your physician (tablets); stopping the drug may lead to worsening of the underlying condition.

Exceeding the dose
An occasional unintentional extra dose is unlikely to cause problems. Large overdoses may cause nausea and vomiting. Notify your physician.

SPECIAL PRECAUTIONS

Cyclophosphamide is prescribed only under close medical supervision, taking account of your present condition and medical history.

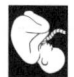

Pregnancy
▼ Not usually prescribed. May cause birth defects or premature birth. Discuss with your physician.

Breast feeding
▼ Discontinue breast feeding. The drug passes into the breast milk and may affect the baby adversely. Discuss with your physician.

Infants and children
▼ Reduced dose necessary.

Over 60
▼ No special problems.

Driving and hazardous work
▼ No known problems.

Alcohol
▼ Avoid. Alcohol consumption may increase nausea and vomiting.

Surgery and general anesthetics
▼ Before any surgery advise your physician, dentist, or anesthetist that you are taking cyclophosphamide.

PROLONGED USE

Prolonged use of this drug may reduce production of blood cells and may impair kidney or liver function.

Monitoring Periodic checks on blood composition and on all effects of the drug are required.

POSSIBLE ADVERSE EFFECTS

Cyclophosphamide often causes nausea and vomiting, which usually diminish as your body adjusts. Also, women may experience irregular periods. Blood in the urine may be a sign of bladder damage and requires prompt medical attention.

Symptom/effect	Frequency		Discuss with physician		Stop taking drug now	Call physician now
	Common	Rare	Only if severe	In all cases		
Nausea/vomiting	●		■			
Hair loss	●		■			
Irregular menstruation		●		■		
Mouth ulcers		●		■		
Fever/chills		●		■		▮
Bloodstained urine		●		■	▲	▮

INTERACTIONS

Allopurinol This drug may increase blood levels of cyclophosphamide, leading to an increased risk of adverse effects.

Phenobarbital Prolonged high doses of this drug may increase the adverse effects of cyclophosphamide.

CYCLOSPORINE

rand names Sandimmune, Neoral
sed in the following combined preparations None

GENERAL INFORMATION

yclosporine was introduced in 1984.
belongs to a group of drugs known as
munosuppressants. These drugs
uppress the body's natural defenses
gainst infection and foreign cells. This
ction is of particular use following
gan transplants, when the immune
stem may start to reject the trans-
anted organ unless the immune
stem is controlled.

Cyclosporine is now widely used
llowing many different types of trans-
ant surgery including heart, kidney,
one marrow, liver, and pancreas. Its

use has considerably reduced the risk of
tissue rejection. Cyclosporine is sometimes used to treat severe psoriasis
when other treatments have failed.

Because cyclosporine reduces the
effectiveness of the immune system,
people being treated with this drug
are more susceptible than usual to
infections. Cyclosporine can also
cause kidney damage.

It is important not to make dose
changes on your own. Ask your
pharmacist for a patient information
leaflet printed by the manufacturer.

QUICK REFERENCE

Drug group Immunosuppressant drug (p.168)

Overdose danger rating Low

Dependence rating Low

Prescription needed Yes

Multi-source suppliers No

INFORMATION FOR USERS

ur drug prescription is tailored for you.
not alter dosage without checking
th your physician.

w taken

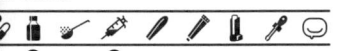

psules, oral liquid, injection.

equency and timing of doses
2 x daily.

sage range
e dosage of this drug is calculated on an
ividual basis according to age and weight.

set of effect
hin 12 hours.

ration of action
to 3 days.

t advice
id high potassium foods and potassium
plements (see p.524).

Storage
Keep liquid at room temperature – do not
store in the refrigerator. Once container has
been opened, contents must be used within
2 months. Capsules should be left in the
blister pack until required for use and may be
stored in the refrigerator. Keep away from
reach of children.

Missed dose
Take as soon as you remember. If your dose
is more than 36 hours late, consult your
physician.

Stopping the drug
Do not stop taking the drug without consulting
with your physician; stopping the drug may
lead to transplant rejection.

Exceeding the dose
An occasional unintentional extra dose is
unlikely to cause problems. Large overdoses
may cause headaches and affect kidney
function. Notify your physician.

SPECIAL PRECAUTIONS

Cyclosporine is prescribed only under
close medical supervision, taking account
of your present condition and medical
history.

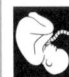

Pregnancy
▼ Safety in pregnancy not
established. Discuss with your
physician.

Breast feeding
▼ Not recommended. The drug
passes into the breast milk and can
affect the baby adversely. Discuss
with your physician.

Infants and children
▼ Safety in infants and children not
established; used only with great
caution.

Over 60
▼ Reduced dose may be
necessary.

Driving and hazardous work
▼ No known problems.

Alcohol
▼ No known problems.

POSSIBLE ADVERSE EFFECTS

most common adverse effects are gum
lling, excessive hair growth, nausea,
iting, and tremor. Headache and muscle

cramps may also occur. Less common effects
are diarrhea, facial swelling, flushing, "pins
and needles" sensations, rash, and itching.

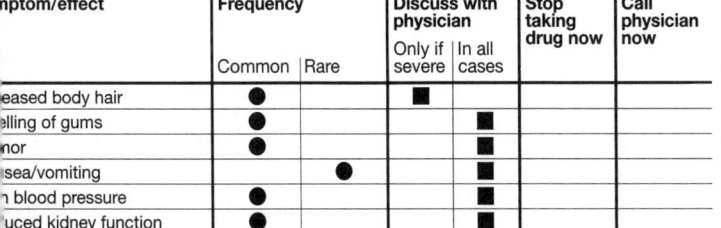

mptom/effect	Frequency		Discuss with physician		Stop taking drug now	Call physician now
	Common	Rare	Only if severe	In all cases		
eased body hair	●		■			
lling of gums	●			■		
mor	●			■		
sea/vomiting		●		■		
blood pressure	●			■		
uced kidney function	●			■		
sitivity to light	●		■			

INTERACTIONS

eneral note Cyclosporine may interact
th a large number of drugs. Check with
ur physician or pharmacist before taking

any prescribed or over-the-counter
medications.

PROLONGED USE

Long-term use of this drug, especially in
high doses, can cause reduced kidney
and/or liver function. It may reduce
numbers of white blood cells, thus
increasing susceptibility to infection.
There is also an increased risk of lymph
gland cancer (lymphomas).

Monitoring Regular checks on blood
samples are normally carried out to
measure cyclosporine levels and to
monitor blood composition, as well as
kidney and liver functions.

DANAZOL

Brand name Cyclomen
Used in the following combined preparations None

GENERAL INFORMATION

Danazol is a synthetic steroid hormone that inhibits certain hormones called pituitary gonadotropins. It is used in a range of conditions including endometriosis (a condition where fragments of endometrial tissue grow outside the uterus) and menorrhagia (excessive menstrual bleeding). Danazol is also used to relieve pain, tenderness, and lumpiness in the breasts caused by fibrocystic disease.

Danazol treatment commonly disrupts normal menstrual periods and in some cases periods may stop altogether. Other adverse effects include nausea, dizziness, rash, back pain, weight gain, and flushing. Women taking high doses may notice unusual hair growth and deepening of the voice.

Nonhormonal contraception should be used during danazol therapy.

QUICK REFERENCE

Drug group Drug for menstrual disorders (p.172)

Overdose danger rating Low

Dependence rating Low

Prescription needed Yes

Multi-source suppliers No

INFORMATION FOR USERS

Your drug prescription is tailored for you. Do not alter dosage without checking with your physician.

How taken

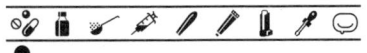

Capsules.

Frequency and timing of doses
2 – 4 x daily with food.

Adult dosage range
200 – 800mg daily, depending on the condition being treated, its severity, and the response to the drug.

Onset of effect
Some effects occur after a few days. Full beneficial effects may take some months.

Duration of action
1 – 2 days.

Diet advice
None.

Storage
Keep in a closed container in a cool, dry place away from reach of children.

Missed dose
Take as soon as you remember. If your next dose is due within 4 hours, take a single dose now and skip the next.

Stopping the drug
Do not stop the drug without consulting your physician; symptoms may recur.

Exceeding the dose
An occasional unintentional extra dose is unlikely to be a cause for concern. But if you notice unusual symptoms, or if a large overdose has been taken, notify your physician.

SPECIAL PRECAUTIONS

Be sure to tell your physician if:
▼ You have impaired liver or kidney function
▼ You have heart disease.
▼ You have had epileptic seizures.
▼ You suffer from unexplained vaginal bleeding.
▼ You have or suspect breast cancer.
▼ You have diabetes mellitus.
▼ You are or may be pregnant.
▼ You are taking other medications.

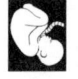

Pregnancy
▼ Not prescribed. May cause masculine characteristics in a female baby. Discuss with your physician.

Breast feeding
▼ The drug passes into the breast milk and may affect the baby. Discuss with your physician.

Infants and children
▼ Safety not established.

Over 60
▼ Unlikely to be required.

Driving and hazardous work
▼ No known problems.

Alcohol
▼ No known problems.

POSSIBLE ADVERSE EFFECTS

Danazol rarely causes adverse effects in low doses. Adverse effects from higher doses – such as acne, weight gain, and nausea – are the result of hormonal changes. Voice changes and unusual hair growth in women are largely reversed after treatment.

Symptom/effect	Frequency		Discuss with physician		Stop taking drug now	Call physician now
	Common	Rare	Only if severe	In all cases		
Swollen feet/ankles	●		■			
Weight gain	●		■			
Nausea	●		■			
Acne/oily skin	●		■			
Unusual hair growth or loss	●			■		
Reduced breast size		●	■			
Voice changes		●		■		
Muscle cramps or spasms		●		■		■

PROLONGED USE

The drug is normally taken for 3 to 9 months depending on the condition being treated. There is a slight risk of liver damage. See also Possible adverse effects, left.

Monitoring Periodic liver function tests may be carried out.

INTERACTIONS

Oral anticoagulants Danazol may increase their effects.

Insulin and oral antidiabetic drugs Danazol may reduce their effects.

Cyclosporine and carbamazepine Blood levels of these drugs may be increased by danazol.

DESIPRAMINE

Brand names Norpramin, Pertofrane
Used in the following combined preparations None

GENERAL INFORMATION

Desipramine is an antidepressant of the tricyclic group. It is used in the treatment of severe, prolonged depression to elevate mood, increase physical activity, improve appetite, and restore interest in everyday activities.

Less sedating than some other antidepressants, desipramine is particularly useful for people who are withdrawn or apathetic. Another advantage of desipramine is that side effects such as dry mouth, dizziness, and blurred vision tend to be less severe than with other similar drugs.

An overdose may cause dangerous heart rhythms and coma, but in normal use serious side effects are rare.

QUICK REFERENCE

Drug group Tricyclic antidepressant drug (p.96)

Overdose danger rating High

Dependence rating Low

Prescription needed Yes

Multi-source suppliers Yes

INFORMATION FOR USERS

Your drug prescription is tailored for you. Do not alter dosage without checking with your physician.

How taken

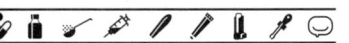

Tablets.

Frequency and timing of doses
1–4 x daily.

Adult dosage range
75–150mg daily (occasionally a higher dose is required).

Onset of effect
Some benefits and effects may appear within a few days of starting treatment, but full benefits may not be felt for 4 weeks or more.

Duration of action
Following prolonged treatment, antidepressant effects may persist for up to 6 weeks. Adverse effects may wear off within days.

Diet advice
None.

Storage
Keep in a closed container in a cool, dry place away from the reach of children. Protect from light.

Missed dose
Take as soon as you remember. If your next dose is due within 3 hours, take a single dose now and skip the next.

Stopping the drug
Do not stop the drug without consulting a physician, who may supervise a gradual reduction in dosage.

OVERDOSE ACTION

Seek immediate medical advice in all cases. Take emergency action if abnormal heart rhythms, seizures, or loss of consciousness occur.

See Drug poisoning emergency guide (p.574).

POSSIBLE ADVERSE EFFECTS

The most common adverse effects of desipramine are the result of its mild *anticholinergic* action. These usually diminish if the dosage is reduced.

Symptom/effect	Frequency		Discuss with physician		Stop taking drug now	Call physician now
	Common	Rare	Only if severe	In all cases		
Sweating/flushing	●		■			
Dry mouth	●		■			
Blurred vision	●			■		
Dizziness/fainting	●			■		
Rash		●		■	▲	▮
Palpitations		●		■	▲	▮

INTERACTIONS

Monoamine oxidase inhibitors (MAOIs) Usually, desipramine is not given with or within 2 weeks of treatment with an MAOI. Serious reactions may occur. These drugs are prescribed together only under strict medical supervision.

Sedatives All drugs, including alcohol, that have a sedative effect on the central nervous system are likely to increase the sedative properties of desipramine.

Antihypertensive drugs Desipramine may reduce the effect of some of these.

SPECIAL PRECAUTIONS

Be sure to tell your physician if:
▼ You have heart problems.
▼ You have impaired liver or kidney function.
▼ You have a thyroid disorder.
▼ You have epilepsy.
▼ You have glaucoma.
▼ You have prostate trouble.
▼ You have a blood disease
▼ You are taking other medications.

Pregnancy
▼ Safety in pregnancy not established. Discuss with your physician.

Breast feeding
▼ The drug passes into the breast milk and may affect the baby. Discuss with your physician.

Infants and children
▼ Not recommended under 12 years. Reduced dose necessary for older children.

Over 60
▼ Increased likelihood of adverse effects. Reduced dose may therefore be necessary.

Driving and hazardous work
▼ Avoid such activities until you have learned how the drug affects you; it can cause drowsiness and blurred vision.

Alcohol
▼ Avoid. Alcohol may increase the sedative effects of this drug.

Surgery and anesthetics
▼ Desipramine treatment may need to be stopped before you have a general anesthetic. Discuss this with your physician or dentist before any operation.

PROLONGED USE

No problems expected.

DEXAMETHASONE

Brand names Decadron, Dexasone, Dexsone, Hexadrol, Maxidex
Used in the following combined preparations Maxitrol, NeoDecadron, Tobradex

GENERAL INFORMATION

Dexamethasone is a long-acting corticosteroid prescribed for a variety of skin and soft tissue conditions caused by allergy or inflammation.

Dexamethasone can be injected into joints to relieve joint pain and stiffness due to rheumatoid arthritis and bursitis (see p.130). It can be injected for the emergency treatment of shock, brain swelling (due to head injury, stroke, or a

tumor), and asthma. Eye/ear preparations are available to treat inflammation of the eyes or ears.

Low doses of dexamethasone taken for short periods rarely cause serious *side effects*. However, as with other corticosteroids, long-term treatment with high doses can cause unpleasant or dangerous side effects.

INFORMATION FOR USERS

Your drug prescription is tailored for you. Do not alter dosage without checking with your physician.

How taken

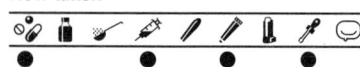

Tablets, injection, eye ointment, eye/ear drops.

Frequency and timing of doses
Considerable variation depending on condition and preparation used.

Dosage range
Wide variation according to preparation and condition. Follow your physician's instructions.

Onset of effect
1 – 4 days.

Duration of action
Some effects may last several days.

Diet advice
You may need to restrict dietary salt and you may need potassium supplements.

Storage
Keep in a closed container in a cool, dry place away from reach of children. Protect from light.

Missed dose
Take as soon as you remember. If your next dose is due within 2 hours, take a single dose now and skip the next.

Stopping the drug
Do not stop taking the drug without consulting your physician. It may be necessary to withdraw the drug gradually.

Exceeding the dose
An occasional unintentional extra dose is unlikely to be cause for concern. But if you notice unusual symptoms, or if a large overdose has been taken, notify your physician.

SPECIAL PRECAUTIONS

Be sure to tell your physician if:
▼ You have had a peptic ulcer.
▼ You have glaucoma.
▼ You have had tuberculosis.
▼ You have suffered from depression or mental illness.
▼ You have an infection.
▼ You are taking other medications.

 Pregnancy
▼ Safety in pregnancy not established. Discuss with your physician.

 Breast feeding
▼ The drug passes into the breast milk and may affect the baby adversely. Discuss with your physician.

 Infants and children
▼ Reduced dose necessary.

 Over 60
▼ Reduced dose may be necessary.

 Driving and hazardous work
▼ No known problems.

 Alcohol
▼ Avoid. Alcohol may increase the risk of peptic ulcer with this drug.

POSSIBLE ADVERSE EFFECTS

The more serious adverse effects only occur when dexamethasone is taken in high doses for long periods of time. These are carefully monitored during prolonged treatment. Other adverse effects tend to become less noticeable as your body adjusts to the drug.

Symptom/effect	Frequency		Discuss with physician		Stop taking drug now	Call physician now
	Common	Rare	Only if severe	In all cases		
Indigestion	●		■			
Weight gain		●	■			
Acne and other skin effects		●	■			
Fluid retention		●		■		
Muscle weakness		●		■		
Mood changes		●		■		

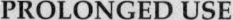

PROLONGED USE

Prolonged use of this drug in high doses can lead to glaucoma, cataracts, diabetes, fragile bones and thin skin, and can retard growth in children.

INTERACTIONS (by mouth or injection only)

Antidiabetic drugs Dexamethasone decreases the action of these drugs.

Barbiturates, phenytoin, and rifampin These drugs may reduce the effectiveness of dexamethasone.

Diuretics Dexamethasone may increase potassium loss.

Oral anticoagulants Dexamethasone may increase or decrease blood clotting.

Vaccines Dexamethasone can interact with some vaccines. Discuss with your physician.

DEXTROMETHORPHAN

Brand names Balminil DM, Benylin DM, Calmylin #1, Delsym, Koffex, Robidex
Used in the following combined preparations Benylin DM-D, Benylin DM-D-E, Robitussin DM, Sudafed DM

GENERAL INFORMATION

Dextromethorphan is a cough suppressant available over the counter in a number of cough remedies. It is useful for suppressing persistent, dry coughing, especially if sleep is disturbed.

It has little general *sedative* effect and, unlike the stronger narcotic cough suppressants, it is unlikely to lead to *dependence* when taken as recommended.

Like other cough suppressants, it should not be used for phlegm-producing coughs because it may prolong a chest infection by preventing the normal elimination of sputum. Although the drug is less sedative than many similar drugs, drowsiness is the principal adverse effect.

INFORMATION FOR USERS

Follow instructions on the label. Call your physician if symptoms worsen.

How taken

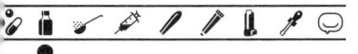

Oral liquid.

Frequency and timing of doses
3 to 4 x daily as required.

Dosage range
Adults 12 years and over, 15 – 30mg per dose up to a maximum of 120mg/24 hours.
Children 6 – 11 years, 15mg per dose up to a maximum of 60mg/24 hours; 2 – 5 years, 5mg per dose up to a maximum of 30mg/24 hours.

Onset of effect
Within 30 minutes.

Duration of action
4 – 8 hours.

Diet advice
None.

Storage
Keep in closed container in a cool, dry place away from reach of children.

Missed dose
Take as soon as you remember if needed to relieve coughing.

Stopping the drug
Can be safely stopped as soon as you no longer need it.

Exceeding the dose
An occasional unintentional extra dose is unlikely to cause problems. Large overdoses may cause nausea, vomiting, stomach pain, dizziness, drowsiness, and breathing problems. Notify your physician.

SPECIAL PRECAUTIONS

Be sure to consult your physician or pharmacist before taking this drug if:
▼ You have a liver disorder.
▼ You suffer from asthma or another serious respiratory problem.
▼ You are taking other medications.

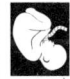

Pregnancy
▼ No evidence of risk to the developing baby when normal doses are used for short periods. Discuss with your physician.

Breast feeding
▼ The drug passes into the breast milk, but at normal doses adverse effects on the baby are unlikely. Discuss with your physician.

Infants and children
▼ Not recommended for children under 2 years of age.

Over 60
▼ Reduced dose necessary.

Driving and hazardous work
▼ Avoid such activities until you have learned how the drug affects you; it may reduce alertness.

Alcohol
▼ Avoid. Alcohol may increase the sedative effects of this drug.

POSSIBLE ADVERSE EFFECTS

Adverse effects are rare when dextromethorphan is taken in recommended doses, and diminish if the dosage is reduced and as your body adjusts to the drug.

Symptom/effect	Frequency		Discuss with physician		Stop taking drug now	Call physician now
	Common	Rare	Only if severe	In all cases		
Dizziness/drowsiness		●	■			
Constipation		●	■			
Nausea/vomiting		●	■			
Abdominal pain		●	■			

INTERACTIONS

Sedatives All drugs, including alcohol, that have a sedative effect on the central nervous system are likely to increase the sedative properties of dextromethorphan. Such drugs include antihistamines, anti-anxiety and sleeping drugs, antidepressants, narcotic analgesics, and antipsychotic drugs.

Monoamine oxidase inhibitors (MAOIs) These drugs may interact dangerously with dextromethorphan to cause excitation and fever.

PROLONGED USE

Dextromethorphan should not be taken for longer than 1 week except on the advice of a physician.

DIAZEPAM

Brand names Valium, Apo-Diazepam, Diazemuls, Vivol
Used in the following combined preparations None

GENERAL INFORMATION

Introduced in 1963, diazepam is the best known and most widely used of a group of drugs known as the benzo-diazepines. These drugs help relieve nervousness and tension, relax muscles, and encourage sleep. The actions and adverse effects of this group of drugs are described more fully on page 95.

Diazepam has a wide range of uses. Besides being commonly used in the treatment of anxiety and anxiety-related

insomnia, it is used in the treatment of alcohol withdrawal, and sometimes as a muscle relaxant. Given intravenously, diazepam is used to sedate people undergoing certain uncomfortable medical procedures and to stop certain kinds of sustained epileptic seizures.

Diazepam can be habit-forming if taken regularly over a long period. Its effects may also diminish with time. Treatment with diazepam is usually reviewed frequently.

INFORMATION FOR USERS

Your drug prescription is tailored for you. Do not alter dosage without checking with your physician.

How taken

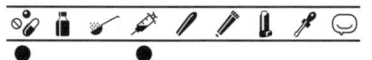

Tablets, capsules, injection.

Frequency and timing of doses
1 – 4 x daily.

Adult dosage range
2 – 40mg daily.

Onset of effect
Immediate effect (intravenously); 30 minutes – 2 hours (other methods of administration).

Duration of action
Up to 24 hours.

Diet advice
None.

Storage
Keep in a closed container in a cool, dry place away from reach of children.

Missed dose
No cause for concern, but take when you next feel you need the drug. If your next dose is due within 2 hours, take a single dose now and skip the next.

Stopping the drug
If you have been taking the drug continuously for less than 2 weeks, it can be safely stopped as soon as you feel you no longer need it. However, if you have been taking it for longer, consult your physician, who will supervise a gradual reduction in dosage. Stopping abruptly may lead to withdrawal symptoms (see p.95).

Exceeding the dose
An occasional unintentional extra dose is unlikely to cause problems. Larger overdoses may cause unusual drowsiness. Notify your physician.

SPECIAL PRECAUTIONS

Be sure to tell your physician if:
▼ You have severe respiratory disease.
▼ You have impaired liver or kidney function
▼ You have had problems with alcohol or drug abuse.
▼ You are taking other medications.

Pregnancy
▼ Safety in pregnancy not established. Discuss with your physician.

Breast feeding
▼ The drug passes into the breast milk. Its effects on the baby are not clearly known. Discuss with your physician.

Infants and children
▼ Reduced dose necessary.

Over 60
▼ Increased likelihood of adverse effects. Reduced dose may therefore be necessary.

Driving and hazardous work
▼ Avoid such activities until you have learned how the drug affects you, because the drug can cause reduced alertness and slowed reactions.

Alcohol
▼ Avoid. Alcohol may increase the sedative effects of this drug.

POSSIBLE ADVERSE EFFECTS

The principal adverse effects of this drug are related to its sedative properties. These effects, including drowsiness and dizziness, normally diminish after the first few days and, if troublesome, can often be reduced by adjustment of the dosage.

Symptom/effect	Frequency		Discuss with physician		Stop taking drug now	Call physician now
	Common	Rare	Only if severe	In all cases		
Daytime drowsiness	●		■			
Dizziness/unsteadiness	●			■		
Headache		●	■			
Blurred vision		●		■		
Forgetfulness/confusion		●		■		
Rash		●		■	▲	

INTERACTIONS

Sedatives All drugs that have a sedative effect on the central nervous system, including alcohol, are likely to increase the sedative properties of diazepam.

Cimetidine Breakdown of diazepam in the liver may be inhibited by cimetidine. This can cause a buildup of diazepam levels in the blood which increases the likelihood of adverse effects.

PROLONGED USE

Regular use of this drug over several weeks can lead to a reduction in its effect as the body adapts. It may also be habit-forming when taken for extended periods. Severe withdrawal reactions have occurred.

DICLOFENAC

Brand names Voltaren, Apo-Diclo, Novo-Difenac, Nu-Diclo
Used in the following combined preparation Arthrotec

GENERAL INFORMATION

Diclofenac, introduced in 1980, is a non-steroidal anti-inflammatory drug (NSAID). Like other drugs of this group, it reduces pain, stiffness, and inflammation. It is used for the symptomatic relief of arthritis and severe osteoarthritis, including degenerative joint disease of the hip, although it does not cure the disease. Diclofenac is also given in the form of eye drops to treat some kinds of eye inflammation. Gastrointestinal, skin and central nervous system *side effects* are the most commonly seen.

Arthrotec is a combination of diclofenac and misoprostol (see p.393). Misoprostol helps prevent gastroduodenal ulceration and may be particularly useful in patients at risk of developing ulcers.

INFORMATION FOR USERS

Your drug prescription is tailored for you. Do not alter dosage without checking with your physician.

How taken

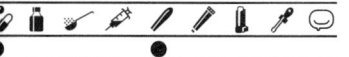

Tablets, slow-release tablets, rectal suppositories.

Frequency and timing of doses
x daily (tablets, rectal suppositories); once daily (slow-release tablets).

Adult dosage range
– 150mg daily.

Onset of effect
in relief within a few hours, but full effect in arthritic conditions may be delayed.

Duration of action
– 12 hours (tablets); up to 36 hours (slow-release tablets).

Diet advice
None.

Storage
Keep in closed container in a cool, dry place away from reach of children.

Missed dose
Take as soon as you remember. If your next dose is due within 2 hours, take a single dose now and skip the next.

Stopping the drug
When taken for short-term pain relief, diclofenac can be safely stopped as soon as you no longer need it. If prescribed for the long-term treatment of arthritis, however, you should seek medical advice before stopping the drug.

Exceeding the dose
An occasional unintentional extra dose is unlikely to be a cause for concern. But if you notice unusual symptoms, or if a large overdose has been taken, notify your physician.

POSSIBLE ADVERSE EFFECTS

The most common adverse effects are the result of gastrointestinal disturbances. Black or bloodstained feces should be reported to your physician without delay. Headaches and dizziness may also occur.

Symptom/effect	Frequency		Discuss with physician		Stop taking drug now	Call physician now
	Common	Rare	Only if severe	In all cases		
Abdominal pain/indigestion	●		■			
Headache	●		■			
Dizziness/lightheadedness	●		■			
Nausea/vomiting	●			■		
Drowsiness/depression		●	■			
Diarrhea		●		■		
Wheezing/breathlessness		●		■	▲	▮
Rash		●		■	▲	
Black/bloodstained feces		●		■	▲	▮

INTERACTIONS

General note Diclofenac may interact with a wide range of drugs to increase the risk of bleeding and/or peptic ulcer. Such drugs include oral anticoagulants, corticosteroids, other non-steroidal anti-inflammatory drugs (NSAIDs), and ASA.

Diclofenac may raise blood levels of digoxin, lithium, and methotrexate. It may also reduce the beneficial effects of antihypertensive drugs and diuretics and may increase the blood sugar, lowering the effects of oral antidiabetics.

SPECIAL PRECAUTIONS

Be sure to tell your physician if:
▼ You have impaired liver or kidney function.
▼ You have heart problems.
▼ You have asthma.
▼ You have high blood pressure.
▼ You have had a peptic ulcer, esophagitis, or acid indigestion.
▼ You are allergic to ASA.
▼ You are taking other medications.

Pregnancy
▼ Safety in pregnancy not established. Discuss with your physician.

Breast feeding
▼ Diclofenac passes into breast milk, but in low concentrations. Discuss with your physician.

Infants and children
▼ Not recommended for children under 16 years.

Over 60
▼ Increased likelihood of adverse effects. Reduced dose may therefore be necessary.

Driving and hazardous work
▼ Avoid such activities until you have learned how the drug affects you; it can cause dizziness and drowsiness.

Alcohol
▼ Avoid. Alcohol may increase the risk of stomach disorders with diclofenac.

Surgery and general anesthetics
▼ Diclofenac may prolong bleeding. Discuss with your physician or dentist before any surgery.

PROLONGED USE

There is an increased risk of bleeding both from peptic ulcers and from the bowel with prolonged use of diclofenac.

DIDANOSINE

Brand name Videx
Used in the following combined preparations None

GENERAL INFORMATION

Didanosine is an antiviral agent used in the treatment of AIDS. Like zidovudine (AZT), it works by blocking the action of the enzyme reverse transcriptase.

Didanosine delays worsening of the disease by temporarily boosting immunity, thereby reducing the frequency and severity of infections, and by helping AIDS patients to gain weight. However, the drug is not a cure for HIV infection, and patients may continue to be afflicted by illnesses associated with AIDS. Didanosine is generally reserved for patients who do not respond to AZT or who are intolerant of it.

The major adverse effects of didanosine are pancreatitis (inflammation of the pancreas) and peripheral neuropathy (impaired function of nerves in the extremities).

QUICK REFERENCE

Drug group Antiviral drug for AIDS (p.169)

Overdose danger rating Medium

Dependence rating Low

Prescription needed Yes

Multi-source suppliers No

INFORMATION FOR USERS

Your drug prescription is tailored for you. Do not alter dosage without checking with your physician.

How taken

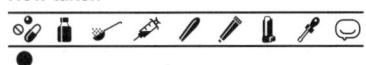

Chewable/dispersible tablets. Tablets should not be swallowed whole: they should be thoroughly chewed, crushed, or dispersed in water before swallowing.

Frequency and timing of doses
Adults Every 12 hours on an empty stomach.
Children Every 8 hours on an empty stomach.

Dosage range
Adults 250 – 600mg daily.
Children 75 – 225mg daily.

Onset of effect
Usually within 48 hours.

Duration of action
8 – 12 hours.

Diet advice
None.

Storage
Keep in a closed container in a cool, dry place away from reach of children. Protect from light.

Missed dose
Take as soon as you remember. If your next dose is due within 4 hours, take a single dose now and skip the next.

Stopping the drug
Do not stop taking the drug without consulting your physician; symptoms may recur.

Exceeding the dose
An occasional unintentional extra dose is unlikely to cause problems. Large overdoses may cause diarrhea and abdominal pain. Notify your physician immediately.

SPECIAL PRECAUTIONS

Be sure to tell your physician if:
▼ You are taking any other drugs to treat AIDS or AIDS complications.
▼ You have impaired liver, kidney, or respiratory function.
▼ You have raised uric acid levels.
▼ You are taking other medications.

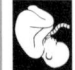
Pregnancy
▼ Safety in pregnancy not established. Discuss with your physician.

Breast feeding
▼ Not recommended. Discuss with your physician.

Infants and children
▼ Not recommended for children under 6 months of age. Reduced dose necessary for older children.

Over 60
▼ Increased likelihood of adverse effects. Reduced dose may therefore be necessary.

Driving and hazardous work
▼ No special problems.

Alcohol
▼ Avoid. May increase the possibility of adverse effects.

POSSIBLE ADVERSE EFFECTS

The major adverse effects are pancreatitis and peripheral neuropathy. Symptoms of pancreatitis include abdominal pain, nausea, and vomiting. Symptoms of peripheral neuropathy include tingling, burning, pain or numbness in hands or feet.

Symptom/effect	Frequency		Discuss with physician		Stop taking drug now	Call physician now
	Common	Rare	Only if severe	In all cases		
Headache/insomnia	●		■			
Nausea/vomiting/diarrhea	●		■			
Pallor/fatigue/weakness	●			■		
Breathlessness/cough	●			■		▌
Joint/muscle pain		●		■		
Hives/chills/fever		●		■	▲	▌
Abdominal pain		●		■	▲	▌
Limb burning/numbness		●		■	▲	▌

INTERACTIONS

General note A wide range of drugs may increase the harmful effects or decrease the absorption of didanosine. Obtain full information from your physician.

PROLONGED USE

The long-term effects of didanosine are unknown at this time. Didanosine therapy has not been shown to reduce the risk of transmission of HIV to others through sexual contact or blood contamination.

Monitoring Regular blood checks are required during treatment. Eye examinations may be recommended.

DIFLUNISAL

Brand names Dolobid, Apo-Diflunisal, Novo-Diflunisal, Nu-Diflunisal
Used in the following combined preparations None

GENERAL INFORMATION

Diflunisal, introduced in 1983, is a non-steroidal anti-inflammatory drug (NSAID) with a prolonged duration of action. Like other members of this group, it reduces pain, stiffness, and inflammation.

Diflunisal is used to relieve discomfort in osteoarthritis and rheumatoid arthritis, although it does not cure the underlying disease. It is also effective for pain relief after minor operations and dental treatment, and may also be given to treat sprains, strains, and some types of back pain.

Serious adverse effects with diflunisal are unusual. However, diarrhea, nausea, indigestion, headache, or a skin rash may occur.

INFORMATION FOR USERS

Your drug prescription is tailored for you. Do not alter dosage without checking with your physician.

How taken

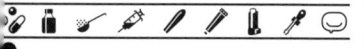

Tablets.

Frequency and timing of doses
x daily with food or milk.

Adult dosage range
90mg – 1g daily.

Onset of effect
Pain relief begins within 1 hour. Full anti-inflammatory effect in arthritic conditions may not be felt for up to 2 weeks.

Duration of action
– 12 hours.

Diet advice
None.

Storage
Keep in a closed container in a cool, dry place away from reach of children.

Missed dose
Take as soon as you remember. If your next dose is due within 2 – 4 hours, take a single dose now and skip the next.

Stopping the drug
When taken for short-term pain relief, diflunisal can be safely stopped as soon as you no longer need it. If prescribed for long-term treatment of arthritis, however, you should seek medical advice before stopping the drug.

Exceeding the dose
An occasional unintentional extra dose is unlikely to cause problems. Large overdoses may cause nausea, drowsiness, and disorientation. Notify your physician.

SPECIAL PRECAUTIONS

Be sure to tell your physician if:
▼ You have impaired liver or kidney function.
▼ You have had a peptic ulcer, esophagitis, or acid indigestion.
▼ You have asthma.
▼ You have heart problems.
▼ You have high blood pressure.
▼ You have bleeding problems.
▼ You are allergic to ASA.
▼ You are taking other medications.

Pregnancy
▼ Safety in pregnancy not established. Discuss with your physician.

Breast feeding
▼ The drug passes into the breast milk and may affect the baby. Discuss with your physician.

Infants and children
▼ Not recommended for children under 12 years.

Over 60
▼ Increased likelihood of adverse effects. Reduced dose may therefore be necessary.

Driving and hazardous work
▼ Avoid such activities until you have learned how the drug affects you; it can cause drowsiness and dizziness.

Alcohol
▼ Avoid. Alcohol may increase the risk of stomach disorders with diflunisal.

Surgery and general anesthetics
▼ Diflunisal may prolong bleeding. Discuss with your physician or dentist before any surgery.

POSSIBLE ADVERSE EFFECTS

Gastrointestinal side effects and headache are not generally serious and may diminish with continued use as your body adapts. The occurrence of black or bloodstained bowel movements should be reported to your physician without delay.

Symptom/effect	Frequency		Discuss with physician		Stop taking drug now	Call physician now
	Common	Rare	Only if severe	In all cases		
Nausea/diarrhea	●		■			
Heartburn/indigestion	●		■			
Abdominal pain	●		■			
Headache	●		■			
Drowsiness/dizziness	●			■		
Rash	●			■	▲	
Wheezing/breathlessness		●		■	▲	▮
Black/bloodstained feces		●		■	▲	▮

INTERACTIONS

General note Diflunisal interacts with a wide range of drugs to increase the risk of bleeding and/or peptic ulcers. Such drugs include oral anticoagulants, corticosteroids, other non-steroidal anti-inflammatory drugs (NSAIDs), ASA, sulfinpyrazone, dipyridamole, some antibiotics, and valproic acid.

Antihypertensive drugs and diuretics
The beneficial effects of these drugs may be reduced by diflunisal.

PROLONGED USE

There is an increased risk of bleeding both from peptic ulcers and in the bowel with prolonged use of diflunisal.

DIGOXIN

Brand name Lanoxin
Used in the following combined preparations None

GENERAL INFORMATION

Digoxin is the most widely used form of digitalis, a drug extracted from the leaves of the foxglove plant. It is sometimes given in the treatment of congestive heart failure and certain alterations of heart rhythm.

Digoxin makes the heart more effective in pumping blood. It also slows the heart. In congestive heart failure, it also helps to control tiredness, breathlessness, and fluid retention. Its

effects are not as long lasting as those of other digitalis drugs, and this makes any adverse reactions easier to control.

For digoxin to be effective, the dose must be very near the toxic dose, and the treatment must be monitored closely. A number of adverse effects (see below) may indicate the toxic level is being reached and should be reported to your physician immediately.

QUICK REFERENCE

Drug group Digitalis drug (p.108)
Overdose danger rating High
Dependence rating Low
Prescription needed Yes
Multi-source suppliers No

INFORMATION FOR USERS

Your drug prescription is tailored for you. Do not alter dosage without checking with your physician.

How taken

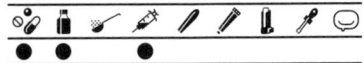

Tablets, oral liquid, injection.

Frequency and timing of doses
Up to 3 x daily while dosage is being established. Once daily for maintenance.

Dosage range
Adults 0.125 – 0.25mg daily (by mouth).
Children Reduced dose according to age and weight.

Onset of effect
Within a few minutes (injection); within 12 hours (by mouth).

Duration of action
Up to 4 days.

Diet advice
This drug may be more toxic if potassium levels are depleted. Include fruit and vegetables in your diet (see p.524).

Storage
Keep in a closed container in a cool, dry place away from reach of children.

Missed dose
Take as soon as you remember. If your next dose is due within 4 hours, take both doses now and skip the next. Return to your normal schedule tomorrow.

Stopping the drug
Do not stop this drug without consulting your physician; stopping the drug may lead to worsening of the underlying condition.

OVERDOSE ACTION

 Seek immediate medical advice in all cases. Take emergency action if palpitations, severe weakness, chest pain, or loss of consciousness occurs.

See Drug poisoning emergency guide (p.574).

SPECIAL PRECAUTIONS

Be sure to tell your physician if:
▼ You have impaired liver or kidney function.
▼ You have a thyroid disorder.
▼ You are taking other medications.

 **Pregnancy**
▼ Safety in pregnancy not established. Discuss with your physician.

 Breast feeding
▼ The drug passes into breast milk, but at normal doses adverse effects on the baby are unlikely. Discuss with your physician.

 Infants and children
▼ Reduced dose necessary.

 Over 60
▼ Increased likelihood of adverse effects. Reduced dose may therefore be necessary.

 Driving and hazardous work
▼ Avoid such activities until you have learned how the drug affects you; it can cause drowsiness and mental confusion.

 Alcohol
▼ No special problems.

PROLONGED USE

No problems expected.

Monitoring Periodic checks on blood levels of digoxin and body salts may be advised.

POSSIBLE ADVERSE EFFECTS

The possible adverse effects of digoxin are usually due to increased levels of the drug in the blood. Any symptoms should be reported to your physician without delay.

Symptom/effect	Frequency		Discuss with physician		Stop taking drug now	Call physician now
	Common	Rare	Only if severe	In all cases		
Tiredness	●		■			
Nausea/loss of appetite	●			■		
Confusion	●			■		
Visual disturbance	●			■		
Palpitations	●			■	▲	▐

INTERACTIONS

General note Many drugs interact with digoxin. Do not take any medication without your physician's advice. Only the most important interactions are described below.

Erythromycin and tetracycline antibiotics may increase the risk of adverse effects from digoxin.

Antacids may reduce the effects of digoxin. The effect of digoxin may increase when such drugs are stopped.

Anti-arrhythmic drugs and calcium channel blockers may increase blood levels of digoxin.

DILTIAZEM

Brand names Cardizem, Apo-Diltiaz, Novo-Diltazem, Nu-Diltiaz, Syn-Diltiazem
Used in the following combined preparations None

GENERAL INFORMATION

Diltiazem belongs to the group of drugs known as calcium channel blockers (p.113). These interfere with the conduction of signals in the muscles of the heart and blood vessels.

Diltiazem is used in the treatment of angina and hypertension. It reduces the frequency of angina attacks but does not work quickly enough to reduce the pain of an angina attack in progress.

Diltiazem does not adversely affect breathing and therefore can be used in people who suffer from asthma, for whom other anti-angina drugs may not be suitable. Adverse effects include headache, ankle swelling, and tiredness.

QUICK REFERENCE

Drug group Anti-angina drug (p.113), antihypertensive drug (p.114)

Overdose danger rating Medium

Dependence rating Low

Prescription needed Yes

Multi-source suppliers Yes

INFORMATION FOR USERS

Your prescription is tailored for you. Do not alter dosage without checking with your physician.

How taken

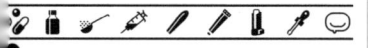

Tablets, slow-release capsules.

Frequency and timing of doses
3 – 4 x daily (tablets); 2 x daily (slow-release capsules).

Adult dosage range
Angina 240 – 360mg daily (tablets). *Hypertension* 120 – 360mg daily (slow-release capsules).

Onset of effect
30 – 60 minutes (tablets); 2 – 3 hours (slow-release capsules).

Duration of action
6 – 8 hours (tablets); 7 – 11 hours (slow-release capsules).

Diet advice
None.

Storage
Keep in a closed container in a cool, dry place away from reach of children.

Missed dose
Take a tablet as soon as you remember. If your next dose is due within 2 hours, take a single dose now and skip the next. If your next slow-release capsule dose is due within 4 hours, take a single dose now and take the next dose 8 hours later, then follow your regular schedule.

Stopping the drug
Do not stop taking the drug without consulting your physician; symptoms may recur.

Exceeding the dose
An occasional unintentional extra dose is unlikely to be cause for concern. Large overdoses may cause dizziness. Notify your physician.

SPECIAL PRECAUTIONS

Be sure to tell your physician if:
▼ You have impaired liver or kidney function.
▼ You have heart failure.
▼ You are taking other medications.

Pregnancy
▼ Safety in pregnancy not established. Discuss with your physician.

Breast feeding
▼ The drug passes into the breast milk and may affect the baby. Discuss with your physician.

Infants and children
▼ Not recommended.

Over 60
▼ Increased likelihood of adverse effects. Reduced dose may therefore be necessary.

Driving and hazardous work
▼ Avoid such activities until you have learned how the drug affects you; it can cause dizziness due to lowered blood pressure.

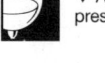
Alcohol
▼ Avoid. Alcohol may reduce blood pressure, causing dizziness.

PROLONGED USE

No problems expected.

Monitoring Periodic tests on liver function may be advised.

POSSIBLE ADVERSE EFFECTS

Diltiazem can cause a variety of minor symptoms that are common to other calcium channel blockers. These include headache and nausea. The most serious effect is the possibility of a slowed heartbeat, which may cause tiredness or dizziness. These effects can sometimes be controlled by an adjustment in dosage.

Symptom/effect	Frequency		Discuss with physician		Stop taking drug now	Call physician now
	Common	Rare	Only if severe	In all cases		
Headache	●		■			
Loss of appetite/nausea	●		■			
Leg and ankle swelling	●		■			
Dry mouth		●	■			
Tiredness		●		■		
Dizziness/fainting		●		■		
Rash		●		■	▲	

INTERACTIONS

Antihypertensive drugs Diltiazem increases their effects, leading to an additional reduction in blood pressure.

Digoxin Blood levels and adverse effects of this drug may be increased if it is taken with diltiazem. The dosage of digoxin may need to be reduced.

DIMENHYDRINATE

Brand names Gravol, Apo-Dimenhydrinate, Novo-Dimenate, PMS Dimenhydrinate, Travel Tabs
Used in the following combined preparation Gravergol

GENERAL INFORMATION

Dimenhydrinate is an antihistamine that is mainly used as an anti-emetic drug. It is especially effective for treating the nausea and vomiting that occur with vertigo. It is also prescribed to relieve the symptoms of inner ear disorders such as Ménière's disease and to prevent and treat motion sickness. Dimenhydrinate is often effective in treating other forms of nausea and vomiting, including those caused by pregnancy and by drug and radiation treatments for cancer.

Like other antihistamines, dimenhydrinate has a sedative effect that can cause problems if you need to drive or operate machinery.

QUICK REFERENCE

Drug group Antihistamine (p.136) and anti-emetic drug (p.102)

Overdose danger rating Medium

Dependence rating Low

Prescription needed No

Multi-source suppliers Yes

INFORMATION FOR USERS

Follow instructions on the label. Call your physician if symptoms worsen.

How taken

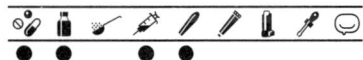

Tablets, slow-release capsules, oral liquid, injection, rectal suppositories.

Frequency and timing of doses
Adults Every 4 hours.
Children Every 6 – 8 hours. To prevent motion sickness the first dose should be taken 30 minutes to 2 hours before travel.

Oral dosage range
Adults 50 – 100mg per dose (maximum 400mg/24 hours).
Children 2 – 6 years, 15 – 25mg per dose (maximum 75mg/24 hours); 6 – 12 years, 25 – 50mg per dose (maximum 150mg/24 hours); 12 years and over, 50mg per dose (maximum 300mg/24 hours).

Onset of effect
Within 30 minutes.

Duration of action
6 – 8 hours.

Diet advice
None.

Storage
Keep in a closed container in a cool, dry place away from reach of children.

Missed dose
Take when you remember. Adjust the timing of your next dose accordingly.

Stopping the drug
Can be safely stopped as soon as you no longer need it.

Exceeding the dose
An occasional unintentional extra dose is unlikely to cause problems. Larger overdoses may cause unusual drowsiness. Notify your physician.

SPECIAL PRECAUTIONS

Be sure to consult your physician or pharmacist before taking this drug if:
▼ You have impaired liver or kidney function.
▼ You have chronic lung disease.
▼ You have had glaucoma.
▼ You have prostate trouble.
▼ You are taking other medications.

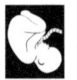

Pregnancy
▼ While there is no evidence of risk to the developing baby, absolute safety in pregnancy has not been established. Discuss with your physician.

Breast feeding
▼ The drug passes into the breast milk. Its effects on the baby are not clearly known. Discuss with your physician.

Infants and children
▼ Only as prescribed by your physician in children under 2 years. Reduced dose necessary in older children.

Over 60
▼ No special problems.

Driving and hazardous work
▼ Because of the possibility of drowsiness, avoid such activities until you have learned how the drug affects you.

Alcohol
▼ Avoid. Alcohol may increase the sedative effects of this drug.

POSSIBLE ADVERSE EFFECTS

The principal adverse effects of this drug are related to its *anticholinergic* properties and, if troublesome, can sometimes be reduced by adjustment of dosage.

Symptom/effect	Frequency		Discuss with physician		Stop taking drug now	Call physician now
	Common	Rare	Only if severe	In all cases		
Drowsiness	●		■			
Dry mouth	●		■			
Blurred vision	●			■		

INTERACTIONS

Alcohol and other sedatives All drugs that have a sedative effect on the central nervous system are likely to increase the sedative properties of dimenhydrinate. Such drugs include alcohol, anti-anxiety and sleeping drugs, antidepressants, narcotic analgesics, and antipsychotics.

PROLONGED USE

No special problems, but this drug should not be used for more than a few days except on medical advice.

Anti-emetics may mask the presence of underlying organic abnormalities or the toxic effects of other drugs.

Antihistamines should be discontinued approximately 48 hours prior to allergy skin testing.

DINOPROSTONE

Brand names Prostin E$_2$, Prepidil Gel
Used in the following combined preparations None

GENERAL INFORMATION

Dinoprostone is a drug derived from a natural chemical substance in the body (prostaglandin E$_2$). This drug softens and opens the cervix, as well as stimulating the full-term pregnant uterus to contract before the onset of normal labor. It is used only in hospital to start a patient into labor for medical reasons such as high blood pressure, toxemia, diabetes, impaired growth of the fetus, and in cases of overdue pregnancy.

Dinoprostone treatment requires close monitoring of the mother and the fetus by a physician and/or a nurse in a labor suite.

The most common *side effects* seen with oral dinoprostone are nausea, vomiting, and diarrhea but these are of short duration and disappear within 1 or 2 hours of the discontinuation of therapy.

QUICK REFERENCE

Drug group Uterine stimulant (p.177)

Overdose danger rating Medium

Dependence rating Low

Prescription needed Yes

Multi-source suppliers No

INFORMATION FOR USERS

This drug is given only in hospital under medical supervision and is not for self-administration.

How taken

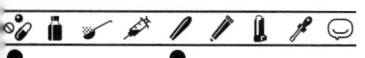

Tablets, vaginal gel, cervical gel.

Frequency and timing of doses
Oral Every hour until labor is established.
Vaginal gel An initial dose which may be repeated in 6 hours.
Cervical gel Single dose only.

Adult dosage range
Oral 0.5 – 1.0mg per dose.
Vaginal gel 1.0 – 2.0mg per dose.
Cervical gel 0.5mg as a single dose.

Onset of effect
5 – 30 minutes.

Duration of action
Up to 6 hours.

Diet advice
None.

Storage
Not applicable. The drug is not kept in the home.

Missed dose
Not applicable. The drug is given only in hospital under medical supervision.

Stopping the drug
Not applicable. The drug is stopped under medical supervision.

Exceeding the dose
The drug is given only in hospital under medical supervision and overdose is extremely unlikely to occur.

POSSIBLE ADVERSE EFFECTS

Nausea, vomiting, and diarrhea are very common with oral dinoprostone. Excessively strong contractions can occur and are controlled by dosage adjustment.

Symptom/effect	Frequency		Discuss with physician		Stop taking drug now	Call physician now
	Common	Rare	Only if severe	In all cases		
Nausea/vomiting (tablets)	●			■		
Diarrhea (tablets)	●			■		
Excessive contractions		●		■	▲	■

INTERACTIONS

Oxytocin Dinoprostone and oxytocin are not given together due to the risk of excessively strong contractions.

SPECIAL PRECAUTIONS

Be sure to tell your physician if:
▼ You suffer from asthma or another lung disease.
▼ You have glaucoma.
▼ You have had epileptic seizures.
▼ You have ever had an operation on your uterus or a cesarean section.
▼ You are taking any other medications.

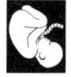

Pregnancy
▼ Not prescribed except for induction of labor.

Breast feeding
▼ Not prescribed.

Infants and children
▼ Not prescribed.

Over 60
▼ Not prescribed.

Driving and hazardous work
▼ Not applicable.

Alcohol
▼ Not applicable.

PROLONGED USE

Not used for prolonged periods.

DIPHENHYDRAMINE

Brand names Benadryl, Allerdryl, Allernix, Nytol, Sleep-Eze D
Used in the following combined preparations Benadryl Decongestant, Caladryl, Ergodryl

GENERAL INFORMATION

Diphenhydramine, one of the oldest antihistamines, is used for treating allergies such as allergic rhinitis and urticaria (hives). Injected diphenhydramine is also used in the treatment of anaphylaxis and hypersensitivity reactions to food, drugs, or insect stings.

Because it has *anticholinergic* properties, it is useful in the treatment of parkinsonism and movement disorders caused by antipsychotic drugs (p.97). It is also an effective anti-emetic, used to prevent and treat vertigo and motion sickness.

Diphenhydramine has a marked sedative action and often causes drowsiness. It is included in several over-the-counter sleeping preparations.

INFORMATION FOR USERS

Follow instructions on the label. Call your physician if symptoms worsen.

How taken

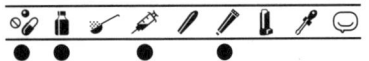

Tablets, capsules, oral liquid, injection, cream.

Frequency and timing of doses
By mouth 3 – 4 x daily (allergic conditions); 30 minutes before traveling and before meals (motion sickness); 20 – 30 minutes before bedtime (insomnia).
Injection Every 2 – 3 hours (adults).
Cream As directed.

Dosage range
Adults 25 – 200mg daily (by mouth); up to 400mg daily (by injection).
Children Reduced dose according to age and weight.

Onset of effect
Within 60 minutes (by mouth); within 20 minutes (injection).

Duration of action
4 – 6 hours.

Diet advice
None.

Storage
Keep in a closed container in a cool, dry place away from reach of children. Do not freeze.

Missed dose
Take as soon as you remember. If your next dose is due within 2 hours, take a single dose now and skip the next.

Stopping the drug
Can be safely stopped as soon as you no longer need it.

Exceeding the dose
An occasional unintentional extra dose is unlikely to cause problems. Large overdoses may cause drowsiness or agitation. Notify your physician.

SPECIAL PRECAUTIONS

Be sure to consult your physician or pharmacist before taken this drug if:
▼ You have impaired liver function.
▼ You have chronic lung disease.
▼ You have had epileptic seizures.
▼ You have glaucoma.
▼ You have urinary difficulties.
▼ You are taking other medications.

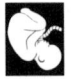

Pregnancy
▼ No evidence of risk to the developing baby when normal doses are used for short periods. Discuss with your physician.

Breast feeding
▼ The drug passes into the breast milk and may make the baby drowsy or irritable. It may also inhibit milk secretion. Discuss with your physician.

Infants and children
▼ Not recommended for newborn or premature infants. Reduced dose necessary for older children.

Over 60
▼ Increased likelihood of adverse effects. Reduced dose may therefore be necessary.

Driving and hazardous work
▼ Avoid such activities until you have learned how the drug affects you; it can cause drowsiness.

Alcohol
▼ Avoid. Alcohol may increase the sedative effects of this drug.

POSSIBLE ADVERSE EFFECTS

Drowsiness is the commonest adverse effect of diphenhydramine. Other side effects, such as dry mouth and blurred vision, are due to its *anticholinergic* action.

Symptom/effect	Frequency		Discuss with physician		Stop taking drug now	Call physician now
	Common	Rare	Only if severe	In all cases		
Drowsiness	●		■			
Dry mouth	●		■			
Nausea/abdominal pain		●	■			
Blurred vision		●	■			
Urinary difficulties		●		■		
Disorientation/excitation		●		■		

INTERACTIONS

Sedatives All sedatives, including alcohol, are likely to enhance the sedative effect of this drug.

Anticholinergic drugs are likely to increase the anticholinergic effects of diphenhydramine.

PROLONGED USE

The effect of this drug may become weaker with prolonged use over a period of weeks or months as the body adapts. Transfer to a different antihistamine may be recommended.

Antihistamines should be discontinued approximately 48 hours prior to allergy skin testing.

DIPHENOXYLATE

Brand name Lomotil Liquid
Used in the following combined preparation Lomotil Tablets

GENERAL INFORMATION

Diphenoxylate, introduced in 1960, is an antidiarrheal drug chemically related to the opiate analgesics. It reduces bowel contractions and consequently the frequency and fluidity of bowel movements. Available as tablets and liquid, it is used for the relief of sudden or recurrent bouts of diarrhea.

It is not suitable for diarrhea caused by infection, antibiotics, or poisons because it may delay recovery by slowing the expulsion of harmful substances from the bowel. In patients with colitis, diphenoxylate can cause toxic megacolon, a dangerous dilation of the bowel that shuts off the blood supply to the wall of the bowel and increases the risk of perforation.

At recommended doses, serious adverse effects are rare. To guard against addiction, atropine is added to diphenoxylate tablets. If these are taken in excessive amounts, the atropine will cause highly unpleasant *anticholinergic* reactions. Diphenoxylate is especially dangerous for young children. Be sure to store it out of their reach.

INFORMATION FOR USERS

Your drug prescription is tailored for you. Do not alter dosage without checking with your physician.

How taken

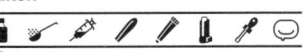

Tablets, oral liquid.

Frequency and timing of doses
3 - 4 x daily.

Dosage range
Adults Up to 20mg/24 hours.
Children Reduced dose necessary according to age and weight.

Onset of effect
Within 1 hour. Control of diarrhea may take several hours.

Duration of action
Up to 24 hours.

Diet advice
Ensure adequate fluid intake during an attack of diarrhea.

Storage
Keep in a closed container in a cool, dry place away from reach of children. Protect from light.

Missed dose
Take as soon as you remember. If your next dose is due within 3 hours, take a single dose now and skip the next.

Stopping the drug
Can be safely stopped as soon as you no longer need it.

Exceeding the dose
An occasional unintentional extra dose is unlikely to cause problems. Large overdoses may cause unusual drowsiness, dryness of the mouth and skin, restlessness, and in extreme cases, loss of consciousness. Notify your physician.

POSSIBLE ADVERSE EFFECTS

Side effects occur infrequently with diphenoxylate. If abdominal pain or distension, nausea, vomiting, or severe constipation occurs, notify your physician.

Symptom/effect	Frequency		Discuss with physician		Stop taking drug now	Call physician now
	Common	Rare	Only if severe	In all cases		
Drowsiness	●		■			
Restlessness		●	■			
Headache		●	■			
Skin rash/itching		●		■		
Dizziness		●		■		
Nausea/vomiting		●		■	▲	
Abdominal swelling/pain		●		■	▲	■

INTERACTIONS

Sedatives All drugs, including alcohol, that have a *sedative* effect on the central nervous system may increase the sedative effect of diphenoxylate.

Monoamine oxidase inhibitors (MAOIs)
There is a risk of a dangerous rise in blood pressure if MAOIs are taken together with diphenoxylate.

SPECIAL PRECAUTIONS

Be sure to tell your physician if:
▼ You have impaired liver function.
▼ You have severe abdominal pain.
▼ You have bloodstained diarrhea.
▼ You have recently taken antibiotics.
▼ You have ulcerative colitis.
▼ You are taking other medications.

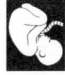

Pregnancy
▼ Safety in pregnancy not established. Discuss with your physician.

Breast feeding
▼ The drug passes into the breast milk and may cause drowsiness in the baby. Discuss with your physician.

Infants and children
▼ Reduced dose necessary. Not recommended for patients under 2 years.

Over 60
▼ Reduced dose may be necessary.

Driving and hazardous work
▼ Avoid such activities until you have learned how the drug affects you, because the drug may cause drowsiness and dizziness.

Alcohol
▼ Avoid. Alcohol may increase the sedative effects of this drug.

PROLONGED USE

Not intended for prolonged use – only for short-term treatment of diarrhea.

DIPYRIDAMOLE

Brand names Persantine, Apo-Dipyridamole, Novo-Dipiradol
Used in the following combined preparation Asasantine

GENERAL INFORMATION

In long-term therapy, dipyridamole may reduce the frequency of angina attacks. Used as an antiplatelet drug, dipyridamole "thins" the blood in patients who have had surgery to replace a heart valve. This reduces the possibility of blood clotting within the circulation.

Dipyridamole is usually given together with other drugs such as ASA or warfarin. The drug can also be given by injection during certain types of diagnostic tests on the heart.

Side effects may occur, especially during the early days of treatment. If they persist, your physician may advise a reduction in dosage.

INFORMATION FOR USERS

Your drug prescription is tailored for you. Do not alter dosage without checking with your physician.

How taken

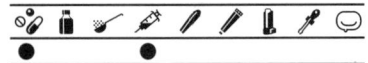

Tablets, injection.

Frequency and timing of doses
3 – 4 x daily with water one hour before meals (tablets).

Adult dosage range
100 – 400mg daily.

Onset of effect
Within an hour. Full therapeutic effect may not be felt for 2 – 3 weeks.

Duration of action
Up to 8 hours.

Diet advice
None.

Storage
Keep in a closed container in a cool, dry place away from reach of children. Protect from light.

Missed dose
Take as soon as you remember. If your next dose is due within 2 hours, take a single dose now and skip the next.

Stopping the drug
Do not stop taking the drug without consulting your physician; withdrawal of the drug could lead to abnormal blood clotting.

Exceeding the dose
An occasional unintentional extra dose is unlikely to cause problems, but you may experience dizziness or vomiting. Notify your physician.

SPECIAL PRECAUTIONS

Be sure to tell your physician if:
▼ You have low blood pressure.
▼ Your suffer from migraine.
▼ You have myasthenia gravis.
▼ You are taking other medications.

 **Pregnancy**
▼ Safety in pregnancy not established. Discuss with your physician.

 Breast feeding
▼ The drug passes into the breast milk but at normal doses adverse effects on the baby are unlikely. Discuss with your physician.

 Infants and children
▼ Not recommended.

 Over 60
▼ No special problems.

 Driving and hazardous work
▼ Avoid such activities until you have learned how the drug affects you, because of the probability of dizziness and faintness.

 Alcohol
▼ No known problems.

POSSIBLE ADVERSE EFFECTS

Adverse effects are rare. Possible symptoms include dizziness, headache, faintness, nausea, and rash. In rare cases, it may aggravate angina.

Symptom/effect	Frequency		Discuss with physician		Stop taking drug now	Call physician now
	Common	Rare	Only if severe	In all cases		
Nausea/vomiting	●		■			
Headache		●	■			
Flushing		●	■			
Dizziness/faintness		●			■	
Rash		●			■	▲

INTERACTIONS

Anticoagulant drugs The effects of these drugs are increased by dipyridamole, increasing the risk of uncontrolled bleeding. The dosage of the anticoagulant should be reduced accordingly.

Antihypertensive drugs Dipyridamole may increase the effects of these drugs in lowering blood pressure.

PROLONGED USE

No known problems.

DISOPYRAMIDE

Brand names Norpace, Rythmodan
Used in the following combined preparations None

GENERAL INFORMATION

Disopyramide is an anti-arrhythmic drug used to treat serious irregularities of heart rhythm, particularly cases of ventricular tachycardia.

It has a mild *anticholinergic* action, and some of its less serious adverse effects are connected to this. Because it reduces the force of the heartbeat, it can worsen existing heart failure and low blood pressure. These effects may be more common with disopyramide than with other anti-arrhythmics. Since disopyramide can lower blood sugar levels, monitoring may be necessary, and people with diabetes must use the drug with caution.

QUICK REFERENCE

Drug group Anti-arrhythmic (p.112)
Overdose danger rating High
Dependence rating Low
Prescription needed Yes
Multi-source suppliers Yes

INFORMATION FOR USERS

Your drug prescription is tailored for you. Do not alter dosage without checking with your physician.

How taken

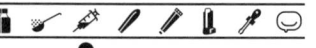

Capsules, slow-release tablets, injection.

Frequency and timing of doses
3 x daily or every 12 hours (slow-release tablets).

Dosage range
300 – 800mg daily (by mouth).

Onset of effect
Within 2 hours.

Duration of action
5 - 7 hours (capsules, injection); up to 12 hours (slow-release tablets).

Diet advice
None.

Storage
Keep in a closed container in a cool, dry place away from reach of children.

Missed dose
Take as soon as you remember. If your next dose is due within 2 hours, take a single dose now and skip the next.

Stopping the drug
Do not stop the drug without consulting your physician; stopping the drug may lead to worsening of the underlying condition.

OVERDOSE ACTION

 Seek immediate medical advice in all cases. Take emergency action if consciousness is lost.

See Drug poisoning emergency guide (p.574).

SPECIAL PRECAUTIONS

Be sure to tell your physician if:
▼ You have impaired liver or kidney function.
▼ You have heart failure.
▼ You have had glaucoma.
▼ You have prostate trouble.
▼ You have diabetes.
▼ You have myasthenia gravis.
▼ You have low blood pressure.
▼ You are taking other medications.

 **Pregnancy**
▼ Safety in pregnancy not established. Discuss with your physician.

 Breast feeding
▼ The drug passes into the breast milk and may affect the baby adversely. Discuss with your physician.

 Infants and children
▼ Safety not established.

 Over 60
▼ Reduced dose may be necessary.

 Driving and hazardous work
▼ Avoid such activities until you have learned how the drug affects you; it can cause dizziness and blurred vision.

 Alcohol
▼ Avoid. Alcohol may increase the adverse effects of this drug.

POSSIBLE ADVERSE EFFECTS

Some of the possible adverse effects of this drug are mainly the result of its *anticholinergic* action. These include dry mouth, constipation, and blurred vision. The most serious adverse effect is the possibility of worsening existing heart failure or low blood pressure. Some of these problems can be overcome by an adjustment in dosage.

Symptom/effect	Frequency		Discuss with physician		Stop taking drug now	Call physician now
	Common	Rare	Only if severe	In all cases		
Dry mouth	●		■			
Constipation/difficult urination	●		■			
Blurred vision	●		■			
Dizziness/feeling faint	●			■		
Rash		●		■	▲	

INTERACTIONS

Phenytoin and rifampin The effects of disopyramide may be reduced by these drugs.

Anticholinergic drugs are likely to increase the anticholinergic effects of disopyramide.

Erythromycin This antibiotic may increase the effect of disopyramide.

Anti-arrhythmic drugs Use of disopyramide with other anti-arrhythmic drugs such as quinidine, procainamide, and/or propranolol may cause abnormal heart rhythms.

PROLONGED USE

No problems expected.

Monitoring Periodic checks on blood sugar levels may be advised.

DISULFIRAM

Brand name Antabuse
Used in the following combined preparations None

GENERAL INFORMATION

Since its introduction, disulfiram has been used to help alcoholics abstain from alcohol. However, evidence for the effectiveness of the drug by itself is not strong. The commitment to take disulfiram often reflects a determination to decrease alcohol use.

If you are taking disulfiram as directed and drink even a small amount of alcohol, serious and highly unpleasant reactions follow. These can include: flushing, throbbing headache, breathlessness, nausea, thirst, palpitations, dizziness, and fainting. Such reactions may last from 30 minutes to several hours, leaving you feeling drowsy and sleepy. Because the reactions can also include unconsciousness, it may be

wise to carry a card indicating that you are taking disulfiram and listing the person to notify in an emergency.

When you take both disulfiram and alcohol, a toxic substance (acetaldehyde) that is manufactured in the body and ordinarily broken down rises to higher concentrations in the blood, thereby triggering the unwelcome reactions. Formerly, some physicians who prescribed disulfiram for alcoholism gave a small test dose of alcohol a few days after starting treatment to give the patient an idea of what might happen. Disulfiram treatment should be combined with other behavioral or alcoholism counseling programs.

INFORMATION FOR USERS

Your drug prescription is tailored for you. Do not alter dosage without checking with your physician.

How taken

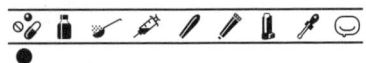

Tablets.

Frequency and timing of doses
Once daily.

Adult dosage range
500mg (starting dose for first week or two), 125 – 500mg (maintenance dose).

Onset of effect
Interaction with alcohol occurs within a few minutes of taking alcohol.

Duration of action
Interaction with alcohol can occur for about 6 days after the last dose of disulfiram.

Diet advice
Avoid all alcoholic drinks even in very small amounts. Food, fermented vinegar, mouthwashes, medicines, and lotions containing alcohol should also be avoided.

Storage
Keep in a closed container in a cool, dry place away from reach of children.

Missed dose
Take as soon as you remember. If your next dose is due within 2 hours, take a single dose now and skip the next.

Stopping the drug
Do not stop taking the drug without consulting your physician.

Exceeding the dose
An occasional unintentional extra dose is unlikely to cause problems. Large overdoses may cause a temporary increase in adverse effects. Notify your physician.

SPECIAL PRECAUTIONS

Be sure to tell your physician if:
▼ You have kidney disease, cirrhosis, or liver insufficiency.
▼ You have heart problems or coronary artery disease.
▼ You have had epileptic seizures.
▼ You have diabetes.
▼ You have an underactive thyroid.
▼ You have a history of depression.
▼ You are taking other medications.

Pregnancy
▼ Safety in pregnancy not established. Discuss with your physician.

Breast feeding
▼ The drug passes into the breast milk and may affect the baby adversely. Discuss with your physician.

Over 60
▼ Reduced dose necessary.

Driving and hazardous work
▼ Avoid such activities until you have learned how the drug affects you, because the drug can cause blurred vision, drowsiness, and dizziness.

Alcohol
▼ Never drink while under treatment with disulfiram and avoid foods and medications that contain alcohol. Alcohol may interact dangerously with this drug.

POSSIBLE ADVERSE EFFECTS

Adverse effects of disulfiram usually disappear when you get used to taking the drug. If they continue indefinitely or become severe, the dosage may need to be adjusted.

Symptom/effect	Frequency		Discuss with physician		Stop taking drug now	Call physician now
	Common	Rare	Only if severe	In all cases		
Headache/drowsiness	●		■			
Metallic or garlic taste	●		■			
Nausea/vomiting		●	■			
Temporary impotence		●	■			
Blurred vision		●		■		

INTERACTIONS

Phenytoin The blood levels of this drug are increased when taken with disulfiram.

Anticoagulants Disulfiram increases the effect of these drugs.

Isoniazid Disulfiram may markedly increase the adverse effects of this drug.

Metronidazole A severe reaction can occur if this drug is taken with disulfiram.

PROLONGED USE

Not usually prescribed for long-term use without review. It is wise to carry a card indicating you are taking disulfiram with instructions as to who should be notified in an emergency.

DOMPERIDONE

Brand name Motilium
Used in the following combined preparations None

GENERAL INFORMATION

Domperidone acts directly on the upper gastrointestinal tract to encourage normal propulsion of food through the stomach and intestine. It is used to help relieve retention of food and acid in the stomach. People with diabetes are among the most likely to experience such gastric retention.

Domperidone has anti-emetic properties and is used to prevent nausea and vomiting caused by levo-dopa, an antiparkinsonism drug. It may also be used to treat the nausea and vomiting caused by anticancer drugs.

Possible side effects of domperidone include dry mouth, headache, dizziness, insomnia, menstrual irregularities, and breast enlargement. It may also stimulate increased secretion of the hormone prolactin which may induce the discharge of a milky fluid by the breasts. Muscle spasms occur in rare cases.

QUICK REFERENCE

Drug group Gastrointestinal motility regulator and anti-emetic drug (p.102)

Overdose danger rating Medium

Dependence rating Low

Prescription needed Yes

Multi-source suppliers Yes

INFORMATION FOR USERS

Your drug prescription is tailored for you. Do not alter dosage without checking with your physician.

How taken

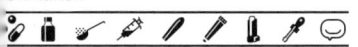

Tablets.

Frequency and timing of doses
1 – 4 x daily, 15 – 30 minutes before meals and at bedtime.

Adult dosage range
30 – 80mg.

Onset of effect
Within 1 hour.

Duration of action
Approximately 6 hours.

Diet advice
None.

Storage
Keep in a closed container in a cool, dry place away from reach of children. Protect from light.

Missed dose
Take as soon as you remember. If your next dose is due within 2 hours, take a single dose now and skip the next.

Stopping the drug
Can be safely stopped as soon as you no longer need it.

Exceeding the dose
An occasional unintentional extra dose is unlikely to cause problems. Large overdoses may cause dizziness. Notify your physician.

POSSIBLE ADVERSE EFFECTS

Adverse effects from this drug are rare, and most resolve spontaneously during continued therapy or are easily tolerated.

Symptom/effect	Frequency		Discuss with physician		Stop taking drug now	Call physician now
	Common	Rare	Only if severe	In all cases		
Breast enlargement		●		■		
Milk secretion from breast		●		■		
Menstrual disturbances		●		■		

INTERACTIONS

General note Domperidone may accelerate absorption of some drugs from the small intestine (for example, acetaminophen, tetracycline antibiotics, levodopa, alcohol) and slow absorption of other drugs from the stomach (for example, digoxin).

Anticholinergic drugs These may reduce the beneficial effects of domperidone.

Monoamine oxidase inhibitors (MAOIs) Caution is required when these agents are administered with domperidone.

SPECIAL PRECAUTIONS

Be sure to tell your physician if:
▼ You have impaired liver or kidney function.
▼ You are taking other medications.

Pregnancy
▼ Safety in pregnancy not established. Discuss with your physician.

Breast feeding
▼ The drug passes into the breast milk but at normal doses adverse effects on the baby are unlikely. Discuss with your physician.

Infants and children
▼ Safety not yet established.

Over 60
▼ No special problems.

Driving and hazardous work
▼ Exercise caution if dizziness occurs.

Alcohol
▼ No special problems, but alcohol is best avoided in cases of nausea and vomiting.

PROLONGED USE

Not prescribed for long-term treatment.

DOXEPIN

Brand names Sinequan, Novo-Doxepin, Triadapin, Zonalon
Used in the following combined preparations None

GENERAL INFORMATION

Doxepin belongs to a class of anti-depressant drugs known as the tricyclics (see Antidepressant drugs, p.96). Used in the treatment of major depressive episodes in severe depression and manic (bipolar) depression, it elevates mood, increases physical activity, improves appetite, and renews interest in everyday activities. Doxepin has a stronger sedative effect than some of the other tricyclic anti-depressants and is therefore particularly useful when depression is accompanied by anxiety and insomnia. Taken at night, it may reduce the need for sleeping drugs.

Doxepin is available in cream form for the relief of itching.

QUICK REFERENCE

Drug group Tricyclic antidepressant drug (p.96)

Overdose danger rating High

Dependence rating Low

Prescription needed Yes

Multi-source suppliers Yes

INFORMATION FOR USERS

Your drug prescription is tailored for you. Do not alter dosage without checking with your physician.

How taken

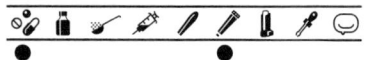

Capsules, cream.

Frequency and timing of doses
1 – 3 x daily.

Adult dosage range
75 – 300mg daily.

Onset of effect
Some benefits and effects may appear within hours, but full antidepressant effect may not be felt for 2 – 6 weeks.

Duration of action
Following prolonged treatment antidepressant effect may persist for up to 6 weeks. Adverse effects may wear off within a few days.

Diet advice
None.

Storage
Keep in a closed container in a cool, dry place away from the reach of children.

Missed dose
Take as soon as you remember. If your next dose is due within 3 hours, take a single dose now and skip the next.

Stopping the drug
Do not stop the drug without consulting your physician.

OVERDOSE ACTION

 Seek immediate medical advice in all cases. Take emergency action if consciousness is lost.

See Drug poisoning emergency guide (p.574).

POSSIBLE ADVERSE EFFECTS

The possible adverse effects of this drug are mainly the result of its *anticholinergic* action and its blocking action on the transmission of signals to the heart. Some problems can be overcome by medically supervised adjustment of dosage.

Symptom/effect	Frequency		Discuss with physician		Stop taking drug now	Call physician now
	Common	Rare	Only if severe	In all cases		
Drowsiness	●		■			
Sweating/flushing	●		■			
Dry mouth	●		■			
Blurred vision	●			■		
Dizziness/fainting	●			■		
Rash		●		■	▲	
Urinary difficulties		●		■	▲	
Palpitations		●		■	▲	■

SPECIAL PRECAUTIONS

Be sure to tell your physician if:
▼ You have heart problems.
▼ You have had epileptic seizures.
▼ You have impaired liver or kidney function.
▼ You have had glaucoma.
▼ You have urinary difficulties.
▼ You have a thyroid disorder.
▼ You have a blood disorder.
▼ You are taking other medications.

 Pregnancy
▼ Safety in pregnancy not established. Discuss with your physician.

 Breast feeding
▼ The drug passes into the breast milk and may affect the baby. Discuss with your physician.

 Infants and children
▼ Not usually prescribed.

 Over 60
▼ Increased likelihood of adverse effects. Reduced dose may therefore be necessary.

 Driving and hazardous work
▼ Avoid until you have learned how the drug affects you, because of the possibility of blurred vision and reduced alertness.

 Alcohol
▼ Avoid. Alcohol may increase the sedative effects of this drug.

Surgery and general anesthetics
▼ Doxepin treatment may need to be stopped before you have a general anesthetic. Discuss this with your physician or dentist before any operation.

PROLONGED USE

No problems expected.

INTERACTIONS

Sedatives All drugs that have a sedative effect are likely to increase the sedative properties of doxepin.

Antihypertensive drugs Doxepin may reduce the effectiveness of some of these drugs, especially guanethidine and clonidine.

Monoamine oxidase inhibitors (MAOIs) Usually, doxepin is not given within 2 weeks of treatment with an MAOI. Serious reactions may occur. These drugs are prescribed together only under strict medical supervision.

DOXYCYCLINE

Brand names Vibramycin, Vibra-Tabs, Apo-Doxy, Doryx, Doxycin, Novo-Doxylin
Used in the following combined preparations None

GENERAL INFORMATION

Doxycycline is a member of the tetracycline group of antibiotics. Longer acting than some other drugs in this group, it is used in the treatment of respiratory and urinary tract infections, and infections of the skin, eye, and gastrointestinal tract. Doxycycline is particularly effective against chlamydial infection.

It is less likely to cause diarrhea as a side effect than other tetracyclines, and absorption of the drug is not significantly impaired by food. It can therefore be taken with meals to reduce side effects such as nausea or indigestion. Doxycycline is also safe (unlike other tetracyclines) for people with impaired kidney function. Like other tetracyclines, doxycycline can damage developing teeth and is therefore usually not prescribed for young children or pregnant women.

INFORMATION FOR USERS

Your drug prescription is tailored for you. Do not alter dosage without checking with your physician.

How taken

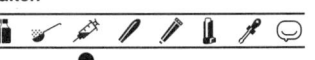

Tablets, capsules, injection.

Frequency and timing of doses
By mouth 1 – 2 x daily with water.

Dosage range
100 – 200mg daily.

Onset of effect
1 – 12 hours.

Duration of action
Up to 24 hours.

Diet advice
You may be advised to avoid milk with this drug.

Storage
Keep in closed container in a cool, dry place away from reach of children.

Missed dose
Take as soon as you remember. If your next dose is due within 6 hours, take a single dose now and skip the next.

Stopping the drug
Take the full course. Even if you feel better, the original infection may still be present and symptoms may recur if treatment is stopped too soon.

Exceeding the dose
An occasional unintentional extra dose is unlikely to be a cause for concern. But if you notice unusual symptoms, or if a large overdose has been taken, notify your physician.

SPECIAL PRECAUTIONS

Be sure to tell your physician if:
▼ You have impaired liver function.
▼ You have previously suffered an allergic reaction to a tetracycline antibiotic.
▼ You are taking other medications.

Pregnancy
▼ Not prescribed. May damage teeth and bones of the developing baby as well as damaging the mother's liver. Discuss with your physician.

Breast feeding
▼ The drug passes into the breast milk and may lead to damage of the baby's teeth. Discuss with your physician.

Infants and children
▼ Not recommended under 8 years. Reduced dose necessary for older children.

Over 60
▼ No special problems.

Driving and hazardous work
▼ No known problems.

Alcohol
▼ Avoid excessive amounts.

Esophageal damage
▼ To prevent retention in the esophagus, a small amount of water should be taken before and a full glass of water taken after each dose of doxycycline. Take this medication in the upright position and do not lie down immediately afterwards.

POSSIBLE ADVERSE EFFECTS

Adverse effects from doxycycline are rare, though some people may experience nausea, vomiting, or diarrhea. Other rare adverse effects include rash, itching, and increased sensitivity of the skin to sunlight, which may cause a rash to develop.

Symptom/effect	Frequency		Discuss with physician		Stop taking drug now	Call physician now
	Common	Rare	Only if severe	In all cases		
Nausea/vomiting		●	■			
Diarrhea		●	■			
Rash/itching		●		■	▲	▮
Light-sensitive rash		●		■	▲	▮

INTERACTIONS

Alcohol, barbiturates, carbamazepine, and phenytoin All these drugs reduce the effectiveness of doxycycline. The doxycycline dosage may need to be increased accordingly.

Oral anticoagulant drugs Doxycycline may increase the anticoagulant action of these drugs.

Iron may reduce the effectiveness of doxycycline.

Penicillin antibiotics Doxycycline interferes with the antibacterial action of these drugs.

Oral contraceptives Doxycycline can reduce the effectiveness of oral contraceptives.

Antacids Antacids interfere with the absorption of doxycycline and may reduce its effectiveness.

PROLONGED USE

No problems expected.

ECONAZOLE

Brand name Ecostatin
Used in the following combined preparations None

GENERAL INFORMATION

Econazole is a relatively new, effective, fast-acting antifungal drug. It is widely used in the form of a cream for the treatment of tinea (ringworm) infections of the skin, athlete's foot, and jock itch. Econazole is also prescribed for candida (thrush) infections of the skin (including some forms of diaper rash)

and the vagina. Its main advantage over similar *topical* antifungal drugs is that it begins to work within two days or so. Also, serious adverse effects with econazole are rare, though local stinging, burning, and skin irritation can sometimes occur.

INFORMATION FOR USERS

Your drug prescription is tailored for you. Do not alter dosage without checking with your physician.

How taken

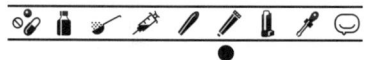

Topical cream, vaginal ovules.

Frequency and timing of doses
2 x daily, morning and evening (topical cream); once daily at bedtime (vaginal ovules).

Dosage range
Topical cream Use sufficient amount to cover the affected and surrounding areas at each application.
Vaginal ovules One ovule for 3 consecutive nights.

Onset of effect
1 – 2 days.

Duration of action
Up to 24 hours.

Diet advice
None.

Storage
Keep in a closed container in a cool, dry place away from reach of children.

Missed dose
No cause for concern, but use as soon as you remember.

Stopping the drug
Apply the full course. Even if symptoms disappear, the original infection may still be present and symptoms may recur if treatment is stopped too soon.

Exceeding the dose
An occasional unintentional extra dose is unlikely to be a cause for concern. But if you notice any unusual symptoms, notify your physician.

SPECIAL PRECAUTIONS

Be sure to tell your physician if:
▼ You have had a previous allergic reaction to this drug.
▼ You are taking other medications.

Pregnancy
▼ No evidence of risk with skin preparations. Vaginal preparations are prescribed with caution in the first 3 months of pregnancy. Use of the vaginal applicator may be undesirable. Discuss with your physician.

Breast feeding
▼ No evidence of risk.

Infants and children
▼ No special problems.

Over 60
▼ No special problems.

Driving and hazardous work
▼ No known problems.

Alcohol
▼ No known problems.

POSSIBLE ADVERSE EFFECTS

Local irritation may occur at the site of application, but always disappears when treatment is stopped. More serious adverse effects rarely occur with econazole.

Symptom/effect	Frequency		Discuss with physician		Stop taking drug now	Call physician now
	Common	Rare	Only if severe	In all cases		
Local burning	●		■			
Redness/itching of skin		●		■		
Rash		●		■	▲	

INTERACTIONS

None.

PROLONGED USE

No problems expected from the drug. However, recurrent or intractable candidiasis may require further assessment by your physician.

ENALAPRIL

Brand names Vasotec, Apo-Enalapril
Used in the following combined preparation Vaseretic

GENERAL INFORMATION

Enalapril belongs to the ACE inhibitor group of *vasodilator* drugs (see p.110) prescribed to treat hypertension (high blood pressure) and heart failure. It is often given in conjunction with a diuretic to increase its effect.

The first dose of enalapril may cause a sudden drop in blood pressure. You should be resting at the time and able to lie down afterwards for 2 – 3 hours.

The more common adverse effects, such as dizziness and headache, usually diminish with long-term treatment. Rashes can also occur during treatment. These usually disappear when the drug is stopped. In some cases they clear up on their own despite continued treatment.

INFORMATION FOR USERS

Your drug prescription is tailored for you. Do not alter dosage without checking with your physician.

How taken

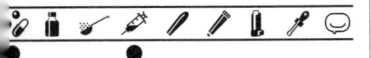

Tablets, injection.

Frequency and timing of doses
Once daily.

Adult dosage range
5 – 5mg daily (starting dose), increased to – 40mg daily (maintenance dose).

Onset of effect
Within 1 hour.

Duration of action
hours.

Diet advice
None.

Storage
Keep in a closed container in a cool, dry place away from reach of children. Protect from light.

Missed dose
Take as soon as you remember. If your next dose is due within 8 hours, do not take the skipped dose. Take your next dose as usual.

Stopping the drug
Do not stop taking the drug without consulting your physician; stopping the drug may lead to worsening of the underlying condition.

Exceeding the dose
An occasional unintentional extra dose is unlikely to cause problems. Large overdoses may cause dizziness or fainting. Notify your physician.

SPECIAL PRECAUTIONS

Be sure to tell your physician if:
▼ You have impaired liver or kidney function.
▼ You have diabetes.
▼ You have an autoimmune disease.
▼ You have coronary artery disease.
▼ You are taking other medications.

Pregnancy
▼ Can cause abnormalities in the unborn baby. Discuss with your physician if planning a pregnancy or **immediately** upon becoming pregnant.

Breast feeding
▼ Effect on breast feeding uncertain. Discuss with your physician.

Infants and children
▼ Not recommended.

Over 60
▼ Reduced dose may be necessary.

Driving and hazardous work
▼ Avoid such activities until you have learned how the drug affects you; it can cause dizziness and fainting.

Alcohol
▼ Avoid. Alcohol increases the likelihood of an excessive drop in blood pressure.

Surgery and general anesthetics
▼ Enalapril treatment may need to be stopped before you have a general anesthetic. Discuss with your physician or dentist before any operation.

POSSIBLE ADVERSE EFFECTS

The more common adverse effects, such as dizziness and headache, usually diminish with long-term treatment. The less common effects may also diminish during long-term treatment, but an adjustment in dosage may be necessary.

Symptom/effect	Frequency		Discuss with physician		Stop taking drug now	Call physician now
	Common	Rare	Only if severe	In all cases		
Dizziness	●		■			
Headache	●		■			
Nausea		●		■		
Persistent cough		●		■		
Diarrhea		●		■		
Rash/urticaria		●		■		
Muscle cramps		●		■		
Swelling of face or tongue		●		■	▲	▮

INTERACTIONS

Antihypertensive drugs are likely to add to the blood pressure-lowering effect of enalapril.

Potassium supplements, potassium-sparing diuretics, and cyclosporine
Enalapril may add to the effect of these drugs leading to raised levels of potassium in the blood.

Lithium Enalapril increases the levels of lithium in the blood, and serious adverse effects from lithium excess may occur.

Non-steroidal anti-inflammatory drugs (NSAIDs) may reduce the effects of enalapril.

PROLONGED USE

No problems expected.

Monitoring Periodic tests on blood and urine should be performed.

EPINEPHRINE

Brand names Adrenalin, Bronkaid, Dysne-Inhal, EpiPen, Sus-Phrine, Vaponefrin
Used in the following combined preparations Ana-Kit, Citanest Forte, E-Pilo, Medihaler-Epi

GENERAL INFORMATION

Epinephrine is a hormone produced in the center (medulla) of the adrenal glands. It has been produced synthetically since 1900. Medically, epinephrine is used to stimulate heart activity and to dilate the airways in order to improve breathing. It also narrows blood vessels in the skin and intestine.

Epinephrine is injected to counteract cardiac arrest and to relieve severe allergic reactions (anaphylaxis) to drugs or insect stings. In the past, epinephrine was used to treat asthma, but newer,

more effective and safer drugs are now used (see Bronchodilators, p.104).

Because it constricts blood vessels, epinephrine is used to control bleeding in surgery, to stop nosebleeds, and to slow the dispersal, and thereby prolong the effect, of local anesthetics. Newer drugs, with fewer side effects, have replaced epinephrine as a nasal decongestant.

As eye drops, it can lower the pressure within the eye, making it useful in glaucoma and eye surgery.

QUICK REFERENCE

Drug group Bronchodilator (p.104) and drug for glaucoma (p.180)

Overdose danger rating High

Dependence rating Low

Prescription needed No

Multi-source suppliers Yes

INFORMATION FOR USERS

Your drug prescription is tailored for you. Do not alter dosage without checking with your physician.

How taken

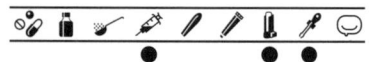

Injection, inhaler, eye drops.

Frequency and timing of doses
As directed according to method of administration and underlying disorder.

Dosage range
As directed according to method of administration and underlying disorder.

Onset of effect
Within 5 minutes (injection, inhaler); within 1 hour (eye drops).

Duration of action
Up to 4 hours (inhaler); up to 4 hours (injection); up to 24 hours (eye drops).

Diet advice
None.

Storage
Keep in a closed container in a cool, dry place away from reach of children. Protect from light.

Missed dose
Do not take the missed dose. Take your next dose as usual.

Stopping the drug
Do not stop taking the drug without consulting your physician; stopping the drug may lead to worsening of the underlying condition.

OVERDOSE ACTION

 Seek immediate medical advice in all cases. Take emergency action if palpitations, breathing difficulties, or loss of consciousness occur.

See Drug poisoning emergency guide (p.574).

SPECIAL PRECAUTIONS

Be sure to tell your physician if:
▼ You have heart problems.
▼ You have high blood pressure.
▼ You have diabetes.
▼ You have an overactive thyroid gland.
▼ You have nervous problems.
▼ You are taking other medications.

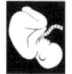 **Pregnancy**
▼ Not usually prescribed. May cause defects in the unborn baby and prolong labor. Discuss with your physician.

 Breast feeding
▼ The drug passes into the breast milk but at normal doses adverse effects on the baby are unlikely. Discuss with your physician.

 Infants and children
▼ Not usually prescribed for asthma in children. Reduced dose necessary.

 Over 60
▼ Increased likelihood of adverse effects. Reduced dose may therefore be necessary.

 Driving and hazardous work
▼ No known problems.

 Alcohol
▼ No known problems.

Surgery and general anesthetics
▼ Epinephrine may need to be stopped before you have a general anesthetic. Discuss this with your physician or dentist before surgery.

POSSIBLE ADVERSE EFFECTS

The principal adverse effects of this drug are related to its stimulant action on the heart and central nervous system. Eye drops may cause local burning or inflammation.

Symptom/effect	Frequency		Discuss with physician		Stop taking drug now	Call physician now
	Common	Rare	Only if severe	In all cases		
Dry mouth	●		■			
Nervousness/restlessness	●		■			
Palpitations	●			■		▮
Headache/blurred vision		●		■		

INTERACTIONS

General note A variety of drugs interact with epinephrine to increase the risk of palpitations and/or high blood pressure. Such drugs include digoxin, quinidine, and tricyclic and monoamine oxidase inhibitor (MAOI) antidepressants.

Beta blockers may block the effects of epinephrine and vice versa.

Antidiabetic drugs The effectiveness of such drugs may be reduced by epinephrine.

PROLONGED USE

Prolonged regular use of similar bronchodilators may be associated with increased asthma severity (see General Information). With eye drops, hypersensitivity as well as pigment deposits on the eyeball and eyelids can occur.

ERGOTAMINE

Brand names Ergomar, Gynergen, Medihaler-Ergotamine
Used in the following combined preparations Bellergal, Cafergot, Ergodryl, Gravergol, Megral, Wigraine

GENERAL INFORMATION

Ergotamine is used in the treatment of migraine headaches (p.101). It constricts blood vessels around the skull and is normally used only by people for whom analgesics such as ASA or acetaminophen fail to provide sufficient relief. It is most effective if taken at the first sign that a migraine is going to occur. Once headache and nausea are established, ergotamine is less likely to be effective and may cause stomach upset and increase the nausea of migraine. It is more effective when taken with caffeine, and combined ergotamine and caffeine preparations are available.

Ergotamine causes temporary narrowing of blood vessels throughout the body and therefore is not prescribed for those with poor circulation or coronary disease. If it is taken too frequently it can dangerously reduce blood circulation to the hands and feet or to the heart muscle; ergotamine should never be taken regularly.

QUICK REFERENCE

Drug group Drug used for migraine (p.101)

Overdose danger rating Medium

Dependence rating Low

Prescription needed Yes

Multi-source suppliers Yes

INFORMATION FOR USERS

Your drug prescription is tailored for you. Do not alter dosage without checking with your physician.

How taken

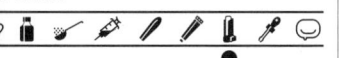

Tablets, inhaler.

Frequency and timing of doses

Once at the onset of a migraine attack, repeated as necessary every 30 minutes (tablets); or 5 minutes (inhaler) up to the maximum dose (below).

Adult dosage range

1–2mg per dose. Take no more than 6mg in 24 hours or 10mg in 1 week (by mouth); 6 inhalations in 24 hours or 15 inhalations in 1 week (inhaler).

Onset of effect

Within 30 minutes.

Duration of action

Up to 48 hours.

Diet advice

Changes in diet are unlikely to affect the action of this drug, but certain foods may provoke migraine attacks in some people (see p.101).

Storage

Keep in a closed container in a cool, dry place away from reach of children. Protect from light. Refrigerate inhaler, but do not freeze.

Missed dose

Regular doses of this drug are not necessary and may be dangerous. Take only when you have symptoms of migraine.

Stopping the drug

Can be safely stopped as soon as you no longer need it.

Exceeding the dose

An occasional unintentional extra dose is unlikely to cause problems. Large overdoses may cause vomiting, dizziness, seizures, or coma. Notify your physician.

SPECIAL PRECAUTIONS

Be sure to tell your physician if:
▼ You have impaired liver or kidney function.
▼ You have heart problems.
▼ You have poor circulation.
▼ You have high blood pressure.
▼ You have had a recent stroke.
▼ You have asthma.
▼ You are taking other medications.

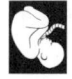

Pregnancy
▼ Not usually prescribed. Ergotamine can cause contractions of the uterus.

Breast feeding
▼ Not recommended during breast feeding. It passes into the milk and may have adverse effects on the baby. It may also reduce your milk supply.

Infants and children
▼ Not usually prescribed.

Over 60
▼ Use with caution. Hidden heart or circulatory problems may be aggravated.

Driving and hazardous work
▼ No special problems.

Alcohol
▼ No special problems, but some drinks may provoke migraine (see p.101).

Surgery and general anesthetics
▼ Notify your physician if you have used ergotamine within 48 hours prior to surgery.

POSSIBLE ADVERSE EFFECTS

The more common symptoms of treatment with ergotamine are digestive disturbances and nausea. An anti-emetic drug may be prescribed to relieve nausea. Rare but serious adverse effects may result from arterial spasm.

Symptom/effect	Frequency		Discuss with physician		Stop taking drug now	Call physician now
	Common	Rare	Only if severe	In all cases		
Nausea and vomiting	●		■			
Diarrhea		●	■			
Muscle pain and stiffness		●		■		
Chest pain		●		■	▲	▮
Leg/groin pain		●		■	▲	▮
Cold/numb fingers/toes		●		■	▲	▮

INTERACTIONS

Erythromycin There is an increased likelihood of adverse effects when this drug is taken with ergotamine.

Beta blockers may increase circulatory problems with ergotamine.

Sumatriptan There is an increased risk of adverse effects on the blood circulation if ergotamine is used with sumatriptan.

PROLONGED USE

Headaches and reduced circulation to the hands and feet may result if doses near to the maximum are taken for a long time. The dosage and length of treatment should not be exceeded.

ERYTHROMYCIN

Brand names Ilotycin, EES-600, Erybid, Eryc, Ilosone, Novo-Rythro Encap
Used in the following combined preparations Pediazole, Sans-Acne, Stievamycin, T-Stat

GENERAL INFORMATION

Introduced in 1952, erythromycin is effective against a wide range of bacteria. It is a useful alternative to penicillins and tetracyclines for people who are allergic to those drugs.

Erythromycin is commonly prescribed for throat, middle ear, and chest infections, including some types of pneumonia such as walking (mycoplasma) pneumonia and Legionnaires' disease, and for some sexually transmitted diseases.

Sometimes given to treat and reduce the likelihood of infecting others with whooping cough, erythromycin may also be given as part of the treatment for diphtheria. *Topical* preparations are used for skin and eye infections and acne.

Erythromycin taken by mouth may sometimes cause abdominal cramping and discomfort, nausea, and vomiting. Other possible adverse effects include rash and a rare risk of liver disorders.

INFORMATION FOR USERS

Your drug prescription is tailored for you. Do not alter dosage without consulting your physician.

How taken

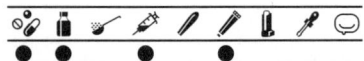

Tablets, capsules, oral liquid, injection, topical lotion, eye ointment.

Frequency and timing of doses
Every 6 – 12 hours.

Dosage range
Wide variation depending on dosage form and the disorder being treated. Follow your physician's instructions.

Onset of effect
Symptoms usually improve within 1 – 3 days, depending on the condition.

Duration of action
6 – 12 hours.

Diet advice
None.

Storage
Keep in a closed container in a cool, dry place away from reach of children.

Missed dose
Take as soon as you remember. If your next dose is within 2 hours, take a single dose now and skip the next.

Stopping the drug
Take the full course. Even if you feel better, the original infection may still be present and symptoms may recur if treatment is stopped too soon.

Exceeding the dose
An occasional unintentional extra dose is unlikely to be a cause for concern. But if you notice unusual symptoms, or if a large overdose has been taken, notify your physician.

SPECIAL PRECAUTIONS

Be sure to tell your physician if:
▼ You have a liver disease or impaired liver function.
▼ You have had a previous allergic reaction to erythromycin.
▼ You are taking other medications.

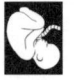

Pregnancy
▼ Safety in pregnancy not established. Discuss with your physician.

Breast feeding
▼ The drug passes into the breast milk, but at normal doses adverse effects on the baby are uncommon. Discuss with your physician.

Infants and children
▼ Reduced dose necessary.

Over 60
▼ No special problems.

Driving and hazardous work
▼ No known problems.

Alcohol
▼ No known problems.

POSSIBLE ADVERSE EFFECTS

Nausea and vomiting are the most common adverse effects and are most likely to occur with large doses taken by mouth. Symptoms such as fever, rash, and jaundice may be a sign of a liver disorder and should always be reported to your physician.

Symptom/effect	Frequency		Discuss with physician		Stop taking drug now	Call physician now
	Common	Rare	Only if severe	In all cases		
Nausea/vomiting	●		■			
Diarrhea		●	■			
Abdominal discomfort	●		■			
Rash/itching		●		■	▲	▌
Jaundice		●		■	▲	▌
Deafness		●		■	▲	▌

PROLONGED USE

Courses of longer than 14 days may increase the risk of liver damage.

INTERACTIONS

Carbamazepine, cyclosporine, digoxin, and theophylline Erythromycin may increase the risk of adverse effects with these drugs.

Triazolam Erythromycin may increase the risk of adverse effects with this drug.

Terfenadine and astemizole Erythromycin increases the risk of adverse effects of these antihistamines on the heart.

Warfarin Erythromycin increases the risk of bleeding with warfarin.

ERYTHROPOIETIN

Brand name Eprex
Used in the following combined preparations None

GENERAL INFORMATION

Erythropoietin is a hormone, produced by the kidneys, which stimulates the body to produce red blood cells. The commercial product is manufactured by recombinant DNA technology using mammalian cells.

It is prescribed to treat anemia in chronic kidney failure patients on dialysis. These patients produce very little erythropoietin themselves so the number of red blood cells is very low. This was previously treatable only by giving regular blood transfusions. When erythropoietin is injected regularly, more red cells will be made by the bone marrow, and this relieves the anemia, making blood transfusions unnecessary. As it is a natural hormone, erythropoietin has few *side effects*, but treatment must be carefully monitored or patients may produce too many red blood cells, causing high blood pressure, or the blood may start clotting too easily.

Erythropoietin has also been used to treat severe anemia related to zidovudine (AZT) therapy in HIV-infected patients, in order to decrease the need for transfusions.

INFORMATION FOR USERS

This drug is given only under medical supervision and is not for self-administration.

How taken

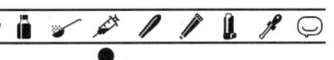

Injection.

Frequency and timing of doses
2 weekly.

Dosage range
Dosage is calculated on an individual basis according to body weight.

Onset of effect
Active inside the body within 2 – 3 hours, but effects may not be noted for 2 – 3 months.

Duration of action
4 – 7 hours. Some effects may persist for several days.

Diet advice
None. However, if you have kidney failure, you may have to follow a special diet.

Storage
Store at 2 – 8°C. Do not freeze or shake. Protect from light.

Missed dose
Do not make up any missed doses.

Stopping the drug
Discuss with your physician.

Exceeding the dose
A single excessive dose is unlikely to cause problems. Too high a dose over a long period can increase the likelihood of adverse effects.

POSSIBLE ADVERSE EFFECTS

The most common effects are increased blood pressure and problems at the site of the injection; all unusual symptoms should be discussed with your physician immediately.

Symptom/effect	Frequency		Discuss with physician		Stop taking drug now	Call physician now
	Common	Rare	Only if severe	In all cases		
Increased blood pressure	●			■		
Problems at injection site	●			■		
Flu symptoms/bone pain	●			■		
Epileptic seizures		●		■		▮
Skin reactions		●		■		
Headache (stabbing pain)	●			■		▮

INTERACTIONS

Iron supplements may increase the effect of erythropoietin if you have a low level of iron in your blood.

SPECIAL PRECAUTIONS

Be sure to tell your physician if:
▼ You have high blood pressure.
▼ You have previously suffered allergic reactions to any drugs.
▼ You have porphyria.
▼ You have gout.
▼ You have peripheral vascular disease.
▼ You have had epileptic seizures.
▼ You are taking other medications.

Pregnancy
▼ Not usually prescribed. Safety in pregnancy not established. Discuss with your physician.

Breast feeding
▼ Safety not established. Discuss with your physician.

Infants and children
▼ Safety and effectiveness not established.

Over 60
▼ No known problems.

Driving and hazardous work
▼ Avoid such activities during erythropoietin therapy.

Alcohol
▼ Follow your physician's advice regarding alcohol.

PROLONGED USE

The long-term effects of the drug are still under investigation, but problems are unlikely if treatment is carefully monitored.

Monitoring Regular blood tests are required to monitor blood composition.

ESTRADIOL

Brand names Delestrogen, Estrace, Estraderm
Used in the following combined preparations Climacteron, Neo-Pause

GENERAL INFORMATION

Estradiol is the principal and most powerful estrogen produced by the ovaries. Synthetically produced since 1940, it is used to supplement or replace the naturally occurring hormone in women who have estrogen deficiency, especially at the time of the menopause.

Estradiol can be injected, given by mouth, or applied to intact skin with a transdermal patch (see p.18). It is effective in controlling menopausal symptoms such as hot flushes. More importantly, replacement estrogen slows postmenopausal bone loss and decreases the risk of fractures. It is also used in the treatment of ovarian failure.

As a replacement therapy, it is often taken in conjunction with a progestin (see p.159). Withdrawal bleeding resembling a menstrual period may occur.

Drug group Female sex hormone (p.159)

QUICK REFERENCE

Drug group Female sex hormone (p.159)

Overdose danger rating Low

Dependence rating Low

Prescription needed Yes

Multi-source suppliers Yes

INFORMATION FOR USERS

Your drug prescription is tailored for you. Do not alter dosage without checking with your physician.

How taken

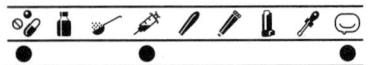

Tablets, injection, transdermal patches.

Frequency and timing of doses
Tablets 1 – 3 x daily with food.
Injection Depending on formulation and condition, from 3 x daily to once every 4 – 6 weeks.
Transdermal patches Twice weekly.

Adult dosage range
Replacement therapy 0.5 – 2mg daily (tablets); injection dosage depends on formulation and condition treated; 0.05 – 0.1mg twice weekly (transdermal patch).

Onset of effect
10 – 20 days.

Duration of action
4 days to 4 weeks.

Diet advice
None.

Storage
Keep in a closed container in a cool, dry place away from reach of children. Protect from light.

Missed dose
Take as soon as you remember.

Stopping the drug
Do not stop the drug without consulting your physician; symptoms may recur.

Exceeding the dose
An occasional unintentional extra dose is unlikely to be a cause for concern. But if you notice unusual symptoms, or if a large overdose has been taken, notify your physician.

POSSIBLE ADVERSE EFFECTS

The most common adverse effects of estradiol are similar to symptoms that occur in the early stages of pregnancy, and generally diminish or disappear after 2 – 3 months of treatment. A sudden, sharp pain in the chest, groin, or legs may indicate an abnormal blood clot and requires urgent medical attention.

Symptom/effect	Frequency		Discuss with physician		Stop taking drug now	Call physician now
	Common	Rare	Only if severe	In all cases		
Nausea/vomiting	●		■			
Breast swelling/tenderness	●		■			
Redness/irritation (skin patch)	●		■			
Depression		●		■		
Abnormal vaginal bleeding		●		■		
Pain in chest/groin/legs		●		■	▲	▮

INTERACTIONS

Tobacco smoking Smoking increases the risk of serious adverse effects on the heart and circulation with estradiol.

Oral anticoagulants and antidiabetic agents Estradiol may reduce the effectiveness of these drugs.

SPECIAL PRECAUTIONS

Be sure to tell your physician if:
▼ You have heart failure or high blood pressure.
▼ You have had blood clots or a stroke.
▼ You have impaired liver or kidney function.
▼ You have had breast or uterine cancer.
▼ You have diabetes.
▼ You are a smoker.
▼ You suffer from migraine or epilepsy.
▼ You are taking other medications.

Pregnancy
▼ Not prescribed. May adversely affect the baby. Discuss with your physician.

Breast feeding
▼ Not prescribed. The drug may inhibit the flow of milk.

Infants and children
▼ Not usually prescribed.

Over 60
▼ No special problems.

Driving and hazardous work
▼ No known problems.

Alcohol
▼ No known problems.

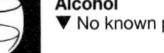

Surgery and general anesthetics
▼ Estradiol may need to be stopped sever weeks before you have major surgery. Discuss this with your physician.

PROLONGED USE

Prolonged use slightly increases the risk of cancer of the uterus after the menopause when used without a progestin. The risk of gallstones also increases.

Monitoring Periodic checks on blood pressure and physical examinations may be performed.

ESTROPIPATE

Brand name Ogen
Used in the following combined preparations None

GENERAL INFORMATION

Estropipate is a natural estrogenic substance used to replace the loss of estrogen from the ovaries at the time of menopause. Symptoms such as sweating, hot flushes, and dryness of the vagina are relieved quickly. Long-term treatment helps prevent osteoporosis, premature bone loss that can result in fractures of the hip, upper arm, and wrist. In order to maintain strong bones, a balanced diet with adequate protein and calcium, as well as regular exercise, is required.

Estropipate is generally taken on a cyclic dosing schedule and, in some cases, with a progestin or androgen to simulate the normal menstrual cycle. Withdrawal bleeding resembling a menstrual period may occur.

INFORMATION FOR USERS

Your drug prescription is tailored for you. Do not alter dosage without checking with your physician.

How taken

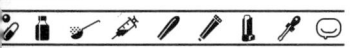

Tablets.

Frequency and timing of doses
Once daily with food.

Dosage range
0.75mg – 3mg daily cyclically (21 – 25 days followed by a 5 – 7 day rest period).

Onset of effect
5 – 20 days.

Duration of action
1 – 2 days.

Diet advice
Maintain balanced diet.

Storage
Keep in a closed container in a cool, dry place away from reach of children.

Missed dose
Take as soon as you remember.

Stopping the drug
Do not stop the drug without consulting your physician; symptoms may recur.

Exceeding the dose
An occasional unintentional extra dose is unlikely to be a cause for concern. But if you notice unusual symptoms, or if a large overdose has been taken, notify your physician.

SPECIAL PRECAUTIONS

Be sure to tell your physician if:
▼ You have heart failure, or high blood pressure.
▼ You have had blood clots or a stroke.
▼ You have impaired liver or kidney function.
▼ You have had breast or uterine cancer.
▼ You have diabetes.
▼ You suffer from migraines or epilepsy.
▼ You are taking any other medications.

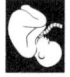

Pregnancy
▼ Not prescribed. May adversely affect the baby. Discuss with your physician.

Breast feeding
▼ Not prescribed. The drug may inhibit the flow of milk. Discuss with your physician.

Infants and children
▼ Not usually prescribed.

Over 60
▼ Reduced dose may be necessary. Discuss with your physician.

Driving and hazardous work
▼ No known problems.

Alcohol
▼ No known problems.

Surgery and general anesthetics
▼ Estropipate may need to be stopped several weeks before you have surgery. Discuss with your physician.

POSSIBLE ADVERSE EFFECTS

The most common adverse effects of estropipate are similar to symptoms that occur in the early stages of pregnancy, and generally diminish or disappear after 2 – 3 months of treatment. A sudden, sharp pain or tenderness in chest, groin, or legs may indicate an abnormal blood clot and requires urgent medical attention.

Symptom/effect	Frequency		Discuss with physician		Stop taking drug now	Call physician now
	Common	Rare	Only if severe	In all cases		
Nausea/vomiting	●		■			
Breast swelling/tenderness	●		■			
Severe headache		●		■	▲	‖
Paralysis/loss of consciousness		●		■	▲	‖
Skin rash/hives/itching		●		■	▲	‖
Abnormal vaginal bleeding		●		■		
Pain in chest/groin/legs		●		■	▲	‖
Visual disturbance		●		■	▲	‖

INTERACTIONS

Oral anticoagulants Estropipate may decrease the action of oral anticoagulants.

Tobacco smoking Smoking increases the risk of serious adverse effects on the heart and circulatory system with estropipate.

PROLONGED USE

There is a slightly increased risk of cancer of the uterus after the menopause, especially when estropipate is used without a progestin.

Monitoring Annual physical examinations and blood tests for glucose, cholesterol, and liver function are recommended.

ETHINYL ESTRADIOL

Brand name Estinyl
Used in the following combined preparations Brevicon, Demulen, Loestrin, Ortho 1/35, Triphasil, Triquilar

GENERAL INFORMATION

Ethinyl estradiol is a powerful synthetic estrogen similar to the natural female sex hormone estradiol. The widest use of ethinyl estradiol is in oral contraceptive tablet formulations, combined with a synthetic progesterone drug (progestin). Ethinyl estradiol is also used to supplement natural estrogen when the body's production is low – for example, during the menopause. In such conditions, it is often given with a progestin.

Ethinyl estradiol is also used to control abnormal bleeding from the uterus and to treat certain inoperable cancers of the breast or the prostate.

INFORMATION FOR USERS

Your drug prescription is tailored for you. Do not alter dosage without checking with your physician.

How taken

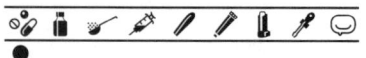

Tablets.

Frequency and timing of doses
1 – 3 x daily with food. Once daily dose for prostate cancers taken at bedtime.

Adult dosage range
Menopausal symptoms 5 – 10mcg daily.
Uterine bleeding 50 – 500mcg daily.
Breast cancer 300mcg daily.
Prostate cancer 0.15 – 3mg daily.

Onset of effect
10 – 20 days.

Duration of action
1 – 2 days.

Diet advice
None.

Storage
Keep in a closed container in a cool, dry place away from reach of children.

Missed dose
Take as soon as you remember. If your next dose is due within 4 hours, take a single dose now and skip the next. If you are taking the drug for contraceptive purposes, see p.173.

Stopping the drug
Do not stop the drug without consulting your physician.

Exceeding the dose
An occasional unintentional extra dose is unlikely to be a cause for concern. But if you notice unusual symptoms, or if a large overdose has been taken, notify your physician.

POSSIBLE ADVERSE EFFECTS

The most common adverse effects are similar to symptoms in the early stages of pregnancy and generally diminish with time. Sudden, sharp pain in the chest, groin, or legs may indicate an abnormal blood clot and needs immediate medical attention.

Symptom/effect	Frequency		Discuss with physician		Stop taking drug now	Call physician now
	Common	Rare	Only if severe	In all cases		
Nausea/vomiting	●			■		
Breast swelling/tenderness	●			■		
Swollen feet/ankles	●			■		
Headache		●		■		
Reduced sex drive		●		■		
Depression		●		■		
Abnormal vaginal bleeding		●		■		
Pain in chest/groin/legs		●		■	▲	■

INTERACTIONS

Tobacco smoking Smoking increases the risk of serious adverse effects on the heart and circulation with ethinyl estradiol.

Antibiotics may reduce the effectiveness of oral contraceptives containing ethinyl estradiol.

Anticonvulsants The effectiveness of these drugs may be reduced by oral contraceptives containing ethinyl estradiol.

SPECIAL PRECAUTIONS

Be sure to tell your physician if:
▼ You have heart failure or high blood pressure.
▼ You have had blood clots or a stroke.
▼ You have impaired liver or kidney function
▼ You have had breast or uterine cancer.
▼ You are a smoker.
▼ You have diabetes.
▼ You suffer from migraine or epilepsy.
▼ You are taking other medications.

Pregnancy
▼ Not prescribed. May adversely affect the baby. Discuss with your physician.

Breast feeding
▼ The drug passes into the breast milk and may inhibit the flow of mil Discuss with your physician.

Infants and children
▼ Safety not established.

Over 60
▼ No special problems.

Driving and hazardous work
▼ No known problems.

Alcohol
▼ No known problems.

Surgery and general anesthetics
▼ Ethinyl estradiol may need to be stoppe several weeks before you have major surge Discuss this with your physician.

PROLONGED USE

Prolonged use of ethinyl estradiol slightly increases the risk of cancer of the uterus after the menopause when used without progestin. The risk of gallstones may also be higher.

Monitoring Periodic checks on blood pressure and physical examinations may be performed.

ETIDRONATE

Brand name Didronel
Used in the following combined preparations None

GENERAL INFORMATION

Etidronate is prescribed for bone disorders such as Paget's disease. It acts only on the bones, reducing the activity of the bone cells thus stopping the progress of the disease. This action also stops calcium from being released from bone into the bloodstream, so it reduces the amount of calcium in the blood. Etidronate by injection is used to treat high levels of blood calcium due to cancer that has spread to bones.

Generally, the *side effects* of etidronate are mild. The most common is diarrhea. If taken at high doses (20mg/kg daily) the drug stops new bone being formed properly, which can lead to thinning of the bones and fractures. Thus, high doses must be carefully monitored and used for as short a time as possible. The effect is reversed on stopping the drug.

INFORMATION FOR USERS

Your drug prescription is tailored for you. Do not alter dosage without checking with your physician.

How taken

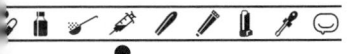

Tablets, injection.

Frequency and timing of doses
Once daily on an empty stomach, 2 hours before meals with fruit juice or water.

Dosage range
Paget's disease 5 – 20mg/kg daily for a maximum of 3 – 6 months (tablets). There may be repeated cycles.
Hypercalcemia 7.5mg/kg daily for 3 days (injection). This may be repeated.

Onset of effect
Paget's disease Beneficial effects may not be felt for several months.
Hypercalcemia Within several hours, but full beneficial effects may take 4 – 7 days.

Duration of action
Up to 24 hours. Some effects may persist for several days or weeks.

Diet advice
Absorption of etidronate is reduced by foods, especially those containing calcium, e.g. dairy products, so the drug should be taken on an empty stomach. The diet must contain adequate calcium and vitamin D; supplements may be given.

Storage
Keep in a closed container in a cool, dry place away from reach of children. Protect from light.

Missed dose
Take as soon as you remember. If your next dose is due within 6 hours, take a single dose now and skip the next.

Stopping the drug
Do not stop the drug without consulting your physician. Stopping the drug may lead to worsening of the underlying condition.

Exceeding the dose
An occasional unintentional extra dose is unlikely to cause problems. Large overdoses may cause numbness and muscle spasm. Notify your physician.

SPECIAL PRECAUTIONS

Be sure to tell your physician if:
▼ You have impaired kidney function.
▼ You have gastrointestinal disease.
▼ You are taking other medications.

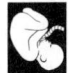

Pregnancy
▼ Safety in pregnancy not established. Discuss with your physician.

Breast feeding
▼ Safety not established. Discuss with your physician.

Infants and children
▼ Not recommended.

Over 60
▼ No special problems.

Driving and hazardous work
▼ No special problems.

Alcohol
▼ No special problems.

POSSIBLE ADVERSE EFFECTS

The most common side effect is diarrhea. This is more likely if the dose is increased above 10mg/kg daily. In some patients with Paget's disease, bone pain may be increased initially, but this usually disappears with further treatment.

Symptom/effect	Frequency		Discuss with physician		Stop taking drug now	Call physician now
	Common	Rare	Only if severe	In all cases		
Diarrhea	●			■		
Nausea	●			■		
Constipation/abdominal pain		●		■		
Rash/itching		●			■	
Bone pain		●			■	▪

INTERACTIONS

General note The effect of etidronate may be increased if given with corticosteroids, phosphate, calcitonin, furosemide, or mithramycin.

Antacids/iron These should be given at least 2 hours before or after etidronate to minimize effects on absorption.

PROLONGED USE

Courses of treatment longer than 3 to 6 months are not usually prescribed, although repeat courses may be required. Continuous use of this drug is not recommended as it may lead to an increased risk of bone fractures.

Monitoring Blood levels of phosphate and alkaline phosphatase (an enzyme found in bones) are sometimes measured. Urine tests for hydroxyproline may also be performed.

ETRETINATE

Brand name Tegison
Used in the following combined preparations None

GENERAL INFORMATION

Etretinate is a drug chemically related to vitamin A that is used in the treatment of severe psoriasis when other drugs have failed to cure the condition.

Etretinate works by reducing production of the protein (keratin) that forms the hard outer layers of skin. This also makes it a useful treatment for certain other rare skin disorders that involve abnormal production of keratin, such as ichthyosis (scaly skin tissue).

Symptoms generally improve after 2 to 4 weeks of treatment. Effects may last for several months after treatment has been stopped, since etretinate accumulates in fatty tissue and is eliminated slowly from the body. *Side effects* are rarely serious, but there is a risk of liver damage and a rise in blood fats.

Etretinate can cause severe birth defects. Women taking the drug must avoid pregnancy during treatment, and for at least 2 years after stopping the drug. Blood should not be donated for at least 1 year after stopping the drug.

INFORMATION FOR USERS

Your drug prescription is tailored for you. Do not alter dosage without checking with your physician.

How taken

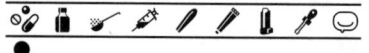

Capsules.

Frequency and timing of doses
2 x daily with or just after a meal.

Adult dosage range
Varies according to individual response and condition treated.

Onset of effect
2 – 4 weeks.

Duration of action
Effects may persist for several months after the drug has been stopped.

Diet advice
None.

Storage
Keep in a closed container in a cool, dry place away from reach of children. Protect from light.

Missed dose
Take as soon as you remember. If your next dose is due within 2 hours, take a single dose now and skip the next.

Stopping the drug
Do not stop the drug without consulting your physician; symptoms may recur.

Exceeding the dose
An occasional unintentional extra dose is unlikely to be a cause for concern. But if you notice unusual symptoms, or if a large overdose has been taken, notify your physician.

POSSIBLE ADVERSE EFFECTS

Dryness and cracking of the lips occur in most people. Dryness of the mouth and nose, nosebleeds, and hair loss are also fairly common. If severe headache accompanied by nausea and vomiting occurs, consult your physician promptly.

Symptom/effect	Frequency		Discuss with physician		Stop taking drug now	Call physician now
	Common	Rare	Only if severe	In all cases		
Dry lips/skin	●		■			
Nosebleeds	●		■			
Hair loss	●		■			
Itching/peeling skin	●		■			
Inflamed eyes		●		■		
Nausea/vomiting/headache		●		■	▲	■

INTERACTIONS

Tetracycline antibiotics increase the risk of high pressure in the skull, leading to headaches and nausea.

Vitamin A supplements increase the risk of adverse effects with etretinate.

Skin-drying preparations Medicated soaps and toiletries increase the likelihood of irritation of the skin with etretinate.

SPECIAL PRECAUTIONS

Be sure to tell your physician if:
▼ You have impaired liver or kidney function.
▼ You have high blood fat levels.
▼ You are taking other medications.

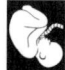
Pregnancy
▼ Etretinate can cause severe birth defects. Women taking the drug must avoid pregnancy during treatment, and for at least 2 years after stopping the drug.

Breast feeding
▼ Do not breast-feed while taking etretinate.

Infants and children
▼ Not usually prescribed.

Over 60
▼ Reduced dose may be necessary.

Driving and hazardous work
▼ No special problems.

Alcohol
▼ Avoid. Regular alcohol consumption may increase the rise in blood fat levels with etretinate, and thus increase the risk of heart and blood vessel disease.

PROLONGED USE

Prolonged use of this drug may increase the risk of liver damage. Courses of treatment are not usually continued for longer than 18 months, and a drug-free holiday is usually allowed between courses.

Monitoring Periodic tests of liver function and fat levels in the blood are usually recommended.

FAMOTIDINE

Brand names Pepcid, Apo-Famotidine, Novo-Famotidine
Used in the following combined preparations None

GENERAL INFORMATION

Famotidine, an anti-ulcer drug, was introduced in 1987 and is mainly used in the prevention and treatment of stomach and duodenal ulcers. It acts by reducing the amount of acid produced by the stomach, allowing the ulcers time to heal. Famotidine is also used in reflux esophagitis, a condition that may cause acid stomach contents to flow partway up the esophagus.

Treatment is usually given in courses lasting from 4 to 8 weeks and maintenance therapy, if required.

Unlike cimetidine, this drug does not affect the actions of certain enzymes in the liver, where many drugs are broken down before being absorbed into the body. This means that famotidine can be taken with other drugs, like anticoagulants and anticonvulsants, without causing an interaction that may reduce the effectiveness of either treatment.

As famotidine promotes healing of the stomach lining, it may mask the symptoms of stomach cancer, delaying diagnosis. Therefore, it is usually prescribed only when the possibility of stomach cancer has been carefully considered.

QUICK REFERENCE

Drug group Anti-ulcer drug (p.121)
Overdose danger rating Low
Dependence rating Low
Prescription needed Yes
Multi-source suppliers Yes

INFORMATION FOR USERS

Your drug prescription is tailored for you. Do not alter dosage without checking with your physician.

How taken

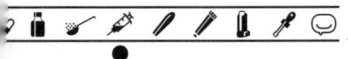

Tablets, injection.

Frequency and timing of doses
1–4 x daily.

Adult dosage range
20–40mg daily.

Onset of effect
Within 1 hour.

Duration of action
6–12 hours.

Diet advice
None.

Storage
Keep in a closed container in a cool, dry place away from reach of children. Protect from light.

Missed dose
Do not take the missed dose. Take your next dose as usual.

Stopping the drug
Do not stop taking the drug without consulting your physician; symptoms may recur.

Exceeding the dose
An occasional unintentional extra dose is unlikely to be a cause for concern. But if you notice unusual symptoms, or if a large overdose has been taken, notify your physician.

POSSIBLE ADVERSE EFFECTS

The adverse effects of famotidine, of which headache is the most common, are usually related to dosage level and almost always disappear when treatment finishes.

Symptom/effect	Frequency		Discuss with physician		Stop taking drug now	Call physician now
	Common	Rare	Only if severe	In all cases		
Headache	●		■			
Dizziness		●	■			
Constipation		●	■			
Diarrhea		●	■			
Nausea/vomiting		●	■			
Itching/rash		●		■		

INTERACTIONS

None.

SPECIAL PRECAUTIONS

Be sure to tell your physician if:
▼ You have impaired liver or kidney function.
▼ You are taking other medications.

Pregnancy
▼ Safety in pregnancy not established. Discuss with your physician.

Breast feeding
▼ Not recommended. The drug passes into the breast milk and may affect the baby. Discuss with your physician.

Infants and children
▼ Safety in children not established.

Over 60
▼ No special problems unless kidney function is reduced, in which case dosage is reduced.

Driving and hazardous work
▼ Avoid such activities until you have learned how the drug affects you; it can cause dizziness.

Alcohol
▼ Avoid. Alcohol may aggravate the underlying condition and counter the beneficial effects of famotidine.

PROLONGED USE

Courses of longer than 12 months are not usually necessary.

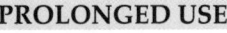

FELODIPINE

Brand names Plendil, Renedil
Used in the following combined preparations None

GENERAL INFORMATION

Felodipine belongs to a group of drugs, known as calcium channel blockers, which interfere with the conduction of signals in the muscles of the heart and blood vessels.

Felodipine is used in the treatment of high blood pressure.

In common with other drugs of its class, felodipine may cause blood pressure to fall too low.

This drug may cause mild to moderate leg and ankle swelling.

QUICK REFERENCE

Drug group Antihypertensive drug (p.114)

Overdose danger rating Medium

Dependence rating Low

Prescription needed Yes

Multi-source suppliers Yes

INFORMATION FOR USERS

Your drug prescription is tailored for you. Do not alter dosage without checking with your physician.

How taken

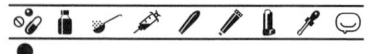

Slow-release tablets.

Frequency and timing of doses
Once daily.

Adult dosage range
5 – 10mg daily.

Onset of effect
2½ – 5 hours.

Duration of action
11 – 16 hours.

Diet advice
Avoid taking felodipine with grapefruit juice.

Storage
Keep in a closed container in a cool, dry place away from reach of children. Protect from light.

Missed dose
If you miss a dose and you remember it within 12 hours, take it as soon as you remember. However, if you do not remember until later, do not take the missed dose at all and do not double up the next one. Instead, go back to your regular schedule.

Stopping the drug
Do not stop taking the drug without consulting your physician; symptoms may recur.

Exceeding the dose
Large overdoses may cause a significant lowering of blood pressure resulting in dizziness. Notify your physician.

SPECIAL PRECAUTIONS

Be sure to tell your physician if:
▼ You have impaired kidney or liver function.
▼ You have heart failure.
▼ You have diabetes.
▼ You are taking other medications.

Pregnancy
▼ Safety in pregnancy not established. Discuss with your physician.

Breast feeding
▼ It is not known if the drug passes into the breast milk. Discuss with your physician.

Infants and children
▼ Not recommended.

Over 60
▼ Increased likelihood of adverse effects. Reduced dose may therefore be necessary.

Driving and hazardous work
▼ Avoid such activities until you have learned how the drug affects you; it can cause dizziness owing lowered blood pressure.

Alcohol
▼ Avoid. Alcohol may further reduce blood pressure, causing dizziness or other symptoms.

POSSIBLE ADVERSE EFFECTS

Felodipine can cause a variety of minor *side effects*, including leg and ankle swelling, headache, dizziness, fatigue, and nausea.

Dizziness, especially on rising, may be caused by an excessive reduction in blood pressure.

Symptom/effect	Frequency		Discuss with physician		Stop taking drug now	Call physician now
	Common	Rare	Only if severe	In all cases		
Leg and ankle swelling	●		■			
Headache	●		■			
Dizziness/fatigue	●		■			
Flushing	●		■			
Nausea/abdominal pain		●		■		
Leg cramps		●	■			
Palpitations		●		■		
Swollen/tender gums		●		■		■

INTERACTIONS

Cimetidine Blood levels of felodipine are increased. Lower doses of felodipine may be required.

Erythromycin Blood levels of felodipine may be increased.

Beta blockers Felodipine may increase the effect of these drugs.

Anticonvulsants Blood levels of felodipine may be decreased.

PROLONGED USE

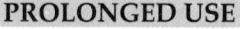

No problems expected.

FENOFIBRATE

Brand names Lipidil, Lipidil Micro
Used in the following combined preparations None

GENERAL INFORMATION

Fenofibrate belongs to a group of drugs that lower lipid levels in the blood. Other drugs in the same chemical group (usually called fibrates) include bezafibrate, clofibrate, and gemfibrozil. These drugs are particularly effective in decreasing blood levels of triglycerides. They also reduce levels of cholesterol.

Raised levels of lipids (fats) in the blood are associated with athero-sclerosis (deposition of fat in blood vessel walls). This can contribute to coronary heart disease (e.g., angina and heart attacks) and cerebrovascular disease (e.g., stroke). There is growing evidence that maintaining normal levels of blood lipids helps prevent heart attacks and strokes.

QUICK REFERENCE

Drug group Lipid-lowering drug (p.115)
Overdose danger rating Low
Dependence rating Low
Prescription needed Yes
Multi-source suppliers No

INFORMATION FOR USERS

Your drug prescription is tailored for you. Do not alter dosage without checking with your physician.

How taken

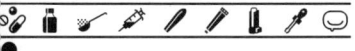

Capsules (regular and micronized).

Frequency and timing of doses
Regular 3 x daily with meals.
Micronized 1 x daily with main meal.

Adult dosage range
100 – 400mg daily (regular).
200mg daily (micronized).

Onset of effect
A beneficial effect on blood fat levels may not occur for weeks.

Duration of action
About 6 – 24 hours. This may vary.

Diet advice
A low-fat diet may be recommended. Follow the advice of your physician.

Storage
Keep in a closed container in a cool, dry place away from reach of children.

Missed dose
Take as soon as you remember. If your next dose is due within 4 hours (and you take once daily), take a single dose now and skip the next. If you take 3 times daily, take the next dose as normal.

Stopping the drug
Do not stop the drug without consulting your physician.

Exceeding the dose
An occasional unintentional extra dose is unlikely to be a cause for concern. But if you notice unusual symptoms, notify your physician.

SPECIAL PRECAUTIONS

Be sure to tell your physician if:
▼ You have impaired liver or kidney function.
▼ You are hypersensitive to fibrates.
▼ You have a history of gallbladder disease.
▼ You are taking other medications.

Pregnancy
▼ Not recommended. If pregnancy occurs despite contraceptive measures, discontinue fenofibrate and inform your physician.

Breast feeding
▼ Not recommended. Discuss with your physician.

Infants and children
▼ Not usually prescribed.

Over 60
▼ No special problems expected.

Driving and hazardous work
▼ Avoid such activities until you have learned how the drug affects you; it can cause dizziness.

Alcohol
▼ No special problems.

POSSIBLE ADVERSE EFFECTS

The most common adverse effects are those on the gastrointestinal tract, such as abdominal pain, diarrhea, and constipation. These effects normally improve as treatment continues.

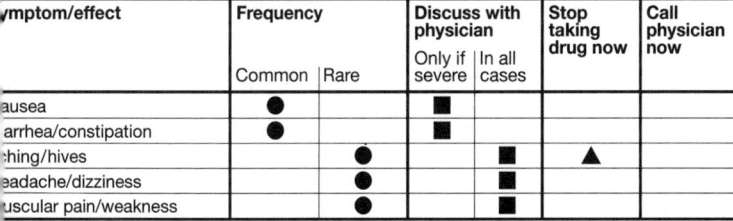

Symptom/effect	Frequency		Discuss with physician		Stop taking drug now	Call physician now
	Common	Rare	Only if severe	In all cases		
Nausea	●		■			
Diarrhea/constipation	●		■			
Itching/hives		●		■	▲	
Headache/dizziness		●		■		
Muscular pain/weakness		●		■		

PROLONGED USE

No problems expected.

Monitoring Blood tests will be undertaken to monitor the effect of the drug on lipids in the blood. Blood tests to monitor liver function may be advised.

INTERACTIONS

Anticoagulants Fenofibrate may increase the effect of anticoagulants such as warfarin.

Monoamine oxidase inhibitors (MAOIs) MAOIs, with a potential for producing liver damage, should not be administered with fenofibrate.

Insulin and oral antidiabetic drugs Fenofibrate may interact with these drugs to lower blood sugar levels.

Lovastatin (and other "statins") and cyclosporine are not usually prescribed with fenofibrate because of the risk of severe muscle inflammation.

FENOTEROL

Brand name Berotec
Used in the following combined preparations None

GENERAL INFORMATION

Fenoterol is a *sympathomimetic* bronchodilator that relaxes the muscles surrounding the bronchioles (airways in the lung).

It is used mainly to relieve the wheezing or shortness of breath caused by asthma, chronic bronchitis, and emphysema. Although fenoterol can be taken by mouth, inhalation is considered more effective because it is delivered directly to the bronchioles, giving rapid relief, allowing smaller doses, and creating fewer *side effects*.

Compared with some similar drugs, it has little stimulant effect on the heart rate and blood pressure, making it safer for those with heart problems or high blood pressure.

The most common side effect of fenoterol is fine tremor of the hands, which may interfere with precise manual work. Dizziness, lightheadedness, nausea, nervousness, and restlessness may also occur.

QUICK REFERENCE

Drug group Bronchodilator (p.104)
Overdose danger rating Low
Dependence rating Low
Prescription needed Yes
Multi-source suppliers No

INFORMATION FOR USERS

Your drug prescription is tailored for you. Do not alter dosage without checking with your physician.

How taken

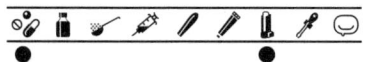

Tablets, inhaler, solution for inhalation.

Frequency and timing of doses
3 – 4 x daily (tablets); 1 – 2 inhalations every 4 – 6 hours as required (inhaler); up to 4 x daily (solution for inhalation).

Adult dosage range
5 – 15mg daily (tablets); 800 – 1,600mcg daily (inhaler); 0.5 – 2.5mg per dose, dilution adjusted to equipment and length of administration (solution for inhalation).

Onset of effect
30 – 60 minutes (tablets); 5 – 15 minutes (inhaler).

Duration of action
Up to 8 hours (tablets); up to 6 hours (inhaler).

Diet advice
None.

Storage
Keep in a closed container in a cool, dry place away from reach of children. Protect from light. Do not puncture or burn inhalers.

Missed dose
Do not take the missed dose. Take your next dose as usual.

Stopping the drug
Do not stop the drug without consulting your physician; symptoms may recur.

Exceeding the dose
An occasional unintentional extra dose is unlikely to cause problems. But if you notice unusual symptoms, or if a large overdose has been taken, notify your physician immediately.

SPECIAL PRECAUTIONS

Be sure to tell your physician if:
▼ You have heart problems.
▼ You have high blood pressure.
▼ You have an overactive thyroid gland.
▼ You have diabetes.
▼ You have glaucoma.
▼ You have difficulty in urination.
▼ You are taking other medications.

Pregnancy
▼ Safety in pregnancy not established. Discuss with your physician.

Breast feeding
▼ Effect on breast feeding uncertain. Discuss with your physician.

Infants and children
▼ Not recommended in patients under 12 years.

Over 60
▼ Increased likelihood of adverse effects. Reduced dose may therefore be necessary.

Driving and hazardous work
▼ Avoid such activities until you have learned how the drug affects you; it can cause tremors and dizziness.

Alcohol
▼ No known problems.

POSSIBLE ADVERSE EFFECTS

Muscle tremor, especially of the hands, dizziness, and restlessness are the most common adverse effects of the drug. Palpitations and headache are rare.

Symptom/effect	Frequency		Discuss with physician		Stop taking drug now	Call physician now
	Common	Rare	Only if severe	In all cases		
Nervousness/lightheadedness	●			■		
Restlessness	●			■		
Tremor	●			■		
Nausea/vomiting		●		■		
Dizziness	●			■		
Headache		●		■		
Palpitations	●				■	

INTERACTIONS

Other sympathomimetics may increase the effect of fenoterol, thus increasing the risk of adverse effects.

Beta blockers may counter the beneficial effects of fenoterol.

Monoamine oxidase inhibitors (MAOIs) can interact with fenoterol to produce a dangerous rise in blood pressure.

PROLONGED USE

Prolonged regular use may result in worsening of asthma and intolerance to the effects of fenoterol. Failure to respond to the drug may be a result of worsening asthma requiring urgent medical attention.

FINASTERIDE

Brand name Proscar
Used in the following combined preparations None

GENERAL INFORMATION

Finasteride is a new drug used to treat benign prostatic hyperplasia (BPH), an enlargement of the prostate gland that commonly occurs in older men. BPH can cause such symptoms as weak stream, frequent urination (daytime and nighttime), and dribbling, as well as incomplete emptying of the bladder, and can lead to urinary blockage.

Severe forms of BPH with blockage are treated with surgery. Medications are used for milder forms of the disease after a thorough examination, including the prostate-specific antigen (PSA) test.

Treatment with finasteride is long-term. The medication works to reduce prostate size, thereby improving urinary flow and reducing symptoms. Benefit may not be noted for 6 months or more after starting treatment.

Finasteride may cause abnormal development of a male fetus. Therefore, while using this drug, a man should not father a child. Also, a pregnant woman should not be exposed to the semen of a man taking finasteride.

INFORMATION FOR USERS

Your drug prescriptions is tailored for you. Do not alter dosage without checking with your physician.

How taken

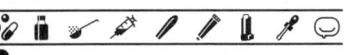

Tablets.

Frequency and timing of doses
Once daily. May be taken with or without food.

Adult dosage range
5mg daily.

Onset of effect
Weeks to many months.

Duration of action
Approximately 24 hours.

Diet advice
None.

Storage
Keep in a closed container in a cool, dry place away from the reach of children.

Missed dose
Take as soon as you remember. If your next dose is due within 8 hours, take a single dose now and skip the next.

Stopping the drug
Do not stop taking the drug without consulting your physician.

Exceeding the dose
An occasional unintentional extra dose is unlikely to cause problems.

POSSIBLE ADVERSE EFFECTS

Adverse effects are generally related to the genitourinary tract and include impotence, decreased libido, and decreased ejaculation.

Symptom/effect	Frequency		Discuss with physician		Stop taking drug now	Call physician now
	Common	Rare	Only if severe	In all cases		
Impotence	●		■			
Decreased libido	●		■			
Decreased ejaculation	●		■			
Breast enlargement	●			■		
Lip swelling/skin rash		●		■	▲	

INTERACTIONS

None.

SPECIAL PRECAUTIONS

Be sure to tell your physician if:
▼ You have impaired kidney function.
▼ You are contemplating a pregnancy or your partner is pregnant.
▼ You are taking other medications.

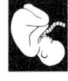 **Pregnancy**
▼ Not prescribed.
However, semen of men taking finasteride may cause abnormal development of a male fetus. Discuss with your physician.

 Breast feeding
▼ Not prescribed.

 Infants and children
▼ Not prescribed.

 Over 60
▼ No special problems.

 Driving and hazardous work
▼ No known problems.

 Alcohol
▼ No known problems.

PROLONGED USE

No known problems, but experience with the drug in long-term use is limited. Discuss with your physician.

Monitoring Periodic checkups are suggested to assess the prostate.

FLUCONAZOLE

Brand name Diflucan
Used in the following combined preparations None

GENERAL INFORMATION

Fluconazole is a relatively new antifungal drug. It is used to treat local candida infections ("thrush") of the vagina and mouth, and also *systemic* candida infection. In addition, it is used to treat some of the more unusual fungal infections including cryptococcal meningitis. Fungal infections in patients with defective immunity may also be prevented by fluconazole. The dosage and length of course will depend on the condition being treated.

Fluconazole is generally well tolerated, the most common *side effects* being those affecting the gastrointestinal tract.

INFORMATION FOR USERS

Your drug prescription is tailored for you. Do not alter dosage without checking with your physician.

How taken

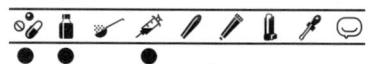

Capsules, oral liquid, injection.

Frequency and timing of doses
Once daily.

Adult dosage range
100 – 400mg daily.

Onset of effect
It begins to work within a few hours but full beneficial effects may take several days.

Duration of action
Up to 24 hours.

Diet advice
None.

Storage
Keep in a closed container in a cool, dry place away from reach of children.

Missed dose
Take as soon as you remember. If your next dose is due within 6 hours, take a single dose now and skip the next.

Stopping the drug
Take the full course. Even if you feel better, the original infection may still be present and may recur if treatment is stopped too soon.

Exceeding the dose
An occasional extra dose is unlikely to be a cause for concern. But if you notice any unusual symptoms, or if a large overdose has been taken, notify your physician.

POSSIBLE ADVERSE EFFECTS

Fluconazole is generally well tolerated. Side effects most commonly affect the gastrointestinal tract.

Symptom/effect	Frequency		Discuss with physician		Stop taking drug now	Call physician now
	Common	Rare	Only if severe	In all cases		
Nausea/vomiting	●		■			
Abdominal discomfort	●		■			
Diarrhea	●		■			
Flatulence	●		■			
Rash		●		■	▲	

INTERACTIONS

Anticoagulants Fluconazole may increase the effect of warfarin.

Oral antidiabetic drugs Fluconazole may increase the risk of hypoglycemia with oral sulfonylureas, e.g., gliclazide, chlorpropamide, glyburide, tolbutamide.

Phenytoin Fluconazole may increase the blood level of phenytoin.

Theophylline Fluconazole may increase the blood level of theophylline.

Cyclosporine Fluconazole may increase the blood level of cyclosporine.

Rifampin The effect of fluconazole may be reduced by rifampin.

Antihistamines Increased risk of terfenadine and astemizole causing adverse effects on the heart.

SPECIAL PRECAUTIONS

Be sure to tell your physician if:
▼ You have impaired liver or kidney function.
▼ You have previously had an allergic reaction to antifungal drugs.
▼ You are taking other medications.

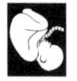

Pregnancy
▼ Safety in pregnancy not established. Discuss with your physician.

Breast feeding
▼ Not recommended. The drug passes into the breast milk. Discuss with your physician.

Infants and children
▼ Not recommended in children under 13 years.

Over 60
▼ Normal dose used as long as kidney function is not impaired.

Driving and hazardous work
▼ No known problems.

Alcohol
▼ No known problems.

PROLONGED USE

Fluconazole is usually given for short courses of treatment. However, for prevention of relapse of cryptococcal meningitis in patients with defective immunity, it may be administered indefinitely.

FLUNISOLIDE

Brand names Bronalide, Rhinalar, Rhinaris F, Syn-Flunisolide
Used in the following combined preparations None

GENERAL INFORMATION

Flunisolide is a corticosteroid drug prescribed to relieve the symptoms of allergic rhinitis (as a nasal inhaler or spray) and to control asthma (as an inhaler). It also helps to reduce symptoms such as wheezing and coughing by reducing inflammation in the bronchi. People who suffer from asthma may take flunisolide to reduce the severity and frequency of attacks. However, once an attack has started, this drug does not relieve symptoms.

Fungal infection (thrush) causing irritation of the mouth and throat is a possible adverse effect of flunisolide asthma treatment that can be minimized by thoroughly rinsing the mouth and gargling with water after each inhalation.

INFORMATION FOR USERS

Your drug prescription is tailored for you. Do not alter dosage without checking with your physician.

How taken

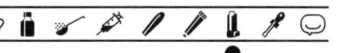

Inhaler, nasal spray.

Frequency and timing of doses
2 x daily (nasal spray, inhaler).

Dosage range
Adults 1 – 2 sprays twice daily (asthma); 2 sprays in each nostril twice daily (allergic rhinitis).
Children Reduced dose according to age and weight.

Onset of effect
Within 1 week (asthma); 1 – 3 days (allergic rhinitis).

Duration of action
Several days after stopping the drug.

Diet advice
None.

Storage
Store away from heat and direct light away from reach of children. Keep the medicine from getting too cold or freezing. This medicine may be less effective if the container is cold when you use it. Do not puncture, break, or burn the aerosol container, even after it is empty.

Missed dose
Take as soon as you remember. However, if it is almost time for your next dose, skip the missed dose and go back to your regular schedule. Do not double doses.

Stopping the drug
Do not stop the drug without consulting your physician; symptoms may recur. It may be necessary to withdraw the drug gradually.

Exceeding the dose
An occasional unintentional extra dose is unlikely to be a cause for concern. But if you do notice unusual symptoms, or if a large overdose has been taken, notify your physician. Adverse effects may occur if the recommended dose is regularly exceeded over a prolonged period.

POSSIBLE ADVERSE EFFECTS

Adverse effects are unlikely as the dose used is low. The main *side effects* are irritation of the nasal passages (nasal spray) and fungal infection of the throat and mouth (inhaler).

Symptom/effect	Frequency		Discuss with physician		Stop taking drug now	Call physician now
	Common	Rare	Only if severe	In all cases		
Nasal discomfort/irritation	●		■			
Cough	●		■			
Breathing difficulties		●		■		■
Nosebleeds		●		■		
Hoarseness/sore throat/mouth	●			■		

INTERACTIONS

None.

SPECIAL PRECAUTIONS

Be sure to tell your physician if:
▼ You have had any nasal ulcers or surgery.
▼ You have had tuberculosis or another respiratory infection.
▼ You are taking other medications.

Pregnancy
▼ Safety in pregnancy not established. Discuss with your physician.

Breast feeding
▼ The drug passes into the breast milk, but at normal doses adverse effects on the baby are unlikely. Discuss with your physician.

Infants and children
▼ Not recommended under 4 years (asthma); under 6 years (allergic rhinitis). Reduced dose necessary in older children.

Over 60
▼ No known problems.

Driving and hazardous work
▼ No known problems.

Alcohol
▼ No known problems.

PROLONGED USE

Monitoring Periodic checks to make sure that the adrenal glands are functioning properly may be required if large doses are being used.

FLUOCINOLONE

Brand names Derma-Smoothe/FS, Fluoderm, Fluonide, Synalar, Synamol
Used in the following combined preparation Synalar Bi-Otic

GENERAL INFORMATION

Fluocinolone, introduced in 1963, is prescribed to relieve the redness, swelling, itching, and discomfort of many skin disorders that occur as a result of inflammation or allergy.

Available in creams, ointments, and solutions, it can be applied directly to relieve the affected area. Fluocinolone is not an appropriate treatment for skin infections caused by bacteria, fungi, or viruses, and may make them worse. It is not prescribed for the treatment of acne, and should not normally be applied to the face. Few people encounter *side effects* when they use fluocinolone for short periods of time because it acts locally and only small amounts are absorbed into the body. Excessive, prolonged use may lead to thinning of the skin, especially in skin folds.

INFORMATION FOR USERS

Your drug prescription is tailored for you. Do not alter dosage without checking with your physician.

How taken

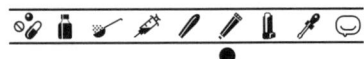

Topical solution, cream, ointment.

Frequency and timing of doses
2 – 4 x daily.

Dosage range
Sufficient cream, ointment, solution to cover the affected area at each application.

Onset of effect
1 – 2 hours.

Duration of action
Up to 24 hours after each dose.

Diet advice
None.

Storage
Keep in a closed container in a cool, dry place away from reach of children.

Missed dose
No cause for concern but apply as soon as you remember.

Stopping the drug
Use as directed by your physician. When symptoms improve, discuss stopping the drug with your physician.

Exceeding the dose
An occasional unintentional extra dose is unlikely to be a cause for concern. But if you notice unusual symptoms, notify your physician.

POSSIBLE ADVERSE EFFECTS

Adverse effects from topical fluocinolone are rare and are restricted to the site of application. Irritation occurs only occasionally.

Thinning of the skin is unlikely and only occurs when the drug is used too frequently or for extended periods of time.

Symptom/effect	Frequency		Discuss with physician		Stop taking drug now	Call physician now
	Common	Rare	Only if severe	In all cases		
Local irritation		●		■		▲
Thinning of the skin		●		■		▲
Reddening of the skin		●		■		▲

INTERACTIONS

None.

SPECIAL PRECAUTIONS

Be sure to tell your physician if:
▼ You are taking other medications.

Pregnancy
▼ No evidence of risk to developing baby.

Breast feeding
▼ No evidence of risk.

Infants and children
▼ No special problems.

Over 60
▼ No special problems.

Driving and hazardous work
▼ No known problems.

Alcohol
▼ No known problems.

PROLONGED USE

Long-term treatment can cause permanent thinning of the skin.

FLUOROURACIL

Brand names Adrucil, Efudex, Fluoroplex
Used in the following combined preparations None

GENERAL INFORMATION

Fluorouracil is an anticancer drug that interferes with the growth of tumor cells. It is given by injection often in conjunction with other anticancer drugs to limit growth of tumors in the colon, rectum, breast, stomach, and pancreas. Other cancers are sometimes treated with this drug, as well.

Fluorouracil is also available as a cream to treat solar keratoses (a skin disorder caused by overexposure to sunlight). It is also effective in the treatment of superficial basal cell carcinoma of the skin. When given by injection, fluorouracil affects healthy as well as cancerous cells, causing a number of *side effects*. Nausea, vomiting, and diarrhea are the most common symptoms.

Fluorouracil taken by injection interferes with the production of blood cells; this may lead to anemia, increased susceptibility to infection, and hair loss. After application of the cream, there may be soreness, itching, burning, and scarring.

QUICK REFERENCE

Drug group Anticancer drug (p.166)

Overdose danger rating Low

Dependence rating Low

Prescription needed Yes

Multi-source suppliers Yes

INFORMATION FOR USERS

Your drug prescription is tailored for you. Do not alter dosage without checking with your physician.

How taken

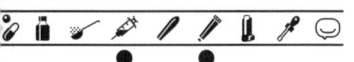

Injection, cream.

Frequency and timing of doses
Once daily (injection); 2 x daily (cream).

Adult dosage range
Injection Dosage is determined individually according to body weight and response.
Cream Apply as directed, avoiding eyes, nose, and mouth. Wash hands after use.

Onset of effect
Some benefits and adverse effects appear within hours of injection. Full beneficial effects may not be felt for up to 4 weeks.

Duration of action
Side effects may last for several weeks.

Diet advice
After injection refrain from foods likely to cause loose bowel movements.

Storage
Keep in a closed container in a cool, dry place away from reach of children. Protect from light.

Missed dose
Injections are given only under close medical supervision. If you are using the cream there is no cause for concern, but apply as soon as you remember.

Stopping the drug
The injection will be stopped under medical supervision. Do not stop the cream without consulting your physician; symptoms may recur.

Exceeding the dose
An occasional unintentional extra application of cream is unlikely to be a cause for concern. But if you notice unusual symptoms, or if a large overdose has been taken, notify your physician.

POSSIBLE ADVERSE EFFECTS

When injected, fluorouracil often causes nausea, vomiting, and diarrhea. Other adverse effects include increased frequency of infections and loss of hair. The cream may occasionally cause blistering and redness of the skin that worsens after exposure to sunlight.

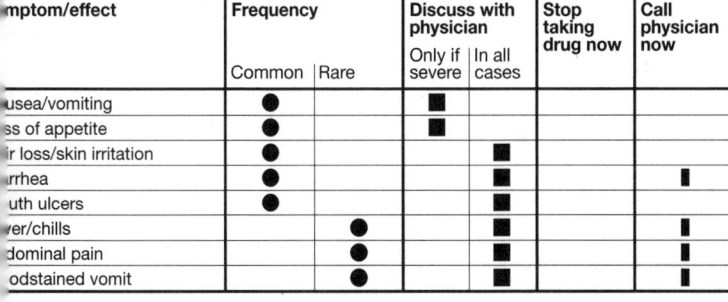

Symptom/effect	Frequency		Discuss with physician		Stop taking drug now	Call physician now
	Common	Rare	Only if severe	In all cases		
Nausea/vomiting	●		■			
Loss of appetite	●		■			
Hair loss/skin irritation	●			■		
Diarrhea	●			■		■
Mouth ulcers	●			■		
Fever/chills		●		■		■
Abdominal pain		●		■		■
Bloodstained vomit		●		■		■

INTERACTIONS

Cimetidine may increase the possibility of adverse effects from fluorouracil. The fluorouracil dosage may need to be adjusted accordingly.

SPECIAL PRECAUTIONS

Be sure to tell your physician if:
▼ You have impaired liver function.
▼ You have a history of heart disease.
▼ You have recently had chickenpox or a herpes infection.
▼ You are taking other medications.

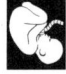

Pregnancy
▼ Discuss treatment with your physician so that you can weigh the benefits of the drugs against its possible risks.

Breast feeding
▼ When given by injection the drug passes into the breast milk and may affect the baby adversely. When applied as a cream, small amounts of the drug pass into the breast milk. Discuss with your physician.

Infants and children
▼ Not usually prescribed.

Over 60
▼ Increased risk of adverse effects. Reduced dose may therefore be necessary.

Driving and hazardous work
▼ No known problems.

Alcohol
▼ No known problems.

PROLONGED USE

Fluorouracil given by injection is likely to reduce resistance to infection and may reduce production of blood cells.

Monitoring Periodic checks on blood composition are advised.

FLUOXETINE

Brand name Prozac
Used in the following combined preparations None

GENERAL INFORMATION

Fluoxetine belongs to a relatively new group of antidepressants called specific serotonin reuptake inhibitors (SSRIs). Drugs of this type tend to cause less sedation and have fewer *side effects* than older antidepressants. Fluoxetine elevates mood, increases physical activity, and restores interest in everyday activities.

Fluoxetine is broken down slowly and remains in the body for several weeks after treatment is stopped. Headache, nausea, restlessness, and insomnia are common side effects. Fluoxetine is also used to reduce binge-eating and purging (bulimia nervosa) as well as in the management of symptoms of obsessive-compulsive disorder.

QUICK REFERENCE

Drug group Antidepressants (p.96)
Overdose danger rating High
Dependence rating Low
Prescription needed Yes
Multi-source suppliers No

INFORMATION FOR USERS

Your drug prescription is tailored for you. Do not alter dosage without checking with your physician.

How taken

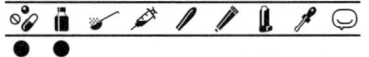

Capsules, liquid.

Frequency and timing of doses
Once daily in the morning.

Adult dosage range
20 – 80mg daily.

Onset of effect
Some benefits and effects may appear within 14 days, but full benefits may not be felt for 4 weeks or more.

Duration of action
Following prolonged treatment, beneficial effects may persist for up to 6 weeks. Adverse effects may wear off within a few days.

Diet advice
None.

Storage
Keep in a closed container in a cool, dry place away from reach of children. Protect from light.

Missed dose
Take as soon as you remember. If your next dose is due within 3 hours, take a single dose now and skip the next.

Stopping the drug
Do not stop the drug without consulting your physician, who may supervise a gradual reduction in dosage.

OVERDOSE ACTION

 Seek immediate medical advice in all cases. Take emergency action if slow or irregular pulse, seizures, or loss of consciousness occurs.

See Drug poisoning emergency guide (p.574).

POSSIBLE ADVERSE EFFECTS

The most common adverse effects are restlessness, insomnia, and gastrointestinal irregularities. Fluoxetine produces fewer *anticholinergic* side effects than the tricyclics.

Symptom/effect	Frequency		Discuss with physician		Stop taking drug now	Call physician now
	Common	Rare	Only if severe	In all cases		
Headache/nervousness	●		■			
Insomnia/anxiety	●			■		
Nausea/diarrhea	●			■		
Appetite decrease	●			■		
Drowsiness		●	■			
Sexual dysfunction		●	■		▲	
Rash		●		■	▲	■

INTERACTIONS

Monoamine oxidase inhibitors (MAOIs)
Leave at least 14 days between stopping an MAOI and starting fluoxetine. Leave at least 5 weeks between stopping fluoxetine and starting an MAOI.

Other antidepressants Fluoxetine may markedly increase blood levels of other antidepressants.

Sedatives All drugs that have a sedative effect are likely to increase the sedative effects of fluoxetine.

Tryptophan A toxic reaction may occur between tryptophan and fluoxetine.

SPECIAL PRECAUTIONS

Be sure to tell your physician if:
▼ You have impaired liver or kidney function.
▼ You have heart problems.
▼ You have diabetes.
▼ You have had epileptic seizures.
▼ You are taking other medications.

 Pregnancy
▼ Safety in pregnancy not established. Discuss with your physician.

 Breast feeding
▼ The drug passes into the breast milk. Discuss with your physician.

 Infants and children
▼ Safety and effectiveness in patients under 18 years not established.

Over 60
▼ Increased likelihood of adverse effects. Reduced dose may therefore be necessary.

Driving and hazardous work
▼ Avoid such activities until you have learned how the drug affects you; it can cause drowsiness.

Alcohol
▼ Avoid. Alcohol may increase the sedative effects of this drug.

Surgery and general anesthetics
▼ Fluoxetine may need to be stopped before you have a general anesthetic. Discuss with your physician or dentist before any operation.

PROLONGED USE

No problems expected. However, fluoxetine is a relatively new drug, and little is known of its long-term effects.

FLUPHENAZINE

Brand names Moditen, Apo-Fluphenazine, Modecate, PMS-Fluphenazine
Used in the following combined preparations None

GENERAL INFORMATION

Introduced in the late 1960s, fluphenazine is the most potent of a group of drugs called the phenothiazines. These are used to suppress abnormal behavior, reduce aggression, and tranquilize those who are agitated. Phenothiazines (see p.97) cannot cure mental disease, but they can control the symptoms of schizophrenia, mania, dementia, and other disorders that cause abnormal or confused behavior.

Fluphenazine's principal advantage is its long-lasting effect. It can be given in the form of a long-acting depot injection. Thus it is valuable for people who cannot remember to take daily medication. It is also available in tablet or liquid form.

The main drawback to the use of fluphenazine is that it often produces abnormal shaking, especially at the start of treatment.

INFORMATION FOR USERS

Your drug prescription is tailored for you. Do not alter dosage without checking with your physician.

How taken

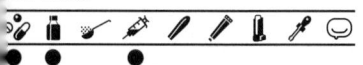

Tablets, oral liquid, injection.

Frequency and timing of doses
1 – 4 x daily (by mouth); every 2 – 4 weeks (depot injection).

Adult dosage range
2.5 – 10mg daily (starting dose), reduced to 1 – 5mg daily (maintenance dose); 5 – 100mg (depot injection).

Onset of effect
1 hour (by mouth); 24 – 72 hours (depot injection).

Duration of action
6 – 8 hours (by mouth); 2 – 6 weeks (depot injection, depending on formulation).

Diet advice
None.

Storage
Keep in a closed container in a cool, dry place away from reach of children. Protect from light.

Missed dose
Take as soon as you remember. If your next dose is due within 2 hours do not take the missed dose. Take the next scheduled dose as usual.

Stopping the drug
Do not stop the drug without consulting your physician; symptoms may recur.

Exceeding the dose
An occasional unintentional extra dose is unlikely to cause problems. Larger overdoses may cause unusual drowsiness, muscle rigidity, and agitation. Notify your physician.

SPECIAL PRECAUTIONS

Be sure to tell your physician if:
▼ You have heart problems.
▼ You have had epileptic seizures.
▼ You have an overactive thyroid gland.
▼ You have impaired liver or kidney function.
▼ You have Parkinson's disease.
▼ You have had glaucoma.
▼ You have prostate trouble.
▼ You are taking other medications.

Pregnancy
▼ Safety in pregnancy not established. Discuss with your physician.

Breast feeding
▼ The drug passes into the breast milk. Its effects on the baby are not clearly known. Discuss with your physician.

Infants and children
▼ Not usually prescribed. Reduced dose necessary.

Over 60
▼ Reduced dose may be necessary.

Driving and hazardous work
▼ Avoid such activities until you have learned how the drug affects you; it can cause drowsiness and slowed reactions.

Alcohol
▼ Avoid. Alcohol may increase the sedative effects of this drug.

POSSIBLE ADVERSE EFFECTS

The most marked adverse effect of this drug is stiffness and abnormal movements of the face and limbs (parkinsonism). This can usually be controlled by medically supervised adjustment of dosage, or a change of drug.

Symptom/effect	Frequency		Discuss with physician		Stop taking drug now	Call physician now
	Common	Rare	Only if severe	In all cases		
Drowsiness/lethargy	●		■			
Parkinsonism	●		■			
Dry mouth		●	■			
Blurred vision		●		■		
Dizziness/faintness		●		■		

INTERACTIONS

Sedatives are likely to increase the sedative properties of fluphenazine.

Anticholinergic drugs Their side effects may be increased by fluphenazine.

Anticonvulsants and antiparkinsonian drugs Fluphenazine may reduce the effectiveness of such drugs.

PROLONGED USE

Use of this drug for more than a few months may lead to the development of *tardive dyskinesia*, and occasionally jaundice may occur.

Monitoring Periodic blood tests may be performed.

FLURAZEPAM

Brand names Dalmane, Apo-Flurazepam, Somnol
Used in the following combined preparations None

GENERAL INFORMATION

Flurazepam is one of a large group of drugs known as the benzodiazepines, generally used to quiet anxieties. The actions and adverse effects of this group of drugs are described on page 95. Flurazepam is primarily used in the short-term management of insomnia.

Because of its long duration of action, flurazepam may cause morning hangover. Taken over a long period, it can be habit-forming. For that reason, and also because the effects of this drug are likely to diminish over time, flurazepam treatment is usually reviewed every two weeks.

QUICK REFERENCE

Drug group Benzodiazepine sleeping drug (p.94)

Overdose danger rating Medium

Dependence rating Medium

Prescription needed Yes

Multi-source suppliers Yes

INFORMATION FOR USERS

Your drug prescription is tailored for you. Do not alter dosage without checking with your physician.

How taken

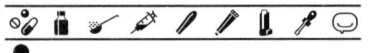

Capsules, tablets.

Frequency and timing of doses
Once daily at bedtime.

Adult dosage range
15 – 30mg daily.

Onset of effect
15 – 45 minutes.

Duration of action
7 – 8 hours, but some effect can last up to 24 hours.

Diet advice
None.

Storage
Keep in a closed container in a cool, dry place away from reach of children. Protect from light.

Missed dose
If you fall asleep without having taken a dose, and wake some hours later, do not take the missed dose. If necessary, return to your normal dose schedule the following night.

Stopping the drug
If you have been taking the drug continuously for less than 2 weeks, it can be safely stopped as soon as you feel you no longer need it. However, if you have been taking the drug for longer, consult your physician, who will supervise a gradual reduction in dosage. Stopping abruptly may lead to withdrawal symptoms (see p.94).

Exceeding the dose
An occasional unintentional extra dose is unlikely to cause problems. Larger overdoses may cause unusual drowsiness. Notify your physician.

SPECIAL PRECAUTIONS

Be sure to tell your physician if:
▼ You have severe respiratory disease.
▼ You have impaired liver or kidney function.
▼ You have glaucoma.
▼ You have myasthenia gravis.
▼ You have had problems with alcohol or drug abuse.
▼ You are taking other medications.

Pregnancy
▼ Safety in pregnancy not established. Discuss with your physician.

Breast feeding
▼ The drug passes into the breast milk and may affect the baby. Discuss with your physician.

Infants and children
▼ Not recommended in children under 15 years.

Over 60
▼ Increased likelihood of adverse effects. Reduced dose may therefore be necessary.

Driving and hazardous work
▼ Avoid such activities until you have learned how the drug affects you; it can cause reduced alertness, slowed reactions, and blurred vision.

Alcohol
▼ Avoid. Alcohol may increase the sedative effects of this drug.

POSSIBLE ADVERSE EFFECTS

The principal adverse effects of this drug are related to its sedative and tranquilizing properties.

Symptom/effect	Frequency		Discuss with physician		Stop taking drug now	Call physician now
	Common	Rare	Only if severe	In all cases		
Daytime drowsiness	●			■		
Dizziness/unsteadiness	●			■		
Headache		●	■			
Blurred vision		●		■		
Forgetfulness/confusion		●		■		
Rash		●		■	▲	

INTERACTIONS

Sedatives All drugs that have a sedative effect on the central nervous system are likely to increase the sedative properties of flurazepam. Such drugs include alcohol, other anti-anxiety and sleeping drugs, antihistamines, antidepressants, narcotic analgesics, and antipsychotics.

Cimetidine Breakdown of flurazepam in the liver may be inhibited by cimetidine. This can cause a buildup of flurazepam levels in the blood, which increases the likelihood of adverse effects.

PROLONGED USE

Regular use of this drug over several weeks can lead to a reduction in its effect as the body adapts. It may also be habit-forming when taken for extended periods, especially if larger-than-average doses are taken.

FLURBIPROFEN

Brand names Ansaid, Apo–Flurbiprofen, Froben, Ocufen
Used in the following combined preparations None

GENERAL INFORMATION

Flurbiprofen, a non-steroidal anti-inflammatory drug (NSAID) introduced in 1985, relieves the pain, stiffness, and inflammation that may accompany a number of disorders. It is similar to other NSAIDs in the way it works and the way it can be used. It acts as an analgesic as well as an anti-inflammatory and is an effective treatment for rheumatoid arthritis, osteoarthritis and ankylosing spondylitis. It is also effective in relieving the mild to moderate pain of menstruation and soft tissue injuries, and pain following operations.

Flurbiprofen is also given in the form of eye drops to reduce inflammation following eye surgery. Any increase in pain or redness in the eye during such treatment should be brought to your physician's attention without delay.

The most common adverse effects of flurbiprofen, as with all NSAIDs, are gastrointestinal disturbances such as indigestion and nausea.

INFORMATION FOR USERS

Your drug prescription is tailored for you. Do not alter dosage without checking with your physician.

How taken

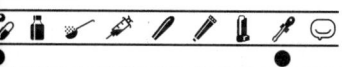

Tablets, eye drops.

Frequency and timing of doses
1 – 4 x daily (by mouth); every 4 hours (eye drops).

Adult dosage range
50 – 200mg daily.

Onset of effect
Pain relief begins in 1 – 2 hours, but full anti-inflammatory effect on arthritic conditions may not be felt for up to 2 weeks.

Duration of action
6 - 12 hours.

Diet advice
None.

Storage
Keep in a closed container in a cool, dry place away from reach of children.

Missed dose
Take as soon as you remember. If your next dose is due within 2 hours, take a single dose now and skip the next.

Stopping the drug
When taken for short-term pain relief, flurbiprofen can be safely stopped as soon as you no longer need it. If prescribed for the long-term treatment of arthritis, however, you should seek medical advice before stopping the drug.

Exceeding the dose
An occasional unintentional extra dose is unlikely to be a cause for concern. But if you notice unusual symptoms, or if a large overdose has been taken, notify your physician.

POSSIBLE ADVERSE EFFECTS

The most common adverse effects of flurbiprofen taken by mouth are the result of gastrointestinal disturbances. Black or bloodstained feces should be reported to your physician without delay.

Symptom/effect	Frequency		Discuss with physician		Stop taking drug now	Call physician now
	Common	Rare	Only if severe	In all cases		
Heartburn/indigestion	●		■			
Nausea/vomiting	●			■		
Diarrhea/constipation	●			■		
Dizziness/lightheadedness		●	■			
Headache		●	■			
Rash		●		■	▲	
Wheezing/breathlessness		●		■	▲	❙
Black/bloodstained feces		●		■	▲	❙

INTERACTIONS

General note Flurbiprofen may interact with a wide range of drugs to increase the risk of bleeding and/or peptic ulcer. Such drugs include oral anticoagulants, corticosteroids, other non-steroidal anti-inflammatory drugs (NSAIDs), and ASA.

Antihypertensive drugs and diuretics The beneficial effects of these drugs may be reduced by flurbiprofen.

Oral antidiabetics Flurbiprofen may increase the blood sugar-lowering effect of these drugs.

SPECIAL PRECAUTIONS

Be sure to tell your physician if:
▼ You have impaired liver or kidney function.
▼ You have heart problems.
▼ You have high blood pressure.
▼ You have asthma.
▼ You have had a peptic ulcer, esophagitis, or acid indigestion.
▼ You are allergic to ASA.
▼ You are taking other medications.

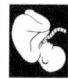

Pregnancy
▼ Not usually prescribed. Safety in pregnancy not established. Discuss with your physician.

Breast feeding
▼ Effects on breast feeding uncertain. Discuss with your physician.

Infants and children
▼ Not recommended in children under 12 years.

Over 60
▼ Increased likelihood of adverse effects. Reduced dose may therefore be necessary.

Driving and hazardous work
▼ Avoid such activities until you have learned how the drug affects you; it can cause dizziness.

Alcohol
▼ Avoid. Alcohol may increase the risk of stomach disorders with flurbiprofen.

Surgery and general anesthetics
▼ Flurbiprofen may prolong bleeding. Discuss with your physician or dentist before any surgery.

PROLONGED USE

There is an increased risk of bleeding, both from peptic ulcers and from the bowel, with prolonged use of flurbiprofen.

FLUTICASONE

Brand names Flonase, Flovent
Used in the following combined preparations None

GENERAL INFORMATION

Fluticasone is a corticosteroid drug used to relieve the symptoms of allergic rhinitis (as a nasal spray – Flonase) and to control asthma (as an inhaler – Flovent). It acts mainly by reducing inflammation. Fluticasone does not produce immediate relief, so it is important to take the drug regularly.

For allergic rhinitis, full effect is achieved after 2 – 3 days. People who suffer from asthma should take fluticasone regularly to prevent attacks from recurring.

There are few serious adverse effects associated with fluticasone as it is administered directly into the lungs (inhalation) and nasal mucosa (nasal spray). However, fungal infection causing irritation of the mouth and throat is a possible *side effect* of inhaled fluticasone. This can be minimized by thoroughly rinsing the mouth and gargling with water after each inhalation.

QUICK REFERENCE

Drug group Corticosteroid (p.153)
Overdose danger rating Low
Dependence rating Low
Prescription needed Yes
Multi-source suppliers No

INFORMATION FOR USERS

Your drug prescription is tailored for you. Do not alter dosage without checking with your physician.

How taken

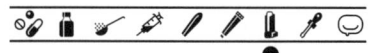

Inhaler, nasal spray.

Frequency and timing of doses
Allergic rhinitis 1 – 2 x daily; *asthma* 2 x daily.

Adult dosage range
Allergic rhinitis 2 sprays into each nostril per dose; *asthma* 100ʹ – 1,000mcg per dose.

Onset of effect
4 – 7 days (asthma); 2 – 3 days (allergic rhinitis).

Duration of action
The effects can last for several days after stopping the drug.

Diet advice
None.

Storage
Keep in a cool, dry place away from reach of children.

Missed dose
Take as soon as you remember.

Stopping the drug
Do not stop the drug without consulting your physician; symptoms may recur. It may be necessary to withdraw the drug gradually.

Exceeding the dose
An occasional unintentional extra dose is unlikely to be a cause for concern. If a large overdose has been taken, notify your physician. Adverse effects may occur if the recommended dose is regularly exceeded over a prolonged period.

SPECIAL PRECAUTIONS

Be sure to tell your physician if:
▼ You have chronic sinusitis.
▼ You have had nasal ulcers or surgery.
▼ You have had tuberculosis or another respiratory infection.
▼ You are taking other medications.

Pregnancy
▼ Safety in pregnancy not established. Discuss with your doctor.

Breast feeding
▼ Safety in breast feeding not established. However, fluticasone is unlikely to pass into breast milk. Discuss with your physician.

Infants and children
▼ Not recommended under 4 years. Reduced dose necessary in older children.

Over 60
▼ No known problems.

Driving and hazardous work
▼ No known problems.

Alcohol
▼ No known problems.

POSSIBLE ADVERSE EFFECTS

Adverse effects are unlikely to occur. The main side effects are irritation of the nasal passages (nasal spray) and fungal infection of the throat and mouth (inhaler).

Symptom/effect	Frequency		Discuss with physician		Stop taking drug now	Call physician now
	Common	Rare	Only if severe	In all cases		
Nasal irritation	●		■			
Nosebleeds		●		■		
Taste/smell disturbances		●	■			
Sore throat/mouth/hoarseness	●			■		
Breathing difficulties		●		■		■

INTERACTIONS

None.

PROLONGED USE

No problems expected. Long-term treatment of children under age 12 is not recommended.

Monitoring Periodic checks to make sure that the adrenal gland is functioning properly may be required if large doses are being taken.

FLUVOXAMINE

Brand name Luvox
Used in the following combined preparations None

GENERAL INFORMATION

Fluvoxamine belongs to a relatively new group of antidepressants called specific serotonin reuptake inhibitors (SSRIs). Drugs of this type tend to cause less sedation and have fewer *anticholinergic side effects* than older antidepressants. Fluvoxamine elevates mood, increases physical activity, and restores interest in everyday life.

Nausea, vomiting, insomnia, headache, and loss of appetite are common adverse effects.

As well as being used to treat the symptoms of depression, fluvoxamine is used to treat the symptoms of obsessive-compulsive disorder (OCD).

QUICK REFERENCE

Drug group Antidepressant (p.96)
Overdose danger rating High
Dependence rating Low
Prescription needed Yes
Multi-source suppliers No

INFORMATION FOR USERS

Your drug prescription is tailored for you. Do not alter dosage without checking with your physician.

How taken

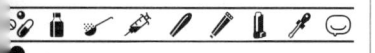

Tablets.

Frequency and timing of doses
1 x daily at bedtime.

Adult dosage range
100 – 300mg daily.

Onset of effect
Some relief from depression has occurred within 4 – 7 days but could take up to 3 weeks.

Duration of action
Effects of fluvoxamine last approximately one day after last dose even if taken for a prolonged period.

Diet advice
None.

Storage
Keep in a tightly closed container in a cool, dry place away from the reach of children. Protect from light.

Missed dose
Take as soon as you remember.

Stopping the drug
Do not stop the drug without consulting your physician, who may supervise a gradual reduction in dosage.

OVERDOSE ACTION

Seek immediate medical advice in all cases. Take emergency action if seizures or loss of consciousness occurs.

See Drug poisoning emergency guide (p.574).

POSSIBLE ADVERSE EFFECTS

Nausea and vomiting are common side effects of fluvoxamine; however, these can be minimized by starting with a low dose and slowly increasing it to the required level.

Symptom/effect	Frequency		Discuss with physician		Stop taking drug now	Call physician now
	Common	Rare	Only if severe	In all cases		
Nausea/vomiting	●			■		
Drowsiness/dizziness	●		■			
Dry mouth/constipation	●		■			
Agitation/insomnia/tremor	●			■		
Headache	●		■			
Loss of appetite	●			■		

INTERACTIONS

Monoamine oxidase inhibitors (MAOIs) Leave at least 14 days between stopping an MAOI and starting fluvoxamine, as serious side effects can occur. Leave 14 days between stopping fluvoxamine and starting an MAOI.

Tryptophan and lithium These drugs may increase the adverse effects of fluvoxamine.

Propranolol, theophylline, phenytoin, and warfarin Fluvoxamine may increase the adverse effects of these drugs.

Sedatives All drugs having a sedative effect on the central nervous system may increase the sedative effects of fluvoxamine.

SPECIAL PRECAUTIONS

Be sure to tell your physician if:
▼ You have impaired liver or kidney function.
▼ You have had epileptic seizures.
▼ You have heart problems.
▼ You are taking other medications.

Pregnancy
▼ Safety in pregnancy not established. Discuss with your physician.

Breast feeding
▼ The drug passes into the breast milk. Discuss with your physician.

Infants and children
▼ Not recommended in patients under 18 years of age.

Over 60
▼ Increased likelihood of adverse effects. Reduced dose may therefore be necessary.

Driving and hazardous work
▼ Avoid such activities until you have learned how the drug affects you; it can cause drowsiness, dizziness, and blurred vision.

Alcohol
▼ Avoid. Alcohol may increase the sedative effects of this drug.

Surgery and general anesthetics
▼ Fluvoxamine may need to be stopped before you have a general anesthetic. Discuss with your physician or dentist before any surgery.

PROLONGED USE

No problems expected. However, fluvoxamine is a new drug and little is known of its long-term effects.

FOSINOPRIL

Brand name Monopril
Used in the following combined preparations None

GENERAL INFORMATION

Fosinopril belongs to the ACE inhibitor group of drugs. It is prescribed to treat hypertension (high blood pressure), achieving its effect by dilating blood vessels. Fosinopril is often given in conjunction with a diuretic to increase its effect.

The first dose of fosinopril may cause a sudden drop in blood pressure. You should therefore be resting at the time of first dose and able to lie down afterward for 2 – 3 hours.

The more common adverse effects, such as dizziness and headache, usually diminish with time. Rashes can also occur during treatment. These usually disappear when the drug is stopped. In some cases they clear up on their own despite continued treatment.

INFORMATION FOR USERS

Your drug prescription is tailored for you. Do not alter dosage without checking with your physician.

How taken

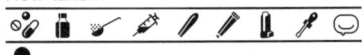

Tablets.

Frequency and timing of doses
1 x daily.

Dosage range
10mg daily (starting dose), increased to 10 – 20mg daily (maintenance dose).

Onset of effect
Within 1 hour.

Duration of action
24 hours.

Diet advice
None.

Storage
Keep in a closed container in a cool, dry place away from reach of children. Protect from light.

Missed dose
Take as soon as you remember. If your next dose is due within 8 hours, do not take the skipped dose. Take your next dose as usual.

Stopping the drug
Do not stop taking the drug without consulting your physician; stopping the drug may lead to worsening of the underlying condition.

Exceeding the dose
An occasional unintentional extra dose is unlikely to cause problems. Large overdoses may cause dizziness or fainting. Notify your physician.

SPECIAL PRECAUTIONS

Be sure to tell your physician if:
▼ You have impaired kidney or liver function.
▼ You have diabetes.
▼ You have an autoimmune disease.
▼ You have coronary artery disease.
▼ You are pregnant or intend to become pregnant.
▼ You are taking other medications.

Pregnancy
▼ Use during pregnancy can cause injury and even death to the developing fetus. Report promptly to your physician if you become pregnant.

Breast feeding
▼ Effect on breast feeding uncertain. Discuss with your physician.

Infants and children
▼ Not recommended.

Over 60
▼ Reduced dose may be necessary.

Driving and hazardous work
▼ Avoid such activities until you have learned how the drug affects you; it can cause dizziness and fainting.

Alcohol
▼ Avoid. Alcohol increases the likelihood of an excessive drop in blood pressure.

Surgery and general anesthetics
▼ Fosinopril treatment may need to be stopped before you have a general anesthetic. Discuss with your physician or dentist before any surgery.

POSSIBLE ADVERSE EFFECTS

The more common adverse effects, such as headache and dizziness, usually diminish with time. The less common effects may also diminish during long-term treatment, but an adjustment in dosage may be necessary.

Symptom/effect	Frequency		Discuss with physician		Stop taking drug now	Call physician now
	Common	Rare	Only if severe	In all cases		
Headache	●		■			
Dizziness	●		■			
Fatigue	●		■			
Cough	●		■			
Diarrhea	●			■		
Nausea/vomiting	●			■		
Fainting		●		■	▲	▮
Swelling of face or tongue		●		■	▲	▮

INTERACTIONS

Antacids interfere with the absorption of fosinopril and may reduce its effectiveness. If needed, take antacids at least 2 hours following fosinopril.

Lithium Fosinopril may increase the level of lithium in the blood, and serious adverse effects from lithium excess may occur.

Potassium supplements and potassium-sparing diuretics Fosinopril may add to the effect of these drugs, leading to raised levels of potassium in the blood.

Antihypertensive drugs are likely to add to the blood pressure-lowering effect of fosinopril.

PROLONGED USE

No problems expected.

Monitoring Periodic tests on blood and urine should be performed.

FUROSEMIDE

Brand names Lasix, Apo-Furosemide, Furoside, Novo-Semide, Uritol
Used in the following combined preparations None

GENERAL INFORMATION

Furosemide is a powerful, short-acting loop diuretic that has been in use for over 25 years. Like other diuretics, it is used to treat the edema (fluid retention) caused by heart failure, kidney disease, or liver cirrhosis. Because it is fast acting, furosemide is often used in emergencies to relieve acute fluid build-up in the lungs. Furosemide is particularly useful for people with impaired kidney function because they do not respond well to thiazide diuretics.

Furosemide increases the loss of potassium, a condition which can result in a wide variety of symptoms. For that reason, supplements of potassium or a potassium-sparing diuretic are often given with this drug.

INFORMATION FOR USERS

Your drug prescription is tailored for you. Do not alter dosage without checking with your physician.

How taken

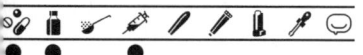

Tablets, oral liquid, injection.

Frequency and timing of doses
1 – 3 x daily.

Adult dosage range
20 – 80mg daily. Dose may be increased considerably if kidney function is impaired.

Onset of effect
Within 1 hour (by mouth); within 5 minutes (injection).

Duration of action
4 – 8 hours (by mouth); 2 hours (injection).

Diet advice
Use of this drug may reduce potassium in the body. Eat plenty of potassium-rich fresh fruit and vegetables (p.162).

Storage
Keep in a closed container in a cool, dry place away from reach of children. Protect from light.

Missed dose
No cause for concern, but take as soon as you remember. However, if it is late in the day do not take the missed dose, or you may need to get up during the night to pass urine. Take the next scheduled dose as usual.

Stopping the drug
Do not stop the drug without consulting your physician; symptoms may recur.

Exceeding the dose
An occasional unintentional extra dose is unlikely to be a cause for concern. But if you notice any unusual symptoms, or if a large overdose has been taken, notify your physician.

SPECIAL PRECAUTIONS

Be sure to tell your physician if:
▼ You have impaired liver or kidney function.
▼ You have gout.
▼ You have diabetes.
▼ You have prostate trouble.
▼ You have hearing problems.
▼ You have had lupus erythematosus.
▼ You are taking other medications.

Pregnancy
▼ Safety in pregnancy not established. Discuss with your physician.

Breast feeding
▼ The drug may reduce milk supply. Discuss with your physician.

Infants and children
▼ Reduced dose necessary.

Over 60
▼ Increased likelihood of adverse effects. Reduced dose may therefore be necessary.

Driving and hazardous work
▼ Avoid these activities until you know how the drug affects you; it can reduce mental alertness.

Alcohol
▼ Keep consumption low. Furosemide increases the likelihood of dehydration and hangovers after the consumption of alcohol.

POSSIBLE ADVERSE EFFECTS

Adverse effects are caused mainly by the rapid fluid loss produced by furosemide. These diminish as the body adjusts to the drug.

Symptom/effect	Frequency		Discuss with physician		Stop taking drug now	Call physician now
	Common	Rare	Only if severe	In all cases		
Dizziness	●		■			
Lethargy		●	■			
Noises in ears (high dose)		●	■			
Cramps		●	■			
Rash		●		■	▲	

PROLONGED USE

Serious problems are unlikely, but levels of salts, such as potassium, sodium, and calcium, may occasionally become depleted during prolonged use.

Monitoring Periodic tests may be performed to check on kidney function and levels of body salts.

INTERACTIONS

Non-steroidal anti-inflammatory drugs (NSAIDs) Some of these drugs may reduce the diuretic effect of furosemide.

Lithium Furosemide may increase the blood level of lithium, leading to an increased risk of lithium poisoning.

Aminoglycoside antibiotics may increase the risk of hearing problems when taken with furosemide.

Cephaloridine Furosemide may increase the risk of kidney damage if given together with cephaloridine.

FUSIDIC ACID

Brand name Fucidin
Used in the following combined preparations None

GENERAL INFORMATION

Fusidic acid, also called sodium fusidate, is an antibiotic. In oral or injection form, it is used mainly to treat serious staphylococcal infections of the skin, skin structures, and bone where other antibiotics have failed (e.g., burns, cystic fibrosis, endocarditis). As a *topical* cream, ointment, or medicated gauze dressing, it is used to treat superficial skin infections, such as impetigo, and infected burns.

Fusidic acid, when given by mouth or injection, must be used with caution in patients with liver impairment since the drug is eliminated from the body mainly via the liver.

INFORMATION FOR USERS

Your drug prescription is tailored for you. Do not alter dosage without checking with your physician.

How taken

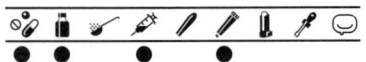

Tablets, oral suspension, injection, ointment, cream, medicated gauze dressing.

Frequency and timing of doses
By mouth and injection 3 x daily.
Skin preparations 3 – 4 x daily.

Dosage range
Adults 1,500 mg daily (by mouth and injection).
Children Reduced dose according to age and weight.

Onset of effect
Within 2 – 4 hours.

Duration of action
Up to 8 hours. Treatment should be continued for 1 to 2 weeks, depending on the type of infection.

Diet advice
None.

Storage
Keep in a closed container in a cool, dry place away from reach of children. Protect from light.

Missed dose
Take a dose (tablet or liquid) as soon as you remember. If your next dose is due within 2 hours, take a single dose now and skip the next, then follow your regular schedule.

Stopping the drug
Take the full course. Even if you feel better, the infection may still be present and symptoms may recur if treatment is stopped too soon.

Exceeding the dose
An occasional unintentional extra dose is unlikely to cause problems. Large overdoses may cause abdominal pain and diarrhea. Notify your physician.

SPECIAL PRECAUTIONS

Be sure to tell your physician if:
▼ You have impaired liver function.
▼ You are taking other medications.

Pregnancy
▼ Safety in pregnancy not established. Discuss with your physician.

Breast feeding
▼ The drug passes into the breast milk. Discuss with your physician.

Infants and children
▼ Reduced dose necessary.

Over 60
▼ Reduced dose may be necessary.

Driving and hazardous work
▼ Avoid such activities until you have learned how the drug affects you; it can cause dizziness and blurred vision.

Alcohol
▼ Avoid. Alcohol may increase the irritative effects of fusidic acid on the liver.

POSSIBLE ADVERSE EFFECTS

Fusidic acid by mouth or injection may cause nausea, vomiting, abdominal pain, and diarrhea. These effects can be lessened if the medication is taken with food.

Symptom/effect	Frequency		Discuss with physician		Stop taking drug now	Call physician now
	Common	Rare	Only if severe	In all cases		
Nausea/vomiting	●		■			
Stomach pain		●		■		
Diarrhea		●	■			
Jaundice		●		■	▲	▐
Skin rashes		●		■	▲	▐
Mild skin irritation (topical)		●	■			

INTERACTIONS

None.

PROLONGED USE

Prolonged ingestion of high doses may produce jaundice and/or abnormal liver function.

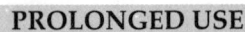

GEMFIBROZIL

Brand names Lopid, Apo-Gemfibrozil
Used in the following combined preparations None

GENERAL INFORMATION

Gemfibrozil is used to lower blood levels of certain types of fats in people with hyperlipidemia and to elevate abnormally low levels of high-density lipoproteins in order to decrease the risk of fatty deposits accumulating in the blood vessels (atherosclerosis). This may help reduce the chance of heart attacks and strokes. With a continued low-fat diet, it is usually given after dietary measures alone have failed to reduce blood fat levels. It is occasionally given with lipid-lowering drugs to treat certain types of inherited hyperlipidemia.

Like similar drugs, gemfibrozil can cause symptoms such as nausea, indigestion, and diarrhea. It is not usually prescribed for people with kidney or liver problems or those with gallstones.

QUICK REFERENCE

Drug group Lipid-lowering drug (p.115)

Overdose danger rating Medium

Dependence rating Low

Prescription needed Yes

Multi-source suppliers Yes

INFORMATION FOR USERS

Your drug prescription is tailored for you. Do not alter dosage without checking with your physician.

How taken

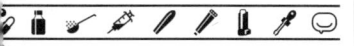

Tablets, capsules.

Frequency and timing of doses
2 daily (morning and evening before meals).

Dosage range
1.2g daily.

Onset of effect
2–5 days. Full beneficial effect may not be felt for several months.

Duration of action
Some effect may last for up to 6 weeks after treatment has stopped.

Diet advice
A low-fat diet is recommended.

Storage
Keep in a closed container in a cool, dry place away from reach of children. Protect from light.

Missed dose
Take as soon as you remember. If your next dose is due within 2 hours, take a single dose now and skip the next.

Stopping the drug
Do not stop taking the drug without consulting your physician; stopping the drug may lead to worsening of the underlying condition.

Exceeding the dose
An occasional unintentional extra dose is unlikely to cause problems. Large overdoses may cause nausea or indigestion. Notify your physician.

POSSIBLE ADVERSE EFFECTS

Gastrointestinal disturbances (especially nausea and diarrhea) and rashes are the most common *side effects* of gemfibrozil. These and other adverse effects are not usually serious and generally go away during treatment. If severe, prolonged abdominal pain and vomiting persist or flu-like symptoms occur, consult your physician.

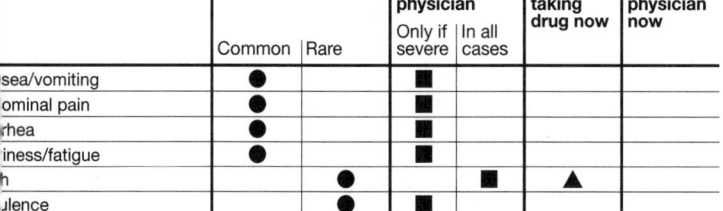

Symptom/effect	Frequency		Discuss with physician		Stop taking drug now	Call physician now
	Common	Rare	Only if severe	In all cases		
Nausea/vomiting	●		■			
Abdominal pain	●		■			
Diarrhea	●		■			
Dizziness/fatigue	●		■			
Rash		●		■	▲	
Flatulence		●	■			
Fever/aching muscles		●		■	▲	

INTERACTIONS

Lipid-lowering drugs Gemfibrozil is not usually given with lipid-lowering statin drugs such as lovastatin or simvastatin because of the risk of severe muscle inflammation.

Oral anticoagulant drugs The effect of these drugs may be increased with gemfibrozil.

SPECIAL PRECAUTIONS

Be sure to tell your physician if:
▼ You have a liver or kidney disorder.
▼ You have gallbladder disease or a history of gallstones.
▼ You have diabetes.
▼ You are taking other medications.

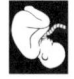
Pregnancy
▼ Not prescribed. The drug should be discontinued several months prior to conception.

Breast feeding
▼ Discontinue breast feeding. The drug passes into the breast milk and may affect the baby adversely.

Infants and children
▼ Not usually prescribed.

Over 60
▼ Reduced dose may be necessary.

Driving and hazardous work
▼ Avoid such activities until you have learned how the drug affects you; it can cause dizziness and blurred vision.

Alcohol
▼ Avoid. Alcohol may reduce the effect of this drug.

PROLONGED USE

The risk of gallstones is increased in people on extended gemfibrozil treatment. The drug may also affect liver function.

Monitoring Regular tests of blood fat levels and liver function may be advised.

GENTAMICIN

Brand names Garamycin, Alcomicin, Cidomycin, Diogent, Garatec, Gentacidin
Used in the following combined preparations Diprogen, Garasone, Valisone-G

GENERAL INFORMATION

Gentamicin is an aminoglycoside antibiotic. Given by injection, it is generally reserved for hospital treatment of serious or complicated infections. These include peritonitis, septicemia, and severe infections of the respiratory and urinary tracts. It is also used with a penicillin for the prevention and treatment of heart valve infections (endocarditis).

Gentamicin is also available as drops and ointments for the treatment of eye and ear infections. Ointment may occasionally be prescribed for infected burns or ulcers.

Development of resistance to the drug, however, is a common problem following treatment with skin preparations.

Gentamicin given by injection can have serious adverse effects on the kidneys and on the ears, leading to damage to the balance mechanism and deafness. Treatment is monitored with care when high doses are needed or when kidney function is poor.

INFORMATION FOR USERS

Your drug prescription is tailored for you. Do not alter dosage without checking with your physician.

How taken

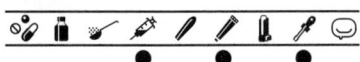

Injection, ointment, eye ointment, cream, eye and ear drops.

Frequency and timing of doses
Every 8 – 24 hours (injection); 3 – 4 x daily (skin preparations); every 6 – 8 hours (eye ointment); every 6 – 8 hours (eye and ear drops).

Adult dosage range
According to condition and response (injection); according to your physician's instructions (eye, ear, and skin preparations).

Onset of effect
Symptoms usually improve within 1 – 3 days, depending on the condition.

Duration of action
8 – 12 hours.

Diet advice
None.

Storage
Keep in closed container in a cool, dry place away from reach of children.

Missed dose
Apply skin, eye, and ear preparations as soon as you remember.

Stopping the drug
Apply the full course. Even if you feel better, the original infection may still be present and may recur if treatment is stopped too soon.

Exceeding the dose
Overdose by injection is unlikely since treatment is carefully monitored. For other preparations, an occasional unintentional extra dose is unlikely to be a cause for concern. If you notice unusual symptoms notify your physician.

SPECIAL PRECAUTIONS

Be sure to tell your physician if:
▼ You have impaired kidney function.
▼ You have a hearing or balance disorder.
▼ You have myasthenia gravis.
▼ You have had a previous allergic reaction to aminoglycosides.
▼ You are taking other medications.

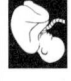

Pregnancy
▼ No evidence of risk with *topical* preparations. Injections are not prescribed, as they cause hearing defects in the baby.

Breast feeding
▼ No evidence of risk with eye, ear, or skin preparations. Given by injection the drug may pass into the breast milk. Discuss with your physician.

Infants and children
▼ Reduced dose necessary for injections.

Over 60
▼ Increased likelihood of adverse effects. Reduced dose may therefore be necessary.

Driving and hazardous work
▼ No known problems from preparations for the skin, eye or ear.

Alcohol
▼ No known problems.

Surgery and general anesthetics
▼ Gentamicin may need to be stopped before you have a general anesthetic.

POSSIBLE ADVERSE EFFECTS

Adverse effects are rare but those that occur with the injectable form may be serious. Dizziness, loss of balance (vertigo), impaired hearing, and changes in the urine should be reported promptly. Allergic reactions, including rash and itching, are symptoms that may occur with all preparations that contain gentamicin.

Symptom/effect	Frequency		Discuss with physician		Stop taking drug now	Call physician now
	Common	Rare	Only if severe	In all cases		
Nausea/vomiting		●	■			
Headache/lethargy		●		■	▲	▌
Dizziness/vertigo		●		■	▲	▌
Rash/itching		●		■	▲	▌
Ringing in the ears		●		■	▲	▌
Loss of hearing		●		■	▲	▌
Bloody, cloudy urine		●		■	▲	▌

INTERACTIONS

General note A wide range of drugs increase the risk of hearing loss and/or kidney failure with gentamicin. Such drugs include other aminoglycoside and polymyxin antibiotics, vancomycin, furosemide, ethacrynic acid, and cisplatin.

PROLONGED USE

Not usually given for longer than 10 days. There is a risk of adverse effects on hearing, balance, and kidney function.

Monitoring Blood levels of the drug are usually checked during injection treatment.

GLICLAZIDE

Brand name Diamicron
Used in the following combined preparations None

GENERAL INFORMATION

Gliclazide is an antidiabetic drug that lowers blood sugar by stimulating insulin secretion from the pancreas. It is used to treat adult (maturity onset) diabetes in conjunction with a balanced diet that limits the intake of carbohydrates and fats and that promotes weight loss. Regular exercise is an essential part of the treatment.

In conditions of severe illness, injury, stress, or surgery, the drug may lose its effectiveness, causing loss of diabetic control and necessitating the use of insulin injections.

QUICK REFERENCE

Drug group Oral antidiabetic drug (p.154)

Overdose danger rating High

Dependence rating Low

Prescription needed Yes

Multi-source suppliers No

INFORMATION FOR USERS

Your drug prescription is tailored for you. Do not alter dosage without checking with your physician.

How taken

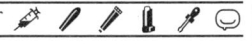

Tablets.

Frequency and timing of doses
2 daily (in the morning and evening with a meal).

Dosage range
40 – 320mg daily.

Onset of effect
Within 1 hour.

Duration of action
12 – 24 hours.

Diet advice
An individualized, low-fat, low-carbohydrate diet must be maintained for the drug to be fully effective. Follow the advice of your physician.

Storage
Keep in a closed container in a cool, dry place away from reach of children.

Missed dose
Take as soon as you remember with the next meal.

Stopping the drug
Do not stop the drug without consulting your physician; stopping the drug may lead to worsening of the underlying condition.

OVERDOSE ACTION

Seek immediate medical advice in all cases. If early warning symptoms of excessively low blood sugar such as faintness, sweating, trembling, confusion, or headache occur, eat or drink something sugary. Take emergency action if seizures or loss of consciousness occurs.

See Drug poisoning emergency guide (p.574).

SPECIAL PRECAUTIONS

Be sure to tell your physician if:
▼ You have or have had a serious trauma or infection recently.
▼ You have impaired liver or kidney function.
▼ You have thyroid problems.
▼ You do not eat properly.
▼ You are planning a pregnancy.
▼ You have Addison's disease.
▼ You are taking other medications.

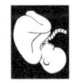

Pregnancy
▼ Not recommended. May cause abnormally low blood sugar in the newborn baby. Insulin is generally substituted in pregnancy because it gives better diabetic control.

Breast feeding
▼ The drug passes into the breast milk and may cause low blood sugar in the baby. Discuss with your physician.

Infants and children
▼ Not prescribed.

Over 60
▼ Signs of low blood sugar may be more difficult to recognize. Reduced dose may be necessary.

Driving and hazardous work
▼ Do not undertake such activities until you know how the drug affects you because it can cause dizziness, drowsiness, and confusion.

Alcohol
▼ Avoid. Alcoholic drinks upset diabetic control and gliclazide may cause intolerance to alcohol.

Surgery and general anesthetics
▼ Notify your physician or dentist that you are diabetic before any type of surgery.

POSSIBLE ADVERSE EFFECTS

Serious adverse effects are rare. Dizziness, confusion, tremors, sweating, and weakness may be signs of low blood sugar due to lack of food or too high a dose of gliclazide.

Symptom/effect	Frequency		Discuss with physician		Stop taking drug now	Call physician now
	Common	Rare	Only if severe	In all cases		
Dizziness/drowsiness/confusion	●			■		
Weakness/lack of energy	●			■		
Tremors/chilliness	●			■		
Sweating/flushing	●			■		
Headache/nervousness	●			■		
Rash/itching		●		■		
Nausea/vomiting/heartburn		●		■		
Thirst		●		■		

INTERACTIONS

General note A variety of drugs may oppose the effect of gliclazide and so may raise blood sugar levels. Such drugs include barbiturates, corticosteroids, birth-control pills, estrogens, diuretics, rifampin, and nicotinic acid.

Other drugs increase the risk of low blood sugar. These include warfarin, ASA, clofibrate, sulfinpyrazone, antituberculosis drugs, sulfonamides, beta blockers, MAO inhibitors, ACE inhibitors, allopurinol, cimetidine, and phenylbutazone.

PROLONGED USE

No problems expected.

Monitoring Regular monitoring of sugar levels in the blood and/or urine is required. Periodic assessment of the eyes, heart, and kidneys may be advised.

GLYBURIDE

Brand names DiaBeta, Euglucon, Apo-Glyburide, Gen-Glybe, Novo-Glyburide
Used in the following combined preparations None

GENERAL INFORMATION

Glyburide is an oral antidiabetic drug. Like other drugs of this class, it stimulates the secretion of insulin from the islet cells in the pancreas and promotes the uptake of sugar into body cells.

It is used in the treatment of adult (maturity-onset) diabetes mellitus in conjunction with a diabetic diet that limits intake of fats and carbohydrates.

Serious adverse effects with glyburide are rare. Unlike some antidiabetic drugs, it has a mild diuretic effect, making it useful for people with a tendency to retain water, such as those with congestive heart failure.

In conditions of severe illness, injury, or stress, the drug may lose its effectiveness in stimulating the pancreas, making insulin injections necessary.

INFORMATION FOR USERS

Your drug prescription is tailored for you. Do not alter dosage without checking with your physician.

How taken

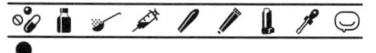

Tablets.

Frequency and timing of doses
Once daily (in the morning) or 2 x daily (in the morning and evening with meals).

Dosage range
2.5 – 20mg daily.

Onset of effect
Within 1 hour.

Duration of action
Approximately 24 hours.

Diet advice
A low-carbohydrate, low-fat diet must be maintained in order for the drug to be fully effective. Follow your physician's advice.

Storage
Keep in a closed container in a cool, dry place away from reach of children.

Missed dose
Take before your next meal.

Stopping the drug
Do not stop taking the drug without consulting your physician; stopping the drug may lead to worsening of your diabetes.

OVERDOSE ACTION

Seek immediate medical advice in all cases. If early warning symptoms of excessively low blood sugar such as faintness, sweating, trembling, confusion, or headache occur, eat or drink something sugary. Take emergency action if seizures or loss of consciousness occurs.

See Drug poisoning emergency guide (p.574).

POSSIBLE ADVERSE EFFECTS

Serious adverse effects are rare. Faintness, sweating, tremor, weakness, and confusion may be signs of low blood sugar due to lack of food or too high a dose of glyburide.

Symptom/effect	Frequency		Discuss with physician		Stop taking drug now	Call physician now
	Common	Rare	Only if severe	In all cases		
Faintness/confusion	●				■	
Weakness/tremor	●				■	
Sweating	●				■	
Nausea/vomiting		●	■			
Thirst		●			■	
Rash/itching		●			■	

INTERACTIONS

General note A variety of drugs may reduce the effect of glyburide and so raise blood sugar levels. Such drugs include corticosteroids, estrogens, diuretics, and rifampin. Other drugs increase the risk of low blood sugar with glyburide. These include warfarin, sulfonamides, salicylates, clofibrate, monoamine oxidase inhibitors (MAOIs), probenecid, and beta blockers.

SPECIAL PRECAUTIONS

Be sure to tell your physician if:
▼ You have impaired liver or kidney function
▼ You are allergic to sulfonamide drugs.
▼ You are taking other medications.

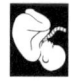

Pregnancy
▼ Not recommended. May cause abnormally low blood sugar in the newborn baby. Insulin is generally substituted in pregnancy because gives better diabetic control.

Breast feeding
▼ The drug passes into the breast milk and may cause low blood sugar in the baby. Discuss with your physician.

Infants and children
▼ Not prescribed.

Over 60
▼ Signs of low blood sugar may more difficult to recognize. Reduced dose may be necessary.

Driving and hazardous work
▼ Usually no problem. Avoid these activities if you have warning signs of low blood sugar.

Alcohol
▼ Avoid. Alcoholic drinks upset diabetic control and glyburide may cause intolerance to alcohol.

Surgery and general anesthetic
▼ Surgery may reduce the response to glyburide. Notify your physician that you are diabetic before any surgery; insulin treatment may need to be substituted.

PROLONGED USE

No problems expected.

Monitoring Regular monitoring of levels of sugar in the urine or blood is required.

GUAIFENESIN

Brand names Robitussin, Balminil Expectorant, Benylin E, Calmylin Expectorant, Resyl
Used in the following combined preparations Benylin DM-E, Entex LA, Formula 44E, Robitussin-DM

GENERAL INFORMATION

Guaifenesin (glyceryl guaiacolate) is the most widely used expectorant. It is claimed to increase the production of phlegm (sputum) in the lungs and to make it easier to expel by coughing. As a result, unproductive (dry) coughs may become more productive and episodes of coughing less frequent.

Unfortunately, the efficacy of guaifenesin in recommended doses is questionable.

Guaifenesin can cause nausea or vomiting, diarrhea, stomach pain, and drowsiness.

INFORMATION FOR USERS

Follow information on the label. Call your physician if symptoms worsen.

How taken

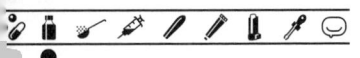

Tablets, syrup.

Frequency and timing of doses
Every 4 hours, with a full glass of water.

Dosage range
Adults and children 12 years and over 200mg per dose to a maximum of 800mg/24 hours; children 6 – 11 years 100mg per dose to a maximum of 400mg/24 hours; 2 – 5 years, 50mg per dose to a maximum of 200mg/24 hours.

Onset of effect
Within a few minutes to an hour.

Duration of action
2 – 4 hours.

Diet advice
None.

Storage
Keep in closed container in a cool, dry place away from reach of children. Protect from light.

Missed dose
No cause for concern. Take your next dose as soon as you remember.

Stopping the drug
Can be safely stopped when symptoms improve.

Exceeding the dose
An occasional unintentional extra dose is unlikely to be a cause for concern. However, larger-than-recommended doses can cause nausea and vomiting.

POSSIBLE ADVERSE EFFECTS

Nausea and vomiting, diarrhea, and drowsiness may occur.

Symptom/effect	Frequency		Discuss with physician		Stop taking drug now	Call physician now
	Common	Rare	Only if severe	In all cases		
Diarrhea		●	■			
Drowsiness		●	■			
Nausea		●	■		▲	
Vomiting		●		■	▲	■

INTERACTIONS

None.

SPECIAL PRECAUTIONS

Be sure to consult your physician or pharmacist before taking this drug if:
▼ You are taking other medications.

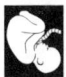

Pregnancy
▼ No evidence of risk to developing baby.

Breast feeding
▼ No evidence of risk.

Infants and children
▼ No special problems in children.

Over 60
▼ No special problems.

Driving and hazardous work
▼ Exercise caution if drowsiness occurs.

Alcohol
▼ No known problems.

PROLONGED USE

Check with your physician if cough persists after medication has been used for 7 days or if high fever, skin rash, continuing headache, or sore throat is present with cough.

HALOPERIDOL

Brand names Haldol, Apo-Haloperidol, Novo-Peridol, Peridol
Used in the following combined preparations None

GENERAL INFORMATION

Introduced in the early 1960s, haloperidol is the most widely used of a group of drugs known as butyrophenones. It is effective in reducing the violent, aggressive manifestations of mental illnesses such as schizophrenia, mania, dementia, and other disorders where hallucinations are experienced. Haloperidol does not cure the underlying disorder, but it does relieve the distressing symptoms. It is also used in the control of Tourette's syndrome and is of benefit in children with severe behavioral problems where other drugs are ineffective.

The main drawback to the use of haloperidol is that it produces disturbing *side effects* – in particular, abnormal, involuntary movements and stiffness of the face and limbs.

INFORMATION FOR USERS

Your drug prescription is tailored for you. Do not alter dosage without checking with your physician.

How taken

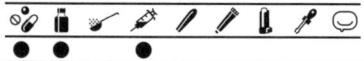

Tablets, oral liquid, injection.

Frequency and timing of doses
1 – 4 x daily with food or milk (by mouth); every 4 weeks (depot injection).

Adult dosage range
2 – 6mg (starting dose), increasing to 12 – 18mg daily (maintenance dose) which may be increased in cases of extreme agitation; 25 – 300mg (depot injection).

Onset of effect
2 – 3 hours (by mouth); within a few days (depot injection).

Duration of action
6 – 24 hours (by mouth). Up to 4 weeks (depot injection).

Diet advice
None.

Storage
Keep in a closed container in a cool, dry place away from reach of children. Protect from light.

Missed dose
Take as soon as you remember. If your next dose is due within 2 hours, take a single dose now and skip the next.

Stopping the drug
Do not stop the drug without consulting your physician; symptoms may recur.

Exceeding the dose
An occasional unintentional extra dose is unlikely to cause problems. Larger overdoses may cause unusual drowsiness, muscle weakness or rigidity, and/or faintness. Notify your physician.

SPECIAL PRECAUTIONS

Be sure to tell your physician if:
▼ You have impaired liver or kidney function.
▼ You have heart or circulation problems.
▼ You have had epileptic seizures.
▼ You have an overactive thyroid gland.
▼ You have Parkinson's disease.
▼ You have had glaucoma.
▼ You have asthma, bronchitis, or another lung disorder.
▼ You are taking other medications.

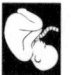

Pregnancy
▼ Safety in pregnancy not established. Discuss with your physician.

Breast feeding
▼ The drug passes into the breast milk. Its effects on the baby are not known. Discuss with your physician.

Infants and children
▼ Rarely required. Reduced dose necessary.

Over 60
▼ Reduced dose may be necessary.

Driving and hazardous work
▼ Avoid such activities until you have learned how the drug affects you; it can cause drowsiness and slowed reactions.

Alcohol
▼ Avoid. Alcohol may increase the sedative effect of this drug.

POSSIBLE ADVERSE EFFECTS

Haloperidol can cause a variety of minor *anticholinergic* symptoms that often become less marked with time. The most significant adverse effect is abnormal movements of the face and limbs (parkinsonism). This may be controlled by dosage adjustment.

Symptom/effect	Frequency		Discuss with physician		Stop taking drug now	Call physician now
	Common	Rare	Only if severe	In all cases		
Drowsiness/lethargy	●		■			
Weight gain	●		■			
Parkinsonism	●			■		
Dizziness/fainting	●			■		
Rash		●		■	▲	
High fever/confusion		●		■	▲	■

INTERACTIONS

Sedatives All drugs, including alcohol, that have sedative effects are likely to increase the sedative properties of haloperidol.

Antiparkinsonism drugs Haloperidol may counter the beneficial effect of such drugs.

Anticholinergic drugs The side effects of drugs with anticholinergic properties may be increased by haloperidol.

Anticonvulsant drugs Dosage may need adjustment.

PROLONGED USE

Use of this drug for more than a few months may lead to *tardive dyskinesia*, i.e., abnormal, involuntary movements of the eyes, face, and tongue. Occasionally, jaundice may occur.

HEPARIN

Brand names Calcilean, Hepalean
Used in the following combined preparation Lipactin

GENERAL INFORMATION

Heparin is an anticoagulant prescribed to prevent and aid in the dispersion of blood clots. Because it acts more quickly than other anticoagulants, it is particularly useful during emergencies – for instance, to prevent the extension of clotting when a clot has already reached the lungs or the brain. People undergoing open heart surgery and kidney dialysis are also given heparin to prevent clotting. A low dose of heparin is sometimes given to elderly, bedridden people after surgery to prevent blood clots from forming in leg veins. Often, heparin is given in conjunction with other slower-acting anticoagulants,

such as warfarin, until they reach their full beneficial effects, usually after a few days. Since it must be injected more than once daily, heparin is not usually given on its own, long term. Its most serious adverse effect, as with all anticoagulants, is the risk of excessive bleeding, usually from overdosage; the ability of the blood to coagulate is watched very carefully under medical supervision. Also, bruising may occur around the site of the injection.

A new form of heparin called low molecular weight (LMW) heparin may be safer and more effective in preventing blood clots after orthopedic surgery.

INFORMATION FOR USERS

This drug is given only under medical supervision and is not for self-administration.

How taken

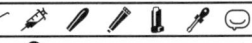

Injection.

Frequency and timing of doses
Every 4 – 12 hours.

Dosage range
Varies according to the condition being treated and individual requirements.

Onset of effect
Within 15 minutes.

Duration of action
12 hours after treatment is stopped.

Diet advice
None.

Storage
Not applicable. This drug is not kept in the home.

Missed dose
Call your physician.

Stopping the drug
Do not stop taking the drug without consulting your physician. Stopping the drug may lead to clotting of blood.

OVERDOSE ACTION

Seek immediate medical advice in all cases. Take emergency action if bleeding, severe headache, or loss of consciousness occurs. Overdose can be reversed under medical supervision by a drug called protamine.

See Drug poisoning emergency guide (p.574).

POSSIBLE ADVERSE EFFECTS

As with all anticoagulants, bleeding is the most common adverse effect with heparin.

The less common effects may occur in long-term treatment.

Symptom/effect	Frequency		Discuss with physician		Stop taking drug now	Call physician now
	Common	Rare	Only if severe	In all cases		
Bleeding/bruising	●			■		▮
Digestive disturbance		●		■		
Aching bones		●		■		
Rash		●		■	▲	

INTERACTIONS

ASA may increase bleeding tendencies. Use only under a physician's direction.

Ethacrynic acid Use of heparin with this drug may increase the risk of gastrointestinal bleeding.

Dipyridamole The anticoagulant effect of heparin may be increased when taken along with this drug.

SPECIAL PRECAUTIONS

Be sure to tell your physician if:
▼ You have impaired liver or kidney function.
▼ You have high blood pressure.
▼ You have stomach ulcers.
▼ You bleed easily.
▼ You have any allergies.
▼ You are taking other medications.

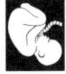

Pregnancy
▼ Careful monitoring is necessary as the drug may cause the mother to bleed excessively if taken near delivery. Discuss with your physician.

Breast feeding
▼ No evidence of risk.

Infants and children
▼ Reduced dose necessary according to age and weight.

Over 60
▼ Reduced dose may be necessary, especially in women.

Driving and hazardous work
▼ Avoid risk of injury, since excessive bruising and bleeding may occur.

Alcohol
▼ No special problems.

Surgery and general anesthetics
▼ Heparin may need to be stopped. Discuss this with your physician or dentist.

PROLONGED USE

Osteoporosis and hair loss may occur; tolerance to heparin may develop.

Monitoring Periodic blood checks will be required.

HUMAN CHORIONIC GONADOTROPIN

Brand names A.P.L., Profasi HP
Used in the following combined preparations None

GENERAL INFORMATION

Human chorionic gonadotropin (HCG) is produced by the placentas of pregnant women and is extracted from their urine. This hormone is used for several purposes.

Its principal value is in the treatment of female infertility. Given by injection, usually with another hormone, HCG stimulates the ovaries to release eggs (ovulate) so that they can be fertilized. Ovulation usually occurs 18 hours after injection, and intercourse should follow within 48 hours. HCG increases the likelihood of multiple births.

It is occasionally used to prevent miscarriage in women who have lost previous pregnancies. The drug is sometimes given to young boys to treat undescended testicles.

In rare cases, HCG is given to men to improve the production of sperm, which can take six to nine months of treatment.

QUICK REFERENCE

Drug group Drug for infertility (p.176)

Overdose danger rating Low

Dependence rating Low

Prescription needed Yes

Multi-source suppliers Yes

INFORMATION FOR USERS

This drug is only given under medical supervision and is not for self-administration.

How taken

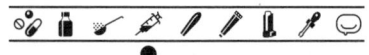

Injection.

Frequency and timing of doses
Every 2 – 3 days.

Dosage range
Dosage varies from person to person, and may need adjustment during treatment.

Onset of effect
1 – 8 days (female infertility); 6 – 9 months (male infertility).

Duration of action
2 – 3 days.

Diet advice
None.

Storage
Not applicable. This drug is not kept in the home.

Missed dose
Arrange to receive the missed dose as soon as possible. Delay of more than 24 hours may reduce the chance of conception.

Stopping the drug
Complete the course of treatment as directed. Stopping the drug prematurely will reduce the chance of conception.

Exceeding the dose
The drug is always injected under close medical supervision. Overdose is unlikely.

SPECIAL PRECAUTIONS

Be sure to tell your physician if:
▼ You have had a previous allergic reaction to this drug.
▼ You have prostate trouble.
▼ You have impaired kidney function.
▼ You have asthma.
▼ You have had seizures.
▼ You suffer from migraine.
▼ You have a heart disorder.
▼ You are taking other medications.

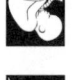

Pregnancy
▼ Not prescribed.

Breast feeding
▼ Not prescribed.

Infants and children
▼ HCG is safely prescribed to treat undescended testicles in boys.

Over 60
▼ Not usually required.

Driving and hazardous work
▼ Avoid such activities until you have learned how the drug affects you; it can cause tiredness.

Alcohol
▼ Avoid. Alcohol increases the likelihood of tiredness, and taken in excess may reduce fertility.

POSSIBLE ADVERSE EFFECTS

When taken for fertility problems, the more common adverse effects of HCG are rarely severe and tend to diminish with time.

Women who take large doses of the drug may experience abdominal pain or swelling due to overstimulation of the ovaries.

Symptom/effect	Frequency		Discuss with physician		Stop taking drug now	Call physician now
	Common	Rare	Only if severe	In all cases		
Headache/tiredness	●		■			
Pain at injection site	●		■			
Mood changes	●			■		
Women only						
Swollen feet/ankles		●		■		
Abdominal pain		●		■		
Men only						
Enlarged breasts		●		■	▲	

INTERACTIONS

None.

PROLONGED USE

No special problems.

Monitoring Women taking HCG to improve fertility usually have regular pelvic examinations and checks on cervical mucus to confirm that ovulation is taking place. Men are given regular sperm counts.

HYDRALAZINE

rand names Apresoline, Apo-Hydralazine, Novo-Hylazin, Nu-Hydral
sed in the following combined preparations None

GENERAL INFORMATION

ydralazine was introduced in 1952 for se as an antihypertensive drug. It is a asodilator (see p.110), i.e., a drug that laxes the muscles of the artery walls d dilates blood vessels. It is used ost often to treat moderate to severe gh blood pressure.

Hydralazine is usually given orally, ten together with a diuretic and/or a eta blocker. When given by injection,

hydralazine has a rapid onset of action. This makes the injectable form particularly useful in emergencies.

The most serious adverse effect is the possibility of drug-induced lupus erythematosus, an autoimmune illness which occurs only with long-term treatment in high doses and usually disappears when the drug is withdrawn.

QUICK REFERENCE

Drug group Antihypertensive drug (p.114)

Overdose danger rating High

Dependence rating Low

Prescription needed Yes

Multi-source suppliers Yes

INFORMATION FOR USERS

ur prescription is tailored for you. Do t alter dosage without checking with ur physician.

ow taken

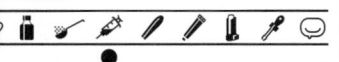

blets, injection.

equency and timing of doses
4 x daily (tablets).

ult dosage range
– 200mg daily, up to a maximum of 300mg ly.

set of effect
minutes – 2 hours (tablets); 10 – 20 minutes ection).

ration of action
8 hours (tablets); 2 – 4 hours (injection).

t advice
ne.

Storage
Keep in a closed container in a cool, dry place away from reach of children.

Missed dose
Take as soon as you remember. If your next dose is due within 2 hours, take a single dose now and skip the next.

Stopping the drug
Do not stop the drug without consulting your physician; stopping the drug may lead to worsening of the underlying condition.

OVERDOSE ACTION

Seek immediate medical advice in all cases. Take emergency action if severe nausea and vomiting, rapid heartbeat, or loss of consciousness occurs.

See Drug poisoning emergency guide (p.574).

POSSIBLE ADVERSE EFFECTS

ny of the common adverse effects inish during long-term treatment.

Dizziness usually occurs when you get up: rising slowly will help.

Symptom/effect	Frequency		Discuss with physician		Stop taking drug now	Call physician now
	Common	Rare	Only if severe	In all cases		
sea/vomiting	●		■			
dache	●		■			
ziness	●		■			
id heartbeat	●			■		
s of appetite		●		■		
h		●		■		
hing		●		■		
t pain		●		■		

INTERACTIONS

cyclic antidepressants and onoamine oxidase inhibitors (MAOIs) ay increase the effects of hydralazine.

SPECIAL PRECAUTIONS

Be sure to tell your physician if:
▼ You have impaired liver or kidney function.
▼ You have heart disease.
▼ You have had a stroke.
▼ You have had lupus erythematosus.
▼ You tend to be allergic.
▼ You are taking other medications.

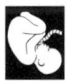

Pregnancy
▼ Sometimes used in an emergency to control very high blood pressure in severe pre-eclampsia (toxemia). Discuss with your physician.

Breast feeding
▼ The drug passes into the breast milk, but at normal doses adverse effects on the baby are unlikely. Discuss with your physician.

Infants and children
▼ Not usually prescribed. Reduced dose necessary.

Over 60
▼ Reduced dose may be necessary.

Driving and hazardous work
▼ Avoid such activities until you have learned how the drug affects you; it can cause dizziness.

Alcohol
▼ Avoid. Alcohol may increase the adverse effects of this drug.

PROLONGED USE

Lupus erythematosus, an autoimmune illness, may occur with prolonged use. This usually disappears when the drug is withdrawn.

Monitoring Periodic blood checks should be performed.

HYDROCHLOROTHIAZIDE

Brand names HydroDiuril, Apo-Hydro, Neo-Codema, Novo-Hydrazide, Urozide
Used in the following combined preparations Aldactazide, Aldoril, Dyazide, Moduret, Prinzide, Vaseretic

GENERAL INFORMATION

Hydrochlorothiazide belongs to the thiazide group of diuretic drugs, which remove excess salt and water from the body and reduce edema (fluid retention) in people with congestive heart failure and cirrhosis of the liver.

Hydrochlorothiazide is frequently used to treat high blood pressure (see Antihypertensive drugs, p.114), and because it reduces the amount of calcium in the urine, it may sometimes be used to prevent the recurrence of certain types of kidney stones.

As with all thiazides, hydrochloro-thiazide increases the loss of potassium in the urine, which, can result in a variety of symptoms (see p.524), and increases the likelihood of irregular heart rhythms, particularly if you are taking drugs such as digoxin for heart failure. Potassium supplements may be prescribed along with it.

INFORMATION FOR USERS

Your prescription is tailored for you. Do not alter dosage without checking with your physician.

How taken

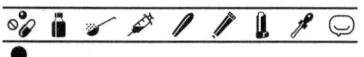

Tablets.

Frequency and timing of doses
Once daily, or every 2 days, early in the day.

Adult dosage range
25 – 100mg daily.

Onset of effect
Within 2 hours.

Duration of action
6 – 12 hours.

Diet advice
Use of this drug may reduce potassium in the body. Eat plenty of fresh fruits and vegetables.

Discuss the advisability of reducing your salt intake with your physician.

Storage
Keep in a closed container in a cool, dry place away from reach of children.

Missed dose
No cause for concern, but take as soon as you remember. However, if it is late in the day do not take the missed dose, or you may have to get up during the night to pass urine. Take the next scheduled dose as usual.

Stopping the drug
Do not stop the drug without consulting your physician; symptoms may recur.

Exceeding the dose
An occasional unintentional extra dose is unlikely to be a cause for concern. But if you notice any unusual symptoms, or if a large overdose has been taken, notify your physician.

SPECIAL PRECAUTIONS

Be sure to tell your physician if:
▼ You have impaired liver or kidney function
▼ You have had gout.
▼ You have diabetes.
▼ You have had lupus erythematosus.
▼ You have a high level of fat in your blood.
▼ You are allergic to sulfonamide drugs.
▼ You are taking other medications.

Pregnancy
▼ Not usually prescribed. May cause jaundice in the newborn baby. Discuss with your physician.

Breast feeding
▼ The drug passes into the breast milk, but at normal doses adverse effects on the baby are unlikely. Discuss with your physician.

Infants and children
▼ Not usually prescribed. Reduced dose necessary.

Over 60
▼ Increased likelihood of adverse effects.

Driving and hazardous work
▼ No special problems, though morning urinary frequency can be anticipated.

Alcohol
▼ Keep consumption low. Hydrochlorothiazide increases the likelihood of dehydration and hangovers after consumption of alcohol.

POSSIBLE ADVERSE EFFECTS

Most effects are caused by excessive loss of potassium. This can usually be put right by taking a potassium supplement. In rare cases gout may occur in susceptible people, and certain forms may become more difficult to control.

Symptom/effect	Frequency		Discuss with physician		Stop taking drug now	Call physician now
	Common	Rare	Only if severe	In all cases		
Leg cramps	●		■			
Lethargy		●	■			
Dizziness		●	■			
Digestive disturbance		●	■			
Temporary impotence		●	■			
Rash		●		■	▲	

INTERACTIONS

Non-steroidal anti-inflammatory drugs (NSAIDs) Some of these drugs may reduce the diuretic effect of hydrochloro-thiazide, whose dosage may need to be adjusted.

Digoxin Adverse effects may be increased if excessive potassium is lost.

Corticosteroids These drugs further increase the loss of potassium from the body when taken with hydrochlorothiazide.

Lithium Hydrochlorothiazide may increase lithium levels in the blood, leading to a risk of serious adverse effects.

PROLONGED USE

Excessive loss of potassium and imbalances of other salts may result.

Monitoring Blood tests may be performed periodically to check kidney function and levels of potassium and other salts.

HYDROCODONE

Brand names Hycodan, Robidone
Used in the following combined preparations Hycomine, Mercodol w/Decapryn, Novahistex DH, Novahistine DH, Tussionex

GENERAL INFORMATION

Hydrocodone is a narcotic antitussive (cough suppressant) drug with a pronounced sedative effect. It is used on its own or in a combined preparation with other drugs (for example, decongestants and antihistamines) to suppress troublesome dry coughs when non-narcotic cough suppressants have not been effective.

Like other narcotic drugs, hydrocodone can be constipating. It may also depress breathing and is therefore unsuitable for people with asthma or emphysema.

Hydrocodone may produce euphoria and has the potential to cause psychological and physical dependence if used in larger-than-recommended doses over an extended period of time. It is therefore recommended only for short-term treatment.

INFORMATION FOR USERS

Your drug prescription is tailored for you. Do not alter dosage without checking with your physician.

How taken

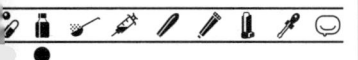

Tablets, oral liquid.

Frequency and timing of doses
3 - 4 times daily with food or milk.

Adult dosage range
5 - 15mg, not to exceed 30mg daily.

Onset of effect
10 – 30 minutes.

Duration of action
4 hours.

Diet advice
None.

Storage
Keep in a closed container in a cool, dry place away from reach of children. Protect from light.

Missed dose
Take as soon as you remember. Adjust the timing of subsequent doses accordingly.

Stopping the drug
Can be safely stopped following short-term treatment.

OVERDOSE ACTION

Seek immediate medical advice in all cases. Take emergency action if there are symptoms such as slow or irregular breathing, severe drowsiness, or loss of consciousness.

See Drug poisoning emergency guide (p.574).

POSSIBLE ADVERSE EFFECTS

All narcotic drugs can produce a variety of adverse effects; these are more frequent in children and older persons.

Symptom/effect	Frequency		Discuss with physician		Stop taking drug now	Call physician now
	Common	Rare	Only if severe	In all cases		
Constipation	●		■			
Drowsiness/dizziness	●		■			
Nausea/vomiting		●		■		
Slow respiration		●		■	▲	▮
Slow heartbeat		●		■	▲	▮
Confusion		●		■	▲	

INTERACTIONS

Sedatives All drugs, including alcohol, that have a sedative effect on the central nervous system are likely to increase sedation with hydrocodone. Such drugs include antidepressants, antipsychotics, sleeping drugs, and antihistamines.

Monoamine oxidase inhibitors (MAOIs) Hydrocodone may interact with these drugs to cause a dangerous rise in blood pressure.

SPECIAL PRECAUTIONS

Be sure to tell your physician if:
▼ You have impaired liver or kidney function.
▼ You have a heart or a circulatory disorder.
▼ You have a lung disorder such as asthma, bronchitis, or emphysema.
▼ You have thyroid disease.
▼ You are taking other medications.

 **Pregnancy**
▼ Safety in pregnancy not established. Discuss with your physician.

 Breast feeding
▼ The drug passes into the breast milk and may affect the baby. Discuss with your physician.

 Infants and children
▼ Reduced dose necessary.

 Over 60
▼ Increased likelihood of adverse effects. Reduced dose necessary.

 Driving and hazardous work
▼ Avoid such activities until you have learned how the drug affects you; it can cause dizziness, drowsiness, or blurred vision.

 Alcohol
▼ Avoid. Alcohol may increase the sedative effects of hydrocodone.

PROLONGED USE

If hydrocodone has been taken in large doses and/or over a long period of time, withdrawal symptoms are likely to occur upon stopping the drug abruptly.

HYDROCORTISONE

Brand names Cortef, Cortate, Cortenema, Emo-Cort, Solu-Cortef, Texacort
Used in the following combined preparations Anusol-HC, Coly-Mycin Otic, Cortisporin, Neo-Cortef, Vioform Hydrocortisone

GENERAL INFORMATION

Hydrocortisone is chemically identical to the hormone cortisol that is produced by the adrenal glands. One use of the drug is in the replacement of natural hormones in adrenal insufficiency (Addison's disease).

Hydrocortisone, however, is mainly used in treating a variety of allergic and inflammatory conditions. Used in *topical* preparations, it provides prompt relief from inflammation of the skin, eye, and outer ear. It is used in oral form to relieve asthma, inflammatory bowel disease, and many other rheumatic and allergic disorders. Injected directly into the joints, it relieves pain and stiffness (see p.130). Injections may also be given to relieve severe attacks of asthma.

Overuse of hydrocortisone skin preparations can rarely lead to permanent thinning of the skin. Long-term treatment with high doses taken by mouth may cause serious *side effects.*

QUICK REFERENCE

Drug group Corticosteroid (p.153)

Overdose danger rating Low

Dependence rating Low

Prescription needed Yes
Creams, lotions, and ointments of 0.5 per cent or less are available without a prescription in pharmacies.

Multi-source suppliers Yes

INFORMATION FOR USERS

Your drug prescription is tailored for you. Do not alter dosage without checking with your physician.

How taken

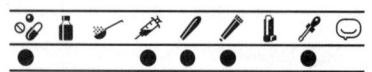

Tablets, injection, rectal suppositories, rectal foam, enema, lotion, ointment, cream, eye/ear drops.

Frequency and timing of doses
Wide variation according to preparation and condition. Follow your physician's instructions.

Dosage range
Wide variation according to preparation and condition. Follow your physician's instructions.

Onset of effect
Within 1 – 4 days.

Duration of action
Up to 12 hours.

Diet advice
Salt intake may need to be restricted when the drug is taken by mouth. It may also be necessary to take potassium supplements.

Storage
Keep in a closed container in a cool, dry place away from the reach of children.

Missed dose
Take as soon as you remember. If your next dose is due within 2 hours, take a single dose now and skip the next.

Stopping the drug
Do not stop the drug without consulting your physician. A gradual reduction in dosage is required following prolonged treatment with oral hydrocortisone.

Exceeding the dose
An occasional unintentional extra dose is unlikely to be cause for concern. But if you notice unusual symptoms, or if a large overdose has been taken, notify your physician.

SPECIAL PRECAUTIONS

Be sure to tell your physician if:
▼ You have had a peptic ulcer.
▼ You have suffered from depression or a mental illness.
▼ You have glaucoma.
▼ You have had tuberculosis.
▼ You have any infection.
▼ You have diabetes.
▼ You are taking other medications.

Pregnancy
▼ No evidence of risk with topical preparations. Oral doses may adversely affect the developing baby. Discuss with your physician.

Breast feeding
▼ The drug passes into the breast milk and may affect the baby. Discuss with your physician.

Infants and children
▼ Reduced dose necessary.

Over 60
▼ Reduced dose may be necessary.

Driving and hazardous work
▼ No special problems, but you may suffer from blurred vision if you are using eye drops.

Alcohol
▼ Avoid. Alcohol may increase the risk of peptic ulcer when this drug is taken by mouth.

POSSIBLE ADVERSE EFFECTS

The most serious adverse effects only occur when hydrocortisone is taken by mouth in high doses for long periods of time. These are carefully monitored during treatment.

Symptom/effect	Frequency		Discuss with physician		Stop taking drug now	Call physician now
	Common	Rare	Only if severe	In all cases		
Indigestion	●		■			
Weight gain	●		■			
Acne	●		■			
Fluid retention		●			■	
Muscle weakness		●			■	
Mood changes		●			■	

INTERACTIONS (by mouth or injection only)

Barbiturates, phenytoin, and rifampin may reduce the effectiveness of hydrocortisone.

Antidiabetic and antihypertensive drugs Hydrocortisone decreases the action of these drugs.

Diuretics Hydrocortisone may increase potassium loss.

Vaccines Hydrocortisone can interact with some vaccines. Discuss with your physician.

PROLONGED USE

Depending on method of administration, prolonged high dosage may cause adverse effects such as diabetes, glaucoma, fragile bones, and thin skin, and may retard growth in children.

Monitoring Periodic checks on blood pressure are usually required when the drug is taken by mouth.

HYDROMORPHONE

rand names Dilaudid, PMS-Hydromorphone
sed in the following combined preparations None

GENERAL INFORMATION

ydromorphone is chemically related
morphine. Small doses produce
fective relief of acute and chronic
ain. The onset of relief is faster
ter injections than after oral doses.
ydromorphone is used to relieve
vere pain and anxiety following
rgery, heart attacks, severe
uries, and in painful diseases
ch as cancer. The drug causes some
gree of drowsiness, although

this is usually not pronounced.
It is habit-forming: dependence and
addiction occur with repeated use,
although this effect should not be used
to justify low or infrequent doses if the
drug is being used to control chronic
pain, such as that associated
with cancer. When used for short
periods of time for acute pain, most
patients can stop taking the drug
without difficulty.

QUICK REFERENCE

Drug group Narcotic analgesic
(p.92)

Overdose danger rating High

Dependence rating High

Prescription needed Yes (no
repeats)

Multi-source suppliers Yes

INFORMATION FOR USERS

ur drug prescription is tailored for you.
not alter dosage without checking
th your physician.

w taken

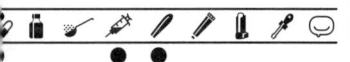

lets, injection, rectal suppositories.

equency and timing of doses
ry 4–6 hours (tablets, injection). Doses by
tal suppository are required less frequently.

ult dosage range
4mg per dose (tablets); 3mg per dose
tal suppository). Dosage by injection varies
siderably between individuals.

set of effect
nin 30 minutes (tablets); within 15 minutes
ction).

ration of action
6 hours.

t advice
elieve constipation, increase intake of
ds and high fiber foods.

Storage
Keep in a closed container in a cool, dry place
that is well secured and away from reach of
children.

Missed dose
Take as soon as you remember. Return to your
normal dosing schedule as soon as possible.

Stopping the drug
If the reason for taking the drug no longer
exists, you may stop taking the drug after
notifying your physician.

OVERDOSE ACTION

 Seek immediate medical advice
in all cases. Take emergency
action if there are symptoms
such as slow or irregular
breathing, severe drowsiness,
loss of consciousness, or slow
or irregular pulse.

**See Drug poisoning
emergency guide (p.574).**

SPECIAL PRECAUTIONS

Be sure to tell your physician if:
▼ You have impaired liver or kidney function.
▼ You have heart or circulatory problems.
▼ You have a lung disorder such as asthma,
bronchitis, or emphysema.
▼ You have thyroid disease.
▼ You are taking other medications.

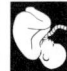 **Pregnancy**
▼ Not recommended. Taken near
the time of delivery, the drug may
cause breathing difficulties in the
newborn baby. Discuss with your
physician.

 Breast feeding
▼ Low levels of narcotic analgesics
have been detected in human milk,
and may affect the baby adversely.
Discuss with your physician.

 Infants and children
▼ Not recommended.

 Over 60
▼ Increased likelihood of adverse
effects. Reduced dose may
therefore be necessary.

 Driving and hazardous work
▼ Persons receiving
hydromorphone are unlikely to be
well enough to undertake such
activities.

 Alcohol
▼ Avoid. Alcohol increases the
sedative effect of hydromorphone.

POSSIBLE ADVERSE EFFECTS

with other narcotics, hydromorphone may
duce nausea, vomiting, dizziness, somno-

lence, loss of appetite, and constipation.
Dosage adjustments may lessen some effects.

nptom/effect	Frequency		Discuss with physician		Stop taking drug now	Call physician now
	Common	Rare	Only if severe	In all cases		
ation	●		■			
stipation	●		■			
sea/vomiting	●			■		
iness/lightheadedness	●			■		
ezing/difficult breathing		●		■	▲	■
fusion/vivid dreams		●		■		

INTERACTIONS

datives Hydromorphone increases the
dative properties of all drugs that have a
dative effect. Such drugs include
ohol, antidepressants, antipsychotics,
eping drugs, and antihistamines.

Monoamine oxidase inhibitors (MAOIs)
may produce a severe rise in blood
pressure when taken with hydromorphone.

PROLONGED USE

The effects of hydromorphone usually
become weaker during prolonged use as
the body adapts. This is known as
tolerance. Other effects of long-term use
include dependence (addiction), sexual
impotence, and loss of sexual desire.

HYDROXYZINE

Brand names Atarax, Apo-Hydroxyzine, Multipax, Novo-Hydroxyzin
Used in the following combined preparations None

GENERAL INFORMATION

Hydroxyzine is an antihistamine drug. It is useful for relieving the itch from allergic skin conditions such as chronic rashes and urticaria (hives). It also has anti-emetic properties and is used to control nausea and vomiting (see Anti-emetic drugs, p.102). Hydroxyzine is occasionally prescribed as an anti-

anxiety drug (p.95). However, although it is most successful in treating mild tension and anxiety, long-term use of this drug is not recommended. The main *side effect* from treatment with hydroxyzine is mild drowsiness. This often subsides after a few days.

QUICK REFERENCE

Drug group Antihistamine (p.136)
Overdose danger rating Medium
Dependence rating Low
Prescription needed Yes
Multi-source suppliers Yes

INFORMATION FOR USERS

Your drug prescription is tailored for you. Do not alter dosage without checking with your physician.

How taken

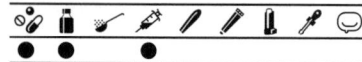

Capsules, oral liquid, injection.

Frequency and timing of doses
3 – 4 x daily.

Dosage range
By mouth 75 – 400mg daily (adults);
50 – 100mg daily (children over 6 years);
30 – 50 mg daily (children under 6 years).
Injection as prescribed.

Onset of effect
15 – 30 minutes.

Duration of action
4 – 6 hours.

Diet advice
None.

Storage
Keep in a closed container in a cool, dry place away from the reach of children.

Missed dose
Take as soon as you remember. If your next dose is due within 3 hours, take a single dose now and skip the next.

Stopping the drug
Do not stop the drug without consulting your physician. Symptoms may recur.

Exceeding the dose
An occasional unintentional extra dose is unlikely to cause problems. Larger overdoses may cause unusual drowsiness. Notify your physician.

SPECIAL PRECAUTIONS

Be sure to tell your physician if:
▼ You have impaired liver or kidney function
▼ You have had epileptic seizures.
▼ You have glaucoma.
▼ You have Parkinson's disease.
▼ You are taking other medications.

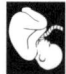

Pregnancy
▼ Contraindicated in early pregnancy. May affect the baby adversely. Discuss with your physician.

Breast feeding
▼ Effect on breast feeding uncertain. Discuss with your physician.

Infants and children
▼ Reduced dose necessary.

Over 60
▼ Reduced dose may be necessary. Increased likelihood of adverse effects.

Driving and hazardous work
▼ Avoid such activities until you have learned how the drug affects you; it can reduce alertness.

Alcohol
▼ Avoid. Alcohol may increase the sedative effects of this drug.

POSSIBLE ADVERSE EFFECTS

When hydroxyzine is used as an anti-emetic or anti-anxiety drug, the possibility of adverse effects is low. The most common symptoms are related to its *anticholinergic* properties and

include drowsiness and dry mouth. Such symptoms may be overcome by an adjustment of dosage or may pass after a few days of usage.

Symptom/effect	Frequency		Discuss with physician		Stop taking drug now	Call physician now
	Common	Rare	Only if severe	In all cases		
Drowsiness	●		■			
Dry mouth		●	■			
Tremor		●		■		
Rash		●		■	▲	

INTERACTIONS

Sedatives All drugs, including alcohol, that have a sedative effect on the central nervous system are likely to increase the sedative properties of hydroxyzine. Such

drugs include anti-anxiety drugs, sleeping drugs, antidepressants, and antipsychotics. This drug should not be taken with barbiturates or narcotic analgesics.

PROLONGED USE

Hydroxyzine is not usually prescribed for prolonged periods.

Discontinue antihistamines approximately 48 hours before allergy skin testing.

IBUPROFEN

Brand names Motrin, Actiprofen, Advil, Apo-Ibuprofen, Medipren, Novo-Profen
Used in the following combined preparation Advil Cold & Sinus

GENERAL INFORMATION

Ibuprofen, introduced in 1972, is a non-steroidal anti-inflammatory drug (NSAID) used to relieve the pain, stiffness, and inflammation that may accompany a number of disorders. It is similar to ASA in the way it works and in the way it can be used. Because it acts as an analgesic as well as an anti-inflammatory, it is an effective treatment for the symptoms of rheumatoid arthritis and osteoarthritis. It also relieves mild to moderate discomfort of headache, menstrual pain, pain from soft tissue injuries, and pain following operations. Sometimes, ibuprofen is given along with slower-acting drugs in the treatment of rheumatoid arthritis.

Ibuprofen has fewer *side effects* than many of the other non-steroidal anti-inflammatory drugs.

INFORMATION FOR USERS

Your drug prescription is tailored for you. Do not alter dosage without checking with your physician.

How taken

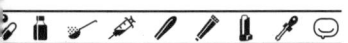

Tablets, capsules.

Frequency and timing of doses
3 – 6 x daily (general pain relief); 3 – 4 x daily with food (arthritis).

Adult dosage range
600mg – 1.2g daily (general pain relief); 1.6 – 2.4g daily (arthritis).

Onset of effect
Pain relief begins in 30 minutes – 2 hours. Full anti-inflammatory effect in arthritic conditions may not be felt for up to 2 weeks.

Duration of action
8 – 10 hours.

Diet advice
None.

Storage
Keep in a closed container in a cool, dry place away from reach of children.

Missed dose
Take as soon as you remember. If your next dose is due within 2 hours, take a single dose now and skip the next.

Stopping the drug
When taken for short-term pain relief, ibuprofen can be safely stopped as soon as you no longer need it. If prescribed for the long-term treatment of arthritis, however, you should seek medical advice before stopping the drug.

Exceeding the dose
An occasional unintentional extra dose is unlikely to be a cause for concern. But if you notice unusual symptoms, or if a large overdose has been taken, notify your physician.

POSSIBLE ADVERSE EFFECTS

The most common adverse effects are the result of gastrointestinal disturbances. Black or bloodstained feces should be reported to your physician without delay.

Symptom/effect	Frequency		Discuss with physician		Stop taking drug now	Call physician now
	Common	Rare	Only if severe	In all cases		
nausea/vomiting	●			■		
diarrhea/constipation	●			■		
heartburn/indigestion			●	■		
dizziness/nervousness			●	■		
headache			●	■		
rash			●	■	▲	
wheezing/breathlessness			●	■	▲	
black/bloodstained feces			●	■	▲	■

INTERACTIONS

General note Ibuprofen interacts with a wide range of drugs to increase the risk of bleeding and/or peptic ulcers. Such drugs include oral anticoagulants, corticosteroids, other non-steroidal anti-inflammatory drugs (NSAIDs), and ASA.

Digoxin Blood levels of digoxin may be increased with ibuprofen.

Lithium Ibuprofen may raise blood levels of lithium, leading to a risk of serious adverse effects.

Antihypertensive drugs and diuretics The beneficial effects of these drugs may be reduced by ibuprofen.

SPECIAL PRECAUTIONS

Be sure to tell your physician if:
▼ You have impaired kidney function.
▼ You have heart problems.
▼ You have high blood pressure.
▼ You have had a peptic ulcer, esophagitis, or acid indigestion.
▼ You are allergic to ASA.
▼ You have asthma.
▼ You are taking other medications.

Pregnancy
▼ Safety in pregnancy not established. Discuss with your physician.

Breast feeding
▼ No evidence of risk.

Infants and children
▼ Not recommended for children under 12 years.

Over 60
▼ Increased likelihood of adverse effects. Reduced dose may therefore be necessary.

Driving and hazardous work
▼ Avoid such activities until you have learned how the drug affects you; it can cause dizziness.

Alcohol
▼ Avoid. Alcohol may increase the risk of stomach disorders with ibuprofen.

Surgery and general anesthetics
▼ Ibuprofen may prolong bleeding. Discuss with your physician or dentist before any surgery.

PROLONGED USE

There is an increased risk of bleeding from peptic ulcers and in the bowel with prolonged use of ibuprofen.

IDOXURIDINE

Brand names Herplex, Herplex-D
Used in the following combined preparations None

GENERAL INFORMATION

Idoxuridine is a *topically* applied drug that is often effective against certain viral infections. As eye drops or ointment, it is used to treat herpes simplex infections of the inner eyelids or the cornea of the eye. Idoxuridine may also be used on infected areas of skin; it may give some relief when used locally for shingles.

For superficial eye infections, idoxuridine is not normally used in combination with corticosteroids because these drugs may accelerate the spread of a viral infection. If such combination therapy is judged necessary for deep infections or in cases complicated by iritis or corneal edema, it is employed with caution under close medical supervision by a specialist. Antibiotics are used with idoxuridine to control bacterial infections. Idoxuridine does not reverse damage to the eye that has resulted from an infection that has already occurred.

Serious adverse effects are rare with idoxuridine, but the risk of eye damage is increased with prolonged treatment or overuse. Courses of treatment longer than 21 days are not usually recommended.

QUICK REFERENCE

Drug group Antiviral drug (p.145)
Overdose danger rating Low
Dependence rating Low
Prescription needed Yes
Multi-source suppliers No

INFORMATION FOR USERS

Your drug prescription is tailored for you. Do not alter your dosage without checking with your physician.

How taken

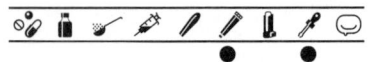

Skin lotion, eye ointment, eye drops.

Frequency and timing of doses
As prescribed.

Dosage range
Eye ointment 1cm strip every 4 hours for 5 applications daily.
Eye drops 1 drop every 2 hours during the day and if possible at night, or 1 drop every minute for 5 minutes, repeated every 4 hours, day and night.
Skin lotion As directed.

Onset of effect
Improvement is usually noted after 7–8 days, sometimes earlier.

Duration of action
A few hours after each application.

Diet advice
None.

Storage
Store eye drops in the refrigerator; eye ointment does not require refrigeration. Store skin lotion in a cool place, away from light. Keep out of reach of children.

Missed dose
Apply as soon as you remember.

Stopping the drug
Apply for 7 days after symptoms disappear, since the original infection may still be active, and symptoms may recur if treatment is stopped too soon.

Exceeding the dose
Do not apply the medication more frequently than prescribed. Efficacy is not improved by more frequent application and corneal damage may occur.

SPECIAL PRECAUTIONS

Be sure to tell your physician if:
▼ You have ever had an allergic reaction to iodine or an iodine-containing preparation.
▼ You are taking other medications.

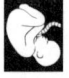

Pregnancy
▼ Not usually prescribed. Safety in pregnancy not established. Discuss with your physician.

Breast feeding
▼ No evidence of risk.

Infants and children
▼ No known problems.

Over 60
▼ No known problems.

Driving and hazardous work
▼ Exercise caution if blurred vision occurs.

Alcohol
▼ No known problems.

POSSIBLE ADVERSE EFFECTS

Serious adverse effects are uncommon with idoxuridine. If you experience unusual sensitivity to light (photophobia), visual impairment, or allergic reactions such as itching, swelling, or pain, consult your physician promptly.

Symptom/effect	Frequency		Discuss with physician		Stop taking drug now	Call physician now
	Common	Rare	Only if severe	In all cases		
Eye irritation	●		■			
Excess flow of tears		●	■			
Unusual sensitivity to light		●		■		
Blurred vision		●		■		
Swollen lids/pain in eye		●		■		▲

PROLONGED USE

Rarely required. Treatment is not normally continued for longer than 21 days, except occasionally for iritis, corneal edema, and deep infections.

INTERACTIONS

Boric acid eye preparations may interact with inactive ingredients or preservatives in idoxuridine preparations, increasing the risk of irritation and of eye damage.

IMIPRAMINE

Brand names Tofranil, Apo-Imipramine, Impril, Novo-Pramine
Used in the following combined preparations None

GENERAL INFORMATION

Imipramine belongs to a class of antidepressant drugs known as the tricyclics. It is mainly used in the long-term treatment of depression to elevate mood, increase physical activity, improve appetite, and restore interest in everyday life. Less sedating than some of the other tricyclic antidepressants, it is particularly useful when a depressed person is withdrawn or apathetic, though it can aggravate insomnia if taken in the evening.

Imipramine may be given for the treatment of bedwetting in children, though proof of benefits is not conclusive. Imipramine can cause a variety of side effects. In overdose it may cause coma and dangerous heart rhythms.

INFORMATION FOR USERS

Your drug prescription is tailored for you. Do not alter dosage without checking with your physician.

How taken

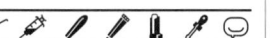

Tablets.

Frequency and timing of doses
1 – 4 x daily.

Dosage range
Adults 75 – 200mg daily (dose may be increased in exceptional circumstances). Children for bedwetting 10 – 75mg daily, before bed, depending on age and response.

Onset of effect
Some benefits and effects may appear within hours, but full antidepressant effect may not be felt for 2 – 6 weeks.

Duration of action
Following prolonged treatment, antidepressant effect may persist for up to 6 weeks. Adverse effects may wear off within days.

Diet advice
None.

Storage
Keep in a closed container in a cool, dry place away from reach of children. Protect from light.

Missed dose
Take as soon as you remember. If your next dose is due within 3 hours, take a single dose now and skip the next.

Stopping the drug
Do not stop taking the drug without consulting your physician, who will supervise a gradual reduction in dosage.

OVERDOSE ACTION

Seek immediate medical advice in all cases. Take emergency action if consciousness is lost.

See Drug poisoning emergency guide (p.574).

POSSIBLE ADVERSE EFFECTS

The possible adverse effects of this drug are mainly the result of its *anticholinergic* action and its blocking action on the transmission of signals in the heart.

Symptom/effect	Frequency		Discuss with physician		Stop taking drug now	Call physician now
	Common	Rare	Only if severe	In all cases		
Sweating/flushing	●		■			
Dry mouth/constipation	●		■			
Blurred vision	●			■		
Dizziness/fainting	●			■		
Rash		●		■	▲	
Palpitations		●		■	▲	■

INTERACTIONS

Sedatives All drugs, including alcohol and anticonvulsants, that have a sedative effect are likely to increase the sedative properties of imipramine.

Antihypertensive drugs Imipramine may reduce the effect of some of these drugs.

Monoamine oxidase inhibitors (MAOIs) Usually, imipramine should not be given with or within two weeks of treatment with an MAOI. Serious reactions may occur. Such drugs are prescribed together only under strict medical supervision.

SPECIAL PRECAUTIONS

Be sure to tell your physician if:
▼ You have had heart problems.
▼ You have impaired liver or kidney function.
▼ You have had epileptic seizures.
▼ You have had glaucoma.
▼ You have prostate trouble.
▼ You have a thyroid disorder.
▼ You have a blood disease.
▼ You are taking other medications.

Pregnancy
▼ Safety in pregnancy not established. Discuss with your physician.

Breast feeding
▼ The drug passes into the breast milk and may affect the baby. Discuss with your physician.

Infants and children
▼ Not recommended for children under 5 years. Reduced dose necessary in older children.

Over 60
▼ Increased likelihood of adverse effects. Reduced dose may therefore be necessary.

Driving and hazardous work
▼ Avoid such activities until you have learned how the drug affects you; it can cause reduced alertness and blurred vision.

Alcohol
▼ Avoid. Alcohol may increase the sedative effects of this drug.

Surgery and general anesthetics
▼ Imipramine treatment may need to be stopped before you have a general anesthetic. Discuss this with your physician or dentist before any operation.

PROLONGED USE

No problems expected. A course of imipramine for bedwetting in children does not usually exceed 4 weeks.

Monitoring Periodic blood tests may be performed.

INDAPAMIDE

Brand name Lozide
Used in the following combined preparations None

GENERAL INFORMATION

Indapamide is a diuretic drug chemically related to the thiazide diuretics. It is, however, longer-acting than many thiazide diuretics and needs only to be given once daily, early in the morning.

Indapamide is most frequently used to treat mildly elevated blood pressure (see Antihypertensives, p.114), and may be given alone or in combination with other antihypertensive drugs.

As with the thiazide diuretics, indapamide increases the loss of potassium and other body salts in the urine which can result in a variety of symptoms (see p.111) and increases the likelihood of irregular heart rhythms, particularly if you are taking drugs such as digoxin for heart failure. For this reason, potassium supplements may be prescribed along with indapamide.

QUICK REFERENCE

Drug group Thiazide-like diuretics (p.111)

Overdose danger rating Low

Dependence rating Low

Prescription needed Yes

Multi-source suppliers No

INFORMATION FOR USERS

Your drug prescription is tailored for you. Do not alter dosage without checking with your physician.

How taken

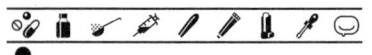

Tablets.

Frequency and timing of doses
Once daily, early in the morning.

Adult dosage range
2.5mg daily.

Onset of effect
1 – 2 hours.

Duration of action
Up to 36 hours.

Diet advice
Use of this drug may reduce potassium in the body. Eat plenty of fresh fruit and vegetables.

Discuss the advisability of reducing your salt intake with your physician.

Storage
Keep in a closed container in a cool, dry place away from reach of children.

Missed dose
No cause for concern, but take as soon as you remember. However, if it is late in the day, do not take the missed dose, or you may have to get up during the night to pass urine. Take the next scheduled dose as usual.

Stopping the drug
Do not stop the drug without consulting your physician; symptoms may recur.

Exceeding the dose
An occasional unintentional extra dose is unlikely to be a cause for concern. But if you notice unusual symptoms, or if a large overdose has been taken, notify your physician.

SPECIAL PRECAUTIONS

Be sure to tell your physician if:
▼ You have impaired liver or kidney function
▼ You have diabetes.
▼ You have gout.
▼ You have a high level of fat in your blood.
▼ You are allergic to sulfonamide drugs.
▼ You are taking other medications.

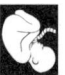

Pregnancy
▼ Safety in pregnancy not established. Discuss with your physician.

Breast feeding
▼ It is not known whether the drug passes into the breast milk. Discuss with your physician.

Infants and children
▼ Not recommended.

Over 60
▼ Increased likelihood of adverse effects. Reduced dose may therefore be necessary.

Driving and hazardous work
▼ Avoid such activities until you have learned how the drug affects you; it can cause drowsiness and blurred vision.

Alcohol
▼ Keep consumption low. Indapamide increases the likelihood of dehydration and hangovers after consumption of alcohol.

POSSIBLE ADVERSE EFFECTS

Most adverse effects are caused by excessive loss of potassium. This can usually be corrected by using a potassium supplement.

In rare cases, gout may occur in susceptible people and certain forms of diabetes may become more difficult to control.

Symptom/effect	Frequency		Discuss with physician		Stop taking drug now	Call physician now
	Common	Rare	Only if severe	In all cases		
Headache	●				■	
Muscle cramps	●				■	
Lethargy	●				■	
Dizziness		●	■			
Digestive disturbance		●	■			
Blurred vision		●			■	

INTERACTIONS

Digoxin The adverse effects of digoxin may be increased if excessive potassium is lost.

Lithium Indapamide may increase blood levels of lithium leading to a risk of serious adverse effects.

Corticosteroids These drugs further increase the loss of potassium from the body when taken with indapamide.

Non-steroidal anti-inflammatory drugs (NSAIDs) Some of these drugs may reduce the diuretic effect of indapamide, dosage of which may need to be adjusted.

PROLONGED USE

Prolonged use of this drug can lead to an excessive loss of potassium and imbalances of other salts, precipitate gout, and worsen diabetes.

Monitoring Blood tests should be done periodically to check kidney function and levels of blood sugar, potassium, and other salts.

INDOMETHACIN

Brand names Indocid, Apo-Indomethacin, Indotec, Novo-Methacin, Nu-Indo
Used in the following combined preparations None

GENERAL INFORMATION

Indomethacin, introduced in 1965, is a non-steroidal anti-inflammatory drug (NSAID). It is used to reduce the pain, stiffness, and inflammation of many arthritic conditions, including rheumatoid arthritis, ankylosing spondylitis, osteoarthritis, and acute attacks of gout. It is sometimes given to treat a heart disorder known as patent ductus arteriosus that occurs in premature infants. Eye drops of indomethacin are sometimes used to prevent swelling following cataract surgery.

Indomethacin has several potentially serious *side effects*, including gastrointestinal disorders, severe headache, and dizziness, and it may mask the symptoms of infections. It is not given to people with poor kidney function.

QUICK REFERENCE

Drug group Non-steroidal anti-inflammatory drug (p.128) and drug for gout (p.131)

Overdose danger rating Medium

Dependence rating Low

Prescription needed Yes

Multi-source suppliers Yes

INFORMATION FOR USERS

Your drug prescription is tailored for you. Do not alter dosage without checking with your physician.

How taken

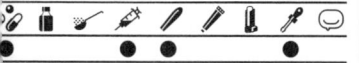

Capsules, slow-release capsules, injection, rectal suppositories, eye drops.

Frequency and timing of doses
1 – 2 x daily (slow-release capsules, rectal suppositories); 2 – 4 x daily (standard capsules). Take with food or milk.

Adult dosage range
0 – 200mg daily.

Onset of effect
Some analgesic effect may be felt within 2 – 4 hours. Full anti-inflammatory effect may not be felt for up to 4 weeks.

Duration of action
5 – 10 hours. Some effect may last for up to 24 hours (slow-release capsules).

Diet advice
None.

Storage
Keep in a closed container in a cool, dry place away from reach of children.

Missed dose
Take as soon as you remember. If your next dose is due within 2 hours, take a single dose now and skip the next.

Stopping the drug
Do not stop the drug without consulting your physician; symptoms may recur.

Exceeding the dose
An occasional unintentional extra dose is unlikely to cause problems. Large overdoses may cause headache, dizziness, confusion, and nausea. Notify your physician.

POSSIBLE ADVERSE EFFECTS

Gastrointestinal disturbances, headaches, and drowsiness are common. Black or bloodstained feces should be reported promptly.

Symptom/effect	Frequency		Discuss with physician		Stop taking drug now	Call physician now
	Common	Rare	Only if severe	In all cases		
Abdominal pain/indigestion	●		■			
Headache	●		■			
Dizziness/lightheadedness	●		■			
Nausea/vomiting	●			■		
Diarrhea		●		■		
Drowsiness/depression		●		■		
Rash		●		■	▲	
Wheezing/breathlessness		●		■	▲	▮
Black/bloodstained feces		●		■	▲	▮

INTERACTIONS

General note Indomethacin interacts with a wide range of drugs to increase the risk of bleeding and/or peptic ulcers. Such drugs include oral anticoagulants, corticosteroids, other non-steroidal anti-inflammatory drugs (NSAIDs), and ASA.

Antihypertensive drugs and diuretics The beneficial effects of these drugs may be reduced by indomethacin.

Lithium and methotrexate Indomethacin may raise blood levels of these drugs leading to an increased risk of adverse effects.

SPECIAL PRECAUTIONS

Be sure to tell your physician if:
▼ You have impaired liver or kidney function.
▼ You have had a peptic ulcer, esophagitis, or acid indigestion.
▼ You have heart problems.
▼ You have high blood pressure.
▼ You have asthma.
▼ You have had epileptic seizures.
▼ You have Parkinson's disease.
▼ You have bleeding problems.
▼ You are allergic to ASA.
▼ You are taking other medications.

Pregnancy
▼ Not usually prescribed. May cause defects in the unborn baby, and taken in late pregnancy, may prolong labor. Discuss with your physician.

Breast feeding
▼ The drug passes into the breast milk and may affect the baby. Discuss with your physician.

Infants and children
▼ Not usually prescribed for children under 14 except for infants with patent ductus arteriosus.

Over 60
▼ Increased likelihood of adverse effects. Reduced dose necessary.

Driving and hazardous work
▼ Avoid such activities until you have learned how the drug affects you; it can cause dizziness and drowsiness.

Alcohol
▼ Never drink while under treatment with indomethacin. Alcohol may interact with this drug to cause peptic ulcers.

Surgery and general anesthetics
▼ Indomethacin may prolong bleeding. Discuss this with your physician or dentist before you are given a general anesthetic.

PROLONGED USE

There is an increased risk of bleeding from peptic ulcers and in the bowel with prolonged use of indomethacin.

INSULIN

Brand names of single and combined preparations
Humulin, Iletin, Novolin

GENERAL INFORMATION

Insulin is a hormone manufactured by the pancreas and vital to the body's ability to use sugar. Introduced as a drug in 1922, it is given by injection to supplement or replace natural insulin in the treatment of diabetes mellitus. It is the only effective treatment in juvenile (insulin-dependent) diabetes and may also be prescribed in adult (maturity-onset) diabetes. It is most effective when used in conjunction with a carefully controlled diet. Illness, vomiting, or alterations in diet or in exercise levels may require dosage adjustment.

A wide variety of different insulin preparations are available. These can be short-, medium-, or long-acting. Combinations of these types are often given together. People receiving insulin should carry a warning card or tag, so that, in case of accident, the appropriate treatment can be given.

QUICK REFERENCE

Drug group Antidiabetic drug (p.154)

Overdose danger rating High

Dependence rating Low

Prescription needed No

Multi-source suppliers Yes

INFORMATION FOR USERS

Your drug prescription is tailored for you. Do not alter dosage or insulin type without checking with your physician.

How taken

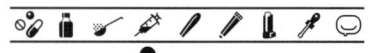

Injection, infusion pump.

Frequency and timing of doses
Varies with preparation or preparations used and individual needs. 1 – 4 x daily usually 30 – 45 minutes before meals and at bedtime.

Dosage range
The dose (and type) of insulin is determined according to the needs of the individual.

Onset of effect
30 – 60 minutes (short-acting); 1 – 4 hours (medium-acting); 4 – 6 hours (long-acting).

Duration of action
6 – 8 hours (short-acting); 18 – 26 hours (medium-acting); 28 – 36 hours (long-acting).

Diet advice
A low-sugar, low-fat diet is needed. Follow your physician's advice.

Storage
Refrigerate, but do not freeze. Follow the instructions on the container.

Missed dose
Discuss with your physician. Appropriate action depends on dose and type of insulin.

Stopping the drug
Do not stop the drug without consulting your physician; stopping the drug may lead to confusion and coma.

OVERDOSE ACTION

Seek immediate medical advice in all cases. You may notice symptoms of low blood sugar such as faintness, hunger, sweating, trembling, confusion, or headache. If these occur, eat or drink something sugary. Take emergency action if a seizure or loss of consciousness occurs.

See Drug poisoning emergency guide (p.574).

POSSIBLE ADVERSE EFFECTS

Symptoms such as dizziness, sweating, weakness, and confusion indicate low blood sugar. Serious allergic reactions (rash, swelling, and shortness of breath) are rare.

Symptom/effect	Frequency		Discuss with physician		Stop taking drug now	Call physician now
	Common	Rare	Only if severe	In all cases		
Injection-site irritation	●			■		
Weakness/sweating	●			■		
Dimpling at injection site		●		■		
Rash/facial swelling		●		■		▮
Shortness of breath		●		■		▮

INTERACTIONS

General note Many drugs increase the risk of low blood sugar, including ASA, phenytoin, some antibiotics, monoamine oxidase inhibitors, and oral antidiabetic drugs.

Corticosteroids and diuretics may oppose the effect of insulin.

Beta blockers may affect insulin needs and mask signs of low blood sugar.

SPECIAL PRECAUTIONS

Be sure to consult your physician or pharmacist before using this drug if:
▼ You have had a previous allergic reaction to insulin.
▼ You have had a thyroid disorder.
▼ You have a liver or kidney disorder.
▼ You are taking other medications, or your other drug treatment is changed.

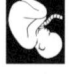

Pregnancy
▼ No evidence of risk to the developing baby from insulin, but poor control of diabetes increases the risk of birth defects. Careful monitoring is required.

Breast feeding
▼ No evidence of risk.

Infants and children
▼ Insulin requirements may vary considerably. Regular monitoring of blood sugar levels is essential.

Over 60
▼ No special problems.

Driving and hazardous work
▼ Usually no problem, but a missed meal or strenuous exercise alters your insulin and sugar requirements. Avoid these activities if you have warning signs of low blood sugar.

Alcohol
▼ Avoid. Alcoholic drinks upset diabetic control.

Surgery and general anesthetics
▼ Insulin requirements may increase during surgery, and blood glucose levels will need be monitored during and after an operation. Notify your physician or dentist that you are diabetic before any surgery.

PROLONGED USE

No problems expected.

Monitoring Regular monitoring of levels of sugar in the urine and/or blood required.

INTERFERON

Brand names Intron-A, Roferon-A, Wellferon
Used in the following combined preparations None

GENERAL INFORMATION

Interferons are a group of substances produced in human and animal cells infected by viruses or stimulated by other substances. They are thought to promote resistance to other types of viral infection (see p.139). Two main types of interferon (interferon-alpha and interferon-gamma) are used to treat a range of diseases. Conditions which may respond to interferon treatment include: hairy cell leukemia, basal-cell carcinoma, chronic non-A, non-B/C hepatitis, and chronic active hepatitis B. It is also used to treat AIDS-related Kaposi's sarcoma. Research is being carried out on the use of interferons in the treatment of life-threatening viral diseases, including those that occur in people who have defective immune systems. Use of interferons is associated with significant adverse effects (see below).

QUICK REFERENCE

Drug group Antiviral drug (p.145) and anticancer drug (p.166).

Overdose danger rating Medium

Dependence rating Low

Prescription needed Yes

Multi-source suppliers Yes

INFORMATION FOR USERS

This drug is given only under medical supervision and is not for self-administration.

How taken

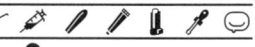

injection.

Frequency and timing of doses
Once daily or on alternate days.

Adult dosage range
The dosage is calculated taking account of the body surface area of the patient, and the condition being treated.

Onset of effect
Active inside the body within 1 hour, but effects may not be noted for 1 to 2 months.

Duration of action
Effects last for about 12 hours.

Diet advice
Do not get dehydrated. Drink fluids regularly.

Storage
The drug is not usually kept in the home.

Missed dose
This drug is usually given only in hospital under close medical supervision.

Stopping the drug
Discuss with your physician.

Exceeding the dose
Overdosage is unlikely since treatment is carefully monitored.

POSSIBLE ADVERSE EFFECTS

The symptoms listed below are the most common problems. All unusual symptoms should be brought to your physician's attention without delay. Some of these symptoms are dose-related; a reduction in dosage may be necessary.

Symptom/effect	Frequency		Discuss with physician		Stop taking drug now	Call physician now
	Common	Rare	Only if severe	In all cases		
Headache	●		■			
Lethargy/depression	●			■		
Dizziness/drowsiness	●			■		
Digestive disturbances	●			■		
Fever/chills	●			■		
Hair loss		●		■		

INTERACTIONS

General note A number of drugs increase the risk of adverse effects on the blood, heart, or nervous system. This is taken into account when prescribing interferon with other drugs.

Theophylline The effects of theophylline may be enhanced.

Sedatives All drugs that have a sedative effect on the nervous system are likely to increase the sedative properties of interferon. Such drugs include anti-anxiety and sleeping drugs, antihistamines, antidepressants, narcotic analgesics, antipsychotics, and alcohol.

SPECIAL PRECAUTIONS

Be sure to tell your physician if:
▼ You have impaired liver or kidney function.
▼ You have heart disease.
▼ You have had epileptic seizures.
▼ You have previously suffered allergic reactions to any drugs.
▼ You have had asthma or psoriasis.
▼ You suffer from depression.
▼ You are taking other medications.

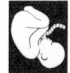

Pregnancy
▼ Not usually prescribed. Safety in pregnancy not established. Discuss with your physician.

Breast feeding
▼ It is not known whether the drug passes into breast milk. Discuss with your physician.

Infants and children
▼ Safety and effectiveness in patients under 18 years not established.

Over 60
▼ Reduced dose may be necessary. Increased likelihood of adverse effects.

Driving and hazardous work
▼ Not applicable.

Alcohol
▼ Avoid. Alcohol may increase the sedative effects of this drug.

PROLONGED USE

There may be an increased risk of liver damage. Blood cell production in the bone marrow may be reduced.

Monitoring Frequent blood tests are required to monitor blood composition and liver function.

IPRATROPIUM BROMIDE

Brand name Atrovent
Used in the following combined preparation Duovent

GENERAL INFORMATION

Ipratropium bromide is an *anticholinergic* bronchodilator that relaxes the muscles surrounding the bronchioles (airways in the lung).

It is used mainly in the maintenance treatment of asthma, chronic bronchitis, and emphysema. Ipratropium bromide can be given only by aerosol or nebulizer spray for inhalation. Although the drug begins to act within 5 – 15 minutes, the maximum effect does not occur until 1 – 2 hours after inhaling. Ipratropium bromide is, therefore, more effective for chronic bronchitis and emphysema than for asthma. Ipratropium bromide is sometimes used together with faster-acting drugs. It is also prescribed as a nasal aerosol to treat a continually runny nose not due to allergy.

Compared with atropine, from which it was developed, ipratropium bromide has fewer effects on other systems such as the heart, eyes, bowel, and bladder. The most common *side effects* are dryness of the mouth or throat, headache, and a bad taste in the mouth. Aerosols must be used with caution by people with glaucoma since accidental direct spraying in the eyes can cause a worsening of the eye problem.

QUICK REFERENCE

Drug group Anticholinergic bronchodilator (p.104)

Overdose danger rating Low

Dependence rating Low

Prescription needed Yes

Multi-source suppliers No

INFORMATION FOR USERS

Your drug prescription is tailored for you. Do not alter dosage without checking with your physician.

How taken

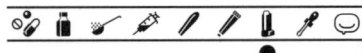

Inhaler, nasal aerosol, liquid for nebulizer.

Frequency and timing of doses
3 – 4 x daily.

Adult dosage range
80 – 320mcg daily (inhaler); 1,000 – 2,000mcg daily (nebulizer); 120 – 160mcg daily (nasal aerosol).

Onset of effect
Within 5 – 15 minutes.

Duration of action
Up to 8 hours.

Diet advice
None.

Storage
Keep in a cool place away from reach of children. Do not puncture or burn containers.

Missed dose
Do not take the missed dose. Take your next dose as usual.

Stopping the drug
Do not stop taking the drug without consulting your physician; symptoms may recur.

Exceeding the dose
An occasional unintentional extra dose is unlikely to be a cause for concern. But if you notice any unusual symptoms, or if a large overdose has been taken, notify your physician.

SPECIAL PRECAUTIONS

Be sure to tell your physician if:
▼ You have heart problems.
▼ You have glaucoma.
▼ You have prostate problems.
▼ You have difficulty in urination.
▼ You are taking other medications.

Pregnancy
▼ Safety in pregnancy not established. Discuss with your physician.

Breast feeding
▼ Effect on breast feeding uncertain. Discuss with your physician.

Infants and children
▼ Not recommended in patients under 12 years (inhaler, nasal aerosol); under 5 years (nebulizer).

Over 60
▼ Increased likelihood of adverse effects. Reduced dose may therefore be necessary.

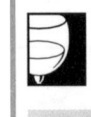

Driving and hazardous work
▼ Avoid such activities until you have learned how the drug affects you; it can cause blurred vision, dizziness, and tremors.

Alcohol
▼ No known problems.

POSSIBLE ADVERSE EFFECTS

Dry mouth or throat, bad taste, and headache are the most common adverse effects with the drug. Palpitations and tremor are rare.

Symptom/effect	Frequency		Discuss with physician		Stop taking drug now	Call physician now
	Common	Rare	Only if severe	In all cases		
Dry mouth/throat/nose	●		■			
Headache	●		■			
Bad taste	●		■			
Stuffy nose		●	■			
Palpitations/tremor		●		■		
Blurred vision		●		■		
Urinary hesitancy		●		■		
Dizziness		●		■		

PROLONGED USE

There is no evidence of tolerance to the effects of this drug with prolonged use.

INTERACTIONS

Other anticholinergic drugs These may increase the effects of ipratropium bromide, thus increasing the risk of adverse effects.

ISONIAZID

Brand names Isotamine, PMS-Isoniazid
Used in the following combined preparations Isotamine B, Rifater

GENERAL INFORMATION

In use for over 30 years, isoniazid (also know as INH) remains an effective drug for tuberculosis. It is given alone to prevent the disease and with other drugs for the treatment of tuberculosis. Treatment usually lasts for at least 1 year, although shorter courses lasting 6 months may sometimes be prescribed.

One of the *side effects* of isoniazid is the increased loss of pyridoxine (vitamin B$_6$) from the body. This effect, which is more likely with high doses, is rare in children, but common among people with poor nutrition. Since pyridoxine deficiency can lead to irreversible nerve damage, supplements are usually given.

INFORMATION FOR USERS

Your drug prescription is tailored for you. Do not alter dosage without checking with your physician.

How taken

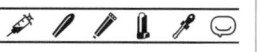

Tablets, oral liquid.

Frequency and timing of doses
Once daily, preferably on an empty stomach.

Dosage range
Adults 300mg daily.
Children According to age and weight.

Onset of effect
Over 2 – 3 days.

Duration of action
Up to 24 hours.

Diet advice
Isoniazid may deplete pyridoxine (vitamin B$_6$) levels in the body, and supplements are usually prescribed. In some people, isoniazid may interact with cheese or fish in the diet, causing redness and itching of the skin, sweating, chills, headache, faintness, and palpitations. This rare reaction requires prompt medical attention.

Storage
Keep in a closed container in a cool, dry place away from reach of children. Protect from light.

Missed dose
Take as soon as you remember. If your next dose is scheduled within 8 hours, take both doses now.

Stopping the drug
Take the full course. Even if you feel better, the infection may still be present and may recur if treatment is stopped too soon.

OVERDOSE ACTION

 Seek immediate medical advice in all cases. Take emergency action if breathing difficulties, loss of consciousness, or seizures occur.

See Drug poisoning emergency guide (p.574).

POSSIBLE ADVERSE EFFECTS

Although serious problems are uncommon, all adverse effects of this drug should receive prompt medical attention because of the possibility of nerve or liver damage.

Symptom/effect	Frequency		Discuss with physician		Stop taking drug now	Call physician now
	Common	Rare	Only if severe	In all cases		
Nausea/vomiting		●	■			
Fatigue/weakness		●		■		
Numbness/tingling		●		■		
Insomnia/restlessness		●		■		
Blurred vision		●		■	▲	
Jaundice		●		■	▲	∎
Twitching/seizures		●		■	▲	∎

INTERACTIONS

Anticonvulsant drugs The effects of these drugs may be increased with isoniazid.

Aluminum-containing antacids These may reduce the absorption of isoniazid.

Disulfiram and isoniazid together may provoke coordination difficulties and/or psychotic episodes.

SPECIAL PRECAUTIONS

Be sure to tell your physician if:
▼ You have impaired liver or kidney function.
▼ You have had liver damage following isoniazid treatment in the past.
▼ You have diabetes.
▼ You have had epileptic seizures.
▼ You are taking other medications.

 **Pregnancy**
▼ Safety in pregnancy not established. Discuss with your physician.

 Breast feeding
▼ The drug passes into the breast milk and may affect the baby. The infant should be monitored for signs of toxic effects. Discuss with your physician.

 Infants and children
▼ Reduced dose necessary.

 Over 60
▼ Increased likelihood of adverse effects.

 Driving and hazardous work
▼ Exercise caution if blurred vision occurs.

 Alcohol
▼ Avoid. Isoniazid may reduce tolerance to alcohol and may increase the risk of liver damage.

PROLONGED USE

Pyridoxine (vitamin B$_6$) deficiency may occur with prolonged use and lead to nerve damage. Supplements are usually prescribed to people at risk. There is also a risk of liver function.

Monitoring Periodic blood tests are usually performed to monitor liver function.

ISOPROTERENOL

Brand name Isuprel
Used in the following combined preparations None

GENERAL INFORMATION

Isoproterenol is a *sympathomimetic* drug that dilates the bronchioles (small air passages in the lungs) and improves the transmission of electrical signals in the heart. Given by aerosol inhaler, it is used as a bronchodilator to relieve the bronchospasm associated with asthma, bronchitis, and emphysema. In rare cases, isoproterenol is given intravenously as an emergency treatment for serious heart disorders and the relief of severe asthma.

Isoproterenol may increase the heart rate, and is used in heart block as an interim treatment before an artificial pacemaker is implanted; it is not suitable for those with angina.

Occasionally, breathing difficulties may be worsened by the drug. Excessive use may cause nervousness, insomnia, headaches, and, in extreme cases, dangerous heart rhythms.

QUICK REFERENCE

Drug group Bronchodilator (p.104)
Overdose danger rating High
Dependence rating Low
Prescription needed Yes
Multi-source suppliers Yes

INFORMATION FOR USERS

Your drug prescription is tailored for you. Do not alter dosage without checking with your physician.

How taken

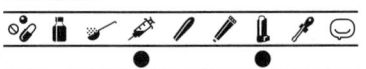

Injection, inhaler, solution for inhalation.

Frequency and timing of doses
As required up to a maximum of 8 doses in 24 hours (inhaler).

Adult dosage range
1 – 2 puffs per dose (inhaler).

Onset of effect
Within 2 – 5 minutes (inhaler).

Duration of action
Up to 6 hours.

Diet advice
None.

Storage
Keep in a closed container in a cool, dry place away from reach of children. Protect from light. Do not puncture or burn inhalers.

Missed dose
Do not take missed dose. Take the next dose as usual.

Stopping the drug
Do not stop taking the drug without consulting your doctor; symptoms may recur.

OVERDOSE ACTION

 Seek immediate medical advice in all cases. Take emergency action if dizziness, fainting, palpitations, or loss of consciousness occurs.

See Drug poisoning emergency guide (p.574).

POSSIBLE ADVERSE EFFECTS

Many of the adverse effects go away during treatment as your body adjusts to the medicine. However, palpitations are a sign of excessive stimulation of the heart, and chest pain always requires prompt medical attention.

Symptom/effect	Frequency		Discuss with physician		Stop taking drug now	Call physician now
	Common	Rare	Only if severe	In all cases		
Dry mouth and throat	●		■			
Nervousness/insomnia	●		■			
Dizziness/fainting	●			■		▮
Headache		●	■			
Chest pain		●		■		▮
Palpitations	●			■		

SPECIAL PRECAUTIONS

Be sure to tell your physician if:
▼ You have heart problems.
▼ You have high blood pressure.
▼ You have an overactive thyroid gland.
▼ You have diabetes.
▼ You suffer from nervous problems.
▼ You are taking other medications.

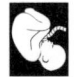 **Pregnancy**
▼ Safety in pregnancy not established. Discuss with your physician.

 Breast feeding
▼ It is not known if the drug passes into breast milk. Discuss with your physician.

 Infants and children
▼ Reduced dose necessary.

 Over 60
▼ Reduced dose may be necessary.

 Driving and hazardous work
▼ Avoid such activities until you have learned how the drug affects you, because the drug can cause dizziness and fainting.

 Alcohol
▼ No known problems.

Surgery and general anesthetics
▼ Inform physician or dentist that you are taking this drug if you need an anesthetic.

INTERACTIONS

Diuretics The antihypertensive effect of these drugs may be reduced.

Monoamine oxidase inhibitors (MAOIs) Isoproterenol may interact with these drugs to cause a dangerous rise in blood pressure.

Tricyclic antidepressant drugs may increase the adverse effects of isoproterenol on heart rhythm.

Beta blockers may reduce the beneficial effects of isoproterenol.

PROLONGED USE

The effect of isoproterenol may wear off with prolonged use. However, reduced benefit from the drug may also indicate a worsening of asthma and should be brought to your physician's attention. The use of sympathomimetic drugs with isoproterenol has been associated with worsening asthma control.

ISOSORBIDE DINITRATE/MONONITRATE

Brand names [Dinitrate] Isordil, Apo-ISDN, Cedocard-SR, Coradur, Coronex, Novo-Sorbide; [Mononitrate] Imdur, ISMO
Used in the following combined preparations None

GENERAL INFORMATION

Isosorbide dinitrate and isosorbide mononitrate are types of vasodilator drugs. Related to nitroglycerin, both these nitrates are most often used to prevent or to relieve angina attacks. Unlike nitroglycerin, both forms of isosorbide can be stored for long periods of time without losing their effectiveness.

Headache, flushing, and dizziness often occur during the early stages of treatment. Small initial doses minimize these symptoms, which generally disappear with time. The effectiveness of isosorbide dinitrate and mononitrate may be reduced after a few months, in which case an alternative treatment may need to be considered.

QUICK REFERENCE

Drug group Nitrate vasodilator (p.110) and anti-angina drug (p.113)

Overdose danger rating Medium

Dependence rating Low

Prescription needed No

Multi-source suppliers Yes

INFORMATION FOR USERS

Your drug prescription is tailored for you. Do not alter dosage without checking with your physician.

How taken

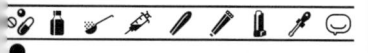

Tablets, slow-release tablets, sublingual tablets.

Frequency and timing of doses
Dinitrate
Relief of angina attacks As needed. Dose may be repeated after 5 minutes if necessary (tablets held under the tongue).
Prevention of angina Every 2 – 4 hours, supplemented by an extra half dose as needed before activities likely to provoke an angina attack (tablets held under the tongue); every 6 hours (swallowed tablets); every hours (slow-release tablets).
Mononitrate
Prevention of angina Once or twice daily.

Adult dosage range
Relief of angina attacks 5 – 10mg per dose.
Prevention of angina 40 – 160mg daily.

Onset of effect
– 5 minutes (held under the tongue);

30 minutes (swallowed); 30 minutes (slow-release tablets).

Duration of action
Up to 2 hours (held under the tongue); 4 – 6 hours (swallowed); up to 8 hours (slow-release tablets).

Diet advice
None.

Storage
Keep in a closed container in a cool, dry place away from reach of children. Protect from light.

Missed dose
Take as soon as you remember. If your next dose is due within 2 hours, take a single dose now and skip the next.

Stopping the drug
Do not stop taking the drug without consulting your physician; stopping the drug may lead to worsening of the underlying condition.

Exceeding the dose
An occasional unintentional extra dose is unlikely to cause problems. Large overdoses may cause dizziness and headache. Notify your physician.

SPECIAL PRECAUTIONS

Be sure to tell your physician if:
▼ You have impaired kidney function.
▼ You have any blood disorders or anemia.
▼ You have had glaucoma.
▼ You have thyroid disease.
▼ You are taking other medications.

Pregnancy
▼ Safety in pregnancy not established. Discuss with your physician.

Breast feeding
▼ It is not known whether the drug passes into the breast milk. Discuss with your physician.

Infants and children
▼ Not usually prescribed.

Over 60
▼ No special problems.

Driving and hazardous work
▼ Avoid such activities until you have learned how the drug affects you; it can cause dizziness.

Alcohol
▼ Avoid. Alcohol may further lower blood pressure, depressing the heart and causing dizziness and faintness.

POSSIBLE ADVERSE EFFECTS

The most serious adverse effect is excessively lowered blood pressure, and this may need to be monitored on a regular basis. Other adverse effects of both forms of the drug usually improve after regular use; dose adjustment may help.

Symptom/effect	Frequency		Discuss with physician		Stop taking drug now	Call physician now
	Common	Rare	Only if severe	In all cases		
Headache	●		■			
Flushing	●		■			
Dizziness	●				■	
Fainting		●		■	■	▪

INTERACTIONS

Antihypertensive drugs A further lowering of blood pressure occurs when antihypertensives are taken with isosorbide dinitrate.

PROLONGED USE

The initial adverse effects may disappear with prolonged use. The effects of the drug become weaker as the body adapts, requiring increased dosage or other drugs.

ISOTRETINOIN

Brand names Accutane, Isotrex
Used in the following combined preparations None

GENERAL INFORMATION

Isotretinoin, chemically related to vitamin A, is used for the treatment of severe acne that has failed to respond to other treatments. It reduces production of the skin's natural oil (sebum) and of the horny protein (keratin) that forms in the outer layers of the skin. A gel form may be used topically for less severe acne. *Side effects* include erythema and peeling.
  Treatment lasting 12 to 16 weeks

often clears acne completely. In the early weeks of treatment, the skin may become unusually dry, flaky, and itchy. This usually improves as treatment continues. Serious adverse effects include liver damage, visual impairment, and inflammation of the bowel. **Because it can cause birth defects, women taking isotretinoin must avoid pregnancy.**

INFORMATION FOR USERS

Your drug prescription is tailored for you. Do not alter dosage without checking with your physician.

How taken

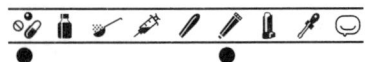

Capsules, gel.

Frequency and timing of doses
1 – 2 x daily (capsules with food).

Adult dosage range
Dosage is determined individually.

Onset of effect
2 – 8 weeks. Acne may worsen during the first few weeks of treatment in some people.

Duration of action
Effects may persist for several weeks after the drug has been stopped.

Diet advice
None.

Storage
Keep in a closed container in a cool, dry place away from reach of children. Protect from light.

Missed dose
Take as soon as you remember. If your next dose is due within 2 hours, take a single dose now and skip the next.

Stopping the drug
Can be safely stopped as soon as you no longer need it, but best results are achieved when the treatment is completed as prescribed.

Exceeding the dose
An occasional unintentional extra dose is unlikely to cause problems. Large overdoses may cause headaches, vomiting, abdominal pain, facial flushing, dizziness, and incoordination. Notify your physician.

SPECIAL PRECAUTIONS

Be sure to tell your physician if:
▼ You have impaired liver or kidney function.
▼ You suffer from arthritis.
▼ You have diabetes.
▼ You wear contact lenses.
▼ You are taking other medications.

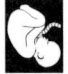

Pregnancy
▼ Isotretinoin can cause severe birth defects. Women taking the drug must avoid pregnancy during treatment and for at least 3 months after stopping the drug.

Breast feeding
▼ Not recommended.

Infants and children
▼ Not prescribed.

Over 60
▼ Not prescribed.

Driving and hazardous work
▼ No special problems.

Alcohol
▼ Regular heavy drinking may raise blood fat levels with isotretinoin, and thus increase the risk of heart and blood vessel disease.

POSSIBLE ADVERSE EFFECTS

Dryness of the nose and mouth, inflammation of the lips, and drying and flaking of the skin occur in most people treated with isotretinoin. If headache accompanied by symptoms such

as nausea and vomiting, abdominal pain with diarrhea, blood in bowel movements, or visual impairment occurs, consult your physician promptly.

Symptom/effect	Frequency		Discuss with physician		Stop taking drug now	Call physician now
	Common	Rare	Only if severe	In all cases		
Inflammation of lips	●		■			
Dry, peeling face	●		■			
Dry nose, eyes/nosebleeds	●		■			
Muscle/joint pain		●	■			
Hair thinning		●	■			
Headache/insomnia		●		■		
Impaired vision		●		■	▲	❙
Nausea/vomiting		●		■	▲	❙
Abdominal pain/diarrhea		●		■	▲	❙

PROLONGED USE

Prolonged use may cause a rise in fat levels in the blood, thereby increasing the risk of heart and blood-vessel disease. Do not donate blood while taking isotretinoin or for at least one month after stopping it.

Monitoring Periodic checks on fat levels in the blood and liver function tests may be recommended.

INTERACTIONS

Tetracycline antibiotics may increase the risk of high pressure in the skull, leading to headaches, nausea, and vomiting.

Vitamin A supplements increase the risk of adverse effects from isotretinoin.

Skin-drying preparations Medicated cosmetics, soaps, toiletries, and anti-acne preparations increase the likelihood of dryness and irritation of the skin with isotretinoin.

KETOCONAZOLE

Brand name Nizoral
Used in the following combined preparations None

GENERAL INFORMATION

Ketoconazole is prescribed mainly for severe internal *systemic* fungal infections – of the lungs, brain, kidneys, and lymph nodes, for example. It is also given to treat serious infections of the skin and mucous membranes caused by the candida yeast. People with rare fungal diseases (paracoccidioidomycosis, histoplasmosis, and blastomycosis) may also be given this drug.

Ketoconazole is applied as a cream to treat fungal skin infections and seborrheic dermatitis, and as a shampoo for the treatment of fungal scalp infections and seborrhea.

The most common *side effect* with oral ketoconazole is nausea, which can be reduced by taking the drug at bedtime or with meals. Ketoconazole may also cause liver damage.

QUICK REFERENCE

Drug group Antifungal drug (p.150)
Overdose danger rating Medium
Dependence rating Low
Prescription needed Yes
Multi-source suppliers No

INFORMATION FOR USERS

Your drug prescription is tailored for you. Do not alter dosage without checking with your physician.

How taken

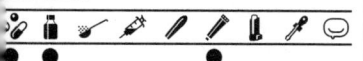

Tablets, oral liquid, topical cream, shampoo.

Frequency and timing of doses
Oral: Once daily with food.
Topical: Apply 1 – 2 x daily.
Shampoo: Apply 1 – 2 times a week.

Dosage range
Oral: *Adults* 200 – 400mg daily. *Children* 20kg or less: 50mg daily; 20 – 40kg: 100mg daily; over 40kg: 200mg daily.
Topical: Apply to affected areas daily for 2 – 6 weeks.

Onset of effect
The drug begins to work within a few hours, but full beneficial effect may take several days.

Duration of action
Up to 24 hours.

Diet advice
None.

Storage
Keep in a closed container in a cool, dry place away from reach of children.

Missed oral dose
Take as soon as you remember. If your next dose is due within 8 hours, take a single dose now and skip the next.

Stopping the drug
Take the full course. Even if you feel better, the original infection may still be present and symptoms may recur if treatment is stopped too soon.

Exceeding the dose
An occasional unintentional extra dose is unlikely to cause problems. Large oral overdoses may cause loss of consciousness. Notify your physician.

SPECIAL PRECAUTIONS

Be sure to tell your physician if:
▼ You have impaired liver or kidney function.
▼ You have had stomach ulcers.
▼ You have previously had an allergic reaction to antifungal drugs.
▼ You are taking other medications.

Pregnancy
▼ Not usually prescribed. May cause defects in the developing baby. Discuss with your physician.

Breast feeding
▼ The drug passes into the breast milk and may affect the baby adversely. Discuss with your physician.

Infants and children
▼ Reduced dose necessary.

Over 60
▼ No special problems.

Driving and hazardous work
▼ Avoid such activities until you have learned how the drug affects you; it can cause dizziness.

Alcohol
▼ Use with caution. Taken with ketoconazole, it rarely causes flushing, nausea, rash, peripheral edema, and headache.

POSSIBLE ADVERSE EFFECTS

Nausea is the most common side effect of oral ketoconazole. Liver damage is a rare but serious effect of oral therapy causing jaundice, and may necessitate stopping the drug.

Symptom/effect	Frequency		Discuss with physician		Stop taking drug now	Call physician now
	Common	Rare	Only if severe	In all cases		
Nausea/vomiting	●		■			
Dizziness		●	■			
Headache		●	■			
Constipation/diarrhea		●	■			
Loss of interest in sex		●	■			
Rash/itching		●		■	▲	
Painful breasts (men)		●		■	▲	
Jaundice		●		■	▲	

INTERACTIONS (by mouth only)

Antacids, cimetidine, and ranitidine These drugs may reduce the effectiveness of ketoconazole if taken within 2 hours.

Rifampin and isoniazid reduce the effect of ketoconazole.

Cyclosporine Ketoconazole increases the level of cyclosporine in the blood.

Antihistamines Increased risk of terfenadine and astemizole causing serious abnormalities of heart rhythm.

Warfarin Oral ketoconazole increases the effect of warfarin.

Phenytoin Oral ketoconazole may increase the effects of phenytoin.

PROLONGED USE

The risk of liver damage increases with long-term use of oral ketoconazole.

Monitoring Periodic blood tests are usually performed to check the effect of oral ketoconazole on the liver.

KETOPROFEN

Brand names Orudis, Apo-Keto, Novo-Keto-EC, Oruvail, PMS-Ketoprofen, Rhodis
Used in the following combined preparations None

GENERAL INFORMATION

Ketoprofen is a non-steroidal anti-inflammatory drug (NSAID). Like other drugs of this group, it relieves pain and reduces inflammation and stiffness in rheumatoid arthritis, osteoarthritis, and ankylosing spondylitis. However, ketoprofen relieves symptoms rather than curing the underlying disease.

Ketoprofen is also effective in relieving the mild to moderate pain of menstruation and soft tissue injuries, and pain following operations.

The most common adverse reactions to ketoprofen, as with all NSAIDs, are gastrointestinal disturbances such as nausea and indigestion. Switching to another NSAID may be recommended if unwanted effects are persistent or troublesome.

INFORMATION FOR USERS

Your drug prescription is tailored for you. Do not alter dosage without checking with your physician.

How taken

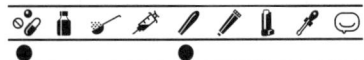

Tablets, capsules, rectal suppositories.

Frequency and timing of doses
3 – 4 x daily with food (by mouth); 2 x daily (rectal suppositories).

Adult dosage range
150 – 200mg daily.

Onset of effect
Pain relief may be felt in 30 minutes to 2 hours. Full anti-inflammatory effect may not be felt for up to 2 weeks.

Duration of action
Up to 8 – 12 hours.

Diet advice
None.

Storage
Keep in a closed container in a cool, dry place away from reach of children.

Missed dose
Take as soon as you remember. If your next dose is due within 4 hours, take a single dose now and skip the next.

Stopping the drug
Seek medical advice before stopping the drug.

Exceeding the dose
An occasional unintentional extra dose is unlikely to cause problems. Large overdoses may cause vomiting, confusion, or irritability. Notify your physician.

SPECIAL PRECAUTIONS

Be sure to tell your physician if:
▼ You have impaired liver or kidney function.
▼ You have heart problems.
▼ You have high blood pressure.
▼ You have asthma.
▼ You have had a peptic ulcer, esophagitis, or acid indigestion.
▼ You have bleeding problems.
▼ You are allergic to ASA.
▼ You are taking other medications.

Pregnancy
▼ Safety in pregnancy not established. Discuss with your physician.

Breast feeding
▼ The drug passes into the breast milk and may affect the baby adversely. Discuss with your physician.

Infants and children
▼ Not recommended for children under 12 years.

Over 60
▼ Increased likelihood of adverse effects. Reduced dose may therefore be necessary.

Driving and hazardous work
▼ Avoid such activities until you have learned how the drug affects you; it can cause dizziness and drowsiness.

Alcohol
▼ Avoid. Alcohol may increase the risk of stomach disorders with ketoprofen.

Surgery and general anesthetics
▼ Ketoprofen may prolong bleeding. Discuss this with your physician or dentist before any surgery.

POSSIBLE ADVERSE EFFECTS

Gastrointestinal disturbances such as nausea and indigestion commonly occur with ketoprofen taken by mouth. Suppositories may cause rectal irritation. Black or bloodstained feces should be reported to your physician without delay.

Symptom/effect	Frequency		Discuss with physician		Stop taking drug now	Call physician now
	Common	Rare	Only if severe	In all cases		
Nausea/vomiting	●			■		
Heartburn	●		■			
Abdominal pain	●			■		
Headache		●	■			
Dizziness/drowsiness		●	■			
Rash/itching		●		■	▲	▎
Wheezing/breathlessness		●		■	▲	▎
Black/bloodstained feces		●		■	▲	▎

INTERACTIONS

General note Ketoprofen interacts with a wide range of drugs to increase the risk of bleeding and/or stomach ulcers. Such drugs include oral anticoagulants, corticosteroids, other non-steroidal anti-inflammatory drugs (NSAIDs), and ASA.

Methotrexate Ketoprofen may raise blood levels of methotrexate leading to an increased risk of adverse effects.

Antihypertensive drugs The beneficial effects of these drugs may be reduced by ketoprofen.

PROLONGED USE

There is an increased risk of bleeding from peptic ulcers and in the bowel with prolonged use of ketoprofen.

KETOROLAC

Brand names Acular, Toradol
Used in the following combined preparations None

GENERAL INFORMATION

Ketorolac, a non-steroidal anti-inflammatory drug (NSAID), has strong analgesic effects. The drug is prescribed for short-term management of moderate to severe acute pain (e.g., following surgery or musculoskeletal trauma). As with all NSAIDs, gastrointestinal *side effects* such as indigestion, heartburn, and nausea are common with ketorolac.

Because the risk of side effects increases with the duration of use, ketorolac tablets should not be used for longer than 5 days for post-surgical pain or 7 days for musculoskeletal pain.

Ketorolac is also given as eye drops for the prevention and relief of inflammation following cataract surgery.

QUICK REFERENCE

Drug group Non-steroidal anti-inflammatory drug (p.128)

Overdose danger rating Low

Dependence rating Low

Prescription needed Yes

Multi-source suppliers Yes

INFORMATION FOR USERS

Your drug prescription is tailored for you. Do not alter dosage without checking with your physician.

How taken

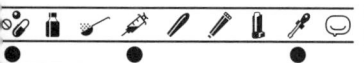

Tablets, injection, eye drops.

Frequency and timing of doses
4 x daily (by mouth); every 6 – 8 hours as prescribed (eye drops).

Adult dosage range
10 – 40mg daily; maximum 10mg every 4 – 6 hours (by mouth). A maximum of 0.75mg (3 drops) – 2mg (8 drops) daily; 1 – 2 drops every 6 – 8 hours (eye drops).

Onset of effect
Within 30 – 60 minutes (tablets); within 10 minutes (injection); within 1 hour (eye drops).

Duration of action
6 – 8 hours.

Diet advice
None.

Storage
Keep in a closed container in a cool, dry place away from children. Protect from light.

Missed dose
Take tablets as soon as you remember if needed for pain relief. If you miss a dose of eye drops, apply it as soon as possible.

Stopping the drug
Ketorolac tablets can be safely stopped as soon as you no longer need them. Do not stop the eye drops without consulting your physician.

Exceeding the dose
An occasional unintentional extra dose is unlikely to cause problems. For large overdoses, notify your physician immediately.

POSSIBLE ADVERSE EFFECTS

The most common adverse effects of ketorolac tablets are the result of gastrointestinal disturbances. Black or bloodstained feces should be reported to your physician without delay. Following instillation of the eye drops, transient stinging and burning, redness, itching and/or swelling, and visual blurring may occur.

Symptom/effect	Frequency		Discuss with physician		Stop taking drug now	Call physician now
	Common	Rare	Only if severe	In all cases		
Heartburn/indigestion	●			■		▮
Nausea/vomiting	●			■		▮
Headache/nervousness	●		■			
Dizziness	●		■			
Ringing in ears/blurred vision		●		■		
Swollen ankles/feet/face		●		■	▲	▮
Rash/itching/hives		●		■	▲	▮
Wheezing/breathlessness		●		■	▲	▮
Black or bloodstained feces		●		■	▲	▮

INTERACTIONS

General note Ketorolac may interact with a wide range of drugs to increase the risk of bleeding and/or peptic ulcer. Such drugs include oral anticoagulants, corticosteroids, other non-steroidal anti-inflammatory drugs (NSAIDs), and ASA.

Other drugs such as probenecid, furosemide, lithium, methotrexate, and ACE inhibitors may interact with ketorolac.

Consult your physician before taking any other drug with ketorolac.

SPECIAL PRECAUTIONS

Be sure to tell your physician if:
▼ You have impaired liver or kidney function.
▼ You have heart problems.
▼ You have high blood pressure.
▼ You have asthma or breathing problems.
▼ You are allergic to ASA or other NSAIDs.
▼ You have had a peptic ulcer, esophagitis, or acid indigestion.
▼ You are taking other medications.

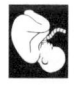

Pregnancy
▼ Not recommended. Discuss with your physician.

Breast feeding
▼ Not recommended. Discuss with your physician.

Infants and children
▼ Not recommended for children under 16 years.

Over 60
▼ Increased likelihood of adverse effects. Reduced dose may therefore be necessary.

Driving and hazardous work
▼ Avoid such activities until you have learned how the drug affects you as it can cause drowsiness and dizziness.

Alcohol
▼ Avoid. Alcohol may increase the risk of stomach irritation associated with ketorolac.

Surgery and general anesthetics
▼ Ketorolac may prolong bleeding. Discuss this with your physician or dentist before any surgery.

PROLONGED USE

Ketorolac (tablets or injection) is indicated for short-term use only (maximum of 5 to 7 days). Close monitoring for signs of serious gastrointestinal side effects is required.

LACTULOSE

Brand names Acilac, Cephulac, Chronulac, Comalose-R, Lactulax
Used in the following combined preparations None

GENERAL INFORMATION

Lactulose is an effective laxative that softens bowel movements by increasing the amount of water in the large intestine. It is useful for the relief of constipation and fecal impaction, especially in the elderly.

Lactulose can also prevent and treat the brain disturbance associated with liver failure known as hepatic encephalopathy.

Because lactulose acts locally in the large intestine and is not absorbed into the body, it is safer than many other laxatives. However, it can cause stomach cramps and flatulence at the start of treatment.

QUICK REFERENCE

Drug group Laxative (p.123)

Overdose danger rating Low

Dependence rating Low

Prescription needed No

Multi-source suppliers Yes

INFORMATION FOR USERS

Follow instructions on the label. Call your physician if symptoms worsen.

How taken

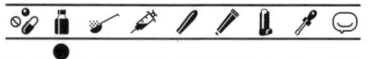

Oral liquid.

Frequency and timing of doses
1 – 2 x daily (chronic constipation);
3 – 4 x daily (liver failure).

Adult dosage range
15 – 60mL daily (chronic constipation);
90 – 180mL daily (liver failure).

Onset of effect
24 – 48 hours.

Duration of action
6 – 18 hours.

Diet advice
It is important to maintain an adequate intake of fluid – up to 8 glasses of water daily.

Storage
Keep in a closed container in a cool, dry place away from reach of children.

Missed dose
Take as soon as you remember. If your next dose is due within 2 hours, take a single dose now and skip the next.

Stopping the drug
In the treatment of constipation, the drug can be stopped as soon as you no longer need it.

Exceeding the dose
An occasional unintentional extra dose is unlikely to be a cause for concern. But if you notice unusual symptoms, or if a large overdose has been taken, notify your physician.

POSSIBLE ADVERSE EFFECTS

Adverse effects are rarely serious and often disappear when your body adjusts to the medicine. Diarrhea indicates that the dosage of lactulose may be too high.

Symptom/effect	Frequency		Discuss with physician		Stop taking drug now	Call physician now
	Common	Rare	Only if severe	In all cases		
Flatulence/belching	●		■			
Stomach cramps	●		■			
Nausea		●	■			
Dizziness/lightheadedness		●		■		
Tiredness/weakness		●		■		
Increased thirst		●		■		
Diarrhea		●		■		

INTERACTIONS

Antibiotics Certain oral antibiotics such as neomycin may have reduced effectiveness when used with lactulose to treat liver failure.

SPECIAL PRECAUTIONS

Be sure to consult your physician or pharmacist before taking this drug if:
▼ You have severe abdominal pain.
▼ You have a kidney disorder.
▼ You have a heart disorder.
▼ You have diabetes.
▼ You are taking other medications.

Pregnancy
▼ Safety in pregnancy not established. Discuss with your physician.

Breast feeding
▼ No evidence of risk.

Infants and children
▼ Not usually prescribed.

Over 60
▼ Increased likelihood of adverse effects.

Driving and hazardous work
▼ No known problems.

Alcohol
▼ No known problems.

PROLONGED USE

People on long-term treatment with this drug, especially the elderly, may develop chemical imbalances in the blood.

Monitoring Monitoring of blood levels of potassium may be advised.

LEVOCABASTINE

Brand name Livostin
Used in the following combined preparations None

GENERAL INFORMATION

Levocabastine is a *topical* antihistamine with a prolonged duration of action. Its main use is in the treatment of allergic conjunctivitis and rhinitis (hay fever). In eye-drop form it is used in management of seasonal allergic eye watering, irritation, and itching. As a spray, it is used in the treatment of symptoms of allergic rhinitis (sneezing, itching, and running nose).

The main difference between this topical antihistamine and the older traditional oral antihistamines is that it has little or no sedative effects on the central nervous system. It is, therefore, useful for people who need to avoid drowsiness, for example at work. It also has fewer *anticholinergic* effects (blurred vision, dry mouth) than older antihistamines.

INFORMATION FOR USERS

Your drug prescription is tailored for you. Do not alter dosage without checking with your physician.

How taken

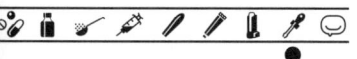

Eye drops, nasal spray.

Frequency and timing of doses
Eye drops 2 – 4 x daily.
Nasal spray 2 – 4 x daily.

Dosage range
Eye drops 1 drop (15mcg) in each eye.
Nasal spray 2 sprays (100mcg) in each nostril.

Onset of effect
Eye drops within 10 – 15 minutes.
Nasal spray within 10 minutes.

Duration of action
– 12 hours.

Diet advice
None.

Storage
Keep in original containers in a cool, dry place away from children. To avoid bacterial contamination, follow instructions on product pamphlets. Discard any unused eye drops 1 month after opening the bottle.

Missed dose
Take as soon as you remember.

Stopping the drug
Can be safely stopped as soon as you no longer need it.

Exceeding the dose
An occasional unintentional extra dose is unlikely to be a cause for concern. But if you notice unusual symptoms, or if a large overdose has been taken, notify your physician.

POSSIBLE ADVERSE EFFECTS

The most frequent *side effect* encountered with levocabastine preparations is transient irritation, which rarely necessitates discontinuation of therapy.

Symptom/effect	Frequency		Discuss with physician		Stop taking drug now	Call physician now
	Common	Rare	Only if severe	In all cases		
Mild eye irritation (drops)	●		■			
Mild nose irritation (spray)	●		■			
Headache	●		■			
Drowsiness/tiredness		●	■			
Dry mouth		●	■			
Rash/itching/swelling		●		■	▲	■

INTERACTIONS

None known.

SPECIAL PRECAUTIONS

Be sure to tell your physician if:
▼ You are using soft (hydrophilic) contact lenses.
▼ You have impaired kidney function.
▼ You are taking other medications.

Pregnancy
▼ Safety in pregnancy not established. Discuss with your physician.

Breast feeding
▼ Effect on breast feeding not established. Discuss with your physician.

Infants and children
▼ Levocabastine is not recommended for use in children under the age of 12 except on the advice of a physician.

Over 60
▼ Safety and efficacy not established. Consult your physician.

Driving and hazardous work
▼ Avoid such activities until you have learned how the drug affects you.

Alcohol
▼ No known problems.

PROLONGED USE

For both the eye drops and nasal spray, it is not useful to continue the treatment for more than 3 days if no improvement is seen. There are no medical studies to support continuous treatment for more than 16 weeks with the eye drops and 10 weeks for the nasal spray.

LEVODOPA

Brand name Larodopa
Used in the following combined preparations Prolopa, Sinemet, Sinemet CR

GENERAL INFORMATION

The treatment of Parkinson's disease underwent dramatic change in the 1960s with the introduction of levodopa. The body transforms levodopa into dopamine, a chemical in the brain whose absence or shortage causes Parkinson's disease (see p.99). Improvements focused not so much on a cure as on symptomatic benefits.

Levodopa, while effective, produced severe *side effects*: nausea, dizziness, palpitations. Even when treatment was initiated gradually, it was difficult to balance the benefits against the adverse reactions. What made the treatment even more difficult was the need for increasingly larger dosages.

Today, when levodopa treatment is prescribed, the drug is combined with carbidopa or benserazide, substances that enhance the effects of levodopa in the brain, enabling lower doses to be given, which reduces the adverse effects of levodopa.

INFORMATION FOR USERS

Your drug prescription is tailored for you. Do not alter dosage without checking with your physician.

How taken

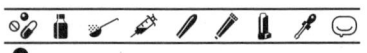

Tablets.

Frequency and timing of doses
2 – 4 x daily with food or milk.

Adult dosage range
500 – 1,000mg (starting dose), gradually increased until maximum benefit permitted by side effects is achieved.

Onset of effect
Within 30 minutes.

Duration of action
2 – 12 hours.

Diet advice
None.

Storage
Keep in a closed container in a cool, dry place away from reach of children. Protect from light.

Missed dose
Take as soon as you remember. If your next dose is due within 2 hours, take a single dose now and skip the next.

Stopping the drug
Do not stop taking the drug without consulting your physician; stopping the drug may lead to worsening of the underlying condition.

Exceeding the dose
An occasional unintentional extra dose is unlikely to cause problems. Larger overdoses may cause vomiting or drowsiness. Notify your physician.

POSSIBLE ADVERSE EFFECTS

Adverse effects of levodopa are closely related to dosage levels. At the start of treatment, when dosage is usually low, unwanted effects are likely to be mild. Such effects may increase in severity as dosage is increased to boost the drug's beneficial effects. All adverse effects of this drug should be discussed with your physician.

Symptom/effect	Frequency		Discuss with physician		Stop taking drug now	Call physician now
	Common	Rare	Only if severe	In all cases		
Digestive disturbance	●			■		
Nervousness/agitation	●			■		
Dizziness/fainting		●		■		
Abdominal movements		●		■		
Confusion/vivid dreams		●		■		
Palpitations		●		■	▲	▮

INTERACTIONS

Antidepressant drugs Levodopa may interact with monoamine oxidase inhibitor antidepressants (MAOIs) to cause a dangerous rise in blood pressure. It may also interact with tricyclic antidepressants.

Methyldopa may reduce the effectiveness of levodopa in Parkinson's disease.

Antipsychotic drugs These may counter the beneficial effects of levodopa.

Pyridoxine (vitamin B$_6$) Excessive intake of this vitamin may reduce the effect of levodopa.

Iron may cause decreased absorption of levodopa.

SPECIAL PRECAUTIONS

Be sure to tell your physician if:
▼ You have heart problems.
▼ You have impaired liver or kidney function.
▼ You have a lung disorder such as asthma, emphysema, or bronchitis.
▼ You have an overactive thyroid gland.
▼ You have a peptic ulcer.
▼ You have diabetes.
▼ You have epilepsy.
▼ You have had glaucoma.
▼ You are taking other medications.

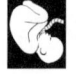

Pregnancy
▼ Safety in pregnancy not established. Discuss with your physician.

Breast feeding
▼ The drug passes into the breast milk. Its effects on the baby are not clearly known. Discuss with your physician.

Infants and children
▼ Not recommended in patients under 12 years.

Over 60
▼ Reduced dose may be necessary.

Driving and hazardous work
▼ Your underlying condition as well as the sedative effects of this drug may make such activities inadvisable. Discuss with your physician.

Alcohol
▼ No known problems.

Surgery and general anesthetics
▼ Discuss the advisability of stopping levodopa with your physician or dentist before any surgery.

PROLONGED USE

Effectiveness usually declines in time, necessitating increased dosage. Also, if adverse effects become more severe, the drug must be stopped.

LEVOTHYROXINE

Brand names Eltroxin, PMS-Levothyroxine Sodium, Synthroid
Used in the following combined preparations None

GENERAL INFORMATION

Levothyroxine, introduced in 1951, is often known as thyroxine, the major hormone produced by the thyroid gland. The drug is used primarily to replace the natural hormone when it is deficient, causing hypothyroidism and sometimes leading to myxedema, characterized by puffiness of the face. Certain types of goiter (enlarged thyroid) are helped by levothyroxine, and it may be given to prevent the development of goiter

during treatment with antithyroid drugs. It is also prescribed for thyroid cancer and its prevention in people undergoing radiation therapy in the neck.

Because adults with severe thyroid deficiency are sensitive to thyroid hormones, treatment is introduced gradually to prevent adverse effects (see below). Particular care is required in those with heart problems.

INFORMATION FOR USERS

Your drug prescription is tailored for you. Do not alter dosage without checking with your physician.

How taken

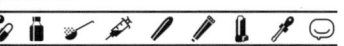

Tablets.

Frequency and timing of doses
Once daily.

Dosage range
Adults Initially 25 – 50mcg daily, increased at 2- or 3-week intervals as required. Usual daily dose: 75 – 150mcg. Maximum daily dose: 200mcg.
Children Reduced dose according to age and weight.

Onset of effect
Within 48 hours. Full beneficial effects may not be felt for several weeks.

Duration of action
1 – 3 weeks.

Diet advice
None.

Storage
Keep tablets in a closed container in a cool, dry place away from reach of children. Protect from light.

Missed dose
Take as soon as you remember. If your next dose is due within 2 hours, take both doses now.

Stopping the drug
Do not stop the drug without consulting your physician; symptoms may recur.

Exceeding the dose
An occasional unintentional extra dose is unlikely to cause problems. Large overdoses may cause palpitations during the next few days. Notify your physician.

SPECIAL PRECAUTIONS

Be sure to tell your physician if:
▼ You have high blood pressure.
▼ You have heart problems.
▼ You are taking other medications.

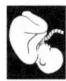

Pregnancy
▼ No evidence of risk to developing baby.

Breast feeding
▼ The drug passes into the breast milk, but at normal doses adverse effects on the baby are unlikely. Discuss with your physician.

Infants and children
▼ Dosage depends on age and weight.

Over 60
▼ Reduced dose usually necessary.

Driving and hazardous work
▼ No known problems.

Alcohol
▼ No known problems.

POSSIBLE ADVERSE EFFECTS

Adverse effects are rare with levothyroxine and are usually the result of overdosage, causing thyroid overactivity. These effects diminish as the dose is lowered. Too low a dose of levothyroxine may cause signs of thyroid underactivity.

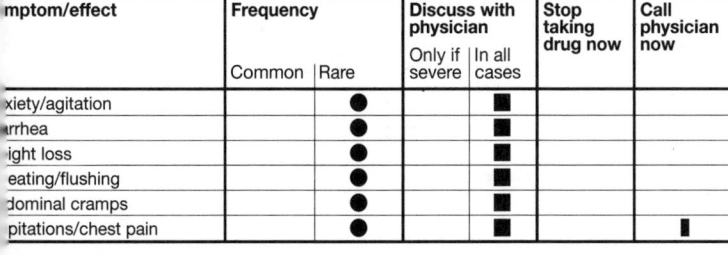

Symptom/effect	Frequency		Discuss with physician		Stop taking drug now	Call physician now
	Common	Rare	Only if severe	In all cases		
Anxiety/agitation	●			■		
Diarrhea	●			■		
Weight loss	●			■		
Sweating/flushing	●			■		
Abdominal cramps	●			■		
Palpitations/chest pain	●			■		▮

PROLONGED USE

No special problems.

Monitoring Periodic tests of thyroid function are required.

INTERACTIONS

General note Levothyroxine can interact with many drugs including cholestyramine, colestipol, salbutamol, phenytoin, tricyclic antidepressants, estrogens, oral contraceptives, beta blockers, and digoxin.

Oral anticoagulants Levothyroxine may increase the effect of these drugs.

Antidiabetic drugs Levothyroxine may increase requirements for insulin or oral antidiabetic drugs.

LIDOCAINE

Brand names Xylocaine, Xylocard
Used in the following combined preparations Depo-Medrol with Lidocaine, EMLA Cream/Patch, Lidosporin Ear Drops

GENERAL INFORMATION

Lidocaine, introduced in 1948, is a powerful local anesthetic with a rapid onset of action. It penetrates tissues well, making it a useful drug for *topical* anesthesia. Available without a prescription, it is used to relieve pain, burning, and itching caused by sunburn, other minor skin disorders, and hemorrhoids. It is also used to relieve pain and discomfort during dental treatment and medical examinations in which a tube is passed down the throat or into the urethra.

Injections of lidocaine are widely used for all types of minor surgery and for epidural or spinal anesthesia during labor. It is also given by injection to treat abnormal heart rhythms after a heart attack, during heart surgery, or after overdosage with digitalis drugs.

QUICK REFERENCE

Drug group Local anesthetic (p.92) and anti-arrhythmic drug (p.112)
Overdose danger rating Medium
Dependence rating Low
Prescription needed No
Multi-source suppliers Yes

INFORMATION FOR USERS

Follow instructions on the label. Call your physician if symptoms worsen.

How taken

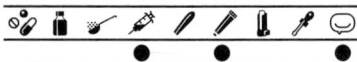

Topical solution, viscous solution, injection, jelly, ointment, patch, spray.

Frequency and timing of doses
As required for anesthetics or pain relief. For hemorrhoids, ointment is applied to the anal area after bowel movement and at night. For arrhythmias, lidocaine is usually given by intravenous injection over 2 – 3 minutes, followed by continuous infusion.

Dosage range
Apply topical preparations thinly to the affected area. Do not exceed the maximum recommended dose. Doses by injection are determined individually.

Onset of effect
2 – 5 minutes (topical preparations); within 2 minutes (intravenous injection).

Duration of action
Up to 1 hour (topical preparations); 10 – 20 minutes (intravenous injection).

Diet advice
Lidocaine by mouth causes numbness of the mouth and throat and may interfere with swallowing. To avoid choking and injury to the inside of your mouth from hot food or drink, do not eat or drink anything for 1 hour after taking lidocaine.

Storage
Keep in a closed container in a cool, dry place away from reach of children.

Missed dose
Apply topical preparations as soon as you remember if still required.

Stopping the drug
Can be safely stopped as soon as you no longer need it.

Exceeding the dose
An occasional unintentional extra application is unlikely to cause problems. Regular overuse may cause anxiety, restlessness, dizziness, trembling, or drowsiness. Notify your physician.

SPECIAL PRECAUTIONS

Be sure to consult your physician or pharmacist before using this drug if:
▼ You have impaired liver function.
▼ You have had an allergic reaction to a local anesthetic.
▼ You have sores or broken skin at the site of application.
▼ You are taking other medications.

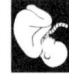

Pregnancy
▼ No evidence of risk with topical preparations. Given for spinal anesthesia during childbirth, it may prolong labor and increase the need for forceps-assisted delivery.

Breast feeding
▼ Topical preparations should not be used around the nipple. No evidence of risk with topical preparations applied at other sites.

Infants and children
▼ Not recommended for children under 3 years except under medical supervision.

Over 60
▼ Increased likelihood of adverse effects. Reduced dose may therefore be necessary.

Driving and hazardous work
▼ No special problems.

Alcohol
▼ No known problems.

POSSIBLE ADVERSE EFFECTS

Adverse effects are rare when lidocaine is used as a topical anesthetic. Central nervous system effects such as agitation, confusion, and drowsiness may occur with excessive use of topical preparations or with injections. High doses, such as those used for treating arrhythmias, may rarely cause tremors and seizures.

Symptom/effect	Frequency		Discuss with physician		Stop taking drug now	Call physician now
	Common	Rare	Only if severe	In all cases		
Anxiety/restlessness		●		■	▲	▮
Confusion/memory loss		●		■	▲	▮
Nausea/vomiting		●		■	▲	▮
Twitching/tremors		●		■	▲	▮
Shallow breathing		●		■	▲	▮
Seizures		●		■	▲	▮

PROLONGED USE

Topical preparations should not be used for prolonged periods. If your symptoms do not improve within a few days, consult your physician.

INTERACTIONS

Cimetidine and propranolol These drugs may increase the adverse effects of intravenous lidocaine injection.

LINDANE

Brand names Kwellada, Hexit, PMS-Lindane
Used in the following combined preparations None

GENERAL INFORMATION

Lindane, introduced in 1952, is an insecticide. Used in the treatment of scabies and lice infestations, it rapidly kills the parasites after being absorbed through their tough outer "skin".

A lotion or cream is used to treat scabies and body lice, while lindane shampoo is highly effective against head and pubic lice.

Adverse effects are rare when recommended doses are applied correctly, although lindane may occasionally cause irritation or a rash. Itching, due to an allergic reaction to residual mite eggs and feces, may persist for several weeks after lindane has been used to treat scabies.

Lindane can be considered a poison because excess use or accidental swallowing may cause seizures. Small children are at particular risk from accidental poisoning by swallowing.

INFORMATION FOR USERS

Read the product information carefully before using lindane. Do not use more than recommended amount without consulting your physician.

How taken

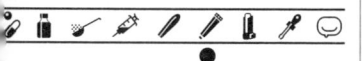

Lotion, cream, shampoo.

Frequency and timing of doses
Single treatment, repeated after one week, as instructed.

Adult dosage range
Use only as directed by package information or your physician. For scabies, the whole body except the head and neck should be covered.

Onset of effect
Within a few minutes.

Duration of action
Active until washed off.

Diet advice
None.

Storage
Keep in a closed container in a cool, dry place away from reach of children.

Missed dose
Not applicable.

Stopping the drug
Follow the advice of your physician. A second treatment is sometimes required to clear the parasites completely.

Exceeding the dose
A single excessive application to the skin or hair is unlikely to cause problems. Frequently repeated applications of the drug may cause agitation, vomiting, muscle cramps, and seizures, requiring prompt medical attention. **If the drug has been swallowed, seek immediate medical help. See Drug poisoning emergency guide (p.574).**

POSSIBLE ADVERSE EFFECTS

Used correctly, lindane rarely causes adverse effects. If you develop skin irritation during treatment, wash off the drug and consult your physician.

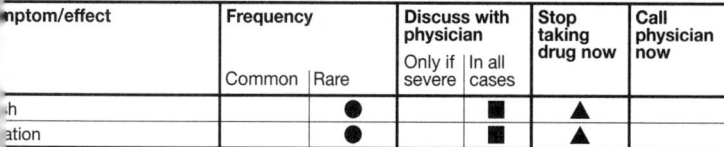

Symptom/effect	Frequency		Discuss with physician		Stop taking drug now	Call physician now
	Common	Rare	Only if severe	In all cases		
Rash		●		■		▲
Irritation		●		■		▲

INTERACTIONS

None.

SPECIAL PRECAUTIONS

Be sure to consult your physician or pharmacist before using this drug if:
▼ You have sensitive skin.
▼ You have had epileptic seizures.
▼ You are taking other medications.

Pregnancy
▼ Not usually prescribed. Safety in pregnancy not established. Discuss with your physician.

Breast feeding
▼ Used as directed, adverse effects on the baby are unlikely. Discuss with your physician.

Infants and children
▼ Not recommended for infants or children under 6 years, except on physician's advice.

Over 60
▼ No special problems.

Driving and hazardous work
▼ No known problems.

Alcohol
▼ No known problems.

PROLONGED USE

Not given for prolonged periods.

LIOTHYRONINE

Brand name Cytomel
Used in the following combined preparations None

GENERAL INFORMATION

Liothyronine, introduced in 1956, is a synthetic form of triiodothyronine, a powerful hormone produced by the thyroid gland. It is used to replace natural thyroid hormones when they are deficient as in hypothyroidism and myxedema. Faster acting than other thyroid hormone preparations, it is used occasionally for initial treatment of severe thyroid deficiency in adults. Taken by mouth, it is better absorbed into the bloodstream than other thyroid drugs and may be prescribed when absorption

of drugs is reduced by bowel disease.

Levels of liothyronine in the blood tend to vary widely between doses. Since this complicates monitoring of treatment, it is not generally given for prolonged periods.

Adults with severe thyroid deficiency are sensitive to thyroid hormones, and treatment needs to be introduced gradually to avoid adverse effects (see below). Since overdosage raises the blood pressure and strains the heart, this drug is given with caution to those with heart problems.

INFORMATION FOR USERS

Your drug prescription is tailored for you. Do not alter dosage without checking with your physician.

How taken

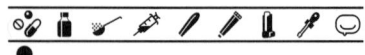

Tablets.

Frequency and timing of doses
As prescribed.

Adult dosage range
Initially 25mcg daily for mild hypothyroidism and 5mcg daily for severe hypothyroidism, increased as required. The usual maintenance dose is 50 – 100mcg daily.

Onset of effect
Within 12 hours. Full beneficial effects may not be felt for several weeks.

Duration of action
Up to 72 hours.

Diet advice
None.

Storage
Keep in a closed container in a cool, dry place away from reach of children.

Missed dose
Take as soon as you remember. If your next dose is due within 2 hours, take a single dose now and postpone your next dose for 4 hours.

Stopping the drug
Do not stop taking the drug without consulting your physician; symptoms may recur.

Exceeding the dose
An occasional unintentional extra dose is unlikely to cause problems. Large overdoses may cause palpitations during the next few days. Notify your physician.

SPECIAL PRECAUTIONS

Be sure to tell your physician if:
▼ You have heart problems.
▼ You have high blood pressure.
▼ You are taking other medications.

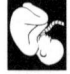 **Pregnancy**
▼ No evidence of risk to developin baby.

 Breast feeding
▼ The drug passes into the breast milk. Discuss with your physician.

 Infants and children
▼ Rarely required.

 Over 60
▼ Reduced dose usually necessar

 Driving and hazardous work
▼ No known problems.

 Alcohol
▼ No known problems.

POSSIBLE ADVERSE EFFECTS

Serious adverse effects are rare with liothyronine. Troublesome symptoms usually indicate that the dose is too high, and generally diminish with adjustment of the dose.

Symptom/effect	Frequency		Discuss with physician		Stop taking drug now	Call physician now
	Common	Rare	Only if severe	In all cases		
Anxiety/agitation	●			■		
Headache	●			■		
Diarrhea	●			■		
Weight loss	●			■		
Sweating/flushing	●			■		
Palpitations/chest pain		●		■		■

PROLONGED USE

Not usually given for prolonged treatment

Monitoring Periodic tests of thyroid function are usually required.

INTERACTIONS

General note Liothyronine can interact with many other drugs including cholestyramine, colestipol, salbutamol, phenytoin, tricyclic antidepressants, estrogens, oral contraceptives, beta blockers, and digoxin.

Oral anticoagulants Liothyronine may increase the effect of these drugs.

Antidiabetic drugs Liothyronine treatment may increase requirements for insulin or oral antidiabetic drugs.

LISINOPRIL

Brand names Prinivil, Zestril
Used in the following combined preparations Prinzide, Zestoretic

GENERAL INFORMATION

Lisinopril belongs to the ACE inhibitor group of vasodilator drugs. It is prescribed to treat hypertension (high blood pressure) and heart failure, achieving its effect by dilating blood vessels. Lisinopril is often given in conjunction with a diuretic to increase its effect.

The first dose of lisinopril may cause a sudden drop in blood pressure. You should therefore be resting at the time of first dose and able to lie down afterward for 2 – 3 hours.

The more common adverse effects, such as dizziness and headache, usually diminish with time. Rashes can also occur during treatment. These usually disappear when the drug is stopped. In some cases they clear up on their own despite continued treatment.

INFORMATION FOR USERS

Your drug prescription is tailored for you. Do not alter dosage without checking with your physician.

How taken

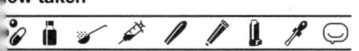

Tablets.

Frequency and timing of doses
Once daily.

Dosage range
5 – 10mg daily (starting dose), increased to 40mg daily (maintenance dose).

Onset of effect
Within 1 hour.

Duration of action
24 hours.

Diet advice
None.

Storage
Keep in a closed container in a cool, dry place away from the reach of children. Protect from light.

Missed dose
Take as soon as you remember. If your next dose is due within 8 hours, do not take the skipped dose. Take your next dose as usual.

Stopping the drug
Do not stop taking the drug without consulting your physician; stopping the drug may lead to worsening of the underlying condition.

Exceeding the dose
An occasional unintentional dose is unlikely to cause problems. Large overdoses may cause dizziness or fainting. Notify your physician.

SPECIAL PRECAUTIONS

Be sure to tell your physician if:
▼ You have impaired kidney or liver function.
▼ You have diabetes.
▼ You have an autoimmune disease.
▼ You have coronary artery disease.
▼ You are pregnant or intend to become pregnant.
▼ You are taking other medications.

Pregnancy
▼ Use during pregnancy can cause injury and even death to the developing fetus. Report promptly to your physician if you become pregnant.

Breast feeding
▼ Effect on breast feeding uncertain. Discuss with your physician.

Infants and children
▼ Not recommended.

Over 60
▼ Reduced dose may be necessary.

Driving and hazardous work
▼ Avoid such activities until you have learned how the drug affects you; it can cause dizziness and fainting.

Alcohol
▼ Avoid. Alcohol increases the likelihood of an excessive drop in blood pressure.

Surgery and general anesthetics
▼ Lisinopril treatment may need to be stopped before you have a general anesthetic. Discuss with your physician or dentist before any surgery.

POSSIBLE ADVERSE EFFECTS

The more common adverse effects, such as headache and dizziness, usually diminish with time. The less common effects may also diminish during long-term treatment, but an adjustment in dosage may be necessary.

Symptom/effect	Frequency		Discuss with physician		Stop taking drug now	Call physician now
	Common	Rare	Only if severe	In all cases		
Headache	●		■			
Dizziness	●		■			
Fatigue	●		■			
Cough	●		■			
Nausea/vomiting	●			■		
Flu-like symptoms		●		■	▲	∎
Increased sweating		●		■		
Swelling of face or tongue		●		■	▲	∎

INTERACTIONS

Antihypertensive drugs are likely to add to the blood pressure-lowering effect of lisinopril.

Lithium Lisinopril may increase the level of lithium in the blood, and serious adverse effects from lithium excess may occur.

Potassium supplements and potassium-sparing diuretics Lisinopril may add to the effect of these drugs, leading to raised levels of potassium in the blood.

Indomethacin may reduce the effect of lisinopril.

PROLONGED USE

No problems expected.

Monitoring Periodic tests on blood and urine should be performed.

LITHIUM

Brand names Carbolith, Duralith, Lithane, Lithizine
Used in the following combined preparations None

GENERAL INFORMATION

A form of the lightest metal we know, the drug lithium has been used since 1949 to help those suffering from a severe mental disturbance, manic depression (bipolar affective disorder). Lithium decreases the intensity and frequency of the episodic swings from extreme excitement to deep depression that are characteristic of that disorder.

A preferred agent for mania alone, it is also sometimes used to prevent and treat severe depression (see p.96).

Treatment with lithium may be started in the hospital for the more seriously ill. Careful monitoring is required because high levels of lithium in the blood can cause serious adverse effects. Since it may take two to three weeks for any benefit of lithium to become apparent, an antipsychotic drug is often given with lithium until the lithium becomes effective.

treat severe depression (see p.96).

QUICK REFERENCE

Drug group Antimanic drug (p.97)
Overdose danger rating High
Dependence rating Low
Prescription needed Yes
Multi-source suppliers Yes

INFORMATION FOR USERS

Your drug prescription is tailored for you. Do not alter dosage without checking with your physician.

How taken

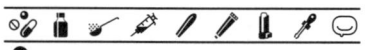

Tablets, slow-release tablets, capsules.

Frequency and timing of doses
2 – 3 x daily with meals (capsules, tablets); every 12 hours (slow-release tablets).

Adult dosage range
900 – 1,800mg daily. Dosage may vary according to individual response.

Onset of effect
Some effects may be noticed in 3 – 5 days, but full benefits may not be felt for 3 weeks.

Duration of action
18 – 36 hours. Some effect may last for several days.

Diet advice
Lithium levels in the blood are affected by the amount of sodium (present in salt) in the body, so you should be careful not to suddenly increase or reduce the amount of salt in your diet. Be sure to drink adequate volumes of fluids, especially in hot weather.

Storage
Keep in a closed container in a cool, dry place away from reach of children. Protect from light.

Missed dose
Take as soon as you remember. If your next dose is due within 2 hours (6 hours for slow-release tablets), do not take the missed dose. Take your next scheduled dose as usual.

Stopping the drug
Do not stop the drug without consulting your physician; symptoms may recur.

OVERDOSE ACTION

Seek immediate medical advice in all cases. Take emergency action if consciousness is lost or if convulsions occur.

See Drug poisoning emergency guide (p.574).

SPECIAL PRECAUTIONS

Be sure to tell your physician if:
▼ You have impaired liver or kidney function.
▼ You have heart or circulation problems.
▼ You have diabetes.
▼ You have had epileptic seizures.
▼ You have an overactive thyroid gland.
▼ You have myasthenia gravis.
▼ You are taking other medications.

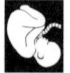

Pregnancy
▼ Not usually prescribed. May cause defects in the unborn baby. Discuss with your physician.

Breast feeding
▼ The drug passes into the breast milk and may affect the baby. Discuss with your physician.

Infants and children
▼ Not recommended.

Over 60
▼ Increased likelihood of adverse effects. Reduced dose may therefore be necessary.

Driving and hazardous work
▼ Avoid such activities until you have learned how the drug affects you; it can cause reduced alertness and blurred vision.

Alcohol
▼ Avoid. Alcohol may increase the sedative effects of this drug.

POSSIBLE ADVERSE EFFECTS

Most adverse effects are related to the blood levels of the drug. Your physician will try to find a dose that is sufficient to control your condition without causing excessive adverse effects. Most of the symptoms listed below are signs of high lithium level in the blood. Seek medical advice if you notice any of these.

Symptom/effect	Frequency		Discuss with physician		Stop taking drug now	Call physician now
	Common	Rare	Only if severe	In all cases		
Nausea/vomiting/diarrhea	●			■	▲	
Trembling	●			■	▲	
Weight gain		●	■			
Drowsiness/lethargy		●		■	▲	
Blurred vision		●		■	▲	
Rash		●		■	▲	
Metallic taste in mouth		●		■		

PROLONGED USE

Prolonged use may lead to kidney problems. Treatment for periods of longer than 5 years is not normally advised unless the benefits are significant and tests show no sign of reduced kidney function.

Monitoring Blood levels of the drug are monitored regularly. In addition, regular blood tests to check blood composition, body salts, and kidney and thyroid function are carried out. Heart function may be assessed by electrocardiograms.

INTERACTIONS

General note Many drugs interact with lithium. Do not take any over-the-counter or prescription drugs without first consulting your physician or pharmacist.

LOPERAMIDE

Brand names Imodium, PMS-Loperamide Hydrochloride
Used in the following combined preparations None

GENERAL INFORMATION

Loperamide is an antidiarrheal drug that is available in capsules or liquid form. It reduces the loss of water and salts from the bowel and slows bowel activity, resulting in the passage of firmer bowel movements at less frequent intervals.

A fast-acting drug, it is widely used to treat both sudden and recurrent bouts of diarrhea. However, it is not generally recommended for diarrhea caused by infection because it may delay the expulsion of harmful substances from the bowel. Loperamide is also used to reduce fluid loss from the stoma (outlet) in people who have had colostomies or ileostomies.

Adverse effects from this drug are rare; unlike the opium-based anti-diarrheals, there is no risk of abuse. It can be purchased without a prescription in a pharmacy.

QUICK REFERENCE

Drug group Antidiarrheal drug (p.122)

Overdose danger rating Medium

Dependence rating Low

Prescription needed No

Multi-source suppliers Yes

INFORMATION FOR USERS

Follow instructions on the label. Call your physician if symptoms worsen.

How taken

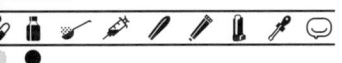

Capsules, oral liquid.

Frequency and timing of doses
Adults 4mg initially, then 2mg after each loose bowel movement; then 2 – 4mg twice daily, as needed.

Dosage range
Adults 4 – 16mg daily.
Children Reduced dose according to age and weight.

Onset of effect
Within 1 – 2 hours.

Duration of action
6 – 18 hours.

Diet advice
None. Ensure adequate fluid, sugar, and salt intake during a diarrheal illness.

Storage
Keep in a closed container in a cool, dry place away from reach of children.

Missed dose
Do not take the missed dose. Take your next dose if needed.

Stopping the drug
Can be safely stopped as soon as you no longer need it.

Exceeding the dose
An occasional unintentional extra dose is unlikely to cause problems. Large overdoses may cause constipation, vomiting, or drowsiness. Notify your physician.

SPECIAL PRECAUTIONS

Be sure to consult your physician or pharmacist before taking this drug if:
▼ You have impaired liver or kidney function.
▼ You have had recent abdominal surgery.
▼ You are taking other medications.

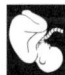

Pregnancy
▼ Safety in pregnancy not established. Discuss with your physician.

Breast feeding
▼ The drug passes into the breast milk and may affect the baby. Discuss with your physician.

Infants and children
▼ Not recommended in children under 12 years except on the advice of a physician.

Over 60
▼ Use with caution as there is an increased risk of blockage of the intestine.

Driving and hazardous work
▼ Avoid such activities until you have learned how the drug affects you; it can cause dizziness, drowsiness, and blurred vision.

Alcohol
▼ No known problems.

POSSIBLE ADVERSE EFFECTS

Adverse effects are rare with loperamide and often difficult to distinguish from the effects of the diarrhea it is used to treat. If symptoms such as bloating, abdominal pain, or fever persist or worsen during treatment with loperamide, consult your physician.

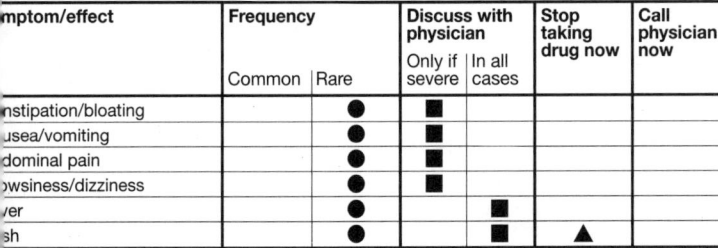

Symptom/effect	Frequency		Discuss with physician		Stop taking drug now	Call physician now
	Common	Rare	Only if severe	In all cases		
Constipation/bloating		●		■		
Nausea/vomiting		●		■		
Abdominal pain		●		■		
Drowsiness/dizziness		●		■		
Fever		●			■	
Rash		●			■	▲

INTERACTIONS

None.

PROLONGED USE

In acute diarrhea, treatment with loperamide should be discontinued after 48 hours if improvement does not occur. This drug is not usually taken for prolonged periods (except for persons with ileostomies), but special problems are not expected during long-term use.

LORATADINE

Brand name Claritin
Used in the following combined preparations Chlor-Tripolon N.D., Claritin Extra

GENERAL INFORMATION

Loratadine is a long-acting antihistamine drug. It is used for the relief of symptoms associated with allergic rhinitis and hay fever such as sneezing, runny nose, and itching and burning of the eyes. Allergic skin conditions such as chronic urticaria (hives) may also be helped by loratadine.

The main difference between this drug and the older, traditional antihistamines is that it has fewer sedative effects. It is therefore less likely to cause drowsiness. It also has fewer *anticholinergic* effects than the older antihistamines.

QUICK REFERENCE

Drug group Antihistamine (p.136)
Overdose danger rating Low
Dependence rating Low
Prescription needed No
Multi-source suppliers No

INFORMATION FOR USERS

Follow instructions on the label. Call your physician if symptoms worsen.

How taken

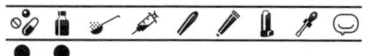

Tablets, oral liquid.

Frequency and timing of doses
Once daily.

Dosage range
Adults and children over 10 years 10mg daily;
Children 2 to 9 years 5mg daily.

Onset of effect
1 – 3 hours.

Duration of action
Up to 24 hours.

Diet advice
None.

Storage
Keep in a closed container in a cool, dry place away from reach of children.

Missed dose
If it is almost time for your next dose, take a single dose now and skip the next.

Stopping the drug
Can be safely stopped as soon as you no longer need it.

Exceeding the dose
An occasional unintentional extra dose is unlikely to be a cause for concern. But if you notice unusual symptoms, or if a large overdose has been taken, notify your physician.

POSSIBLE ADVERSE EFFECTS

Fatigue, headache, dry mouth, sedation, and other *side effects* are rare. A rash may be a sign of an unusual allergic reaction.

Symptom/effect	Frequency		Discuss with physician		Stop taking drug now	Call physician now
	Common	Rare	Only if severe	In all cases		
Drowsiness/fatigue		●		■		
Headache		●		■		
Dry mouth		●		■		
Rash		●			■	▲

INTERACTIONS

Sedatives Loratadine may increase the *sedative* effects on the central nervous system of anti-anxiety drugs, sleeping drugs, antidepressants, and antipsychotics.

Anticholinergic drugs The anticholinergic effects of loratadine are likely to be increased by all drugs that have anticholinergic effects including antipsychotics and tricyclic antidepressants.

SPECIAL PRECAUTIONS

Be sure to consult your physician or pharmacist before taking this drug if:
▼ You have glaucoma.
▼ You have impaired liver function.
▼ You are taking other medications.

Pregnancy
▼ Safety in pregnancy not established. Discuss with your physician.

Breast feeding
▼ Safety in breast feeding not established. Discuss with your physician.

Infants and children
▼ Not recommended in patients under 2 years.

Over 60
▼ Reduced dose may be necessary.

Driving and hazardous work
▼ Avoid such activities until you have learned how the drug affects you; it can occasionally cause sedation.

Alcohol
▼ No known problems.

PROLONGED USE

Antihistamines should be discontinued approximately 48 hours prior to allergy skin testing.

LORAZEPAM

Brand names Ativan, Apo-Lorazepam, Novo-Lorazem, Nu-Loraz
Used in the following combined preparations None

GENERAL INFORMATION

Lorazepam belongs to a group of drugs known as the benzodiazepines, which help to relieve anxiety and encourage sleep. The actions and adverse effects of this group of drugs are described more fully on page 95.

Lorazepam is used for the short-term treatment of excessive anxiety. The injectable form of the drug may be used as an anticonvulsant for the control of status epilepticus (see p.98). Lorazepam is less likely than some of the other benzodiazepines to accumulate in the body.

In common with other benzodiazepines, lorazepam can be habit-forming if taken regularly over a long period. Its effects may also diminish with time. For those reasons, treatment with lorazepam should be reviewed regularly.

(see p.98)

QUICK REFERENCE

Drug group Benzodiazepine anti-anxiety drug (p.95)

Overdose danger rating Medium

Dependence rating High

Prescription needed Yes

Multi-source suppliers Yes

INFORMATION FOR USERS

Your drug prescription is tailored for you. Do not alter dosage without checking with your physician.

How taken

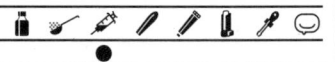

Tablets, sublingual tablets, injection.

Frequency and timing of doses
1–4 x daily.

Adult dosage range
1–6mg daily (by mouth); varies with condition under treatment (injection).

Onset of effect
30–60 minutes (oral tablets); 5–10 minutes (intravenous injection); less than 30 minutes (intramuscular injection, sublingual tablets).

Duration of action
6 to 8 hours.

Diet advice
None.

Storage
Keep in a closed container in a cool, dry place away from reach of children. Protect from light.

Missed dose
If you are taking the drug once daily for insomnia, a missed dose is no cause for concern. Return to your normal dose schedule the following night, if necessary. On a daytime schedule, take the missed dose when you remember. If your next dose is due within 2 hours, take a single dose now and skip the next.

Stopping the drug
If you have been taking the drug continuously for less than 2 weeks, it can be safely stopped as soon as you feel you no longer need it. However, if you have been taking the drug for longer, consult your physician, who will supervise a gradual reduction in dosage. Stopping abruptly may lead to withdrawal symptoms (see p.94).

Exceeding the dose
An occasional unintentional extra dose is unlikely to cause problems. Larger overdoses may cause unusual drowsiness. Notify your physician.

(see p.94)

SPECIAL PRECAUTIONS

Be sure to tell your physician if:
▼ You have severe respiratory disease.
▼ You have impaired liver or kidney function.
▼ You have myasthenia gravis.
▼ You have glaucoma.
▼ You have problems with alcohol or drug abuse.
▼ You are taking other medications.

Pregnancy
▼ Safety in pregnancy not established. Discuss with your physician.

Breast feeding
▼ The drug passes into the breast milk. Its effects on the baby are not clearly known. Discuss with your physician.

Infants and children
▼ Not recommended for those under 18 years.

Over 60
▼ Increased likelihood of adverse effects. Reduced dose may therefore be necessary.

Driving and hazardous work
▼ Avoid such activities until you have learned how the drug affects you; it can cause reduced alertness and slowed reactions.

Alcohol
▼ Avoid. Alcohol increases the sedative effects of this drug.

POSSIBLE ADVERSE EFFECTS

The principal adverse effects of this drug are related to its sedative and tranquilizing properties. These effects normally diminish after the first few days of treatment and, if troublesome, can often be reduced by adjustment of dosage.

Symptom/effect	Frequency		Discuss with physician		Stop taking drug now	Call physician now
	Common	Rare	Only if severe	In all cases		
Drowsiness/unsteadiness	●		■			
Dizziness/weakness	●		■			
Headache		●		■		
Nausea/vomiting		●		■		
Amnesia		●		■	▲	
Confusion/disorientation		●		■		▮
Rash		●		■	▲	▮

PROLONGED USE

Regular use of this drug over several weeks can lead to a reduction in its effect as the body adapts. It may also be habit-forming when taken for extended periods, especially if large doses are taken.

INTERACTIONS

Sedatives All drugs, including alcohol, that have a sedative effect on the central nervous system are likely to increase the sedative properties of lorazepam. Such drugs include other anti-anxiety and sleeping drugs, antihistamines, antidepressants, narcotic analgesics, scopolamine, and antipsychotics.

LOVASTATIN

Brand name Mevacor
Used in the following combined preparations None

GENERAL INFORMATION

Lovastatin is a lipid-lowering drug for reducing blood levels of cholesterol. It works by blocking an enzyme needed in the formation of cholesterol and by increasing *receptors* on cells, thereby allowing removal of cholesterol from the bloodstream. In particular, lovastatin significantly lowers the harmful low-density lipoprotein (LDL) component of cholesterol. A high blood level of cholesterol has been shown to be a risk factor in the development of athero-sclerosis (narrowing of arteries).

To be fully effective, lovastatin needs to be used in conjunction with a low-fat, low-cholesterol diet and adequate exercise. Studies are underway to determine whether lovastatin reduces established atherosclerosis.

Lovastatin is usually well tolerated with few adverse effects.

QUICK REFERENCE

Drug group Lipid-lowering drug (p.115)

Overdose danger rating Low

Dependence rating Low

Prescription needed Yes

Multi-source suppliers No

INFORMATION FOR USERS

Your drug prescription is tailored for you. Do not alter dosage without checking with your physician.

How taken

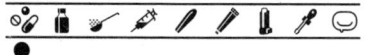

Tablets.

Frequency and timing of doses
1 – 2 x daily with food.

Adult dosage range
20 – 80mg daily.

Onset of effect
2 – 4 hours. Maximum effect on lipids within 4 – 6 weeks.

Duration of action
12 – 24 hours.

Diet advice
A low-fat, low-cholesterol diet must be maintained for the drug to be fully effective. Follow your physician's advice.

Storage
Keep in a closed container in a cool, dry place away from reach of children. Protect from light.

Missed dose
Take as soon as you remember. If your next dose is due within 2 hours, take a single dose now and skip the next.

Stopping the drug
Do not stop the drug without consulting your physician; stopping the drug may lead to worsening of the underlying condition.

Exceeding the dose
An occasional unintentional extra dose is unlikely to be a cause for concern. But if you notice unusual symptoms, or if a large over-dose has been taken, notify your physician.

SPECIAL PRECAUTIONS

Be sure to tell your physician if:
▼ You have impaired liver function.
▼ You have had problems with alcohol abuse.
▼ You have had epileptic seizures.
▼ You have cataracts.
▼ You have muscle pain or tenderness.
▼ You are taking other medications.

Pregnancy
▼ Not prescribed.

Breast feeding
▼ Not recommended. It is not known if the drug passes into breast milk. Discuss with your physician.

Infants and children
▼ Not recommended.

Over 60
▼ No special problems.

Driving and hazardous work
▼ Exercise caution if blurred vision or dizziness occurs.

Alcohol
▼ Avoid excessive alcohol, as it may affect levels of fats in the blood and liver function.

Surgery and general anesthetics
▼ Discuss with your physician or dentist before any operation.

POSSIBLE ADVERSE EFFECTS

The drug is usually well tolerated. Adverse effects that may occur include headache, aching muscles, muscle cramping, or weakness.

Symptom/effect	Frequency		Discuss with physician		Stop taking drug now	Call physician now
	Common	Rare	Only if severe	In all cases		
Headache	●		■			
Nausea	●		■			
Cramps/diarrhea/constipation	●		■			
Rash		●		■		
Muscle pain/tenderness		●		■		▮
Blurred vision		●		■		▮

INTERACTIONS

Lipid-lowering drugs Lovastatin and gemfibrozil or other fibrate derivatives are not usually prescribed together because of the risk of severe muscle inflammation.

Oral anticoagulants Lovastatin may increase bleeding with warfarin. Therefore the dose of warfarin must be monitored.

PROLONGED USE

The drug may alter liver function during long-term use. In rare cases, the drug may encourage cataract formation. ·

Monitoring Regular checks on levels of lipids in blood are usually required, as well as checks on liver function and muscle enzymes. A yearly eye examination is recommended.

LOXAPINE

Brand name Loxapac
Used in the following combined preparations None

GENERAL INFORMATION

Loxapine is a relatively new tricyclic antipsychotic drug used to treat schizophrenia. It is chemically different from previous drugs used to treat this condition.

A transient drowsiness may occur when starting the drug or increasing the dose, but this usually subsides as therapy continues.

Loxapine can cause a variety of *side effects* (see below). However, in overdose it is less likely to cause abnormal heart rhythms than other tricyclic agents, though it carries a greater risk of causing seizures.

INFORMATION FOR USERS

Your drug prescription is tailored for you. Do not alter dosage without checking with your physician.

How taken

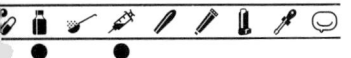

Tablets, oral liquid, injection.

Frequency and timing of doses
1 – 4 x daily.

Adult dosage range
20 – 250mg daily.

Onset of effect
1 – 3 hours; full clinical effect in some patients may not be felt for weeks or months.

Duration of action
Sedative effect lasts for 12 hours, or longer, particularly with the injection.

Diet advice
None.

Storage
Keep in a closed container in a cool, dry place away from reach of children. Protect from light. Protect the liquid from freezing.

Missed dose
Take as soon as you remember. If your next dose is due within 1 hour, skip the missed dose and go back to your regular dosing schedule. Do not double doses.

Stopping the drug
Do not stop taking the drug without consulting your physician, who may supervise a gradual reduction in dosage.

OVERDOSE ACTION

 Seek immediate medical advice in all cases. Do not induce vomiting. Take emergency action if seizures occur.

See Drug poisoning emergency guide (p.574).

SPECIAL PRECAUTIONS

Be sure to tell your physician if:
▼ You have heart problems.
▼ You have had prostate trouble.
▼ You have glaucoma.
▼ You have a history of blood disorders.
▼ You have difficulty urinating.
▼ You have impaired liver function.
▼ You have had epileptic seizures.
▼ You are taking other medications.

 **Pregnancy**
▼ Safety in pregnancy not established. Discuss with your physician.

 Breast feeding
▼ It is not known whether the drug passes into the breast milk. Discuss with your physician.

 Infants and children
▼ Not recommended for use in children under 16 years.

 Over 60
▼ Increased likelihood of adverse effects. Reduced dose may therefore be necessary.

 Driving and hazardous work
▼ Avoid such activities until you have learned how the drug affects you; it can cause drowsiness, dizziness, and blurred vision.

 Alcohol
▼ Avoid. Alcohol may increase the sedative effects of this drug.

Surgery and anesthetics
▼ Loxapine may need to be stopped before you have a general anesthetic. Discuss this with your physician or dentist before any surgery.

POSSIBLE ADVERSE EFFECTS

The possible adverse effects of the drug are mainly the result of its *anticholinergic* action and its blocking effect on the transmission of signals through the heart. Some problems can be overcome by medically supervised adjustment of dosage.

Symptom/effect	Frequency		Discuss with physician		Stop taking drug now	Call physician now
	Common	Rare	Only if severe	In all cases		
Drowsiness/dizziness	●		■			
Dry mouth	●		■			
Constipation	●		■			
Involuntary movements	●			■	▲	▌
Nipple discharge		●		■		
Palpitations/seizures		●		■	▲	▌
Rash/itching		●		■	▲	

INTERACTIONS

Sedatives All drugs, including alcohol, that have a sedative effect on the central nervous system are likely to increase the sedative effects of loxapine.

Antacids or antidiarrheal medications Do not take loxapine within an hour or two of these medications as they may decrease the effect of loxapine.

PROLONGED USE

Loxapine may produce tremors and abnormal movements (*parkinsonism* or *tardive dyskinesia*) when used for periods of several months or longer.

MAGNESIUM HYDROXIDE

Brand names Phillips' Milk of Magnesia
Used in the following combined preparations Amphojel 500, Diovol Ex, Maalox, Neutralca-S, Phillips' Gelcaps

GENERAL INFORMATION

Magnesium hydroxide is a fast-acting antacid used to neutralize stomach acid. It is available in a number of over-the-counter preparations for the treatment of indigestion, heartburn, and pain due to stomach and duodenal ulcers, gastritis, and reflux esophagitis. It also acts as a laxative by pulling water into the intestine from surrounding blood vessels to soften the feces.

Magnesium hydroxide is not often used alone as an antacid because of this laxative effect. However, this is countered when the drug is combined with aluminum hydroxide, which tends to be constipating.

INFORMATION FOR USERS

Follow the instructions on the label. Call your physician if symptoms worsen.

How taken

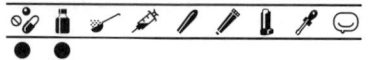

Tablets, oral liquid.

Frequency and timing of doses
4 x daily with water.

Adult dosage range
Antacid 5 – 20 mL per dose (liquid); 0.6 – 1.2g per dose (tablets).
Laxative 30 – 60mL per dose (liquid); 1.8 – 2.4g per dose (tablets).

Onset of effect
Within 15 minutes (antacid); 2 – 8 hours (laxative).

Duration of action
2 – 4 hours

Diet advice
None.

Storage
Keep in a closed container in a cool, dry place away from reach of children.

Missed dose
Take as soon as you remember.

Stopping the drug
When used as an antacid, can be safely stopped as soon as you no longer need it. When given as ulcer treatment, follow your physician's advice.

Exceeding the dose
An occasional unintentional extra dose is unlikely to be a cause for concern. But if you notice unusual symptoms, or if a large overdose has been taken, notify your physician.

SPECIAL PRECAUTIONS

Be sure to consult your physician or pharmacist before taking this drug if:
▼ You have impaired kidney function.
▼ You have a bowel disorder.
▼ You are taking other medications.

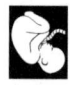
Pregnancy
▼ No evidence of risk to developing baby in normal doses.

Breast feeding
▼ No evidence of risk.

Infants and children
▼ Not recommended under 6 years except on the advice of a physician. Reduced dose necessary for older children.

Over 60
▼ No special problems.

Driving and hazardous work
▼ No known problems.

Alcohol
▼ Avoid excess alcohol as it irritates the stomach and may reduce the benefits of this drug.

POSSIBLE ADVERSE EFFECTS

Diarrhea is the most common adverse effect of this drug. Dizziness and muscle weakness due to absorption of excess magnesium in the body are likely to occur only in people with poor kidney function.

Symptom/effect	Frequency		Discuss with physician		Stop taking drug now	Call physician now
	Common	Rare	Only if severe	In all cases		
Diarrhea	●		■			
Nausea	●		■			
Vomiting		●			■	
Dizziness		●			■	

PROLONGED USE

Magnesium hydroxide should not be used for longer than 4 weeks without consulting your physician. Prolonged use in people with kidney damage may cause nausea, dizziness, and weakness, due to accumulation of magnesium in the body.

INTERACTIONS

General note Magnesium hydroxide interferes with the absorption of a wide range of drugs taken by mouth, including tetracycline antibiotics, iron supplements, penicillamine, and digoxin.

Enteric-coated tablets As with other antacids, magnesium hydroxide may allow breakup of the enteric coating of tablets such as bisacodyl, sometimes leading to stomach irritation.

MAPROTILINE

Brand name Ludiomil
Used in the following combined preparations None

GENERAL INFORMATION

Maprotiline was the first of a group of antidepressant drugs known as the tetracyclics to be introduced in Canada. Tetracyclics help lift mood, restore appetite, and renew interest in everyday activities. Maprotiline is used to treat many types of depression including manic depression (bipolar affective disorder).

In common with the tricyclic antidepressants, maprotiline can cause abnormal heart rhythms. It is therefore used with caution in those with heart problems or thyroid disorders. At higher doses there may be an increased risk of convulsions.

QUICK REFERENCE

Drug group Tetracyclic antidepressant drug (p.96)

Overdose danger rating High

Dependence rating Low

Prescription needed Yes

Multi-source suppliers No

INFORMATION FOR USERS

Your drug prescription is tailored for you. Do not alter dosage without checking with your physician.

How taken

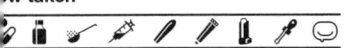

Tablets.

Frequency and timing of doses
1 – 3 x daily.

Adult dosage range
25 – 150mg daily. Dose may be increased in exceptional circumstances.

Onset of effect
Some effects may appear within a couple of days, but full antidepressant effect may not be felt for 2 – 6 weeks.

Duration of action
Beneficial effects may persist after discontinuation, sometimes in diminishing degrees, for up to 6 weeks. Adverse effects may wear off within days.

Diet advice
None.

Storage
Keep in a closed container in a cool, dry place away from the reach of children. Protect from light.

Missed dose
Take as soon as you remember. If your next dose is due within 3 hours, take a single dose now and skip the next.

Stopping the drug
Do not stop the drug without consulting your physician.

OVERDOSE ACTION

 Seek immediate medical advice in all cases. Take emergency action if consciousness is lost.

See Drug poisoning emergency guide (p.574).

POSSIBLE ADVERSE EFFECTS

The possible adverse effects of this drug are mainly the result of its *anticholinergic* action and its blocking action on the transmission of signals in the heart.

Symptom/effect	Frequency		Discuss with physician		Stop taking drug now	Call physician now
	Common	Rare	Only if severe	In all cases		
Drowsiness	●		■			
Dry mouth/blurred vision	●		■			
Rash	●			■	▲	
Dizziness/fainting		●		■		
Difficulty in passing urine		●		■		
Palpitations		●		■	▲	■
Seizures		●		■	▲	■

INTERACTIONS

Sedatives All drugs, including alcohol, that have a sedative effect on the central nervous system are likely to increase the sedative properties of maprotiline.

Antihypertensive drugs Maprotiline may reduce the beneficial effects of some of these drugs.

Monoamine oxidase inhibitors (MAOIs) There is a possibility of a serious interaction, producing seizures and delirium. Two weeks should elapse between maprotiline and MAOI treatments.

SPECIAL PRECAUTIONS

Be sure to tell your physician if:
▼ You have heart problems.
▼ You have had epileptic seizures.
▼ You have impaired liver or kidney function.
▼ You have had glaucoma.
▼ You have had prostate trouble.
▼ You have a thyroid disorder.
▼ You have a blood disease.
▼ You are taking other medications.

Pregnancy
▼ Safety in pregnancy not established. Discuss with your physician.

Breast feeding
▼ The drug passes into the breast milk and may affect the baby adversely. Discuss with your physician.

Infants and children
▼ Not recommended.

Over 60
▼ Increased likelihood of adverse effects, particularly dizziness or unsteadiness on standing. Reduced dose necessary.

Driving and hazardous work
▼ Avoid such activities until you have learned how the drug affects you; it can cause blurred vision and reduced alertness.

Alcohol
▼ Avoid. Alcohol may increase the sedative effects of this drug.

Surgery and general anesthetics
▼ Maprotiline treatment may need to be stopped before you have a general anesthetic. Discuss this with your physician or dentist before any operation.

PROLONGED USE

No problems expected.

MEBENDAZOLE

Brand name Vermox
Used in the following combined preparations None

GENERAL INFORMATION

Mebendazole is an anthelmintic that is effective in the treatment of pinworm, roundworm, whipworm, and hookworm infestations of the bowel. It has also been used to treat infestations due to large tapeworms. Because it has a wide range of activity, it is sometimes prescribed for multiple worm infestations and may be useful when the worm cannot be identified.

Taken as tablets, mebendazole kills worms by blocking their energy supply. Pinworm infestations are usually cleared up by a single dose, while other worm infestations of the bowel require treatment for three consecutive days. Treatment may be repeated after three weeks if the infestation has not completely cleared up. For pinworms, which are highly infectious, all members of a household are usually treated.

Because mebendazole is absorbed into the bloodstream only in small amounts, it rarely causes side effects other than diarrhea and abdominal pain.

INFORMATION FOR USERS

Your drug prescription is tailored for you. Do not alter dosage without checking with your physician.

How taken

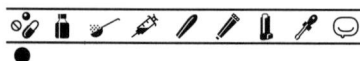

Chewable tablets.

Frequency and timing of doses
2 x daily morning and evening for 3 days (hookworm, common roundworm, whipworm); single dose (pinworm).

Dosage range
100mg in the morning and evening (hookworm, common roundworm, whipworm); one 100mg dose (pinworm).

Onset of effect
2 – 4 hours.

Duration of action
2 – 3 days.

Diet advice
None.

Storage
Keep in a closed container in a cool, dry place away from reach of children.

Missed dose
Take as soon as you remember. If your next dose is due at this time, take the two doses together. Return to your normal schedule thereafter.

Stopping the drug
Take the full course. Even if you feel better, the original infection may still be present and may recur if treatment is stopped too soon.

Exceeding the dose
An occasional unintentional extra dose is unlikely to cause problems. Large overdoses may cause abdominal cramps, nausea, vomiting, and diarrhea. Notify your physician.

SPECIAL PRECAUTIONS

Be sure to tell your physician if:
▼ You have impaired kidney or liver function.
▼ You have a bowel disorder.
▼ You are taking other medications.

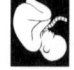
Pregnancy
▼ Safety in pregnancy not established. Discuss with your physician.

Breast feeding
▼ Effect on breast feeding unknown. Discuss with your physician.

Infants and children
▼ Not recommended for children under 2 years.

Over 60
▼ No special problems.

Driving and hazardous work
▼ Avoid such activities until you have learned how the drug affects you; it can cause drowsiness and dizziness.

Alcohol
▼ No known problems.

POSSIBLE ADVERSE EFFECTS

Abdominal pain and diarrhea may occur occasionally with mebendazole, but are rarely serious and generally disappear as treatment continues.

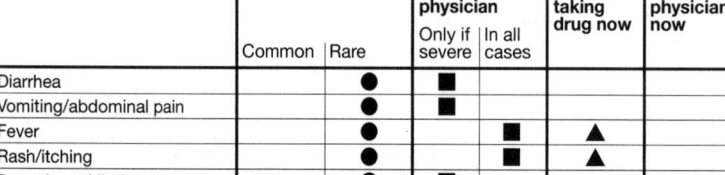

Symptom/effect	Frequency		Discuss with physician		Stop taking drug now	Call physician now
	Common	Rare	Only if severe	In all cases		
Diarrhea		●	■			
Vomiting/abdominal pain		●	■			
Fever		●		■	▲	
Rash/itching		●		■	▲	
Drowsiness/dizziness		●	■			

PROLONGED USE

High-dose therapy may increase the risk of a blood disorder.

Monitoring Periodic white blood cell counts are usually performed.

INTERACTIONS

Cimetidine may increase blood levels of mebendazole. The dose of mebendazole may need to be adjusted.

MECLIZINE

Brand name Bonamine
Used in the following combined preparation Antivert

GENERAL INFORMATION

Meclizine is an antihistamine that is used as an anti-emetic drug (see p.102). It is effective in preventing and treating motion sickness. Meclizine has slower onset of action and its effects last longer than those of many similar drugs; therefore it needs to be taken less frequently.

Meclizine is used to treat the vertigo, vomiting, and nausea caused by inner ear disorders. It is also occasionally used to relieve nausea and vomiting caused by drug or radiation therapy for cancer.

Meclizine has adverse effects similar to those of other antihistamines and *anticholinergic* drugs, including drowsiness, dry mouth, and blurred vision.

INFORMATION FOR USERS

Your drug prescription is tailored for you. Do not alter dosage without checking with your physician.

How taken

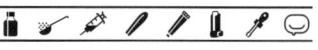

Tablets.

Frequency and timing of doses
Nausea and vertigo 1 – 2 x daily.
Motion sickness Once daily at least 1 hour before travel.
Radiation sickness Single dose 2 – 12 hours prior to treatment.

Adult dosage range
25 – 100mg daily.

Onset of effect
Within 1 hour.

Duration of action
8 – 24 hours.

Diet advice
None.

Storage
Keep in a closed container in a cool, dry place away from reach of children. Protect from light.

Missed dose
Take as soon as you remember. If your next dose is due within 2 hours, take a single dose now and skip the next.

Stopping the drug
Can be safely stopped as soon as you no longer need it.

Exceeding the dose
An occasional unintentional extra dose is unlikely to cause problems. Large overdoses may cause drowsiness or agitation. Notify your physician.

SPECIAL PRECAUTIONS

Be sure to tell your physician if:
▼ You have impaired liver or kidney function.
▼ You have glaucoma.
▼ You have had epileptic seizures.
▼ You have urinary difficulties.
▼ You are about to undergo allergy skin tests.
▼ You are taking other medications.

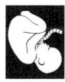

Pregnancy
▼ Safety in pregnancy not established. Discuss with your physician.

Breast feeding
▼ The drug passes into the breast milk in small amounts and may inhibit lactation. Discuss with your physician.

Infants and children
▼ Not recommended.

Over 60
▼ No special problems.

Driving and hazardous work
▼ Avoid such activities until you have learned how the drug affects you, because the drug can cause drowsiness and/or blurred vision.

Alcohol
▼ Avoid. Alcohol may increase the sedative effects of this drug.

POSSIBLE ADVERSE EFFECTS

The adverse effects of meclizine are similar to those of other antihistamines. The most common effect, drowsiness, may be controlled by an adjustment in dosage.

Symptom/effect	Frequency		Discuss with physician		Stop taking drug now	Call physician now
	Common	Rare	Only if severe	In all cases		
Drowsiness	●		■			
Dry mouth	●		■			
Blurred vision		●		■		

INTERACTIONS

Sedatives All drugs that have a sedative effect on the central nervous system are likely to increase the sedative effect of meclizine. Such drugs include alcohol, anti-anxiety drugs, sleeping drugs, narcotic analgesics, antihistamines, and antidepressants.

Anticonvulsant drugs Taking meclizine in conjunction with anticonvulsants may increase its sedation.

Monoamine oxidase inhibitors (MAOIs) may prolong and intensify meclizine's anticholinergic effects.

PROLONGED USE

Continuous use of this drug for more than a few days is unlikely to be necessary.

Antihistamines should be discontinued approximately 48 hours before allergy skin testing.

MEDROXYPROGESTERONE

Brand names Depo-Provera, Provera
Used in the following combined preparations None

GENERAL INFORMATION

Medroxyprogesterone is a progestin, a synthetic female sex hormone similar to the natural hormone progesterone. It is used to treat menstrual disorders such as mid-cycle bleeding and amenorrhea (absence of menstruation).

The drug may also be given in conjunction with estrogen replacement therapy for menopausal symptoms or underdeveloped ovaries. This reduces the risk of cancer of the uterus with estrogen treatment.

Medroxyprogesterone is often used to treat endometriosis, a condition in which there is abnormal growth of the uterine-lining tissue in the pelvic cavity.

Depot injections of the drug are used as a contraceptive in some foreign countries. However, since it may cause serious *side effects* including persistent bleeding from the uterus, amenorrhea, and prolonged infertility, this use remains controversial. It is not approved for general use as a contraceptive in Canada.

Medroxyprogesterone may be used to treat some types of cancer of the breast or uterus.

QUICK REFERENCE

Drug group Female sex hormone (p.159)

Overdose danger rating Low

Dependence rating Low

Prescription needed Yes

Multi-source suppliers No

INFORMATION FOR USERS

Your drug prescription is tailored for you. Do not alter dosage without checking with your physician.

How taken

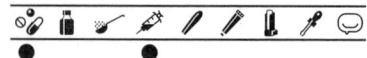

Tablets, injection.

Frequency and timing of doses
1 – 4 x daily with food (by mouth).

Adult dosage range
Cancer 200 – 400mg daily (by mouth).
Other conditions 5 – 10mg daily (by mouth).

Onset of effect
1 – 2 months (cancer); 1 – 2 weeks (other conditions).

Duration of action
1 – 2 days (by mouth); up to some months (injection).

Diet advice
None.

Storage
Keep in a closed container in a cool, dry place away from reach of children.

Missed dose
Take as soon as you remember. If your next dose is due within 12 hours, take a single dose now and skip the next.

Stopping the drug
Do not stop the drug without consulting your physician; symptoms may recur.

Exceeding the dose
An occasional unintentional extra dose is unlikely to be a cause for concern. But if you notice unusual symptoms, or if a large overdose has been taken, notify your physician.

SPECIAL PRECAUTIONS

Be sure to tell your physician if:
▼ You have high blood pressure.
▼ You have diabetes.
▼ You have had blood clots or a stroke.
▼ You have impaired liver or kidney function.
▼ You have a history of depression.
▼ You are taking other medications.

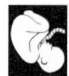

Pregnancy
▼ Not prescribed.

Breast feeding
▼ The drug passes into the breast milk and may affect the baby. Discuss with your physician.

Infants and children
▼ Not usually prescribed.

Over 60
▼ No special problems.

Driving and hazardous work
▼ No known problems.

Alcohol
▼ No known problems.

POSSIBLE ADVERSE EFFECTS

Medroxyprogesterone rarely causes serious adverse effects. Fluid retention may lead to weight gain, swollen feet or ankles, and breast tenderness. Long-term treatment may cause irregular menstrual bleeding or spotting between periods.

Symptom/effect	Frequency		Discuss with physician		Stop taking drug now	Call physician now
	Common	Rare	Only if severe	In all cases		
Weight gain	●		■			
Swollen ankles	●		■			
Breast tenderness		●	■			
Acne		●	■			
Irregular menstruation		●		■		
Rash/itching/jaundice		●		■	▲	

INTERACTIONS

None.

PROLONGED USE

Long-term use of this drug may slightly increase the risk of blood clots in the leg veins.

Monitoring Periodic checks on blood pressure, yearly cervical smear tests, and breast examinations are usually required.

MEFENAMIC ACID

Brand name Ponstan
Used in the following combined preparations None

GENERAL INFORMATION

Mefenamic acid, introduced in 1966, is a non-steroidal anti-inflammatory drug (NSAID). Like other NSAIDs, it relieves pain and inflammation. It is an effective analgesic, and is used to treat headache, toothache, and menstrual pains (dysmenorrhea). Mefenamic acid is also used for long-term relief of pain and stiffness in rheumatoid arthritis and osteoarthritis. The most common *side effects* of mefenamic acid are gastrointestinal: abdominal pain, indigestion, nausea, and vomiting. Other more serious adverse effects include kidney problems and blood disorders.

INFORMATION FOR USERS

Your drug prescription is tailored for you. Do not alter dosage without checking with your physician.

How taken

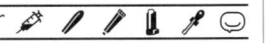

Capsules.

Frequency and timing of doses
Every 6 hours with food.

Adult dosage range
500mg (starting dose), then 250mg per dose as required.

Onset of effect
1 – 2 hours.

Duration of action
Up to 6 hours.

Diet advice
None.

Storage
Keep in a closed container in a cool, dry place away from reach of children.

Missed dose
Take as soon as you remember. If your next dose is due within 2 hours, take a single dose now and skip the next.

Stopping the drug
Can be safely stopped as soon as you no longer need it.

Exceeding the dose
An occasional unintentional extra dose is unlikely to cause problems. Large overdoses may cause muscle twitching, poor coordination, or seizures. Notify your physician.

SPECIAL PRECAUTIONS

Be sure to tell your physician if:
▼ You have impaired liver or kidney function.
▼ You have had a peptic ulcer, esophagitis, or acid indigestion.
▼ You have inflammatory bowel disease.
▼ You have asthma.
▼ You have heart problems.
▼ You have high blood pressure.
▼ You are allergic to ASA.
▼ You are taking other medications.

Pregnancy
▼ Not usually prescribed. May cause defects in the unborn baby and, taken in late pregnancy, may prolong labor. Discuss with your physician.

Breast feeding
▼ The drug passes into the breast milk, and may affect the baby adversely. Discuss with your physician.

Infants and children
▼ Not recommended for children under 14 years.

Over 60
▼ Increased likelihood of adverse effects. Reduced dose may therefore be necessary.

Driving and hazardous work
▼ Avoid such activities until you have learned how the drug affects you; it can cause drowsiness and dizziness.

Alcohol
▼ Avoid. Alcohol may increase the risk of stomach irritation with mefenamic acid.

Surgery and general anesthetics
▼ Mefenamic acid may prolong bleeding. Discuss with your physician or dentist before any surgery.

POSSIBLE ADVERSE EFFECTS

Gastrointestinal disturbances are the most common side effects of mefenamic acid. The drug should be stopped if diarrhea or a rash occurs, and not used thereafter. Black or bloodstained feces should be reported to your physician without delay.

Symptom/effect	Frequency		Discuss with physician		Stop taking drug now	Call physician now
	Common	Rare	Only if severe	In all cases		
Indigestion	●		■			
Dizziness/drowsiness		●	■			
Abdominal pain	●			■		
Diarrhea	●			■	▲	
Nausea/vomiting	●		■			
Headache		●		■		
Rash		●		■	▲	
Wheezing/breathlessness		●		■	▲	▮
Black/bloodstained feces		●		■	▲	▮

INTERACTIONS

General note Mefenamic acid interacts with a wide range of drugs to increase the risk of bleeding and/or peptic ulcers. Such drugs include oral anticoagulants, corticosteroids, other non-steroidal anti-inflammatory drugs (NSAIDs), ASA, some antibiotics, sulfinpyrazone, dipyridamole, and valproic acid.

Lithium Mefenamic acid may raise blood levels of lithium, leading to a risk of serious adverse effects.

Antihypertensive drugs and diuretics The beneficial effects of these drugs may be reduced by mefenamic acid.

Oral antidiabetic drugs Mefenamic acid may increase the blood sugar-lowering effect of these drugs.

PROLONGED USE

There is an increased risk of bleeding from peptic ulcers and in the bowel during long-term use. In rare cases, the drug may affect the liver and blood. Blood tests should be carried out during prolonged use. Kidney damage has occurred in elderly patients.

MEPERIDINE

Brand name Demerol
Used in the following combined preparation Pamergan

GENERAL INFORMATION

Similar to morphine, meperidine is a strong *narcotic* analgesic that was introduced in 1944. It is used almost exclusively in hospitals to relieve the severe pain felt during labor, and to relieve pain after an operation. It takes effect quickly, but its effect lasts for a short time compared to some other analgesics. This means that doses can be timed during labor to minimize adverse effects on the baby.

Meperidine is habit-forming. Both *tolerance* and *dependence* can develop if the drug is used inappropriately or excessively. When taken for pain relief of the appropriate conditions for brief periods of time, it is unlikely that drug dependence will occur.

QUICK REFERENCE

Drug group Narcotic analgesic (see pp.92, 177)

Overdose danger rating High

Dependence rating High

Prescription needed Yes

Multi-source suppliers Yes

INFORMATION FOR USERS

Your drug prescription is tailored for you. Do not alter dosage without checking with your physician.

How taken

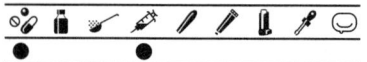

Tablets, injection.

Frequency and timing of doses
Every 3 – 4 hours as needed for pain.

Adult dosage range
50 – 150mg per dose.

Onset of effect
Within 1 hour (by mouth); within 15 minutes (injection).

Duration of action
2 – 4 hours.

Diet advice
None.

Storage
Keep in a closed container in a cool, dry place away from reach of children. Protect from light.

Missed dose
Take only if required for pain relief.

Stopping the drug
If you have been given the drug for pain relief, it can be safely stopped as soon as you no longer need it.

OVERDOSE ACTION

 Seek immediate medical advice in all cases. Take emergency action if there are symptoms such as muscle twitching, nervousness, shallow breathing, severe drowsiness, or loss of consciousness.

See Drug poisoning emergency guide (p.574).

SPECIAL PRECAUTIONS

Be sure to tell your physician if:
▼ You have impaired kidney or liver function.
▼ You have heart problems.
▼ You have had epileptic seizures.
▼ You have a lung disorder such as asthma or bronchitis.
▼ You have a thyroid disorder.
▼ You have urinary difficulties.
▼ You have a head injury.
▼ You are taking other medications.

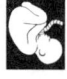 **Pregnancy**
▼ Not usually prescribed before the onset of labor. Safety in pregnancy not established. Meperidine is often used to relieve pain during labor but is given with care as it may cause breathing difficulties in the newborn baby.

 Breast feeding
▼ The drug passes into the breast milk and may affect the baby. Discuss with your physician.

 Infants and children
▼ Reduced dose necessary.

 Over 60
▼ Increased likelihood of adverse effects. Reduced dose may therefore be necessary.

 Driving and hazardous work
▼ It is unlikely that someone requiring this drug will be engaging in these activities.

 Alcohol
▼ Avoid. Alcohol may increase the sedative effects of this drug.

POSSIBLE ADVERSE EFFECTS

Adverse effects of meperidine are common but may wear off with continued use of the drug as your body adjusts. Discuss any symptoms with your physician.

Symptom/effect	Frequency		Discuss with physician		Stop taking drug now	Call physician now
	Common	Rare	Only if severe	In all cases		
Dizziness	●		■			
Nausea/vomiting	●		■			
Drowsiness	●		■			
Constipation	●			■		
Confusion	●			■		
Shortness of breath		●		■	▲	▮

INTERACTIONS

Sedatives All drugs, including alcohol, that have a sedative effect on the central nervous system may dangerously increase the sedative properties of meperidine.

Monoamine oxidase inhibitors (MAOIs) If taken within 14 days of these drugs, meperidine may cause dangerous adverse reactions.

PROLONGED USE

The effects of the drug usually become weaker during prolonged use as the body adapts. It may also be habit-forming if taken for extended periods.

MEPROBAMATE

Brand names Equanil, Apo-Meprobamate, Meditran, Novo-Mepro
Used in the following combined preparations Equagesic, 282 Mep

GENERAL INFORMATION

Introduced in the 1950s, meprobamate was first used as a muscle relaxant, then later as a short-term treatment for the symptoms generally associated with anxiety and stress (see Anti-anxiety drugs, p.95).

In addition to its use in anxiety, meprobamate has been combined with ASA for the treatment of pain, anxiety, and tension that may accompany injuries and arthritic conditions affecting the muscles, bones, and joints.

Now rarely used, meprobamate has largely been replaced in the treatment of anxiety by benzodiazepines (p.95), which have proved to be safer and more effective.

INFORMATION FOR USERS

Your drug prescription is tailored for you. Do not alter dosage without checking with your physician.

How taken

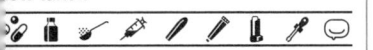

Tablets.

Frequency and timing of doses
1 – 4 x daily.

Adult dosage range
1,200 – 1,600mg daily. May be increased if required, but should not exceed 2.4g daily.

Onset of effect
Within 1 hour.

Duration of action
6 hours.

Diet advice
None.

Storage
Keep in a closed container in a cool, dry place away from reach of children. Protect from light.

Missed dose
Take as soon as you remember. If your next dose is due within 2 hours, take a single dose now and skip the next.

Stopping the drug
If you have been taking the drug for less than 2 weeks, it can be safely stopped as soon as you feel you no longer need it. If you have been taking it regularly for longer than 2 weeks, sudden discontinuation may be accompanied by severe withdrawal reactions. Consult your physician, who will supervise a gradual reduction in dosage.

OVERDOSE ACTION

 Seek immediate medical advice in all cases. Take emergency action if loss of consciousness occurs.

See Drug poisoning emergency guide (p.574).

POSSIBLE ADVERSE EFFECTS

The main adverse effects of this drug are related to its sedative properties. Drowsiness and dizziness normally diminish after the first few days of treatment, and can often be reduced by medically supervised adjustment of dosage.

Symptom/effect	Frequency		Discuss with physician		Stop taking drug now	Call physician now
	Common	Rare	Only if severe	In all cases		
Drowsiness/dizziness	●		■			
Nausea/vomiting/diarrhea		●		■		
Unusual excitement		●		■		
Rash		●		■	▲	∎

INTERACTIONS

Sedatives All drugs, including alcohol, that have a sedative effect on the central nervous system are likely to increase the sedative properties of meprobamate. Such drugs include anti-anxiety and sleeping drugs, antihistamines, antidepressants, narcotic analgesics, and antipsychotics.

Anticoagulant drugs Meprobamate may reduce the effect of anticoagulant drugs. The anticoagulant dose may need to be adjusted accordingly.

SPECIAL PRECAUTIONS

Be sure to tell your physician if:
▼ You have impaired kidney or liver function.
▼ You suffer from porphyria.
▼ You have had problems with alcohol or drug abuse.
▼ You are taking other medications.

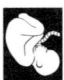 **Pregnancy**
▼ Not usually prescribed. May cause defects in the unborn baby. Discuss with your physician.

 Breast feeding
▼ The drug passes into the breast milk and may affect the baby adversely. Discuss with your physician.

 Infants and children
▼ Not usually prescribed. Reduced dose necessary.

 Over 60
▼ Reduced dose may be necessary.

 Driving and hazardous work
▼ Avoid such activities until you have learned how the drug affects you: it can cause drowsiness.

 Alcohol
▼ Avoid. Alcohol may increase the sedative effects of this drug.

PROLONGED USE

Regular use of this drug may lead to dependence and severe withdrawal reactions if suddenly discontinued. Courses of longer than 2 weeks are not usually recommended.

MESALAMINE

Brand names Asacol, Mesasal, Pentasa, Salofalk, Quintasq
Used in the following combined preparations None

GENERAL INFORMATION

Mesalamine (also known as 5-amino-salicylic acid) is used in the treatment and prevention of relapse of ulcerative colitis. It may also be used in selected patients with Crohn's disease. Mesal-amine is the major active component of sulfasalazine, another drug commonly used in the treatment or prevention of relapse of inflammatory bowel disease. Mesalamine differs from sulfasalazine in that it does not contain sulfa.

Because of this difference, mesal-amine therapy generally produces fewer and less severe *side effects* than sulfasalazine. A specially coated tablet formulation of mesalamine delays the release of the drug until the tablet reaches the affected part of the colon. A rectal retention enema (drug in suspension form inserted at bedtime and retained overnight) and suppositories of mesalamine are also available for self-administration.

QUICK REFERENCE

Drug group Drug for inflammatory bowel disease (p.124)

Overdose danger rating Low

Dependence rating Low

Prescription needed Yes

Multi-source suppliers Yes

INFORMATION FOR USERS

Your drug prescription is tailored for you. Do not alter dosage without checking with your physician.

How taken

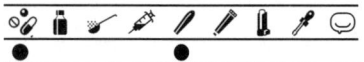

Tablets, retention enema, suppositories.

Frequency and timing of doses
3 – 4 x daily after food (tablets). Do not chew or crush the tablets; once daily at bedtime (retention enema); 1 – 3 x daily (suppositories).

Adult dosage range
0.8 – 4g daily in divided doses (tablets); 1 – 4g (retention enema); 1 – 1.5g daily (suppositories).

Onset of effect
Several days (tablets); within 1 – 2 hours (retention enema, suppositories).

Duration of action
6 – 8 hours.

Diet advice
Your physician may counsel you about diet, depending on the severity of your condition.

Storage
Keep in a closed container in a cool, dry place away from reach of children. Protect from light.

Missed dose
Take as soon as you remember. If your next dose is due within 2 hours, take a single dose now and skip the next.

Stopping the drug
Do not stop taking the drug without consulting your physician; symptoms may recur.

Exceeding the dose
An occasional unintentional extra dose is unlikely to cause problems. But if you notice unusual symptoms, or if a large overdose has been taken, notify your physician.

SPECIAL PRECAUTIONS

Be sure to tell your physician if:
▼ You have impaired kidney or liver function.
▼ You are allergic to salicylates.
▼ You have a peptic ulcer.
▼ You have a bleeding or clotting disorder.
▼ You have pyloric stenosis (a narrowing of the opening between the stomach and the small intestine).
▼ You are taking other medications.

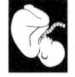 **Pregnancy**
▼ Safety in pregnancy not established. Discuss with your physician.

 Breast feeding
▼ Small amounts pass into the breast milk. However, safety not established. Discuss with your physician.

 Infants and children
▼ Not recommended in children under 2 years.

 Over 60
▼ No special problems.

 Driving and hazardous work
▼ No special problems.

 Alcohol
▼ No known problems.

POSSIBLE ADVERSE EFFECTS

Side effects are generally less frequent and less severe than with sulfasalazine. Some of the listed side effects may resemble the symptoms or the complications of inflammatory bowel disease. Consult with your physician regarding specific concerns.

Symptom/effect	Frequency		Discuss with physician		Stop taking drug now	Call physician now
	Common	Rare	Only if severe	In all cases		
Nausea/vomiting	●		■			
Diarrhea/abdominal cramps	●		■			
Headache	●		■			
Rash	●			■	▲	
Tingling/numbness		●		■	▲	
Chest pain		●		■	▲	▮
Fever		●		■	▲	▮
Hives		●		■	▲	▮
Jaundice		●		■	▲	▮

INTERACTIONS

General note Mesalamine may have interactions similar to those of ASA (p.200).

Lactulose may interfere with the beneficial effects of mesalamine.

PROLONGED USE

No problems expected.

METFORMIN

Brand names Glucophage, Novo-Metformin
Used in the following combined preparations None

GENERAL INFORMATION

Metformin, an antidiabetic drug taken by mouth, is used to treat adult (maturity-onset) diabetes in which insulin-secreting cells are still active in the pancreas.

Metformin lowers blood sugar by reducing the absorption of glucose from the digestive tract into the bloodstream, by reducing glucose production by cells in the liver and kidneys, and by increasing the sensitivity of cells to insulin so that they take up glucose more effectively from the blood.

Metformin is administered in conjunction with a special diabetic diet that limits the intake of carbohydrates and fats. It is often prescribed with another antidiabetic drug that stimulates insulin secretion by the pancreas. Metformin is not used in people with kidney or liver disease because of the risk of increased blood acidity.

INFORMATION FOR USERS

Your drug prescription is tailored for you. Do not alter dosage without checking with your physician.

How taken

Tablets.

Frequency and timing of doses
× daily with food.

Adult dosage range
5 – 2.5g daily.

Onset of effect
Within 2 hours.

Duration of action
- 12 hours.

Diet advice
An individualized low-fat, low-carbohydrate diet must be maintained in order for the drug to be fully effective. Follow your physician's advice.

Storage
Keep in a closed container in a cool, dry place away from reach of children.

Missed dose
Take as soon as you remember. If your next dose is due within 2 hours, take a single dose now and skip the next.

Stopping the drug
Do not stop taking the drug without consulting your physician; stopping the drug may lead to worsening of the underlying condition.

OVERDOSE ACTION

Seek immediate medical advice in all cases. Take emergency action if seizures or loss of consciousness occurs.

See Drug poisoning emergency guide (p.574).

POSSIBLE ADVERSE EFFECTS

Minor gastrointestinal symptoms such as loss of appetite, nausea, and vomiting are often stopped by taking the drug with food. Diarrhea usually settles after a few days of continued treatment. Symptoms such as dizziness, sweating, weakness, and confusion require prompt medical attention because they could indicate excessive lowering of blood sugar or an increase in blood acidity.

Symptom/effect	Frequency		Discuss with physician		Stop taking drug now	Call physician now
	Common	Rare	Only if severe	In all cases		
Loss of appetite	●		■			
Metallic taste	●		■			
Nausea/vomiting	●		■			
Diarrhea		●	■			
Dizziness/confusion		●		■		
Weakness/sweating		●		■		
Rash		●		■		

INTERACTIONS

General note A number of drugs reduce the effects of metformin. These include corticosteroids, estrogens and diuretics. Other drugs, notably monoamine oxidase inhibitors (MAOIs) and beta blockers, increase its effects.

The dose of any anticoagulant may have to be adjusted.

SPECIAL PRECAUTIONS

Be sure to tell your physician if:
▼ You have impaired kidney or liver function.
▼ You have heart failure.
▼ You are a heavy drinker.
▼ You are taking other medications.

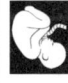 **Pregnancy**
▼ Not recommended. Insulin is usually substituted because it provides better diabetic control during pregnancy. Discuss with your physician.

 Breast feeding
▼ The drug passes into the breast milk and may affect the baby. Discuss with your physician.

 Infants and children
▼ Not recommended.

 Over 60
▼ Increased likelihood of adverse effects. Reduced dose may therefore be necessary.

 Driving and hazardous work
▼ Usually no problems. Avoid such activities if you have warning signs of low blood sugar.

 Alcohol
▼ Avoid. Alcohol increases the risk of low blood sugar and can cause coma by increasing the acidity of the blood.

Surgery and general anesthetics
▼ Surgery may reduce the response to this drug. Notify your physician that you are diabetic before any surgery; insulin treatment may need to be substituted.

PROLONGED USE

Prolonged treatment with metformin can deplete reserves of vitamin B_{12}, and this may cause anemia.

Monitoring Regular checks on levels of sugar in the urine and/or blood are usually required. An annual check on vitamin B_{12} levels may also be carried out.

METHOCARBAMOL

Brand name Robaxin
Used in the following combined preparations Robaxacet, Robaxacet-8, Robaxisal, Robaxisal-C

GENERAL INFORMATION

Methocarbamol acts on nerve cells in the central nervous system to relieve muscle spasm, rigidity, and pain arising from muscle injury. Because the drug does not help the underlying damage, treatment usually includes rest and physical therapy. Methocarbamol is also sometimes injected to relieve the symptoms of tetanus. Muscle spasm from other serious causes, such as disease of or injury to the spinal cord, or multiple sclerosis, rarely responds effectively to methocarbamol.

Drowsiness is the most common adverse effect, but there is also a slight risk of liver damage.

QUICK REFERENCE

Drug group Muscle-relaxant drug (p.132)

Overdose danger rating Medium

Dependence rating Medium

Prescription needed No

Multi-source suppliers No

INFORMATION FOR USERS

Follow instructions on the label. Call your physician if symptoms worsen.

How taken

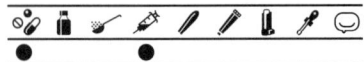

Tablets, injection.

Frequency and timing of doses
4 x daily.

Adult dosage range
6 – 8g daily for 2 – 3 days, then 4g daily.

Onset of effect
Within 30 minutes.

Duration of action
Up to 8 hours.

Diet advice
None.

Storage
Keep in a closed container in a cool, dry place away from reach of children.

Missed dose
Take as soon as you remember. If your next dose is due within 2 hours, take a single dose now and skip the next.

Stopping the drug
If you have been taking the drug for less than 6 weeks, it can be safely stopped as soon as you feel that you no longer need it. However, if you have been taking the drug for longer, consult your physician.

Exceeding the dose
An occasional unintentional extra dose is unlikely to cause problems. Large overdoses may cause severe drowsiness and muscle weakness. Notify your physician.

SPECIAL PRECAUTIONS

Be sure to consult your physician or pharmacist before taking this drug if:
▼ You have impaired liver or kidney function.
▼ You have had epileptic seizures.
▼ You have a history of allergies.
▼ You are taking other medications.

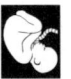

Pregnancy
▼ Safety in pregnancy not established. Discuss with your physician.

Breast feeding
▼ Safety during breast feeding has not been established. Discuss with your physician.

Infants and children
▼ Not recommended for children under 12 years.

Over 60
▼ Increased likelihood of adverse effects. Reduced dose may therefore be necessary.

Driving and hazardous work
▼ Avoid such activities until you have learned how this drug affects you; it can cause drowsiness and dizziness.

Alcohol
▼ Avoid. Alcohol may increase the sedative effects of this drug.

Surgery and general anesthetics
▼ Methocarbamol may need to be stopped before you have a general anesthetic. Discuss this with your physician or dentist before any surgery.

POSSIBLE ADVERSE EFFECTS

The most common adverse effects of methocarbamol are due to the drug's action on the central nervous system. These usually diminish as your body adjusts to the drug, and they disappear when treatment with methocarbamol is stopped.

Symptom/effect	Frequency		Discuss with physician		Stop taking drug now	Call physician now
	Common	Rare	Only if severe	In all cases		
Drowsiness	●		■			
Dizziness	●		■			
Nausea		●	■			
Headache		●	■			
Loss of appetite		●	■			
Flushing		●	■			
Metallic taste		●	■			
Rash/itching		●		■		

INTERACTIONS

Sedatives All drugs, including alcohol, that have a sedative effect on the central nervous system are likely to increase the sedative properties of methocarbamol. Such drugs include anti-anxiety and sleeping drugs, antihistamines, antidepressants, narcotic analgesics, and antipsychotic drugs.

PROLONGED USE

There is a slight risk of liver damage during long-term treatment.

Monitoring Periodic blood tests to check liver function are usually required.

METHOTREXATE

Brand name Rheumatrex
Used in the following combined preparations None

GENERAL INFORMATION

Methotrexate, introduced in 1955, is effective against a wide range of cancers. Used with other anticancer drugs, it is particularly effective against a rare cancer of placental tissue in the uterus (choriocarcinoma), certain forms of leukemia (cancer of the blood), and lymph node cancer (lymphoma). This drug is also sometimes given to treat cancer of the testicle, ovary, breast, neck, bone, bladder, and lung. In addition, methotrexate is prescribed cautiously for people with severe psoriasis. It has occasionally been used for rheumatoid arthritis that has not responded to other treatment.

As with other anticancer drugs, methotrexate affects healthy as well as cancerous cells, creating a number of side effects. Nausea and vomiting, diarrhea, and mouth ulcers are common.

The drug may also increase the risk of anemia and bleeding disorders. There may be an increased susceptibility to infection.

QUICK REFERENCE

Drug group Anticancer drug (p.166)

Overdose danger rating High

Dependence rating Low

Prescription needed Yes

Multi-source suppliers Yes

INFORMATION FOR USERS

Your drug prescription is tailored for you. Do not alter dosage without checking with your physician.

How taken

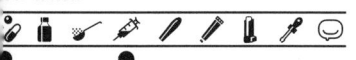

Tablets, injection.

Frequency and timing of doses
Varies according to condition being treated and route of administration.

Adult dosage range
Dosage is determined individually according to body weight and response.

Onset of effect
Some effects such as nausea and vomiting may appear within hours of starting the drug treatment. Full beneficial effect may not be felt for up to 6 weeks.

Duration of action
Adverse reactions may last for several weeks after stopping treatment.

Diet advice
Drink at least 2 litres of water daily.

Storage
Keep in a closed container in a cool, dry place away from reach of children.

Missed dose
Take as soon as you remember. If your next dose is due within 6 hours, take a single dose now and skip the next. Tell your physician that you missed a dose.

Stopping the drug
Do not stop taking the drug without consulting your physician; stopping the drug may lead to worsening of the underlying condition.

OVERDOSE ACTION

 Seek immediate medical advice in all cases.

See Drug poisoning emergency guide (p.574).

POSSIBLE ADVERSE EFFECTS

Nausea and vomiting generally occur within a few hours of taking methotrexate. Diarrhea and mouth ulcers are also common *side effects* of methotrexate.

Symptom/effect	Frequency		Discuss with physician		Stop taking drug now	Call physician now
	Common	Rare	Only if severe	In all cases		
Nausea/vomiting	●		■			
Diarrhea/abdominal pain	●		■		▲	
Mouth ulcers	●			■	▲	
Chills/fever	●			■	▲	■
Hair loss		●		■		
Rash		●		■	▲	
Jaundice		●		■	▲	■

INTERACTIONS

General note A number of drugs increase the adverse effects of methotrexate including ASA and other non-steroidal anti-inflammatory drugs (NSAIDs), anticonvulsant drugs, sulfonamides, corticosteroids, folic acid, and some antibiotics.

SPECIAL PRECAUTIONS

Methotrexate is prescribed only under close medical supervision, taking account of your present condition and medical history.

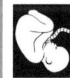 **Pregnancy**
▼ Not usually prescribed. Methotrexate may cause birth defects, premature birth, or stillbirth. Discuss with your physician.

 Breast feeding
▼ Discontinue breast feeding. The drug passes into the breast milk and may affect the baby adversely.

 Infants and children
▼ Prescribed only when absolutely necessary.

 Over 60
▼ Increased risk of adverse effects. Reduced dose may therefore be necessary.

 Driving and hazardous work
▼ No special problems.

 Alcohol
▼ Avoid. Alcohol may increase the adverse effects of this drug.

PROLONGED USE

Prolonged use of this drug may lead to an increased risk of damage to the liver, kidneys, and bone marrow.

Monitoring Periodic checks on liver and kidney function are required. A liver biopsy may be required. Chest X rays may be necessary.

METHOTRIMEPRAZINE

Brand name Nozinan
Used in the following combined preparations None

GENERAL INFORMATION

Methotrimeprazine belongs to a group of drugs called the phenothiazines that act on the brain to modify abnormal behavior (see Antipsychotics, p.97). It is effective in suppressing abnormal behavior, reducing aggression, and tranquilizing agitation.

Methotrimeprazine is used in the treatment of schizophrenia, dementia, and other disorders where confusion, aggression, hallucinations, and abnormal behavior may occur. It is also used as a pain killer and to increase the effects of anesthesia.

The main drawback to the use of methotrimeprazine is that it often produces drowsiness and abnormal shaking movements (*parkinsonism*).

INFORMATION FOR USERS

Your drug prescription is tailored for you. Do not alter dosage without checking with your physician.

How taken

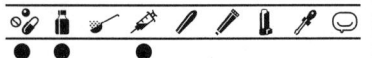

Tablets, oral liquid, injection.

Frequency and timing of doses
1 – 3 x daily with food.

Adult dosage range
Mental illness 25 – 75mg daily (starting dose); 70 – 200mg daily (maintenance dose). Dose may be increased in cases of extreme agitation.
Analgesia 6 – 25mg daily.

Onset of effect
15 – 20 minutes (injection); 30 – 60 minutes (by mouth).

Duration of action
10 – 12 hours. Some effects may persist for several weeks after stopping the drug following regular use.

Diet advice
None.

Storage
Keep in a closed container in a cool, dry place away from reach of children. Protect from light.

Missed dose
Take as soon as you remember. If your next dose is due within 2 hours, take a single dose now and skip the next.

Stopping the drug
Do not stop the drug without consulting your physician; symptoms may recur. Insomnia may be experienced after stopping the drug.

Exceeding the dose
An occasional unintentional extra dose is unlikely to cause problems. Larger overdoses may cause unusual drowsiness, muscle weakness or rigidity, and/or faintness. Notify your physician.

SPECIAL PRECAUTIONS

Be sure to tell your physician if:
▼ You have impaired liver or kidney function.
▼ You have heart or circulation problems.
▼ You have had epileptic seizures.
▼ You have an overactive thyroid gland.
▼ You have Parkinson's disease.
▼ You have had glaucoma.
▼ You have prostate trouble.
▼ You are taking other medications.

Pregnancy
▼ Safety in pregnancy not established. Discuss with your physician.

Breast feeding
▼ The drug passes into the breast milk and effects on the baby are not known. Discuss with your physician.

Infants and children
▼ Reduced dose necessary.

Over 60
▼ Reduced dose may be necessary.

Driving and hazardous work
▼ Avoid such activities until you have learned how the drug affects you; it can cause drowsiness and slowed reactions.

Alcohol
▼ Avoid. Alcohol may increase the sedative effects of this drug.

POSSIBLE ADVERSE EFFECTS

Methotrimeprazine can cause a variety of minor *anticholinergic* symptoms that often become less marked with time. The most significant adverse effect is abnormal movement of the face and limbs (parkinsonism). This may be controlled by dosage adjustment.

Symptom/effect	Frequency		Discuss with physician		Stop taking drug now	Call physician now
	Common	Rare	Only if severe	In all cases		
Drowsiness/lethargy	●		■			
Weight gain	●		■			
Parkinsonism	●			■		
Dizziness/fainting	●			■		
Blurred vision	●			■		
Infrequent periods		●		■		
Rash		●		■	▲	
High fever/confusion		●		■	▲	■

PROLONGED USE

Use of this drug for more than a few months may lead to *tardive dyskinesia*, i.e., abnormal, involuntary movements of the eyes, face, and tongue. Occasionally jaundice may occur.

Monitoring Periodic blood tests may be performed.

INTERACTIONS

Sedatives All drugs, including alcohol, that have a sedative effect on the central nervous system are likely to increase the sedative properties of methotrimeprazine.

Anticholinergic drugs Their side effects may be increased by methotrimeprazine.

Anticonvulsants and antiparkinsonian drugs Methotrimeprazine may reduce the effectiveness of these drugs.

METHOXSALEN

Brand names Oxsoralen, Oxsorolen-Ultra, Ultra MOP
Used in the following combined preparations None

GENERAL INFORMATION

Methoxsalen belongs to a group of substances called psoralens. These occur naturally in plants and have been used historically to correct vitiligo, a condition in which patches of skin lose their color, or pigmentation. Today, methoxsalen is more often given for severe psoriasis that has failed to improve with other treatments. It is also used for the treatment of atopic eczema.

Used in conjunction with ultraviolet light treatment, it stimulates the production of the skin pigment and, in psoriasis, halts the accelerated growth of skin cells. Methoxsalen lotion is used for small areas of vitiligo, while capsules are given for widespread depigmentation and severe psoriasis.

The pigment-promoting effect of methoxsalen has led to its inclusion in some countries in preparations for the promotion of suntanning. This use is prohibited in Canada. After taking methoxsalen, a person should limit his or her exposure to sunlight.

INFORMATION FOR USERS

Your drug prescription is tailored for you. Do not alter dosage without checking with your physician.

How taken

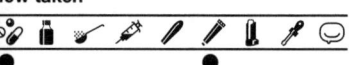

Capsules, topical lotion.

Frequency and timing of doses
By mouth Varies. Should not be taken more often than every second day.
Lotion Once weekly under medical supervision.

Adult dosage range
By mouth Varies with condition being treated and type of capsule prescribed.
Lotion Applied to the affected area under medical supervision.

Onset of effect
Within 1 hour (by mouth); within 15 minutes (lotion). Full benefit may not be seen for 10 weeks (psoriasis) or 6 months (vitiligo).

Duration of action
Sensitivity of the skin to sunlight is increased for 24 – 48 hours after drug is taken.

Diet advice
Certain foods, such as limes, figs, parsley, parsnips, mustard, carrots, and celery may increase the sensitivity of the skin to light with methoxsalen.

Storage
Keep in a closed container in a cool, dry place away from heat and direct light and out of reach of children.

Missed dose
No cause for concern. Consult your physician.

Stopping the drug
Can be safely stopped as soon as you no longer need it.

Exceeding the dose
If accidental overdose or overexposure occurs, stay in a darkened room for 8 hours or until the skin reaction subsides. Treat for burns if needed.

POSSIBLE ADVERSE EFFECTS

Slight redness of the skin normally occurs for a day or two after treatment. High doses of methoxsalen or overexposure to ultraviolet light may cause severe redness, soreness, blistering, or peeling of skin and swelling of the feet or lower legs.

Symptom/effect	Frequency		Discuss with physician		Stop taking drug now	Call physician now
	Common	Rare	Only if severe	In all cases		
Redness/soreness/itching	●			■		
Nausea		●	■			
Dizziness/headache		●	■			
Depression/insomnia		●	■			
Blistering/peeling		●		■		
Swollen feet/ankles		●		■		

INTERACTIONS

General note Any drug that increases the sensitivity of the skin to light, as methoxsalen does, may increase the risk of redness, blistering, and peeling. Such drugs include griseofulvin, coal tar derivatives, thiazide diuretics, phenothiazines, sulfonamides, and tetracyclines.

SPECIAL PRECAUTIONS

Be sure to tell your physician if:
▼ You have impaired liver function.
▼ You are regularly exposed or about to be exposed to intense sunlight, X rays, or industrial or laboratory chemicals.
▼ You have porphyria or systemic lupus erythematosus.
▼ You have had skin cancer.
▼ You have recently received anticancer drugs or radiation therapy.
▼ You have cataracts.
▼ You are taking other medications.

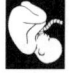

Pregnancy
▼ Safety in pregnancy not established. Discuss with your physician.

Breast feeding
▼ The effects of this drug during breast feeding are not established. Discuss with your physician.

Infants and children
▼ Not recommended for children under 12 years.

Over 60
▼ No special problems.

Driving and hazardous work
▼ No known problems.

Alcohol
▼ No known problems.

PROLONGED USE

Prolonged use may increase the risk of premature aging of the skin and skin cancer in fair-skinned people. Cataracts are a risk of ultraviolet light treatment.

METHYLDOPA

Brand names Aldomet, Apo-Methyldopa, Novo-Medopa, Nu-Medopa
Used in the following combined preparations Aldoril, Apo-Methazide, Supres

GENERAL INFORMATION

Methyldopa, introduced in the 1960s, is one of the best known antihypertensive drugs. People take this drug to deal with varying degrees of high blood pressure. A diuretic is usually prescribed along with methyldopa in order to enhance its effect and to reduce fluid retention. Other antihypertensive drugs are sometimes added to increase effect. The usefulness of methyldopa may be limited by frequent adverse effects.

Women with high blood pressure during late pregnancy often take methyldopa, as it will not affect the unborn child.

The most common adverse effect of methyldopa is that it often causes drowsiness and, sometimes, depression. Methyldopa is less likely than other antihypertensive drugs to cause dizziness due to a fall in blood pressure. Also, because this drug does not reduce blood flow to the kidneys, it is sometimes given to people with kidney disorders.

INFORMATION FOR USERS

Your drug prescription is tailored for you. Do not alter dosage without checking with your physician.

How taken

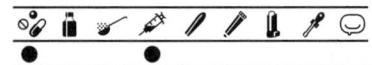

Tablets, injection.

Frequency and timing of doses
2 – 4 x daily.

Dosage range
Adults 500mg – 2g daily.
Children Reduced dose necessary according to age and weight.

Onset of effect
3 – 6 hours. Full effect begins after 2 – 3 days.

Duration of action
6 – 12 hours. Some effects may last for 1 – 2 days after stopping the drug.

Diet advice
None.

Storage
Keep in a closed container in a cool, dry place away from reach of children.

Missed dose
Take as soon as you remember. If your next dose is due within 2 hours, take a single dose now and skip the next.

Stopping the drug
Do not stop the drug without consulting your physician, who will gradually reduce your dose. Suddenly stopping methyldopa may lead to an increase in blood pressure.

Exceeding the dose
An occasional unintentional extra dose is unlikely to cause problems. Larger overdoses may cause drowsiness or palpitations. Notify your physician.

SPECIAL PRECAUTIONS

Be sure to tell your physician if:
▼ You have impaired liver function.
▼ You have anemia.
▼ You have angina.
▼ You suffer from depression.
▼ You are taking other medications.

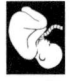

Pregnancy
▼ Effects on developing baby are uncertain. It is taken during late pregnancy to treat high blood pressure with no serious effects on the baby.

Breast feeding
▼ The drug passes into the breast milk, but at normal doses adverse effects on the baby are unlikely. Discuss with your physician.

Infants and children
▼ Reduced dose necessary.

Over 60
▼ Reduced dose may be necessary.

Driving and hazardous work
▼ Avoid such activities until you have learned how the drug affects you; it can cause drowsiness.

Alcohol
▼ Avoid. Alcohol may increase the sedative effects of this drug.

Surgery and general anesthetics
▼ Discuss the possibility of stopping methyldopa with your physician or dentist before any surgery.

POSSIBLE ADVERSE EFFECTS

Most adverse effects are uncommon and diminish in time. The fluid retention that occurs during treatment with methyldopa is counteracted by taking a diuretic.

Symptom/effect	Frequency		Discuss with physician		Stop taking drug now	Call physician now
	Common	Rare	Only if severe	In all cases		
Drowsiness	●		■			
Depression	●			■		
Fever	●			■		
Stuffy nose		●		■		
Dizziness/fainting		●		■		
Nausea/vomiting		●		■		
Rash		●		■	▲	
Jaundice		●		■	▲	■

PROLONGED USE

Liver and blood problems may occur in rare cases.

Monitoring Periodic checks on blood and urine are usually required.

INTERACTIONS

Monoamine oxidase inhibitors (MAOIs) may lead to serious adverse effects when taken with methyldopa.

Tricyclic antidepressants may reduce the effects of methyldopa.

Levodopa Methyldopa may reduce control of Parkinson's disease.

Lithium Methyldopa may increase the adverse effects of lithium.

METHYLPHENIDATE

Brand names Ritalin, Ritalin SR, PMS-Methylphenidate
Used in the following combined preparations None

GENERAL INFORMATION

Methylphenidate is a mild central nervous system stimulant used in the treatment of attention-deficit hyper-activity disorder (ADHD). Children and adults with this disorder have difficulty concentrating and are easily distracted. The use of medication is only one part of an ongoing treatment program also involving psychological, social, and educational interventions.

Methylphenidate is a short-acting drug that is often given 2 or 3 times daily. Once its effect has worn off there are no residual effects. A slow-release tablet formulation starts working more slowly and may have a longer action.

The main problems seen with the use of methylphenidate in children are sleep difficulties (insomnia) and decreased appetite; these can improve with time. Even though growth may be slowed in children while they are taking methylphenidate, the eventual height does not seem to be compromised.

QUICK REFERENCE

Drug group Nervous system stimulant (p.100)

Overdose danger rating High

Dependence rating Medium

Prescription needed Yes

Multi-source suppliers Yes

INFORMATION FOR USERS

Your drug prescription is tailored for you. Do not alter dosage without checking with your physician.

How taken

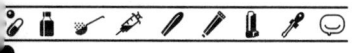

Tablets, slow-release tablets.

Frequency and timing of doses
2 – 3 x daily (tablets), once daily (slow-release tablets).

Dosage range
10 – 30mg daily, adjusted according to weight and response.

Onset of effect
30 – 60 minutes (tablets).

Duration of action
3 – 5 hours (tablets).

Diet advice
None.

Storage
Keep in a closed container in a cool, dry place away from the reach of children.

Missed dose
Take as needed. Allow at least 4 hours between doses of regular tablets.

Stopping the drug
Can safely be stopped. Consult your physician re overall management of your ADHD.

OVERDOSE ACTION

 Seek immediate medical advice in all cases. Take emergency action if confusion, palpitations, seizures, or loss of conscious-ness occurs.

See Drug poisoning emergency guide (p.574).

SPECIAL PRECAUTIONS

Be sure to tell your physician if:
▼ You have high blood pressure.
▼ You have heart problems.
▼ You have thyroid disease.
▼ You have glaucoma.
▼ You have a history of seizures.
▼ You are taking other medications.

 **Pregnancy**
▼ Safety in pregnancy not established. Discuss with your physician.

 Breast feeding
▼ It is not known if the drug passes into the breast milk. Discuss with your physician.

 Infants and children
▼ Not recommended for children under 6 years.

 Over 60
▼ Increased likelihood of adverse effects. Reduced dose may therefore be necessary.

 Driving and hazardous work
▼ Avoid such activities until you have learned how the drug affects you; it can cause dizziness.

 Alcohol
▼ No known problems.

POSSIBLE ADVERSE EFFECTS

The main adverse effects in children are insomnia and decreased appetite; these may improve with time. Abdominal pain, headache, and irritability may occur at the start of treatment.

Symptom/effect	Frequency		Discuss with physician		Stop taking drug now	Call physician now
	Common	Rare	Only if severe	In all cases		
Decreased appetite	●		■			
Insomnia	●		■			
Abdominal pain	●			■		
Headache	●			■		
Fatigue	●			■		
Irritability/anxiety		●		■		
Sadness/social withdrawal		●		■		

INTERACTIONS

General note Methylphenidate may interact with many drugs to increase their effects. These drugs include anticoagulants, anticonvulsants, and tricyclic antidepressants.

Antihypertensive drugs Methylphenidate may interact with these drugs to reverse their effect.

PROLONGED USE

Continuous, long-term use may impair growth. "Drug holidays" may be recommended by your physician.

Monitoring Your physician will assess growth and blood pressure at regular intervals. In addition, periodic checks of blood count may be advised.

METHYLPREDNISOLONE

Brand names Depo-Medrol, Medrol, Solu-Medrol
Used In the following combined preparations Depo-Medrol with Lidocaine, Neo-Medrol

GENERAL INFORMATION

Methylprednisolone, introduced in 1957, is a synthetic corticosteroid drug derived from prednisolone. It is prescribed as an ointment to relieve skin conditions such as dermatitis, eczema, and psoriasis, or in a lotion form to control acne. Methylprednisolone can be injected into joints to relieve rheumatoid arthritis and other types of joint inflammation (see p.130). It is also prescribed by mouth to replace hormones in pituitary or adrenal gland disorders that reduce the body's natural corticosteroid production. Occasionally, methylprednisolone tablets are given for the long-term control of severe asthma.

Side effects are rare when the drug is administered short-term. However, long-term treatment by mouth can cause adverse effects such as fluid retention, indigestion, fragile bones, and muscle weakness. It may also induce diabetes.

INFORMATION FOR USERS

Your drug prescription is tailored for you. Do not alter dosage without checking with your physician.

How taken

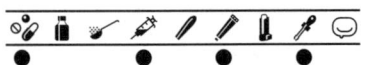

Tablets, injection, ointment, topical lotion, eye/ear drops.

Frequency and timing of doses
Varies according to preparation and condition. Follow your physician's instructions.

Dosage range
Considerable variation. Follow your physician's instructions.

Onset of effect
2 – 4 days.

Duration of action
12 – 36 hours.

Diet advice
A low-sodium, high-potassium diet may be recommended when the oral or injectable form of the drug is prescribed for extended periods. Follow the advice of your physician.

Storage
Keep in a closed container in a cool, dry place away from reach of children.

Missed dose
Take as soon as you remember. If your next dose is due within 6 hours, take a single dose now and skip the next.

Stopping the drug
Do not stop tablets without consulting your physician, who may supervise a gradual reduction in dosage. Abrupt cessation may cause adrenal collapse.

Exceeding the dose
An occasional unintentional extra dose is unlikely to be a cause for concern. But if you notice unusual symptoms, or if a large overdose has been taken, notify your physician.

SPECIAL PRECAUTIONS

Be sure to tell your physician if:
▼ You have had glaucoma.
▼ You have high blood pressure.
▼ You have diabetes.
▼ You have had a peptic ulcer.
▼ You have suffered from depression.
▼ You have a herpes infection.
▼ You are taking other medications.

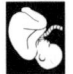

Pregnancy
▼ No evidence of risk with topical preparations or joint injections. Prescribed in tablet form in low doses, harm to the baby is unlikely. Discuss with your physician.

Breast feeding
▼ No evidence of risk with topical solutions or joint injections. Taken regularly by mouth, the drug may adversely affect the baby's growth. Discuss with your physician.

Infants and children
▼ Reduced dose necessary.

Over 60
▼ Reduced dose may be necessary.

Driving and hazardous work
▼ No known problems.

Alcohol
▼ Alcohol may increase the risk of peptic ulcers with methylprednisolone tablets. No special problems with other dosage forms.

POSSIBLE ADVERSE EFFECTS

The rare, but more serious, adverse effects occur only when methylprednisolone is taken by mouth in high doses for long periods of time.

Symptom/effect	Frequency		Discuss with physician		Stop taking drug now	Call physician now
	Common	Rare	Only if severe	In all cases		
Indigestion/weight gain	●		■			
Muscle weakness		●		■		
Mood changes		●		■		
Seizures		●		■	▲	❙
Black/bloody feces		●		■	▲	❙

INTERACTIONS (by mouth or injection only)

Oral anticoagulants Methylprednisolone may decrease the effect of anticoagulants.

Vaccines Serious reactions can occur when vaccinations are given with methylprednisolone. Discuss with your physician.

Barbiturates, phenytoin, and rifampin These drugs may reduce the effect of methylprednisolone.

Antidiabetic drugs Methylprednisolone reduces the actions of these drugs.

Antihypertensive drugs Methylprednisolone may reduce the effect of antihypertensive drugs.

Diuretics Methylprednisolone may increase potassium loss.

PROLONGED USE

Prolonged use of methylprednisolone in high doses by mouth can lead to serious adverse effects, such as diabetes, glaucoma, muscle weakness, cataracts, and fragile bones. The drug may retard growth in children.

METOCLOPRAMIDE

Brand names Maxeran, Apo-Metoclop, Reglan
Used in the following combined preparations None

GENERAL INFORMATION

Metoclopramide acts directly on the upper gastrointestinal tract to encourage normal propulsion of food through the stomach and intestine. It is used to help relieve retention of food and acid in the stomach following ulcer surgery or other operations of the stomach. It may also be used in other medical conditions (for example, diabetes) where gastric retention occurs.

Metoclopramide has anti-emetic properties and is commonly used for the prevention of vomiting caused by anticancer drugs. It is sometimes administered as *premedication* before surgery to prevent the vomiting caused by anesthetics. Metoclopramide is useful as an aid in some diagnostic X-ray procedures.

Side effects of metoclopramide include drowsiness, fatigue, insomnia, *parkinsonism*, and the increased secretion of the hormone prolactin, which may cause the breasts to discharge a milky fluid.

INFORMATION FOR USERS

Your drug prescription is tailored for you. Do not alter dosage without checking with your physician.

How taken

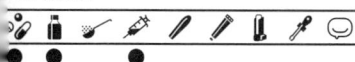

Tablets, oral liquid, injection.

Frequency and timing of doses
3 – 4 x daily before meals and at bedtime (by mouth).

Adult dosage range
5 – 40mg daily (by mouth); according to the condition being treated and body weight (injection).

Onset of effect
Within 1 hour.

Duration of action
6 – 8 hours.

Diet advice
Fatty and spicy foods and alcohol are best avoided if nausea is a problem.

Storage
Keep in a closed container in a cool, dry place away from reach of children.

Missed dose
Take as soon as you remember. If your next dose is due within 2 hours, take a single dose now and skip the next.

Stopping the drug
Can be safely stopped as soon as you no longer need it.

Exceeding the dose
An occasional unintentional extra dose is unlikely to be cause for concern. Large overdoses may cause drowsiness and muscle spasms. Notify your physician.

SPECIAL PRECAUTIONS

Be sure to tell your physician if:
▼ You have impaired liver or kidney function.
▼ You have pheochromocytoma.
▼ You have had epileptic seizures.
▼ You have Parkinson's disease.
▼ You have a prior history of depression.
▼ You are taking other medications.

Pregnancy
▼ Safety in pregnancy not established. Discuss with your physician.

Breast feeding
▼ The drug passes into the breast milk but in normal doses adverse effects on the baby are unlikely. Discuss with your physician.

Infants and children
▼ Reduced dose necessary.

Over 60
▼ Reduced dose may be necessary.

Driving and hazardous work
▼ Avoid such activities until you have learned how the drug affects you; it can cause dizziness and drowsiness.

Alcohol
▼ Avoid. Alcohol may oppose the beneficial effects and increase the sedative effects of this drug.

POSSIBLE ADVERSE EFFECTS

The adverse effects of metoclopramide include drowsiness, restlessness, dizziness, headache, parkinsonism, and menstrual disorders.

Symptom/effect	Frequency		Discuss with physician		Stop taking drug now	Call physician now
	Common	Rare	Only if severe	In all cases		
Drowsiness/fatigue	●		■			
Restlessness		●		■		
Diarrhea		●		■		
Parkinsonism		●		■		
Muscle spasm of face		●		■	▲	■

PROLONGED USE

Tardive dyskinesia, which in some cases appears to be irreversible, has been reported in association with metoclopramide therapy.

INTERACTIONS

General note Metoclopramide may decrease the absorption of some drugs from the stomach (for example, digoxin) whereas absorption of other drugs from the small bowel may be accelerated (for example, acetaminophen, tetracycline antibiotics, levodopa, and alcohol).

Anticholinergic drugs may reduce the beneficial effects of metoclopramide.

Sedatives All drugs, including alcohol, that have a sedative effect on the central nervous system are likely to increase the sedative properties of metoclopramide. Such drugs include anti-anxiety and sleeping drugs, antidepressants, antihistamines, narcotic analgesics, and antipsychotics.

Monoamine oxidase inhibitors (MAOIs) Use with care in conjunction with metoclopramide.

METOPROLOL

Brand names Lopresor, Apo-Metoprolol, Betaloc, Novo-Metoprol, Nu-Metop
Used in the following combined preparations None

GENERAL INFORMATION

Introduced in 1977, metoprolol is a beta blocker used in the treatment of angina and, in combination with a diuretic, hypertension. It is also prescribed to relieve palpitations and tremor caused by overactivity of the thyroid gland. Metoprolol may be given following a heart attack to prevent further damage.

Unlike similar drugs that act on the heart and lungs, metoprolol is cardio-selective, acting mainly on the heart. This makes it less dangerous for people with asthma, bronchitis, or other lung problems. Caution is still required. Metoprolol masks the body's response to low blood sugar, a problem in diabetics.

It can also reduce circulation to the hands and feet, making them feel cold.

INFORMATION FOR USERS

Your drug prescription is tailored for you. Do not alter dosage without checking with your physician.

How taken

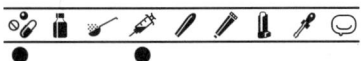

Tablets, slow-release tablets, injection.

Frequency and timing of doses
2 – 3 x daily (tablets): once daily (slow-release tablets).

Dosage range
100 – 400mg daily.

Onset of effect
Within 2 hours.

Duration of action
Up to 4 weeks (hypertension); up to 12 hours (angina).

Diet advice
None.

Storage
Keep in a closed container in a cool, dry place away from reach of children. Protect from light.

Missed dose
Take as soon as you remember. If your next dose is due within 2 hours (if you take the drug 2 – 3 times daily), or 5 hours (if you take the drug once daily) take a single dose now and skip the next.

Stopping the drug
Do not stop the drug without consulting your physician; stopping the drug suddenly may lead to dangerous worsening of the underlying condition or precipitate a heart attack.

OVERDOSE ACTION

 Seek immediate medical advice in all cases. Take emergency action if breathing difficulties, collapse, or loss of consciousness occur.

See Drug poisoning emergency guide (p.574).

POSSIBLE ADVERSE EFFECTS

Metoprolol has adverse effects that are common to most beta blockers. Symptoms such as fatigue and nausea are usually temporary and diminish with long-term use. Metoprolol can occasionally provoke or worsen asthma and some heart problems.

Symptom/effect	Frequency		Discuss with physician		Stop taking drug now	Call physician now
	Common	Rare	Only if severe	In all cases		
Lethargy	●		■			
Cold hands and feet		●	■			
Nausea/nightmares/dreams		●	■			
Rash		●		■	▲	
Breathing difficulties		●		■	▲	▮
Fainting		●		■	▲	▮

INTERACTIONS

Non-steroidal anti-inflammatory drugs (NSAIDs) may reduce the antihypertensive effect of metoprolol.

Cimetidine may increase the levels of metoprolol in the blood.

Nifedipine may lower the blood pressure excessively if taken with metoprolol.

Ergotamine may aggravate circulation problems in hands and feet if taken with metoprolol.

SPECIAL PRECAUTIONS

Be sure to tell your physician if:
▼ You have impaired liver or kidney function.
▼ You have heart failure.
▼ You have poor circulation in the legs.
▼ You have a lung disorder such as asthma, emphysema, or bronchitis.
▼ You have allergies.
▼ You have diabetes.
▼ You are taking other medications.

 **Pregnancy**
▼ Safety in pregnancy not established. Discuss with your physician.

 Breast feeding
▼ The drug may pass into the breast milk and may affect the baby. Discuss with your physician.

 Infants and children
▼ Not usually prescribed.

 Over 60
▼ Increased likelihood of adverse effects.

 Driving and hazardous work
▼ Avoid such activities until you have learned how the drug affects you, because the drug can cause dizziness and tiredness.

 Alcohol
▼ No known problems with moderate intake.

Surgery and general anesthetics
▼ Metoprolol may need to be stopped before you have a general anesthetic. Discuss this with your physician or dentist before any surgery.

PROLONGED USE

No special problems expected.

METRONIDAZOLE

Brand names Flagyl, Apo-Metronidazole, Metrogel, NidaGel, Novo-Nidazol, Trikacide
Used in the following combined preparation Flagystatin

GENERAL INFORMATION

Metronidazole is an antibiotic that is effective against both protozoal infections and a variety of bacterial infections. It is widely used in the treatment of bacterial vaginosis and trichomonas infection of the vagina. Because the trichomonas organism is sexually transmitted and may not cause any symptoms, a simultaneous course of treatment may be advised for sexual partners.

Serious anaerobic infections of the abdomen and pelvis respond well to metronidazole. The drug is also prescribed for amebic dysentery and giardiasis, protozoal infections causing diarrhea.

Metronidazole is available in the form of a gel for topical treatment of rosacea, a skin condition marked by redness of the nose and cheeks.

The most common adverse effects that occur with metronidazole are nausea and abdominal pain.

QUICK REFERENCE

Drug group Antibiotic (p.143) and antiprotozoal drug (p.148)

Overdose danger rating Low

Dependence rating Low

Prescription needed Yes

Multi-source suppliers Yes

INFORMATION FOR USERS

Your drug prescription is tailored for you. Do not alter dosage without checking with your physician.

How taken

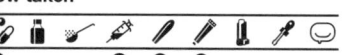

Tablets, capsules, injection, vaginal inserts, vaginal cream or gel, topical gel.

Frequency and timing of doses
Usually 3 x daily for 5 – 10 days, depending on condition being treated. Occasionally a single large dose may be prescribed.

Adult dosage range
5 – 2.25g daily (by mouth); 1.5g daily (injection).

Onset of effect
The drug starts to work within an hour or so, but beneficial effects may not be apparent for 1 – 2 days.

Duration of action
6 – 12 hours.

Diet advice
None.

Storage
Keep in a closed container in a cool, dry place away from reach of children. Protect from light.

Missed dose
Take as soon as you remember. If your next dose is due within 2 hours, take a single dose now and skip the next.

Stopping the drug
Take the full course. Even if you feel better, the infection may still be present and symptoms may recur if the treatment is stopped too soon.

Exceeding the dose
An occasional unintentional extra dose is unlikely to be a cause for concern. But if you notice unusual symptoms, especially numbness or tingling, or if a large overdose has been taken, notify your physician.

SPECIAL PRECAUTIONS

Be sure to tell your physician if:
▼ You have impaired liver or kidney function.
▼ You have a blood disorder.
▼ You have a disorder of the central nervous system, such as epilepsy.
▼ You are taking other medications.

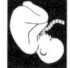

Pregnancy
▼ Safety in pregnancy not established. Discuss with your physician.

Breast feeding
▼ The drug passes into the breast milk, but at normal doses adverse effects on the baby are unlikely. However, metronidazole may give a bitter taste to the milk. Discuss with your physician.

Infants and children
▼ Clinical experience in children is very limited.

Over 60
▼ No special problems.

Driving and hazardous work
▼ Avoid such activities until you have learned how the drug affects you; it can cause dizziness, drowsiness, and headache.

Alcohol
▼ Avoid. Taken with metronidazole, alcohol may cause flushing, nausea, vomiting, abdominal pain, and headache.

POSSIBLE ADVERSE EFFECTS

The most common problems are minor gastro-intestinal disturbances that tend to diminish as your body adjusts to the drug. It commonly causes a darkening of the urine, which is of no concern. More serious adverse effects affecting the central nervous system, causing numbness or tingling, are extremely rare.

Symptom/effect	Frequency		Discuss with physician		Stop taking drug now	Call physician now
	Common	Rare	Only if severe	In all cases		
Nausea/loss of appetite	●		■			
Abdominal pain/dark urine	●		■			
Dry mouth/metallic taste		●	■			
Headache/dizziness		●	■			
Numbness/tingling		●		■		

INTERACTIONS

Oral anticoagulants Metronidazole may increase the effect of oral anticoagulants.

Lithium Metronidazole increases the risk of adverse effects on the kidney.

Phenytoin Metronidazole may increase the effects of phenytoin.

Cimetidine may increase the levels of metronidazole in the body.

PROLONGED USE

Not usually prescribed for longer than 10 days. Prolonged treatment may cause temporary loss of sensation in the hands and feet and may also reduce production of white blood cells.

MICONAZOLE

Brand names Micatin, Monistat
Used in the following combined preparations None

GENERAL INFORMATION

Miconazole is prescribed for yeast and fungal infections. It is effective for treating tinea infections of the skin (ringworm) and athlete's foot. It is also effective for treating candida (thrush) infections of the vagina and of the skin (jock itch) and some forms of diaper rash. The drug is applied to the skin as a cream and to the vagina as a cream, medicated tampon, suppository, or ovule (gelatin shell filled with concentrated cream).

Adverse effects from miconazole are very rare, although some people may experience local burning and irritation.

INFORMATION FOR USERS

Follow instructions on the label. Call your physician if symptoms worsen.

How taken

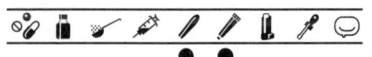

Vaginal suppositories, vaginal ovules, cream.

Frequency and timing of doses
2 x daily (skin infection); once daily at bedtime (vaginal infections).

Adult dosage range
Skin infections Sufficient cream to cover the affected skin and surrounding area at each application.
Vaginal infections 100mg daily for 7 nights (vaginal suppositories); 400mg daily for 3 nights (vaginal ovules); one applicatorful daily for 7 nights (vaginal cream).

Onset of effect
2 – 7 days.

Duration of action
Up to 24 hours after each dose.

Diet advice
None.

Storage
Keep in a closed container in a cool, dry place away from reach of children.

Missed dose
No cause for concern, but make up the missed dose or application as soon as you remember.

Stopping the drug
Use the full course. Even if symptoms disappear, the original infection may still be present and symptoms may recur if treatment is stopped too soon.

Exceeding the dose
An occasional unintentional extra dose when using the topical or intravaginal preparations is unlikely to be cause for concern. But if you notice unusual symptoms, consult your physician.

SPECIAL PRECAUTIONS

Be sure to consult your physician or pharmacist before using this drug if:
▼ You have previously had an allergic reaction to this drug.
▼ You are taking other medications.

Pregnancy
▼ No evidence of risk with skin preparations. Vaginal preparations should be used with caution in the first 3 months of pregnancy. Use of the vaginal applicator may be undesirable. Discuss with your physician.

Breast feeding
▼ No evidence of risk.

Infants and children
▼ Reduced dose necessary.

Over 60
▼ No special problems.

Driving and hazardous work
▼ No known problems.

Alcohol
▼ No known problems.

POSSIBLE ADVERSE EFFECTS

Miconazole applied to the skin or used intravaginally rarely causes troublesome adverse effects. Irritation at the site of application is unusual.

Symptom/effect	Frequency		Discuss with physician		Stop taking drug now	Call physician now
	Common	Rare	Only if severe	In all cases		
Irritation/burning		●	■			
Rash		●		■	▲	
Hives		●		■	▲	

INTERACTIONS

None.

PROLONGED USE

No problems expected from the drug. However, recurrent or intractable candidiasis may require further assessment by your physician.

MINOCYCLINE

and name Minocin
ed in the following combined preparations None

GENERAL INFORMATION

nocycline is a member of the tetra-cline group of antibiotics but has a ostantially longer duration of action an tetracycline itself. It is most mmonly used to treat acne. Minocycline may be used in the atment of pneumonia or in the evention of infection in people with ronic bronchitis. It is prescribed for e treatment of gonorrhea and non-nococcal urethritis and may be eful in the treatment of other sexually transmitted diseases.

This drug's most frequent *side effects* are nausea, vomiting, and diarrhea. A problem peculiar to minocycline is interference with the balance mechanism in the inner ear with resultant nausea, dizziness, and unsteadiness, but these symptoms generally disappear after the drug is stopped. Minocycline is not prescribed for people with poor kidney function.

INFORMATION FOR USERS

ur drug prescription is tailored for you. not alter dosage without checking h your physician.

w taken

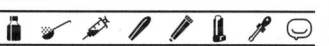

sules.

quency and timing of doses
4 x daily.

sage range
ults 200mg daily.
ldren Reduced dose according to age and ght.

set of effect
12 hours.

ration of action
to 24 hours.

t advice
products may impair absorption of this drug. Avoid these from one hour before to two hours after dosage.

Storage
Keep in a closed container in a cool, dry place that is well secured and away from reach of children.

Missed dose
Take as soon as you remember. If your next dose is due within 4 hours, take a single dose now and skip the next.

Stopping the drug
Use the full course. Even if you feel better, the original infection may still be present and symptoms may recur if treatment is stopped too soon.

Exceeding the dose
An occasional unintentional extra dose is unlikely to cause problems. But if you notice unusual symptoms, or if a larger overdose has been taken, notify your physician.

POSSIBLE ADVERSE EFFECTS

ocycline may occasionally cause nausea, iting, or diarrhea. Other less common erse effects are rashes, an increased sensitivity of the skin to sunlight and, occasionally, dizziness and loss of balance (vertigo).

nptom/effect	Frequency		Discuss with physician		Stop taking drug now	Call physician now
	Common	Rare	Only if severe	In all cases		
sea/vomiting/diarrhea	●		■			
ziness/vertigo	●			■	▲	
h/itching		●		■	▲	
t-sensitive rash		●		■	▲	

INTERACTIONS

ral anticoagulants Minocycline may crease the anticoagulant action of these ugs.

ral contraceptives Minocycline can duce the effectiveness of oral ntraceptives.

on may reduce the effectiveness of inocycline.

Penicillin antibiotics Minocycline interferes with the antibacterial action of these drugs.

Antacids interfere with the absorption of minocycline and may reduce its effectiveness.

SPECIAL PRECAUTIONS

Be sure to tell your physician if:
▼ You have impaired liver or kidney function.
▼ You have previously suffered an allergic reaction to a tetracycline antibiotic.
▼ You are taking other medications.

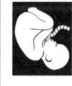

Pregnancy
▼ Not prescribed. May damage the teeth and bones of the developing baby, as well as damaging the mother's liver. Discuss with your physician.

Breast feeding
▼ The drug passes into the breast milk and may lead to discoloration of the baby's teeth. Discuss with your physician.

Infants and children
▼ Not recommended for children under 13 years old. Reduced dose necessary in older children.

Over 60
▼ No special problems.

Driving and hazardous work
▼ Avoid such activities until you have learned how the drug affects you; it can cause dizziness and drowsiness.

Alcohol
▼ No known problems.

Esophageal damage
▼ To prevent retention in the esophagus, a small amount of water should be taken before, and a full glass of water taken after, each dose of minocycline. Take this medication in the upright position and do not lie down immediately afterward.

PROLONGED USE

No problems expected.

MINOXIDIL

Brand names Loniten, Apo-Gain, Gen-Minoxidil, Minoxigain, Rogaine
Used in the following combined preparations None

GENERAL INFORMATION

Minoxidil, a *vasodilator* drug (see p.110), relaxes the muscles of artery walls and dilates blood vessels. It is effective in controlling dangerously high blood pressure or pressure that is rising very rapidly. Because it is stronger acting than many other antihypertensive drugs, it is particularly useful for people whose blood pressure has not been controlled by other treatment. Because minoxidil can cause fluid retention and increased heart rate, it is usually prescribed with a

diuretic and a beta blocker to increase effectiveness and counteract *side effects*.

If taken orally for longer than two months, it may increase hair growth, especially on the face. While some find the abnormal growth distressing, others may view this "side effect" positively. Minoxidil *topical* solution is used for the treatment of early male pattern baldness, though the resulting hair growth is highly variable.

INFORMATION FOR USERS

Your drug prescription is tailored for you. Do not alter dosage without checking with your physician.

How taken

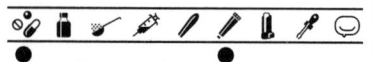

Tablets, topical solution.

Frequency and timing of doses
1 – 2 x daily (tablets); 2 x daily (topical solution).

Adult dosage range
5 – 40mg daily (tablets).

Onset of effect
Within 1 hour.

Duration of action
Up to 24 hours. Some effect may last for 2 – 5 days after the drug has stopped (tablets); hair growth may not appear for 3 – 4 months (topical solution).

Diet advice
None.

Storage
Keep in a closed container in a cool, dry place away from reach of children. Protect from light.

Missed dose
Take a missed oral dose as soon as you remember. If your next dose is due within 6 hours, take a single dose now and skip the next.

Stopping the drug
Do not stop the tablets without consulting your physician; stopping the drug may lead to worsening of the underlying condition.

OVERDOSE ACTION

Seek immediate medical advice in all cases of overdose by mouth. Take emergency action if palpitations, nausea, vomiting, dizziness, or loss of consciousness occurs.

See Drug poisoning emergency guide (p.574).

SPECIAL PRECAUTIONS

Be sure to tell your physician if:
▼ You have impaired kidney or liver function.
▼ You have heart problems.
▼ You retain fluid.
▼ You are taking other medications.

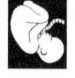

Pregnancy
▼ Safety in pregnancy not established. Discuss with your physician.

Breast feeding
▼ The drug passes into the breast milk, but at normal doses adverse effects on the baby are unlikely. Discuss with your physician.

Infants and children
▼ Not usually prescribed. Reduced dose necessary.

Over 60
▼ Reduced dose may be necessary.

Driving and hazardous work
▼ Avoid such activities until you have learned how the drug affects you; it can cause dizziness and lightheadedness.

Alcohol
▼ Avoid. Alcohol may further reduce blood pressure.

POSSIBLE ADVERSE EFFECTS

Fluid retention is a common adverse effect of oral minoxidil, which may lead to an increase

in weight. Diuretics are often prescribed to control this.

Symptom/effect	Frequency		Discuss with physician		Stop taking drug now	Call physician now
	Common	Rare	Only if severe	In all cases		
Increased hair growth	●			■		
Fluid retention/ankle swelling	●			■		
Breast tenderness		●		■		
Rash		●		■		
Shortness of breath		●		■		▮
Dizziness/lightheadedness		●		■		▮
Nausea		●		■		▮
Fast heartbeat		●		■		▮

PROLONGED USE

Prolonged oral therapy may lead to swelling of the ankles and increased hair growth. If systemic effects (for example, dizziness, palpitations, chest pain) occur with topical use, discontinue the drug and call your physician. If scalp itching, burning, rash, or hives occurs, call your physician.

INTERACTIONS

Guanethidine increases the risk of dizziness and lightheadedness when taken with minoxidil. Whenever possible,

guanethidine will be discontinued before treatment with minoxidil begins.

MISOPROSTOL

Brand name Cytotec
Used in the following combined preparation Arthrotec

GENERAL INFORMATION

Misoprostol is a synthetic version of a naturally occurring body chemical, prostaglandin E$_1$. It reduces the secretion of stomach acid, and protects the lining cells of the stomach against that acid. Since alcohol, and some medications employed to treat arthritis and some other forms of inflammation, can irritate the stomach, misoprostol can be used to protect the stomach lining. Misoprostol is also used in the treatment of duodenal ulcers, which usually heal rapidly when acid levels are reduced. It may sometimes be given concurrently with aluminum-based antacids.

Prostaglandins, however, affect muscle fibers in other parts of the body, including the muscle tissues of the uterus (womb). As this effect could jeopardize a pregnancy, women of childbearing potential should employ reliable contraception while receiving misoprostol. Women who are pregnant must not use this drug. If you think you might be pregnant, do not take the risk of using misoprostol, as it can cause miscarriage. Some diarrhea is common at the start of treatment and is no cause for concern; it usually clears up in a day or two.

QUICK REFERENCE

Drug group Prostaglandin anti-ulcer drug (p.121)
Overdose danger rating High
Dependence rating Low
Prescription needed Yes
Multi-source suppliers No

INFORMATION FOR USERS

Your drug prescription is tailored for you. Do not alter dosage without checking with your physician.

How taken

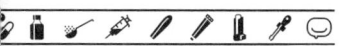

Tablets.

Frequency and timing of doses
1 - 4 x daily after food.

Adult dosage range
Drug-induced gastric ulceration
400 – 800mcg daily.
Duodenal ulcer 800mcg daily, usually for 4 – 8 weeks.

Onset of effect
Symptoms usually improve after a few doses.

Duration of action
Usually 3 – 6 hours.

Diet advice
None.

Storage
Keep in a closed container in a cool, dry place away from reach of children.

Missed dose
Take as soon as you remember with a light snack, and space out your remaining doses, always after food, until bedtime.

Stopping the drug
Do not stop the drug without consulting your physician; symptoms may recur.

OVERDOSE ACTION

 Seek immediate medical advice in all cases. Take emergency action if breathing difficulties, unconsciousness, convulsions, loss of blood pressure, or very slow heart rate occurs.

See Drug poisoning emergency guide (p.574).

POSSIBLE ADVERSE EFFECTS

The most common adverse effect is diarrhea, but it usually improves with time. Headaches may occur, and some women may experience menstrual cramps and spotting.

Symptom/effect	Frequency		Discuss with physician		Stop taking drug now	Call physician now
	Common	Rare	Only if severe	In all cases		
Abdominal cramps/diarrhea	●		■			
Flatulence	●		■			
Headache	●		■			
Nausea/vomiting	●			■		
Menstrual disorders		●	■			
Constipation		●	■			

INTERACTIONS

None known at present.

SPECIAL PRECAUTIONS

Be sure to tell your physician if:
▼ You think you could be pregnant, or know that you are pregnant.
▼ You have impaired kidney or liver function.
▼ You have had epilepsy.
▼ You have heart problems.
▼ You have high blood pressure.
▼ You have had blood clots or stroke.
▼ You have a history of bowel disease such as colitis or diverticulitis.
▼ You have had an alcohol problem.
▼ You are taking other medications.

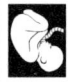 **Pregnancy**
▼ Not prescribed. The drug may cause a miscarriage, and its effects on the developing baby are not known.

 Breast feeding
▼ Effects on breast feeding unknown. Discuss with your physician.

 Infants and children
▼ Safety in children not established.

 Over 60
▼ No special problems.

 Driving and hazardous work
▼ Avoid such activities until you have learned how the drug affects you.

 Alcohol
▼ Avoid. Alcohol aggravates peptic ulcers.

PROLONGED USE

No known problems, but experience with the drug in long-term use is limited. Discuss with your physician.

MOCLOBEMIDE

Brand name Manerix
Used in the following combined preparations None

GENERAL INFORMATION

Moclobemide is the first of a new class of antidepressants known as reversible inhibitors of monoamine oxidase A (RIMA). By relieving depressive illness, moclobemide helps to elevate mood and restore interest in everyday activities. Like all antidepressants, it takes at least one to two weeks before moclobemide starts to lift depression.

Unlike traditional monoamine oxidase inhibitors (MAOIs), such as phenelzine and tranylcypromine, moclobemide is unlikely to interact with foods that contain tyramine, e.g. matured cheeses and yeast extracts. However, it is advisable to avoid large quantities of tyramine-rich foods as some people may be particularly sensitive.

Moclobemide is well tolerated, although nausea and dizziness may be experienced early in treatment. These should soon wear off.

QUICK REFERENCE

Drug group MAOI antidepressant drug (p.96)

Overdose danger rating Medium

Dependence rating Medium

Prescription needed Yes

Multi-source suppliers No

INFORMATION FOR USERS

Your drug prescription is tailored for you. Do not alter dosage without checking with your physician.

How taken

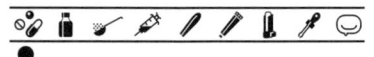

Tablets.

Frequency and timing of doses
2 – 3 x daily.

Adult dosage range
300 – 600mg daily.

Onset of effect
1 – 4 weeks.

Duration of action
Up to 24 hours.

Diet advice
Avoid very large amounts of tyramine-rich foods (e.g. matured cheeses, yeast extracts, fermented soya bean products).

Storage
Keep in a closed container in a cool, dry place away from reach of children.

Missed dose
Take as soon as you remember. If your next dose is due within 2 hours, take a single dose now and skip the next.

Stopping the drug
Do not stop the drug without consulting your physician; symptoms may recur.

Exceeding the dose
An occasional unintentional extra dose is unlikely to be a cause for concern. If a large overdose has been taken, seek immediate medical advice.

POSSIBLE ADVERSE EFFECTS

Moclobemide is generally well tolerated. Adverse *side effects* such as sleep disturbances, nausea, and headache usually disappear after a while.

Symptom/effect	Frequency		Discuss with physician		Stop taking drug now	Call physician now
	Common	Rare	Only if severe	In all cases		
Sleep disturbances	●		■			
Dizziness	●			■		
Nausea	●		■			
Headache	●		■			
Confusion		●			■	
Restlessness/agitation		●			■	

INTERACTIONS

General note A number of drugs interact with moclobemide. If you take other medications, discuss this with your physician or pharmacist.

Cimetidine The levels of moclobemide may be increased by cimetidine, requiring an adjustment in dosage.

Opiate analgesics Drugs such as meperidine, codeine, and morphine should not be taken with moclobemide.

Antidepressants Other antidepressants are not normally taken together with moclobemide. In some cases a time lapse is required before moclobemide is taken.

Ephedrine, pseudoephedrine, phenylpropanolamine These are contained in certain cold remedies. They should not be taken while on moclobemide.

SPECIAL PRECAUTIONS

Be sure to tell your physician if:
▼ You have impaired liver or kidney function
▼ You have pheochromocytoma.
▼ You have an overactive thyroid.
▼ You are taking other medications.

Pregnancy
▼ Safety in pregnancy not established. Discuss with your physician.

Breast feeding
▼ Small amounts of the drug pass into breast milk. Discuss with your physician.

Infants and children
▼ Safety and effectiveness in patients under 18 years not established.

Over 60
▼ No special problems.

Driving and hazardous work
▼ Avoid such activities until you have learned how the drug affects you because the drug can cause dizziness and confusion.

Alcohol
▼ Avoid excessive consumption.

Surgery and general anesthetics
▼ Moclobemide treatment should be stopped at least 2 days before you have a general anesthetic. Discuss with your physician or dentist before any surgery.

PROLONGED USE

No problems expected, but care should be taken to avoid interactions with food or other drugs, as the risk does not diminish with time.

MORPHINE

Brand names Epimorph, M-Eslon, M.O.S., MS Contin, Oramorph SR, Statex
Used in the following combined preparations None

GENERAL INFORMATION

Morphine, a narcotic analgesic (see p.93), relieves the severe pain that can be caused by injury, surgery, heart attack, or such chronic diseases as cancer. Also, to make a patient feel sleepy and less anxious, morphine may be given as *premedication* before surgery.

After a single intravenous injection or a single oral dose of tablet or liquid, morphine's painkilling effect wears off quickly. However, a slow-release tablet

may be given just twice daily to relieve continuous, severe pain. Such tablets should be swallowed whole and not chewed, crushed or broken.

It is habit-forming; *dependence* and *addiction* can occur. However, most patients taking morphine for pain relief over brief periods of time do not become dependent and are able to stop the drug without difficulty. Cancer patients may require morphine long term to control severe, unrelenting pain.

QUICK REFERENCE

Drug group Narcotic analgesic (p.92)

Overdose danger rating High

Dependence rating High

Prescription needed Yes

Multi-source suppliers Yes

INFORMATION FOR USERS

Your drug prescription is tailored for you. Do not alter your dosage without checking with your physician.

How taken

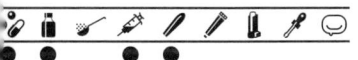

Tablets, slow-release tablets, oral liquid, injection, rectal suppositories.

Frequency and timing of doses
Every 4 hours; every 12 hours (slow-release tablets).

Adult dosage range
5 – 25mg per dose. However, doses vary considerably for every individual; some patients may need 75mg or more per dose.

Onset of effect
Within 1 hour; within 4 hours (slow-release tablets).

Duration of action
4 hours. Up to 12 hours (slow-release tablets).

Diet advice
To relieve constipation, increase intake of

fluids and high-fiber foods.

Storage
Keep in a closed container in a cool, dry place away from reach of children.

Missed dose
Take as soon as you remember. Return to your normal dosing schedule as soon as possible.

Stopping the drug
If the reason for taking the drug no longer exists, you may stop the drug and notify your physician.

OVERDOSE ACTION

 Seek immediate medical advice in all cases. Take emergency action if there are symptoms such as slow or irregular breathing, severe drowsiness, or loss of consciousness.

See Drug poisoning emergency guide (p.574).

SPECIAL PRECAUTIONS

Be sure to tell your physician if:
▼ You have impaired kidney or liver function.
▼ You have heart or circulatory problems.
▼ You have a lung disorder such as asthma or bronchitis.
▼ You have thyroid disease.
▼ You have a history of convulsions.
▼ You are taking other medications.

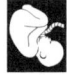 **Pregnancy**
▼ Not usually prescribed. May cause breathing difficulties in the newborn baby. Discuss with your physician.

 Breast feeding
▼ The drug passes into the breast milk in small amounts and may affect the baby adversely. Discuss with your physician.

 Infants and children
▼ Reduced dose necessary.

 Over 60
▼ Increased likelihood of adverse effects. Reduced dose may therefore be necessary.

 Driving and hazardous work
▼ Persons on morphine treatment are unlikely to be well enough to undertake such activities.

 Alcohol
▼ Avoid. Alcohol may increase the sedative effects of this drug.

POSSIBLE ADVERSE EFFECTS

Nausea, vomiting, constipation, drowsiness, and sweating are common, especially with high doses. Other drugs may be needed to counteract these symptoms.

Symptom/effect	Frequency		Discuss with physician		Stop taking drug now	Call physician now
	Common	Rare	Only if severe	In all cases		
Drowsiness	●		■			
Nausea/vomiting	●		■			
Constipation	●		■			
Dizziness	●			■		
Confusion		●		■		
Breathing difficulties		●		■	▲	▮

PROLONGED USE

The effects of the drug usually become weaker during prolonged use as the body adapts. But it is likely to produce dependence if taken for extended periods.

INTERACTIONS

Sedatives Morphine increases the sedative properties of all drugs that have a sedative effect. Such drugs include alcohol, antidepressants, antipsychotics, sleeping drugs, and antihistamines.

Monoamine oxidase inhibitors (MAOIs) These drugs may produce a severe rise in blood pressure when taken with morphine.

MUPIROCIN

Brand name Bactroban
Used in the following combined preparations None

GENERAL INFORMATION

Mupirocin is a relatively new *topical* antibiotic which kills bacteria responsible for skin infections. It is used to treat impetigo, folliculitis (infected hair follicles), furunculosis (boils), as well as infected eczema, and infected cuts and scrapes.

Adverse effects of mupirocin occur rarely and are limited to the skin. These effects, which may be due to the non-active ingredients (base) of the ointment rather than the active drug itself, tend to be mild and short-lived.

Do not apply in or near the eyes, mouth, or on burns. Wash your hands after contact with the affected area.

INFORMATION FOR USERS

Follow instructions on the label. Consult your physician if symptoms worsen.

How taken

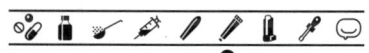

Ointment.

Frequency and timing of doses
3 x daily.

Dosage range
Sufficient to cover the affected area at each application.

Onset of effect
1 – 3 days.

Duration of action
At least 24 hours.

Diet advice
None.

Storage
Keep in a closed container in a cool, dry place away from reach of children. Protect from freezing and direct heat.

Missed dose
Apply as soon as you remember.

Stopping the drug
Apply the full course. Even if symptoms disappear, the original infection may still be present and symptoms may recur if treatment is stopped too soon.

POSSIBLE ADVERSE EFFECTS

Adverse effects that include itching, burning, stinging, and dryness occur rarely during therapy with mupirocin.

Symptom/effect	Frequency		Discuss with physician		Stop taking drug now	Call physician now
	Common	Rare	Only if severe	In all cases		
Dry skin		●	■			
Skin rash		●	■			
Redness		●	■			
Swelling		●	■			
Burning		●	■			
Itching		●	■			
Stinging		●	■			
Pain at site of infection		●	■			

INTERACTIONS

None.

SPECIAL PRECAUTIONS

Be sure to consult your physician or pharmacist before taking this drug if:
▼ You have impaired kidney function.

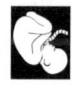
Pregnancy
▼ Safety in pregnancy not established. Discuss with your physician.

Breast feeding
▼ Effect on breast feeding uncertain. Discuss with your physician.

Infants and children
▼ No special problems.

Over 60
▼ No special problems.

Driving and hazardous work
▼ No known problems.

Alcohol
▼ No known problems.

PROLONGED USE

Not intended for prolonged use. Consult your physician if infections have not improved after 10 days of treatment.

NABUMETONE

Brand name Relafen
Used in the following combined preparations None

GENERAL INFORMATION

Nabumetone is a non-steroidal anti-inflammatory drug (NSAID) used for its analgesic and anti-inflammatory effects to relieve joint pain, swelling, and stiffness. Therefore, it is used to relieve the symptoms of acute and chronic rheumatoid arthritis and osteoarthritis (degenerative arthritis), although it does not cure the underlying disease.

Gastrointestinal *side effects* such as diarrhea, indigestion, abdominal pain, and nausea are fairly common. Peptic ulcer, with or without bleeding, rarely occurs.

INFORMATION FOR USERS

Your drug prescription is tailored for you. Do not alter dosage without checking with your physician.

How taken

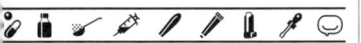

Tablets.

Frequency and timing of doses
1 - 2 x daily with or without food.

Adult dosage range
1,000 – 2,000mg daily.

Onset of effect
Within 1 – 4 hours, but full anti-inflammatory effect may not be felt for 3 – 6 days.

Duration of action
Up to 24 hours or more.

Diet advice
None.

Storage
Keep in a closed container in a cool, dry place away from reach of children.

Missed dose
As nabumetone is taken usually only once daily, take as soon as you remember. If your next dose is due within 6 hours, take a single dose now and skip the next.

Stopping the drug
When taken for a short period of time, there should be no problem. If prescribed for long-term treatment, you should seek medical advice before stopping the drug.

Exceeding the dose
An occasional unintentional extra dose is unlikely to be a cause for concern. But if you notice any unusual symptoms, or if a large overdose has been taken, notify your physician immediately.

SPECIAL PRECAUTIONS

Be sure to tell your physician if:
▼ You are allergic to ASA or other NSAIDs.
▼ You have impaired liver or kidney function.
▼ You have a heart problem or high blood pressure.
▼ You have had esophagitis, inflammatory bowel disease, or a peptic ulcer disease.
▼ You have a bleeding disorder.
▼ You have asthma.
▼ You are taking other medications.

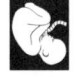

Pregnancy
▼ Not recommended. Discuss with your physician.

Breast feeding
▼ Not recommended.

Infants and children
▼ Not recommended.

Over 60
▼ Increased likelihood of adverse effects. Reduced dosage may therefore be necessary.

Driving and hazardous work
▼ Avoid such activities until you have learned how the drug affects you; it can cause drowsiness and dizziness.

Alcohol
▼ Avoid. Alcohol may increase the risk of stomach irritation with nabumetone.

Surgery and general anesthetics
Nabumetone may prolong bleeding. Discuss with your physician or dentist before any surgery.

POSSIBLE ADVERSE EFFECTS

Most adverse effects are not serious and may diminish with time. The most common adverse effects are the result of gastrointestinal disturbances, such as diarrhea, indigestion, abdominal pain, nausea, and constipation.

Headache, tiredness, dizziness, drowsiness, and insomnia may also occur. Black and/or bloodstained feces should be reported to your physician without delay.

Symptom/effect	Frequency		Discuss with physician		Stop taking drug now	Call physician now
	Common	Rare	Only if severe	In all cases		
Gastrointestinal disturbance	●		■			
Headache	●		■			
Dizziness/drowsiness	●		■			
Ringing in ears/blurred vision		●		■		
Swollen feet/ankles/face		●		■	▲	‖
Rash/hives/itching		●		■	▲	‖
Breathlessness/wheezing		●		■	▲	‖
Bloodstained/black feces		●		■	▲	‖

INTERACTIONS

General note Nabumetone may interact with a wide range of drugs and thereby increase their adverse effects. Such drugs include warfarin, phenytoin, oral hypoglycemics, methotrexate, digoxin, lithium, other NSAIDs, and ASA.

Antihypertensive drugs and diuretics
The beneficial effects of these drugs may be reduced by nabumetone.

PROLONGED USE

There is an increased risk of bleeding, both from peptic ulcers and from the bowel, with prolonged use of nabumetone.

NADOLOL

Brand names Corgard, Apo-Nadol, Syn-Nadolol
Used in the following combined preparation Corzide

GENERAL INFORMATION

Nadolol is a beta blocker prescribed for hypertension (high blood pressure) and angina. When nadolol is prescribed for hypertension, the prescription is sometimes for a combined preparation containing a diuretic. One advantage nadolol has over some other beta blockers is that it needs to be taken only once daily.

Because it can cause breathing difficulties, nadolol should not be taken by asthmatics or people suffering from chronic bronchitis or emphysema. In common with all beta blockers, nadolol has a slowing effect on the heart rate and masks the body's response to low blood sugar; it should be used with caution by diabetics.

QUICK REFERENCE

Drug group Beta blocker (p.109)
Overdose danger rating High
Dependence rating Low
Prescription needed Yes
Multi-source suppliers Yes

INFORMATION FOR USERS

Your drug prescription is tailored for you. Do not alter dosage without checking with your physician.

How taken

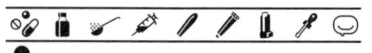

Tablets.

Frequency and timing of doses
Once daily.

Dosage range
Hypertension 80 – 320mg daily.
Angina 40 – 240mg daily.

Onset of effect
2 – 4 hours. For high blood pressure, it may be several weeks before full benefit is felt.

Duration of action
Over 24 hours.

Diet advice
None.

Storage
Keep in a closed container in a cool, dry place away from reach of children. Protect from light.

Missed dose
Take as soon as you remember. If your next dose is due within 6 hours, take a single dose now and skip the next.

Stopping the drug
Do not stop the drug without consulting your physician; stopping the drug may lead to dangerous worsening of your underlying condition or may precipitate a heart attack.

OVERDOSE ACTION

Seek immediate medical advice in all cases. Take emergency action if collapse or loss of consciousness occurs.

See Drug poisoning emergency guide (p.574).

POSSIBLE ADVERSE EFFECTS

Nadolol has a number of adverse effects which are usually temporary and diminish with long-term use. Breathing difficulties, fainting, and rash require medical attention.

Symptom/effect	Frequency		Discuss with physician		Stop taking drug now	Call physician now
	Common	Rare	Only if severe	In all cases		
Cold hands and feet	●		■			
Lethargy/fatigue	●		■			
Fainting/dizziness	●			■		▮
Slow heartbeat	●			■		▮
Insomnia		●	■			
Impotence		●		■		
Breathing difficulties		●		■		
Rash		●		■		▮

SPECIAL PRECAUTIONS

Be sure to tell your physician if:
▼ You have impaired liver or kidney function
▼ You have poor circulation in the legs.
▼ You have heart failure.
▼ You have a lung disorder such as asthma, emphysema, or bronchitis.
▼ You have allergies.
▼ You have diabetes.
▼ You are taking other medications.

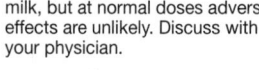

Pregnancy
▼ Safety in pregnancy not established. Discuss with your physician.

Breast feeding
▼ The drug passes into the breast milk, but at normal doses adverse effects are unlikely. Discuss with your physician.

Infants and children
▼ Not usually prescribed.

Over 60
▼ Increased likelihood of adverse effects.

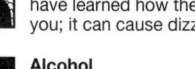

Driving and hazardous work
▼ Avoid such activities until you have learned how the drug affects you; it can cause dizziness.

Alcohol
▼ No special problems with moderate intake.

Surgery and general anesthetics
▼ Nadolol may need to be stopped before you have a general anesthetic. Discuss with your physician or dentist before any surgery.

INTERACTIONS

Non-steroidal anti-inflammatory drugs may reduce the antihypertensive effect of nadolol.

Sympathomimetic decongestants used with nadolol may increase blood pressure and/or heart rate.

Calcium channel blockers Taken with nadolol, some of these drugs may further decrease blood pressure and/or heart rate and may also reduce the force of the heart's pumping action.

PROLONGED USE

No special problems expected.

NANDROLONE

Brand names Deca-Durabolin, Durabolin
Used in the following combined preparations None

GENERAL INFORMATION

Nandrolone is an anabolic steroid, a synthetic hormone related to the male sex hormone testosterone. Given by injection, it encourages growth in boys whose development has been slowed because of hormone disturbances. It has been used to help people gain weight after a serious illness or injury and to treat certain types of anemia. Violating the rules of most athletic organizations, athletes have taken nandrolone and other anabolic steroids to increase body weight and muscle strength. But scientific studies indicate that the weight gain may be caused by fluid retention; the evidence of increased strength is equivocal. The use of these agents in sport should be strongly discouraged.

Because the testosterone-like properties cannot be completely separated from the anabolic effects, women taking nandrolone are likely to suffer from excessive hair growth and disturbed menstrual periods. Liver damage and liver tumors have been reported, but are more common with oral anabolic steroids.

QUICK REFERENCE

Drug group Anabolic steroid (p.158)

Overdose danger rating Low

Dependence rating Low

Prescription needed Yes

Multi-source suppliers No

INFORMATION FOR USERS

This drug is given only under medical supervision and is not for self-administration.

How taken

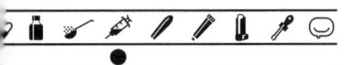

Action.

Frequency and timing of doses
Once a week (some anemias); once every 2–4 weeks (other uses).

Dosage range
Dosage varies according to preparation and condition being treated.

Onset of effect
Within a few hours.

Duration of action
2–4 weeks.

Diet advice
Drug treatment for weight gain and growth needs to be accompanied by a nourishing balanced diet. Excessive intake of protein may cause a buildup of nitrogen waste in the body. Your physician will give detailed advice.

Storage
Not applicable. This drug is not normally kept in the home.

Missed dose
Arranged for a missed injection to be administered as soon as possible.

Stopping the drug
Treatment can be safely stopped when it has effectively dealt with the disorder.

Exceeding the dose
Overdose is unlikely, since treatment is carefully monitored.

SPECIAL PRECAUTIONS

Be sure to tell your physician if:
▼ You have impaired kidney or liver function.
▼ You have heart problems.
▼ You have urinary difficulties.
▼ You have diabetes.
▼ You are taking other medications.

Pregnancy
▼ Not prescribed.

Breast feeding
▼ Not prescribed.

Infants and children
▼ Reduced dose necessary.

Over 60
▼ Increased risk of prostate problems in men. Reduced dose may be necessary.

Driving and hazardous work
▼ No known problems.

Alcohol
▼ No known problems.

POSSIBLE ADVERSE EFFECTS

Most of the more serious adverse effects are likely to occur only with long-term treatment with nandrolone, and may be helped by a reduction in dosage.

Symptom/effect	Frequency		Discuss with physician		Stop taking drug now	Call physician now
	Common	Rare	Only if severe	In all cases		
Swollen feet/ankles	●		■			
Nausea/vomiting		●	■			
Aggressive behavior		●		■		
Jaundice		●	■	▲		
Men only						
Difficulty passing urine		●	■	▲		
Women only						
Irregular menstruation	●		■			
Unusual hair growth		●	■			

PROLONGED USE

Prolonged use of this drug may lead to early stopping of growth in children and masculinization in women. Long-term use may also raise blood cholesterol levels, thereby increasing the chances of coronary heart disease. Because the benefits are doubtful, athletes taking anabolic steroids over long periods of time run a needless risk.

Monitoring Periodic checks on the level of salts in the blood are usually needed.

INTERACTIONS

Anticoagulant drugs Nandrolone increases the effects of these drugs. Anticoagulant dosage may need to be adjusted accordingly.

Antidiabetic drugs Because nandrolone may lower blood sugar levels, dosage of these drugs may need to be reduced.

NAPROXEN

Brand names Naprosyn, Anaprox (naproxen sodium), Apo-Naproxen, Naxen, Novo-Naprox
Used in the following combined preparations None

GENERAL INFORMATION

Naproxen was introduced in 1974. Like other non-steroidal anti-inflammatory drugs (NSAIDs), it reduces pain, stiffness, and inflammation.

It is used to relieve symptoms of adult and juvenile rheumatoid arthritis, osteoarthritis, and ankylosing spondylitis, although it does not cure the underlying disease.

Naproxen may also be prescribed short term for pain relief after childbirth, orthopedic surgery, dental treatment, strains and sprains. It is also effective for treating headaches and painful menstrual cramps.

Gastrointestinal *side effects* are fairly common, and there is an increased risk of bleeding. In long-term use naproxen needs to be taken only twice daily.

QUICK REFERENCE

Drug group Non-steroidal anti-inflammatory drug (p.128)

Overdose danger rating Low

Dependence rating Low

Prescription needed Yes

Multi-source suppliers Yes

INFORMATION FOR USERS

Your drug prescription is tailored for you. Do not alter dosage without checking with your physician.

How taken

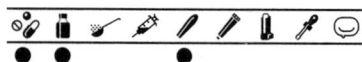

Tablets, oral liquid, suppositories.

Frequency and timing of doses
2 x daily (muscular pain and arthritis); every 6 – 8 hours as required (general pain relief). All doses should be taken with food.

Adult dosage range
Mild to moderate pain, menstrual cramps 500mg (starting dose), then 250mg every 6 – 8 hours as required up to 1g daily.
Muscular pain and arthritis 0.5 – 1g daily.

Onset of effect
Pain relief begins within 1 hour. Full anti-inflammatory effect may take 2 weeks.

Duration of action
Up to 12 hours.

Diet advice
None.

Storage
Keep in a closed container in a cool, dry place away from reach of children.

Missed dose
Take as soon as you remember. If your next dose is due within 6 hours, take a single dose now and skip the next.

Stopping the drug
When taken for short-term pain relief, naproxen can be safely stopped as soon as you no longer need it. If prescribed for long-term treatment, however, you should seek medical advice before stopping the drug.

Exceeding the dose
An occasional unintentional extra dose is unlikely to be a cause for concern. But if you notice any unusual symptoms, or if a large overdose has been taken, notify your physician.

SPECIAL PRECAUTIONS

Be sure to tell your physician if:
▼ You have impaired kidney or liver function
▼ You have heart problems.
▼ You have a bleeding disorder.
▼ You have high blood pressure.
▼ You have had a peptic ulcer, esophagitis, or acid indigestion.
▼ You are allergic to ASA.
▼ You have asthma.
▼ You are taking other medications.

Pregnancy
▼ Safety in pregnancy not established. When taken in the last trimester of pregnancy, may affect the heart of the fetus and may prolong labor. Discuss with your physician.

Breast feeding
▼ The drug passes into the breast milk, but at normal doses adverse effects on the baby are unlikely. Discuss with your physician.

Infants and children
▼ Reduced dose necessary. Suppositories are contraindicated children under 12.

Over 60
▼ Increased likelihood of adverse effects. Reduced dose may therefore be necessary.

Driving and hazardous work
▼ Avoid such activities until you have learned how the drug affects you; it can cause dizziness and drowsiness.

Alcohol
▼ Avoid. Alcohol may increase the risk of stomach irritation with naproxen.

Surgery and general anesthetics
▼ Naproxen may prolong bleeding. Discuss with your physician or dentist before any surgery.

POSSIBLE ADVERSE EFFECTS

Most adverse effects are not serious and may diminish with time. Black or bloodstained feces should be reported to your physician without delay.

Symptom/effect	Frequency		Discuss with physician		Stop taking drug now	Call physician now
	Common	Rare	Only if severe	In all cases		
Gastrointestinal disorders	●		■			
Headache	●		■			
Dizziness/drowsiness	●		■			
Ringing in the ears		●		■		
Swollen feet/ankles		●		■		
Rash/itching		●		■	▲	
Wheezing/breathlessness		●		■	▲	▐
Black, bloodstained feces		●		■	▲	▐

INTERACTIONS

General note Naproxen interacts with a wide range of drugs to increase the risk of bleeding and/or peptic ulcers. It may also increase the toxic effects of lithium and digoxin.

Antihypertensive drugs and diuretics The beneficial effects of these drugs may be reduced by naproxen.

PROLONGED USE

There is an increased risk of bleeding from peptic ulcers and in the bowel with prolonged use of naproxen.

NEDOCROMIL

Brand name Tilade
Used in the following combined preparations None

GENERAL INFORMATION

Nedocromil is used in the treatment of asthma. Taken by *inhaler* on a regular basis, it helps to prevent asthmatic exacerbations. It may also reduce the frequency and severity of asthmatic attacks induced by inhaled allergens, atmospheric pollutants, exercise, and cold air.

Nedocromil has a slow onset of action, taking up to a week, or longer, to produce its asthma-stabilizing effects. It is therefore not effective in the relief of acute asthmatic attacks. Although nedocromil is not intended to be an alternative to *bronchodilators,* it may lessen the need for them.

Adverse effects, including unpleasant taste, headache, and upper gastrointestinal upset, are mild. They usually do not require discontinuation of treatment.

QUICK REFERENCE

Drug group Anti-inflammatory drug (p.136)

Overdose danger rating Low

Dependence rating Low

Prescription needed Yes

Multi-source suppliers No

INFORMATION FOR USERS

Your drug prescription is tailored for you. Do not alter dosage without checking with your physician.

How taken

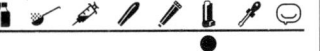

Inhaler.

Frequency and timing of doses
2 - 4 x daily.

Dosage range
8 - 16mg daily (by mouth).

Onset of effect
Benefits of repeated doses will be apparent within 1 week, but it may take longer in some cases.

Duration of action
Up to 6 hours. Some effects persist for several days after treatment is stopped.

Diet advice
None.

Storage
Keep in original container in a cool, dry place away from reach of children. Protect from light.

Missed dose
Take as soon as you remember. If your next dose is due within 2 hours, take a single dose now and skip the next.

Stopping the drug
Do not stop the drug without consulting your physician; symptoms may recur.

Exceeding the dose
An occasional unintentional extra dose is unlikely to be a cause for concern. But if you notice unusual symptoms, or if a large overdose has been taken, notify your physician.

SPECIAL PRECAUTIONS

Be sure to tell your physician if:
▼ You have impaired kidney or liver function.
▼ You have a known problem of abuse with propellants in inhalers.
▼ You are taking other medications.

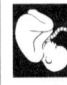

Pregnancy
▼ Safety in pregnancy not established. Discuss with your physician.

Breast feeding
▼ Safety in breast feeding not established. Discuss with your physician.

Infants and children
▼ Not recommended in children under 12 years.

Over 60
▼ No known problems but reduced dose may be necessary.

Driving and hazardous work
▼ Exercise caution if headache occurs.

Alcohol
▼ No known problems.

POSSIBLE ADVERSE EFFECTS

Few adverse effects have been reported, principally headache and upper gastrointestinal symptoms, that have been mild and transient. They rarely require discontinuation of treatment.

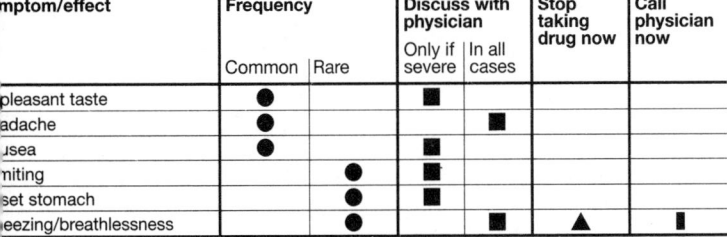

Symptom/effect	Frequency		Discuss with physician		Stop taking drug now	Call physician now
	Common	Rare	Only if severe	In all cases		
Unpleasant taste	●		■			
Headache	●			■		
Nausea	●		■			
Vomiting		●	■			
Upset stomach		●	■			
Wheezing/breathlessness		●		■	▲	∎

INTERACTIONS

None.

PROLONGED USE

No problems expected.

NEOMYCIN

Brand names Mycifradin, Myciguent
Used in the following combined preparations Coly-Mycin Otic, Cortisporin, Neo-Cortef, Neo-Medrol, Neosporin

GENERAL INFORMATION

Neomycin, introduced in 1951, is one of the oldest aminoglycoside antibiotics. It is most commonly prescribed in the form of drops, cream, or ointment, often in combination with other drugs for ear and skin infections. It is not given by injection because it is more damaging to the kidneys than other aminoglycosides.

Given by mouth, neomycin is minimally absorbed, but is effective in killing bacteria inside the intestine and may be used prior to bowel surgery to prevent infections. It is prescribed in the treatment of hepatic coma caused by high blood levels of ammonia in people with liver failure.

QUICK REFERENCE

Drug group Aminoglycoside antibiotic (p.140)

Overdose danger rating Low

Dependence rating Low

Prescription needed Yes

Multi-source suppliers No

INFORMATION FOR USERS

Your drug prescription is tailored for you. Do not alter dosage without checking with your physician.

How taken

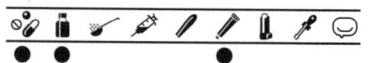

Tablets, oral liquid, ointment.

Frequency and timing of doses
By mouth 4 x daily (hepatic coma); 3 x daily (bowel sterilization).
Skin preparations 2 – 5 x daily.
Eye preparations Every 3 – 4 hours.
Ear drops Every 6 – 8 hours.

Adult dosage range
By mouth 3g daily (bowel sterilization); 4 – 12g daily (hepatic coma);
Skin, eye, and ear preparations As directed.

Onset of effect
1 – 2 days.

Duration of action
6 – 8 hours (by mouth); up to 24 hours (on skin).

Diet advice
A low-protein diet is usually recommended in hepatic coma.

Storage
Keep in a closed container in a cool, dry place away from reach of children. Protect liquid preparations from light.

Missed dose
Take as soon as you remember. If your next dose is due within 2 hours, take a single dose now and skip the next.

Stopping the drug
Do not stop the drug without consulting your physician.

Exceeding the dose
An occasional unintentional extra dose is unlikely to be a cause for concern. But if you notice unusual symptoms, or if a large overdose has been taken, notify your physician.

SPECIAL PRECAUTIONS

Be sure to tell your physician if:
▼ You have impaired kidney function.
▼ You have inflammatory or ulcerative bowel disease.
▼ You have a hearing or balance disorder.
▼ You have myasthenia gravis or Parkinson's disease.
▼ You are taking other medications.

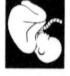

Pregnancy
▼ Safety in pregnancy of oral form not established. Discuss with your physician.

Breast feeding
▼ Taken by mouth, the drug passes into the breast milk. Discuss with your physician.

Infants and children
▼ Safety of oral neomycin therapy in patients under 18 years not established.

Over 60
▼ Increased likelihood of adverse effects.

Driving and hazardous work
▼ No special problems. However, exercise caution if dizziness occurs.

Alcohol
▼ No known problems.

Surgery and general anesthetics
▼ Neomycin may need to be stopped before you have a general anesthetic. Discuss this with your physician or dentist before any surgery.

POSSIBLE ADVERSE EFFECTS

Allergic reactions including rash and itching occur commonly with skin, eye, and ear preparations. Taken by mouth, the drug may cause diarrhea and abdominal cramps. Dizziness, loss of balance, or ringing in the ears should be reported promptly.

Symptom/effect	Frequency		Discuss with physician		Stop taking drug now	Call physician now
	Common	Rare	Only if severe	In all cases		
Mild diarrhea	●		■			
Nausea/vomiting	●		■			
Rash/itching	●			■	▲	
Hearing loss/disturbance		●		■	▲	
Dizziness/vertigo		●		■	▲	
Severe bloody diarrhea		●		■	▲	■

INTERACTIONS

General note Any drug that has adverse effects on hearing and/or kidney function increases the risk of such effects with neomycin. Such drugs include other aminoglycosides, furosemide, polymyxin antibiotics, and cisplatin.

Oral contraceptives Possible decreased contraceptive effect.

Oral anticoagulant drugs Neomycin by mouth may increase the effect of these drugs.

Digoxin, penicillin V, oral vitamin B_{12}, methotrexate Oral neomycin may reduce the absorption of these drugs.

PROLONGED USE

There is a rare risk of adverse effects on hearing, balance, and kidney function with prolonged high-dose neomycin therapy.

NEOSTIGMINE

Brand name Prostigmin
Used in the following combined preparations None

GENERAL INFORMATION

Shorter acting and more potent than some other drugs in its field, neostigmine has been used for over 50 years to treat myasthenia gravis, a rare auto-immune condition (see p.133). The disorder involves muscle weakness caused by faulty transmission of nerve impulses. By prolonging them, neostigmine improves muscle strength, though it does not cure the disease. In severe cases it may be prescribed in conjunction with corticosteroids.

The injectable form of neostigmine is also used to relieve urinary retention or temporary paralysis of the bowel (paralytic ileus).

QUICK REFERENCE

Drug group Drug for myasthenia gravis (p.133)

Overdose danger rating High

Dependence rating Low

Prescription needed Yes

Multi-source suppliers No

INFORMATION FOR USERS

Your drug prescription is tailored for you. Do not alter dosage without checking with your physician.

How taken

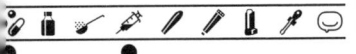

Tablets, injection.

Frequency and timing of doses
Every 3 – 4 hours initially. Thereafter according to the needs of the individual.

Dosage range
Adults 75 – 300mg daily (by mouth); 5 – 15mg daily (injection).
Children Reduced dose necessary according to age and weight.

Onset of effect
45 – 75 minutes (by mouth); within 20 minutes (injection).

Duration of action
2 – 4 hours.

Diet advice
None.

Storage
Keep in a closed container in a cool, dry place away from children. Protect from light.

Missed dose
Take as soon as you remember. If your next dose is due within 2 hours, take a single dose now and skip the next.

Stopping the drug
Do not stop the drug without consulting your physician; symptoms may recur.

OVERDOSE ACTION

Seek immediate medical advice in all cases. You may experience severe abdominal cramps, diarrhea, vomiting, increased salivation, weakness, and tremor. Take emergency action if unusually slow heartbeat, troubled breathing, seizures, or loss of consciousness occur.

See Drug poisoning emergency guide (p.574).

SPECIAL PRECAUTIONS

Be sure to tell your physician if:
▼ You have heart problems.
▼ You have had epileptic seizures.
▼ You have asthma.
▼ You have difficulty passing urine.
▼ You have Parkinson's disease.
▼ You are taking other medications.

Pregnancy
▼ No evidence of risk to developing baby with neostigmine taken in the first 6 months of pregnancy. Large doses near the time of delivery may cause premature labor and lead to temporary muscle weakness in the newborn baby. Discuss with your physician.

Breast feeding
▼ The drug may pass into the breast milk. Discuss with your physician.

Infants and children
▼ Reduced dose necessary.

Over 60
▼ Increased likelihood of adverse effects.

Driving and hazardous work
▼ Your underlying condition may make such activities inadvisable. Discuss with your physician.

Alcohol
▼ Avoid. Alcohol may cause breathing difficulties in myasthenia gravis sufferers.

Surgery and general anesthetics
▼ Neostigmine may interact with some anesthetics. Make sure your treatment is known to your physician or dentist before any surgery.

POSSIBLE ADVERSE EFFECTS

Most of the common adverse effects of neostigmine are dose-related and due to overstimulation of the parasympathetic nervous system (see p.107).

Symptom/effect	Frequency		Discuss with physician		Stop taking drug now	Call physician now
	Common	Rare	Only if severe	In all cases		
Increased salivation	●		■			
Diarrhea	●			■		
Abdominal cramps	●			■		
Nausea/vomiting	●			■		
Blurred vision/sweating	●			■		
Muscle cramps/twitching	●			■		
Rash		●		■	▲	■

INTERACTIONS

General note Drugs that suppress the transmission of nerve signals in muscles may aggravate myasthenia gravis and oppose the effect of neostigmine. Such drugs include atropine, quinidine, procainamide, phenytoin, lithium, and aminoglycoside antibiotics.

PROLONGED USE

Reduced effectiveness may occur during prolonged use. This may be restored by stopping the drug for a few days or by adjusting the dose. But this should be done only under the direction of your physician.

NIFEDIPINE

Brand names Adalat, Apo-Nifed, Gen-Nifedipine, Novo-Nifedin, Nu-Nifed
Used in the following combined preparations None

GENERAL INFORMATION

Nifedipine, introduced in 1982, belongs to a group of drugs known as calcium channel blockers (p.113), which interfere with the conduction of signals in the muscles of the heart and blood vessels.

Nifedipine is used in the treatment of angina to help prevent attacks of chest pain. Unlike some other anti-angina drugs (i.e., beta blockers), it can be used safely by asthmatics. Nifedipine is also used to lower high blood pressure,
and may be helpful in improving circulation to the limbs, e.g., in Raynaud's disease.

In common with other drugs of its class, nifedipine may cause blood pressure to fall too low. In rare cases, angina may become worse at the start of nifedipine therapy. This drug may cause mild to moderate leg and ankle swelling.

INFORMATION FOR USERS

Your drug prescription is tailored for you. Do not alter dosage without checking with your physician.

How taken

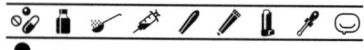

Slow-release tablets, capsules.

Frequency and timing of doses
Capsules 3 – 4 x daily (angina).
Slow-release tablets 1 x daily (angina and hypertension).

Adult dosage range
Angina 30 – 120mg daily (capsules);
30 – 90mg (slow-release tablets).
Hypertension 30 – 120mg daily (slow-release tablets).

Onset of effect
30 – 60 minutes (capsules); 1 – 2 hours (slow-release tablets).

Duration of action
6 – 8 hours (capsules); 10 – 12 hours (slow-release tablets).

Diet advice
None.

Storage
Keep in a closed container in a cool, dry place away from reach of children. Protect from light.

Missed dose
Take a capsule as soon as you remember, or when needed. If your next dose is due within 2 hours, take a single dose now and skip the next. If your next slow-release tablet is due within 4 hours, take a single dose now and take the next dose 8 hours later, then follow your regular schedule.

Stopping the drug
Do not stop the drug without consulting your physician; symptoms may recur.

Exceeding the dose
An occasional unintentional extra dose is unlikely to cause problems. Large overdoses may cause dizziness. Notify your physician.

SPECIAL PRECAUTIONS

Be sure to tell your physician if:
▼ You have impaired kidney or liver function.
▼ You have heart failure.
▼ You have diabetes.
▼ You are taking other medications.

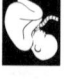

Pregnancy
▼ Not usually prescribed. Discuss with your physician.

Breast feeding
▼ Not usually prescribed. Discuss with your physician.

Infants and children
▼ Not recommended.

Over 60
▼ Increased likelihood of adverse effects. Reduced dose may therefore be necessary.

Driving and hazardous work
▼ Avoid such activities until you have learned how the drug affects you; it can cause dizziness owing to lowered blood pressure.

Alcohol
▼ Avoid. Alcohol may further reduce blood pressure, causing dizziness or other symptoms.

POSSIBLE ADVERSE EFFECTS

Nifedipine can cause a variety of minor symptoms, including leg and ankle swelling, headache, dizziness, fatigue, and nausea. Dizziness, especially on rising, may be caused by an excessive reduction in blood pressure.

The most serious effect is the rare possibility of angina becoming worse after starting nifedipine treatment. This should always be reported to your physician.

Symptom/effect	Frequency		Discuss with physician		Stop taking drug now	Call physician now
	Common	Rare	Only if severe	In all cases		
Leg and ankle swelling	●		■			
Headache	●		■			
Dizziness/fatigue	●		■			
Flushing	●		■			
Leg cramps		●	■			
Nausea		●		■		
Swollen, tender gums		●		■		■

INTERACTIONS

Antihypertensive drugs Nifedipine may increase the effects of these drugs.

Digoxin Blood levels of digoxin may be increased when it is taken with nifedipine.

PROLONGED USE

No problems expected.

NILUTAMIDE

Brand name Anandron
Used in the following combined preparations None

GENERAL INFORMATION

Nilutamide is used in the treatment of advanced prostate cancer that has spread to other parts of the body.

Normally, androgenic hormones stimulate both normal cells and cancer cells in the prostate gland. Surgical castration (removal of the testicles) eliminates a major source of androgens. Another source, the adrenal glands, cannot be removed because they supply other essential hormones. However, nilutamide blocks the action of adrenal androgens on the prostate gland.

Studies have shown that, in advanced prostate cancer, nilutamide decreases cancerous bone pain, slows the progression of the cancer, and prolongs survival time.

INFORMATION FOR USERS

Your drug prescription is tailored for you. Do not alter dosage without checking with your physician.

How taken

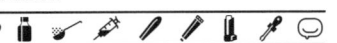

Tablets.

Frequency and timing of doses
Once daily.

Dosage range
300mg daily.

Onset of effect
Can appear within hours, but optimal effect is reached approximately 2 weeks after starting the drug.

Duration of action
1 – 4 days.

Diet advice
None.

Storage
Keep in a closed container in a cool, dry place away from reach of children.

Missed dose
Take as soon as you remember.

Stopping the drug
Do not stop taking the drug without consulting your physician.

Exceeding the dose
An occasional unintentional extra dose is unlikely to be a cause for concern. But if you notice unusual symptoms, or if a large overdose has been taken, notify your physician.

SPECIAL PRECAUTIONS

Be sure to tell your physician if:
▼ You have impaired liver or kidney function.
▼ You have a lung disorder.
▼ You have any blood disorders, especially anemia.
▼ You are taking other medications.

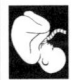

Pregnancy
▼ Not prescribed.

Breast feeding
▼ Not prescribed.

Infants and children
▼ Not prescribed.

Over 60
▼ No special problems.

Driving and hazardous work
▼ Avoid such activities until you have learned how the drug affects you; it can cause dizziness and visual disturbances.

Alcohol
▼ Avoid. Taken with nilutamide, alcohol may cause flushing, nausea, vomiting, abdominal pain, and headache.

PROLONGED USE

Monitoring Regular blood tests are advised to monitor the blood count and liver function. Periodic chest X rays and/or eye examinations may be recommended.

POSSIBLE ADVERSE EFFECTS

The important adverse effect is visual disturbance marked by an increase in adaptation time when passing from a well-lit to a more dimly-lit area. Other more serious adverse effects are the onset or worsening of shortness of breath and signs of liver problems (including itching, dark urine, loss of appetite, jaundice, and/or unexplained "flu-like" symptoms) which may lead to discontinuation of the drug. Discuss these effects with your physician immediately.

Symptom/effect	Frequency		Discuss with physician		Stop taking drug now	Call physician now
	Common	Rare	Only if severe	In all cases		
Visual disturbances	●			■		
Nausea/vomiting	●			■		
Dizziness	●		■			
Hot flushes	●		■			
Impotence/decreased libido	●		■			
Rash/itching		●		■	▲	∎
Difficult, labored breathing		●		■	▲	∎
Fatigue/malaise		●		■	▲	∎
Jaundice		●		■	▲	∎

INTERACTIONS

General note Nilutamide may increase the effects of a number of drugs including phenytoin, propranolol, chlordiazepoxide, diazepam, lidocaine, and theophylline.

Anticoagulant drugs Nilutamide may increase the effects of these drugs. The dosage of anticoagulant may need to be reduced.

NITRAZEPAM

Brand name Mogadon
Used in the following combined preparations None

GENERAL INFORMATION

Nitrazepam belongs to a group of drugs known as the benzodiazepines. The actions and adverse effects of this group of drugs are described more fully under Anti-anxiety drugs (p.95).

Nitrazepam is used in the short-term treatment of insomnia. Because it is a long-acting drug compared with some other benzodiazepines, the drug is effective for preventing early wakening. However, it is more likely to cause drowsiness and/or lightheadedness the following day. Nitrazepam is also used in the prevention and treatment of certain kinds of seizures, especially in children.

Like other benzodiazepines, nitrazepam can be habit-forming if taken regularly over a long period for insomnia. Its effects may also grow weaker with time. For these reasons, treatment with nitrazepam is usually reviewed at least every two weeks.

INFORMATION FOR USERS

Your drug prescription is tailored for you. Do not alter dosage without checking with your physician.

How taken

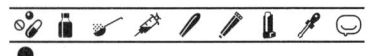

Tablets.

Frequency and timing of doses
Insomnia Once daily immediately before bedtime.
Seizures 3 x daily.

Adult dosage range
5 – 10mg daily.

Onset of effect
30 – 60 minutes.

Duration of action
6 – 8 hours. Some effects may persist for 24 – 36 hours.

Diet advice
None.

Storage
Keep in a closed container in a cool, dry place away from reach of children. Protect from light.

Missed dose
Insomnia If you fall asleep without having taken a dose and wake some hours later, do not take the missed dose.

Seizures Take as soon as you remember. Take your next dose when it is due.

Stopping the drug
If you have been taking the drug continuously for less than 2 weeks, it can be safely stopped as soon as you feel you no longer need it. However, if you have been taking the drug for longer, consult your physician who may supervise a gradual reduction in dosage. Stopping abruptly may lead to *withdrawal symptoms*.

Exceeding the dose
An occasional unintentional extra dose is unlikely to cause problems. Large overdoses may cause unusual drowsiness. Notify your physician.

SPECIAL PRECAUTIONS

Be sure to tell your physician if:
▼ You have severe respiratory disease.
▼ You have long-term liver or kidney problems.
▼ You have had problems with alcohol or drug abuse.
▼ You have myasthenia gravis.
▼ You are taking other medications.

Pregnancy
▼ Safety in pregnancy not established. Discuss with your physician.

Breast feeding
▼ The drug passes into the breast milk and may affect the baby. Discuss with your physician.

Infants and children
▼ Dose according to weight and response (seizures).

Over 60
▼ Increased likelihood of adverse effects. Reduced dose may therefore be necessary.

Driving and hazardous work
▼ Avoid such activities until you have learned how the drug affects you because the drug can cause reduced alertness and slowed reactions (even the following day).

Alcohol
▼ Avoid. Alcohol may increase the sedative effects of this drug.

POSSIBLE ADVERSE EFFECTS

The principal adverse effects of this drug are related to its sedative and tranquilizing properties. These effects normally diminish after the first few days of treatment.

Symptom/effect	Frequency		Discuss with physician		Stop taking drug now	Call physician now
	Common	Rare	Only if severe	In all cases		
Daytime drowsiness	●		■			
Dizziness/unsteadiness	●			■		
Forgetfulness/confusion	●			■		
Headache		●		■		
Blurred vision		●		■		
Rash		●		■		▲

INTERACTIONS

Sedatives All drugs that have a sedative effect on the central nervous system are likely to increase the sedative effects of nitrazepam.

PROLONGED USE

Regular use of this drug over several weeks can lead to a reduction in its effect as the body adapts. It may also be habit-forming when taken for extended periods, especially if larger-than-average doses are taken.

NITROFURANTOIN

and names Macrodantin, Apo-Nitrofurantoin, Macrobid
ed in the following combined preparations None

GENERAL INFORMATION

rofurantoin is a fast-acting antibiotic scribed to treat urinary tract ctions such as cystitis. The drug ches high levels in the urinary tract, ere the bacteria are concentrated. Unfortunately, nitrofurantoin produces erse effects in about 10 per cent of ople taking it, the most common of ch are nausea, vomiting, and rhea. These can be alleviated to

some extent if the drug is taken with food or if the macrocrystalline form of the drug is prescribed. Nitrofurantoin occasionally causes inflammation of the lungs and/or nervous system; it may also affect liver function, leading to jaundice. Serious adverse effects are much more likely in people with reduced kidney function, causing drug levels to build up in the body.

INFORMATION FOR USERS

r drug prescription is tailored for you.
not alter dosage without checking
your physician.

v taken

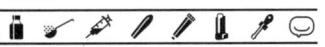

ets, capsules.

quency and timing of doses
x daily with food or milk.

age range
ts 200 – 400mg daily.
ren Reduced dose according to age and ht.

et of effect
hours.

ation of action
2 hours.

Diet advice
None.

Storage
Keep in a closed container in a cool, dry place away from reach of children. Protect from light.

Missed dose
Take as soon as you remember. If it is almost time for your next dose, space the missed dose and the next dose 2 to 4 hours apart.

Stopping the drug
Take the full course. Even if you feel better, the original infection may still be present, and symptoms may recur if treatment is stopped too soon.

Exceeding the dose
An occasional unintentional extra dose is unlikely to be a cause for concern. But if you notice unusual symptoms, or if a large overdose has been taken, notify your physician.

SPECIAL PRECAUTIONS

Be sure to tell your physician if:
▼ You have impaired liver or kidney function.
▼ You have diabetes.
▼ You have anemia.
▼ You have a lung disorder.
▼ You have glucose-6-phosphate dehydrogenase (G6PD) deficiency.
▼ You are taking other medications.

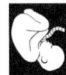
Pregnancy
▼ While there is no evidence of risk to the developing baby, absolute safety in pregnancy has not been established. Avoid at term. Discuss with your physician.

Breast feeding
▼ The drug passes into the breast milk and may cause anemia in G6PD-deficient infants. Discuss with your physician.

Infants and children
▼ The drug should not be used in infants under 1 month of age. Reduced dose necessary in infants and older children.

Over 60
▼ No special problems.

Driving and hazardous work
▼ Avoid such activities until you have learned how the drug affects you; it can cause dizziness and drowsiness.

Alcohol
▼ No known problems.

OSSIBLE ADVERSE EFFECTS

furantoin has a number of serious rse effects that may make it necessary op taking the drug. The more common

adverse effects, such as loss of appetite, nausea, and vomiting, tend to diminish as your body adjusts to the drug.

ptom/effect	Frequency		Discuss with physician		Stop taking drug now	Call physician now
	Common	Rare	Only if severe	In all cases		
of appetite	●		■			
sea/vomiting	●		■			
nea	●		■			
ache/dizziness	●		■			
dice		●		■	▲	
b/tingling face		●		■	▲	
plained fever		●		■	▲	
ness of breath		●		■	▲	■

INTERACTIONS

benecid, sulfinpyrazone These drugs y increase the risk of adverse effects en taken in conjunction with ofurantoin.

tacids may decrease the effects of ofurantoin.

Nalidixic acid Nitrofurantoin interferes with the therapeutic effects of nalidixic acid; the two drugs should not be used together.

PROLONGED USE

If nitrofurantoin is prescribed for long periods, close monitoring by your physician is necessary to detect possible changes in the lungs.

NITROGLYCERIN

Brand names Nitro-Dur, Nitrogard-SR, Nitrol, Nitrolingual, Nitrong SR, Nitrostat, Transderm-Nitro, Tridil
Used in the following combined preparations None

GENERAL INFORMATION

Introduced in the late 1800s, nitroglycerin is one of the oldest drugs in continual use. It belongs to a group of vasodilator drugs called nitrates, which are used to relieve the pain of angina attacks. Nitroglycerin is not a cure for heart disease; it can only relieve symptoms, and it may have to be taken for long periods of time. Vasodilator drugs are sometimes used to lower blood pressure during surgery and in treatment for heart failure.

Nitroglycerin acts very quickly but for a short time only. It may cause a variety of minor symptoms, such as flushing and headache, most of which can be controlled by adjusting the dosage. Nitroglycerin is best taken for the first time while you are sitting. Fainting may follow the drop in blood pressure.

INFORMATION FOR USERS

Follow instructions on the label. Call your physician if symptoms worsen.

How taken

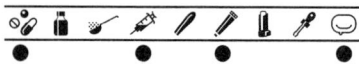

Tablets, injection, ointment, transdermal patch, sublingual spray.

Frequency and timing of doses
Prevention of angina attacks 3 x daily (tablets); every 3 – 8 hours (ointment); 12 – 14 hours/day (patch).
Relief of angina attacks Use spray, buccal or sublingual tablets at the onset of attack or immediately prior to exercise. Dose of sublingual tablets or spray may be repeated within 5 minutes if further relief is required.

Adult dosage range
0.3 – 0.6mg per dose, up to 10mg daily (sublingual tablets); 1 – 5mg per dose, up to 10mg daily (buccal tablets); 7.8 – 15.6mg daily (slow-release tablets); 2.5 – 5cm of 2 per cent ointment per dose, up to 12.5cm daily (ointment); 0.4 – 0.8mg per dose, up to 1.2mg daily (spray); 0.2 – 0.8mg per dose once daily (patch).

Onset of effect
1 – 2 minutes (sublingual/buccal); 2 – 4 minutes (spray); 15 minutes (ointment). Within 2 hours (patch).

Duration of action
30 – 60 minutes (sublingual tablets and spray); 3 – 8 hours (ointment); 5 hours (buccal tablets); 8 hours (slow-release tablets); 12–14 hours (patch).

Diet advice
None.

Storage
Keep sublingual tablets in a tightly closed container fitted with a metal screw-on cap in a cool, dry place away from reach of children. Protect from light. Do not expose to heat. Discard within 8 weeks of opening. Check labels of other preparations for storage conditions.

Missed dose
Take as soon as you remember, or when needed. It your next dose is due within 2 hours, take a single dose now and skip the next.

Stopping the drug
Do not stop taking the drug without consulting your physician.

Exceeding the dose
An occasional unintentional extra dose is unlikely to cause problems. Larger overdoses may cause dizziness, vomiting, severe headache, seizures, or loss of consciousness. Notify your physician.

SPECIAL PRECAUTIONS

Be sure to consult your physician or pharmacist before taking this drug if:
▼ You have any blood disorders or anemia.
▼ You have had glaucoma.
▼ You have thyroid disease.
▼ You are taking other medications.

Pregnancy
▼ Safety in pregnancy not established. Discuss with your physician.

Breast feeding
▼ Effects on breast milk are uncertain. Discuss with your physician.

Infants and children
▼ Not usually prescribed.

Over 60
▼ No special problems.

Driving and hazardous work
▼ Avoid such activities until you have learned how the drug affect you; it can cause dizziness.

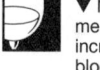

Alcohol
▼ Never drink while under treatment with nitroglycerin. Alcohol increase dizziness due to lowere blood pressure.

PROLONGED USE

The effects of the drug usually become slightly weaker during prolonged use as the body adapts.

Monitoring Periodic checks on blood pressure are usually required.

POSSIBLE ADVERSE EFFECTS

The most serious adverse effect is lowered blood pressure, and this should be monitored periodically. Other adverse effects usually disappear after regular use, and they can also be controlled by an adjustment in dosage.

Symptom/effect	Frequency		Discuss with physician		Stop taking drug now	Call physician now
	Common	Rare	Only if severe	In all cases		
Headache	●		■			
Flushing	●		■			
Dizziness	●			■		

INTERACTIONS

Antihypertensive drugs These drugs increase the possibility of lowered blood pressure or fainting when taken with nitroglycerin.

Sympathomimetics Because of their effect in speeding up the heart rate, these drugs reduce the effect of nitroglycerin.

NIZATIDINE

...and name Axid
...sed in the following combined preparations None

GENERAL INFORMATION

...zatidine, an anti-ulcer drug introduced ...1988, is used in the prevention and ...atment of stomach and duodenal ...cers. It acts by reducing the amount of ...id produced by the stomach, allowing ...e ulcers time to heal.

...Nizatidine is also used in reflux ...ophagitis, a condition that may cause ...d stomach contents to flow partway ...the esophagus.

...Unlike some other similar anti-ulcer ...ugs, this drug does not affect the ...tions of certain enzymes in the liver, ...ere many drugs are broken down ...fore being absorbed into the body.

This means that nizatidine can be taken with other drugs, like anticoagulants and anticonvulsants, without causing an interaction that may reduce the effectiveness of either treatment.

Most people do not experience any serious effects during a course of treatment with nizatidine. As nizatidine promotes healing of the stomach lining, there is a risk that it may mask stomach cancer, delaying diagnosis. It is therefore usually prescribed only when the possibility of stomach cancer has been carefully considered.

...NFORMATION FOR USERS

...ur drug prescription is tailored for you.
...not alter dosage without checking
...h your physician.

...w taken

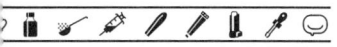

...sules.

...quency and timing of doses
...2 x daily.

...lt dosage range
...– 300mg daily.

...set of effect
...in 1 hour.

...ation of action
...ours.

Diet advice
None.

Storage
Keep in a closed container in a cool, dry place away from reach of children.

Missed dose
Do not take the missed dose. Take your next dose as usual.

Stopping the drug
Do not stop taking the drug without consulting your physician; symptoms may recur.

Exceeding the dose
An occasional unintentional extra dose is unlikely to be a cause for concern. But if you notice unusual symptoms, or if a large over-dose has been taken, notify your physician.

...OSSIBLE ADVERSE EFFECTS

...adverse effects of nizatidine, of which ...wsiness is the most common, are usually related to dosage level and almost always disappear when treatment finishes.

...ptom/effect	Frequency		Discuss with physician		Stop taking drug now	Call physician now
	Common	Rare	Only if severe	In all cases		
...wsiness	●		■			
...ating		●	■			
...w/hives		●		■	▲	
...dice		●	■		▲	▮
...st enlargement (men)		●	■			

...TERACTIONS

...ne.

SPECIAL PRECAUTIONS

Be sure to tell your physician if:
▼ You have impaired liver or kidney function.
▼ You are taking other medications.

Pregnancy
▼ Safety in pregnancy not established. Discuss with your physician.

Breast feeding
▼ The drug passes into the breast milk, but at normal doses adverse effects on the baby are unlikely. Discuss with your physician.

Infants and children
▼ Safety not established.

Over 60
▼ No special problems unless kidney function is reduced, in which case dosage is decreased.

Driving and hazardous work
▼ Avoid such activities until you have learned how the drug affects you; it can cause drowsiness.

Alcohol
▼ Avoid. Alcohol may aggravate the underlying condition and counter the beneficial effects of nizatidine.

PROLONGED USE

Courses of longer than 12 months are not usually necessary.

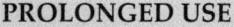

NORFLOXACIN

Brand names Noroxin, Noroxin Ophthalmic
Used in the following combined preparations None

GENERAL INFORMATION

Norfloxacin, a quinolone antibiotic, is effective against several types of bacteria that tend to be resistant to older, more commonly used antibiotics. It is particularly effective against bacteria responsible for urinary tract infections, and it is for this purpose that norfloxacin is usually prescribed. It is also used to treat uncomplicated gonorrhea. The eye drops are used to treat acute superficial eye infections.

Norfloxacin is generally well tolerated, but occasional *side effects* occur, the most common of which involves gastrointestinal upset. Allergic reactions may also occur, and those with a history of allergies to quinolone antibiotics are not usually given this drug. Headache, dizziness, and drowsiness sometimes occur. Seizures are a rare possibility.

INFORMATION FOR USERS

Your drug prescription is tailored for you. Do not alter dosage without checking with your physician.

How taken

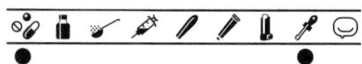

Tablets, eye drops.

Frequency and timing of doses
1 – 2 x daily at least 1 hour before or 2 hours after meals (tablets); 4 x daily (eye drops).

Adult dosage range
800mg daily for 7 – 10 days (acute infections); doses of 400mg daily are used for longer courses of treatment if kidney function is impaired; 800mg as a single dose (gonorrhea).

Onset of effect
1 – 2 days.

Duration of action
12 – 24 hours.

Diet advice
Do not get dehydrated. Ensure that you drink fluids regularly.

Storage
Keep in a closed container in a cool, dry place away from reach of children.

Missed dose
Take as soon as you remember. If your next dose is due within 4 hours, take a single dose now and skip the next.

Stopping the drug
Take full course. Even if you feel better, the infection may still be present and symptoms may recur if treatment is stopped too soon.

Exceeding the dose
An occasional unintentional extra dose is unlikely to cause problems. If a large overdose has been taken, or if you notice unusual symptoms, notify your physician.

SPECIAL PRECAUTIONS

Be sure to tell your physician if:
▼ You have impaired kidney function.
▼ You have had epileptic seizures.
▼ You are allergic to quinolone antibiotics.
▼ You are taking other medications.

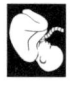
Pregnancy
▼ Safety in pregnancy not established. Discuss with your physician.

Breast feeding
▼ The drug passes into the breast milk and may affect the baby. Discuss with your physician.

Infants and children
▼ Not recommended.

Over 60
▼ Reduced dose may be necessary.

Driving and hazardous work
▼ Avoid such activities until you have learned how the drug affects you; it can cause dizziness, drowsiness, and blurred vision.

Alcohol
▼ Avoid. Alcohol may increase the sedative effects of this drug.

POSSIBLE ADVERSE EFFECTS

The most common side effects with norfloxacin tablets are nausea, headache, dizziness, and lightheadedness. It can also cause fatigue, rash, and drowsiness.

Symptom/effect	Frequency		Discuss with physician		Stop taking drug now	Call physician now
	Common	Rare	Only if severe	In all cases		
Nausea/vomiting	●		■			
Dizziness/lightheadedness	●		■			
Headache		●	■			
Drowsiness/fatigue		●	■			
Rash/itching		●		■		
Light-sensitive rash		●		■		
Burning of the eyes (drops)	●		■			

INTERACTIONS

Oral anticoagulants Norfloxacin may increase the anticoagulant action of these drugs.

Theophylline Norfloxacin may increase the adverse effects with theophylline.

Cyclosporine Norfloxacin may increase the blood levels of cyclosporine.

Caffeine Norfloxacin may increase the effects of caffeine: avoid excessive intake.

Antacids, iron, sucralfate These drugs decrease the absorption of norfloxacin. Avoid taking these within 2 hours of each other.

PROLONGED USE

No problems expected.

NORTRIPTYLINE

Brand name Aventyl
Used in the following combined preparations None

GENERAL INFORMATION

Nortriptyline belongs to a class of antidepressant drugs known as the tricyclics. It is mainly used in the long-term treatment of depression. It elevates mood, increases physical activity, improves appetite, and restores interest in everyday activities.

It is also used in the treatment of post-stroke depression and depression associated with Parkinson's disease. Nortriptyline is less likely to cause dizziness than some of the other tricyclics.

In overdose, nortriptyline may cause coma, seizures, and dangerously abnormal heart rhythms, but in normal use serious *side effects* are rare.

INFORMATION FOR USERS

Your drug prescription is tailored for you. Do not alter dosage without checking with your physician.

How taken

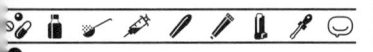

Capsules.

Frequency and timing of doses
Single dose at bedtime or 3 - 4 x daily.

Dosage range
Adults 30 – 100mg daily.
Children Reduced dosage according to age and weight.

Onset of effect
Some benefits and effects may appear within hours, but full antidepressant effect may not be felt for 2 – 6 weeks.

Duration of action
Following prolonged treatment antidepressant effect may persist for up to 6 weeks. Adverse effects wear off within a few days.

Diet advice
None.

Storage
Keep in a closed container in a cool, dry place away from reach of children.

Missed dose
If taken once at bedtime, take next dose as usual. If taken 3 – 4 x daily and your next dose is due within 3 hours, take a single dose now and skip the next; otherwise take as soon as you remember.

Stopping the drug
Do not stop the drug without consulting your physician.

OVERDOSE ACTION

 Seek immediate medical advice in all cases. Take emergency action if consciousness is lost.

See Drug poisoning emergency guide (p.574).

SPECIAL PRECAUTIONS

Be sure to tell your physician if:
▼ You have heart problems.
▼ You have a thyroid disorder.
▼ You have had epileptic seizures.
▼ You have impaired liver or kidney function.
▼ You have had glaucoma.
▼ You have urinary difficulties.
▼ You are taking other medications.

 **Pregnancy**
▼ Safety in pregnancy not established. Discuss with your physician.

 Breast feeding
▼ The drug passes into the breast milk and may affect the baby. Discuss with your physician.

 Infants and children
▼ Not recommended under 12 years. Reduced dose necessary in older children.

 Over 60
▼ Increased likelihood of adverse effects. Reduced dose may therefore be necessary.

 Driving and hazardous work
▼ Avoid such activities until you have learned how the drug affects you; it can cause blurred vision and drowsiness.

 Alcohol
▼ Avoid. Alcohol may increase the sedative effects of this drug.

Surgery and general anesthetics
▼ Nortriptyline treatment may need to be stopped before you have a general anes-thetic. Discuss this with your physician or dentist before any operation.

POSSIBLE ADVERSE EFFECTS

The possible adverse effects of this drug are mainly the result of its *anticholinergic* action and its blocking action on the transmission of signals in the heart.

Symptom/effect	Frequency		Discuss with physician		Stop taking drug now	Call physician now
	Common	Rare	Only if severe	In all cases		
Drowsiness	●		■			
Constipation	●		■			
Dry mouth	●		■			
Blurred vision	●			■		
Dizziness/fainting	●			■		
Rash		●		■	▲	
Difficulty passing urine		●		■	▲	
Palpitations		●		■	▲	■

INTERACTIONS

Sedatives All drugs, including alcohol, that have a sedative effect on the central nervous system are likely to increase the sedative properties of nortriptyline.

Antihypertensive drugs Nortriptyline may reduce the effectiveness of some of these drugs.

Monoamine oxidase inhibitors (MAOIs)
Usually, nortriptyline should not be given during or within 14 days of treatment with an MAOI. Serious reactions may occur. Such drugs are prescribed together only under strict medical supervision.

PROLONGED USE

No problems expected.

Monitoring Periodic blood tests may be performed.

NYSTATIN

Brand names Mycostatin, Nadostine, Nilstat, Nyaderm
Used in the following combined preparations Flagystatin, Kenacomb, Lidecomb, Viaderm K.C.

GENERAL INFORMATION

Introduced in 1955, the antifungal drug nystatin was named after the New York State Institute of Health, where it was developed. It is effective against candidiasis (thrush), an infection caused by the Candida yeast. Available in a variety of dosage forms, it is used to treat infections of the skin, mouth, throat, esophagus, and vagina.

Poorly absorbed from the digestive tract into the bloodstream, it is of little use against *systemic* infections. It is not given by injection.

Resistance to nystatin is uncommon. It rarely causes adverse effects and has been used during pregnancy to treat vaginal candidiasis.

QUICK REFERENCE

Drug group Antifungal drug (p.150)

Overdose danger rating Low

Dependence rating Low

Prescription needed Only for vaginal and oral products

Multi-source suppliers Yes

INFORMATION FOR USERS

Your drug prescription is tailored for you. Do not alter dosage without checking with your physician.

How taken

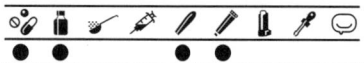

Tablets, oral suspension, topical powder, vaginal tablets, topical cream, topical ointment, vaginal cream.

Frequency and timing of doses
Mouth or throat infections 4 x daily. Liquid should be held in the mouth for several minutes before swallowing.
Skin infections 2 – 4 x daily.
Vaginal infections 1 – 2 x daily for 2 or more weeks.

Adult dosage range
1.5 million – 3 million units daily (oral); 100,000 – 200,000 units daily (vaginal tablets); 1 – 2 applicatorfuls (vaginal cream); as directed (skin preparations).

Onset of effect
1 – 3 days. Full beneficial effect may not be felt for 7 – 14 days.

Duration of action
Up to 6 hours.

Diet advice
None.

Storage
Keep in a closed container in a cool, dry place away from reach of children. Protect from light.

Missed dose
Take as soon as you remember. Take your next dose as usual.

Stopping the drug
Take the full course. Even if the affected area seems to be cured, the original infection may still be present, and symptoms may recur if treatment is stopped too soon.

Exceeding the dose
An occasional unintentional extra dose is unlikely to be a cause for concern. But if you notice unusual symptoms, or if a large overdose has been taken, notify your physician.

SPECIAL PRECAUTIONS

Be sure to tell your physician if:
▼ You have had a previous allergic reaction to nystatin.
▼ You are taking other medications.

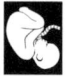

Pregnancy
▼ No evidence of risk to developing baby. Use of vaginal applicator may not be considered desirable during pregnancy. Consult your physician.

Breast feeding
▼ No evidence of risk.

Infants and children
▼ Reduced dose necessary.

Over 60
▼ No special problems.

Driving and hazardous work
▼ No known problems.

Alcohol
▼ No known problems.

POSSIBLE ADVERSE EFFECTS

Adverse effects are uncommon, and are usually mild and transient. Nausea, vomiting, and abdominal pain may occur with high doses of nystatin taken by mouth.

Symptom/effect	Frequency		Discuss with physician		Stop taking drug now	Call physician now
	Common	Rare	Only if severe	In all cases		
Diarrhea	●		■			
Nausea/vomiting	●		■			
Abdominal pain	●		■			
Local irritation	●			■	▲	∎

PROLONGED USE

No problems expected.

INTERACTIONS

None.

OMEPRAZOLE

Brand name Losec
Used in the following combined preparations None

GENERAL INFORMATION

Omeprazole is an anti-ulcer drug which was introduced in 1989. It is used mainly to treat stomach and duodenal ulcers that have not responded to other treatment. It reduces (by about 70 per cent) the amount of acid produced by the stomach and works in a different way from other anti-ulcer drugs which reduce acid secretion. Omeprazole is very effective for treating pain and inflammation caused by reflux esophagitis.

Treatment is usually given for 4 to 8 weeks, depending on where the ulcer is situated. The drug is not used long term to prevent ulcers developing.

Most people do not have serious *side effects* with omeprazole. However, it may affect the actions of enzymes in the liver, where many drugs are broken down, so treatment should be monitored if it is used with phenytoin or warfarin. As with other anti-ulcer drugs, it may mask signs of stomach cancer, so it is used only when the possibility of this disease has been carefully considered.

QUICK REFERENCE

Drug group Anti-ulcer drug (p.121)
Overdose danger rating Low
Dependence rating Low
Prescription needed Yes
Multi-source suppliers No

INFORMATION FOR USERS

Your drug prescription is tailored for you. Do not alter dosage without checking with your physician.

How taken

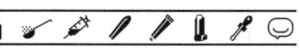

Capsules.

Frequency and timing of doses
Once daily.

Adult dosage range
20 – 40mg daily and sometimes up to 120mg daily.

Onset of effect
2 – 5 hours.

Duration of action
24 hours.

Diet advice
None.

Storage
Keep in the original closed container in a cool, dry place away from reach of children. Omeprazole is very sensitive to moisture. It must not be transferred to another container.

Missed dose
Take as soon as you remember. If your next dose is due within 8 hours, take a single dose now, and skip the next.

Stopping the drug
Do not stop the drug without consulting your physician. Symptoms may recur.

Exceeding the dose
An occasional unintentional extra dose is unlikely to be a cause for concern. But if you notice unusual symptoms or if a large over-dose has been taken, notify your physician.

SPECIAL PRECAUTIONS

Be sure to tell your physician if:
▼ You have impaired kidney or liver function.
▼ You are taking other medications.

Pregnancy
▼ Safety in pregnancy not established. Discuss with your physician.

Breast feeding
▼ Safety of breast feeding not established. Discuss with your physician.

Infants and children
▼ Not recommended.

Over 60
▼ Increased likelihood of adverse effects. The daily dose should not exceed 20mg.

Driving and hazardous work
▼ No special problems.

Alcohol
▼ Avoid. Alcohol may aggravate your underlying condition and reduce the beneficial effects of this drug.

POSSIBLE ADVERSE EFFECTS

Adverse effects are usually mild, and often diminish with continued use of the drug.

Symptom/effect	Frequency		Discuss with physician		Stop taking drug now	Call physician now
	Common	Rare	Only if severe	In all cases		
Nausea	●			■		
Headache	●			■		
Diarrhea	●			■		
Constipation		●		■		
Rash		●			■	

PROLONGED USE

Courses of longer than 8 weeks are not usually prescribed for anti-ulcer therapy.

INTERACTIONS

Warfarin The effects of warfarin may be increased by omeprazole.

Phenytoin The effects of phenytoin may be increased by omeprazole.

Cyclosporine Blood levels of cyclosporine are raised by omeprazole.

Diazepam The effects of diazepam may be increased by omeprazole.

ONDANSETRON

Brand name Zofran
Used in the following combined preparations None

GENERAL INFORMATION

Ondansetron is an anti-emetic particularly useful for treating nausea and vomiting associated with anti-cancer drugs, such as cisplatin, and radiotherapy. It may also be used for nausea and vomiting that occur after an operation.

The dose given and the frequency will depend on the anti-cancer drug prescribed and the dose of that drug.

Generally, a dose of ondansetron will be given either by mouth or by injection before infusion of the anti-cancer agent and then tablets for up to five days after the treatment has finished.

Sometimes, other drugs, such as dexamethasone, are taken with ondansetron as this can enhance its effectiveness. Serious adverse effects are unlikely to occur.

QUICK REFERENCE

Drug group Anti-emetic (p.102)
Overdose danger rating Low
Dependence rating Low
Prescription needed Yes
Multi-source suppliers No

INFORMATION FOR USERS

Your drug prescription is tailored for you. Do not alter dosage without checking with your physician.

How taken

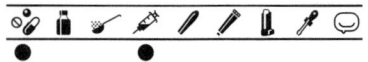

Tablets, injection.

Frequency and timing of doses
Normally 2 x daily but the frequency will depend on the reason for which it is being used.

Adult dosage range
8 – 32mg daily depending on the reason for which it is being used.

Onset of effect
Within 1 hour.

Duration of action
Approximately 12 hours.

Diet advice
None.

Storage
Keep in a closed container in a cool, dry place away from reach of children. Protect from light.

Missed dose
If you miss a dose and do not feel sick, take the next dose when it is due. If you forget to take your medicine and feel sick or vomit, take a tablet as soon as possible.

Stopping the drug
Can be safely stopped as soon as you no longer need it.

Exceeding the dose
An occasional unintentional extra dose is unlikely to be a cause for concern. But if you notice unusual symptoms, or if a large overdose has been taken, notify your physician.

POSSIBLE ADVERSE EFFECTS

Ondansetron is generally well tolerated. It is less likely to cause sedation and movement disorders than some other anti-emetics.

Symptom/effect	Frequency		Discuss with physician		Stop taking drug now	Call physician now
	Common	Rare	Only if severe	In all cases		
Constipation	●		■			
Headache	●		■			
Warm feeling in head/stomach		●	■			

INTERACTIONS

None.

SPECIAL PRECAUTIONS

Be sure to tell your physician if:
▼ You have impaired liver function.
▼ You are taking other medications.

Pregnancy
▼ Safety in pregnancy not established. Discuss with your physician.

Breast feeding
▼ The drug may pass into the breast milk. Discuss with your physician.

Infants and children
▼ Reduced dose necessary.

Over 60
▼ No special problems.

Driving and hazardous work
▼ No problems expected.

Alcohol
▼ No known problems.

PROLONGED USE

Not generally prescribed for long-term treatment.

ORCIPRENALINE

Brand name Alupent
Used in the following combined preparations None

GENERAL INFORMATION

Orciprenaline is a *sympathomimetic bronchodilator* that acts selectively to dilate the airways in the lungs while having little stimulant effect on the heart.

Used in the prevention and treatment of attacks of bronchospasm occurring in asthma, bronchitis, and emphysema, it is generally given by inhalation, and sometimes by mouth.

Anxiety and restlessness may occur, as with all other sympathomimetics. Fine tremor of the hands is common, although it may be controlled by reducing the dose. Heart palpitations as well as tolerance to its beneficial effects occur less often with orciprenaline than with similar drugs.

QUICK REFERENCE

Drug group Bronchodilator (p.104)
Overdose danger rating Low
Dependence rating Low
Prescription needed Yes
Multi-source suppliers No

INFORMATION FOR USERS

Your drug prescription is tailored for you. Do not alter dosage without checking with your physician.

How taken

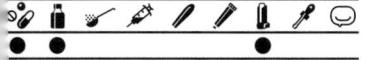

Tablets, oral liquid, inhaler, solution for inhalation.

Frequency and timing of doses
3 – 4 x daily (tablets, liquid); every 4 – 6 hours (inhaler, solution for inhalation).

Adult dosage range
30 – 80mg daily (tablets, liquid); 1.5mg (2 puffs) per dose (inhaler); according to instructions depending on preparation and equipment (solution for inhalation).

Onset of effect
Within 15 minutes (inhaler, solution for inhalation); within 30 minutes (tablets, liquid).

Duration of action
3 – 6 hours.

Diet advice
None.

Storage
Keep in a closed container in a cool, dry place away from reach of children. Protect from light. Do not puncture or burn aerosol container.

Missed dose
Do not take the missed dose. Take your next dose as usual.

Stopping the drug
People with mild or infrequent attacks should take orciprenaline as needed. If you have severe asthma, do not stop your treatment without consulting your physician.

Exceeding the dose
An occasional unintentional extra dose is unlikely to be a cause for concern. But if you notice any unusual symptoms or if a large overdose has been taken, notify your physician.

POSSIBLE ADVERSE EFFECTS

Muscle tremor, anxiety, and restlessness are the most common adverse effects.

Palpitations and headache due to stimulation of the heart are rare.

Symptom/effect	Frequency		Discuss with physician		Stop taking drug now	Call physician now
	Common	Rare	Only if severe	In all cases		
Nausea	●			■		
Tremor	●			■		
Anxiety/restlessness	●			■		
Headache		●		■		
Bad taste in mouth		●		■		
Palpitations		●			■	

INTERACTIONS

Beta blockers should not be used by asthmatics.

Other sympathomimetic drugs, such as those listed on page 104, may increase the effect of orciprenaline, thus increasing the risks of adverse effects.

Monoamine oxidase inhibitors (MAOIs) can interact with orciprenaline to produce a dangerous rise in blood pressure.

SPECIAL PRECAUTIONS

Be sure to tell your physician if:
▼ You have heart problems.
▼ You have high blood pressure.
▼ You have an overactive thyroid.
▼ You have glaucoma.
▼ You have urinary difficulties.
▼ You have diabetes.
▼ You are taking other medications.

Pregnancy
▼ Safety in pregnancy not established. Discuss with your physician.

Breast feeding
▼ Effect of breast feeding unknown. Discuss with your physician.

Infants and children
▼ Not usually prescribed for inhalation for children under 12 years. Reduced oral dose necessary.

Over 60
▼ Increased likelihood of adverse effects. Reduced dose may therefore be necessary.

Driving and hazardous work
▼ Avoid such activities until you have learned how the drug affects you; it can cause trembling.

Alcohol
▼ No special problems.

PROLONGED USE

Prolonged use may result in tolerance to the effects of orciprenaline. However, failure to respond can also be a sign of worsening asthma, requiring urgent medical treatment.

ORPHENADRINE

Brand names Disipal, Norflex
Used in the following combined preparations Norgesic, Norgesic Forte

GENERAL INFORMATION

Orphenadrine hydrochloride, an *anticholinergic* drug related chemically to the *antihistamines*, is used to reduce the muscle rigidity that often occurs in Parkinson's disease. However, it has little effect on the slowing of movement or tremor that are also prominent features of this condition.

Orphenadrine citrate possesses muscle-relaxant properties. It produces this effect by blocking nerve pathways responsible for muscle rigidity and spasm. It is sometimes used as an adjunct to rest, physical therapy, and other measures for the relief of painful muscle spasm associated with sprains and strains.

INFORMATION FOR USERS

Follow instructions on the label. Call your physician if symptoms worsen.

How taken

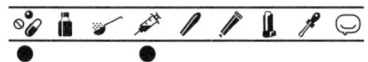

Tablets, slow-release tablets, injection.

Frequency and timing of doses
2 – 3 x daily.

Adult dosage range
150 – 200mg daily.

Onset of effect
Within 60 minutes (tablets); within 5 minutes (injection).

Duration of action
12 hours (orphenadrine citrate); 8 hours (orphenadrine hydrochloride).

Diet advice
None.

Storage
Keep in a closed container in a cool, dry place away from reach of children. Protect from light.

Missed dose
Take as soon as you remember. If your next dose is due within 2 hours take a single dose now and skip the next.

Stopping the drug
Do not stop the drug without consulting your physician; symptoms may recur.

OVERDOSE ACTION

 Seek immediate medical advice in all cases. Take emergency action if palpitations, seizures, or loss of consciousness occurs.

See Drug poisoning emergency guide (p.574).

SPECIAL PRECAUTIONS

Be sure to consult your physician or pharmacist before taking this drug if:
▼ You have impaired kidney or liver function.
▼ You have heart problems.
▼ You have had glaucoma.
▼ You have difficulty passing urine.
▼ You have had peptic ulcers.
▼ You have myasthenia gravis.
▼ You are taking other medications.

 Pregnancy
▼ Safety in pregnancy not established. Discuss with your physician.

 Breast feeding
▼ It is not known whether the drug passes into the breast milk. Discuss with your physician.

 Infants and children
▼ Not recommended.

 Over 60
▼ Increased likelihood of adverse effects. Reduced dose may therefore be necessary.

 Driving and hazardous work
▼ Avoid such activities until you have learned how the drug affects you; it can cause dizziness and lightheadedness.

 Alcohol
▼ Avoid. Alcohol may increase the sedative effects of this drug.

Surgery and general anesthetics
▼ Orphenadrine may need to be stopped before you have a general anesthetic. Discuss this with your physician or dentist before any surgery.

POSSIBLE ADVERSE EFFECTS

The adverse effects of orphenadrine are similar to those of other anticholinergic drugs. The more common symptoms, such as dryness of the mouth and blurred vision, can often be overcome by an adjustment in dosage.

Symptom/effect	Frequency		Discuss with physician		Stop taking drug now	Call physician now
	Common	Rare	Only if severe	In all cases		
Dry mouth/skin	●		■			
Difficulty passing urine	●		■			
Constipation	●		■			
Dizziness	●		■			
Blurred vision	●			■		
Confusion/agitation		●		■		
Rash/itching		●		■	▲	
Palpitations		●		■	▲	■

INTERACTIONS

Anticholinergic drugs The anticholinergic effects of orphenadrine are likely to be increased by these drugs.

Propoxyphene Confusion, anxiety, and tremors may occur if this drug is given together with orphenadrine.

Sedatives The effects of all drugs, including alcohol, that have a sedative effect on the central nervous system are likely to be increased with orphenadrine.

PROLONGED USE

No problems expected. Effectiveness in treating Parkinson's disease may diminish with time.

OXAZEPAM

Brand names Serax, Apo-Oxazepam, Novo-Oxapam, Oxpam
Used in the following combined preparations None

GENERAL INFORMATION

Oxazepam belongs to a group of drugs known as the benzodiazepines. These drugs help to relieve anxiety and tension, and encourage sleep. Their actions and adverse effects are described more fully on page 95.

Oxazepam is used in the short-term symptomatic relief of anxiety and insomnia, and may be of value in relieving the symptoms of acute alcohol withdrawal. Because of its relatively slow onset of effect and long duration of action, it may be more effective for treating early waking than for difficulty falling asleep. Oxazepam is less likely than similar drugs to accumulate in the body.

In common with other benzodiazepines, oxazepam can be habit-forming if taken regularly over a long period. Its effects may also become weaker with time. For these reasons, treatment with oxazepam should be limited to a few weeks and then reviewed.

QUICK REFERENCE

Drug group Benzodiazepine anti-anxiety drug (p.95)

Overdose danger rating Medium

Dependence rating Medium

Prescription needed Yes

Multi-source suppliers Yes

INFORMATION FOR USERS

Your drug prescription is tailored for you. Do not alter dosage without checking with your physician.

How taken

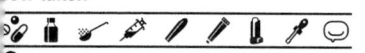

Tablets.

Frequency and timing of doses
1 – 4 x daily.

Adult dosage range
30 – 120mg daily.

Onset of effect
1 – 2 hours.

Duration of action
Up to 12 hours.

Diet advice
None.

Storage
Keep in a closed container in a cool, dry place away from reach of children.

Missed dose
If you are taking the drug once daily for insomnia, a missed dose is no cause for concern. Return to your normal dose schedule the following night, if necessary. Otherwise, take the missed dose when you remember. If your next dose is due within 2 hours, take a single dose now and skip the next.

Stopping the drug
If you have been taking the drug continuously for less than 2 weeks, it can be safely stopped as soon as you feel you no longer need it. However, if you have been taking it for longer, consult your physician, who will supervise a gradual reduction in dosage. Stopping abruptly may lead to withdrawal symptoms.

Exceeding the dose
An occasional unintentional extra dose is unlikely to cause problems. Larger overdoses may cause unusual drowsiness. Notify your physician.

SPECIAL PRECAUTIONS

Be sure to tell your physician if:
▼ You have impaired kidney function.
▼ You have had problems with alcohol or drug abuse.
▼ You have myasthenia gravis.
▼ You have glaucoma.
▼ You are taking other medications.

Pregnancy
▼ Safety in pregnancy not established. Discuss with your physician.

Breast feeding
▼ The drug passes into the breast milk and may affect the baby adversely. Discuss with your physician.

Infants and children
▼ Not prescribed under 6 years of age. Dosage uncertain for older children.

Over 60
▼ Increased likelihood of adverse effects. Reduced dose may therefore be necessary.

Driving and hazardous work
▼ Avoid such activities until you have learned how the drug affects you; it can cause reduced alertness, slowed reactions, and blurred vision.

Alcohol
▼ Avoid. Alcohol may increase the sedative effects of this drug.

POSSIBLE ADVERSE EFFECTS

The principal adverse effects of this drug are related to its sedative and tranquilizing properties. These effects normally diminish after the first few days of treatment.

Symptom/effect	Frequency		Discuss with physician		Stop taking drug now	Call physician now
	Common	Rare	Only if severe	In all cases		
Daytime drowsiness	●		■			
Dizziness/unsteadiness	●		■			
Headache		●	■			
Blurred vision		●	■			
Forgetfulness/confusion		●		■		▮
Rash		●		■	▲	▮

PROLONGED USE

Regular use of this drug over several weeks can lead to a reduction in its effect as the body adapts. It may also be habit-forming when taken for extended periods, especially if larger-than-average doses are taken.

INTERACTIONS

Sedatives All drugs, including alcohol, that have a sedative effect on the central nervous system are likely to increase the sedative properties of oxazepam. Such drugs include other anti-anxiety and sleeping drugs, antihistamines, antidepressants, narcotic analgesics, and antipsychotics.

417

OXYBUTYNIN

Brand name Ditropan
Used in the following combined preparations None

GENERAL INFORMATION

Oxybutynin is an *anticholinergic* drug that reduces spasm of the bladder muscle. It is used in conjunction with bladder training procedures, for example timed voiding, to relieve the symptoms associated with an overactive bladder such as urgency, frequency, urinary leakage, and incontinence. Improvement of symptoms is a result of increased bladder capacity, decreased nerve signals from the bladder, and diminished frequency of bladder contractions.

The most common adverse effects of oxybutynin are blurred vision and dry mouth. These are the result of the drug's anticholinergic actions.

INFORMATION FOR USERS

Your drug prescription is tailored for you. Do not alter dosage without checking with your physician.

How taken

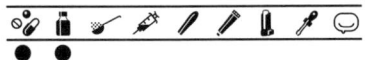

Tablets, oral liquid.

Frequency and timing of doses
2 – 4 x daily with water on an empty stomach. If stomach upset occurs, take with food or milk.

Dosage range
Adults 5 – 20mg daily.
Children over 5 years 5 – 15mg daily.

Onset of effect
Within 1 hour; maximum effect within 3 – 6 hours.

Duration of action
Up to 10 hours.

Diet advice
None.

Storage
Keep in a closed container in a cool, dry place away from reach of children.

Missed dose
Take as soon as you remember. If your next dose is due within 2 hours, take a single dose now and skip the next.

Stopping the drug
Do not stop taking the drug without consulting your physician; symptoms may recur.

Exceeding the dose
An occasional unintentional extra dose is unlikely to cause problems. Large overdoses may cause tremors, convulsions, hallucinations, and palpitations. Notify your physician.

SPECIAL PRECAUTIONS

Be sure to tell your physician if:
▼ You have impaired liver or kidney function.
▼ You have glaucoma.
▼ You have heart or blood pressure problems.
▼ You have prostate trouble.
▼ You have thyroid disease.
▼ You have reflux esophagitis, gastrointestinal blockage, or other stomach or intestinal problems.
▼ You have colitis.
▼ You have myasthenia gravis.
▼ You are taking other medications.

Pregnancy
▼ Safety in pregnancy not established. Discuss with your physician.

Breast feeding
▼ Oxybutynin may reduce milk production. Discuss with your physician.

Infants and children
▼ Rarely prescribed. Not recommended under 5 years of age.

Over 60
▼ Increased likelihood of adverse effects. Reduced dose may therefore be necessary.

Driving and hazardous work
▼ Avoid such activities until you have learned how the drug affects you; it can cause dizziness, drowsiness, or blurred vision.

Alcohol
▼ Avoid. Alcohol may increase any drowsiness caused by this drug.

POSSIBLE ADVERSE EFFECTS

Adverse effects of oxybutynin are typical of those produced by anticholinergic agents and are occasionally severe enough to require discontinuation of therapy.

Symptom/effect	Frequency		Discuss with physician		Stop taking drug now	Call physician now
	Common	Rare	Only if severe	In all cases		
Dry mouth	●		■			
Drowsiness/lethargy		●	■			
Nausea/vomiting/constipation		●	■			
Headache		●		■		
Blurred vision		●		■		
Urinary retention		●		■	▲	▮
Confusion		●		■	▲	▮

INTERACTIONS

Sedatives All drugs, including alcohol, that have a sedative effect on the central nervous system may enhance any drowsiness caused by oxybutynin.

Anticholinergic drugs The anticholinergic effects of oxybutynin are likely to be enhanced by all drugs that have anticholinergic effects, including some antihistamines, antiparkinsonian drugs, antipsychotics, and tricyclic antidepressants.

PROLONGED USE

Oxybutynin has been taken for up to 2 years without problems.

OXYCODONE

Brand name Supeudol
Used in the following combined preparations Endocet, Oxycocet, Oxycodan, Percocet, Percodan

GENERAL INFORMATION

Oxycodone is a semi-synthetic narcotic analgesic used for the treatment of pain when milder analgesics such as ASA or acetaminophen are not sufficient to maintain adequate relief. It produces sedation along with pain relief.

As with all narcotics, constipation is a common adverse effect; those on regular treatment may be advised to increase their intake of high-fiber foods.

Stimulant laxatives may sometimes be required.

Psychological and physical *dependence* may occur with long-term use, but this should not rule out the drug's use when necessary for relief of chronic pain such as that caused by cancer.

INFORMATION FOR USERS

Your drug prescription is tailored for you. Do not alter dosage without checking with your physician.

How taken

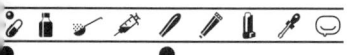

Tablets, rectal suppositories.

Frequency and timing of doses
Every 4 – 6 hours.

Dosage range
Adults 5 – 10mg per dose. Larger doses may be required in some cases.
Children Reduced dose according to age.

Onset of effect
Within 30 minutes.

Duration of action
4 - 6 hours.

Diet advice
A high-fiber diet may be advised to prevent constipation.

Storage
Keep in a closed container in a cool, dry place away from reach of children. Protect from light.

Missed dose
If you are taking the drug for chronic pain and have missed a dose, take the next dose right away and recalculate a new 4 – 6 hour regular schedule. For acute pain, take the missed dose if discomfort has returned and follow your physician's instructions thereafter.

Stopping the drug
When taken short term for acute pain, the drug can be safely stopped as soon as you no longer need it. If you have been taking the drug regularly for chronic pain, do not stop taking the drug without consulting your physician who may supervise a gradual reduction in dosage.

OVERDOSE ACTION

Seek immediate medical advice in all cases. Take emergency action if there are symptoms such as slow or irregular breathing, severe drowsiness, or loss of consciousness.

See Drug poisoning emergency guide (p.574).

SPECIAL PRECAUTIONS

Be sure to tell your physician if:
▼ You have impaired kidney or liver function.
▼ You have heart or circulatory problems.
▼ You have a lung disorder such as asthma, emphysema, or bronchitis.
▼ You have thyroid disease.
▼ You have had problems with alcohol or drug abuse.
▼ You are taking other medications.

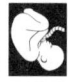

Pregnancy
▼ Not usually prescribed. Discuss with your physician.

Breast feeding
▼ Safety not established. Discuss with your physician.

Infants and children
▼ Safety not established in children under 6 years. Reduced dose necessary in older children.

Over 60
▼ Increased likelihood of adverse effects. Reduced dose may therefore be necessary.

Driving and hazardous work
▼ Avoid such activities until you have learned how the drug affects you; it can cause dizziness and drowsiness.

Alcohol
▼ Avoid. Alcohol increases the sedative effects of oxycodone.

PROLONGED USE

Tolerance to the drug's effects is likely to occur. Some degree of dependence is common with long-term use, but this should not prevent you taking the drug in order to achieve adequate pain control.

POSSIBLE ADVERSE EFFECTS

Adverse effects are more prominent in ambulatory patients. Some can be alleviated by lying down. Euphoria, unpleasant mood changes, and constipation are usual.

Symptom/effect	Frequency		Discuss with physician		Stop taking drug now	Call physician now
	Common	Rare	Only if severe	In all cases		
Nausea/vomiting	●		■			
Drowsiness	●		■			
Dizziness/lightheadedness	●		■			
Constipation	●		■			
Itching		●		■		
Rash/swelling of face		●		■	▲	■

INTERACTIONS

Sedatives All drugs, including alcohol, that have a sedative effect on the central nervous system are likely to increase sedation with oxycodone. Such drugs include antidepressants, antipsychotics, sleeping drugs, and antihistamines.

Monoamine oxidase inhibitors (MAOIs) Oxycodone may interact with these drugs to produce a dangerous rise in blood pressure.

OXYMETAZOLINE

Brand names Dristan Long Lasting Nasal Mist/Spray, Drixoral Nasal, Ocuclear
Used in the following combined preparations None

GENERAL INFORMATION

Oxymetazoline is an over-the-counter topical decongestant that relieves the symptoms of hay fever, sinusitis, and head colds. By constricting the small blood vessels in the nose, it reduces swelling and congestion in the nasal passages. Oxymetazoline eye drops act in a similar way to relieve redness caused by minor irritations.

Because oxymetazoline has a longer-lasting effect than other nasal decongestants, it needs to be taken only twice daily. However, it should not be taken for more than a few days at a time; prolonged use can lead to a rebound of nasal congestion and stuffiness.

Discomfort in the nasal passages may occur if the recommended dose is exceeded.

INFORMATION FOR USERS

Follow instructions on the label. Call your physician if symptoms worsen.

How taken

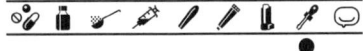

Eye drops, nasal spray.

Frequency and timing of doses
1 – 3 x daily (nasal spray); 3 – 4 x daily (eye drops).

Dosage range
Nasal spray 2 – 3 sprays in each nostril per application (adults and children over 6 years).
Eye drops 1 – 2 drops in each eye per application (adults and children over 6 years).

Onset of effect
Within 5 – 10 minutes.

Duration of action
Up to 12 hours (nasal spray); 6 hours (eye drops).

Diet advice
None.

Storage
Keep in a closed container in a cool, dry place away from reach of children. Protect from light.

Missed dose
No cause for concern. If still needed, take your next dose as usual.

Stopping the drug
Can be safely stopped as soon as you no longer need it. Seek medical advice if symptoms persist for more than a few days.

Exceeding the dose
An occasional unintentional extra dose is unlikely to cause problems. Large overdoses or accidental swallowing may cause palpitations, headache, or sleeplessness. Notify your physician.

SPECIAL PRECAUTIONS

Be sure to consult your physician or pharmacist before using this drug if:
▼ You have heart problems.
▼ You have had glaucoma.
▼ You have an eye infection or other eye disease.
▼ You have high blood pressure.
▼ You are taking other medications.

Pregnancy
▼ No evidence of risk to the developing baby when used sparingly for short periods. However, overuse can cause a rise in blood pressure that could harm the developing baby. Discuss with your physician.

Breast feeding
▼ The drug passes into the breast milk, but at normal doses adverse effects on the baby are unlikely. Discuss with your physician.

Infants and children
▼ Not recommended for use in children under 6 years.

Over 60
▼ Increased likelihood of adverse effects. Reduced dose may therefore be necessary.

Driving and hazardous work
▼ Exercise caution if dizziness or eye irritation occurs.

Alcohol
▼ No known problems.

POSSIBLE ADVERSE EFFECTS

The adverse effects of oxymetazoline nose drops or spray are milder than those of many other drugs of the same group. Eye drops rarely cause irritation, eyelid retraction, or nervous system effects.

Symptom/effect	Frequency		Discuss with physician		Stop taking drug now	Call physician now
	Common	Rare	Only if severe	In all cases		
Rebound nasal congestion	●		■			
Sneezing		●	■			
Dizziness		●		■		
Lightheadedness		●		■		
Palpitations		●		■	▲	
Headache		●		■	▲	
Sleeplessness		●		■	▲	

INTERACTIONS

Antihypertensive drugs Oxymetazoline may interact with these drugs to reverse their effect and should be used with caution by people under treatment for high blood pressure.

Monoamine oxidase inhibitors (MAOIs) may interact dangerously with oxymetazoline to raise blood pressure.

PROLONGED USE

Prolonged use of this drug may lead to worsening of the condition. Courses of longer than a few days (nasal spray) or 1 days (eye drops) are not recommended.

OXYTOCIN

Brand name Toesen
Used in the following combined preparations None

GENERAL INFORMATION

Oxytocin is a hormone secreted by the pituitary gland. It causes contraction of the uterus during labor and stimulates the flow of milk in nursing mothers. It is used to induce labor when overdue or when other medical problems make early delivery necessary. It may be given to stimulate labor when contractions are weak or absent and to help expel the placenta after birth. It is also given to expel the contents of the uterus after an incomplete miscarriage or a fetal death. Given after delivery, it makes the uterine muscles contract, thereby controlling bleeding.

Oxytocin is sometimes used to test the well-being of the fetus if the mother is at high risk because of diabetes or high blood pressure. In such cases the response of the baby's heart rate to the drug-induced contractions is monitored. If there are fetal difficulties, labor may be induced or a cesarean section performed.

Oxytocin does not actually cause troublesome *side effects* for mother or baby. However, induced labor may be more painful because the contractions are more powerful. Oxytocin dosage is carefully controlled to avoid excessively strong contractions.

QUICK REFERENCE

Drug group Uterine stimulant used in labor (p.177)

Overdose danger rating Medium

Dependence rating Low

Prescription needed Yes

Multi-source suppliers Yes

INFORMATION FOR USERS

Your drug prescription is tailored for you. Do not alter dosage without checking with your physician.

How taken

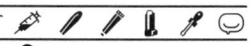

Injection.

Frequency and timing of doses
Continuously during labor.

Adult dosage range
Dosage is determined by individual response.

Onset of effect
Within 10 minutes.

Duration of action
Up to 1 hour.

Diet advice
None.

Storage
Not applicable. The drug is not kept in the home.

Missed dose
Not applicable. The drug is given only in hospital under medical supervision.

Stopping the drug
Not applicable. The drug is stopped as soon as regular strong contractions of the uterus are established.

Exceeding the dose
Overdosage is unlikely, since treatment is carefully monitored.

POSSIBLE ADVERSE EFFECTS

Oxytocin does not usually cause lasting adverse effects on mother or baby. The major effect is an increase in the strength and frequency of contractions of the uterus.

Additional pain relief may be needed. Since the drug is only given in hospital, all adverse effects are closely monitored and quickly dealt with.

Symptom/effect	Frequency		Discuss with physician		Stop taking drug now	Call physician now
	Common	Rare	Only if severe	In all cases		
Nausea/vomiting		●	■			
Painful spasm of the uterus		●		■		
Palpitations		●		■		
Seizures/coma		●		■		■

INTERACTIONS

None.

SPECIAL PRECAUTIONS

Be sure to tell your physician if:
▼ You have high blood pressure.
▼ You have heart disease.
▼ You have had a previous difficult delivery or a cesarean section.
▼ You have had an operation on the uterus.
▼ You are taking other medications.

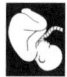

Pregnancy
▼ Not usually prescribed in early or mid-pregnancy.

Breast feeding
▼ No evidence of risk.

Infants and children
▼ Not prescribed.

Over 60
▼ Not prescribed.

Driving and hazardous work
▼ Not applicable.

Alcohol
▼ Not applicable.

PROLONGED USE

Not used for prolonged periods.

PAROXETINE

Brand name Paxil
Used in the following combined preparations None

GENERAL INFORMATION

Paroxetine belongs to a new class of antidepressants known as selective serotonin reuptake inhibitors (SSRIs). It is used in the treatment of mild to moderate depression to elevate mood, increase physical activity, and restore interest in everyday activities. It also helps to control anxiety that often accompanies depression.

Compared to the older tricyclic antidepressants, SSRIs are less likely to cause *anticholinergic side effects* such as dry mouth, blurred vision, and difficulty urinating. SSRIs are also much less dangerous in overdose.

The most common adverse effects of paroxetine include nausea, drowsiness, sweating, tremor, weakness, insomnia, and sexual dysfunction.

INFORMATION FOR USERS

Your drug prescription is tailored for you. Do not alter dosage without checking with your physician.

How taken

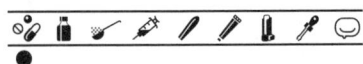

Tablets.

Frequency and timing of doses
Once daily, in the morning.

Dosage range
20 – 40mg daily.

Onset of effect
Onset of therapeutic response usually occurs within 7 – 14 days, but full antidepressant effect may not be felt for 3 – 4 weeks.

Duration of action
Up to 24 hours.

Diet advice
None.

Storage
Keep in a closed container in a cool, dry place away from reach of children.

Missed dose
Take as soon as you remember.

Stopping the drug
Do not stop the drug without consulting your physician; symptoms may recur.

Exceeding the dose
An occasional unintentional extra dose is unlikely to cause problems. Large doses may cause unusual drowsiness. Notify your physician immediately.

POSSIBLE ADVERSE EFFECTS

The most commonly observed adverse effects are nausea, somnolence, sweating, tremor, weakness, insomnia, and sexual dysfunction (lack of orgasm, male ejaculation problems).

Symptom/effect	Frequency		Discuss with physician		Stop taking drug now	Call physician now
	Common	Rare	Only if severe	In all cases		
Gastrointestinal disturbance	●			■		
Drowsiness/dizziness	●			■		
Insomnia	●			■		
Sexual dysfunction (both sexes)	●			■		
Nervousness/anxiety/agitation		●		■		
Weakness	●			■		
Rash/itching/hives		●		■	▲	▮

INTERACTIONS

General note Any drug that affects the breakdown of other drugs in the liver may alter blood levels of paroxetine or vice versa. Such other drugs include cimetidine, digoxin, and phenytoin.

Anticoagulants Paroxetine may increase the effects of these drugs, necessitating an adjustment of dose.

Monoamine oxidase inhibitors (MAOIs) Paroxetine should not be used in combination with MAOIs or within 2 weeks of terminating treatment with these drugs.

MAOIs should not be introduced within 2 weeks of cessation of therapy with paroxetine.

Sedatives All drugs that have a sedative effect on the central nervous system are likely to increase the sedative effects of paroxetine. Such drugs include alcohol, antihistamines, sleeping drugs, narcotic analgesics, and antipsychotics.

Tricyclic antidepressants When taken together, paroxetine may increase the toxicity of these drugs.

SPECIAL PRECAUTIONS

Be sure to tell your physician if:
▼ You have impaired liver or kidney function.
▼ You have a heart problem.
▼ You have a history or a family history of seizures.
▼ You are taking other medications.

 **Pregnancy**
▼ Safety in pregnancy not established. Discuss with your physician.

 Breast feeding
▼ The drug passes into the breast milk. Discuss with your physician.

 Infants and children
▼ Not recommended in patients under 18 years.

 Over 60
▼ No special problems.

 Driving and hazardous work
▼ Avoid such activities until you have learned how the drug affects you; it can cause drowsiness.

 Alcohol
▼ Avoid. Alcohol may increase the sedative effects of this drug.

PROLONGED USE

No problems expected. However, paroxetine is a new drug and little is known of its long-term effects.

PENICILLAMINE

Brand names Cuprimine, Depen
Used in the following combined preparations None

GENERAL INFORMATION

Penicillamine has two principal uses. It is an antirheumatic drug, given to adults and juveniles to slow or even halt the progression of rheumatoid arthritis. Because of its potentially serious side effects on the blood and kidneys, it is used only when the inflammation of the joints is disabling or when other drugs have proven ineffective.

Penicillamine is also a *chelating* agent, used in cases of metal poisoning to eliminate copper, mercury, lead, or arsenic from the body. Penicillamine binds (i.e., combines) with those substances, forming a chemical compound that the body can excrete. It is also prescribed in Wilson's disease, a rare disorder involving copper deposits in the liver and brain, and prevents a certain rare type of urinary stone (cystine).

QUICK REFERENCE

Drug group Antirheumatic drug (p.129)

Overdose danger rating Medium

Dependence rating Low

Prescription needed Yes

Multi-source suppliers Yes

INFORMATION FOR USERS

Your drug prescription is tailored for you. Do not alter dosage without checking with your physician.

How taken

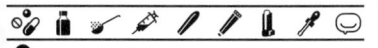

Tablets, capsules.

Frequency and timing of doses
Once daily one hour before meals (rheumatoid arthritis); 4 x daily one hour before meals (Wilson's disease, kidney stones, metal poisoning).

Dosage range
Adults 125 – 250mg daily (starting dose), increasing to 500 – 750mg over 6 – 12 months (rheumatoid arthritis); 125 – 250mg daily (starting dose), increasing to up to 1 – 2g daily over 4 – 8 weeks (Wilson's disease); 1 – 4g daily (kidney stones); according to size or weight (metal poisoning).
Children Reduced dose necessary according to age and weight.

Onset of effect
Full effect may not be felt for 2 – 3 months.

Duration of action
Some effect may last for 1 – 3 months after the drug has been stopped.

Diet advice
People with Wilson's disease may be advised to follow a low-copper diet. Discuss with your physician.

Storage
Keep in a closed container in a cool, dry place away from reach of children.

Missed dose
Take as soon as you remember.

Stopping the drug
Do not stop the drug without consulting your physician; symptoms may recur.

Exceeding the dose
An occasional unintentional extra dose is unlikely to cause problems. Large overdoses may cause joint pain, fever, or a rash. Consult your physician.

POSSIBLE ADVERSE EFFECTS

Adverse effects are frequent. Allergic rashes and itching, gastrointestinal disturbances (nausea, vomiting, abdominal pain), and loss of taste are common and often dose-related. More serious, life-threatening reactions may occur.

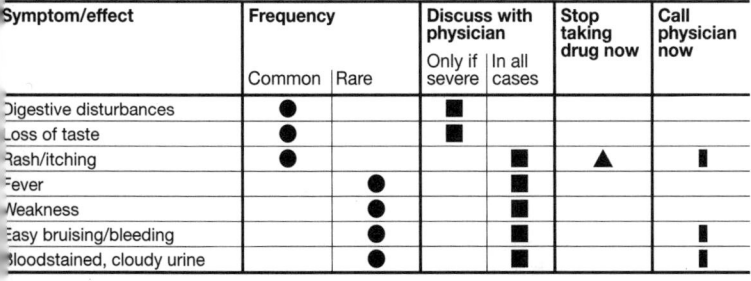

Symptom/effect	Frequency		Discuss with physician		Stop taking drug now	Call physician now
	Common	Rare	Only if severe	In all cases		
Digestive disturbances	●		■			
Loss of taste	●		■			
Rash/itching	●			■	▲	▮
Fever		●		■		
Weakness		●		■		
Easy bruising/bleeding		●		■		▮
Bloodstained, cloudy urine		●		■		▮

INTERACTIONS

Iron preparations may interfere with the effects of penicillamine.

Antacids may reduce the absorption of penicillamine.

Digoxin Penicillamine may reduce the effect of digoxin.

SPECIAL PRECAUTIONS

Be sure to tell your physician if:
▼ You have impaired kidney or liver function.
▼ You have a blood disorder.
▼ You have a skin disorder.
▼ You are taking other medications.

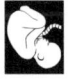

Pregnancy
▼ Not usually prescribed. May cause defects in the baby. Discuss with your physician.

Breast feeding
▼ The drug may pass into the breast milk and may affect the baby. Discuss with your physician.

Infants and children
▼ Reduced dose necessary.

Over 60
▼ Increased likelihood of adverse effects.

Driving and hazardous work
▼ No known problems.

Alcohol
▼ No known problems.

PROLONGED USE

Prolonged use may deplete pyridoxine (vitamin B_6) and iron; supplements may be advised. In rare cases, blood disorders or impaired kidney function may develop.

Monitoring Blood and urine are regularly tested for liver or kidney damage or blood abnormalities.

PENICILLIN G

Brand names Wycillin, Ayercillin, Bicillin, Crystapen, Megacillin, Novo-Pen G
Used in the following combined preparations None

GENERAL INFORMATION

Also known as benzylpenicillin, penicillin G was one of the first antibiotics to be discovered, purified, and used in medicine. Because it is broken down in the digestive tract, penicillin G is less effective when taken by mouth. Almost always given by injection, it is used to treat a variety of bacterial infections when the organisms are shown to be susceptible. These infections include certain types of tonsillitis, bronchitis, and pneumonia. It is effective in a gum infection known as Vincent's gingivitis,

and may be used to treat certain sexually transmitted diseases, including gonorrhea and syphilis.

Penicillin G is also prescribed for less common conditions caused by streptococcal infections, such as scarlet fever and erysipelas (a skin infection). The drug is also used to treat bacterial endocarditis.

As with other penicillin antibiotics, the most common *side effect* is a rash, but more serious allergic reactions can cause wheezing or anaphylactic shock.

INFORMATION FOR USERS

Your drug prescription is tailored for you. Do not alter dosage without checking with your physician.

How taken

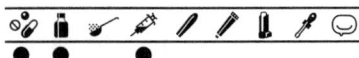

Tablets, oral liquid, injection.

Frequency and timing of doses
3 – 4 x daily at least one hour before or two hours after eating (by mouth); up to 6 x daily depending on preparation (by injection).

Dosage range
Adults 1 – 2g daily (by mouth).
Children Reduced dose according to age and weight.

Onset of effect
Symptoms usually improve within 1 – 2 days, depending on the condition.

Duration of action
Up to 12 hours.

Diet advice
None.

Storage
Keep in a closed container in a cool, dry place away from reach of children.

Missed dose
Take as soon as you remember. If your next dose is due within 2 hours, take a single dose now and skip the next.

Stopping the drug
Take the full course. Even if you feel better, the original infection may still be present and may recur if treatment is stopped too soon.

Exceeding the dose
An occasional unintentional extra dose is unlikely to be a cause for concern. But if you notice unusual symptoms, or if a large overdose has been taken, notify your physician.

SPECIAL PRECAUTIONS

Be sure to tell your physician if:
▼ You have impaired kidney function.
▼ You have an allergic disorder such as asthma or hives.
▼ You have had a previous allergic reaction to a penicillin or cephalosporin antibiotic.
▼ You are taking other medications.

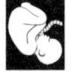

Pregnancy
▼ No evidence of risk.

Breast feeding
▼ The drug passes into the breast milk, but at normal doses adverse effects on the baby are unlikely. Discuss with your physician.

Infants and children
▼ Reduced dose necessary.

Over 60
▼ Increased likelihood of adverse effects. Reduced dose may therefore be necessary.

Driving and hazardous work
▼ No known problems.

Alcohol
▼ May reduce effect of the drug.

POSSIBLE ADVERSE EFFECTS

Most people do not experience any serious adverse effects with penicillin G. Allergic reactions that produce a rash are uncommon, but necessitate stopping the drug.

Symptom/effect	Frequency		Discuss with physician		Stop taking drug now	Call physician now
	Common	Rare	Only if severe	In all cases		
Nausea/vomiting	●		■			
Diarrhea	●		■			
Breathing difficulties		●		■	▲	▌
Rash/itching		●		■	▲	▌

INTERACTIONS

Probenecid increases the level of penicillin G in the blood.

Tetracycline antibiotics may reduce the effectiveness of penicillin G.

Oral contraceptives Penicillin G may reduce the contraceptive effect of these drugs.

PROLONGED USE

Prolonged use may increase the risk of diarrhea and yeast infections of the mouth or vagina.

PENICILLIN V

Brand names Pen-Vee, Apo-Pen-VK, Nadopen-V, Novo-Pen-VK, PVF K, V-Cillin K
Used in the following combined preparations None

GENERAL INFORMATION

Penicillin V, introduced in 1956, is a synthetic antibiotic prescribed for a wide range of infections. Taken by mouth, it is better absorbed than penicillin G.

Various commonly occurring respiratory tract infections – some types of tonsillitis and pharyngitis, for example – often respond well to treatment with penicillin V. It is also effective for the treatment of the gum disease known as Vincent's gingivitis.

Less common infections caused by the streptococcus bacterium, such as scarlet fever and erysipelas (a skin infection), may also be treated with penicillin V. It is also prescribed long term to prevent the recurrence of rheumatic fever, a rare though potentially serious condition.

As with other penicillin antibiotics the most common adverse effect is a rash. More serious allergic reactions involving wheezing, hives, or anaphylactic shock are much rarer.

QUICK REFERENCE

Drug group Penicillin antibiotic (p.140)

Overdose danger rating Low

Dependence rating Low

Prescription needed Yes

Multi-source suppliers Yes

INFORMATION FOR USERS

Your drug prescription is tailored for you. Do not alter dosage without checking with your physician.

How taken

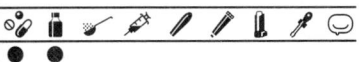

Tablets, capsules, oral liquid.

Frequency and timing of doses
2 – 4 x daily.

Dosage range
Adults 500mg – 2g daily.
Children Reduced dose according to age and weight.

Onset of effect
Symptoms usually improve within 1 – 2 days, depending on the condition.

Duration of action
Up to 12 hours.

Diet advice
None.

Storage
Keep in a closed container in a cool, dry place away from reach of children.

Missed dose
Take as soon as you remember. If your next dose is due within 2 hours, take a single dose now and skip the next.

Stopping the drug
Take the full course. Even if you feel better the original infection may still be present and may recur if treatment is stopped too soon.

Exceeding the dose
An occasional unintentional extra dose is unlikely to be a cause for concern. But if you notice unusual symptoms, or if a large overdose has been taken, notify your physician.

SPECIAL PRECAUTIONS

Be sure to tell your physician if:
▼ You have impaired kidney function.
▼ You have had a previous allergic reaction to a penicillin or cephalosporin antibiotic.
▼ You have an allergic disorder such as asthma or hives.
▼ You are taking other medications.

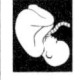
Pregnancy
▼ No evidence of risk.

Breast feeding
▼ The drug passes into the breast milk, but at normal doses adverse effects on the baby are unlikely. Discuss with your physician.

Infants and children
▼ Reduced dose necessary.

Over 60
▼ Increased likelihood of adverse effects. Reduced dose may therefore be necessary.

Driving and hazardous work
▼ No known problems.

Alcohol
▼ No known problems.

POSSIBLE ADVERSE EFFECTS

Most people do not experience any serious adverse effects when taking penicillin V.

However, this drug may occasionally provoke an allergic rash in susceptible people.

Symptom/effect	Frequency		Discuss with physician		Stop taking drug now	Call physician now
	Common	Rare	Only if severe	In all cases		
Nausea/vomiting	●		■			
Diarrhea	●		■			
Rash/itching		●		■	▲	▮
Breathing difficulties		●		■	▲	▮

INTERACTIONS

Probenecid increases the level of penicillin V in the blood.

Tetracycline antibiotics may reduce the effectiveness of penicillin V.

Oral contraceptives Penicillin V may reduce the contraceptive effect of these drugs.

PROLONGED USE

Prolonged use may increase the risk of yeast infections and diarrhea.

PENTOXIFYLLINE

Brand name Trental
Used in the following combined preparations None

GENERAL INFORMATION

Pentoxifylline, a drug related to caffeine, may be prescribed for the symptomatic treatment of peripheral vascular disease, a group of conditions caused by poor circulation in the limbs, such as intermittent claudication (pain in the legs during exercise) and trophic ulcers. It is not, however, recommended for the treatment of severe arterial obstructive disease, including conditions such as gangrene.

Pentoxifylline, it is claimed, makes the red blood cells more flexible and improves their ability to pass through the smallest capillaries. This enables the blood to flow through narrowed arteries and increases the supply of blood and oxygen to all parts of the body.

The most frequent adverse effects from this drug are dizziness, light-headedness, nausea, and vomiting. It may not be suitable for people who react adversely to caffeine.

INFORMATION FOR USERS

Your drug prescription is tailored for you. Do not alter dosage without checking with your physician.

How taken

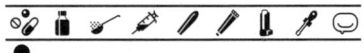

Slow-release tablets.

Frequency and timing of doses
2 – 3 x daily after meals.

Adult dosage range
800 – 1,200mg daily.

Onset of effect
Some effects may occur within a few hours, but full benefits may not be felt for 2 months.

Duration of action
8 – 12 hours.

Diet advice
None.

Storage
Keep in a closed container in a cool, dry place away from reach of children. Protect from light.

Missed dose
Take as soon as you remember. If your next dose is due within 2 hours, take a single dose now and skip the next.

Stopping the drug
Do not stop taking the drug without consulting your physician; symptoms may recur.

Exceeding the dose
An occasional unintentional extra dose is unlikely to cause problems. Larger overdoses may cause agitation, fever, flushing, convulsions, and faintness. Seek immediate medical advice.

SPECIAL PRECAUTIONS

Be sure to tell your physician if:
▼ You have impaired kidney or liver function.
▼ You have heart problems.
▼ You have a blood clotting disorder.
▼ You have a peptic ulcer.
▼ You have low or unstable blood pressure.
▼ You are taking other medications.

Pregnancy
▼ Safety in pregnancy not established. Discuss with your physician.

Breast feeding
▼ The drug passes into the breast milk and may affect the baby adversely. Discuss with your physician.

Infants and children
▼ Not recommended in patients under 18 years.

Over 60
▼ Increased likelihood of adverse effects. Reduced dose may therefore be necessary.

Driving and hazardous work
▼ Avoid such activities until you have learned how the drug affects you, because the drug can cause dizziness and blurred vision.

Alcohol
▼ No known problems.

POSSIBLE ADVERSE EFFECTS

Severe adverse effects are rare with pentoxifylline. Dizziness, headaches, and gastrointestinal disturbances may be controlled by reducing the dose. If chest pain or palpitations occur, consult your physician at once.

Symptom/effect	Frequency		Discuss with physician		Stop taking drug now	Call physician now
	Common	Rare	Only if severe	In all cases		
Nausea/vomiting	●		■			
Flushing	●		■			
Dizziness/lightheadedness	●		■			
Headache	●		■			
Chest pain		●		■	▲	▌
Palpitations		●		■	▲	▌

PROLONGED USE

No known problems.

INTERACTIONS

Antihypertensive drugs Pentoxifylline may increase the effect of antihypertensive drugs, and the dosages of both may need to be adjusted accordingly.

Theophylline and sympathomimetic drugs Combined use of pentoxifylline with theophylline or *sympathomimetic* drugs may cause excessive central nervous system stimulation.

Anticoagulants Pentoxifylline may increase the risk of bleeding if given with anticoagulants.

Oral antidiabetic drugs Dosage adjustment of these agents may be necessary when they are taken with pentoxifylline.

PERMETHRIN

Brand name Nix
Used in the following combined preparations None

GENERAL INFORMATION

Permethrin is a synthetic insecticide. A creme rinse formulation is used in the treatment of infestation with head lice and their nits (eggs).

Permethrin *topical* cream is used to treat scabies infestation.

The drug destroys the infesting parasites through its disruptive action on the nervous system of the insects.

Adverse effects are infrequent and confined to the skin.

QUICK REFERENCE

Drug group Topical antiparasitic drug (p.188)

Overdose danger rating Low

Dependence rating Low

Prescription needed No

Multi-source suppliers No

INFORMATION FOR USERS

Follow instructions on the label. Call your physician if symptoms worsen.

How taken

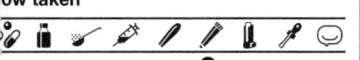

Topical cream, creme rinse.

Frequency and timing of doses
A single treatment after shampooing the hair for the creme rinse or a single skin application for the topical cream. May need to be repeated in 7 – 10 days but only if live lice or mites or new lesions appear.

Dosage range
Use only as directed by package information or your physician. For scabies, the whole body from the head to the soles of the feet should be covered.

Onset of effect
Within a few minutes.

Duration of action
Active until washed off.

Diet advice
None.

Storage
Keep in a cool, dry place away from reach of children. Protect from freezing and direct heat. Discard unused portions of the medication.

Missed dose
Not applicable.

Stopping the drug
Follow the advice of your physician. A second treatment is sometimes required to clear the parasite completely.

Exceeding the dose
If the drug has been swallowed, seek medical attention immediately. If it makes contact with the eyes, flush with water.

POSSIBLE ADVERSE EFFECTS

Mild temporary skin irritation and itching may occur following the use of permethrin products.

Symptom/effect	Frequency		Discuss with physician		Stop taking drug now	Call physician now
	Common	Rare	Only if severe	In all cases		
Rash or swelling		●			■	▲
Itching	●		■			
Skin redness		●	■			
Numbness		●	■			
Tingling		●	■			
Burning/stinging		●	■			

INTERACTIONS

None.

SPECIAL PRECAUTIONS

Be sure to consult your physician or pharmacist before using this drug if:
▼ You are sensitive to chrysanthemums, pyrethroids, or pyrethrin.
▼ You are taking other medications.

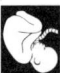

Pregnancy
▼ Discuss with your physician to ensure that permethrin treatment is required.

Breast feeding
▼ Discontinue nursing while using permethrin or discuss with your physician to ensure that permethrin treatment is required.

Infants and children
▼ Safe for children over 2 years. For children under 2 years of age, discuss with your physician.

Over 60
▼ No special problems.

Driving and hazardous work
▼ No known problems.

Alcohol
▼ No known problems.

PROLONGED USE

Not given for prolonged periods.

PERPHENAZINE

Brand names Trilafon, Apo-Perphenazine
Used in the following combined preparations Elavil Plus, Etrafon, PMS-Levazine, Triavil

GENERAL INFORMATION

Perphenazine was introduced in 1957 and belongs to a group of drugs called the phenothiazines. These drugs act on the brain to modify abnormal behavior (see Antipsychotic drugs, p.97).

Perphenazine is used in the treatment of schizophrenia, mania, dementia, and other disorders where confused or agitated behavior may occur. It does not cure the disorders but does relieve some of the distressing symptoms of these illnesses.

Another use of perphenazine is in the treatment of nausea and vomiting, especially if caused by drug treatment, radiation therapy, or anesthetics.

The main drawback to the use of this drug is that it often produces drowsiness and may cause abnormal shaking movements (*parkinsonism*).

INFORMATION FOR USERS

Your drug prescription is tailored for you. Do not alter dosage without checking with your physician.

How taken

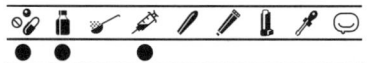

Tablets, oral liquid, injection.

Frequency and timing of doses
3 x daily.

Adult dosage range
12 – 24mg daily (antipsychotic); 8 – 24mg daily (nausea and vomiting).

Onset of effect
30 minutes – 1 hour; full effect in mental illness may not be felt for several weeks.

Duration of action
6 – 8 hours.

Diet advice
None.

Storage
Keep in a closed container in a cool, dry place away from reach of children. Protect from light.

Missed dose
Take as soon as you remember. If your next dose is due within 2 hours, take a single dose now and skip the next.

Stopping the drug
Do not stop the drug without consulting your physician; symptoms may recur.

Exceeding the dose
An occasional unintentional extra dose is unlikely to cause problems. Large overdoses may cause drowsiness, muscle stiffness, or trembling. Notify your physician.

SPECIAL PRECAUTIONS

Be sure to tell your physician if:
▼ You have impaired kidney or liver function.
▼ You have heart problems.
▼ You have poor circulation.
▼ You have had epileptic seizures.
▼ You have thyroid disease.
▼ You have had glaucoma.
▼ You have prostate trouble.
▼ You have Parkinson's disease.
▼ You are taking other medications.

Pregnancy
▼ Safety in pregnancy not established. Discuss with your physician.

Breast feeding
▼ The drug passes into the breast milk. Its effects on the baby are not known. Discuss with your physician.

Infants and children
▼ Safety and effectiveness in patients under 12 not established.

Over 60
▼ Increased likelihood of adverse effects. Reduced dose may therefore be necessary.

Driving and hazardous work
▼ Avoid such activities until you have learned how the drug affects you; it can cause drowsiness and slowed reactions.

Alcohol
▼ Avoid. Alcohol may increase the sedative effects of this drug.

POSSIBLE ADVERSE EFFECTS

When used as an antipsychotic, drowsiness is the most common adverse effect of perphenazine. This effect usually weakens after long-term treatment, and adjusting the dosage often helps. Other adverse effects, such as blurred vision, stuffy nose, and headache, are more common when the drug is used as an anti-emetic.

Symptom/effect	Frequency		Discuss with physician		Stop taking drug now	Call physician now
	Common	Rare	Only if severe	In all cases		
Drowsiness	●		■			
Stuffy nose	●		■			
Constipation	●		■			
Parkinsonism	●			■		
Dizziness	●			■		
Blurred vision	●			■		
Muscle rigidity and stupor		●		■	▲	▮

INTERACTIONS

Sedatives All drugs, including alcohol, that have a sedative effect on the central nervous system are likely to increase the sedative effect of perphenazine.

Antacids reduce the absorption of perphenazine if the two drugs are taken less than 1 hour apart.

Anticonvulsants and antiparkinsonian drugs Perphenazine may reduce the effectiveness of these drugs.

Anticholinergic drugs Perphenazine may increase the side effects of these drugs.

PROLONGED USE

Use of this drug for more than a few months may lead to the development of abnormal movements of the face and limbs (*tardive dyskinesia*), and occasionally jaundice may occur. Sometimes a reduction in dosage may be recommended.

PHENAZOPYRIDINE

...nd names Pyridium, Phenazo
...d in the following combined preparation Azo Gantrisin

ENERAL INFORMATION

...oduced in 1927, phenazopyridine is ...nalgesic that passes quickly into ...urine and relieves pain or discomfort ...e urinary tract for up to 48 hours. ...h symptoms can result from ...ction, injury, surgery, catheterization, ...cystoscopy. ...ith urinary tract infection, other ...gs are given to cure the infection. ...ugh phenazopyridine is available in ...bination with sulfa drugs, most ...sicians prefer separate prescrip-

tions. Because the use of phenazopyridine can delay proper diagnosis of an underlying problem, it is best to consult your physician before starting the drug.

Gastrointestinal disturbance is a fairly common *side effect*. Because this drug is a dye, it colors the urine orange or red, and this may stain clothing.

Headache, dizziness, and skin discoloration occur only occasionally. Diabetics may have false readings of urine sugar tests.

INFORMATION FOR USERS

...r drug prescription is tailored for you. ...not alter dosage without checking ...your physician.

...w taken

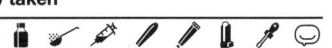

...ets.

...quency and timing of doses
...aily after meals.

...age range
...ts 600mg daily.
...dren 9 to 12 years 300mg daily.

...et of effect
...in 4 hours.

...ation of action
...2 hours.

Diet advice
None.

Storage
Keep in a closed container in a cool, dry place away from reach of children.

Missed dose
Take as soon as you remember. If your next dose is due within 2 hours, take a single dose now and skip the next.

Stopping the drug
Can be safely stopped as soon as you no longer need it.

Exceeding the dose
An occasional unintentional extra dose is unlikely to be a cause for concern. But if you notice unusual symptoms, or if a large overdose has been taken, notify your physician.

SPECIAL PRECAUTIONS

Be sure to tell your physician if:
▼ You have impaired kidney or liver function.
▼ You are taking other medications.

Pregnancy
▼ Not usually prescribed. Safety in pregnancy not established. Discuss with your physician.

Breast feeding
▼ No evidence of risk.

Infants and children
▼ Not recommended in patients under 9 years.

Over 60
▼ No special problems.

Driving and hazardous work
▼ Phenazopyridine occasionally causes dizziness and this possibility should be kept in mind.

Alcohol
▼ No known problems.

POSSIBLE ADVERSE EFFECTS

...ominal pain is the most common adverse ...t. Discoloration of the urine may be

inconvenient, but it is no cause for concern. Other adverse effects are rare.

...ptom/effect	Frequency		Discuss with physician		Stop taking drug now	Call physician now
	Common	Rare	Only if severe	In all cases		
...ominal pain	●		■			
...or orange urine	●		■			
...dache		●	■			
...ness		●		■		
...discoloration		●		■		

INTERACTIONS

...ne.

PROLONGED USE

No problems expected. Phenazopyridine is not usually prescribed for long periods because it tends to lose its effect after 48 hours when used for urinary tract infections.

PHENOBARBITAL

Brand name Barbilixir
Used in the following combined preparations Dilantin with Phenobarbital, Donnatal, Phenaphen with Codeine

GENERAL INFORMATION

Introduced over 75 years ago, phenobarbital belongs to the group of drugs known as barbiturates. It is mainly used in the treatment of epilepsy. Before the development of safer drugs, it was also used as a sedative and sleeping drug.

In the treatment of epilepsy, phenobarbital is often given with other anticonvulsant drugs such as phenytoin. It is also included in some *anti-spasmodic* preparations for the treatment of irritable bowel syndrome, although this use is no longer widely recommended.

The main disadvantage of phenobarbital is that it often causes unwanted sedation. In children and the elderly, however, it may occasionally cause excessive excitement.

QUICK REFERENCE

Drug group Barbiturate anticonvulsant drug (p.98)

Overdose danger rating High

Dependence rating High

Prescription needed Yes

Multi-source suppliers Yes

INFORMATION FOR USERS

Your drug prescription is tailored for you. Do not alter dosage without checking with your physician.

How taken

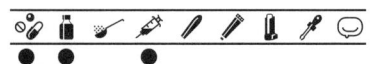

Tablets, oral liquid, injection.

Frequency and timing of doses
2 – 4 x daily.

Dosage range
Adults 30 – 200mg daily; up to 300mg daily may be used to control seizures.
Children Reduced dose according to age and weight.

Onset of effect
30 – 60 minutes (by mouth).

Duration of action
24 – 48 hours (some effect may persist for up to 6 days).

Diet advice
None.

Storage
Keep in a closed container in a cool, dry place away from reach of children.

Missed dose
Take as soon as you remember for seizure control. If your next dose is due within 2 hours, do not take the missed dose. Take the next dose as usual. For other purposes take a dose at the next scheduled time.

Stopping the drug
Do not stop taking the drug without consulting your physician, who may supervise a gradual reduction in dosage. Abrupt cessation may cause seizures or lead to restlessness, trembling, and insomnia.

OVERDOSE ACTION

 Seek immediate medical advice in all cases. Take emergency action if unsteadiness, severe weakness, confusion, or loss of consciousness occurs.

See Drug poisoning emergency guide (p.574).

SPECIAL PRECAUTIONS

Be sure to tell your physician if:
▼ You have impaired kidney or liver function
▼ You have heart problems.
▼ You have poor circulation.
▼ You have respiratory problems.
▼ You have porphyria.
▼ You have persistent pain.
▼ You are taking other medications.

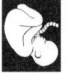 **Pregnancy**
▼ Safety in pregnancy not established. Discuss with your physician.

 Breast feeding
▼ The drug passes into the breast milk and may affect the baby adversely. Discuss with your physician.

 Infants and children
▼ Reduced dose necessary.

 Over 60
▼ Reduced dose may be necessary.

 Driving and hazardous work
▼ Your underlying condition, as well as the possibility of reduced alertness while taking this drug, m make such activities inadvisable. Discuss with your physician.

 Alcohol
▼ Never drink alcohol while under treatment with phenobarbital, as i may interact dangerously with this drug.

POSSIBLE ADVERSE EFFECTS

Most of the adverse effects of phenobarbital are the result of its sedative effect on the brain. They can sometimes be minimized by medically supervised reduction of dosage.

Symptom/effect	Frequency		Discuss with physician		Stop taking drug now	Call physician now
	Common	Rare	Only if severe	In all cases		
Drowsiness	●		■			
Dizziness/faintness	●		■			
Clumsiness/unsteadiness	●			■		▐
Rash		●		■	▲	
Confusion		●		■		▐

INTERACTIONS

General note Phenobarbital may decrease the blood levels and reduce the effects of a wide range of drugs requiring careful monitoring if given concurrently. Such drugs include warfarin, theophylline, corticosteroids, digoxin, beta blockers, oral contraceptives, griseofulvin, oral anticoagulants, anticonvulsants, quinidine, testosterone, and tricyclic antidepressants.

Sedatives All drugs, including alcohol, that have a sedative effect on the central nervous system are likely to increase the sedative effects of phenobarbital.

PROLONGED USE

The sedative effect of phenobarbital can build up during prolonged use, causing excessive drowsiness and lethargy. However, *tolerance* may develop and reduce these effects. In rare cases it may cause deficiency of vitamin D.

Monitoring Blood samples may be take periodically to test blood levels of the drug.

PHENYLEPHRINE

Brand names Neo-Synephrine, Dionephrine, Mydrin, Novahistine Decongestant, Prefrin
Used in the following combined preparations Dimetapp, Dristan, Novahistex C, Novahistine DH, Vasosulf

GENERAL INFORMATION

Phenylephrine is one of the most common nasal decongestants. It relieves the symptoms of hay fever and head colds. Less potent but longer acting than other nasal decongestants, it seems to cause fewer adverse effects. By constricting blood vessels in the lining of the eye, small doses of the drug can also reduce the pain of conjunctivitis. Combined with local anesthetics, it constricts the blood vessels around an injection site, prolonging the anesthetic's effect by delaying its absorption. Phenylephrine is also used to dilate the pupil during eye examinations and eye surgery.

Care should be taken not to exceed the dose, because this may cause increased eye irritation (eye drops) and produce congestion and swelling in the nasal passages. High or prolonged doses of phenylephrine are liable to cause a rebound of nasal stuffiness and a rise in blood pressure and heart rate, and should be avoided by people with heart trouble or high blood pressure.

INFORMATION FOR USERS

Follow instructions on the label. Call your physician if symptoms worsen.

How taken

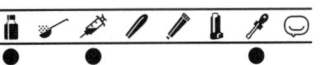

Pill, liquid, injection, nasal drops, nasal spray, eye drops.

Frequency and timing of doses
As directed according to preparation.

Dosage range
As directed according to preparation.

Onset of effect
Within a few minutes.

Duration of action
4–6 hours.

Diet advice
None.

Storage
Keep in a closed container in a cool, dry place away from reach of children. Protect from light.

Missed dose
Take as soon as you remember. If your next dose is due within 2 hours, take a single dose now and skip the next.

Stopping the drug
Can be safely stopped as soon as you no longer need it. Seek medical advice if symptoms persist for more than a few days.

Exceeding the dose
An occasional unintentional extra dose is unlikely to cause problems. Large overdoses may cause irritation of the eyes or palpitations. Notify your physician.

SPECIAL PRECAUTIONS

Be sure to consult your physician or pharmacist before taking this drug if:
▼ You have angina.
▼ You have high blood pressure.
▼ You have had glaucoma.
▼ You have an eye infection or other eye disease.
▼ You are taking other medications.

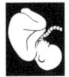
Pregnancy
▼ No evidence of risk to the developing baby when used sparingly for short periods. However, overuse can cause a rise in blood pressure that could harm the developing baby. Discuss with your physician.

Breast feeding
▼ The drug passes into the breast milk, but at normal doses adverse effects on the baby are unlikely. Discuss with your physician.

Infants and children
▼ Reduced dose necessary.

Over 60
▼ Increased likelihood of adverse effects. Reduced dose may therefore be necessary.

Driving and hazardous work
▼ Avoid such activities until you have learned how the drug affects you; when used in the eye it can cause blurred vision.

Alcohol
▼ No known problems.

POSSIBLE ADVERSE EFFECTS

Phenylephrine has fewer adverse effects than many other drugs of the same group because it has little stimulating effect on the central nervous system. Most of the symptoms are related to frequent use, and should be reported promptly.

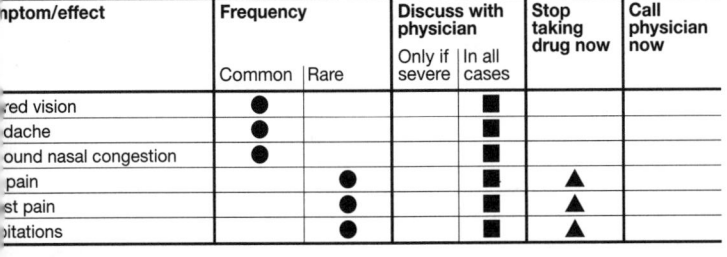

Symptom/effect	Frequency		Discuss with physician		Stop taking drug now	Call physician now
	Common	Rare	Only if severe	In all cases		
Blurred vision	●			■		
Headache	●			■		
Rebound nasal congestion	●			■		
Eye pain		●		■	▲	
Chest pain		●		■	▲	
Palpitations		●		■	▲	

INTERACTIONS

Monoamine oxidase inhibitors (MAOIs) There is a risk of a dangerous rise in blood pressure if phenylephrine is taken with these drugs. It should not be taken during or within 14 days of MAOI treatment.

Antihypertensive drugs Phenylephrine may interact with these drugs to reverse their effect.

PROLONGED USE

Prolonged continuous use may lead to worsening of the underlying condition.

Monitoring Periodic eye examinations may be required.

PHENYTOIN

Brand names Dilantin, Novo-Phenytoin
Used in the following combined preparation Dilantin with phenobarbital

GENERAL INFORMATION

By reducing electrical discharges within the brain, phenytoin reduces the likelihood of convulsions (see Anticonvulsant drugs, p.98). Introduced in 1938, it has been widely prescribed for the long-term treatment of several types of epilepsy, including grand mal and temporal lobe seizures.

Over the years other uses for phenytoin have been found: for the pain of trigeminal neuralgia, and for correction of certain types of abnormal heart rhythms.

Because some adverse effects of phenytoin (such as overgrowth of the gums) are more pronounced in children, it is prescribed for children only when other drugs are unsuitable. However, careful dental hygiene can delay or minimize the gum problems.

QUICK REFERENCE

Drug group Anticonvulsant drug (p.98)

Overdose danger rating Medium

Dependence rating Low

Prescription needed Yes

Multi-source suppliers Yes

INFORMATION FOR USERS

Your drug prescription is tailored for you. Do not alter dosage without checking with your physician.

How taken

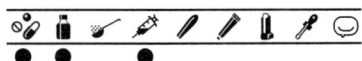

Tablets, capsules, oral liquid, injection.

Frequency and timing of doses
1 – 3 x daily (depending on preparation) with food or water.

Dosage range
Adults 300 – 400mg daily.
Children According to age and weight.

Onset of effect
Full anticonvulsant effect may not be felt for 7 – 10 days.

Duration of action
24 hours.

Diet advice
Folic acid and vitamin D deficiency may occasionally occur while phenytoin is taken. Make sure you eat a balanced diet containing fresh, green vegetables.

Storage
Keep in a tightly closed container in a cool, dry place away from reach of children.

Missed dose
Take as soon as you remember.

Stopping the drug
Do not stop the drug without consulting your physician; symptoms may recur.

Exceeding the dose
An occasional, unintentional extra dose is unlikely to cause problems. You may notice unusual drowsiness, slurred speech, or confusion. Notify your physician.

POSSIBLE ADVERSE EFFECTS

Phenytoin has a number of adverse effects, many of which appear only after prolonged use. If they become severe, your physician may prescribe a different anticonvulsant.

Symptom/effect	Frequency		Discuss with physician		Stop taking drug now	Call physician now
	Common	Rare	Only if severe	In all cases		
Slurred speech	●		■			
Dizziness/headache	●		■			
Confusion	●		■			
Insomnia	●		■			
Overgrowth of gums	●			■		
Increased body hair		●	■			
Rash		●			■	▲

INTERACTIONS

General note Many drugs may interact with phenytoin, causing either an increase or a reduction in the blood level of phenytoin. The dosage of phenytoin may need to be adjusted while you are taking other medications. Consult your physician.

Oral contraceptives Phenytoin may reduce the effectiveness of oral contraceptives. An alternative form of contraception may need to be used. Discuss with your physician.

SPECIAL PRECAUTIONS

Be sure to tell your physician if:
▼ You have impaired kidney or liver function.
▼ You have diabetes.
▼ You are taking other medications.

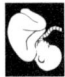

Pregnancy
▼ The drug may be associated with malformation and a tendency to bleeding in the newborn baby. Folate supplements should be taken by the mother. Discuss with your physician.

Breast feeding
▼ The drug passes into the breast milk, but at normal doses adverse effects on the baby are unlikely. Discuss with your physician.

Infants and children
▼ Reduced dose necessary. Increased likelihood of overgrowth of the gums and excessive growth of body hair.

Over 60
▼ Reduced dose may be necessary.

Driving and hazardous work
▼ Your underlying condition, as well as the sedative effects of this drug, may make such activities inadvisable. Discuss with your physician.

Alcohol
▼ Avoid. Alcohol increases the sedative effects of this drug.

PROLONGED USE

There is a slight risk of blood abnormalities occurring. Prolonged use may also lead to adverse effects on skin, gums, and bones. It may also disrupt control of diabetes.

Monitoring Periodic blood tests may be performed to monitor levels of the drug in the body and composition of the blood cells and blood chemistry.

PILOCARPINE

Brand names Isopto Carpine, Miocarpine, Ocusert Pilo, Pilopine HS, R.O. Carpine
Used in the following combined preparations E-Pilo, Timpilo

GENERAL INFORMATION

Pilocarpine, in use since 1875, is a pupil-constricting drug (miotic) used to treat glaucoma. Obtained from the leaves of a plant, Pilocarpus, it is frequently prescribed for chronic glaucoma and, less often, for emergency treatment of severe glaucoma prior to surgery. It may also be given to counteract the dilation of the pupil induced by drugs given during surgery or eye examination.

It is prescribed most frequently in the form of eye drops. These are quick-acting but have to be re-applied every 4 to 8 hours in chronic glaucoma. A long-acting gel formulation, applied once daily, and a slow-release formulation (Ocusert) inserted under the eyelid once weekly, may be more convenient for long-term use.

Like other similar drugs, pilocarpine frequently causes blurred vision. Excessive spasm of eye muscles may cause headaches, particularly at the start of treatment. However, serious adverse effects are rare.

INFORMATION FOR USERS

Your drug prescription is tailored for you. Do not alter dosage without checking with your physician.

How taken

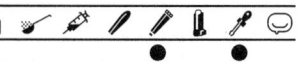

Gel, eye drops, slow-release inserts (Ocuserts).

Frequency and timing of doses
Eye drops 3 – 6 x daily (chronic glaucoma); every 5 minutes until the condition is controlled (acute glaucoma).
Gel Once daily at bedtime.
Ocusert Once every 7 days at bedtime.

Dosage range
According to formulation and condition. In general, 1 or 2 eye drops are used per application. Gel is applied as a 1.5cm strip daily.

Onset of effect
10 – 30 minutes.

Duration of action
4 – 8 hours (eye drops); 18 – 24 hours (gel); about 7 days (Ocusert).

Diet advice
None.

Storage
Keep in a closed container in a cool, dry place away from reach of children (eye drops, gel). Refrigerate but do not freeze (Ocusert).

Missed dose
Use as soon as you remember. If not remembered until the next day (gel) or until 2 hours before your next dose (eye drops), skip the missed dose and take your next dose now.

Stopping the drug
Do not stop the drug without consulting your physician; symptoms may recur.

Exceeding the dose
An occasional unintentional extra application is unlikely to cause problems. Excessive use may cause facial flushing, an increase in the flow of saliva, and sweating. If accidentally swallowed, seek medical attention immediately.

SPECIAL PRECAUTIONS

Be sure to tell your physician if:
▼ You have asthma.
▼ You have inflamed eyes.
▼ You wear contact lenses.
▼ You are taking other medications.

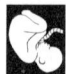

Pregnancy
▼ No evidence of risk at the doses used for chronic glaucoma. Discuss with your physician.

Breast feeding
▼ The drug passes into the breast milk, but at normal doses adverse effects on the baby are unlikely. Discuss with your physician.

Infants and children
▼ Not usually prescribed.

Over 60
▼ Reduced night vision is particularly noticeable.

Driving and hazardous work
▼ Avoid such activities, especially in poor light, until you have learned how the drug affects you; it may cause nearsightedness and poor night vision.

Alcohol
▼ No known problems.

POSSIBLE ADVERSE EFFECTS

Gel applied overnight may cause sticking of the eyelids the following morning. The Ocuserts may cause irritation if they move out of position. Brow ache and eye pain are common at the start of treatment, but effects usually wear off after a few days.

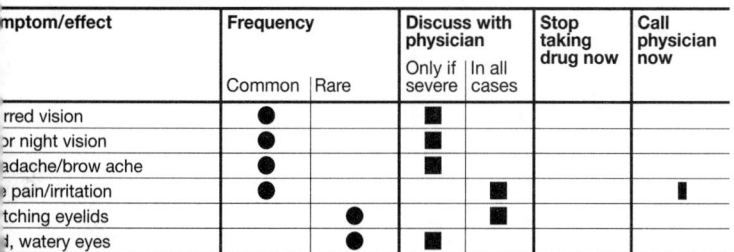

Symptom/effect	Frequency		Discuss with physician		Stop taking drug now	Call physician now
	Common	Rare	Only if severe	In all cases		
Blurred vision	●		■			
Poor night vision	●		■			
Headache/brow ache	●		■			
Eye pain/irritation	●			■		■
Stinging eyelids		●		■		
Red, watery eyes		●	■			

INTERACTIONS

Atropine and cyclopentolate Eye drops containing these drugs may interfere with the antiglaucoma action of pilocarpine.

PROLONGED USE

The effect of the drug may occasionally wear off with prolonged use as the body adapts, but may be restored by changing to another antiglaucoma drug temporarily.

PINDOLOL

Brand names Visken, Apo-Pindol, Novo-Pindol, Nu-Pindol, Syn-Pindolol
Used in the following combined preparation Viskazide

GENERAL INFORMATION

Pindolol is a beta blocker used to treat angina and mild to moderate high blood pressure (hypertension). When prescribed for hypertension, pindolol is sometimes prescribed in a combined preparation that also contains a diuretic.

Because it can cause breathing difficulties, pindolol is not normally prescribed for anyone suffering from asthma, emphysema, or chronic bronchitis. In common with all beta blockers, pindolol has a slowing effect on the heart rate and affects the body's response to low blood sugar; it should be used with caution by diabetics.

QUICK REFERENCE

Drug group Beta blocker (p.109)

Overdose danger rating High

Dependence rating Low

Prescription needed Yes

Multi-source suppliers Yes

INFORMATION FOR USERS

Your drug prescription is tailored for you. Do not alter dosage without checking with your physician.

How taken

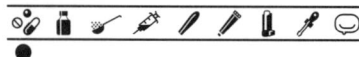

Tablets.

Frequency and timing of doses
2 – 4 x daily with food.

Adult dosage range
15 – 40mg daily.

Onset of effect
Within 24 hours.

Duration of action
Short; most of the drug is gone within 24 hours of stopping.

Diet advice
None.

Storage
Keep in a closed container in a cool, dry place away from reach of children. Protect from light.

Missed dose
Take as soon as you remember. If your next dose is due within 3 hours (4 x daily schedule), 4 hours (3 x daily schedule), or 6 hours (2 x daily schedule), do not take the missed dose. Take your next scheduled dose as usual.

Stopping the drug
Do not stop the drug without consulting your physician; stopping the drug may lead to a dangerous worsening of your underlying condition or precipitation of a heart attack.

OVERDOSE ACTION

Seek immediate medical advice in all cases. Take emergency action if breathing difficulties, collapse, or loss of consciousness occurs.

See Drug poisoning emergency guide (p.574).

SPECIAL PRECAUTIONS

Be sure to tell your physician if:
▼ You have impaired kidney or liver function.
▼ You have heart failure.
▼ You have a lung disorder such as asthma, bronchitis, or emphysema.
▼ You have diabetes.
▼ You have allergies.
▼ You have poor circulation in the legs.
▼ You are taking other medications.

Pregnancy
▼ Safety in pregnancy not established. Discuss with your physician.

Breast feeding
▼ The drug passes into the breast milk but adverse effects on the baby are unlikely. Discuss with your physician.

Infants and children
▼ Not usually prescribed.

Over 60
▼ No special problems.

Driving and hazardous work
▼ No known problems.

Alcohol
▼ No known problems.

Surgery and general anesthetics
▼ Pindolol may need to be stopped before you have a general anesthetic. Discuss with your physician or dentist before any surgery.

PROLONGED USE

No problems expected.

POSSIBLE ADVERSE EFFECTS

Pindolol has adverse effects common to most beta blockers. Symptoms such as fatigue and nausea are usually temporary and diminish with use. Fainting may be a sign that the drug has slowed the heart excessively.

symptom/effect	Frequency		Discuss with physician		Stop taking drug now	Call physician now
	Common	Rare	Only if severe	In all cases		
Lethargy	●			■		
Cold hands and feet		●		■		
Nausea/diarrhea		●		■		
Nightmares		●	■		▲	▮
Rash		●	■		▲	▮
Fainting/breathlessness		●	■		▲	▮

INTERACTIONS

General note Pindolol may interact with many drugs, most notably non-steroidal anti-inflammatory drugs (reduced antihypertensive effect), calcium channel blockers (decreased blood pressure and/or heart rate, and/or force of heart pumping action), cimetidine (increased blood levels of pindolol), *sympathomimetic* decongestants (increased blood pressure and/or heart rate).

PIROXICAM

Brand names Feldene, Apo-Piroxicam, Novo-Pirocam, Nu-Pirox
Used in the following combined preparations None

GENERAL INFORMATION

Piroxicam is a non-steroidal anti-inflammatory drug (NSAID). Like other drugs of this group, it reduces pain, stiffness, and inflammation. Blood levels of the drug remain high for many hours after a dose, so that it need be taken only once daily.

It is prescribed for rheumatoid arthritis, osteoarthritis, and ankylosing spondylitis. Although piroxicam gives lasting relief of the symptoms of arthritis, it does not cure the disease. It is sometimes prescribed in conjunction with the slow-acting drugs in rheumatoid arthritis to relieve pain and inflammation while these drugs take effect. It may be given for pain relief in bursitis and tendinitis.

INFORMATION FOR USERS

Your drug prescription is tailored for you. Do not alter dosage without checking with your physician.

How taken

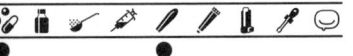

Capsules, rectal suppositories.

Frequency and timing of doses
Once daily with food.

Adult dosage range
0 – 20mg daily.

Onset of effect
Pain relief begins in 3 – 4 hours. Used for arthritis, the full anti-inflammatory effect develops over 2 – 4 weeks.

Duration of action
Up to 2 days. Some effect may last for 7 – 10 days after treatment has been stopped.

Diet advice
None.

Storage
Keep in a closed container in a cool, dry place away from reach of children. Protect from light.

Missed dose
Take as soon as you remember. If your next dose is due within 6 hours, take a single dose now and skip the next.

Stopping the drug
When taken for short-term pain relief, piroxicam can be safely stopped as soon as you no longer need it. If prescribed for the long-term treatment of arthritis, however, you should seek medical advice before stopping the drug.

Exceeding the dose
An occasional unintentional extra dose is unlikely to cause problems. Large overdoses may cause nausea and vomiting. Notify your physician.

SPECIAL PRECAUTIONS

Be sure to tell your physician if:
▼ You have impaired liver or kidney function.
▼ You have heart problems.
▼ You have high blood pressure.
▼ You have had a peptic ulcer, esophagitis, or acid indigestion.
▼ You have asthma.
▼ You are allergic to ASA.
▼ You are taking other medications.

Pregnancy
▼ Safety in pregnancy not established. Discuss with your physician.

Breast feeding
▼ The drug passes into the breast milk but at normal doses adverse effects are unlikely. Discuss with your physician.

Infants and children
▼ Not recommended for infants and children under 16 years.

Over 60
▼ Increased likelihood of adverse effects. Reduced dose may therefore be necessary.

Driving and hazardous work
▼ Avoid such activities until you have learned how the drug affects you; it can cause dizziness.

Alcohol
▼ Avoid. Alcohol may increase the risk of stomach disorders with piroxicam.

Surgery and general anesthetics
▼ Piroxicam may prolong bleeding. Discuss this with your physician or dentist before any surgery.

POSSIBLE ADVERSE EFFECTS

The most common adverse effects are the result of gastrointestinal disturbances. Black or bloodstained feces should be reported to your physician promptly.

Symptom/effect	Frequency		Discuss with physician		Stop taking drug now	Call physician now
	Common	Rare	Only if severe	In all cases		
Nausea/indigestion	●			■		▮
Abdominal pain	●			■		▮
Dizziness/headache		●	■			
Rash/itching		●		■	▲	
Swollen feet/ankles		●		■	▲	▮
Wheezing/breathlessness		●		■	▲	▮
Black/bloodstained feces		●		■	▲	▮

INTERACTIONS

General note Piroxicam interacts with a wide range of drugs to increase the risk of bleeding and/or peptic ulcers. Such drugs include oral anticoagulants, corticosteroids, other NSAIDs, and ASA.

Lithium Piroxicam may raise blood levels of lithium, leading to a risk of serious adverse effects.

Antihypertensive drugs and diuretics
The beneficial effects of these drugs may be reduced by piroxicam.

PROLONGED USE

There is an increased risk of bleeding from peptic ulcers and in the bowel with prolonged use of piroxicam.

PIVAMPICILLIN

Brand name Pondocillin
Used in the following combined preparations None

GENERAL INFORMATION

Pivampicillin, a penicillin antibiotic, is converted in the body to ampicillin. It is prescribed to treat a variety of infections.

In common with other penicillin antibiotics, it is particularly useful for treating ear, nose, and throat infections, infections in the respiratory tract, cystitis, uncomplicated gonorrhea, and certain skin and soft tissue infections. Gastrointestinal infections caused by salmonella and shigella bacteria may sometimes by treated with pivampicillin.

As with other penicillin antibiotics, rashes are not uncommon. More severe allergic reactions are also possible.

QUICK REFERENCE

Drug group Penicillin antibiotic (p.140)

Overdose danger rating Low

Dependence rating Low

Prescription needed Yes

Multi-source suppliers No

INFORMATION FOR USERS

Your drug prescription is tailored for you. Do not alter dosage without checking with your physician.

How taken

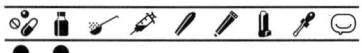

Tablets, oral liquid.

Frequency and timing of doses
2 x daily.

Dosage range
Adults 1 – 2g daily.
Children Reduced dose according to age and weight.

Onset of effect
Symptoms usually improve within 1 – 2 days, depending on the condition.

Duration of action
12 hours.

Diet advice
None.

Storage
Keep tablets in a closed container in a cool, dry place away from reach of children. Refrigerate oral liquid, but do not freeze and do not keep for longer than 14 days.

Missed dose
Take as soon as you remember. If your next dose is due within 4 hours, take a single dose now and skip the next.

Stopping the drug
Take the full course. Even if you feel better, the original infection may still be present and symptoms may recur if treatment is stopped too soon.

Exceeding the dose
An occasional unintentional extra dose is unlikely to be a cause for concern. But if you notice unusual symptoms, or if a large overdose has been taken, notify your physician.

SPECIAL PRECAUTIONS

Be sure to tell your physician if:
▼ You have impaired kidney function.
▼ You have an allergy (for example, asthma, hay fever, eczema, or hives).
▼ You have had a previous reaction to a penicillin or cephalosporin antibiotic.
▼ You have had ulcerative colitis.
▼ You have recently had infectious mono-nucleosis.
▼ You have a deficiency of carnitine.
▼ You are taking other medications.

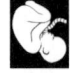

Pregnancy
▼ Safety in pregnancy not established. Discuss with your physician.

Breast feeding
▼ It is not known if pivampicillin passes into the breast milk. Discuss with your physician.

Infants and children
▼ Reduced dose necessary. Not recommended for children under 3 months.

Over 60
▼ No known problems.

Driving and hazardous work
▼ No known problems.

Alcohol
▼ No known problems.

POSSIBLE ADVERSE EFFECTS

If you develop a rash, wheezing, itching, fever, or joint swelling, this may indicate an allergy. Call your physician, who may prescribe a different antibiotic.

Symptom/effect	Frequency		Discuss with physician		Stop taking drug now	Call physician now
	Common	Rare	Only if severe	In all cases		
Diarrhea	●			■		
Rash	●			■	▲	▮
Nausea/vomiting		●	■			
Tiredness/weakness		●	■			
Wheezing		●		■	▲	▮
Itching		●		■	▲	▮
Swollen mouth, tongue		●		■	▲	▮

PROLONGED USE

Pivampicillin is usually given only for short courses of treatment.

INTERACTIONS

Oral contraceptives Pivampicillin may reduce the effectiveness of oral contraceptive tablets and also increase the risk of breakthrough bleeding. Discuss with your physician.

PRAVASTATIN

Brand name Pravachol
Used in the following combined preparations None

GENERAL INFORMATION

Pravastatin is a lipid-lowering drug for reducing blood levels of cholesterol. It works by blocking an enzyme needed in the formation of cholesterol, and by increasing *receptors* on the cell, thereby allowing removal of cholesterol from the bloodstream. In particular, pravastatin significantly lowers the harmful low-density lipoprotein (LDL) component of cholesterol. A high blood level of cholesterol has been shown to be a risk factor in the development of atherosclerosis (narrowing of arteries). There is ongoing research to determine to what extent, if any, existing atherosclerosis can be reversed by lowering blood cholesterol.

Pravastatin is usually well tolerated with few adverse effects. It is usually reserved for use in people with important elevations of blood cholesterol who have been unsuccessfully treated with other drugs, exercise, weight control, and other measures.

QUICK REFERENCE

Drug group Lipid-lowering drug (p.115)

Overdose danger rating Low

Dependence rating Low

Prescription needed Yes

Multi-source suppliers No

INFORMATION FOR USERS

Your drug prescription is tailored for you. Do not alter dosage without checking with your physician.

How taken

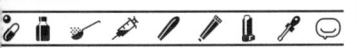

Tablets.

Frequency and timing of doses
Taken as a single dose at bedtime.

Dosage range
10 – 40mg daily.

Onset of effect
1 – 2 hours. Maximum effects on lipids within 4 weeks.

Duration of action
12 – 24 hours.

Diet advice
A low-fat, low-cholesterol diet must be maintained during treatment for the drug to be fully effective. Follow your physician's advice.

Storage
Keep in a closed container in a cool, dry place away from reach of children. Protect from light.

Missed dose
Take as soon as you remember.

Stopping the drug
Do not stop the drug without consulting your physician; stopping the drug may lead to worsening of the underlying condition.

Exceeding the dose
An occasional unintentional extra dose is unlikely to be a cause for concern. But if you notice unusual symptoms, or if a large overdose has been taken, notify your physician.

SPECIAL PRECAUTIONS

Be sure to tell your physician if:
▼ You have had epileptic seizures.
▼ You have impaired liver function.
▼ You have had problems with alcohol abuse.
▼ You have cataracts.
▼ You have muscle pains or tenderness.
▼ You are taking other medications.

Pregnancy
▼ Not prescribed.

Breast feeding
▼ Not recommended. Discuss with your physician.

Infants and children
▼ Not recommended.

Over 60
▼ The lowest possible initial dose should be administered and monitored.

Driving and hazardous work
▼ Exercise caution if dizziness or blurred vision occurs.

Alcohol
▼ Although this drug does not interact with alcohol, your underlying condition may make it inadvisable to take alcohol.

Surgery and general anesthetics
▼ Notify your physician or dentist that you are taking this drug as you may need careful monitoring or discontinuation of the drug before surgery.

POSSIBLE ADVERSE EFFECTS

Adverse effects are usually mild and transient. They may include abdominal cramps, constipation, diarrhea, nausea, headache, dizziness, and skin rashes. More severe adverse effects may include aching or cramping muscles, tiredness or weakness, fever, and blurred vision.

Symptom/effect	Frequency		Discuss with physician		Stop taking drug now	Call physician now
	Common	Rare	Only if severe	In all cases		
Cramps/diarrhea/constipation	●		■			
Nausea	●		■			
Headache/dizziness	●		■			
Skin rashes		●		■		
Muscle aches or cramping		●		■	▲	‖
Tiredness or weakness		●		■	▲	‖
Fever		●		■	▲	‖
Blurred vision		●		■	▲	‖

INTERACTIONS

Erythromycin, cyclosporine, and fibrates (e.g., gemfibrozil) Pravastatin and these drugs are not usually prescribed together because of the risk of severe muscle inflammation.

Cholestyramine and colestipol Pravastatin should not be taken together with these two drugs. Pravastatin should be given 1 hour or more before or at least 4 hours following cholestyramine and colestipol.

Oral anticoagulants Pravastatin may increase bleeding with warfarin, therefore the prothrombin time must be monitored.

PROLONGED USE

Monitoring: Regular checks on lipid blood levels, on liver function, and muscle enzymes are recommended. Periodic eye tests may also be performed.

PRAZOSIN

Brand names Minipress, Apo-Prazo, Novo-Prazin, Nu-Prazo
Used in the following combined preparations None

GENERAL INFORMATION

Prazosin is an antihypertensive drug that relieves high blood pressure by relaxing the muscles in the walls of the blood vessels, dilating them and easing the flow of blood.

In moderate to severe high blood pressure, prazosin may be given with beta blockers or other antihypertensive drugs. Prazosin may also be given in low doses to relieve symptoms caused by an enlarged prostate gland.

Dizziness and fainting are common at the onset of treatment with prazosin because of the dramatic drop in blood pressure. For this reason, the initial dose is usually low and given when the person is lying down. Dosage levels may later be increased as necessary.

INFORMATION FOR USERS

Your drug prescription is tailored for you. Do not alter dosage without checking with your physician.

How taken

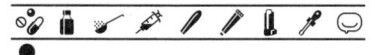

Tablets.

Frequency and timing of doses
2 – 3 x daily with food.

Adult dosage range
High blood pressure 0.5mg daily (starting dose), increased as necessary to 20mg daily (maintenance dose).
Enlarged prostate 1 – 4mg daily.

Onset of effect
Within 2 hours.

Duration of action
6 – 8 hours.

Diet advice
None.

Storage
Keep in a closed container in a cool, dry place away from reach of children.

Missed dose
Take as soon as you remember. If your next dose is due within 2 hours, take a single dose now and skip the next.

Stopping the drug
Do not stop taking the drug without consulting your physician; stopping the drug may lead to a rise in blood pressure.

Exceeding the dose
An occasional unintentional extra dose is unlikely to cause problems. Large overdoses may cause dizziness or fainting. Notify your physician.

SPECIAL PRECAUTIONS

Be sure to tell your physician if:
▼ You have impaired kidney or liver function
▼ You have heart failure.
▼ You are taking other medications.

Pregnancy
▼ Safety in pregnancy not established. Discuss with your physician.

Breast feeding
▼ The drug passes into the breast milk in small amounts. Discuss with your physician.

Infants and children
▼ Not recommended in children under 12 years.

Over 60
▼ Reduced dose may be necessary.

Driving and hazardous work
▼ Avoid such activities until you have learned how the drug affects you; it can cause drowsiness, dizziness, and fainting.

Alcohol
▼ Avoid. Alcohol may increase the adverse effects of this drug.

PROLONGED USE

No problems expected.

POSSIBLE ADVERSE EFFECTS

Prazosin may cause dizziness and fainting on rising, so it is important that the first dose is taken at bedtime. You should remain in bed for at least 3 hours after taking the drug.

Some of the minor symptoms, such as headache and nausea, will diminish after long-term therapy, although this may take up to 3 months.

Symptom/effect	Frequency		Discuss with physician		Stop taking drug now	Call physician now
	Common	Rare	Only if severe	In all cases		
Nausea	●		■			
Headache	●		■			
Dizziness/faintness	●		■			
Dry mouth	●		■			
Stuffy nose		●	■			
Weakness/drowsiness	●		■			
Palpitations	●				■	
Rash		●			■	■

INTERACTIONS

Other antihypertensive agents Beta blockers and diuretics may enhance the blood pressure-lowering effect of prazosin.

PREDNISOLONE

Brand names Diopred, Inflamase, Ophtho-Tate, Pediapred, Pred Forte, Pred Mild
Used in the following combined preparations Dioptimyd, Blephamide, Metimyd, Vasocidin

GENERAL INFORMATION

Prednisolone is a powerful cortico-steroid. It can be given by mouth for a wide range of conditions including rheumatic disorders, certain skin diseases, and allergic states.

Available as eye drops or ointment, it reduces eye inflammation in conjunctivitis and iritis.

As with other corticosteroids, low doses taken by mouth over a short term or *topical* applications rarely cause serious *side effects*. However, long-term treatment with large doses by mouth can cause fluid retention, indigestion, acne, and hypertension. Prednisolone may also induce diabetes.

QUICK REFERENCE

Drug group Corticosteroid (p.153)
Overdose danger rating Low
Dependence rating Low
Prescription needed Yes
Multi-source suppliers Yes

INFORMATION FOR USERS

Your drug prescription is tailored for you. Do not alter dosage without checking with your physician.

How taken

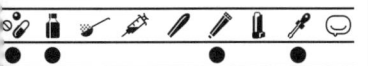

Tablets, oral solution, eye ointment, eye and ear drops.

Frequency and timing of doses
1 – 4 x daily (eye/ear preparations); single or divided doses (tablets or oral solution).

Dosage range
Considerable variation. Follow your physician's instructions.

Onset of effect
1 – 4 days.

Duration of action
12 – 72 hours.

Diet advice
A low-sodium, high-potassium diet is recommended when the oral form of the drug

is prescribed for extended periods. Follow the advice of your physician.

Storage
Keep in a closed container in a cool, dry place away from reach of children.

Missed dose
Take as soon as you remember. If your next dose is due within 6 hours, take a single dose now and skip the next.

Stopping the drug
Do not stop the drug without consulting your physician. Abrupt cessation of long-term treatment by mouth may cause severe hormonal imbalance.

Exceeding the dose
An occasional unintentional extra dose is unlikely to be a cause for concern. But if you notice unusual symptoms, or if a large overdose has been taken, notify your physician.

POSSIBLE ADVERSE EFFECTS

The rare but more serious adverse effects occur only when prednisolone is taken by mouth in high doses or for long periods of time.

Symptom/effect	Frequency		Discuss with physician		Stop taking drug now	Call physician now
	Common	Rare	Only if severe	In all cases		
Indigestion	●			■		
Acne	●			■		
Weight gain		●		■		
Muscle weakness		●		■		
Mood changes		●		■		
Bloody, black feces		●		■	▲	▮

INTERACTIONS (by mouth only)

Oral anticoagulants Prednisolone may decrease the effect of anticoagulants.

Vaccines Serious reactions can occur when vaccinations are given while taking this drug. Discuss with your physician.

Barbiturates, phenytoin, and rifampin These drugs may reduce the effect of prednisolone.

Antidiabetic drugs Prednisolone reduces the actions of these drugs.

Antihypertensive drugs Prednisolone may reduce the effect of antihypertensive drugs.

Diuretics Prednisolone may increase potassium loss with these drugs.

SPECIAL PRECAUTIONS

Be sure to tell your physician if:
▼ You have had a peptic ulcer.
▼ You have had glaucoma.
▼ You have had tuberculosis.
▼ You suffer from depression.
▼ You have a herpes infection.
▼ You have diabetes.
▼ You are taking other medications.

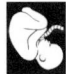

Pregnancy
▼ No evidence of risk with eye/ear preparations. Given as tablets in low doses, harm to the baby is unlikely. Discuss with your physician.

Breast feeding
▼ No evidence of risk with eye/ear preparations. Taken by mouth, the drug passes into the breast milk and if taken regularly may adversely affect the baby. Discuss with your physician.

Infants and children
▼ Reduced dose may be necessary.

Over 60
▼ Increased likelihood of adverse effects. Reduced dose may therefore be necessary.

Driving and hazardous work
▼ No known problems.

Alcohol
▼ Alcohol may increase the risk of peptic ulcers with prednisolone by mouth. No special problems with eye/ear preparations.

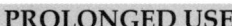

PROLONGED USE

Prolonged use of prednisolone in high doses by mouth is recommended only when essential because it can lead to adverse conditions such as diabetes, glaucoma, cataracts, and fragile bones, and may retard growth in children.

PREDNISONE

Brand names Deltasone, Apo-Prednisone, Novo-Prednisone, Winpred
Used in the following combined preparations None

GENERAL INFORMATION

Prednisone, introduced in 1955, is a long-acting, synthetic corticosteroid drug used in the treatment of a variety of inflammatory disorders, including inflammatory bowel disease, and connective tissue diseases and joint disorders such as rheumatoid arthritis. Severe asthma may also be controlled by regular administration of prednisone.

Less common uses of the drug include the prevention of organ transplant rejection, replacement therapy in Addison's disease, and treatment of blood disorders such as thrombocytopenia and leukemia, when it is often used in conjunction with other drugs.

Used in low doses, prednisone seldom causes troublesome *side effects*. However, large doses taken over a prolonged period can cause adverse effects such as indigestion, mood changes, muscle weakness, bone damage and fractures, fluid retention, acne, diabetes mellitus, facial rounding, excessive hair, cataracts, and hypertension.

INFORMATION FOR USERS

Your drug prescription is tailored for you. Do not alter dosage without checking with your physician.

How taken

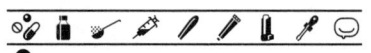

Tablets.

Frequency and timing of doses
Varies according to condition.

Dosage range
Varies according to condition.

Onset of effect
1 – 4 days.

Duration of action
Up to 24 hours.

Diet advice
A low-sodium and high-potassium diet may be required when prednisone is taken for extended periods. Follow your physician's advice.

Storage
Keep in a closed container in a cool, dry place away from reach of children.

Missed dose
Take as soon as you remember. If your next dose is scheduled within 4 hours, take both doses now.

Stopping the drug
Do not stop the drug without consulting your physician. A gradual reduction in dose is required following prolonged treatment.

Exceeding the dose
An occasional unintentional extra dose is unlikely to be a cause for concern. But if you notice unusual symptoms, or if a large overdose has been taken, notify your physician.

SPECIAL PRECAUTIONS

Be sure to tell your physician if:
▼ You have had a peptic ulcer.
▼ You have glaucoma.
▼ You have any infection.
▼ You have suffered from depression or psychotic illness.
▼ You have diabetes.
▼ You have had tuberculosis.
▼ You are taking other medications.

Pregnancy
▼ Not usually prescribed. Safety in pregnancy not established. Discuss with your physician.

Breast feeding
▼ The drug passes into the breast milk and may affect the baby adversely. Discuss with your physician.

Infants and children
▼ Only given when essential. Reduced dose necessary.

Over 60
▼ Increased likelihood of adverse effects. Reduced dose may therefore be necessary.

Driving and hazardous work
▼ No known problems.

Alcohol
▼ Avoid. Alcohol may increase the risk of developing peptic ulcers.

POSSIBLE ADVERSE EFFECTS

Adverse effects are uncommon at low doses; serious adverse effects occur only when prednisone is taken in high doses or for long periods.

Symptom/effect	Frequency		Discuss with physician		Stop taking drug now	Call physician now
	Common	Rare	Only if severe	In all cases		
Indigestion	●			■		
Acne	●			■		
Weight gain		●		■		
Muscle weakness		●		■		
Mood changes		●		■		
Black/bloodstained feces		●		■	▲	▮

INTERACTIONS

Antidiabetic drugs Prednisone reduces the actions of these drugs.

Antihypertensive drugs Prednisone may reduce the effect of antihypertensives.

Oral anticoagulant drugs Prednisone may increase or decrease blood clotting.

Barbiturates, phenytoin, and rifampin These drugs reduce the effectiveness of prednisone.

Vaccines Serious reactions can occur when vaccinations are given with this drug. Discuss with your physician.

PROLONGED USE

Prolonged use of this drug in high doses is recommended only when essential because it can lead to adverse effects such as diabetes, glaucoma, cataracts, and fragile bones, and may retard growth in children.

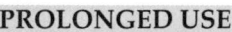

PRIMIDONE

Brand names Mysoline, Apo-Primidone
Used in the following combined preparations None

GENERAL INFORMATION

Introduced in 1954, primidone belongs to a group of drugs known as anti-convulsants. It is chemically related to the barbiturates (see Sleeping drugs, p.94) and is partially converted to phenobarbital in the body. Primidone is mainly used for its effect in suppressing epileptic seizures. However, it is also occasionally prescribed to treat people who suffer from benign tremors.

Though it may be prescribed on its own, it is more frequently taken with another anticonvulsant. Its major adverse effects are due to its sedative action on the central nervous system.

QUICK REFERENCE

Drug group Anticonvulsant (p.98)
Overdose danger rating High
Dependence rating Medium
Prescription needed Yes
Multi-source suppliers Yes

INFORMATION FOR USERS

Your drug prescription is tailored for you. Do not alter dosage without checking with your physician.

How taken

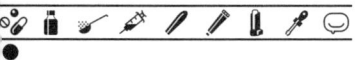

Tablets, chewable tablets.

Frequency and timing of doses
1 – 4 x daily.

Adult dosage range
250mg – 2g daily.

Onset of effect
Within 30 minutes.

Duration of action
Up to 24 hours.

Diet advice
None.

Storage
Keep in a closed container in a cool, dry place away from reach of children.

Missed dose
Take as soon as you remember. If your next dose is due within 2 hours, wait for 6 hours to take it.

Stopping the drug
Do not stop the drug without consulting your physician; symptoms may recur and withdrawal reactions can result.

OVERDOSE ACTION

Seek immediate medical advice in all cases. Take emergency action if consciousness is lost.

See Drug poisoning emergency guide (p.574).

POSSIBLE ADVERSE EFFECTS

Most people experience very few adverse effects with this drug, but when blood levels get too high, adverse effects are common and the dose may need to be reduced.

Symptom/effect	Frequency		Discuss with physician		Stop taking drug now	Call physician now
	Common	Rare	Only if severe	In all cases		
Drowsiness	●		■			
Clumsiness/unsteadiness	●		■			
Dizziness/lightheadedness	●		■			
Headache	●		■			
Nausea/vomiting		●	■			
Rash		●		■	▲	■

INTERACTIONS

Sedatives All drugs that have a sedative effect on the central nervous system are likely to increase the sedative effects of primidone. Such drugs include other anticonvulsants, antihistamines, sleeping drugs, narcotic analgesics, antipsychotics, and antidepressants.

Anticoagulant drugs Primidone may reduce the effect of anticoagulant drugs. The anticoagulant dose may need to be adjusted accordingly.

Tricyclic antidepressants Use of tricyclic antidepressants may counteract the effect of primidone.

Oral contraceptives Primidone may reduce the effectiveness of oral contraceptives. An alternative form of contraception may need to be used. Discuss with your physician.

Corticosteroids Primidone opposes the action of some of these drugs. The corticosteroid dose may need to be adjusted accordingly.

SPECIAL PRECAUTIONS

Be sure to tell your physician if:
▼ You have impaired kidney or liver function.
▼ You have heart problems.
▼ You have poor circulation.
▼ You have a lung disorder such as asthma or bronchitis.
▼ You have porphyria.
▼ You are taking other medications.

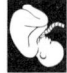

Pregnancy
▼ Not usually prescribed. May cause abnormalities in the unborn baby. Discuss with your physician.

Breast feeding
▼ The drug passes into the breast milk and may affect the baby. Discuss with your physician.

Infants and children
▼ Reduced dose necessary.

Over 60
▼ May cause unusual excitement in the elderly. Reduced dose may be necessary.

Driving and hazardous work
▼ Your underlying condition, as well as the possibility of reduced alertness while taking this drug, may make such activities inadvisable. Discuss with your physician.

Alcohol
▼ Avoid. Alcohol may dangerously increase the sedative effects of this drug.

PROLONGED USE

Continued use of this drug may sometimes lead to *dependence*.

Monitoring Regular blood tests may be performed to measure blood levels of primidone.

PROBENECID

Brand names Benemid, Benuryl
Used in the following combined preparations None

GENERAL INFORMATION

Probenecid is prescribed for people who suffer from recurrent attacks of gout. It reduces the level of uric acid in the body by increasing the amount excreted in the urine. It is used for the long-term prevention of gout attacks, not for the inflammation and pain once an attack has begun. During the first 6 months of treatment, attacks may even be more frequent, and another drug may be given in addition to probenecid during this period.

Probenecid is occasionally prescribed to boost the effect of penicillin or cephalosporin antibiotics in the treatment of certain infections, since it blocks excretion of these antibiotics by the kidneys, thereby increasing their levels in the blood.

Serious adverse reactions are rare, though by increasing uric acid excretion, probenecid can increase the risk of uric acid kidney stones.

INFORMATION FOR USERS

Your drug prescription is tailored for you. Do not alter dosage without checking with your physician.

How taken

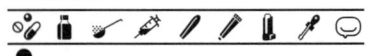

Tablets.

Frequency and timing of doses
1 – 2 x daily with food (gout); 4 x daily or as a single dose treatment (with penicillin or cephalosporin antibiotics).

Dosage range
Gout 0.5g daily for 1 week then 1 – 2g daily. *With penicillin or cephalosporin antibiotics* 2g daily.

Onset of effect
Within 2 – 4 hours. Full beneficial effects in gout may not be seen for several weeks.

Duration of action
4 – 16 hours.

Diet advice
Drink at least 2 litres of fluids daily.

Storage
Keep in a closed container in a cool, dry place away from reach of children. Protect from light.

Missed dose
Take as soon as you remember. If your next dose is due within 4 hours, take a single dose now and skip the next.

Stopping the drug
Do not stop the drug without consulting your physician; symptoms may recur.

Exceeding the dose
An occasional unintentional extra dose is unlikely to cause problems. Large overdoses may cause nausea, vomiting, or tremors. Notify your physician.

POSSIBLE ADVERSE EFFECTS

Most people do not feel any severe adverse effects when taking probenecid. The more common ones usually diminish as your body adjusts to the medicine. However, excretion of uric acid crystals can lead to the passing of blood and painful urination.

Symptom/effect	Frequency		Discuss with physician		Stop taking drug now	Call physician now
	Common	Rare	Only if severe	In all cases		
Nausea/vomiting	●		■			
Headache/dizziness	●		■			
Flushing		●		■		
Blood in urine		●		■	▲	▮
Painful urination		●		■		▮
Rash/itching		●		■	▲	▮

INTERACTIONS

General note Many drugs affect the action of probenecid and may require an adjustment of dosage. Some may reduce the effect of probenecid (for example, thiazide diuretics, ASA, and alcohol); and others may have their effects and/or

toxicity increased by probenecid (for example, oral antidiabetic drugs, indomethacin, sulfonamides, acyclovir, and methotrexate). Do not take any over-the-counter products containing ASA while on probenecid therapy.

SPECIAL PRECAUTIONS

Be sure to tell your physician if:
▼ You have impaired kidney function.
▼ You have had a blood disorder.
▼ You have had kidney stones.
▼ You have had a peptic ulcer.
▼ You are taking other medications.

Pregnancy
▼ Safety in pregnancy not established. Discuss with your physician.

Breast feeding
▼ The drug passes into the breast milk and may affect the baby. Discuss with your physician.

Infants and children
▼ Not recommended for children under 2 years. Reduced dose necessary in older children.

Over 60
▼ Reduced dose may be necessary.

Driving and hazardous work
▼ No known problems.

Alcohol
▼ Avoid excessive amounts.

PROLONGED USE

No problems expected.

Monitoring Periodic blood tests may be carried out to ensure that blood levels of uric acid are normal and that anemia does not occur.

PROCAINAMIDE

Brand names Pronestyl, Apo-Procainamide, Procan SR
Used in the following combined preparations None

GENERAL INFORMATION

Procainamide was introduced in the 1940s as an anti-arrhythmic drug. It is used to treat abnormal heart rhythms of the ventricles that cause important symptoms or that are life-threatening. It may be administered when lidocaine, a more commonly used anti-arrhythmic, is unsuccessful.

Procainamide is often given initially in the hospital, where its effect on the heartbeat can be carefully monitored.

Many of the adverse effects common to anti-arrhythmics occur less often with procainamide. However, when taken over a long period, a drug-induced lupus erythematosus-like syndrome may occur in some people, thus limiting procainamide's usefulness.

QUICK REFERENCE

Drug group Anti-arrhythmic drug (p.112)

Overdose danger rating Medium

Dependence rating Low

Prescription needed Yes

Multi-source suppliers Yes

INFORMATION FOR USERS

Your drug prescription is tailored for you. Do not alter dosage without checking with your physician.

How taken

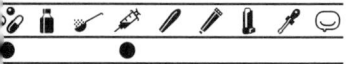

Slow-release tablets, capsules, injection.

Frequency and timing of doses
Every 4 – 6 hours (capsules); every 6 – 8 hours (slow-release tablets).

Adult dosage range
2 – 4g daily (by mouth).

Onset of effect
30 – 60 minutes.

Duration of action
4 – 6 hours (capsules); 6 – 8 hours (slow-release tablets).

Diet advice
No special problems.

Storage
Keep in a closed container in a cool, dry place away from reach of children. Protect from light.

Missed dose
Take as soon as you remember. If your next dose is due within 2 hours (4 hours for slow-release tablets), take a single dose now and skip the next.

Stopping the drug
Do not stop the drug without consulting your physician; symptoms may recur.

Exceeding the dose
An occasional unintentional extra dose is unlikely to cause problems. Large overdoses may cause palpitations, lethargy, confusion, nausea, and vomiting. Notify your physician.

POSSIBLE ADVERSE EFFECTS

Some of the minor symptoms, such as loss of appetite, nausea, and vomiting are common to many anti-arrhythmic drugs. The more serious effects occur much less frequently with procainamide than with other similar drugs (see also Prolonged Use).

Symptom/effect	Frequency		Discuss with physician		Stop taking drug now	Call physician now
	Common	Rare	Only if severe	In all cases		
Nausea/vomiting/diarrhea	●		■			
Loss of appetite	●		■			
Fever/chills		●		■		
Joint pain and swelling		●		■		
Confusion/lethargy		●		■		
Rash		●		■	▲	▮

SPECIAL PRECAUTIONS

Be sure to tell your physician if:
▼ You have impaired kidney or liver function.
▼ You have a lung disorder such as asthma or bronchitis.
▼ You have myasthenia gravis.
▼ You have had lupus erythematosus.
▼ You are taking other medications.

Pregnancy
▼ Safety in pregnancy not established. Discuss with your physician.

Breast feeding
▼ The drug passes into the breast milk and may affect the baby. Discuss with your physician.

Infants and children
▼ Safety and effectiveness not established in children.

Over 60
▼ Reduced dose may be necessary.

Driving and hazardous work
▼ No special problems.

Alcohol
▼ No special problems.

Surgery and general anesthetics
▼ Procainamide may interact with some anesthetic agents. Make sure your treatment is known to your physician or dentist and anesthetist before any surgery.

INTERACTIONS

General note Many drugs may interact with procainamide. Check with your physician or pharmacist before taking any medication.

Antihypertensive drugs These drugs increase the likelihood of excessively lowered blood pressure.

Anticholinergic drugs Procainamide enhances the effect of *anticholinergic* drugs. Such a combination should be used with extreme caution.

PROLONGED USE

Prolonged use of this drug may lead to lupus erythematosus-like symptoms, including fever, joint pain, swelling, and rash. These effects usually disappear when the drug is discontinued.

PROCHLORPERAZINE

Brand names Stemetil, Nu-Prochlor, PMS-Prochlorperazine
Used in the following combined preparations None

GENERAL INFORMATION

Prochlorperazine, introduced in the late 1950s, belongs to a group of drugs called phenothiazines, which act on the central nervous system.

In small doses, it controls nausea and vomiting, especially when they occur as the aftereffects of medical treatment by drugs, radiation, or anesthesia. In large doses, it is effective as an antipsychotic, suppressing abnormal behavior, reducing aggressiveness, and producing a generally tranquilizing effect (see p.97). It thus minimizes and controls the abnormal behavior associated with schizophrenia, mania, dementia, and other mental disorders. It does not cure these diseases but helps relieve symptoms.

INFORMATION FOR USERS

Your drug prescription is tailored for you. Do not alter dosage without checking with your physician.

How taken

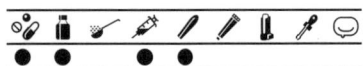

Tablets, oral liquid, injection, rectal suppositories.

Frequency and timing of doses
3 – 4 x daily (tablets); 2 x daily (rectal suppositories); every 2 – 4 hours (injection).

Adult dosage range
Nausea and vomiting 5 – 10mg per dose (tablets); 25mg per dose (rectal suppositories). *Mental illness* 15 – 40mg daily. Larger doses may be given in exceptional circumstances.

Onset of effect
Within 60 minutes by suppository, 30 – 40 minutes by mouth, 10 – 20 minutes by injection.

Duration of action
3 – 4 hours.

Diet advice
None.

Storage
Keep in a closed container in a cool, dry place away from reach of children. Protect from light.

Missed dose
Take as soon as you remember. If your next dose is due within 2 hours, do not take the missed dose; take the next scheduled dose as usual.

Stopping the drug
Do not stop the drug without consulting your physician; symptoms may recur.

Exceeding the dose
An occasional unintentional extra dose is unlikely to cause problems. Large overdoses may cause unusual drowsiness. Notify your physician.

SPECIAL PRECAUTIONS

Be sure to tell your physician if:
▼ You have heart problems.
▼ You have impaired kidney or liver function.
▼ You have prostate trouble.
▼ You have glaucoma.
▼ You have had epileptic seizures.
▼ You have Parkinson's disease.
▼ You have an overactive thyroid gland.
▼ You are taking other medications.

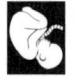

Pregnancy
▼ Safety in pregnancy not established. Discuss with your physician.

Breast feeding
▼ The drug passes into the breast milk and may affect the baby. Discuss with your physician.

Infants and children
▼ Not recommended in patients under 2 years. Reduced dose necessary in older children.

Over 60
▼ Increased likelihood of adverse effects. Reduced dose may therefore be necessary.

Driving and hazardous work
▼ Avoid such activities until you have learned how the drug affects you; it can cause drowsiness and reduced alertness.

Alcohol
▼ Avoid. Alcohol may increase and prolong the sedative effects of this drug.

POSSIBLE ADVERSE EFFECTS

Prochlorperazine has a strong *anticholinergic* effect, which can cause a variety of minor adverse effects. These often become less marked with time. The most significant adverse effect with high doses is abnormal movements of the face and limbs (*parkinsonism*) caused by changes in the balance of chemicals in the brain.

Symptom/effect	Frequency		Discuss with physician		Stop taking drug now	Call physician now
	Common	Rare	Only if severe	In all cases		
Drowsiness/lethargy	●		■			
Dry mouth	●		■			
Blurred vision	●			■		
Dizziness/fainting	●			■		
Parkinsonism	●			■		
Rash		●		■	▲	

PROLONGED USE

Use of this drug for more than a few months may lead to the development of involuntary, potentially irreversible movements of the eyes, mouth, and tongue (*tardive dyskinesia*). Occasionally jaundice may occur.

Monitoring Periodic blood tests may be performed.

INTERACTIONS

Sedatives All drugs, including alcohol, that have a sedative effect on the central nervous system are likely to increase the sedative effects of prochlorperazine.

Anticonvulsants and antiparkinsonian drugs Prochlorperazine may reduce the effectiveness of these drugs.

Anticholinergic drugs Prochlorperazine may increase the side effects of these drugs.

PROCYCLIDINE

Brand names Kemadrin, PMS Procyclidine, Procyclid
Used in the following combined preparations None

GENERAL INFORMATION

Introduced in 1956, procyclidine is an *anticholinergic* drug that is used to treat Parkinson's disease. It is particularly helpful in the early stages of the disorder for treating muscle rigidity. It also helps to reduce excess salivation and to some extent the tremor. However, it has little effect on the shuffling gait and slow muscular movements that are also characteristic of Parkinson's disease.

Procyclidine may also be used to treat *parkinsonism* resulting from treatment with antipsychotic drugs.

The drug may cause a number of minor adverse effects (see below), but these are rarely sufficiently serious to warrant stopping treatment.

INFORMATION FOR USERS

Your drug prescription is tailored for you. **Do not alter dosage without checking with your physician.**

How taken

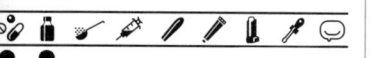

Tablets, oral liquid.

Frequency and timing of doses
3 x daily after meals.

Adult dosage range
2.5 – 20mg daily. Dosage with this drug has to be determined individually in order to find the best balance between effective relief of symptoms and the occurrence of adverse effects.

Onset of effect
Within 30 minutes.

Duration of action
8 – 12 hours.

Diet advice
None.

Storage
Keep in a closed container in a cool, dry place away from reach of children.

Missed dose
Take as soon as you remember. If your next dose is due within 2 hours, take a single dose now and skip the next.

Stopping the drug
Do not stop the drug without consulting your physician; symptoms may recur.

OVERDOSE ACTION

 Seek immediate medical advice in all cases. Take emergency action if palpitations, seizures, or unconsciousness occurs.

See Drug poisoning emergency guide (p.574).

POSSIBLE ADVERSE EFFECTS

The possible adverse effects of procyclidine are mainly the result of its anticholinergic action. Some of the more common symptoms, such as dry mouth, constipation, and blurred vision, may be overcome by adjustment of dosage.

Symptom/effect	Frequency		Discuss with physician		Stop taking drug now	Call physician now
	Common	Rare	Only if severe	In all cases		
Dry mouth	●		■			
Constipation	●		■			
Nervousness	●		■			
Blurred vision	●			■		
Confusion		●		■		
Nausea/vomiting		●		■		
Rash		●		■	▲	
Difficulty in passing urine		●		■		
Palpitations		●		■	▲	■

INTERACTIONS

Anticholinergic drugs and antihistamines These drugs may increase the adverse effects of procyclidine.

Alcohol may increase the sedative effect of procyclidine.

SPECIAL PRECAUTIONS

Be sure to tell your physician if:
▼ You have impaired kidney or liver function.
▼ You have had glaucoma.
▼ You have high blood pressure.
▼ You suffer from constipation.
▼ You have prostate trouble.
▼ You have had peptic ulcers.
▼ You are taking other medications.

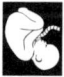 **Pregnancy**
▼ Safety in pregnancy not established. Discuss with your physician.

 Breast feeding
▼ The drug passes into the breast milk and may affect the baby. Discuss with your physician.

 Infants and children
▼ Not recommended.

 Over 60
▼ Increased likelihood of adverse effects. Reduced dose may therefore be necessary.

 Driving and hazardous work
▼ Avoid such activities until you have learned how the drug affects you; it can cause drowsiness, blurred vision, and mild confusion.

 Alcohol
▼ Avoid. Alcohol may increase the adverse effects of this drug.

PROLONGED USE

Prolonged use of this drug may provoke the onset of glaucoma.

Monitoring Periodic eye examinations are usually required.

PROMETHAZINE

Brand names Phenergan, Histantil, PMS Promethazine
Used in the following combined preparations Pamergan, Phenergan Expectorant, Phenergan VC Expectorant

GENERAL INFORMATION

Promethazine is one of the pheno-thiazines, a class of drugs developed in the 1950s for their beneficial effect on abnormal behavior arising from mental illnesses (see Antipsychotic drugs, p.97). Promethazine was, however, found to have effects more like the antihistamines used to treat allergies (see p.136) and some types of nausea and vomiting (see Anti-emetic drugs, p.102). It is primarily used for such conditions, though it is sometimes combined with certain narcotics to increase their effect.

Promethazine is widely used to reduce itching in a variety of skin conditions including urticaria (hives), chickenpox, and eczema. It can also relieve the nausea and vomiting caused by inner ear disturbances such as motion sickness and Ménière's disease. Because of its sedative effect, promethazine is sometimes given as *premedication* before surgery.

Promethazine is sometimes combined with codeine or other ingredients for the relief of allergy-related coughs and nasal congestion.

INFORMATION FOR USERS

Follow instructions on the label. Call your physician if symptoms worsen.

How taken

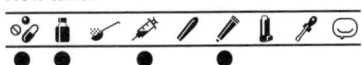

Tablets, oral liquid, injection, cream.

Frequency and timing of doses
Allergic symptoms 1 – 4 x daily or as a single dose at night.
Nausea and vomiting Every 4 – 6 hours as necessary.

Dosage range
Adults 10 – 25mg per dose – up to 100mg/24 hours.
Children Reduced dose according to age and weight.
Topical Apply cream 2 or 3 times daily to affected area. Avoid application to extensive skin areas.

Onset of effect
Within 1 hour. If dose is taken after nausea has started, the onset of effect is delayed.

Duration of action
12 – 24 hours.

Diet advice
None.

Storage
Keep in a closed container in a cool, dry place away from reach of children. Protect from light.

Missed dose
No cause for concern, but take as soon as you remember. Adjust the timing of your next dose accordingly.

Stopping the drug
Can be safely stopped as soon as symptoms disappear.

Exceeding the dose
An occasional unintentional extra dose is unlikely to cause problems. Large overdoses may cause drowsiness, unsteadiness, or agitation. Notify your physician.

SPECIAL PRECAUTIONS

Be sure to consult your physician or pharmacist before taking this drug if:
▼ You have impaired kidney or liver function.
▼ You have had epileptic seizures.
▼ You have heart disease.
▼ You have glaucoma.
▼ You have Parkinson's disease.
▼ You have urinary difficulties.
▼ You are taking other medications.

Pregnancy
▼ Safety in pregnancy not established. Discuss with your physician.

Breast feeding
▼ The drug passes into the breast milk, but at normal doses adverse effects on the baby are unlikely. Discuss with your physician.

Infants and children
▼ Not recommended in patients under 2 years. Reduced dose necessary for older children.

Over 60
▼ No special problems.

Driving and hazardous work
▼ Avoid such activities until you have learned how the drug affects you; it can cause drowsiness.

Alcohol
▼ Avoid. Alcohol may increase the sedative effects of this drug.

POSSIBLE ADVERSE EFFECTS

Promethazine usually causes only minor *anticholinergic* effects. More serious adverse effects generally occur only during long-term use or with abnormally high doses.

Symptom/effect	Frequency		Discuss with physician		Stop taking drug now	Call physician now
	Common	Rare	Only if severe	In all cases		
Drowsiness/lethargy	●		■			
Dry mouth	●		■			
Blurred vision	●		■			
Light-sensitive rash		●		■		▲

INTERACTIONS

Alcohol and other sedatives All drugs, including alcohol, that have a sedative effect are likely to increase the sedative effects of promethazine. Such drugs include antihistamines, sleeping drugs, and antipsychotics.

Antacids may reduce the absorption of promethazine from the stomach, thus preventing its full effect from being felt. Antacids and promethazine should be taken at least 1 hour apart.

PROLONGED USE

Use of this drug for extended periods is rarely necessary, but may sometimes cause abnormal movements of the face and limbs (*parkinsonism*). The problem normally disappears when the drug is stopped.

PROPOXYPHENE

Brand names Darvon-N, Novo-Propoxyn, 642 Tablets
Used in the following combined preparations Darvon-N with ASA, Darvon-N Compound, 692 Tablets

GENERAL INFORMATION

Propoxyphene is a weak narcotic analgesic used to relieve mild or moderate pain. It is not useful for severe pain. Longer-lasting than many other drugs of this class, it may be more convenient for relief of chronic pain. It may sometimes be given in combination with another analgesic, such as ASA or acetaminophen, to boost its effect.

High doses of propoxyphene taken for prolonged periods may lead to physical *dependence* on the drug. However, it is less addictive than other similar drugs, and most people are able to stop treatment without difficulty.

Side effects such as dizziness, drowsiness, and nausea are more common in active people and can often be overcome by rest.

INFORMATION FOR USERS

Your drug prescription is tailored for you. Do not alter dosage without checking with your physician.

How taken

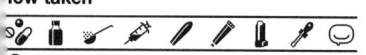

Tablets, capsules.

Frequency and timing of doses
1 – 4 x daily.

Adult dosage range
65mg or 100mg per dose depending on preparation, up to a maximum of 6 doses in 24 hours.

Onset of effect
15 – 60 minutes.

Duration of action
6 – 12 hours.

Diet advice
None.

Storage
Keep in a closed container in a cool, dry place away from reach of children. Protect from light.

Missed dose
Take as soon as you remember if required for pain.

Stopping the drug
If you have been taking the drug for less than 2 weeks, it can be safely stopped as soon as you no longer need it. However, if you have been regularly taking it for longer than this, consult your physician, who may supervise a gradual reduction in dosage.

OVERDOSE ACTION

 Seek immediate medical advice in all cases. Take emergency action if breathing difficulties, seizures, or loss of consciousness occurs.

See Drug poisoning emergency guide (p.574).

SPECIAL PRECAUTIONS

Be sure to tell your physician if:
▼ You have impaired kidney or liver function.
▼ You have a lung disorder such as asthma or bronchitis.
▼ You have had problems with alcohol or drug abuse.
▼ You are taking other medications.

 **Pregnancy**
▼ Safety in pregnancy not established. Discuss with your physician.

 Breast feeding
▼ The drug passes into the breast milk, but at normal doses adverse effects on the baby are unlikely. Discuss with your physician.

 Infants and children
▼ Not recommended.

 Over 60
▼ Reduced dose may be necessary.

 Driving and hazardous work
▼ Avoid such activities until you have learned how the drug affects you; it can cause drowsiness and dizziness.

 Alcohol
▼ Avoid. Alcohol may markedly increase the sedative effects of this drug.

PROLONGED USE

The effects of the drug may become weaker during prolonged use as the body adapts. It may also be habit-forming if taken for extended periods in higher-than-recommended doses.

POSSIBLE ADVERSE EFFECTS

Minor side effects are common with propoxyphene, but often wear off with continued use. Dizziness, drowsiness, and nausea are often relieved by lying down and resting. Serious adverse effects are rare except in overdose.

Symptom/effect	Frequency		Discuss with physician		Stop taking drug now	Call physician now
	Common	Rare	Only if severe	In all cases		
Dizziness/drowsiness	●			■		
Nausea/vomiting	●			■		
Headache		●		■		
Constipation		●		■		
Confusion		●			■	▮
Rash		●		■	▲	▮

INTERACTIONS

Sedatives All drugs, including alcohol, that have a *sedative* effect on the central nervous system are likely to increase sedation with propoxyphene.

PROPRANOLOL

Brand names Inderal, Apo-Propranolol, Novo-Pranol, PMS Propranolol
Used in the following combined preparation Inderide

GENERAL INFORMATION

Propranolol was the first of the beta blockers to become widely available. It is most often used to treat hypertension, angina, and abnormal heart rhythms, and to prevent further damage to the heart following a heart attack. It is also helpful in controlling symptoms caused by overactivity of the thyroid gland and in reducing the palpitations, sweating, and tremor caused by severe anxiety. It is used to prevent migraine as well.

Because propranolol can cause breathing difficulties, it is not prescribed to anyone suffering from asthma, chronic bronchitis, or emphysema. Propranolol, like all beta blockers, affects the body's response to low blood sugar; it should be used with caution by diabetics.

INFORMATION FOR USERS

Your drug prescription is tailored for you. Do not alter dosage without checking with your physician.

How taken

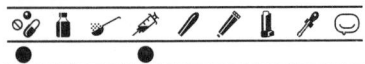

Tablets, slow-release capsules, injection.

Frequency and timing of doses
2 – 4 x daily (tablets); once daily (slow-release capsules).

Adult dosage range
Abnormal heart rhythms 30 – 120mg daily.
Angina 40 – 80mg daily (starting dose); 160 – 400mg daily (maintenance dose).
Hypertension 160 – 320mg daily.
Migraine prevention 80 – 160mg daily.

Onset of effect
1 – 2 hours (tablets); after 6 hours (slow-release capsules). In hypertension and migraine, it may be several weeks before full benefits of this drug are felt.

Duration of action
6 – 12 hours (tablets); 24 – 30 hours (slow-release capsules).

Diet advice
None.

Storage
Keep in a closed container in a cool, dry place away from reach of children. Protect from light.

Missed dose
Take as soon as you remember. If your next dose is due within 2 hours (tablets) or 12 hours (slow-release capsules), take a single dose now and skip the next.

Stopping the drug
Do not stop the drug without consulting your physician. Abrupt cessation may lead to dangerous worsening of the underlying condition or precipitate a heart attack.

OVERDOSE ACTION

Seek immediate medical advice in all cases. Take emergency action if breathing difficulties, collapse, or loss of consciousness occurs.

See Drug poisoning emergency guide (p.574).

SPECIAL PRECAUTIONS

Be sure to tell your physician if:
▼ You have impaired kidney or liver function.
▼ You have a lung disorder such as asthma, bronchitis, or emphysema.
▼ You have allergies.
▼ You have heart failure.
▼ You have diabetes.
▼ You have poor circulation in the legs.
▼ You are taking other medications.

Pregnancy
▼ Safety in pregnancy not established. Discuss with your physician.

Breast feeding
▼ The drug passes into breast milk, but at normal doses adverse effects on the baby are unlikely. Discuss with your physician.

Infants and children
▼ Reduced dose necessary.

Over 60
▼ Increased risk of adverse effects.

Driving and hazardous work
▼ Avoid such activities until you have learned how the drug affects you because the drug can cause dizziness and lightheadedness.

Alcohol
▼ No special problems with moderate intake.

Surgery and general anesthetics
▼ Propranolol may need to be stopped before you have a general anesthetic. Discuss this with your physician or dentist before any surgery.

PROLONGED USE

No problems expected.

POSSIBLE ADVERSE EFFECTS

Propranolol has adverse effects that are common to most beta blockers. Symptoms such as fatigue, nausea, and vomiting are usually temporary and diminish with long-term use. Fainting may be a sign that the drug has slowed the heartbeat excessively.

Symptom/effect	Frequency		Discuss with physician		Stop taking drug now	Call physician now
	Common	Rare	Only if severe	In all cases		
Lethargy/fatigue	●		■			
Nightmares/vivid dreams	●			■		
Cold hands and feet	●		■			
Impotence		●		■		
Rash		●		■		
Fainting/breathlessness		●		■	▲	■

INTERACTIONS

General note Propranolol may interact with many drugs, most notably NSAIDs (reduced antihypertensive effect), calcium channel blockers (decreased blood pressure and/or heart rate and/or force of pumping action), cimetidine (increased blood levels of propranolol).

PROPYLTHIOURACIL

Brand name Propyl-Thyracil
Used in the following combined preparations None

GENERAL INFORMATION

Propylthiouracil is an antithyroid drug used to manage an overactive thyroid gland (thyrotoxicosis). In some people, particularly those with Grave's disease (the commonest form of this disorder), drug treatment alone may bring on a remission. It may also be prescribed for long-term treatment of the disease in those who may be at special risk from surgery, such as children and pregnant women.

Propylthiouracil is also employed in the following circumstances: to restore the normal functioning of the gland before its partial removal by surgery, to intensify its absorption of radioactive iodine when that cell-destroying drug is used, or to prevent a harmful release of hormones that can sometimes follow the use of radioactive iodine. More effective than other antithyroid drugs in the treatment of thyrotoxic crisis (thyroid storm), propylthiouracil is also thought to cross the placenta less readily than similar drugs do, and it is preferred when treatment is essential during pregnancy.

The major possible adverse effect of this drug is a reduction in white blood cells, leading to risk of infection.

QUICK REFERENCE

Drug group Antithyroid drug (p.156)

Overdose danger rating Medium

Dependence rating Low

Prescription needed Yes

Multi-source suppliers No

INFORMATION FOR USERS

Your drug prescription is tailored for you. Do not alter dosage without consulting your physician.

How taken

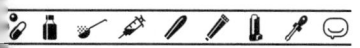

Tablets.

Frequency and timing of doses
Every 6 – 8 hours. May be given every 4 – 6 hours for treatment of thyrotoxic crisis.

Dosage range
Adults 100 – 900mg daily depending on the condition under treatment.
Children Reduced dose according to age and weight.

Onset of effect
1 – 20 days. Full beneficial effects may not be felt for 6 – 10 weeks.

Duration of action
24 – 36 hours.

Diet advice
Your physician may advise you to avoid foods that are high in iodine (see p.522).

Storage
Keep in a closed container in a cool, dry place away from reach of children. Protect from light.

Missed dose
Take as soon as you remember. If your next dose is due, take the missed dose and the next scheduled dose together.

Stopping the drug
Do not stop the drug without consulting your physician; stopping the drug may lead to a recurrence of thyrotoxicosis.

Exceeding the dose
An occasional unintentional extra dose is unlikely to cause problems. Large overdoses may cause nausea, vomiting, and headache. Notify your physician.

SPECIAL PRECAUTIONS

Be sure to tell your physician if:
▼ You have impaired kidney or liver function.
▼ You are taking other medications.

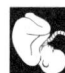

Pregnancy
▼ Prescribed with caution. May cause goiter and thyroid hormone deficiency (hypothyroidism) in the newborn infant if too high a dose is used. Discuss with your physician.

Breast feeding
▼ The drug passes into the breast milk and may affect the baby. Discuss with your physician.

Infants and children
▼ Reduced dose necessary.

Over 60
▼ No special problems.

Driving and hazardous work
▼ Avoid such activities until you have learned how the drug affects you, because the drug may cause dizziness and drowsiness.

Alcohol
▼ No known problems.

POSSIBLE ADVERSE EFFECTS

Serious *side effects* are rare with propylthiouracil. Skin rashes and itching are fairly common, although itching may sometimes be caused by overactivity of the thyroid gland. Sore throat or fever may indicate reduced white blood cell production.

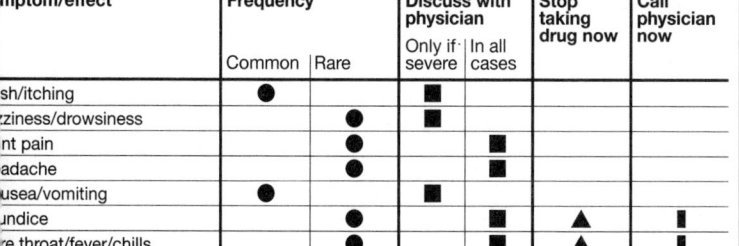

Symptom/effect	Frequency		Discuss with physician		Stop taking drug now	Call physician now
	Common	Rare	Only if severe	In all cases		
Rash/itching	●		■			
Dizziness/drowsiness		●	■			
Joint pain		●		■		
Headache		●		■		
Nausea/vomiting	●		■			
Jaundice		●		■	▲	▐
Sore throat/fever/chills		●		■	▲	▐

PROLONGED USE

High doses of propylthiouracil over a prolonged period may reduce the number of white blood cells. Hypothyroidism may also result from prolonged therapy.

Monitoring Periodic tests of thyroid function are usually required, and blood cell counts may also be carried out.

INTERACTIONS

Anticoagulant drugs Propylthiouracil may enhance the effects of these drugs.

PSEUDOEPHEDRINE

Brand names Sudafed, Balminil Decongestant Syrup, Maxenal, Robidrine
Used in the following combined preparations Actifed, Benylin DM-D, Claritin Extra, Drixoral N.D., Sudafed DM, Trinalin

GENERAL INFORMATION

Pseudoephedrine, a component of many nonprescription remedies, is a *sympathomimetic* nasal decongestant. It reduces congestion of the nasal passages and sinuses by narrowing blood vessels in the nose.

Apart from its use in nasal congestion, it is also useful for reducing congestion of the eustachian tube (the tube connecting the middle ear with the cavity at the back of the nose). This often occurs with inflammation and infection of the middle ear.

Pseudoephedrine is less likely than other decongestants to cause anxiety, tremor, and restlessness by stimulating the central nervous system. But, in common with other drugs in this group, it may cause rebound congestion (worsening of congestion after prolonged use).

QUICK REFERENCE

Drug group Decongestant (p.105)
Overdose danger rating High
Dependence rating Low
Prescription needed No
Multi-source suppliers Yes

INFORMATION FOR USERS

Follow instructions on the label. Call your physician if symptoms worsen.

How taken

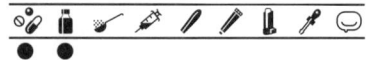

Tablets, capsules, oral liquid.

Frequency and timing of doses
Every 4 – 6 hours (tablets, liquid); every 12 hours (slow-release preparations).

Dosage range
Adults and children 12 years and over Up to 240mg daily.
Children 6 – 11 years Up to 120mg daily.
Children 2 – 5 years Up to 60mg daily.
120mg slow-release preparations are not recommended under 12 years.

Onset of effect
15 – 30 minutes (tablets and liquid).

Duration of action
4 – 6 hours (tablets and liquid); 8 – 12 hours (slow-release preparations).

Diet advice
None.

Storage
Keep in a closed container in a cool, dry place away from reach of children. Protect from light.

Missed dose
Take as soon as you remember. If your next dose is due within 2 hours, take a single dose now and skip the next.

Stopping the drug
Can be safely stopped as soon as you no longer need it.

OVERDOSE ACTION

 Seek immediate medical advice in all cases. Take emergency action if delirium, seizures, or loss of consciousness occur.

See Drug poisoning emergency guide (p.574).

SPECIAL PRECAUTIONS

Be sure to consult your physician or pharmacist before taking this drug if:
▼ You have heart problems.
▼ You have high blood pressure.
▼ You have had glaucoma.
▼ You have diabetes.
▼ You have an overactive thyroid.
▼ You have urinary difficulties.
▼ You are taking other medications.

 Pregnancy
▼ Safety in pregnancy not established. Discuss with your physician.

 Breast feeding
▼ The drug passes into the breast milk and may affect the baby. Discuss with your physician.

 Infants and children
▼ Not recommended for children under 2 years. Reduced dose necessary in older children.

 Over 60
▼ Increased likelihood of adverse effects. Reduced dose may therefore be necessary.

 Driving and hazardous work
▼ Avoid such activities until you have learned how the drug affects you; it can cause dizziness.

 Alcohol
▼ No known problems.

POSSIBLE ADVERSE EFFECTS

High doses may cause anxiety, nausea, dizziness, and, rarely, a marked rise in blood pressure, causing palpitations, headache, and breathlessness.

Symptom/effect	Frequency		Discuss with physician		Stop taking drug now	Call physician now
	Common	Rare	Only if severe	In all cases		
Nausea/vomiting		●	■			
Dizziness/lightheadedness		●	■			
Nervousness/insomnia		●	■			
Hallucinations		●		■		
Rash		●		■	▲	
Palpitations/breathlessness		●		■		∎
Headache		●		■		∎

PROLONGED USE

Pseudoephedrine is not normally taken for prolonged periods. It should not be taken for longer than 7 days except on the advice of your physician.

INTERACTIONS

Antihypertensive drugs Pseudoephedrine counteracts the lowered blood pressure from antihypertensive drugs.

Other sympathomimetic drugs increase the risk of adverse effects with this drug.

Monoamine oxidase inhibitors (MAOIs) There is a risk of a dangerous rise in blood pressure if pseudoephedrine is taken with these drugs.

PSYLLIUM

Brand names Metamucil, Fibrepur, Novo-Mucilax, Prodiem Plain
Used in the following combined preparation Prodiem Plus

GENERAL INFORMATION

This bulk-forming laxative has been extracted from the seeds of Plantago plants since 1934. It is used in the treatment of constipation. Taken by mouth, as powder or granules dissolved in water, psyllium passes through the stomach to the intestines, where it absorbs up to 25 times its volume in water, softening and increasing the volume of bowel movements. It may take several days for improved bowel habits to be established.

Psyllium is also used to reduce the frequency and increase the firmness of bowel movements of people with persistent watery diarrhea or those who have had intestinal surgery such as colostomies or ileostomies. Psyllium may dry up and plug the bowel if the intake of fluids is insufficient.

Side effects are rare, but the drug may sometimes cause bloating and excess gas, especially at the start of treatment. It should not be taken without medical advice for constipation that is accompanied by severe abdominal pain because of the risk of obstructing the bowel. People sensitive to inhaled psyllium may experience allergic reactions while mixing it.

QUICK REFERENCE

Drug group Bulk-forming laxative (p.123)

Overdose danger rating Low

Dependence rating Low

Prescription needed No

Multi-source suppliers Yes

INFORMATION FOR USERS

Follow instructions on label. Call your physician if symptoms worsen.

How taken

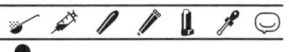

Powder, granules.

Frequency and timing of doses
1 – 3 x daily with at least 240mL of water or fruit juice.

Adult dosage range
Adults 2.5g – 30g daily.
Children over 6 years 1.25g – 15g daily.

Onset of effect
12 – 24 hours.

Duration of action
Up to 24 hours.

Diet advice
Drink plenty of fluids, at least 240mL with each dose plus additional liquid during the day.

Storage
Keep in a closed container in a cool, dry place away from reach of children.

Missed dose
Take as soon as you remember. Resume normal dose thereafter.

Stopping the drug
Can be safely stopped as soon as you no longer need it.

Exceeding the dose
An occasional unintentional extra dose is unlikely to be a cause for concern. But if you notice unusual symptoms, or if a large overdose has been taken, notify your physician.

POSSIBLE ADVERSE EFFECTS

Serious adverse effects are rare, but persistent or severe abdominal pain following the use of this (or any) laxative should always receive medical attention.

Symptom/effect	Frequency		Discuss with physician		Stop taking drug now	Call physician now
	Common	Rare	Only if severe	In all cases		
Excess gas	●		■			
Bloating	●		■			
Abdominal pain		●		■		
Wheezing/breathlessness		●		■	▲	■

INTERACTIONS

General note Psyllium may reduce the absorption of oral anticoagulant drugs, digoxin, and salicylates. Spacing of doses may be recommended.

SPECIAL PRECAUTIONS

Be sure to consult your physician or pharmacist before taking this drug if:
▼ You have severe constipation and/or nausea, vomiting, or abdominal pain.
▼ You have unexplained rectal bleeding.
▼ You have difficulty swallowing.
▼ You are allergic to psyllium products.
▼ You have a known narrowing of the bowel.
▼ You are taking other medications.

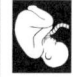

Pregnancy
▼ No evidence of risk to developing baby.

Breast feeding
▼ No evidence of risk.

Infants and children
▼ Given to children over 6 years only on medical advice.

Over 60
▼ No special problems.

Driving and hazardous work
▼ No known problems.

Alcohol
▼ No known problems.

PROLONGED USE

No problems expected.

PYRANTEL

Brand name Combantrin
Used in the following combined preparations None

GENERAL INFORMATION

Pyrantel is an anthelmintic used in the treatment of worm infestation of the bowel. It works by paralyzing the worms so that they let go and pass in the bowel movements.

Common roundworm or pinworm infestations, which are caused by fecal contamination of hands or food or by eating contaminated soil (on raw vegetables, for example), are usually cleared with a single dose. Since pinworms are highly infectious, all members of a household are usually treated at the same time. Dosing may be repeated after two or three weeks if the infestation has not cleared.

For hookworm infestation, which is much less common in Canada, the drug may be prescribed for three consecutive days. Laxatives are usually necessary prior to or during therapy. Iron supplements may also be given to treat any anemia resulting from the hookworm infestation.

Pyrantel is ineffective in tapeworm infestations.

QUICK REFERENCE

Drug group Anthelmintic drug (p.151)

Overdose danger rating Low

Dependence rating Low

Prescription needed No

Multi-source suppliers No

INFORMATION FOR USERS

Follow instructions on the label. Call your physician if symptoms worsen.

How taken

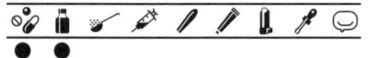

Tablets, oral liquid.

Frequency and timing of doses
A single dose that may be repeated after 2 – 3 weeks.

Dosage range
According to body weight up to a maximum dose of 1g daily.

Onset of effect
1 – 3 hours.

Duration of action
2 – 3 days.

Diet advice
None.

Storage
Keep in a closed container in a cool, dry place away from reach of children. Protect from light. Do not freeze.

Missed dose
If you are taking multiple-day therapy, take as soon as you remember, spacing the missed dose and the next dose 10 – 12 hours apart.

Stopping the drug
If multiple-day therapy is required, complete the course of treatment. If the drug is stopped prematurely, the infestation may persist.

Exceeding the dose
An occasional unintentional extra dose is unlikely to be a cause for concern. But if you notice unusual symptoms, or if a large overdose has been taken, notify your physician.

POSSIBLE ADVERSE EFFECTS

Side effects are rarely serious with pyrantel. Gastrointestinal disturbances, including nausea, loss of appetite, and abdominal pain, are the most common problems.

Symptom/effect	Frequency		Discuss with physician		Stop taking drug now	Call physician now
	Common	Rare	Only if severe	In all cases		
Nausea/vomiting	●		■			
Diarrhea	●		■			
Abdominal cramps	●		■			
Drowsiness/dizziness	●		■			
Headache	●		■			
Rash	●			■	▲	▮

INTERACTIONS

Piperazine may reduce the effect of pyrantel.

SPECIAL PRECAUTIONS

Be sure to consult your physician or pharmacist before taking this drug if:
▼ You have impaired liver function.
▼ You are taking other medications.

 **Pregnancy**
▼ Not usually prescribed. Safety in pregnancy not established. Discuss with your physician.

 Breast feeding
▼ No evidence of risk.

 Infants and children
▼ Not prescribed in infants under 1 year.

 Over 60
▼ No known problems.

 Driving and hazardous work
▼ Avoid such activities until you have learned how the drug affects you; it can cause drowsiness and dizziness.

 Alcohol
▼ No known problems.

PROLONGED USE

Not taken for prolonged periods.

PYRIDOSTIGMINE

Brand names Mestinon, Regonol
Used in the following combined preparations None

GENERAL INFORMATION

Pyridostigmine is used to treat myasthenia gravis, a rare autoimmune condition involving the faulty transmission of nerve impulses to the muscles (p.133). By prolonging nerve signals, pyridostigmine improves muscle strength, though it does not cure the disease. In severe cases it may be prescribed with corticosteroids. Because the response to pyridostigmine is predictable, it may also be used to help diagnose the disease: lack of a response rules out myasthenia gravis. Pyridostigmine may also be given to reverse temporary paralysis of the bowel.

Side effects such as abdominal cramps, nausea, and diarrhea generally disappear when the dose of pyridostigmine is reduced.

INFORMATION FOR USERS

Your drug prescription is tailored for you. Do not alter dosage without checking with your physician.

How taken

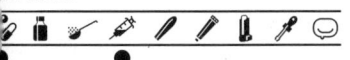

Tablets, slow-release tablets, injection.

Frequency and timing of doses
Tablets 2 – 4 x daily.
Slow-release tablets 1 – 2 x daily.

Dosage range
Adults 120 – 1,080mg daily (by mouth).
Children Reduced dose necessary according to age and weight.

Onset of effect
30 – 60 minutes (by mouth); within 2 – 5 minutes (injection).

Duration of action
3 – 6 hours (tablets); about 4 hours (injection); 6 – 12 hours (slow-release tablets).

Diet advice
None.

Storage
Keep in a closed container in a cool, dry place away from reach of children. Protect from light.

Missed dose
Take as soon as you remember. If your next dose is due within 2 hours, take a single dose now and skip the next.

Stopping the drug
Do not stop the drug without consulting your physician; symptoms may recur.

OVERDOSE ACTION

Seek immediate medical advice in all cases. You may experience severe abdominal cramps, vomiting, weakness and tremor. Take emergency action if unusually slow heartbeat, troubled breathing, seizures, or loss of consciousness occurs.

See Drug poisoning emergency guide (p.574).

POSSIBLE ADVERSE EFFECTS

Adverse effects of pyridostigmine, due to parasympathetic overstimulation (p.91), are usually dose-related. Rarely, an allergic skin rash may occur.

Symptom/effect	Frequency		Discuss with physician		Stop taking drug now	Call physician now
	Common	Rare	Only if severe	In all cases		
Nausea/vomiting	●			■		
Increased salivation	●			■		
Sweating	●			■		
Abdominal cramps/diarrhea	●			■		
Watering eyes/small pupils		●		■		
Injection site pain/swelling		●			■	
Rash		●			■	▲

INTERACTIONS

General note Drugs that affect transmission of nerve signals may oppose the effect of pyridostigmine. Such drugs include digoxin, aminoglycoside antibiotics, chlorpromazine, quinidine, and procainamide.

SPECIAL PRECAUTIONS

Be sure to tell your physician if:
▼ You have heart problems.
▼ You have had epileptic seizures.
▼ You have asthma.
▼ You have difficulty passing urine.
▼ You have Parkinson's disease.
▼ You are taking other medications.

Pregnancy
▼ No evidence of risk to developing baby in the first 6 months of pregnancy. Large doses near the time of delivery may cause premature labor and lead to temporary muscle weakness in the newborn baby. Discuss with your physician.

Breast feeding
▼ Not recommended. Discuss with your physician.

Infants and children
▼ Reduced dose necessary.

Over 60
▼ Increased likelihood of adverse effects.

Driving and hazardous work
▼ Your underlying condition may make such activities inadvisable. Discuss with your physician.

Alcohol
▼ Avoid. Alcohol may cause breathing difficulties in myasthenia gravis sufferers.

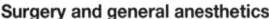

Surgery and general anesthetics
▼ Pyridostigmine will interact with some anesthetic agents. Make sure your treatment is known to your physician, dentist, and anesthetist before any surgery.

PROLONGED USE

The effects of the drug may diminish with time. Benefits may be restored by stopping the drug for a few days or by adjusting the dose. But this should be done only under the direction of your physician.

PYRIMETHAMINE

Brand name Daraprim
Used in the following combined preparation Fansidar

GENERAL INFORMATION

Pyrimethamine is an antimalarial drug generally used against types of malaria resistant to other drugs. It is valuable as a suppressive agent, and it effectively relieves the chills-and-fever symptoms of malaria attacks.

Because malaria parasites can readily develop resistance to pyrimethamine, the drug is usually given with a sulfonamide such as sulfadoxine. This dual

activity exceeds that of either drug alone.

Pyrimethamine is also prescribed with sulfonamides to treat human toxoplasmosis, a protozoal infection endemic in cats whose feces can be infective. Because blood disorders can arise during prolonged use, regular blood counts are made and vitamin supplements are given, especially to pregnant women receiving the drug.

INFORMATION FOR USERS

Your drug prescription is tailored for you. Do not alter dosage without checking with your physician.

How taken

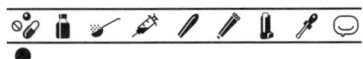

Tablets.

Frequency and timing of doses
Once weekly starting 1 week before travel continuing for at least 10 weeks after leaving malarial area (suppression of malaria); 2 x daily for 2 days (treatment of malaria); 1 – 2 x daily with sulfonamide (toxoplasmosis). Doses are best taken with food.

Adult dosage range
25mg once weekly (suppression of malaria); 25mg daily for 2 days with other antimalarials (treatment of malaria); 50mg initially, then 25mg daily with a sulfonamide for 3 – 6 weeks (toxoplasmosis).

Onset of effect
24 hours.

Duration of action
Up to 1 week.

Diet advice
None.

Storage
Keep in a closed container in a cool, dry place away from reach of children. Protect from light.

Missed dose
Take as soon as you remember. If your next dose is due within 24 hours (once weekly schedule), 12 hours (once daily schedule), or 2 hours (more than once daily schedule), take a single dose now and skip the next.

Stopping the drug
Take the full course. If stopped too soon, treatment may fail.

Exceeding the dose
An occasional unintentional extra dose is unlikely to cause problems. Large overdoses may cause trembling, breathing difficulties, unsteadiness, and seizures. Notify your physician immediately. The drug is very toxic to children.

SPECIAL PRECAUTIONS

Be sure to tell your physician if:
▼ You have impaired liver or kidney function.
▼ You have had epileptic seizures.
▼ You have anemia.
▼ You are taking other medications.

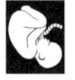 **Pregnancy**
▼ Not prescribed unless absolutely necessary. May cause defects in the unborn baby. Discuss with your physician.

 Breast feeding
▼ The drug passes into the breast milk, but at normal doses adverse effects on the baby are unlikely. Discuss with your physician.

 Infants and children
▼ Reduced dose necessary.

 Over 60
▼ No special problems.

 Driving and hazardous work
▼ No special problems.

 Alcohol
▼ No known problems.

POSSIBLE ADVERSE EFFECTS

Side effects of pyrimethamine occur only rarely with the low doses given for suppression of malaria. Vomiting may be minimized by taking the drug with food.

Unusual tiredness, weakness, bleeding, bruising, and sore throat may be signs of a blood disorder. Notify your physician promptly if they occur.

| Symptom/effect | Frequency | | Discuss with physician | | Stop taking drug now | Call physician now |
	Common	Rare	Only if severe	In all cases		
Loss of appetite		●	■			
Nausea/vomiting	●		■			
Weakness/fatigue		●		■		
Rash		●		■		▮
Unusual bleeding/bruising		●		■		▮
Sore throat/fever		●		■		▮

PROLONGED USE

Prolonged use of this drug may cause folic acid deficiency, leading to serious blood disorders. Supplements of folic acid may be recommended.

Monitoring Regular blood cell counts are required during high-dose treatment for toxoplasmosis.

INTERACTIONS

General note Drugs that suppress the bone marrow or cause folic acid deficiency may increase the risk of serious blood disorders. Such drugs include anticancer and antirheumatic drugs, phenylbutazone,

sulfasalazine, cotrimoxazole, and phenytoin.

Lorazepam and pyrimethamine together may produce liver damage.

QUINAPRIL

Brand name Accupril
Used in the following combined preparations None

GENERAL INFORMATION

Quinapril belongs to the ACE inhibitor group of drugs. It is prescribed to treat hypertension (high blood pressure) and heart failure, achieving its effect by dilating blood vessels. Quinapril is often given in conjunction with a diuretic to increase its effect.

The first dose of quinapril may cause a sudden drop in blood pressure. You should therefore be resting at the time of the first dose and able to lie down afterwards for 2 – 3 hours.

The more common adverse effects, such as dizziness and headache, usually diminish with time. Rashes can also occur during treatment. These usually disappear when the drug is stopped. In some cases they clear up on their own despite continued treatment.

INFORMATION FOR USERS

Your drug prescription is tailored for you. Do not alter dosage without checking with your physician.

How taken

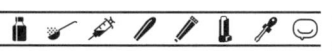

Tablets.

Frequency and timing of doses
Once daily.

Dosage range
_mg daily (starting dose), increased to _ – 20mg daily (maintenance dose).

Onset of effect
Within 1 hour.

Duration of action
_ hours.

Diet advice
None.

Storage
Keep in a closed container in a cool, dry place away from reach of children. Protect from light.

Missed dose
Take as soon as you remember. If your next dose is due within 8 hours, do not take the skipped dose. Take your next dose as usual.

Stopping the drug
Do not stop taking the drug without consulting your physician; stopping the drug may lead to worsening of the underlying condition.

Exceeding the dose
An occasional unintentional extra dose is unlikely to cause problems. Large overdoses may cause dizziness or fainting. Notify your physician.

SPECIAL PRECAUTIONS

Be sure to tell your physician if:
▼ You have impaired kidney or liver function.
▼ You have diabetes.
▼ You have an autoimmune disease.
▼ You have coronary artery disease.
▼ You are pregnant or intend to become pregnant.
▼ You are taking other medications.

Pregnancy
▼ Use during pregnancy can cause injury or even death to the developing fetus. Report promptly to your physician if you become pregnant.

Breast feeding
▼ Effect on breast feeding uncertain. Discuss with your physician.

Infants and children
▼ Not recommended.

Over 60
▼ Reduced dose may be necessary.

Driving and hazardous work
▼ Avoid such activities until you have learned how the drug affects you; it can cause dizziness and fainting.

Alcohol
▼ Avoid. Alcohol increases the likelihood of an excessive drop in blood pressure.

Surgery and general anesthetics
▼ Quinapril treatment may need to be stopped before you have a general anesthetic. Discuss with your physician or dentist before any surgery.

PROLONGED USE

No problems expected.

Monitoring Periodic tests on blood and urine should be performed.

POSSIBLE ADVERSE EFFECTS

The more common adverse effects, such as headache and dizziness, usually diminish with time. The less common effects may also diminish during long-term treatment, but an adjustment in dosage may be necessary.

Symptom/effect	Frequency		Discuss with physician		Stop taking drug now	Call physician now
	Common	Rare	Only if severe	In all cases		
Headache	●		■			
Dizziness	●		■			
Fatigue	●		■			
Cough	●		■			
Abdominal pain	●			■		
Nausea/vomiting	●			■		
Increased sweating		●		■		
Swelling of face or tongue		●		■	▲	■

INTERACTIONS

Antihypertensive drugs are likely to add to the blood pressure-lowering effect of quinapril.

Lithium Quinapril may increase the level of lithium in the blood, and serious adverse effects from lithium excess may occur.

Potassium supplements and potassium-sparing diuretics Quinapril may add to the effect of these drugs, leading to raised levels of potassium in the blood.

Tetracycline antibiotics Quinapril decreases the absorption of tetracyclines.

QUINIDINE

Brand names Biquin, Cardioquin, Quinate, Quinidex
Used in the following combined preparations None

GENERAL INFORMATION

Although quinidine is one of the oldest of the anti-arrhythmic drugs, it is still used to treat many different abnormal heart rhythms, particularly in cases where a rapid heartbeat causes important symptoms or is life-threatening.

When taken by mouth, the onset of action is slow. It can be given by injection in emergencies when rapid control

of an abnormal heart rhythm is required.

Quinidine has several possible adverse effects. Diarrhea, nausea, and vomiting, which are common, may be due to its irritant effect. Serious allergic reactions have also occurred. The most serious adverse effect is the possibility of further abnormal heart rhythms that may give rise to palpitations.

INFORMATION FOR USERS

Your drug prescription is tailored for you. Do not alter the dosage without checking with your physician.

How taken

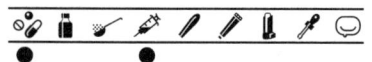

Tablets, slow-release tablets, injection.

Frequency and timing of doses
Every 6 hours (tablets); every 8 – 12 hours (slow-release tablets).

Dosage range
Adults 600mg – 4g daily.
Children Reduced dose necessary according to age and weight.

Onset of effect
Within 3 hours.

Duration of action
6 – 8 hours (tablets); up to 12 hours (slow-release tablets).

Diet advice
None.

Storage
Keep in a closed container in a cool, dry place away from reach of children. Protect from light.

Missed dose
Take as soon as you remember. If your next dose is due within 2 hours, take a single dose now and skip the next.

Stopping the drug
Do not stop taking the drug without consulting your physician; symptoms may recur.

OVERDOSE ACTION

 Seek immediate medical advice in all cases. Take emergency action if breathing difficulties, seizures, or collapse occurs.

See Drug poisoning emergency guide (p.574).

SPECIAL PRECAUTIONS

Be sure to tell your physician or pharmacist before taking this drug if:
▼ You have impaired kidney or liver function
▼ You have heart failure.
▼ You have myasthenia gravis.
▼ You have had a rash following quinidine on a previous occasion.
▼ You are taking other medications.

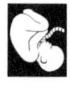 **Pregnancy**
▼ Safety in pregnancy not established. Discuss with your physician.

 Breast feeding
▼ The drug passes into the breast milk and may affect the baby. Discuss with your physician.

 Infants and children
▼ Not usually prescribed.

 Over 60
▼ Reduced dose necessary.

 Driving and hazardous work
▼ Avoid such activities until you have learned how the drug affects you; it can cause dizziness and blurred vision.

 Alcohol
▼ No known problems.

POSSIBLE ADVERSE EFFECTS

The most common adverse effects are diarrhea, nausea, and vomiting. If they become severe, a change of drug may be necessary. Vertigo or palpitations may indicate the dose is too high; notify your physician promptly.

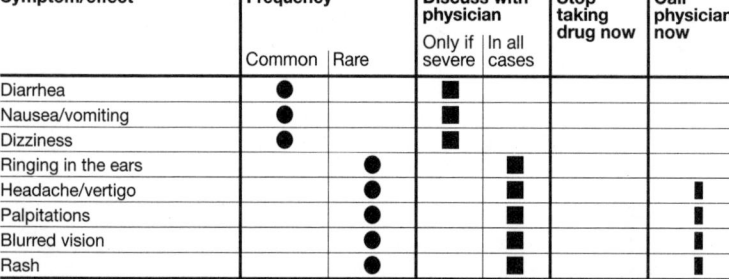

Symptom/effect	Frequency		Discuss with physician		Stop taking drug now	Call physician now
	Common	Rare	Only if severe	In all cases		
Diarrhea	●			■		
Nausea/vomiting	●			■		
Dizziness	●			■		
Ringing in the ears		●		■		
Headache/vertigo		●		■		▌
Palpitations		●		■		▌
Blurred vision		●		■		▌
Rash		●		■		▌

PROLONGED USE

Sudden onset of abnormal heart rhythms or abnormalities of the blood may occur.

Monitoring Periodic checks on blood levels of the drug may be required.

INTERACTIONS

Digoxin Quinidine increases the effects of digoxin, requiring that blood levels be checked.

Anticoagulant drugs Quinidine increases the effect of these drugs.

Phenobarbital and phenytoin reduce the effect of quinidine.

Antihypertensive drugs Quinidine may increase the blood pressure-lowering effects of antihypertensive drugs such as beta blockers and vasodilators.

QUININE

Brand name Legatrin
Used in the following combined preparations None

GENERAL INFORMATION

Quinine is the earliest antimalarial drug. It is no longer widely used, but it is still occasionally given for malaria that is resistant to safer treatments. In some of these cases, it is administered by mouth in conjunction with other drugs. In serious cases of malaria affecting the brain, it may be given intravenously. Quinine is given in low doses for prevention of leg cramps during the night. It has also been used to reduce fever, and to help diagnose myasthenia gravis.

At doses used to treat malaria, quinine may cause ringing in the ears, headaches, nausea, hearing loss, and blurred vision. Rarely, the drug may also cause subcutaneous bleeding due to a reduction in blood platelets or blood prothrombin.

INFORMATION FOR USERS

Follow instructions on the label. Call your physician if symptoms worsen.

How taken

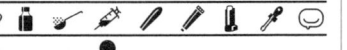

Capsules, injection.

Frequency and timing of doses
Malaria Every 8 hours for 3 – 7 days (by mouth).
Muscle cramps Once daily at bedtime or twice daily after evening meal and at bedtime.

Dosage range
Adults 1.8g daily (malaria); 200 – 300mg daily (cramps).
Children Reduced dose according to age and weight.

Onset of effect
1 – 3 hours (cramps); 1 – 2 days (malaria).

Duration of action
Up to 24 hours.

Diet advice
None.

Storage
Keep in a closed container in a cool, dry place

away from reach of children. Protect from light.

Missed dose
Take as soon as you remember. If your next dose is due within 4 hours, skip the missed dose and resume your normal dosing schedule thereafter.

Stopping the drug
If prescribed for malaria, take the full course. Even if you feel better, the original infection may still be present and may recur if treatment is stopped too soon. If taken for muscle cramps, the drug can safely be stopped as soon as you no longer need it.

OVERDOSE ACTION

 Seek immediate medical advice in all cases. Take emergency action if breathing problems, seizures, delirium, lowered blood pressure, or loss of consciousness occurs.

See Drug poisoning emergency guide (p.574).

POSSIBLE ADVERSE EFFECTS

Adverse effects are unlikely with low doses. At antimalarial doses, hearing disturbances, headache, and blurred vision are more common. Nausea and diarrhea may occur.

Symptom/effect	Frequency		Discuss with physician		Stop taking drug now	Call physician now
	Common	Rare	Only if severe	In all cases		
Itching/flushing	●			■	▲	▮
Nausea/diarrhea		●	■			
Headache		●		■		
Ringing in ears/hearing loss		●		■	▲	
Asthma		●●		■		▮
Blurred vision		●		■	▲	

INTERACTIONS

Digoxin Quinine increases the blood levels of digoxin.

Oral anticoagulant drugs Quinine may enhance the action of oral anticoagulants.

Muscle-relaxant drugs Quinine may enhance the action of muscle-relaxant drugs such as succinylcholine and tubocurarine.

SPECIAL PRECAUTIONS

Be sure to consult your physician or pharmacist before taking this drug if:
▼ You have impaired kidney function.
▼ You have tinnitus (ringing in the ears).
▼ You have optic neuritis.
▼ You have myasthenia gravis.
▼ You have glucose-6-phosphate dehydrogenase (G6PD) deficiency.
▼ You have heart problems.
▼ You are taking other medications.

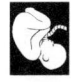 **Pregnancy**
▼ Not prescribed. May cause defects in the unborn baby. Discuss with your physician.

 Breast feeding
▼ The drug passes into the breast milk and may affect the baby. Discuss with your physician.

 Infants and children
▼ Reduced dose necessary.

 Over 60
▼ No special problems.

 Driving and hazardous work
▼ Blurring of vision and other eye problems may impair these activities.

 Alcohol
▼ No known problems.

PROLONGED USE

Reactions to continued antimalarial use include disturbed color perception, intolerance to light, double vision, night blindness, blurred vision, and chest wheezing. After large doses, profuse sweating and, rarely, swelling of the mouth and throat (angioedema) may occur.

No problems expected with low doses used to control nighttime leg cramps.

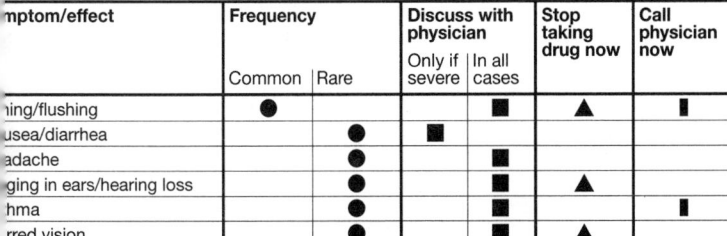

RANITIDINE

Brand names Zantac, Apo-Ranitidine, Novo-Ranidine, Nu-Ranit
Used in the following combined preparations None

GENERAL INFORMATION

Ranitidine, a drug similar to cimetidine, was introduced in 1982 and is mainly used in the prevention and treatment of stomach and duodenal ulcers. It acts by reducing the amount of acid produced by the stomach, allowing the ulcers time to heal. Ranitidine also reduces discomfort and inflammation from reflux esophagitis.

Treatment is usually given in courses lasting from 4 to 12 weeks, with further courses if symptoms recur.

Unlike cimetidine, this drug does not affect the actions of certain enzymes in the liver, where many drugs are broken down before being absorbed into the body. This means that ranitidine can be taken with other drugs, such as anti-coagulants and anticonvulsants, without causing an interaction that may reduce the effectiveness of either treatment.

Most people do not experience any serious effects during a course of treatment with ranitidine. As ranitidine promotes healing of the stomach lining, there is a risk that it may mask stomach cancer, delaying diagnosis. It is therefore usually prescribed only when the possibility of stomach cancer has been carefully considered.

QUICK REFERENCE

Drug group Anti-ulcer drug (p.121)
Overdose danger rating Low
Dependence rating Low
Prescription needed Yes
Multi-source suppliers Yes

INFORMATION FOR USERS

Your drug prescription is tailored for you. Do not alter dosage without checking with your physician.

How taken

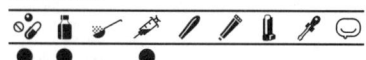

Tablets, capsules, oral liquid, injection.

Frequency and timing of doses
Once daily at bedtime or 2 – 3 x daily.

Adult dosage range
150mg – 6g daily depending on the condition being treated.

Onset of effect
Within 1 hour.

Duration of action
12 hours.

Diet advice
None.

Storage
Keep in a closed container in a cool, dry place away from reach of children. Protect from light.

Missed dose
Take as soon as you remember. If your next dose is due within 3 hours, take a single dose now and skip the next.

Stopping the drug
Do not stop the drug without consulting your physician; symptoms may recur.

Exceeding the dose
An occasional unintentional extra dose is unlikely to be a cause for concern. But if you notice unusual symptoms, or if a large overdose has been taken, notify your physician.

SPECIAL PRECAUTIONS

Be sure to tell your physician if:
▼ You have impaired liver or kidney function
▼ You are taking other medications.

Pregnancy
▼ Safety in pregnancy not established. Discuss with your physician.

Breast feeding
▼ The drug passes into the breast milk and may affect the baby. Discuss with your physician.

Infants and children
▼ Reduced dose necessary.

Over 60
▼ No special problems.

Driving and hazardous work
▼ No known problems. Dizziness can occur in a very small proportion of patients.

Alcohol
▼ Avoid. Alcohol may aggravate your underlying condition and reduce the beneficial effects of the drug.

PROLONGED USE

No problems expected.

POSSIBLE ADVERSE EFFECTS

The adverse effects of ranitidine, of which headache is the most common, are usually related to dosage level and almost always disappear when treatment finishes.

Symptom/effect	Frequency		Discuss with physician		Stop taking drug now	Call physician now
	Common	Rare	Only if severe	In all cases		
Headache/dizziness	●		■			
Nausea/vomiting		●	■			
Constipation		●	■			
Diarrhea		●	■			
Rash/jaundice		●		■	▲	▮

INTERACTIONS

Sucralfate The absorption of ranitidine may be reduced if the drug is taken with high doses (2g) of sucralfate. Take sucralfate at least 2 hours after ranitidine.

Ketoconazole Ranitidine may reduce the absorption of ketoconazole. Take ranitidine at least 2 hours after ketoconazole.

RIFAMPIN

Brand names Rimactane, Rifadin, Rofact
Used in the following combined preparation Rifater

GENERAL INFORMATION

Rifampin, introduced in 1972, is an antibiotic that is highly effective in the treatment of tuberculosis. Taken by mouth, it is well absorbed in the intestine and widely distributed throughout the body, including the brain. It is very useful in the treatment of active pulmonary tuberculosis. Rifampin is always prescribed with at least one other antituberculosis drug; this enhances its effect and prevents the development of resistance to the drug.

Treatment may continue for 6 months to 2 years or more. Rifampin is also used to prevent infection in anyone in close contact with certain kinds of bacterial meningitis.

Although rifampin is generally well tolerated at usual doses, it may damage the liver. Gastrointestinal disturbances, rashes, and a flu-like illness may also occur. Rifampin may decrease the effects of many other drugs, including oral contraceptives.

INFORMATION FOR USERS

Your drug prescription is tailored for you. Do not alter dosage without checking with your physician.

How taken

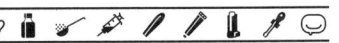

Capsules.

Frequency and timing of doses
1 daily in the morning 1 hour before breakfast (tuberculosis); 2 x daily (prevention of meningitis).

Adult dosage range
According to weight, usually 450 – 600mg daily (tuberculosis); 1.2g daily for 2 days (prevention of meningitis).

Onset of effect
Several days.

Duration of action
Up to 72 hours.

Diet advice
None.

Storage
Keep in a closed container in a cool, dry place away from reach of children. Protect from light.

Missed dose
Take as soon as you remember. If your next dose is due within 6 hours, take both doses now and return to normal dosing thereafter.

Stopping the drug
Take the full course. Even if you feel better, the original infection may still be present and symptoms may recur if treatment is stopped too soon. In rare cases stopping the drug suddenly after high-dose treatment can lead to a severe flu-like illness.

Exceeding the dose
An occasional unintentional extra dose is unlikely to cause problems. Large overdoses may cause nausea, vomiting, and lethargy. Notify your physician.

POSSIBLE ADVERSE EFFECTS

Rifampin normally causes a harmless red-orange discoloration of the feces, urine, and other body fluids. Serious adverse effects are rare. Jaundice usually improves during treatment but should nevertheless be reported to your physician. Symptoms such as headache and breathing difficulties may occur after stopping high-dose treatment.

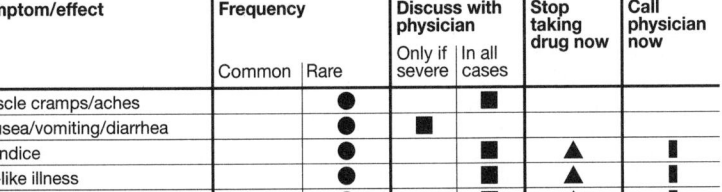

Symptom/effect	Frequency		Discuss with physician		Stop taking drug now	Call physician now
	Common	Rare	Only if severe	In all cases		
Muscle cramps/aches		●			■	
Nausea/vomiting/diarrhea		●	■			
Jaundice		●		■	▲	▮
Flu-like illness		●		■	▲	▮
Rash/itching		●		■	▲	▮

INTERACTIONS

General note Rifampin may reduce the effectiveness of a wide variety of drugs. Such drugs include digoxin, oral contraceptives, corticosteroids, oral antidiabetics, disopyramide, cyclosporine, phenytoin, and oral anticoagulants.

Ketoconazole may impair the absorption of rifampin. Separation of doses by 12 hours may be recommended.

SPECIAL PRECAUTIONS

Be sure to tell your physician if:
▼ You have impaired liver function.
▼ You have porphyria.
▼ You wear contact lenses.
▼ You are taking other medications.

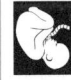

Pregnancy
▼ Safety in pregnancy not established. Discuss with your physician.

Breast feeding
▼ The drug passes into the breast milk, but at normal doses adverse effects on the baby are unlikely. Discuss with your physician.

Infants and children
▼ Reduced dose necessary.

Over 60
▼ Increased risk of adverse effects. Reduced dose may therefore be necessary.

Driving and hazardous work
▼ Avoid such activities until you have learned how the drug affects you, because the drug may cause dizziness.

Alcohol
▼ No special problems. Avoid excessive amounts.

PROLONGED USE

Prolonged use of rifampin may cause liver damage. Staining of soft contact lenses may occur.

Monitoring Periodic blood tests may be performed to monitor liver function.

RITODRINE

Brand name Yutopar
Used in the following combined preparations None

GENERAL INFORMATION

Ritodrine, introduced in 1984, is a *sympathomimetic* drug that relaxes the muscles of the uterus. It is used to prevent premature labor. After contractions are initially stopped by continuous intravenous infusion of the drug, ritodrine may be given by mouth until the physician considers it safe for the baby to be born, usually at or after 36 weeks.

Ritodrine may also be used to halt labor temporarily while corticosteroid drugs are given to hasten development of the baby's lungs and lessen the risk of breathing problems after delivery.

Stimulation of the heart, leading to palpitations, is the most common *side effect* of ritodrine. Given by injection, it may also increase blood sugar levels and aggravate diabetes.

INFORMATION FOR USERS

Your drug prescription is tailored for you. Do not alter dosage without checking with your physician.

How taken

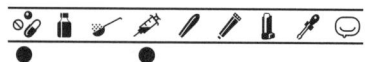

Tablets, injection.

Frequency and timing of doses
By continuous infusion until contractions stop; then by mouth as prescribed.

Adult dosage range
Up to 120mg daily (by mouth).

Onset of effect
Within a few minutes (injection); 30 – 60 minutes (tablets).

Duration of action
6 – 8 hours.

Diet advice
Eat nothing and drink only clear fluids until drug treatment has halted contractions.

Storage
Keep in a closed container in a cool, dry place away from reach of children. Protect from light.

Missed dose
Take as soon as you remember. If your doses are scheduled every 4 – 6 hours and your next dose is due within 2 hours, take a single dose now and skip the next.

Stopping the drug
Do not stop taking the drug without consulting your physician; stopping the drug may lead to the onset of labor.

Exceeding the dose
An occasional unintentional extra dose is unlikely to cause problems. Large overdoses may cause palpitations and breathing difficulty. Notify your physician.

SPECIAL PRECAUTIONS

Be sure to tell your physician if:
▼ You have heart problems.
▼ You suffer from migraine headaches.
▼ You have high blood pressure.
▼ You have an overactive thyroid.
▼ You have diabetes.
▼ You have asthma.
▼ You are taking other medications.

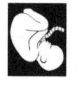

Pregnancy
▼ Used in pregnancy of over 20 weeks, there is no proven risk to the health of the baby. Ritodrine is not prescribed in pregnancies of less than 20 weeks, since its safety is not established.

Breast feeding
▼ Not applicable. Ritodrine is not used during breast feeding.

Infants and children
▼ Not prescribed.

Over 60
▼ Not prescribed.

Driving and hazardous work
▼ Your underlying condition may make such activities inadvisable. Discuss with your physician.

Alcohol
▼ Not advisable.

Surgery and general anesthetics
▼ Ritodrine may increase the risk of adverse effects on the heart with a general anesthetic. Discuss with your physician before any surgery.

POSSIBLE ADVERSE EFFECTS

Adverse effects are dose-related and are more severe when ritodrine is given by injection. By mouth, adverse effects other than palpitations are rare. Breathlessness due to fluid in the lungs may occasionally occur.

Symptom/effect	Frequency		Discuss with physician		Stop taking drug now	Call physician now
	Common	Rare	Only if severe	In all cases		
Trembling/agitation	●		■			
Palpitations	●			■		
Nausea/vomiting		●		■		
Chest pain/breathlessness		●		■	▲	▌
Rash/flushing		●		■	▲	▌

INTERACTIONS

Diuretics Ritodrine may increase the risk of side effects with some diuretics.

Beta blockers reduce the effect of ritodrine.

Other sympathomimetic drugs Ritodrine may increase the effects of these drugs.

Antidepressant drugs may increase the likelihood of adverse effects from ritodrine.

Corticosteroids There is an increased risk of high blood sugar and shortness of breath when ritodrine is taken with corticosteroids.

Antidiabetic drugs Ritodrine may increase blood sugar. Antidiabetic drug dosage may need to be increased.

PROLONGED USE

No special problems.

SALBUTAMOL

Brand names Ventolin, Ventodisk, Apo-Salvent, Asmavent, Gen-Salbutamol, Novo-Salmol
Used in the following combined preparations None

GENERAL INFORMATION

Salbutamol is a *sympathomimetic bronchodilator* that relaxes the muscle surrounding the bronchioles (airways in the lungs).

It is used mainly in the treatment of asthma, chronic bronchitis, and emphysema. Although salbutamol can be taken by mouth, inhalation is considered more effective because the drug is delivered directly to the bronchioles, giving rapid relief, allowing smaller doses, and creating fewer *side effects*.

Compared with some similar drugs, it has little stimulant effect on the heart rate and blood pressure, making it safer for those with heart problems or high blood pressure.

The most common side effect of salbutamol is fine tremor of the hands, which may interfere with precise manual work. Nervousness, headache, and restlessness may also occur.

INFORMATION FOR USERS

Your drug prescription is tailored for you. Do not alter dosage without checking with your physician.

How taken

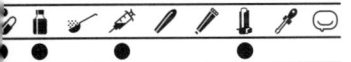

Tablets, oral liquid, injection, inhaler, solution inhalation.

Frequency and timing of doses
Varies according to preparation used, method of administration, and underlying disorder.

Dosage range
Varies according to preparation used, method of administration, and underlying disorder.

Onset of effect
Within 5 – 15 minutes (by inhalation); within 30 – 60 minutes (by mouth).

Duration of action
4 to 6 hours (by inhalation); up to 8 hours (by mouth).

Diet advice
None.

Storage
Keep in a closed container in a cool, dry place away from reach of children. Protect from light. Do not puncture or burn inhalers.

Missed dose
Do not take the missed dose. Take your next dose as usual.

Stopping the drug
Do not stop the drug without consulting your physician; symptoms may recur.

Exceeding the dose
An occasional unintentional extra dose is unlikely to be cause for concern. But if you notice any unusual symptoms, or if a large overdose has been taken, notify your physician.

POSSIBLE ADVERSE EFFECTS

Muscle tremor, especially of the hands, anxiety, and restlessness are the most common adverse effects. Palpitations and headache are rare.

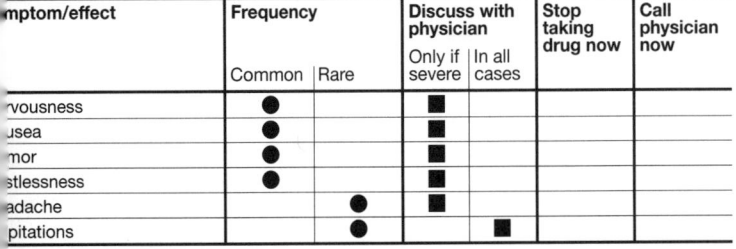

Symptom/effect	Frequency		Discuss with physician		Stop taking drug now	Call physician now
	Common	Rare	Only if severe	In all cases		
Nervousness	●		■			
Nausea	●		■			
Tremor	●		■			
Restlessness	●		■			
Headache		●	■			
Palpitations		●			■	

INTERACTIONS

Other sympathomimetic drugs may increase the effects of salbutamol, increasing the risk of adverse effects.

Beta blockers may reduce the action of salbutamol.

Tricyclic antidepressants and monoamine oxidase inhibitors (MAOIs) can interact with salbutamol to produce a dangerous rise in blood pressure.

SPECIAL PRECAUTIONS

Be sure to tell your physician if:
▼ You have heart problems.
▼ You have high blood pressure.
▼ You have an overactive thyroid gland.
▼ You have diabetes.
▼ You are taking other medications.

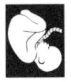 **Pregnancy**
▼ No evidence of risk when used to treat asthma, or to treat or prevent premature labor. Discuss with your physician.

 Breast feeding
▼ The drug passes into the breast milk, but at normal doses adverse effects on the baby are unlikely. Discuss with your physician.

 Infants and children
▼ Reduced dose necessary.

 Over 60
▼ Increased likelihood of adverse effects. Reduced dose may therefore be necessary.

 Driving and hazardous work
▼ Avoid such activities until you have learned how the drug affects you; it can cause tremors and dizziness.

 Alcohol
▼ No known problems.

PROLONGED USE

Prolonged use may result in tolerance to the effects of salbutamol. However, failure to respond to the drug may be a result of worsening asthma that requires urgent medical attention.

SALMETEROL

Brand name Serevent
Used in the following combined preparations None

GENERAL INFORMATION

Salmeterol is a long-acting *sympatho-mimetic bronchodilator* that relaxes the muscle surrounding the bronchioles (airways in the lungs). It is used in the daily treatment of asthma, chronic bronchitis, and emphysema.

Unlike fast-acting bronchodilators – such as fenoterol, salbutamol, and terbutaline – which can be used as needed for rapid relief of acute bronchospasm, salmeterol is used for maintenance treatment only. Because of its slower onset of action, salmeterol is

not intended to relieve acute asthma symptoms. Should acute broncho-spasm occur in a person already taking salmeterol, then the temporary addition of a fast-acting bronchodilator is required. However, regular use of a fast-acting bronchodilator with salmeterol increases the risk of adverse cardiovascular effects.

The most common *side effects* of salmeterol are headache, fine tremor of the hands, and palpitations.

QUICK REFERENCE

Drug group Bronchodilator (p.104)
Overdose danger rating Medium
Dependence rating Low
Prescription needed Yes
Multi-source suppliers No

INFORMATION FOR USERS

Your drug prescription is tailored for you. Do not alter dosage without checking with your physician.

How taken

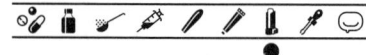

Inhaler (aerosol, dry powder).

Frequency and timing of doses
2 x daily.

Dosage range
100mcg daily.

Onset of effect
10 – 20 minutes.

Duration of action
12 hours.

Diet advice
None.

Storage
Keep in a cool, dry place away from reach of children. Do not puncture or burn inhalers.

Missed dose
Take as soon as you remember. If your next dose is scheduled within 3 hours, take a single dose now and skip the next.

Stopping the drug
Do not stop the drug without consulting your physician; symptoms may recur.

Exceeding the dose
An occasional unintentional extra dose is unlikely to be a cause for concern. But if you notice any unusual symptoms, or if a large overdose has been taken, notify your physician.

SPECIAL PRECAUTIONS

Be sure to tell your physician if:
▼ You have heart problems.
▼ You have high blood pressure.
▼ You have diabetes.
▼ You have an overactive thyroid.
▼ You are taking other medications.

Pregnancy
▼ Safety in pregnancy not established. Discuss with your physician.

Breast feeding
▼ It is not known if the drug passes into the breast milk. Discuss with your physician.

Infants and children
▼ Not recommended for children under 12 years.

Over 60
▼ Increased likelihood of adverse effects. Reduced dose may therefore be necessary.

Driving and hazardous work
▼ Avoid such activities until you have learned how the drug affects you; it can cause tremor and dizziness.

Alcohol
▼ No known problems.

POSSIBLE ADVERSE EFFECTS

Tremor, headache, and palpitations are the most common adverse effects. Tremor, which is dose-related, tends to decrease with continued use.

Symptom/effect	Frequency		Discuss with physician		Stop taking drug now	Call physician now
	Common	Rare	Only if severe	In all cases		
Headache	●		■			
Tremor	●		■			
Palpitations	●		■			
Rash/hives	●		■		▲	∎

INTERACTIONS

Other sympathomimetic drugs may add to the effects of salmeterol and vice versa, so increasing the risk of adverse effects.

Tricyclic antidepressants and monoamine oxidase inhibitors (MAOIs) Salmeterol may interact with these drugs to cause a dangerous rise in blood pressure.

Beta blockers may counter the beneficial effects of salmeterol.

PROLONGED USE

Prolonged use may result in tolerance to the effects of salmeterol. However, failure to respond to the drug may be a result of worsening asthma that requires urgent medical attention.

SCOPOLAMINE

Brand names Buscopan, Transderm-V
Used in the following combined preparations None

GENERAL INFORMATION

Scopolamine (hyoscine) is an *anticholinergic* drug. It increases heart rate, decreases salivary and sweat secretions, dilates the pupils, and alters near-vision. Scopolamine also exerts an *antispasmodic* activity on the gastrointestinal tract and urinary bladder. Because of this the drug is used orally, rectally, and by injection for the relief of gastrointestinal and genitourinary smooth muscle

disorders. Scopolamine also reduces motion sickness. Transdermal patches (see p.18) containing scopolamine are applied to the skin behind the ear 12 hours before departure to decrease motion sickness in adults.

Scopolamine has a number of classic anticholinergic adverse effects, including heart palpitations and dryness of the mouth (see below).

QUICK REFERENCE

Drug group Drug for irritable bowel syndrome (p.122) and anti-emetic drugs (p.102).

Overdose danger rating Medium

Dependence rating Low

Prescription needed No

Multi-source suppliers Yes

INFORMATION FOR USERS

Follow instructions on the label. Call your physician if symptoms worsen.

How taken

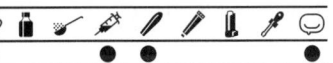

Tablets, injection, rectal suppositories, transdermal patches.

Frequency and timing of doses
1–4 x daily (tablets, rectal suppositories); every 72 hours (transdermal patch).

Dosage range
10–20mg (oral, rectal, injection); 1mg (transdermal patch), limit of 2 consecutive patches.

Onset of effect
Within an hour (oral, rectal, injection); up to 6 hours (transdermal patch).

Duration of action
6–8 hours (oral, rectal, injection); up to 72 hours (transdermal patch).

Diet advice
None.

Storage
Keep in a closed container in a cool, dry place away from reach of children.

Missed dose
Take when you remember. Adjust the timing of your next dose accordingly.

Stopping the drug
Do not stop the drug without consulting your physician, who may supervise a gradual reduction in dosage.

Exceeding the dose
An occasional unintentional extra dose is unlikely to cause problems. Large overdoses may cause drowsiness or agitation. Notify your physician.

SPECIAL PRECAUTIONS

Be sure to consult your physician or pharmacist before taking this drug if:
▼ You have impaired liver or kidney function.
▼ You have heart problems.
▼ You have high blood pressure.
▼ You have had glaucoma.
▼ You have prostate trouble.
▼ You have myasthenia gravis.
▼ You have reflux esophagitis.
▼ You are taking other medications.

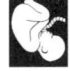 **Pregnancy**
▼ Not usually prescribed. Safety in pregnancy not established. Discuss with your physician.

 Breast feeding
▼ The drug passes into the breast milk. Discuss with your physician.

 Infants and children
▼ Safety and effectiveness not established.

 Over 60
▼ Reduced dose may be necessary.

 Driving and hazardous work
▼ Avoid such activities until you have learned how the drug affects you; it can cause drowsiness and blurred vision, and may impair your concentration.

 Alcohol
▼ Keep consumption low. Alcohol may increase the sedative effect of this drug.

POSSIBLE ADVERSE EFFECTS

Scopolamine has a strong anticholinergic effect on the body, causing a variety of minor symptoms. These can sometimes be minimized by a reduction in dosage.

Symptom/effect	Frequency		Discuss with physician		Stop taking drug now	Call physician now
	Common	Rare	Only if severe	In all cases		
Drowsiness	●		■			
Dry mouth	●		■			
Blurred vision	●			■		
Constipation		●	■			
Difficulty passing urine		●		■		
Headache/eye pain		●		■		
Palpitations		●		■		

INTERACTIONS

Sedatives All drugs, including alcohol, that have a sedative effect on the central nervous system are likely to increase the sedative properties of scopolamine. Such drugs include anti-anxiety and sleeping drugs, antidepressants, narcotic analgesics, and antipsychotics.

Antacids may reduce the absorption of scopolamine. Doses should be spaced 1 hour apart.

Amantadine, quinidine, tricyclic antidepressants These drugs can increase the anticholinergic effect of scopolamine injection.

PROLONGED USE

Use of this drug for longer than a few days is unlikely to be necessary. However, since the body adapts to this drug, a gradual reduction in dose is usually recommended when stopping the drug after prolonged use.

SELEGILINE

Brand names Eldepryl, Novo-Selegiline
Used in the following combined preparations None

GENERAL INFORMATION

Selegiline, also known as deprenyl, is an inhibitor of an enzyme in the brain called monoamine oxidase type B (MAO-B). It is used alone or together with levodopa or levodopa-carbidopa combination to treat Parkinson's disease. In patients newly diagnosed with Parkinson's disease, selegiline may delay the need to start levodopa treatment and may help to slow the progress of the disease itself. In combination with levodopa, it works to increase and extend the effects of levodopa.

At usual doses of up to 10mg, there are no dietary restrictions. However, if the maximum recommended daily dose of 10mg is exceeded, the risk of dangerous reactions, such as sudden elevation of blood pressure, is increased if selegiline is taken with foods that are high in tyramine content. These foods include mature cheeses, pickled herring, red wine, and other foods that are aged or fermented, including beer.

QUICK REFERENCE

Drug group Antiparkinsonism drugs (p.99)

Overdose danger rating High

Dependence rating Low

Prescription needed Yes

Multi-source suppliers Yes

INFORMATION FOR USERS

Your drug prescription is tailored for you. Do not alter dosage without checking with your physician.

How taken

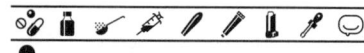

Tablets.

Frequency and timing of doses
2 x daily (breakfast and lunch).

Dosage range
2.5 – 10mg daily.

Onset of effect
30 minutes to 2 hours.

Duration of action
Variable.

Diet advice
No restrictions on food or beverages when taken in doses of 10mg/day or less.

Storage
Keep in a closed container in a cool, dry place away from reach of children. Protect from light.

Missed dose
Take a tablet as soon as you remember. If your next dose is due within 2 hours, take a single dose now and skip the next, then follow your regular schedule.

Stopping the drug
Do not stop taking the drug without consulting your physician; symptoms may recur.

OVERDOSE ACTION

 Seek immediate medical advice in all cases. Take emergency action if chest pains or loss of consciousness occurs.

See Drug poisoning emergency guide (p.574).

POSSIBLE ADVERSE EFFECTS

The adverse effects associated with selegiline, when taken in combination with levodopa, are usually related to excess levodopa and may require a dosage adjustment. Some of the most serious adverse reactions occurring with the combination are hallucinations and confusion, particularly visual hallucinations.

Severe headache, nausea and/or vomiting or unexplained sweating require immediate medical attention.

Symptom/effect	Frequency		Discuss with physician		Stop taking drug now	Call physician now
	Common	Rare	Only if severe	In all cases		
Nausea	●		■			
Dizziness//faintness	●		■			
Hallucinations		●		■		∎
Dry mouth		●	■			
Severe headache/chest pains		●		■	▲	∎
Diarrhea		●		■		

INTERACTIONS

General note Because of the wide range of possible drug interactions with selegiline, do not take any medication, whether prescription or nonprescription, without first consulting your physician or pharmacist.

Meperidine, fluoxetine The combination of fluoxetine with either of these drugs may cause severe and dangerous reactions. Allow at least 14 days after stopping selegiline before taking fluoxetine.

SPECIAL PRECAUTIONS

Be sure to tell your physician if:
▼ You have impaired liver function.
▼ You have a peptic ulcer.
▼ You are taking other medications.

 **Pregnancy**
▼ Safety in pregnancy not established. Discuss with your physician.

 Breast feeding
▼ It is not known if the drug passes into the breast milk. Discuss with your physician.

 Infants and children
▼ Not recommended.

 Over 60
▼ Increased likelihood of adverse effects. Reduced dose may therefore be necessary.

 Driving and hazardous work
▼ Avoid such activities until you have learned how the drug affects you; it can cause dizziness.

 Alcohol
▼ Avoid. Alcohol may increase the risk of adverse effects.

Surgery and general anesthetics
▼ Selegiline treatment should be withdrawn at least 2 weeks before you have a general anesthetic and some dental treatments. Discuss this with your physician or dentist before any surgery.

PROLONGED USE

No problems expected.

SERTRALINE

Brand name Zoloft
Used in the following combined preparations None

GENERAL INFORMATION

Sertraline belongs to the relatively new group of antidepressants called specific serotonin reuptake inhibitors (SSRIs). It elevates mood, increases physical activity, and restores interest in everyday life. Sertraline is generally well tolerated and any gastrointestinal adverse effects, such as nausea or diarrhea, are usually dose-related and decrease with continued use. It is less sedating and causes fewer *anticholinergic side effects* than tricyclic antidepressants.

INFORMATION FOR USERS

Your drug prescription is tailored for you. Do not alter dosage without checking with your physician.

How taken

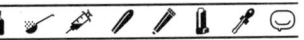

Capsules.

Frequency and timing of doses
Once daily with food.

Adult dosage range
50 – 200mg daily.

Onset of effect
2 – 4 weeks are usually necessary for full antidepressant activity.

Duration of action
Following prolonged treatment, antidepressant effects may persist for some weeks. Adverse effects may wear off within a few days.

Diet advice
None.

Storage
Keep in a closed container at room temperature (15 – 30°C), away from reach of children.

Missed dose
Take as soon as you remember. If your next dose is due within 8 hours, take a single dose now and skip the next.

Stopping the drug
Do not stop taking the drug without consulting your physician; symptoms may recur.

Exceeding the dose
An occasional unintentional extra dose is unlikely to cause problems. But if you notice any unusual symptoms, or if a large overdose has been taken, notify your physician.

POSSIBLE ADVERSE EFFECTS

Adverse effects on the gastrointestinal tract, such as nausea, indigestion, and diarrhea, may decrease with a reduction in dosage. Other adverse effects are rarely a problem.

Symptom/effect	Frequency		Discuss with physician		Stop taking drug now	Call physician now
	Common	Rare	Only if severe	In all cases		
Dry mouth/increased sweating	●		■			
Nausea/diarrhea	●			■		
Indigestion	●		■			
Sexual difficulty		●	■		▲	
Tremor		●	■			
Insomnia		●		■		
Dizziness		●	■			

INTERACTIONS

Monoamine oxidase inhibitors (MAOIs) Sertraline should not be given within 14 days of treatment with an MAOI.

Tryptophan Taken together, tryptophan and sertraline may cause agitation and nausea.

Lithium Taken with sertraline, lithium can increase the risk of unwanted effects.

Cimetidine Taken with sertraline, cimetidine may increase the risk of unwanted effects.

Sedatives These may increase any sedative effect of sertraline.

SPECIAL PRECAUTIONS

Be sure to tell your physician if:
▼ You have impaired liver or kidney function.
▼ You have had epileptic seizures.
▼ You are taking other medications.

Pregnancy
▼ Safety in pregnancy not established. Discuss with your physician.

Breast feeding
▼ Safety not established. Discuss with your physician.

Infants and children
▼ Not recommended in patients under 18 years.

Over 60
▼ No special problems.

Driving and hazardous work
▼ Avoid such activities until you have learned how the drug affects you because the drug can cause drowsiness.

Alcohol
▼ Avoid. Alcohol may increase the sedative effects of this drug.

Surgery and general anesthetics
▼ Sertraline may need to be stopped before you have a general anesthetic. Discuss this with your physician or dentist before any surgery.

PROLONGED USE

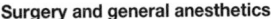

No problems expected.

SILVER SULFADIAZINE

Brand names Flamazine, SSD
Used in the following combined preparation Flamazine C

GENERAL INFORMATION

Silver sulfadiazine is an antibacterial agent applied as cream to prevent infections in burns. The silver in the drug contributes to its antibacterial action, and it is effective against a wide range of bacteria and yeasts. It is sometimes prescribed to prevent the infection of a skin graft. Poorly absorbed from the wound surface, the drug has a long-lasting effect, one daily application generally being sufficient. The most common adverse effect of silver sulfadiazine is a local hypersensitivity reaction that may be difficult to distinguish from the burn itself. When treatment is prolonged or involves large areas of skin, more of the drug may be absorbed, increasing the risk of adverse effects to the kidneys. Monitoring of blood levels of the drug may be advised in those cases.

QUICK REFERENCE

Drug group Anti-infective skin preparation (p.187)

Overdose danger rating Low

Dependence rating Low

Prescription needed Yes

Multi-source suppliers Yes

INFORMATION FOR USERS

Your drug prescription is tailored for you. Do not alter dosage without checking with your physician.

How taken

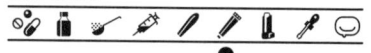

Cream.

Frequency and timing of doses
Usually once daily.

Dosage range
Apply to affected area to a depth of 3 – 5mm.

Onset of effect
Immediately.

Duration of action
24 hours or more.

Diet advice
None.

Storage
Keep in a closed container in a cool, dry place away from reach of children. Protect from light.

Missed dose
Apply as soon as you remember, then return to your once-daily routine.

Stopping the drug
Do not stop taking the drug without consulting your physician. If treatment is stopped before the affected area has healed, infection may occur.

Exceeding the dose
An occasional extra application is unlikely to be cause for concern. If you notice any unusual symptoms, notify your physician.

SPECIAL PRECAUTIONS

Be sure to tell your physician if:
▼ You have impaired liver or kidney functio
▼ You have previously had an allergic reaction to a sulfonamide drug.
▼ You have glucose-6-phosphate dehydrogenase (G6PD) deficiency.
▼ You are taking other medications.

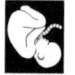

Pregnancy
▼ Should not be used near term.

Breast feeding
▼ At normal doses, adverse effec on the baby are unlikely. Discuss with your physician.

Infants and children
▼ Not recommended for infants under 2 months.

Over 60
▼ No special problems.

Driving and hazardous work
▼ No known problems.

Alcohol
▼ No known problems.

POSSIBLE ADVERSE EFFECTS

Adverse effects occur rarely with silver sulfadiazine and are more likely in those being treated for extensive burns. Sore throat, fever, or jaundice may be early signs of a serious blood disorder, and blood in the urine may indicate kidney problems.

Symptom/effect	Frequency		Discuss with physician		Stop taking drug now	Call physician now
	Common	Rare	Only if severe	In all cases		
Burning sensation		●		■		▮
Rash/itching		●		■		▮
Jaundice		●		■		▮
Blood in urine		●		■		▮
Sore throat/fever		●		■		▮

INTERACTIONS

Enzyme debriding agents The effects of these agents, used to remove dead or infected tissue from a wound or burn, may be negated if used in conjunction with silver sulfadiazine.

Oral antidiabetic agents, phenytoin The effects of these drugs may be increased in patients with large-area burns treated with silver sulfadiazine.

Cimetidine The use of cimetidine in patients with a large-area burn treated with silver sulfadiazine may cause a serious decrease in the white blood cell count.

PROLONGED USE

May increase the risk of serious blood disorders and kidney problems.

Monitoring In treatment of extensive burns, blood levels of the drug and kidney function may be monitored.

SIMVASTATIN

and name Zocor
ed in the following combined preparations None

GENERAL INFORMATION

nvastatin is a new lipid-lowering drug reducing blood cholesterol. It blocks e action of an *enzyme* that is needed cholesterol to be manufactured in e liver, and as a result the blood levels cholesterol are lowered. It is pre-ibed for people with hypercholes-olemia (high levels of cholesterol in e blood) who have not responded to er forms of therapy, such as a ecial diet, and are at risk of developing heart disease. However, if another disease, such as diabetes or hypothyroidism, is responsible for elevated cholesterol, the underlying disease is first treated before using simvastatin.

Side effects are usually mild and often wear off with time. In the body, simvastatin is found mainly in the liver, and it may mildly elevate the levels of various liver enzymes.

INFORMATION FOR USERS

ur drug prescription is tailored for you. not alter dosage without checking h your physician.

w taken

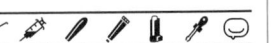

lets.

quency and timing of doses
ce daily at night.

ult dosage range
- 40mg daily.

set of effect
hin 2 weeks; full beneficial effects may not elt for 4 – 6 weeks.

ration of action
to 24 hours.

t advice
ow-fat diet is usually recommended.

Storage
Keep in a closed container in a cool dry place away from reach of children. Protect from light.

Missed dose
Take as soon as you remember. If your next dose is due within 8 hours, do not take the missed dose, but take the next dose on schedule.

Stopping the drug
Do not stop taking the drug without consulting your physician. Stopping the drug may lead to worsening of the underlying condition.

Exceeding the dose
An occasional unintentional extra dose is unlikely to cause problems. Large overdoses may cause liver problems. Notify your physician.

POSSIBLE ADVERSE EFFECTS

e effects are usually mild and do not last g. The most common are those affecting gastrointestinal system. Simvastatin very rarely may cause muscle problems, and any muscle pain or weakness should be reported at once.

nptom/effect	Frequency		Discuss with physician		Stop taking drug now	Call physician now
	Common	Rare	Only if severe	In all cases		
dominal pain		●	■			
stipation/diarrhea		●	■			
sea		●	■			
ulence		●	■			
adache		●		■		
h		●		■	▲	
scle pain/weakness		●		■		▮

INTERACTIONS

nticoagulants Simvastatin may increase e effect of anticoagulants. Dosage djustment may be necessary, and rothrombin time should be monitored egularly.

Cyclosporine, erythromycin, other lipid-lowering drugs Simvastatin and these drugs are not usually prescribed together because of the risk of severe muscle inflammation.

SPECIAL PRECAUTIONS

Be sure to tell your physician if:
▼ You have impaired liver function.
▼ You have had problems with alcohol abuse.
▼ You have eye or vision problems.
▼ You have muscle weakness.
▼ You are taking other medications.

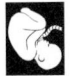

Pregnancy
▼ Not prescribed.

Breast feeding
▼ Not recommended. Discuss with your physician.

Infants and children
▼ Not recommended.

Over 60
▼ No special problems.

Driving and hazardous work
▼ No special problems.

Alcohol
▼ Avoid excessive amounts. Alcohol may increase the risk of developing liver problems with this drug.

Surgery and general anesthetics
▼ Simvastatin may need to be stopped before you have a general anesthetic. Discuss with your physician or dentist before any surgery.

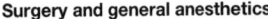

PROLONGED USE

Prolonged treatment can adversely affect liver function.

Monitoring Regular liver function tests are recommended. Periodic eye tests may also be performed.

SOTALOL

Brand name Sotacor
Used in the following combined preparations None

GENERAL INFORMATION

Sotalol is an anti-arrhythmic drug with beta-blocking properties. It is used to prevent and to treat abnormal heart rhythms, particularly life-threatening arrhythmias that originate in the ventricles of the heart. Paradoxically, sotalol can also cause new arrhythmias or worsen existing ones so that a physician must monitor the drug treatment very closely.

Because sotalol can cause breathing difficulties, it should not be prescribed to anyone suffering from asthma, chronic bronchitis, or emphysema. Like all beta blockers, sotalol affects the body's response to low blood sugar; it should therefore be used with caution by diabetics.

INFORMATION FOR USERS

Your drug prescription is tailored for you. Do not alter dosage without checking with your physician.

How taken

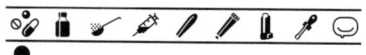

Tablets.

Frequency and timing of doses
2 – 3 x daily on an empty stomach.

Dosage range
160 – 320mg daily.

Onset of effect
2½ – 4 hours.

Duration of action
15 hours.

Diet advice
None.

Storage
Keep in a closed container in a cool, dry place away from reach of children. Protect from light.

Missed dose
Take a tablet as soon as you remember. If your next dose is due within 2 hours, take a single dose now and skip the next, then follow your regular schedule.

Stopping the drug
Do not stop taking the drug without consulting your physician; symptoms may recur.

OVERDOSE ACTION

Seek immediate medical advice in all cases. Take emergency action if breathing difficulties, collapse, or loss of consciousness occurs.

See Drug poisoning emergency guide (p.574).

SPECIAL PRECAUTIONS

Be sure to tell your physician if:
▼ You have impaired liver or kidney function.
▼ You have a lung disorder such as asthma, emphysema, or bronchitis.
▼ You have diabetes.
▼ You are taking other medications.

Pregnancy
▼ Safety in pregnancy not established. Discuss with your physician.

Breast feeding
▼ The drug passes into the breast milk and may affect the baby. Discuss with your physician.

Infants and children
▼ Safety and effectiveness not established.

Over 60
▼ Increased likelihood of adverse effects. Reduced dose may therefore be necessary.

Driving and hazardous work
▼ Avoid such activities until you have learned how the drug affects you; it can cause dizziness.

Alcohol
▼ No special problems with moderate intake.

Surgery and general anesthetics
▼ Sotalol may need to be stopped before you have a general anesthetic. Discuss with your physician or dentist before any surgery.

POSSIBLE ADVERSE EFFECTS

Sotalol has adverse effects that are common to most beta blockers. Symptoms such as fatigue, nausea, and vomiting are usually temporary and diminish with long-term use. Fainting may be a sign that the drug has slowed the heartbeat excessively.

Symptom/effect	Frequency		Discuss with physician		Stop taking drug now	Call physician now
	Common	Rare	Only if severe	In all cases		
Fatigue	●		■			
Slowed heartbeat		●		■		▮
Breathing difficulty		●		■		▮
Fast or irregular heartbeat		●		■		▮
Weakness		●	■			
Dizziness		●				

INTERACTIONS

General note Sotalol may interact with many drugs to cause or worsen abnormal heart rhythms. Such drugs include other anti-arrhythmics, astemizole, terfenadine, tricyclic antidepressants, and phenothiazines.

PROLONGED USE

No special problems expected.

Monitoring Electrocardiograms and periodic tests of body salts are required.

SPIRONOLACTONE

Brand names Aldactone, Novo-Spiroton
Used in the following combined preparations Aldactazide, Apo-Spirozide, Novo-Spirozine

GENERAL INFORMATION

Spironolactone belongs to the class of drugs known as potassium-sparing diuretics. It is used alone or combined with thiazide or loop diuretics in the treatment of hypertension and edema (fluid retention) resulting from congestive heart failure. On its own or, more commonly, in combination with a thiazide diuretic, it may be used to treat edema associated with cirrhosis of the liver, nephrotic syndrome (a kidney disease), and a rare disease called Conn's syndrome, caused by a tumor of the adrenal glands.

Spironolactone is relatively slow to act, and its effects may appear only after several days of treatment. As with other potassium-sparing diuretics, there is a risk of unusually high levels of potassium in the blood if the kidneys are functioning abnormally. For that reason spironolactone is prescribed with caution for people with kidney failure. The drug does not worsen diabetes or gout, as do some other diuretics. The major *side effect* is nausea; abnormal breast enlargement may sometimes occur in men if high doses are given.

INFORMATION FOR USERS

Your drug prescription is tailored for you. Do not alter dosage without checking with your physician.

How taken

Tablets.

Frequency and timing of doses
In single or divided doses, with food.

Adult dosage range
100 – 400mg daily.

Onset of effect
Within 1 – 3 days, but full effect may take up to 2 weeks.

Duration of action
2 – 3 days.

Diet advice
Avoid foods that are high in potassium, e.g. dried fruit and salt substitutes.

Storage
Keep in a closed container in a cool, dry place away from reach of children. Protect from light.

Missed dose
Take as soon as you remember.

Stopping the drug
Do not stop the drug without consulting your physician; symptoms may recur.

Exceeding the dose
An occasional unintentional extra dose is unlikely to be cause for concern. But if you notice any unusual symptoms, or if a large overdose has been taken, notify your physician.

POSSIBLE ADVERSE EFFECTS

Spironolactone has few adverse effects; the main problem is the possibility that potassium may be retained in the body, causing muscle weakness and numbness.

Symptom/effect	Frequency		Discuss with physician		Stop taking drug now	Call physician now
	Common	Rare	Only if severe	In all cases		
Nausea/vomiting	●		■			
Diarrhea		●	■			
Lethargy/drowsiness		●	■			
Irregular menstruation		●		■		
Breast enlargement (men)		●		■		
Impotence		●		■		
Rash		●		■		■

INTERACTIONS

Digoxin Adverse effects may result from increased digoxin levels.

ACE inhibitors may increase the risk of raised blood levels of potassium.

Lithium Spironolactone may increase the blood levels of lithium, leading to an increased risk of lithium poisoning.

SPECIAL PRECAUTIONS

Be sure to tell your physician if:
▼ You have impaired liver or kidney function.
▼ You have Addison's disease.
▼ You have diabetes.
▼ You are taking other medications.

Pregnancy
▼ Safety in pregnancy not established. Discuss with your physician.

Breast feeding
▼ The drug passes into the breast milk but it is not known to be harmful. Discuss with your physician.

Infants and children
▼ Not often prescribed. Reduced dose necessary.

Over 60
▼ Increased likelihood of adverse effects. Reduced dose may therefore be necessary.

Driving and hazardous work
▼ Avoid such activities until you have learned how the drug affects you because it may occasionally cause drowsiness.

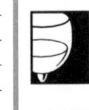

Alcohol
▼ No known problems.

PROLONGED USE

Monitoring Blood tests may be performed to check on kidney function and levels of body salts.

STREPTOKINASE

Brand name Streptase
Used in the following combined preparations None

GENERAL INFORMATION

Streptokinase, an enzyme produced by streptococcus bacteria, is used in hospitals to dissolve the fibrin (see p.117) of blood clots, especially those in the arteries of the heart and lungs. It is also used on the clots formed in shunts during kidney dialysis.

A fast-acting drug, streptokinase is most effective in dissolving newly formed clots, and it is often released at the site of the clot via a catheter inserted into an artery. Administered in the early stages of a heart attack to dissolve a clot in the coronary arteries (thrombosis), it can reduce the amount of damage to heart muscle.

Because excessive bleeding is a common *side effect*, treatment is closely supervised. Since streptokinase is a protein, it can cause allergic reactions. To reduce this risk it is given in a highly purified form, and antihistamines may also be administered at the start of treatment.

INFORMATION FOR USERS

The drug is only given under medical supervision and is not for self-administration.

How taken

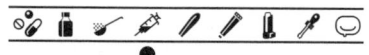

Injection.

Frequency and timing of doses
By a single injection or continuously over a period of 24 – 72 hours.

Dosage range
Dosage is determined individually by the condition and response.

Onset of effect
As soon as streptokinase reaches the blood clot, which begins to dissolve within minutes. Most of the clot will be dissolved within 1 – 2 hours.

Duration of action
Effects disappear within a few minutes of stopping the drug.

Diet advice
None.

Storage
Not applicable. This drug is not normally kept in the home.

Missed dose
Not applicable. This drug is given only in a hospital under close medical supervision.

Stopping the drug
The drug is stopped as soon as the clot has dissolved.

Exceeding the dose
Overdosage is unlikely, since treatment is carefully monitored.

SPECIAL PRECAUTIONS

Streptokinase is prescribed only under close medical supervision, usually only in life-threatening circumstances.

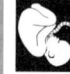

Pregnancy
▼ Not usually prescribed. If used during the first 18 weeks of pregnancy there is a risk that the placenta may separate from the wall of the uterus.

Breast feeding
▼ Effect on breast feeding uncertain. Discuss with your physician.

Infants and children
▼ Not recommended.

Over 60
▼ Increased likelihood of bleeding.

Driving and hazardous work
▼ Not applicable.

Alcohol
▼ Not applicable.

POSSIBLE ADVERSE EFFECTS

Streptokinase is given under strict supervision and all adverse effects are closely monitored so that any of the symptoms below can be quickly dealt with.

Symptom/effect	Frequency		Discuss with physician		Stop taking drug now	Call physician now
	Common	Rare	Only if severe	In all cases		
Excessive bleeding	●			■		
Fever	●			■		
Rash		●		■		
Wheezing		●		■		
Abnormal heart rhythms		●		■		
Collapse		●		■		

PROLONGED USE

Streptokinase is never used long term.

INTERACTIONS

Anticoagulant drugs There is an increased risk of bleeding when these are taken at the same time as streptokinase.

Antiplatelet drugs increase the risk of bleeding if given with streptokinase.

STREPTOMYCIN

Brand names None
Used in the following combined preparations None

GENERAL INFORMATION

Although it is one of the oldest amino-glycoside antibiotics, streptomycin is used with considerable restraint. For one thing, many bacteria have developed open resistance to it since its introduction in 1946. It can also damage the nerves in the ears, upsetting the human balance system and even causing deafness. It is generally reserved for serious infections that do not respond to general antibiotics. Its greatest value is in the early treatment of tuberculosis. Given by injection, it rapidly reaches effective blood levels

and enhances the antibacterial effects of other antituberculous drugs. With some people, it may be given twice weekly on an outpatient basis, and it is usually taken for about two months, after which other drugs are used.

In shorter courses, streptomycin is effective in the treatment of such rare diseases as tularemia, plague, severe brucellosis, rat-bite fever, and glanders. With a penicillin antibiotic it is occasionally used to treat bacterial infection of the heart valves (endocarditis).

QUICK REFERENCE

Drug group Aminoglycoside antibiotic (p.140) and antituberculous drug (p.144).

Overdose danger rating Medium

Dependence rating Low

Prescription needed Yes

Multi-source suppliers No

INFORMATION FOR USERS

The drug is only given under medical supervision and is not for self-administration.

How taken

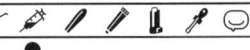

injection.

Frequency and timing of doses
Once daily for 2 – 3 weeks, then every alternate day or 3 x weekly, reduced to 2 x weekly (tuberculosis); 2 x daily (tularemia, plague, brucellosis); 2 x daily for 7 – 10 days, then once daily (other bacterial infections).

Dosage range
Dosage is determined individually according to the condition and response.

Onset of effect
1 – 3 days.

Duration of action
Up to 24 hours. Some beneficial effect may last for several days.

Diet advice
None.

Storage
Not applicable. The drug is not kept in the home.

Missed dose
If you miss a streptomycin injection, contact your physician as soon as possible to arrange for the missed dose to be made up.

Stopping the drug
Take the full course. Even if you feel better, the original infection may still be present and may recur if treatment is stopped too soon.

Exceeding the dose
Overdose is unlikely, since treatment is carefully monitored.

SPECIAL PRECAUTIONS

Be sure to tell your physician if:
▼ You have impaired kidney function.
▼ You have a hearing or a balance disorder.
▼ You have myasthenia gravis or Parkinson's disease.
▼ You are taking other medications.

Pregnancy
▼ Not prescribed. May cause hearing defects in the baby.

Breast feeding
▼ The drug passes into the breast milk and may affect the baby adversely. Discuss with your physician.

Infants and children
▼ Not usually prescribed. Reduced dose necessary.

Over 60
▼ Increased likelihood of adverse effects. Reduced dose may therefore be necessary.

Driving and hazardous work
▼ No known problems.

Alcohol
▼ No known problems.

Surgery and general anesthetics
▼ Streptomycin may need to be stopped before you have a general anesthetic. Discuss this with your physician or dentist before any surgery.

POSSIBLE ADVERSE EFFECTS

The most common side effect of streptomycin is transient facial numbness, sometimes accompanied by tingling in the hands. Headache or malaise also occur occasionally after injection. Dizziness, loss of balance (vertigo), ringing in the ears, and any loss of hearing should be reported to your physician promptly.

Symptom/effect	Frequency		Discuss with physician		Stop taking drug now	Call physician now
	Common	Rare	Only if severe	In all cases		
Headache/malaise	●		■			
Numbness/tingling	●		■			
Nausea/vomiting		●		■		
Dizziness/vertigo		●		■	▲	▮
Ringing in the ears		●		■	▲	▮
Loss of hearing		●		■	▲	▮

INTERACTIONS

General note A wide range of drugs increase the risk of hearing loss and/or kidney failure with streptomycin. Such drugs include other aminoglycosides, furosemide, polymyxin antibiotics, amphotericin B, cisplatin, and cyclosporine.

PROLONGED USE

There is a risk of adverse effects on hearing and balance with prolonged use.

Monitoring Blood levels of the drug may be measured. Periodic hearing and balance tests are usually needed.

SUCRALFATE

Brand names Sulcrate, Sulcrate Suspension Plus, Novo-Sucralate
Used in the following combined preparations None

GENERAL INFORMATION

Sucralfate is prescribed to treat gastric and duodenal ulcers. It does not neutralize stomach acid, but sucralfate forms a protective barrier over the ulcer that prevents it from being attacked by digestive juices, thus giving the ulcer time to heal.

If it is necessary during treatment to take antacids to relieve pain, they should be taken at least half an hour before or after sucralfate, or they will reduce its effectiveness.

Sucralfate in liquid form may be given to prevent gastrointestinal bleeding due to stress ulceration.

Apart from constipation, sucralfate does not have any common adverse effects. However, it interferes with the absorption of fats and may therefore reduce absorption of vitamins that are dissolved in fat – notably vitamins A, D, E, and K. During prolonged treatment it may be necessary to take supplements of these vitamins.

INFORMATION FOR USERS

Your drug prescription is tailored for you. Do not alter dosage without checking with your physician.

How taken

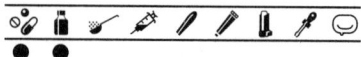

Tablets, oral liquid.

Frequency and timing of doses
2 – 4 x daily, one hour before each meal and at bedtime on an empty stomach; occasionally, up to 6 x daily.

Dosage range
4 – 6g daily.

Onset of effect
Some improvement may be noted after one or two doses, but it takes a few weeks for the ulcer to heal.

Duration of action
Up to 5 hours.

Diet advice
During prolonged treatment make sure your diet includes foods containing vitamins A, D, E, and K (see pp.527–30). Your physician will advise you if supplements are necessary.

Storage
Keep in a closed container in a cool, dry place away from reach of children.

Missed dose
Do not make up the drug you missed. Take your next dose on your original schedule.

Stopping the drug
Do not stop the drug without consulting your physician; symptoms may recur.

Exceeding the dose
An occasional unintentional extra dose is unlikely to be a cause for concern. But if you notice any unusual symptoms, or if a large overdose has been taken, notify your physician.

SPECIAL PRECAUTIONS

Be sure to tell your physician if:
▼ You have impaired kidney function.
▼ You are taking other medications.

Pregnancy
▼ Safety in pregnancy not established. Discuss with your physician.

Breast feeding
▼ No evidence of risk.

Infants and children
▼ Not recommended in patients under 18 years.

Over 60
▼ No special problems.

Driving and hazardous work
▼ Usually no problem, but the drug may cause dizziness in some patients.

Alcohol
▼ Avoid. Alcohol may counteract the beneficial effect of this drug.

POSSIBLE ADVERSE EFFECTS

Most people do not feel any adverse effects while they are taking sucralfate. The most common is constipation, which diminishes as your body adjusts to the drug.

Symptom/effect	Frequency		Discuss with physician		Stop taking drug now	Call physician now
	Common	Rare	Only if severe	In all cases		
Constipation	●			■		
Diarrhea		●		■		
Abdominal pain		●		■		
Dizziness/lightheadedness		●			■	
Nausea		●			■	
Dry mouth		●		■		
Itching/skin rash		●			■	

PROLONGED USE

Not usually prescribed for periods longer than 12 weeks at a time. Prolonged use may lead to deficiencies of vitamins A, D, E, and K.

INTERACTIONS

Phenytoin The effect of this drug may be reduced if taken with sucralfate.

Tetracyclines, ciprofloxacin, norfloxacin, ofloxacin Sucralfate may reduce the effect of these antibiotics.

Antacids and other anti-ulcer drugs These reduce the effectiveness of sucralfate and should be taken at least half an hour before or after sucralfate.

SULFACETAMIDE

Brand names Sodium Sulamyd, AK-Sulf, Bleph-10, Cetamide, Sulfex
Used in the following combined preparations AK-Cide, Blephamide, Cetapred, Metimyd, Vasosulf

GENERAL INFORMATION

Sulfacetamide, an antibacterial drug, is a derivative of the sulfonamide drugs developed in the 1930s. Available as eye drops or ointment, it is used to treat bacterial conjunctivitis. It is also sometimes prescribed to prevent infection after an eye injury or the removal of a foreign body.

Although effective against a wide range of bacteria, the development of resistance to the drug during prolonged treatment is a common problem. Sulfacetamide is therefore most useful for short-term treatment. When given for chronic blepharitis (inflammation of the eyelids) and conjunctivitis, it is not always effective, and other treatments may be preferred. One reason for this is that pus may contain an acid that inactivates sulfonamides.

Fixed-dose combinations of sulfacetamide and a corticosteroid, sometimes with a decongestant, may be used to treat conditions in which there is inflammation or allergy.

INFORMATION FOR USERS

Your drug prescription is tailored for you. Do not alter dosage without checking with your physician.

How taken

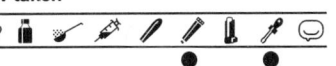

Ointment, eye drops.

Frequency and timing of doses
Every 1 – 3 hours (eye drops); every 6 hours and at bedtime (ointment).

Dosage range
1 – 2 drops per application (eye drops); 1.25 – 2.5cm per application (ointment).

Onset of effect
12 – 24 hours.

Duration of action
1 – 3 hours (drops); up to 6 hours (ointment).

Diet advice
None.

Storage
Keep in a closed container in a cool, dry place away from reach of children. Protect from light. Discard 4 weeks after opening.

Missed dose
Take as soon as you remember. If your next dose is due within 1 hour (eye drops) or within 2 hours (ointment), take a single dose now and skip the next.

Stopping the drug
Use the full course. Even if the affected area seems cured, the original infection may still be present and may recur if treatment is stopped too soon.

Exceeding the dose
An occasional unintentional extra dose is unlikely to be a cause for concern. But if you notice unusual symptoms, or if a large overdose has been taken, notify your physician.

POSSIBLE ADVERSE EFFECTS

Eye drops may cause stinging or burning on application. Itching, redness, or other signs of irritation may be symptoms of an allergic reaction to the drug.

Symptom/effect	Frequency		Discuss with physician		Stop taking drug now	Call physician now
	Common	Rare	Only if severe	In all cases		
Stinging/burning	●		■			
Itching/redness		●		■	▲	▌
Swelling of eyelids		●		■	▲	▌

INTERACTIONS

Silver eye preparations Sulfacetamide is incompatible with these preparations and they should not be used together.

Zinc sulfate Sulfacetamide interacts with zinc sulfate eye drops and the two should not be used together.

SPECIAL PRECAUTIONS

Be sure to tell your physician if:
▼ You have had a previous allergic reaction to sulfonamides.
▼ You wear contact lenses.
▼ You are taking other medications.

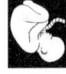

Pregnancy
▼ No evidence of risk to the developing baby when the drug is used in the manner prescribed.

Breast feeding
▼ No evidence of risk when the drug is used in the manner prescribed.

Infants and children
▼ No special problems.

Over 60
▼ No special problems.

Driving and hazardous work
▼ No known problems.

Alcohol
▼ No known problems.

PROLONGED USE

Not usually given for longer than 10 days.

SULFAMETHOXAZOLE

Brand name Apo-Sulfamethoxazole
Used in the following combined preparations Apo-Sulfatrim, Bactrim, Novo-Trimel, Roubac, Septra

GENERAL INFORMATION

Sulfamethoxazole, a sulfonamide drug, is prescribed for the treatment of many bacterial infections. It is available alone or in combination with trimethoprim, another antibiotic.

Alone, sulfamethoxazole is used to treat urinary tract infections. Combined with trimethoprim, it is thought by some physicians to be less likely to produce drug-resistant infections, and is widely used for bacterial infections of the respiratory and urinary tracts,

gastroenteritis, typhoid fever, and pneumocystis pneumonia.

A long-acting drug, sulfamethoxazole does not have to be taken as often as many other sulfonamides. Its *side effects* are like those of similar drugs, rash and digestive upset being among the most common. An adequate fluid intake must be maintained to prevent the damaging formation of crystals in the urine.

INFORMATION FOR USERS

Your drug prescription is tailored for you. Do not alter dosage without checking with your physician.

How taken

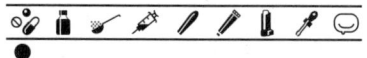

Tablets.

Frequency and timing of doses
2 – 3 x daily with water.

Dosage range
Adults 2 – 3g daily.
Children Reduced dose according to age and weight.

Onset of effect
Symptoms usually improve within 1 – 3 days, depending on the condition.

Duration of action
10 – 12 hours.

Diet advice
It is important to drink plenty of fluids (at least 1.5 litres a day) during treatment.

Storage
Keep in a closed container in a cool, dry place away from reach of children. Protect from light.

Missed dose
Take as soon as you remember. If your next dose is due at this time, double the usual dose to make up for the missed dose.

Stopping the drug
Take the full course. Even if you feel better, the original infection may still be present and symptoms may recur if treatment is stopped too soon.

Exceeding the dose
An occasional unintentional extra dose is unlikely to be a cause for concern. But if you notice unusual symptoms, or if a large overdose has been taken, notify your physician.

SPECIAL PRECAUTIONS

Be sure to tell your physician if:
▼ You have impaired liver or kidney function.
▼ You have a blood disorder.
▼ You suffer from porphyria.
▼ You are allergic to sulfonamides.
▼ You have glucose-6-phosphate dehydrogenase (G6PD) deficiency.
▼ You are taking other medications.

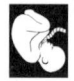

Pregnancy
▼ No evidence of risk in early pregnancy, but if taken in late pregnancy it may cause jaundice and liver problems in the newborn baby. Discuss with your physician.

Breast feeding
▼ The drug passes into the breast milk and may affect the baby adversely. Discuss with your physician.

Infants and children
▼ Not usually prescribed for infants under 2 months. Reduced dose necessary in older children.

Over 60
▼ Reduced dose may be necessary.

Driving and hazardous work
▼ No known problems.

Alcohol
▼ No known problems.

POSSIBLE ADVERSE EFFECTS

Sulfamethoxazole has a number of common adverse effects. When taken with trimethoprim, these effects may become slightly more severe.

Symptom/effect	Frequency		Discuss with physician		Stop taking drug now	Call physician now
	Common	Rare	Only if severe	In all cases		
Nausea/vomiting	●			■		
Loss of appetite	●			■		
Diarrhea		●		■		
Headache/dizziness		●		■		
Fever		●		■		▮
Aching joints/muscles		●		■		▮
Rash		●		■	▲	▮

INTERACTIONS

Oral anticoagulants Sulfamethoxazole may increase the effects of these drugs.

Phenytoin Sulfamethoxazole may cause a buildup of phenytoin in the body.

Oral antidiabetic drugs Sulfamethoxazole may increase the effect of these drugs in lowering blood sugar.

PROLONGED USE

Use of this drug over an extended period can lead to blood disorders in rare cases.

Monitoring Periodic blood samples may be taken to check blood composition during prolonged treatment.

SULFASALAZINE

Brand names Salazopyrin, PMS Sulfasalazine, SAS-500
Used in the following combined preparations None

GENERAL INFORMATION

Sulfasalazine, chemically related to the sulfonamide antibacterial drugs, is used to treat two inflammatory disorders of the bowel. One is ulcerative colitis which mainly affects the large intestine); the other is Crohn's disease (which typically affects the small intestine). In recent years, sulfasalazine has also been found to be effective in the treatment of rheumatoid arthritis.

Adverse effects such nausea, loss of appetite, and general discomfort are more likely when higher doses are taken. *Side effects* caused by stomach irritation may be reduced by a change to a specially coated tablet formulation of the drug. Allergic reactions such as fever and skin rash may be avoided or minimized by low initial doses that are gradually increased. Adequate fluid intake is important while taking this drug. In rare cases, temporary sterility in men may occur.

INFORMATION FOR USERS

Your drug prescription is tailored for you. Do not alter dosage without checking with your physician.

How taken

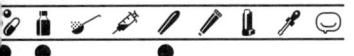

Tablets, oral liquid, enema.

Frequency and timing of doses
1 – 4 x daily after meals with a glass of water (tablets, oral liquid); once daily, usually at bedtime (enema).

Adult dosage range
1 – 4g daily (Crohn's disease, ulcerative colitis); 1 – 3g daily (rheumatoid arthritis).

Onset of effect
Adverse effects may be noticed within a few days but beneficial effects may not be felt for 1 – 3 weeks, depending on the severity of the condition.

Duration of action
About 24 hours.

Diet advice
It is important to drink plenty of liquids (at least 1.5 litres a day) during treatment. Sulfasalazine may reduce the absorption of folic acid from the intestine, leading to a deficiency of this vitamin. Eat plenty of green vegetables.

Storage
Keep in a closed container in a cool, dry place away from reach of children.

Missed dose
Take as soon as you remember. If your next dose is due within 2 hours, take a single dose now and skip the next.

Stopping the drug
Do not stop the drug without consulting your physician; symptoms may recur.

Exceeding the dose
An occasional unintentional extra dose is unlikely to be a cause for concern. But if you notice unusual symptoms, or if a large overdose has been taken, notify your physician.

SPECIAL PRECAUTIONS

Be sure to tell your physician if:
▼ You have impaired liver or kidney function.
▼ You have intestinal or urinary obstruction.
▼ You wear soft contact lenses.
▼ You have glucose-6-phosphate dehydrogenase (G6PD) deficiency.
▼ You have a blood disorder.
▼ You suffer from porphyria.
▼ You are allergic to sulfonamides or salicylates.
▼ You are taking other medications.

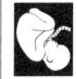

Pregnancy
▼ No evidence of risk to the developing baby, but caution is warranted, especially near term. Folic acid supplements may be required.

Breast feeding
▼ The drug passes into the breast milk and may affect the baby. Discuss with your physician.

Infants and children
▼ Not recommended for children under 2 years. Reduced dose necessary for older children, according to body weight.

Over 60
▼ No special problems.

Driving and hazardous work
▼ No special problems.

Alcohol
▼ No known problems.

POSSIBLE ADVERSE EFFECTS

Adverse effects are common with high doses, but may disappear with a reduction in the dose. Symptoms such as nausea, vomiting, and diarrhea may be helped by taking the drug with food. Orange or yellow discoloration of the urine is no cause for alarm.

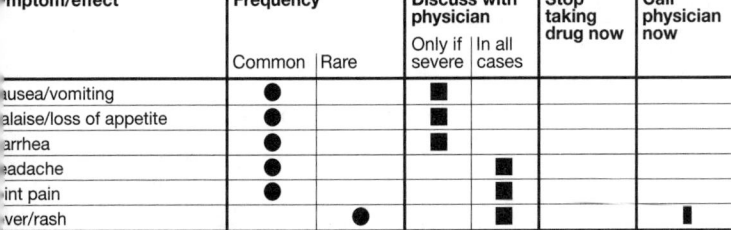

Symptom/effect	Frequency		Discuss with physician		Stop taking drug now	Call physician now
	Common	Rare	Only if severe	In all cases		
Nausea/vomiting	●		■			
Malaise/loss of appetite	●		■			
Diarrhea	●		■			
Headache	●			■		
Joint pain	●			■		
Fever/rash		●		■	■	■

PROLONGED USE

Prolonged use of this drug may lead to blood disorders.

Monitoring Periodic tests of blood composition and liver function are usually required.

INTERACTIONS

General note Sulfasalazine may increase the effects of a variety of drugs, including oral anticoagulant, oral antidiabetic, and anticonvulsant drugs, and methotrexate.

Digoxin and folic acid Sulfasalazine may reduce the absorption of these drugs.

SULFINPYRAZONE

Brand names Anturan, Apo-Sulfinpyrazone, Novo-Pyrazone
Used in the following combined preparations None

GENERAL INFORMATION

Sulfinpyrazone is prescribed for people who suffer from frequent attacks of gout. It reduces the amount of uric acid in the body by increasing the amount excreted in the urine.

Prescribed for the long-term prevention of gout attacks, it is not helpful for relieving the pain and inflammation of gout once an attack has started.

During the first months of treatment attacks may be more frequent, and colchicine may be prescribed to reduce the frequency and severity of gout attacks during this period.

Sulfinpyrazone may sometimes be used to prevent the formation of abnormal blood clots caused by excessive platelet stickiness (see Drugs that affect blood clotting, p.116), for example, transient ischemic attacks. The drug may occasionally be prescribed following a first heart attack to prevent further attacks.

INFORMATION FOR USERS

Your drug prescription is tailored for you. Do not alter dosage without checking with your physician.

How taken

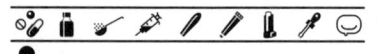

Tablets.

Frequency and timing of doses
1 – 4 x daily with meals or milk.

Adult dosage range
200 – 800mg daily, depending on condition and response.

Onset of effect
Some response in 1 – 2 weeks, but full beneficial effects may not be felt for 3 – 6 months.

Duration of action
Up to 10 hours.

Diet advice
Drink plenty of fluids.

Storage
Keep in a closed container in a cool, dry place away from reach of children.

Missed dose
Take as soon as you remember. If your next dose is due within 3 hours, take a single dose now and skip the next.

Stopping the drug
Do not stop the drug without consulting your physician; symptoms may recur.

Exceeding the dose
An occasional unintentional extra dose is unlikely to cause problems. Large overdoses may cause nausea, vomiting, or unsteadiness. Notify your physician.

SPECIAL PRECAUTIONS

Be sure to tell your physician if:
▼ You have impaired liver or kidney function
▼ You have kidney stones.
▼ You have asthma.
▼ You have had a peptic ulcer.
▼ You have a blood disorder.
▼ You are allergic to ASA.
▼ You are taking other medications.

Pregnancy
▼ Safety in pregnancy not established. Discuss with your physician.

Breast feeding
▼ It is not known whether the drug passes into the breast milk. Discuss with your physician.

Infants and children
▼ Not recommended.

Over 60
▼ No special problems.

Driving and hazardous work
▼ No known problems.

Alcohol
▼ Avoid. Alcohol may reduce the effect of this drug. It may also worsen gout.

POSSIBLE ADVERSE EFFECTS

Most people do not notice any severe adverse effects when taking sulfinpyrazone. The more common adverse effects usually diminish during treatment as your body adjusts to the drug. A peptic ulcer may be reactivated.

Symptom/effect	Frequency		Discuss with physician		Stop taking drug now	Call physician now
	Common	Rare	Only if severe	In all cases		
Nausea/vomiting	●		■			
Headache		●		■		
Flushing		●		■		
Bloodstained/cloudy urine		●		■		▌
Rash/itching		●		■	▲	▌
Wheezing/breathlessness		●		■		▌

INTERACTIONS

General note Many drugs affect the action of sulfinpyrazone and may require an adjustment of dosage. Some may reduce the effect of sulfinpyrazone (for example, thiazide diuretics and alcohol). Others may have their effects increased by sulfinpyrazone (for example, oral diabetic drugs, insulin, indomethacin, sulfonamides, and oral anticoagulant drugs).

ASA and other salicylates may reduce the effect of sulfinpyrazone in the treatment of gout, and may also cause bleeding.

PROLONGED USE

In rare cases blood disorders may occur.

Monitoring Periodic checks on blood cells and uric acid levels in the blood are usually required.

SULFISOXAZOLE

Brand names Apo-Sulfisoxazole, Novo-Soxazole, Sulfizole
Used in the following combined preparations Azo Gantrisin, Pediazole

GENERAL INFORMATION

Sulfisoxazole, introduced in 1951, is prescribed to treat a variety of bacterial infections. When taken by mouth, it is rapidly absorbed from the intestine. Unlike many other sulfonamide antibacterial drugs, it does not build up in the body in excessive amounts.

The main use of sulfisoxazole is in the short-term treatment of lower urinary tract infections which involve the bladder but do not affect the kidneys. In combination with erythromycin, it is used to treat middle ear infections in children.

Although serious adverse effects are uncommon, sulfisoxazole sometimes causes nausea, vomiting, and loss of appetite. Allergic rashes can also occur.

INFORMATION FOR USERS

Your drug prescription is tailored for you. Do not alter dosage without checking with your physician.

How taken

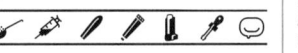

Tablets.

Frequency and timing of doses
3 – 6 x daily with water.

Dosage range
Adults 2 – 4g (starting dose), then 4 – 8g daily (maintenance dose).
Children Reduced dose according to age and weight.

Onset of effect
Symptoms usually improve within 1 – 2 days, depending on the condition.

Duration of action
4 – 6 hours.

Diet advice
It is important to drink plenty of fluids (at least 1.5 litres a day) during sulfisoxazole treatment.

Storage
Keep in a closed container in a cool, dry place away from reach of children. Protect from light.

Missed dose
Take as soon as you remember. If your next dose is due at this time, double the usual dose to make up for the missed dose.

Stopping the drug
Take the full course. Even if you feel better, the original infection may still be present and symptoms may recur if treatment is stopped too soon.

Exceeding the dose
An occasional unintentional extra dose is unlikely to be a cause for concern. But if you notice unusual symptoms, or if a large overdose has been taken, notify your physician.

POSSIBLE ADVERSE EFFECTS

Sulfisoxazole commonly causes digestive upsets such as nausea and loss of appetite. If more serious adverse reactions such as rash occur, the drug may have to be stopped.

Symptom/effect	Frequency		Discuss with physician		Stop taking drug now	Call physician now
	Common	Rare	Only if severe	In all cases		
Nausea/vomiting	●		■			
Loss of appetite	●		■			
Diarrhea		●	■			
Headache/dizziness		●	■			
Rash		●		■	▲	▮

INTERACTIONS

Oral antidiabetic drugs Sulfisoxazole may increase the effect of these drugs in lowering blood sugar.

Oral anticoagulant drugs Sulfisoxazole may increase the effect of oral anticoagulants.

Phenytoin Sulfisoxazole may cause a buildup of phenytoin in the body.

SPECIAL PRECAUTIONS

Be sure to tell your physician if:
▼ You have impaired liver or kidney function.
▼ You have a blood disorder.
▼ You suffer from porphyria.
▼ You have glucose-6-phosphate dehydrogenase (G6PD) deficiency.
▼ You are allergic to sulfonamides.
▼ You are taking other medications.

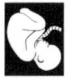

Pregnancy
▼ No evidence of risk in early pregnancy, but if taken in late pregnancy it may cause jaundice and liver problems in the newborn baby. Discuss with your physician.

Breast feeding
▼ The drug passes into the breast milk and may affect the baby adversely. Discuss with your physician.

Infants and children
▼ Not usually prescribed for infants under 2 months. Reduced dose necessary in older children.

Over 60
▼ Reduced dose may be necessary.

Driving and hazardous work
▼ No known problems.

Alcohol
▼ No known problems.

PROLONGED USE

Can lead to blood disorders in rare cases.

SULINDAC

Brand names Clinoril, Apo-Sulin, Novo-Sundac
Used in the following combined preparations None

GENERAL INFORMATION

Sulindac, introduced in 1979, is a non-steroidal anti-inflammatory drug (NSAID) that reduces pain, stiffness, and inflammation.

It is used in the treatment of many arthritic conditions, including rheumatoid arthritis, osteoarthritis, and ankylosing spondylitis. It is sometimes prescribed for psoriatic arthritis and Reiter's syndrome, a disorder that affects the joints, urinary tract, and eyes. Acute attacks of gout and bursitis or tendinitis of the shoulder usually respond to one or two weeks of treatment.

Indigestion, nausea, diarrhea, and constipation are fairly common with this drug. There is also a risk of stomach bleeding or peptic ulcer. Sulindac may be preferred to certain other NSAIDs for long-term use as it requires only two doses a day.

QUICK REFERENCE

Drug group Non-steroidal anti-inflammatory drug (p.128)

Overdose danger rating Low

Dependence rating Low

Prescription needed Yes

Multi-source suppliers Yes

INFORMATION FOR USERS

Your drug prescription is tailored for you. Do not alter dosage without checking with your physician.

How taken

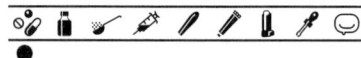

Tablets.

Frequency and timing of doses
2 x daily with food or milk.

Adult dosage range
300 – 400mg daily.

Onset of effect
Pain relief begins within 2 hours. Full anti-inflammatory effect may not be felt for 2 – 3 weeks.

Duration of action
12 – 24 hours.

Diet advice
None.

Storage
Keep in a closed container in a cool, dry place away from reach of children.

Missed dose
Take as soon as you remember. If your next dose is due within 2 hours, take a single dose now and skip the next.

Stopping the drug
For short-term pain relief, the drug can be safely stopped when you no longer need it. For rheumatoid arthritis, do not stop the drug without consulting your physician.

Exceeding the dose
An occasional unintentional extra dose is unlikely to be a cause for concern. But if you notice unusual symptoms, or if a large overdose has been taken, notify your physician.

SPECIAL PRECAUTIONS

Be sure to tell your physician if:
▼ You have heart problems or high blood pressure.
▼ You have a bleeding disorder.
▼ You have impaired liver or kidney function.
▼ You have asthma.
▼ You have had a peptic ulcer, esophagitis, or gastritis.
▼ You are allergic to ASA or other NSAIDs.
▼ You are taking other medications.

Pregnancy
▼ Not usually prescribed. Safety in pregnancy not established. Discuss with your physician.

Breast feeding
▼ The drug passes into the breast milk and may affect the baby. Discuss with your physician.

Infants and children
▼ Not usually prescribed.

Over 60
▼ Increased likelihood of adverse effects. Reduced dose may therefore be necessary.

Driving and hazardous work
▼ Avoid such activities until you have learned how the drug affects you, because the drug may occasionally cause dizziness and drowsiness.

Alcohol
▼ Avoid. Alcohol increases the risk of peptic ulcers with this drug.

POSSIBLE ADVERSE EFFECTS

Most adverse effects are not serious and may disappear as treatment continues. Black or bloodstained feces should be reported without delay.

Symptom/effect	Frequency		Discuss with physician		Stop taking drug now	Call physician now
	Common	Rare	Only if severe	In all cases		
Nausea/vomiting	●		■			
Constipation/diarrhea	●		■			
Abdominal pain/indigestion	●			■		
Dizziness/drowsiness		●		■		
Rash/itching		●		■	▲	▮
Black/bloodstained feces		●		■	▲	▮
Wheezing/breathlessness		●		■	▲	▮

INTERACTIONS

General note Sulindac interacts with a wide range of drugs to increase the risk of bleeding and/or peptic ulcers. Such drugs include oral anticoagulants, corticosteroids, other non-steroidal anti-inflammatory drugs (NSAIDs), and ASA.

Antihypertensive and diuretic drugs The beneficial effects of these drugs may be reduced by sulindac.

Surgery and general anesthetics
▼ Sulindac may prolong bleeding. Discuss with your physician or dentist before any surgery.

PROLONGED USE

There is an increased risk of bleeding from peptic ulcers and in the bowel with prolonged use of sulindac.

SUMATRIPTAN

Brand name Imitrex
Used in the following combined preparations None

GENERAL INFORMATION

Sumatriptan is a highly effective new drug for migraine, generally used when people fail to respond to simple analgesics (e.g., ASA, acetaminophen). It is of considerable value in the treatment of acute migraine attacks, with or without aura, but it is not meant to be taken regularly to prevent attacks.

Sumatriptan should be taken as soon as possible after the onset of the attack, although, unlike other drugs used in migraine, it will still be of benefit at whatever stage of the attack it is taken.

Sumatriptan relieves symptoms by preventing the dilation of blood vessels in the brain, which causes the migraine attack.

INFORMATION FOR USERS

Your drug prescription is tailored for you. Do not alter dosage without checking with your physician.

How taken

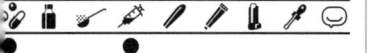

Tablets, injection.

Frequency and timing of doses
Should be taken as soon as possible after the onset of an attack. However, it is equally effective at whatever stage it is taken. DO NOT take a second dose for the same attack. The tablets should be swallowed whole with water.

Adult dosage range
Tablets 100mg per attack. This can be repeated if another attack occurs up to a maximum of 300mg in 24 hours.
Injection 6mg per attack. For a second attack the injection may be repeated after at least 1 hour. Maximum 12mg (two injections) in 24 hours.

Onset of effect
Tablets 30 minutes. *Injection* 10 – 15 minutes.

Duration of action
Tablets The maximum effect occurs after 2 – 4 hours.
Injection The maximum effect occurs after 1½ – 2 hours.

Diet advice
None unless otherwise advised.

Storage
Keep in a closed container in a cool, dry place away from reach of children. Protect from light.

Missed dose
Not applicable.

Stopping the drug
Only taken to treat a migraine attack.

Exceeding the dose
An occasional unintentional extra tablet/ injection is unlikely to be a cause for concern. But if you notice unusual symptoms, or if a large overdose has been taken, notify your physician.

POSSIBLE ADVERSE EFFECTS

Many of the adverse effects will disappear after about 1 hour as your body adjusts to the medication. If the symptoms persist and are severe, contact your physician.

Symptom/effect	Frequency		Discuss with physician		Stop taking drug now	Call physician now
	Common	Rare	Only if severe	In all cases		
Pain at injection site	●			■		
Tingling/heat sensation	●			■		
Muscle weakness	●			■		
Nausea/vomiting	●			■		
Heaviness/pressure sensation		●		■	▲	▌
Dizziness/flushing		●	■			
Fatigue/drowsiness		●	■			
Chest pain		●		■	▲	▌

INTERACTIONS

Antidepressants Monoamine oxidase inhibitors (MAOIs) and some other antidepressants, such as fluvoxamine, fluoxetine, paroxetine, and sertraline, increase the risk of adverse effects with sumatriptan.

Lithium Sumatriptan should not be given to patients taking lithium, due to an increased risk of adverse effects.

Ergotamine There is an increased risk of adverse effects on the blood circulation if ergotamine is used with sumatriptan.

SPECIAL PRECAUTIONS

Be sure to tell your physician if:
▼ You have impaired liver or kidney function.
▼ You have angina or other heart problems.
▼ You have had epileptic seizures.
▼ You have high blood pressure.
▼ You are allergic to sulfonamides.
▼ You are taking other medications.

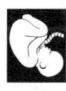

Pregnancy
▼ Safety in pregnancy not established. Discuss with your physician.

Breast feeding
▼ Safety not established. Discuss with your physician.

Infants and children
▼ Not recommended in patients under 18 years.

Over 60
▼ Not recommended.

Driving and hazardous work
▼ Avoid such activities until you have learned how the drug affects you because the drug can cause drowsiness.

Alcohol
▼ No special problems, but some drinks may provoke migraine in some people.

Surgery and general anesthetics
▼ Notify your physician or dentist if you have used sumatriptan within 48 hours prior to surgery.

PROLONGED USE

Sumatriptan should not be used continuously to prevent migraine but only to treat migraine attacks as prescribed.

TAMOXIFEN

Brand names Nolvadex, Alpha-Tamoxifen, Apo-Tamoxifen, Novo-Tamoxifen, Tamofen, Tamone
Used in the following combined preparations None

GENERAL INFORMATION

Tamoxifen is an anticancer drug used in the treatment of breast cancer, both before and after the menopause. It works against cancers whose growth is stimulated by female sex hormones called estrogens. By latching on to cells that recognize these hormones, it can slow the growth of the tumor and even shrink it. Tamoxifen can be used either alone or with other anticancer drugs to treat breast cancer.

Because its effect is specific, tamoxifen has fewer adverse effects than most other drugs used to treat breast cancer. However, it may cause eye damage if high doses are taken for long periods. When used to treat cancer that has spread to the bones, tamoxifen may cause pain in the affected site at first. This discomfort is often a good sign of response to treatment.

INFORMATION FOR USERS

Your drug prescription is tailored for you. Do not alter dosage without checking with your physician.

How taken

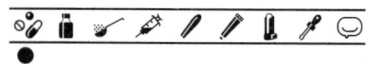

Tablets.

Frequency and timing of doses
1 – 2 x daily.

Adult dosage range
20 – 40mg daily.

Onset of effect
Side effects may be felt within days, but beneficial effects may take 4 – 10 weeks.

Duration of action
Effects may be felt for several weeks after stopping the drug.

Diet advice
None.

Storage
Keep in a closed container in a cool, dry place away from reach of children. Protect from light.

Missed dose
Take as soon as you remember. If your next dose is due within 2 hours, take a single dose now and skip the next.

Stopping the drug
Do not stop the drug without consulting your physician; stopping the drug may lead to worsening of the underlying condition.

Exceeding the dose
An occasional unintentional extra dose is unlikely to be a cause for concern. But if you notice unusual symptoms, or if a large overdose has been taken, notify your physician.

SPECIAL PRECAUTIONS

Be sure to tell your physician if:
▼ You have cataracts or poor eyesight.
▼ You are taking other medications.

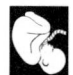

Pregnancy
▼ Not prescribed.

Breast feeding
▼ Not usually prescribed. Discuss with your physician.

Infants and children
▼ Not prescribed.

Over 60
▼ No special problems.

Driving and hazardous work
▼ Do not drive until you have learned how the drug affects you; it can cause blurred vision and dizziness.

Alcohol
▼ No known problems.

POSSIBLE ADVERSE EFFECTS

These are rarely serious and do not usually require treatment to be stopped. Nausea, vomiting, and hot flushes are the most common reactions.

Symptom/effect	Frequency		Discuss with physician		Stop taking drug now	Call physician now
	Common	Rare	Only if severe	In all cases		
Hot flushes	●		■			
Irregular vaginal bleeding	●			■		
Nausea/vomiting	●		■			
Swollen feet/ankles		●	■			
Bone and tumor pain		●			■	
Rash/itching		●			■	
Blurred vision/headache		●			■	

PROLONGED USE

There is a risk of damage to the eyes with long-term high-dose treatment.

Monitoring Eyesight may be tested periodically. Blood tests to measure calcium may be done periodically.

INTERACTIONS

Anticoagulants Patients treated with anticoagulants such as warfarin will usually need a lower dose of the anticoagulant.

TEMAZEPAM

Brand name Restoril
Used in the following combined preparations None

GENERAL INFORMATION

Temazepam belongs to a group of drugs known as the benzodiazepines. The actions and adverse effects of this group of drugs are described more fully under Anti-anxiety drugs (p.95).

Temazepam is used in the short-term treatment of insomnia. It seems well suited to prevent early awakening. However, because of its slow onset of effect, it may be less helpful to patients having trouble falling asleep. Mild morning hangover is possible.

Like other benzodiazepines, temazepam can be habit-forming if taken regularly over a long period. Its effects may also grow weaker with time. For those reasons, treatment with temazepam is usually reviewed every two weeks.

INFORMATION FOR USERS

Your drug prescription is tailored for you. Do not alter dosage without checking with your physician.

How taken

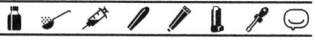

Capsules.

Frequency and timing of doses
Once daily at bedtime.

Adult dosage range
15 – 30mg.

Onset of effect
30 – 60 minutes, or longer.

Duration of action
6 – 8 hours.

Diet advice
None.

Storage
Keep in a closed container in a cool, dry place away from reach of children. Protect from light.

Missed dose
If you fall asleep without having taken a dose and wake some hours later, do not take the missed dose. If necessary, return to your normal dose schedule the following night.

Stopping the drug
If you have been taking the drug continuously for less than 2 weeks, it can be safely stopped as soon as you feel you no longer need it. However, if you have been taking the drug for longer, consult your physician, who may supervise a gradual reduction in dosage. Stopping abruptly may lead to withdrawal symptoms (see p.94).

Exceeding the dose
An occasional unintentional extra dose is unlikely to cause problems. Large overdoses may cause unusual drowsiness. Notify your physician.

SPECIAL PRECAUTIONS

Be sure to tell your physician if:
▼ You have a severe respiratory disease.
▼ You have impaired liver or kidney function.
▼ You have myasthenia gravis.
▼ You have had problems with alcohol or drug abuse.
▼ You suffer from depression.
▼ You are taking other medications.

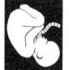

Pregnancy
▼ Safety in pregnancy not established. Discuss with your physician.

Breast feeding
▼ Not usually prescribed. Discuss with your physician.

Infants and children
▼ Not recommended in patients under 18 years.

Over 60
▼ Increased likelihood of adverse effects. Reduced dose may therefore be necessary.

Driving and hazardous work
▼ Avoid such activities until you have learned how the drug affects you; it can cause blurred vision, reduced alertness, and slowed reactions.

Alcohol
▼ Avoid. Alcohol increases the sedative effects of this drug.

POSSIBLE ADVERSE EFFECTS

The principal adverse effects of this drug are related to its sedative and tranquilizing properties. These effects normally diminish after the first few days of treatment.

Symptom/effect	Frequency		Discuss with physician		Stop taking drug now	Call physician now
	Common	Rare	Only if severe	In all cases		
Daytime drowsiness	●		■			
Dizziness/unsteadiness	●		■			
Shortness of breath		●		■		
Blurred vision		●		■		
Forgetfulness/confusion		●		■		■
Rash		●		■	▲	■

INTERACTIONS

Sedatives All drugs, including alcohol, that have a sedative effect on the central nervous system are likely to increase the sedative properties of temazepam. Such drugs include other anti-anxiety and sleeping drugs, antihistamines, antidepressants, narcotic analgesics, and antipsychotics.

PROLONGED USE

Regular use of this drug over several weeks can lead to a reduction in its effect as the body adapts. It may also be habit-forming when taken for extended periods, especially if larger-than-average doses are taken.

TENOXICAM

Brand name Mobiflex
Used in the following combined preparations None

GENERAL INFORMATION

Tenoxicam is a non-steroidal anti-inflammatory drug (NSAID). Like other drugs of this group, it reduces pain, stiffness, and inflammation. Blood levels of the drug remain high for many hours after a dose, so that it needs to be taken only once daily.

It is prescribed for rheumatoid arthritis, osteoarthritis, and ankylosing spondylitis. Although tenoxicam gives lasting relief of the symptoms of arthritis, it does not cure the disease. It is sometimes prescribed in conjunction with slow-acting drugs in rheumatoid arthritis to relieve pain and inflammation while these drugs take effect. It may be given for pain relief in bursitis and tendinitis.

QUICK REFERENCE

Drug group Non-steroidal anti-inflammatory drug (p.128)

Overdose danger rating Medium

Dependence rating Low

Prescription needed Yes

Multi-source suppliers No

INFORMATION FOR USERS

Your drug prescription is tailored for you. Do not alter dosage without checking with your physician.

How taken

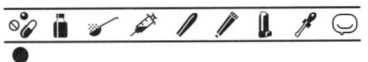

Tablets.

Frequency and timing of doses
Once daily with food.

Dosage range
10 – 20mg daily.

Onset of effect
Pain relief begins within 1 – 3 hours. Used for arthritis, full anti-inflammatory effect develops over 2 weeks or longer.

Duration of action
Up to 2 days. Some effect may last for 7 – 10 days after treatment has been stopped.

Diet advice
None.

Storage
Keep in a closed container in a cool, dry place away from reach of children.

Missed dose
Take as soon as you remember. If your next dose is due within 6 hours, take a single dose now and skip the next.

Stopping the drug
When taken for short-term pain relief, tenoxicam can be safely stopped as soon as you no longer need it. If prescribed for the long-term treatment of arthritis, however, you should seek medical advice before stopping the drug.

Exceeding the dose
An occasional unintentional extra dose is unlikely to be a cause for concern. But if you notice any unusual symptoms, or if a large overdose has been taken, notify your physician immediately.

SPECIAL PRECAUTIONS

Be sure to tell your physician if:
▼ You are allergic to ASA or other NSAIDs.
▼ You have impaired liver or kidney function.
▼ You have had a peptic ulcer, esophagitis, or inflammatory disease of the gastrointestinal tract.
▼ You have asthma.
▼ You have heart problems or high blood pressure.
▼ You are taking other medications.

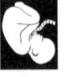

Pregnancy
▼ Not recommended. Discuss with your physician.

Breast feeding
▼ Not recommended as effect on breast feeding is uncertain. Discuss with your physician.

Infants and children
▼ Not recommended for patients under 16 years.

Over 60
▼ Increased likelihood of adverse effects. Reduced dose may therefore be necessary.

Driving and hazardous work
▼ Avoid such activities until you have learned how the drug affects you; it can cause dizziness and drowsiness.

Alcohol
▼ Avoid. Alcohol may increase the risk of stomach disorders with tenoxicam.

Surgery and general anesthetics:
▼ Tenoxicam may prolong bleeding. Discuss this with your physician or dentist before any surgery.

POSSIBLE ADVERSE EFFECTS

The most common adverse effects with tenoxicam are gastrointestinal, of which ulceration and perforation are the most severe. Fatalities have occurred on occasion, particularly in the elderly. Black or blood-stained feces should be reported to your physician promptly.

Symptom/effect	Frequency		Discuss with physician		Stop taking drug now	Call physician now
	Common	Rare	Only if severe	In all cases		
Nausea/indigestion	●			■		
Abdominal pain	●			■		
Dizziness/headache		●	■			
Swollen feet/ankles		●		■	▲	
Rash/itching/hives		●		■	▲	
Wheezing/breathlessness		●		■	▲	▮
Black/bloodstained feces		●		■	▲	▮

INTERACTIONS

General note Tenoxicam interacts with a wide range of drugs to increase the risk of bleeding and/or peptic ulcers. Such drugs include oral anticoagulants, corticosteroids, ASA, and other NSAIDs.

Antihypertensive drugs and diuretics
The beneficial effects of these drugs may be reduced by tenoxicam.

Lithium, methotrexate Tenoxicam may raise blood levels of these drugs, leading to a risk of serious adverse effects.

PROLONGED USE

There is an increased risk of bleeding from peptic ulcers and in the bowel with prolonged use of tenoxicam.

TERAZOSIN

Brand name Hytrin
Used in the following combined preparations None

GENERAL INFORMATION

Terazosin is an antihypertensive drug that relieves high blood pressure by relaxing the muscles in the walls of the blood vessels, dilating them and easing the flow of blood. Terazosin is usually prescribed with a diuretic, and may also be given with beta blockers or other antihypertensive drugs.

Terazosin is also used in the treatment of benign prostatic hyperplasia (BPH), an enlargement of the prostate gland. Symptoms of BPH include weak or interrupted urinary stream, inability to completely empty the bladder, delay or hesitation on starting urination, and the need to urinate often, especially at night. Terazosin works by decreasing the tone of the muscles surrounding the prostate and urinary bladder. Unlike finasteride, it does not reduce the size of the prostate.

Dizziness and fainting are common at the onset of treatment with terazosin because of the dramatic drop in blood pressure or elevation of pulse rate. For this reason, the initial dose is usually low and given at bedtime upon lying down. Dosage levels may later be increased as necessary.

QUICK REFERENCE

Drug group Antihypertensive drug (p.114), urinary disorders drug (p.178)

Overdose danger rating Medium

Dependence rating Low

Prescription needed Yes

Multi-source suppliers No

INFORMATION FOR USERS

Your drug prescription is tailored for you. **Do not alter dosage without checking with your physician.**

How taken

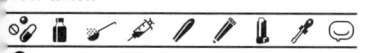

Tablets.

Frequency and timing of doses
Once daily, at bedtime (hypertension and BPH).

Dosage range
1mg (starting dose), increased as necessary to 10mg (BPH) or 20mg (hypertension).

Onset of effect
Within 2 hours. Improvement in the symptoms of BPH may appear as early as 2 weeks, but may be delayed as late as 6 weeks or more.

Duration of action
Up to 24 hours.

Diet advice
None.

Storage
Keep in a closed container in a cool, dry place away from reach of children.

Missed dose
Take as soon as you remember. If your next dose is due within 6 hours, take a single dose now and skip the next.

Stopping the drug
Do not stop taking the drug without consulting your physician; stopping the drug may lead to a rise in blood pressure or the return of the symptoms of BPH.

Exceeding the dose
An occasional unintentional extra dose is unlikely to cause problems. Large overdoses may cause dizziness or fainting. Notify your physician.

SPECIAL PRECAUTIONS

Be sure to tell your physician if:
▼ You have impaired liver or kidney function.
▼ You have heart failure.
▼ You have urinary or bladder problems (in addition to BPH).
▼ You are taking other medications.

 Pregnancy
▼ Safety in pregnancy not established. Discuss with your physician.

 Breast feeding
▼ Effect on breast feeding unknown. Discuss with your physician.

 Infants and children
▼ Not recommended.

 Over 60
▼ Increased likelihood of adverse effects. Reduced dose may therefore be necessary.

 Driving and hazardous work
▼ Avoid such activities until you have learned how the drug affects you; it can cause drowsiness, dizziness, and faintness.

 Alcohol
▼ Avoid. Alcohol may increase the adverse effects of this drug.

POSSIBLE ADVERSE EFFECTS

Terazosin may cause dizziness and fainting on rising, so it is important that the drug be taken at bedtime. Some of the minor adverse effects, such as headache and nausea, will diminish with time.

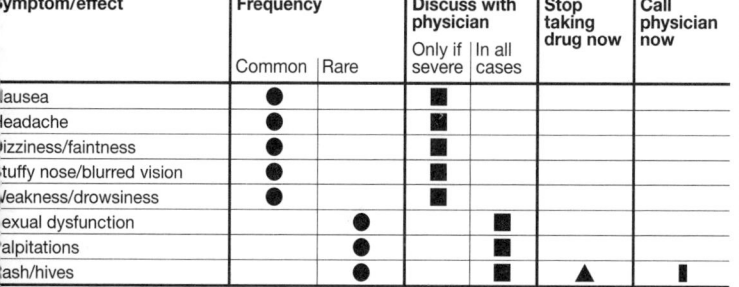

Symptom/effect	Frequency		Discuss with physician		Stop taking drug now	Call physician now
	Common	Rare	Only if severe	In all cases		
Nausea	●		■			
Headache	●		■			
Dizziness/faintness	●		■			
Stuffy nose/blurred vision	●		■			
Weakness/drowsiness	●		■			
Sexual dysfunction		●		■		
Palpitations		●		■		
Rash/hives		●		■	▲	▮

PROLONGED USE

No problems expected. However, as this is a new medication for the treatment of BPH, the long-term effects of terazosin on the need for surgery or on complications of BPH are yet to be determined.

Monitoring Following 18 months of treatment, the status of the BPH should be completely reevaluated.

INTERACTIONS

Diuretics, beta blockers, verapamil These drugs may increase the blood pressure-lowering effect of terazosin.

TERBINAFINE

Brand name Lamisil
Used in the following combined preparations None

GENERAL INFORMATION

Terbinafine is an antifungal drug available in both *topical* and oral forms. The cream is used in the treatment of common fungal infections of the skin. The tablets are used to treat more difficult fungal infections of thick skin – scalp, palms, soles – and the nails.

Adverse effects from terbinafine are rare. Some people may experience irritation on the skin surface where the cream has been applied. Gastro-intestinal symptoms – abdominal cramps and nausea – are the most common adverse effects with the oral form.

INFORMATION FOR USERS

Your drug prescription is tailored for you. Do not alter dosage without checking with your physician.

How taken

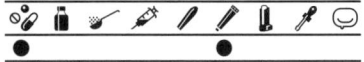

Tablets, cream.

Frequency and timing of doses
1 – 2 x daily (oral and topical).

Dosage range
250mg daily (oral).

Onset of effect
Within 3 – 7 days (common skin conditions); weeks – months (fungal infection of toenails).

Duration of action
12 – 24 hours.

Diet advice
None.

Storage
Keep in a closed container in a cool, dry place away from reach of children. Protect from light.

Missed dose
No cause for concern but make up the missed dose or application as soon as you remember.

Stopping the drug
Take the full course. Even if you feel better, the original infection may still be present and symptoms may recur if treatment is stopped.

Exceeding the dose
An occasional unintentional extra dose is unlikely to cause problems. Large oral overdoses may cause nausea and vomiting. Notify your physician.

SPECIAL PRECAUTIONS

Be sure to tell your physician if:
▼ You have impaired liver or kidney function.
▼ You are taking other medications.

Pregnancy
▼ Safety in pregnancy not established. Discuss with your physician.

Breast feeding
▼ Terbinafine passes into the breast milk. Discuss with your physician.

Infants and children
▼ Not recommended.

Over 60
▼ No special problems.

Driving and hazardous work
▼ No known problems.

Alcohol
▼ No known problems.

POSSIBLE ADVERSE EFFECTS (tablets only)

Terbinafine is generally well tolerated. The most common adverse effects of the tablets are gastrointestinal symptoms and simple rash. Although very rare, there have been reports of serious skin reactions and of a decrease in the white blood cell count. If progressive skin rash occurs or if you develop a sore throat and/or fever, notify your physician immediately.

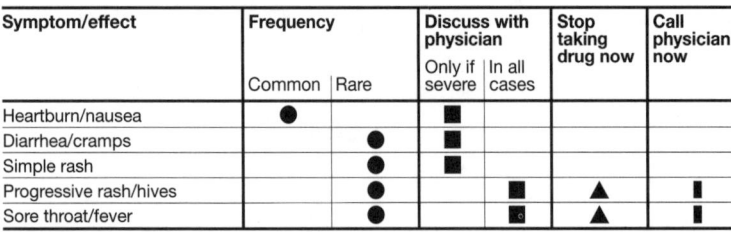

Symptom/effect	Frequency		Discuss with physician		Stop taking drug now	Call physician now
	Common	Rare	Only if severe	In all cases		
Heartburn/nausea	●		■			
Diarrhea/cramps		●	■			
Simple rash		●	■			
Progressive rash/hives		●		■	▲	▌
Sore throat/fever		●		■	▲	▌

INTERACTIONS

None.

PROLONGED USE

As this is a new medication, the effects of prolonged use are as yet unknown.

Monitoring Periodic blood tests may be performed to check the effect of oral terbinafine on the white blood cell count and on the liver.

TERBUTALINE

Brand name Bricanyl
Used in the following combined preparations None

GENERAL INFORMATION

Terbutaline is a *sympathomimetic bronchodilator* that dilates the small airways in the lungs. It is used in the treatment and prevention of the bronchospasm occurring with asthma, chronic bronchitis, and emphysema. It may be given orally or by inhaler when rapid relief of breathlessness is required.

Muscle tremor, especially of the hands, is common with terbutaline and usually disappears on reduction of the dosage or with continued use as the body adapts. In common with other sympathomimetics, it may produce nervousness and restlessness.

INFORMATION FOR USERS

Your drug prescription is tailored for you. Do not alter dosage without checking with your physician.

How taken

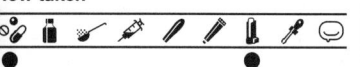

Tablets, inhaler.

Frequency and timing of doses
3 x daily (tablets); as necessary (inhaler).

Dosage range
Adults 7.5 – 15mg daily (tablets); 5mg (inhaler).
Children Reduced dose according to age and weight.

Onset of effect
Within a few minutes (inhaler); within 1 – 2 hours (tablets).

Duration of action
4 – 8 hours (tablets).

Diet advice
None.

Storage
Keep in a closed container in a cool, dry place away from reach of children. Protect from light. Do not puncture or burn aerosol containers.

Missed dose
Do not take the missed dose. Take your next dose as usual.

Stopping the drug
Do not stop the drug without consulting your physician; symptoms may recur.

Exceeding the dose
An occasional unintentional extra dose is unlikely to be a cause for concern. But if you notice any unusual symptoms, or if a large overdose has been taken, notify your physician.

SPECIAL PRECAUTIONS

Be sure to tell your physician if:
▼ You have heart problems.
▼ You have high blood pressure.
▼ You have diabetes.
▼ You have an overactive thyroid.
▼ You are taking other medications.

Pregnancy
▼ Safety in pregnancy not established. Discuss with your physician.

Breast feeding
▼ The drug passes into the breast milk and may affect the baby adversely. Discuss with your physician.

Infants and children
▼ Not recommended in children under 6 years of age. Reduced dose necessary in older children.

Over 60
▼ Increased likelihood of adverse effects. Reduced dose may therefore be necessary.

Driving and hazardous work
▼ Avoid such activities until you have learned how the drug affects you; it can cause tremor of the hands.

Alcohol
▼ No special problems.

POSSIBLE ADVERSE EFFECTS

Possible adverse effects include tremor, nervousness, restlessness, and nausea. These may be reduced by adjustment of dosage.

Palpitations and headache, resulting from stimulation of the heart and narrowing of the blood vessels, are rare.

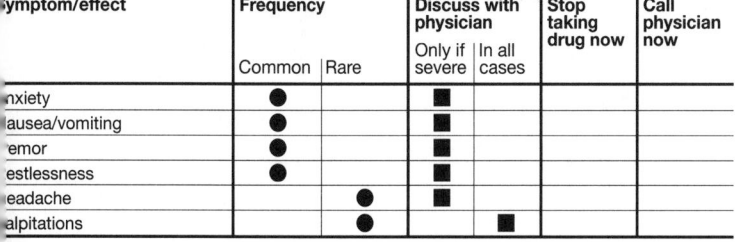

Symptom/effect	Frequency		Discuss with physician		Stop taking drug now	Call physician now
	Common	Rare	Only if severe	In all cases		
Anxiety	●		■			
Nausea/vomiting	●		■			
Tremor	●		■			
Restlessness	●		■			
Headache		●	■			
Palpitations		●		■		

PROLONGED USE

Prolonged use may result in tolerance to the effects of terbutaline. However, failure to respond to the drug may be a result of worsening asthma, requiring prompt medical attention.

INTERACTIONS

Other sympathomimetic drugs may add to the effects of terbutaline and vice versa, so increasing the risk of adverse effects.

Monoamine oxidase inhibitors (MAOIs) Terbutaline may interact with these drugs to cause a dangerous rise in blood pressure.

Beta blockers may reduce the beneficial effects of terbutaline.

TERCONAZOLE

Brand name Terazol
Used in the following combined preparations None

GENERAL INFORMATION

Terconazole is a new, fast-acting *topical* antifungal drug used for the treatment of candidal infection of the vagina (also called thrush or monilial infection). The therapeutic effect of terconazole is not affected by birth-control pills, menstruation, or previous monilial infections.

Terconazole comes in two vaginal forms, cream and ovules. The base contained in the ovule formulation may interact with certain natural rubber products, such as those used in vaginal contraceptive diaphragms or condoms. Therefore, the cream is preferred when using barrier contraceptive devices made of rubber.

Serious adverse effects with terconazole are rare, though local stinging, burning, and skin irritation can sometimes occur.

INFORMATION FOR USERS

Your drug prescription is tailored for you. Do not alter dosage without checking with your physician.

How taken

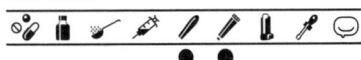

Vaginal ovules, cream.

Frequency and timing of doses
Once daily, at bedtime.

Dosage range
80mg (vaginal ovules); 1 applicatorful per dose (vaginal cream).

Onset of effect
Within 1 – 2 days.

Duration of action
Up to 24 hours.

Diet advice
None.

Storage
Keep in a closed container in a cool, dry place away from reach of children.

Missed dose
No cause for concern, but make up the missed application as soon as you remember.

Stopping the drug
Apply the full course. Even if symptoms disappear, the original infection may still be present and symptoms may recur if treatment is stopped too soon.

Exceeding the dose
An occasional unintentional extra dose is unlikely to be a cause for concern. But if you notice any unusual symptoms, notify your physician immediately.

SPECIAL PRECAUTIONS

Be sure to tell your physician if:
▼ You are taking other medications.

Pregnancy
▼ Terconazole should not be used in the first 3 months of pregnancy. Use of the vaginal applicator may be undesirable. Discuss with your physician.

Breast feeding
▼ It is not known if terconazole passes into the breast milk. Discuss with your physician.

Infants and children
▼ Safety and effectiveness not established.

Over 60
▼ No known problems.

Driving and hazardous work
▼ No known problems.

Alcohol
▼ No known problems.

POSSIBLE ADVERSE EFFECTS

Terconazole rarely causes adverse effects. Vaginal burning or skin irritation may occasionally occur with this drug.

Symptom/effect	Frequency		Discuss with physician		Stop taking drug now	Call physician now
	Common	Rare	Only if severe	In all cases		
Local irritation	●		■			
Headache	●		■			
Rash/fever/chills		●		■	▲	▐

PROLONGED USE

No problems expected from the drug. However, recurrent or intractable vaginal infections require further assessment by your physician.

INTERACTIONS

None.

TERFENADINE

Brand names Seldane, Apo-Terfenadine, Novo-Terfenadine
Used in the following combined preparations None

GENERAL INFORMATION

Terfenadine is a long-acting antihistamine. Its main use is in the treatment of allergic rhinitis, particularly hay fever. Taken as tablets or liquid, it reduces sneezing and irritation of the eyes and nose. Allergic skin conditions such as urticaria (hives) may also be helped by terfenadine.

The main difference between this drug and the older antihistamines is that it has little sedative effect. It is therefore particularly suitable for people who need to avoid drowsiness – for example, at work.

Terfenadine rarely produces dangerous changes in heart rhythm. If palpitations develop and you feel faint, seek medical help at once.

INFORMATION FOR USERS

Follow instructions on the label. Call your physician if symptoms worsen.

How taken

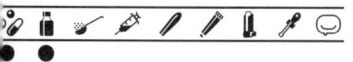

Tablets, oral liquid.

Frequency and timing of doses
1 – 2 x daily.

Dosage range
Adults 120mg daily.
Children Reduced dose according to age.

Onset of effect
1 – 3 hours. Some effects may not be felt for 1 – 2 days.

Duration of action
Up to 12 hours.

Diet advice
None.

Storage
Keep in a closed container in a cool, dry place away from reach of children.

Missed dose
No cause for concern, but take as soon as you remember. If your next dose is due within 5 hours, take a single dose now and skip the next.

Stopping the drug
Can be safely stopped as soon as you no longer need it.

Exceeding the dose
An occasional unintentional extra dose is unlikely to cause problems. Large overdoses may cause nausea or drowsiness and have an adverse effect on the heart. Notify your physician.

SPECIAL PRECAUTIONS

Be sure to consult your physician or pharmacist before taking this drug if:
▼ You have impaired liver function.
▼ You have had epileptic seizures.
▼ You have any heart problems.
▼ You have a metabolic disease.
▼ You are taking other medications.

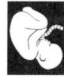

Pregnancy
▼ Safety in pregnancy not established. Discuss with your physician.

Breast feeding
▼ No evidence of risk. Discuss with your physician.

Infants and children
▼ Not recommended for children under 3 years. Reduced dose necessary in older children.

Over 60
▼ Reduced dose may be necessary.

Driving and hazardous work
▼ Problems are unlikely. However, avoid such activities until you have learned how the drug affects you because it can cause drowsiness in some people.

Alcohol
▼ No known problems.

POSSIBLE ADVERSE EFFECTS

Abdominal distress, nausea, and vomiting occur occasionally with terfenadine; other *side effects* are uncommon. Terfenadine can have adverse effects on the heart; if you have palpitations and feel faint, seek medical help without delay.

Symptom/effect	Frequency		Discuss with physician		Stop taking drug now	Call physician now
	Common	Rare	Only if severe	In all cases		
Abdominal distress	●		■			
Headache	●		■			
Drowsiness	●		■			
Fatigue	●		■			
Fainting/palpitations		●		■	▲	▮
Rash		●		■	▲	

INTERACTIONS

Sedatives Terfenadine may increase the sedative effects on the central nervous system of anti-anxiety drugs, sleeping drugs, antidepressants, and antipsychotic drugs.

Anticholinergic drugs The *anticholinergic* effects of terfenadine are likely to be increased by all drugs that have anticholinergic effects, including antipsychotic drugs and tricyclic antidepressant drugs.

Erythromycin This antibiotic may increase levels of terfenadine and lead to adverse effects on the heart.

Antifungal drugs Ketoconazole, itraconazole, and possibly other antifungal drugs increase levels of terfenadine and may lead to adverse effects on the heart.

PROLONGED USE

Use in children should be limited to periods of 1 week unless otherwise directed by a physician.

Antihistamines should be discontinued approximately 48 hours before allergy skin testing.

TESTOSTERONE

Brand names Depo-Testosterone, Andriol, Delatestryl, PMS-Testosterone Enanthate
Used in the following combined preparations Climacteron, Duogex, Neo-Pause

GENERAL INFORMATION

Testosterone is a male sex hormone (androgen) produced by the testicles, and also in small quantities by the ovaries in women. It encourages bone and muscle growth in both men and women and stimulates sexual development in men. A shortage of testosterone may be caused by a disorder of the testicles or pituitary gland. When this happens, synthetic testosterone supplements may be given by injection or by mouth.

Testosterone is used to initiate puberty in male adolescents if it has been delayed because of a hormone deficiency. The drug may help to increase male fertility in men who suffer from pituitary or testicular disorders. It does not, however, increase sperm production in men with normally developed testicles. Rarely, testosterone is used for breast cancer.

Testosterone has a number of adverse effects. Dosages for treating delayed puberty need to be controlled with particular care because it can interfere with growth or cause over-rapid sexual development. High doses may cause voice changes, excessive hair growth, or hair loss in women.

QUICK REFERENCE

Drug group Male sex hormone (p.158)

Overdose danger rating Low

Dependence rating Low

Prescription needed Yes

Multi-source suppliers Yes

INFORMATION FOR USERS

Your drug prescription is tailored for you. Do not alter dosage without checking with your physician.

How taken

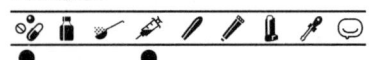

Capsules, injection.

Frequency and timing of doses
2 x daily (capsules); once every 2 – 4 weeks (injection) depending on condition being treated.

Dosage range
Varies with condition being treated and method of administration.

Onset of effect
2 – 3 days.

Duration of action
3 – 4 days (capsules); 3 – 4 weeks (injection).

Diet advice
None.

Storage
Varies according to preparation. See manufacturer's package insert.

Missed dose
No cause for concern but take as soon as you remember. If your next dose (by mouth) is due within 3 hours, take a single dose now and skip the next.

Stopping the drug
Do not stop taking the drug without consulting your physician.

Exceeding the dose
An occasional unintentional extra dose is unlikely to be a cause for concern. But if you notice unusual symptoms, or if a large overdose has been taken, notify your physician.

SPECIAL PRECAUTIONS

Be sure to tell your physician if:
▼ You have impaired liver or kidney function.
▼ You have heart problems.
▼ You have prostate cancer.
▼ You have diabetes.
▼ You are taking other medications.

 **Pregnancy**
▼ Not prescribed.

 Breast feeding
▼ Not prescribed.

 Infants and children
▼ Not prescribed for infants and young children. Reduced dose necessary in adolescents.

 Over 60
▼ Rarely required. Increased risk of prostate problems in elderly males.

 Driving and hazardous work
▼ No special problems.

 Alcohol
▼ No special problems.

POSSIBLE ADVERSE EFFECTS

Most of the more serious adverse effects are likely to occur only with long-term treatment with testosterone, and may be helped by a reduction in dosage.

Symptom/effect	Frequency		Discuss with physician		Stop taking drug now	Call physician now
	Common	Rare	Only if severe	In all cases		
Jaundice		●		■	▲	
Men only						
Difficulty in passing urine		●		■		
Abnormal erection		●		■		
Women only						
Unusual hair growth		●	■			
Voice changes		●		■		
Enlarged clitoris		●		■		

PROLONGED USE

Prolonged use of this drug may lead to reduced growth in adolescents.

Monitoring Regular checks of the effects of testosterone treatment are required.

INTERACTIONS

Anticoagulant drugs Testosterone may increase the effect of these drugs. Dosage of anticoagulant drugs may need to be adjusted accordingly.

Antidiabetic agents Because testosterone may lower the blood sugar, dosage of antidiabetic drugs and insulin may need to be reduced.

TETRACYCLINE

Brand names Achromycin V, Apo-Tetra, Novo-Tetra, Nu-Tetra, Tetracyn
Used in the following combined preparation Achrocidin

GENERAL INFORMATION

Tetracyclines were a widely used group of antibiotics. However, the development of bacterial resistances to these drugs has reduced their effectiveness in many types of infection. Tetracycline is still used for chest infections caused by chlamydia (e.g. psittacosis) and mycoplasma microorganisms. It is used in nonspecific urethritis and a number of rare conditions, which include Q fever, Rocky Mountain spotted fever,

cholera, and brucellosis. Acne usually improves following long-term treatment with oral tetracyclines.

Common *side effects* are nausea, vomiting, and diarrhea. Rashes may also occur. Tetracycline may discolor developing teeth if taken by children or by the mother during pregnancy. It is not prescribed for people with poor kidney function, as it can cause further deterioration.

INFORMATION FOR USERS

Your drug prescription is tailored for you. Do not alter your dosage without checking with your physician.

How taken

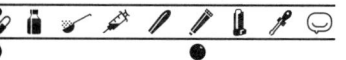

Capsules, eye ointment.

Frequency and timing of doses
By mouth 2 – 4 x daily, at least 1 hour before or 2 hours after meals. Long-term treatment of acne may require only a single dose daily.
Eye ointment Apply every 2 hours or as directed.

Adult dosage range
Infections 1 – 2g daily.
Acne 250mg – 1g daily.

Onset of effect
8 – 12 hours. Improvement in acne may not be noticed for up to 4 weeks.

Duration of action
Up to 12 hours.

Diet advice
Milk products should be avoided for one hour before and two hours after taking the drug, since they may impair its absorption.

Storage
Keep in a closed container in a cool, dry place away from reach of children.

Missed dose
Take as soon as you remember. If your next dose is due within 2 hours, take a single dose now and skip the next.

Stopping the drug
Take the full course. Even if you feel better, the original infection may still be present and may recur if treatment is stopped too soon.

Exceeding the dose
An occasional unintentional extra dose is unlikely to be a cause for concern. But if you notice unusual symptoms, or if a larger overdose has been taken, notify your physician.

SPECIAL PRECAUTIONS

Be sure to tell your physician if:
▼ You have impaired liver or kidney function.
▼ You have previously suffered an allergic reaction to a tetracycline antibiotic.
▼ You are taking other medications.

Pregnancy
▼ Not prescribed. May damage teeth and bones of the developing baby, as well as damaging the mother's liver. Discuss with your physician.

Breast feeding
▼ The drug passes into the breast milk and may lead to discoloration of the baby's teeth. Discuss with your physician.

Infants and children
▼ Not recommended under 8 years of age. Reduced dose necessary for older children.

Over 60
▼ No special problems.

Driving and hazardous work
▼ No known problems.

Alcohol
▼ No known problems.

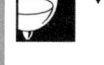

Esophageal damage
▼ To prevent irritation to the esophagus, each dose of the drug should be taken with a full glass of water while standing.

POSSIBLE ADVERSE EFFECTS

Adverse effects from tetracycline eye ointment are rare. Taken *systemically* the drug may occasionally cause nausea, vomiting, or diarrhea.

Symptom/effect	Frequency		Discuss with physician		Stop taking drug now	Call physician now
	Common	Rare	Only if severe	In all cases		
Nausea/vomiting	●		■			
Diarrhea	●		■			
Light-sensitive rash		●		■	▲	▮
Rash/itching		●		■	▲	▮

INTERACTIONS

Oral contraceptives Tetracycline can reduce the effectiveness of oral contraceptives.

Iron may reduce the effectiveness of tetracycline.

Penicillins Tetracycline interferes with the antibacterial action of penicillins.

Antacids Antacids interfere with the absorption of tetracycline and may reduce its effectiveness.

Oral anticoagulants Tetracycline may increase the action of these drugs.

PROLONGED USE

No problems expected.

THEOPHYLLINE (AMINOPHYLLINE)

Brand names Apo-Theo LA, Jaa Aminophylline, Phyllocontin, Pulmophylline, Quibron-T/SR, Slo-Bid, Somophyllin-12, Theochron, Theo-Dur, Theolair, Theolair-SR, Theolixir, Theo-SR, Uniphyl
Used in the following combined preparations Asbron, Tedral, Theo-Dronc, Theophylline KI

GENERAL INFORMATION

Theophylline (and aminophylline, which breaks down to theophylline in the body) belongs to the xanthine group of *bronchodilator* drugs. These agents open up the airways to the lungs and increase the flow of air through them. Theophylline is used mainly in the treatment of asthma, emphysema, and chronic bronchitis. It relieves cough, wheezing, shortness of breath, and difficult breathing.

Theophylline can be used either alone or in conjunction with *sympathomimetic* or *anticholinergic bronchodilators* and/or inhaled corticosteroids. While it is not very useful for the treatment of acute symptoms, theophylline helps people with chronic asthma by reducing the severity of symptoms during the night.

INFORMATION FOR USERS

Your drug prescription is tailored for you. Do not alter dosage without checking with your physician.

How taken

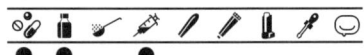

Tablets, slow-release tablets and capsules, oral liquid, injection.

Frequency and timing of doses
3 – 4 x daily (tablets, liquid); every 12 hours (slow-release capsules or tablets); continuous infusion (injection).

Dosage range
Considerable variation among different formulations and methods of administration.

Onset of effect
Within a few minutes (intravenous infusion); within 45 – 60 minutes (tablets, liquid); within 90 minutes (slow-release tablets and capsules).

Duration of action
6 – 8 hours (tablets, liquid); 12 hours (slow-release tablets and capsules).

Diet advice
Avoid barbecued foods and caffeine-containing foods or beverages.

Storage
Keep in a closed container in a cool, dry place away from reach of children.

Missed dose
Take as soon as you remember. If your next dose is due within 2 hours, take half the dose now (short-acting preparations) or take your next dose now (long-acting preparations). Return to your normal dose schedule thereafter.

Stopping the drug
Do not stop taking the drug without consulting your physician.

OVERDOSE ACTION

 Seek immediate medical advice in all cases. Take emergency action if chest pains, confusion, or loss of consciousness occurs.

See Drug poisoning emergency guide (p.574).

SPECIAL PRECAUTIONS

Be sure to tell your physician if:
▼ You have impaired liver or kidney function.
▼ You have angina or irregular heartbeat.
▼ You have epilepsy.
▼ You have gastrointestinal ulcers.
▼ You have an overactive thyroid gland.
▼ You smoke.
▼ You are taking other medications.

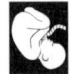 **Pregnancy**
▼ Safety in pregnancy has not been established. Discuss with your physician.

 Breast feeding
Theophylline passes into the breast milk and may affect the baby. Discuss with your physician.

 Infants and children
▼ Reduced dose necessary according to age and weight.

 Over 60
▼ Reduced dose may be necessary.

 Driving and hazardous work
▼ Avoid such activities until you have learned how the drug affects you; it can cause dizziness.

 Alcohol
▼ Avoid excess use as this may alter levels of the drug and may increase gastrointestinal symptoms.

PROLONGED USE

No problems expected.

Monitoring Periodic checks on blood levels of the drug are required because the effective dose is very close to the toxic dose.

POSSIBLE ADVERSE EFFECTS

Most adverse effects of this drug are related to dosage and to theophylline's (aminophylline's) effect on the central nervous system.

Symptom/effect	Frequency		Discuss with physician		Stop taking drug now	Call physician now
	Common	Rare	Only if severe	In all cases		
Nausea/vomiting	●		■			
Headache/dizziness	●			■		
Diarrhea		●	■			
Irritability/insomnia		●	■			
Palpitations		●		■	▲	▮
Seizures		●		■	▲	▮

INTERACTIONS

General note Many drugs increase the effect of theophylline (e.g., erythromycin, cimetidine, propranolol); many others reduce its effect (e.g., carbamazepine, phenytoin, rifampin). Discuss with your physician.

THIORIDAZINE

Brand names Mellaril, Apo-Thioridazine, Novo-Ridazine
Used in the following combined preparations None

GENERAL INFORMATION

Thioridazine belongs to the phenothiazine antipsychotic group of drugs (see p.97).

Thioridazine is an important tranquilizer widely used to treat a variety of psychotic conditions. Its tranquilizing effect suppresses abnormal behavior and reduces aggression. It is used in the treatment of schizophrenia, mania, dementia, and other disorders where confused or abnormal behavior may occur. Thioridazine does not cure the underlying disorder, but it does relieve the distressing symptoms. It also helps to relieve the anxiety and depression associated with serious mental disorders.

Thioridazine is sometimes chosen for treating the elderly because it is less likely to cause abnormal shaking movements than some of the other drugs in this group.

A drawback to the use of thioridazine, as with other phenothiazines, is that when given in high doses it can cause eye problems. If large doses are required for long periods, other antipsychotic drugs are usually substituted.

INFORMATION FOR USERS

Your drug prescription is tailored for you. Do not alter your dosage without checking with your physician.

How taken

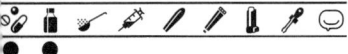

Tablets, liquid.

Frequency and timing of doses
– 4 x daily.

Adult dosage range
50 – 400mg daily.

Onset of effect
– 3 hours.

Duration of action
– 10 hours. Some effects may last up to 16 hours.

Diet advice
None.

Storage
Keep in a closed container in a cool, dry place away from the reach of children. Protect from light.

Missed dose
Take as soon as you remember. If your next dose is due within 2 hours, do not take the missed dose. Take your next scheduled dose as usual.

Stopping the drug
Do not stop the drug without consulting your physician; symptoms may recur.

Exceeding the dose
An occasional unintentional extra dose is unlikely to cause problems. Large overdoses may cause unusual drowsiness, fainting, muscle rigidity, and agitation. Notify your physician.

POSSIBLE ADVERSE EFFECTS

Thioridazine has a strong *anticholinergic* effect that can cause a variety of minor symptoms (see p.91). These often become less marked with time. The most significant adverse effect is eye problems. This can occasionally be controlled by medically supervised adjustment of dosage, or a change of drug.

Symptom/effect	Frequency		Discuss with physician		Stop taking drug now	Call physician now
	Common	Rare	Only if severe	In all cases		
Drowsiness	●		■			
Dry mouth	●		■			
Stuffy nose	●			■		
Blurred vision		●		■		
Muscle stiffness		●		■		
Unsteadiness		●		■		
Dizziness/fainting		●		■	▲	

INTERACTIONS

Sedatives All drugs, including alcohol, that have a sedative effect on the central nervous system are likely to increase the sedative properties of thioridazine.

Anticonvulsants and antiparkinsonian drugs Thioridazine may reduce the effectiveness of these drugs.

Anticholinergic drugs Thioridazine may increase the side effects of these drugs.

SPECIAL PRECAUTIONS

Be sure to tell your physician if:
▼ You have impaired liver or kidney function.
▼ You have heart or circulation problems.
▼ You have prostate trouble.
▼ You have had epileptic seizures.
▼ You have had glaucoma.
▼ You have an overactive thyroid gland.
▼ You have Parkinson's disease.
▼ You are taking other medications.

Pregnancy
▼ Safety in pregnancy not established. Discuss with your physician.

Breast feeding
▼ The drug passes into the breast milk and may affect the baby. Discuss with your physician.

Infants and children
▼ Not recommended under 2 years of age. Reduced dose is necessary for older children.

Over 60
▼ There is an increased likelihood of adverse effects. Reduced dose may therefore be necessary.

Driving and hazardous work
▼ Avoid such activities until you have learned how this drug affects you; it can cause drowsiness and blurred vision.

Alcohol
▼ Avoid. Alcohol may increase the sedative effects of this drug.

Surgery and general anesthetics
▼ Thioridazine treatment may need to be stopped before you have a general anesthetic. Discuss this with your physician or dentist before any operation.

PROLONGED USE

Use of this drug for more than a few months may lead to eye problems and *tardive dyskinesia*. Occasionally jaundice may occur.

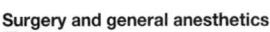

TIAPROFENIC ACID

Brand names Surgam, Surgam SR, Albert Tiafen
Used in the following combined preparations None

GENERAL INFORMATION

Tiaprofenic acid, a non-steroidal anti-inflammatory drug (NSAID), was introduced in 1986. Like other NSAIDs, it reduces pain, stiffness, and inflammation. Therefore, it is used to relieve symptoms of rheumatoid arthritis and osteoarthritis (degenerative joint diseases), although it does not cure the underlying disease. Gastrointestinal *side effects* such as indigestion, heartburn, and nausea are fairly common. Many of the other side effects of tiaprofenic acid are similar to those of other NSAIDs (see p.128).

(see p.128).

QUICK REFERENCE

Drug group Non-steroidal anti-inflammatory drug (p.128)

Overdose danger rating Low

Dependence rating Low

Prescription needed Yes

Multi-source suppliers Yes

INFORMATION FOR USERS

Your drug prescription is tailored for you. Do not alter dosage without checking with your physician.

How taken

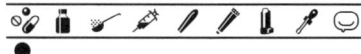

Tablets, slow-release tablets.

Frequency and timing of doses
2 – 3 x daily (tablets); once daily (slow-release tablets).

Adult dosage range
600mg daily.

Onset of effect
Pain relief may begin within a few hours, but full anti-inflammatory effect in arthritic conditions may not be felt for 2 weeks.

Duration of action
5 – 12 hours.

Diet advice
None.

Storage
Keep in a closed container in a cool, dry place away from reach of children.

Missed dose
Take as soon as you remember. If your next dose is due within 2 hours, take a single dose now and skip the next.

Stopping the drug
When taken for short-term pain relief, tiaprofenic acid can be safely stopped as soon as you no longer need it. If prescribed for the long-term treatment of arthritis, however, you should seek medical advice before stopping the drug.

Exceeding the dose
An occasional unintentional extra dose is unlikely to be a cause for concern. But if you notice unusual symptoms, or if a large overdose has been taken, notify your physician.

SPECIAL PRECAUTIONS

Be sure to tell your physician if:
▼ You have impaired liver or kidney function.
▼ You have asthma.
▼ You have heart problems.
▼ You have high blood pressure.
▼ You have had a peptic ulcer, esophagitis, or acid indigestion.
▼ You are allergic to ASA or other NSAIDs.
▼ You are taking other medications.

Pregnancy
▼ Not usually prescribed. Safety in pregnancy not established. Discuss with your physician.

Breast feeding
▼ Tiaprofenic acid passes into breast milk, but in low concentrations. Discuss with your physician.

Infants and children
▼ Not recommended under 12 years.

Over 60
▼ Increased likelihood of adverse effects. Reduced dose may therefore be necessary.

Driving and hazardous work
▼ Avoid such activities until you have learned how the drug affects you; it can cause dizziness and drowsiness.

Alcohol
▼ Avoid. Alcohol may increase the risk of stomach disorders with tiaprofenic acid.

▼ **Surgery and general anesthetics**
Tiaprofenic acid may prolong bleeding. Discuss with your physician or dentist before any surgery.

POSSIBLE ADVERSE EFFECTS

The most common adverse effects are the result of gastrointestinal disturbances. Black or bloodstained feces should be reported to your physician without delay. Headaches and dizziness may also occur.

Symptom/effect	Frequency		Discuss with physician		Stop taking drug now	Call physician now
	Common	Rare	Only if severe	In all cases		
Gastrointestinal disorders	●		■			
Headache	●		■			
Dizziness/drowsiness	●		■			
Ringing in ears		●		■		
Swollen feet/ankles		●		■		
Rash/itching		●		■	▲	
Wheezing/breathlessness		●		■	▲	■
Black/bloodstained feces		●		■	▲	■

PROLONGED USE

There is an increased risk of bleeding, both from peptic ulcers and from the bowel, with prolonged use of tiaprofenic acid.

INTERACTIONS

General note Tiaprofenic acid may interact with a wide range of drugs to increase the risk of bleeding and/or peptic ulcer. Such drugs include oral anticoagulants, corticosteroids, other non-steroidal anti-inflammatory drugs (NSAIDs), and ASA.

Antihypertensive drugs and diuretics The beneficial effects of these drugs may be reduced by tiaprofenic acid.

TICLOPIDINE

Brand name Ticlid
Used in the following combined preparations None

GENERAL INFORMATION

Ticlopidine is used as an antiplatelet drug (see Drugs that affect blood clotting, p.116). It reduces the ability of platelets to stick to each other and to walls of the blood vessels, thereby preventing blood clotting within the arteries.

Ticlopidine is usually prescribed to patients who have had a previous stroke or who experienced one or more warning episodes indicating an increased risk of stroke. The drug has been shown to decrease both the stroke mortality and the occurrence of first or repeat strokes in such patients.

QUICK REFERENCE

Drug group Antiplatelet drug (p.116)

Overdose danger rating Medium

Dependence rating Low

Prescription needed Yes

Multi-source suppliers No

INFORMATION FOR USERS

Your drug prescription is tailored for you. Do not alter dosage without checking with your physician.

How taken

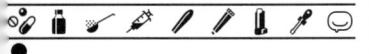

Tablets.

Frequency and timing of doses
2 x daily with food.

Dosage range
500mg daily.

Onset of effect
Within 2 hours. Full therapeutic effect may not be present for 8 to 11 days.

Duration of action
Up to 12 hours.

Diet advice
None.

Storage
Keep in a closed container in a cool, dry place away from reach of children. Protect from light.

Missed dose
Take as soon as you remember.

Stopping the drug
Do not stop taking the drug without consulting your physician; stopping the drug could lead to abnormal blood clotting.

Exceeding the dose
An occasional unintentional extra dose is unlikely to cause problems, but you may experience gastric upset or nausea. Notify your physician.

POSSIBLE ADVERSE EFFECTS

Most *side effects* are mild, transient, and occur during the first 3 months of treatment; these usually disappear within 1 – 2 weeks after the drug is stopped. More common side effects are upset stomach, diarrhea, and skin rashes.

Symptom/effect	Frequency		Discuss with physician		Stop taking drug now	Call physician now
	Common	Rare	Only if severe	In all cases		
Upset stomach	●		■			
Diarrhea	●		■			
Rash	●			■	▲	❙
Fever/chills/sore throat		●		■	▲	❙
Bleeding/bruising		●		■	▲	❙
Jaundice		●		■	▲	❙

INTERACTIONS

ASA, antipyrine, theophylline Ticlopidine may increase the effects of these drugs.

Cimetidine Chronic administration of cimetidine may increase the effects of ticlopidine.

Antacids Administration of antacids may reduce the blood levels of ticlopidine.

Anticoagulants Avoid simultaneous administration with ticlopidine; safety and tolerance not established.

SPECIAL PRECAUTIONS

Be sure to tell your physician if:
▼ You have peptic ulcer disease.
▼ You have any abnormal bleeding or bruising disorders.
▼ You have impaired liver or kidney function.
▼ You have certain blood disorders (neutropenia, thrombocytopenia).
▼ You are taking anticoagulants or other medications.

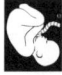

Pregnancy
▼ Safety in pregnancy not established. Discuss with your physician.

Breast feeding
▼ Safety in breast feeding not established. Discuss with your physician.

Infants and children
▼ Not recommended.

Over 60
▼ Increased likelihood of adverse effects. Reduced dose may therefore be necessary.

Driving and hazardous work
▼ Avoid such activities until you have learned how the drug affects you because of the possibility of dizziness.

Alcohol
▼ Avoid. Alcohol may increase the likelihood of stomach irritation with this drug.

Surgery and general anesthetics
▼ Be sure to tell your physician or dentist that you are taking ticlopidine. This drug may cause prolonged bleeding.

PROLONGED USE

Monitoring Periodic blood cell counts and liver function testing are required.

TIMOLOL

Brand names Blocadren, Timoptic, Apo-Timol, Apo-Timop, Gen-Timolol, Novo-Timol
Used in the following combined preparations Timolide, Timpilo

GENERAL INFORMATION

Timolol is a beta blocker prescribed to treat hypertension (high blood pressure) and angina. It may also be given to a person after a heart attack to prevent further damage to the heart muscle. Timolol is also administered in the form of eye drops to people suffering from certain types of glaucoma.

It is given in tablet form to prevent migraine.

Taken *systemically*, timolol can cause breathing difficulties, especially in individuals with asthma, chronic bronchitis, or emphysema. As with other beta blockers, timolol may mask the body's response to low blood sugar and, for that reason, is prescribed with caution to diabetics.

Given as eye drops for glaucoma, timolol may be absorbed systemically, causing the adverse effects noted above.

QUICK REFERENCE

Drug group Beta blocker (p.109) and drug for glaucoma (p.180)

Overdose danger rating High

Dependence rating Low

Prescription needed Yes

Multi-source suppliers Yes

INFORMATION FOR USERS

Your drug prescription is tailored for you. Do not alter dosage without checking with your physician.

How taken

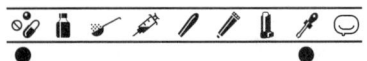

Tablets, eye drops.

Frequency and timing of doses
2 – 3 x daily.

Adult dosage range
By mouth 20 – 60mg daily (hypertension); 10 – 45mg daily (angina); 10 – 20mg daily (after a heart attack); 10 – 30mg daily (migraine prevention).
Eye drops 2 drops daily.

Onset of effect
1 – 2 hours (by mouth); within 20 minutes (eye drops).

Duration of action
12 – 36 hours.

Diet advice
None.

Storage
Keep in a closed container in a cool, dry place away from reach of children.

Missed dose
Take as soon as you remember. If your next dose is due within 3 hours, take a single dose now and skip the next.

Stopping the drug
Do not stop the drug without consulting your physician; stopping the drug may lead to worsening of the underlying condition.

OVERDOSE ACTION

Seek immediate medical advice in all cases of overdose by mouth. Take emergency action if palpitations, breathing difficulties, and/or loss of consciousness occur.

See Drug poisoning emergency guide (p.574).

POSSIBLE ADVERSE EFFECTS

Timolol taken by mouth can occasionally provoke or worsen asthma and heart problems. Fainting may be a sign that the drug has slowed the heartbeat excessively. Eye drops cause these problems only rarely; headache or blurred vision is more likely.

Symptom/effect	Frequency		Discuss with physician		Stop taking drug now	Call physician now
	Common	Rare	Only if severe	In all cases		
Lethargy/fatigue	●		■			
Blurred vision (eye drops)	●		■			
Headache/dizziness	●		■			
Fainting/breathlessness		●		■	▲	▮
Cold hands/feet		●	■			
Nightmares/vivid dreams		●		■		

INTERACTIONS

General note Timolol may interact with numerous drugs, most notably non-steroidal anti-inflammatory drugs (NSAIDs), calcium channel blockers, cimetidine, and *sympathomimetic* decongestants.

SPECIAL PRECAUTIONS

Be sure to tell your physician if:
▼ You have a lung disorder such as asthma, bronchitis, or emphysema.
▼ You have diabetes.
▼ You have poor circulation.
▼ You have allergies.
▼ You are taking other medications.

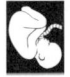

Pregnancy
▼ Safety in pregnancy not established. Discuss with your physician.

Breast feeding
▼ The drug passes into the breast milk, but at normal doses adverse effects on the baby are unlikely. Discuss with your physician.

Infants and children
▼ Not usually prescribed.

Over 60
▼ Reduced dose may be necessary.

Driving and hazardous work
▼ Avoid such activities until you have learned how the drug affects you; tablets may cause drowsiness and eye drops may cause blurred vision.

Alcohol
▼ May enhance lowering of blood pressure; avoid excessive amounts

Surgery and general anesthetics
▼ Timolol by mouth may need to be stopped before you have a general anesthetic. Discuss with your physician or dentist before any surgery.

PROLONGED USE

No problems expected.

TISSUE PLASMINOGEN ACTIVATOR

Brand name Activase rt-PA
Used in the following combined preparations None

GENERAL INFORMATION

Tissue plasminogen activator (tPA or alteplase) is an enzyme involved in the breakdown of blood clots. Manufactured or cloned by genetic engineering techniques, it is used in the treatment of heart attacks in which a blood clot (thrombus) forms in one of the blood vessels of the heart muscle, cutting off its blood supply.

Given by infusion into a vein or directly into the coronary artery, tPA acts quickly to dissolve the clot and restore the blood supply to the heart muscle. Used within a few hours of an

attack, it can dramatically reduce the amount of damage to the heart muscle. Infusion is usually continued for a few hours after the clot has dissolved to prevent further clot formation.

As with other thrombolytic drugs, there is a risk of internal bleeding with tPA, and bleeding or bruising at the injection site is common. As a naturally occurring substance, however, it is less likely to produce an allergic reaction than other thrombolytic drugs, such as streptokinase.

QUICK REFERENCE

Drug group Thrombolytic drug (p.117)

Overdose danger rating Medium

Dependence rating Low

Prescription needed No

Multi-source suppliers No

INFORMATION FOR USERS

This drug is given only under medical supervision and is not for self-administration.

How taken

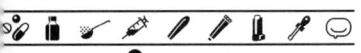

Injection.

Frequency and timing of doses
By continuous infusion over several hours.

Dosage range
Dosage is determined individually by condition and response.

Onset of effect
The blood clot begins to dissolve as soon as the drug reaches it. Most of the clot is dissolved within 1 hour.

Duration of action
The effect of the drug disappears a few minutes after it is stopped.

Diet advice
None.

Storage
Not applicable. This drug is not kept in the home.

Missed dose
Not applicable. This drug is given only in a hospital under close medical supervision.

Stopping the drug
The drug is stopped under medical supervision a few hours after the clot has dispersed.

Exceeding the dose
Overdosage is unlikely, since treatment is carefully monitored in the hospital.

SPECIAL PRECAUTIONS

tPA is administered only under close medical supervision, taking account of your present condition and medical history.

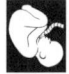

Pregnancy
▼ Used only when the life of the mother is at risk.

Breast feeding
▼ Used only when the life of the mother is at risk.

Infants and children
▼ Not recommended.

Over 60
▼ Increased likelihood of bruising at injection site.

Driving and hazardous work
▼ Not applicable.

Alcohol
▼ Not applicable.

POSSIBLE ADVERSE EFFECTS

There is a risk of internal bleeding with tPA, particularly in the stomach and intestinal tract.

All adverse effects are closely monitored under strict medical supervision.

Symptom/effect	Frequency		Discuss with physician		Stop taking drug now	Call physician now
	Common	Rare	Only if severe	In all cases		
Nausea/vomiting	●			■		▮
Abnormal bleeding	●			■		▮

INTERACTIONS

Anticoagulant drugs There is an increased risk of bleeding when these are taken at the same time as tPA.

Antiplatelet drugs increase the risk of bleeding if given with tPA.

PROLONGED USE

The drug is not used long term.

TOBRAMYCIN

Brand names Nebcin, Tobrex Ophthalmic
Used in the following combined preparation Tobradex

GENERAL INFORMATION

Tobramycin, introduced in 1975, is an aminoglycoside antibiotic. Given by injection, it is generally reserved for serious, complicated infections treated in hospital. These include peritonitis and meningitis; severe infections of the lungs, kidneys, skin, bones, and joints; and burn and wound infections. It is frequently used together with a penicillin, since combined treatment maximizes the antibacterial effect of both drugs.

Tobramycin eye drops and ointment are sometimes prescribed for external eye infections such as conjunctivitis and blepharitis (inflammation of the eyelids).

Tobramycin given by injection may have serious adverse effects on the kidneys and on the inner ear, leading to damage to the balance mechanism and deafness. However, the risk of kidney problems is thought to be lower than with other aminoglycoside antibiotics, and tobramycin may be preferred when kidney function is poor. Blood levels of the drug are usually monitored during injection treatment.

QUICK REFERENCE

Drug group Aminoglycoside antibiotic (p.140)

Overdose danger rating Medium

Dependence rating Low

Prescription needed Yes

Multi-source suppliers Yes

INFORMATION FOR USERS

Your drug prescription is tailored for you. Do not alter dosage without checking with your physician.

How taken

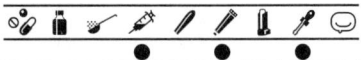

Injection, eye ointment, eye drops.

Frequency and timing of doses
Every 6 – 24 hours (injection); between 2 x daily and every 3 – 4 hours as directed (eye drops or ointment).

Adult dosage range
According to condition and response (injection); according to your physician's instructions (eye drops or ointment).

Onset of effect
2 – 3 days.

Duration of action
8 hours.

Diet advice
None.

Storage
Keep ointment in a closed container in a cool, dry place away from reach of children.

Missed dose
Apply eye drops or ointment as soon as you remember.

Stopping the drug
Apply the full course of ointment. Even if you feel better, the original infection may still be present and may recur if treatment is stopped too soon.

Exceeding the dose
Overdose by injection is unlikely, since treatment is carefully monitored in hospital. For eye preparations, an occasional unintentional extra dose is unlikely to be a cause for concern. If you notice unusual symptoms, notify your physician.

SPECIAL PRECAUTIONS

Be sure to tell your physician if:
▼ You have impaired kidney function.
▼ You have a hearing or balance disorder.
▼ You have myasthenia gravis.
▼ You have had a previous allergic reaction to aminoglycosides.
▼ You are taking other medications.

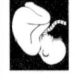

Pregnancy
▼ Injections are not prescribed as safety in pregnancy has not been established. No evidence of risk with topical preparations.

Breast feeding
▼ No evidence of risk with topical preparations. Given by injection, the drug passes into the breast milk, but at normal doses adverse effects on the baby are unlikely. Discuss with your physician.

Infants and children
▼ Injection used with caution in premature infants and newborn babies. Reduced dose may be necessary.

Over 60
▼ Increased likelihood of adverse effects with injections. Reduced dose may be necessary.

Driving and hazardous work
▼ Not usually applicable, but no known problems.

Alcohol
▼ No known problems.

POSSIBLE ADVERSE EFFECTS

Adverse effects are rare, but those that occur with the injectable form may be serious. Dizziness, loss of balance (vertigo), impaired hearing, and changes in the urine should be reported promptly. Rash and itching may occur with all preparations.

Symptom/effect	Frequency		Discuss with physician		Stop taking drug now	Call physician now
	Common	Rare	Only if severe	In all cases		
Nausea/vomiting	●		■			
Headache/lethargy	●			■	▲	
Dizziness/vertigo	●			■	▲	
Ringing in the ears	●			■	▲	
Rash/itching	●			■	▲	
Bloody/cloudy urine	●			■	▲	
Loss of hearing	●			■	▲	

INTERACTIONS

General note A wide range of drugs increase the risk of hearing loss and/or kidney failure with tobramycin. Such drugs include other aminoglycosides, furosemide, polymyxin antibiotics, amphotericin B, cisplatin, and cyclosporine.

PROLONGED USE

Injection is not usually given for longer than 10 days. There is a risk of adverse effects on hearing, balance, and kidney function.

Monitoring Blood levels of the drug are usually checked during injection treatment.

TOLBUTAMIDE

Brand names Orinase, Apo-Tolbutamide, Mobenol, Novo-Butamide
Used in the following combined preparations None

GENERAL INFORMATION

Tolbutamide, introduced in 1957, is an antidiabetic agent that lowers blood sugar by stimulating insulin secretion from the pancreas. Taken by mouth, it is used to treat adult (maturity-onset) diabetes in which active insulin-excreting cells are still present. Where these are lacking, as in juvenile diabetes, the drug is ineffective.

Tolbutamide does not work in isolation, but is given in conjunction with a special diabetic diet that limits intake of sugar and fats.

Shorter acting than many oral antidiabetic drugs, tolbutamide may help in the initial control of diabetes. It may also be used in those with impaired kidney function because it is less likely to build up in the body and cause excessive lowering of blood sugar. As with other oral antidiabetic drugs, it may need to be replaced with insulin during serious illnesses, injury, or surgery, when diabetic control is lost.

QUICK REFERENCE

Drug group Antidiabetic drug (p.154)

Overdose danger rating High

Dependence rating Low

Prescription needed Yes

Multi-source suppliers Yes

INFORMATION FOR USERS

Your drug prescription is tailored for you. Do not alter dosage without checking with your physician.

How taken

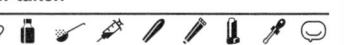

Tablets.

Frequency and timing of doses
Taken with meals either once daily in the morning, or 2 x daily in the morning and evening.

Adult dosage range
500mg – 2g daily.

Onset of effect
Within 1 hour.

Duration of action
6 – 12 hours.

Diet advice
An individualized low-fat, low-sugar diet must be maintained for the drug to be fully effective. Follow the advice of your physician.

Storage
Keep in a closed container in a cool, dry place away from reach of children. Protect from light.

Missed dose
Take as soon as you remember. If your next dose is due within 2 hours, take a single dose now and skip the next.

Stopping the drug
Do not stop the drug without consulting your physician; stopping the drug may lead to worsening of the underlying condition.

OVERDOSE ACTION

Seek immediate medical advice in all cases. If faintness, confusion, or headache occurs, eat something sugary. Take emergency action if a seizure or loss of consciousness occurs.

See Drug poisoning emergency guide (p.574).

POSSIBLE ADVERSE EFFECTS

Serious adverse effects are rare with tolbutamide. Symptoms such as dizziness, sweating, weakness, and confusion, indicate low blood sugar levels.

Symptom/effect	Frequency		Discuss with physician		Stop taking drug now	Call physician now
	Common	Rare	Only if severe	In all cases		
Dizziness/confusion	●			■		
Weakness/sweating	●			■		
Headache		●	■			
Nausea/vomiting		●		■		
Jaundice		●		■	▲	▮
Rash/itching		●		■	▲	

SPECIAL PRECAUTIONS

Be sure to tell your physician if:
▼ You have impaired liver or kidney function.
▼ You are allergic to sulfonamides.
▼ You have thyroid problems.
▼ You are taking other medications.

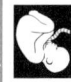 **Pregnancy**
▼ Not recommended. May cause birth defects if taken in the first 3 months of pregnancy. Furthermore, insulin is substituted in pregnancy because it gives better diabetic control. Discuss with your physician.

 Breast feeding
▼ The drug passes into the breast milk and may affect the baby. Discuss with your physician.

 Infants and children
▼ Not prescribed.

 Over 60
▼ Increased likelihood of low blood sugar. Reduced dose is therefore usually necessary.

 Driving and hazardous work
▼ Usually no problem. Avoid these activities if you have warning signs of low blood sugar.

 Alcohol
▼ Avoid. Alcohol may upset diabetic control.

Surgery and general anesthetics
▼ Surgery may reduce the beneficial effect of tolbutamide on diabetes. Notify your physician that you are diabetic before any surgery; insulin treatment may need to be substituted.

INTERACTIONS

General note A variety of drugs may oppose the effect of tolbutamide and so may raise blood sugar levels. Such drugs include corticosteroids, estrogens, diuretics, and rifampin. Other drugs increase the risk of low blood sugar. These include warfarin, ASA, clofibrate, chloramphenicol, sulfonamides, non-steroidal anti-inflammatory drugs, beta blockers, probenecid, and monoamine oxidase inhibitors.

PROLONGED USE

No problems expected.

Monitoring Regular monitoring of urine and/or blood sugar is required.

TOLNAFTATE

Brand names Tinactin, Pitrex, Zedsorb AF
Used in the following combined preparations None

GENERAL INFORMATION

Tolnaftate, introduced in 1964, was the first antifungal drug found to be effective when applied topically. Available over the counter as a cream, powder, solution, aerosol powder, and aerosol liquid, it is used to treat tinea (ringworm) infections of the skin, although it may not work as well as some other antifungal drugs that are taken by mouth. However, its effectiveness as a cream is increased if it is used in conjunction with salicylic acid ointment, which improves its absorption. Though useful for athlete's foot, it does not help fungal infections of the scalp, nails, palms, and soles. Tolnaftate can be used long-term to prevent recurrence of infections in susceptible people.

Side effects are rare, and unlike other antifungal drugs, tolnaftate does not generally cause skin irritation or rash. Occasionally, stinging may occur when this drug is sprayed onto the skin.

INFORMATION FOR USERS

Follow the instructions on the label. Call your physician if symptoms worsen.

How taken

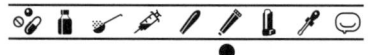

Topical powder, cream, topical solution, aerosol powder, aerosol liquid.

Frequency and timing of doses
2 x daily.

Dosage range
Follow manufacturer's instructions.

Onset of effect
Within 1 – 2 days. Full beneficial effects may not be felt for 2 – 6 weeks.

Duration of action
Up to 12 hours.

Diet advice
None.

Storage
Keep in a closed container in a cool, dry place away from reach of children.

Missed dose
No cause for concern, but apply as soon as you remember.

Stopping the drug
Use the full course. Even if symptoms disappear, the original infection may still be present and may recur if treatment is stopped too soon.

Exceeding the dose
An occasional unintentional extra dose is unlikely to be a cause for concern. But if you notice unusual symptoms, or if a large amount has been swallowed, notify your physician.

POSSIBLE ADVERSE EFFECTS

Adverse effects occur rarely with tolnaftate. If this antifungal drug irritates the skin, discontinue use and consult your physician about these symptoms.

Symptom/effect	Frequency		Discuss with physician		Stop taking drug now	Call physician now
	Common	Rare	Only if severe	In all cases		
Itching/irritation		●		■		▲
Rash		●		■		▲

INTERACTIONS

None.

SPECIAL PRECAUTIONS

Be sure to consult your physician or pharmacist before using this drug if:
▼ You have had a rash when using this drug in the past.
▼ You are taking other medications.

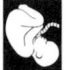
Pregnancy
▼ No evidence of risk to developing baby.

Breast feeding
▼ No evidence of risk.

Infants and children
▼ Not usually prescribed for infants. No special problems in older children.

Over 60
▼ No known problems.

Driving and hazardous work
▼ No known problems.

Alcohol
▼ No known problems.

PROLONGED USE

No problems expected.

TRAZODONE

rand names Desyrel, PMS-Trazodone, Syn-Trazodone
sed in the following combined preparations None

GENERAL INFORMATION

azodone is one of many drugs used to eat depression. It helps to elevate ood, improve appetite, and restore terest in everyday activities. But ecause it has a strong sedative effect, s particularly useful when the depreson is accompanied by anxiety or somnia or both. Taken at night, it

helps to reduce the need for additional sleeping drugs.

Trazodone is less likely to cause adverse effects than the tricyclic antidepressants. It is also somewhat safer for people with heart problems and is therefore used to treat depression in elderly patients.

QUICK REFERENCE

Drug group Antidepressant (p.96)
Overdose danger rating Medium
Dependence rating Low
Prescription needed Yes
Multi-source suppliers Yes

INFORMATION FOR USERS

ur drug prescription is tailored for you. not alter dosage without checking th your physician.

w taken

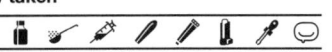

lets.

equency and timing of doses
3 x daily with food.

ult dosage range
0 – 400mg daily. Dose may be increased in ceptional circumstances.

set of effect
me benefits and adverse effects may pear within hours of starting treatment, but antidepressant effect may not be felt for 4 weeks.

ration of action
verse effects may last up to 24 hours after pping the drug. Following cessation of

prolonged treatment, the antidepressant effect may persist for up to 6 weeks.

Diet advice
None.

Storage
Keep in a closed container in a cool, dry place away from reach of children. Protect from light.

Missed dose
Take as soon as you remember. If your next dose is due within 3 hours, take a single dose now and skip the next.

Stopping the drug
Do not stop the drug without consulting your physician; symptoms may recur.

Exceeding the dose
An occasional unintentional extra dose is unlikely to cause problems. Large doses may cause unusual drowsiness. Notify your physician.

SPECIAL PRECAUTIONS

Be sure to tell your physician if:
▼ You have had epileptic seizures.
▼ You have impaired liver or kidney function.
▼ You have heart disease or are recovering from a recent heart attack.
▼ You are taking other medications.

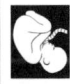

Pregnancy
▼ Safety in pregnancy not established. Discuss with your physician.

Breast feeding
▼ Safety in lactation not established. Discuss with your physician.

Infants and children
▼ Not recommended in patients under 18 years.

Over 60
▼ Increased likelihood of adverse effects. Reduced dose necessary.

Driving and hazardous work
▼ Avoid such activities until you have learned how the drug affects you; it can cause drowsiness.

Alcohol
▼ Avoid. Alcohol may increase the sedative effects of this drug.

Surgery and general anesthetics
▼ Trazodone may need to be stopped before you have a general anesthetic. Discuss this with your physician or dentist before any surgery.

POSSIBLE ADVERSE EFFECTS

zodone has fewer common adverse effects n some of the other antidepressants,

mainly because it has a much weaker *anticholinergic* action.

mptom/effect	Frequency		Discuss with physician		Stop taking drug now	Call physician now
	Common	Rare	Only if severe	In all cases		
wsiness	●		■			
usea/vomiting	●		■			
mouth	●		■			
ziness/fainting		●		■		
adache	●			■		
sh		●		■	▲	
nful/prolonged erection		●		■	▲	■

PROLONGED USE

No problems expected.

INTERACTIONS

ntihypertensive drugs Trazodone may crease the effects of these drugs and quire dosage adjustment of the ntihypertensive drugs.

Monoamine oxidase inhibitors (MAOIs) pecial caution is advised if coministration of trazodone with an MAOI being considered.

Digoxin and phenytoin Trazodone may increase the blood levels and *side effects* of these drugs.

Sedatives All drugs that have a sedative effect on the central nervous system are likely to increase the sedative properties of trazodone. Such drugs include alcohol, antihistamines, sleeping drugs, narcotic analgesics, and antipsychotics.

TRETINOIN

Brand names Retin-A, Retisol-A, StieVA-A, Vitamin A Acid
Used in the following combined preparation Stievamycin

GENERAL INFORMATION

Tretinoin is an anti-acne drug that is chemically related to vitamin A. It is available in various skin preparations. Tretinoin works by loosening the outer layers of skin, speeding up the process of skin renewal. This also makes it a useful treatment for certain other skin disorders in which the skin thickens abnormally, causing scaling.

Given for acne, tretinoin generally produces an improvement within 3 to 4 months, although there may be apparent worsening of the condition in the first few weeks of treatment.

Serious adverse *systemic* effects do not occur with tretinoin, but it sometimes causes skin irritation and peeling, particularly if overused. Excessive washing and exposure to sunlight may aggravate any irritation and lead to sunburn.

If excessive irritation occurs, a reduction in the frequency of application or strength of formulation may be advised.

QUICK REFERENCE

Drug group Drug for acne (p.189)
Overdose danger rating Low
Dependence rating Low
Prescription needed Yes
Multi-source suppliers Yes

INFORMATION FOR USERS

Your drug prescription is tailored for you. Do not alter dosage without checking with your physician.

How taken

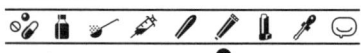

Gel, cream, solution.

Frequency and timing of doses
Apply to dry, clean skin once daily at bedtime, 15 – 30 minutes after washing.

Dosage range
Apply to cover affected area lightly. Avoid contact with eyes, lips, and nostril area.

Onset of effect
2 – 3 weeks. Maximum improvement may not be apparent for 8 – 12 weeks. Acne may worsen during the first 2 – 3 weeks of treatment in some people.

Duration of action
Effects may persist for several weeks after the drug has been stopped.

Diet advice
None.

Storage
Keep in a closed container in a cool, dry place away from reach of children. Protect from light.

Missed dose
Do not apply the missed dose. Apply your next dose as usual.

Stopping the drug
The drug can be safely stopped as soon as you no longer need it.

Exceeding the dose
A single extra application is unlikely to cause problems. Regular overuse may cause redness, stinging, or peeling of skin.

SPECIAL PRECAUTIONS

Be sure to tell your physician if:
▼ You have eczema.
▼ Your skin is sensitive to sunlight.
▼ You have sunburn.
▼ You are taking other medications.

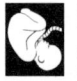
Pregnancy
▼ Safety in pregnancy not established. Discuss with your physician.

Breast feeding
▼ At normal doses, adverse effec on the baby are unlikely. Discuss with your physician.

Infants and children
▼ Not usually prescribed.

Over 60
▼ Not usually required.

Driving and hazardous work
▼ No known problems.

Alcohol
▼ No known problems.

PROLONGED USE

No special problems.

POSSIBLE ADVERSE EFFECTS

Application of tretinoin may cause temporary burning or stinging. Redness, peeling of the skin, and sometimes blistering, crusting, or swelling may occur with overuse but generally clear up if the treatment is stopped temporarily or its use is reduced. Bleaching or darkening of the skin occurs rarely, and usually disappears when the drug is stopped.

Symptom/effect	Frequency		Discuss with physician		Stop taking drug now	Call physician now
	Common	Rare	Only if severe	In all cases		
Stinging/redness		●	■			
Peeling of the skin		●	■			
Sensitivity of skin to sunlight		●	■			
Bleaching or darkening of skin		●		■		
Blistering/crusting/swelling		●		■	▲	∎

INTERACTIONS

Skin-drying preparations Medicated cosmetics, soaps, toiletries, and anti-acne preparations increase the likelihood of dryness and irritation of the skin with tretinoin.

TRIAMCINOLONE

Brand names Aristocort, Aristospan, Kenalog in Orabase, Nasocort, Oracort, Triaderm
Used in the following combined preparations Aristoform "R", Kenacomb, Triacomb, Viaderm K.C.

GENERAL INFORMATION

Triamcinolone, introduced in 1958, is a corticosteroid with a wide variety of uses and forms. It comes in *topical* preparations for dermatitis, eczema, and psoriasis. There is also a dental paste for mouth and gum inflammation. Taken orally, it can correct corticosteroid hormone deficiency caused by pituitary or adrenal gland disorders. Injected into the affected joints, it relieves rheumatoid arthritis and other forms of inflammation. Triamcinolone is also prescribed for certain blood disorders, such as thrombocytopenia and leukemia.

As with other corticosteroids, low doses taken by mouth over a short term or topical applications rarely cause *side effects*. However, long-term treatment, or large doses by mouth or injection, can cause indigestion, fluid retention, mood changes, acne, and muscle weakness. The drug may also induce diabetes.

INFORMATION FOR USERS

Your drug prescription is tailored for you. Do not alter dosage without checking with your physician.

How taken

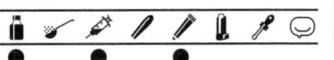

Tablets, syrup, injection, cream, ointment, dental paste, topical spray.

Frequency and timing of doses
2 – 4 x daily (by mouth); 2 – 4 x daily (topically); 2 – 3 x daily after meals and at bedtime (dental paste); considerable variation, depending on the condition (injection).

Dosage range
Considerable variation. Follow your physician's instructions.

Onset of effect
This may vary between a day and several weeks, depending on the condition.

Duration of action
Several days.

Diet advice
A low-sodium, high-potassium diet may be recommended when the oral form of the drug is prescribed for extended periods. Follow the advice of your physician.

Storage
Keep in a closed container in a cool, dry place away from reach of children. Protect from light.

Missed dose
Take as soon as you remember. If your next dose is due at this time, double the usual dose to make up the missed dose.

Stopping the drug
Do not stop tablets without consulting your physician. A gradual reduction in dose is required following prolonged treatment.

Exceeding the dose
An occasional unintentional extra dose is unlikely to be a cause for concern. But if you notice unusual symptoms, or if a large overdose has been taken, notify your physician.

POSSIBLE ADVERSE EFFECTS

The more serious adverse effects usually occur only when triamcinolone is taken by mouth. *Topical* preparations are highly unlikely to cause any problems.

Symptom/effect	Frequency		Discuss with physician		Stop taking drug now	Call physician now
	Common	Rare	Only if severe	In all cases		
Indigestion	●		■			
Weight gain/acne	●		■			
Muscle weakness		●		■		
Mood changes		●		■		

SPECIAL PRECAUTIONS

Be sure to tell your physician if:
▼ You suffer from depression.
▼ You have or have had a herpes infection.
▼ You have a peptic ulcer.
▼ You have had tuberculosis.
▼ You have high blood pressure.
▼ You have diabetes.
▼ You have had glaucoma.
▼ You are taking other medications.

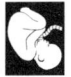

Pregnancy
▼ No evidence of risk with topical preparations or joint injections. Prescribed by mouth in low doses, harm to the baby is unlikely. Discuss with your physician.

Breast feeding
▼ No evidence of risk with topical preparations or joint injections. Taken by mouth, the drug passes into the breast milk. Discuss with your physician.

Infants and children
▼ Reduced dose necessary.

Over 60
▼ Increased likelihood of adverse effects. Reduced dose may therefore be necessary.

Driving and hazardous work
▼ No known problems.

Alcohol
▼ Avoid. Alcohol may increase the risk of a peptic ulcer with this drug.

INTERACTIONS (by mouth or injection only)

Oral anticoagulants Triamcinolone may decrease the effect of anticoagulants.

Vaccines Serious reactions can occur when vaccinations are given with this drug. Discuss with your physician.

Barbiturates, phenytoin, and rifampin may reduce the effect of triamcinolone.

Antidiabetic drugs Triamcinolone reduces the actions of these drugs.

Antihypertensive drugs Triamcinolone may reduce the effect of antihypertensive drugs.

Diuretics Triamcinolone may increase potassium loss with these drugs.

PROLONGED USE

Prolonged use of high doses of triamcinolone by mouth or injection can lead to adverse effects such as diabetes, glaucoma, cataracts, bone damage, and may retard growth in children.

TRIAMTERENE

Brand name Dyrenium
Used in the following combined preparations Apo-Triazide, Dyazide, Novo-Triamzide, Nu-Triazide

GENERAL INFORMATION

Triamterene, introduced in 1965, belongs to the class of drugs known as potassium-sparing diuretics. In combination with thiazide or loop diuretics, it is used in the treatment of hypertension and edema (fluid retention).

On its own, or more commonly in combination with a thiazide diuretic, triamterene may be used to treat edema as a complication of heart failure, nephrotic syndrome, or liver cirrhosis.

Triamterene is quick to act; its effect on urine flow is apparent within 2 hours. As with other potassium-sparing diuretics, there is a risk of unusually high levels of potassium building up in the blood if the kidneys are functioning abnormally. Consequently, triamterene is prescribed with caution for people with kidney failure.

QUICK REFERENCE

Drug group Potassium-sparing diuretic (p.111)

Overdose danger rating Low

Dependence rating Low

Prescription needed Yes

Multi-source suppliers No

INFORMATION FOR USERS

Your drug prescription is tailored for you. Do not alter dosage without checking with your physician.

How taken

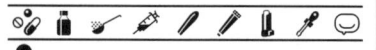

Tablets.

Frequency and timing of doses
1 – 2 x daily after meals or on alternate days.

Adult dosage range
100 – 300mg daily.

Onset of effect
2 – 4 hours.

Duration of action
9 – 12 hours.

Diet advice
Avoid foods that are high in potassium, e.g., dried fruit and salt substitutes.

Storage
Keep in a closed container in a cool, dry place away from reach of children.

Missed dose
Take as soon as you remember. However, if it is late in the day, do not take the missed dose, or you may need to get up at night to pass urine. Take the next scheduled dose as usual.

Stopping the drug
Do not stop the drug without consulting your physician; symptoms may recur.

Exceeding the dose
An occasional unintentional extra dose is unlikely to be a cause for concern. But if you notice unusual symptoms, or if a large overdose has been taken, notify your physician.

POSSIBLE ADVERSE EFFECTS

Triamterene has few adverse effects; the main problem is the possibility that potassium may be retained by the body, causing muscle weakness and numbness.

Symptom/effect	Frequency		Discuss with physician		Stop taking drug now	Call physician now
	Common	Rare	Only if severe	In all cases		
Digestive disturbance		●	■			
Headache		●	■			
Muscle weakness		●		■		
Rash		●		■		
Dry mouth		●	■			

INTERACTIONS

Lithium Triamterene may increase the blood levels of lithium, leading to an increased risk of lithium poisoning.

Spironolactone, amiloride, ACE inhibitors These agents may increase the risk of raised blood levels of potassium with triamterene.

Non-steroidal anti-inflammatory drugs (NSAIDs) may increase the risk of raised blood levels of potassium.

SPECIAL PRECAUTIONS

Be sure to tell your physician if:
▼ You have impaired liver or kidney function
▼ You have had kidney stones.
▼ You have a blood disease.
▼ You have gout.
▼ You have diabetes.
▼ You are taking other medications.

Pregnancy
▼ Safety in pregnancy not established. Discuss with your physician.

Breast feeding
▼ The drug may pass into breast milk. Discuss with your physician.

Infants and children
▼ Not usually prescribed.

Over 60
▼ Increased likelihood of adverse effects. Reduced dose may therefore be necessary.

Driving and hazardous work
▼ No special problems.

Alcohol
▼ No known problems.

PROLONGED USE

Serious problems are unlikely, but levels of salts such as sodium and potassium may occasionally become disrupted during prolonged use.

Monitoring Blood tests may be performed to check on kidney function and levels of body salts.

TRIAZOLAM

Brand names Halcion, Apo-Triazo, Gen-Triazolam, Novo-Triolam, Nu-Triazo
Used in the following combined preparations None

GENERAL INFORMATION

Triazolam, a benzodiazepine drug, is used for the occasional, short-term treatment of insomnia marked by difficulty falling asleep. It is not recommended for early morning wakenings. When using this drug, it is especially important to ensure a full night's sleep (7 – 8 hours).

In general, sleeping drugs should only be used when non-drug measures have not been effective and where sleep disturbance causes impairment of daytime functioning.

The most common adverse effects of triazolam are related to its sedative and tranquilizing properties. Of special importance are the rare instances of confusion, disorientation, short-term loss of memory, and hallucinations. These particular problems may be more likely to occur in the elderly.

In common with other benzodiazepines, triazolam can be habit-forming if taken regularly for even a few weeks. Its effects also become weaker with time. For these reasons, treatment with triazolam should be reviewed every 7 to 10 days.

INFORMATION FOR USERS

Your drug prescription is tailored for you. Do not alter dosage without checking with your physician.

How taken

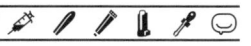

Tablets.

Frequency and timing of doses
Once daily at bedtime.

Adult dosage range
0.125 – 0.25mg daily. Physicians usually prescribe the lowest possible dose and increase gradually, if needed.

Onset of effect
0 – 30 minutes.

Duration of action
6 hours.

Diet advice
None.

Storage
Keep in a closed container in a cool, dry place away from reach of children.

Missed dose
If you fall asleep without having taken a dose and wake some hours later, do not take the missed dose. If necessary, return to your normal dose schedule the next night.

Stopping the drug
If you have been taking the drug continuously for less than 2 weeks, it can be safely stopped as soon as you feel you no longer need it. However, if you have been taking the drug for longer, consult your physician, who may supervise a gradual reduction in dosage. Stopping abruptly may lead to withdrawal symptoms (see p.94).

Exceeding the dose
An occasional, unintentional extra dose is unlikely to cause problems. Large overdoses may cause unusual drowsiness. Notify your physician.

POSSIBLE ADVERSE EFFECTS

The most common adverse effects of this drug are related to its sedative and tranquilizing properties.

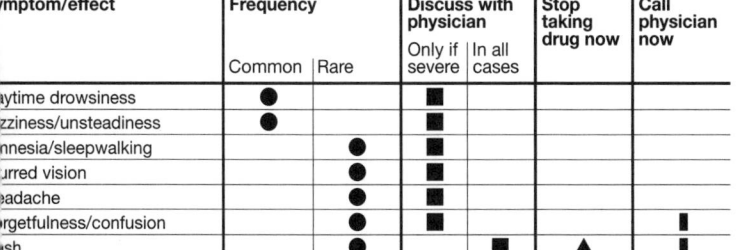

Symptom/effect	Frequency		Discuss with physician		Stop taking drug now	Call physician now
	Common	Rare	Only if severe	In all cases		
Daytime drowsiness	●			■		
Dizziness/unsteadiness	●			■		
Amnesia/sleepwalking		●		■		
Blurred vision		●		■		
Headache		●		■		
Forgetfulness/confusion		●		■		▌
Rash		●			■	▲	▌

INTERACTIONS

Sedatives All drugs, including alcohol, that have a sedative effect on the central nervous system are likely to increase the sedative properties of triazolam.

Cimetidine and erythromycin These drugs may increase the blood levels of triazolam.

SPECIAL PRECAUTIONS

Be sure to tell your physician if:
▼ You have impaired liver or kidney function.
▼ You have had problems with alcohol or drug abuse.
▼ You have myasthenia gravis.
▼ You have glaucoma.
▼ You are taking other medications.

Pregnancy
▼ Safety in pregnancy not established. Discuss with your physician.

Breast feeding
▼ Not recommended. The drug passes into the breast milk and may affect the baby adversely. Discuss with your physician.

Infants and children
▼ Not recommended in patients under 18 years.

Over 60
▼ Increased likelihood of adverse effects. Reduced dose may therefore be necessary.

Driving and hazardous work
▼ Avoid such activities until you have learned how the drug affects you; it can cause blurred vision, reduced alertness, and slowed reactions.

Alcohol
▼ Avoid. Alcohol increases the sedative effects of this drug.

PROLONGED USE

Regular use of this drug over even a few weeks can lead to a reduction in its effect as the body adapts. It may also be habit-forming when taken for extended periods, especially if larger-than-average doses are taken. The drug should not be used for more than 10 consecutive days.

TRIFLUOPERAZINE

Brand names Stelazine, Apo-Trifluoperazine, Novo-Flurazine, Terfluzine
Used in the following combined preparation Stelabid

GENERAL INFORMATION

Trifluoperazine belongs to a group of drugs called the phenothiazines. These drugs act on the brain to modify abnormal behavior (see Antipsychotics, p.97). It is effective in suppressing abnormal behavior, reducing aggression, and tranquilizing agitation.

Trifluoperazine is used in the treatment of schizophrenia, mania, dementia, and other disorders where confusion, aggression, hallucinations, or abnormal behavior may occur. It is sometimes used to treat nausea and vomiting caused by drug or radiation therapy.

Trifluoperazine causes less drowsiness and *anticholinergic side effects* than most phenothiazines, but it can produce stiffness and shaking *(parkinsonism)*, and abnormal movements of the face, limbs, and body *(tardive dyskinesia)*.

QUICK REFERENCE

Drug group Antipsychotic (p.97), anti-emetic drug (p.102)

Overdose danger rating Medium

Dependence rating Low

Prescription needed Yes

Multi-source suppliers Yes

INFORMATION FOR USERS

Your drug prescription is tailored for you. Do not alter dosage without checking with your physician.

How taken

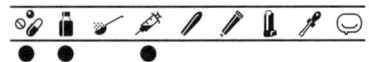

Tablets, oral liquid, injection.

Frequency and timing of doses
2 – 4 x daily.

Adult dosage range
Mental illness 2 – 10mg daily (starting dose), increasing to 20mg daily (maintenance dose). Dose may be increased in cases of extreme agitation.
Nausea and vomiting 2 – 4mg daily.

Onset of effect
20 – 30 minutes (by injection); 2 – 3 hours (by mouth).

Duration of action
6 – 24 hours. Some effects may persist for weeks when stopping the drug after regular use.

Diet advice
None.

Storage
Keep in a closed container in a cool, dry place away from reach of children. Protect from light and from freezing.

Missed dose
Take as soon as you remember. If your next dose is due within 2 hours, take a single dose now and skip the next.

Stopping the drug
Do not stop the drug without consulting your physician; symptoms may recur.

Exceeding the dose
An occasional unintentional extra dose is unlikely to be a cause for concern. Larger overdoses may cause unusual drowsiness, muscle weakness or rigidity, and/or faintness. Notify your physician.

SPECIAL PRECAUTIONS

Be sure to tell your physician if:
▼ You have impaired liver or kidney function.
▼ You have heart or circulation problems.
▼ You have had epileptic seizures.
▼ You have an overactive thyroid gland.
▼ You have Parkinson's disease.
▼ You have had glaucoma.
▼ You have prostate trouble.
▼ You are taking other medications.

Pregnancy
▼ Safety in pregnancy not established. Discuss with your physician.

Breast feeding
▼ The drug passes into the breast milk. Its effects on the baby are not known. Discuss with your physician

Infants and children
▼ Rarely required. Reduced dose necessary.

Over 60
▼ Reduced dose may be necessary.

Driving and hazardous work
▼ Avoid such activities until you have learned how the drug affects you; it can cause drowsiness and slowed reactions.

Alcohol
▼ Avoid. Alcohol may increase the sedative effect of this drug.

POSSIBLE ADVERSE EFFECTS

Trifluoperazine can cause a variety of minor anticholinergic symptoms that often become less marked with time. The most significant adverse effect is abnormal movements of the face and limbs (parkinsonism). This may be controlled by dosage adjustment.

Symptom/effect	Frequency		Discuss with physician		Stop taking drug now	Call physician now
	Common	Rare	Only if severe	In all cases		
Drowsiness/lethargy	●		■			
Parkinsonism	●			■		
Dizziness/fainting	●			■		
Infrequent periods		●		■		
Rash		●		■	▲	
High fever/confusion		●		■	▲	■

INTERACTIONS

Anticonvulsants and antiparkinsonian drugs Trifluoperazine may reduce the effectiveness of such drugs.

Anticholinergic drugs Their *side effects* may be increased by trifluoperazine.

Sedatives All drugs, including alcohol, that have a sedative effect on the central nervous system are likely to increase the sedative effects of trifluoperazine.

PROLONGED USE

Use of this drug for more than a few months may lead to tardive dyskinesia, i.e., abnormal, involuntary movements of the eyes, face, and tongue. Occasionally, jaundice may occur.

Monitoring Periodic blood tests may be performed.

TRIHEXYPHENIDYL

Brand names Artane, Aparkane, Apo-Trihex, Novo-Hexidyl, PMS Trihexyphenidyl
Used in the following combined preparations None

GENERAL INFORMATION

Trihexyphenidyl is an *anticholinergic* drug that was introduced for the treatment of Parkinson's disease in the 1940s. It continues to be used, especially in the early stages of the disease. It is particularly effective for relieving rigidity and tremor, but it has little effect on the shuffling gait and slow muscular movements that are also characteristic of Parkinson's disease.

For further information on antiparkinsonism drugs, see page 99. Trihexyphenidyl is also occasionally used to counter the adverse effects of antipsychotic drugs (p.97).

Like all anticholinergic drugs, trihexyphenidyl can cause a variety of adverse effects (see below). These symptoms have to be balanced against the benefits of the drug.

INFORMATION FOR USERS

Your drug prescription is tailored for you. Do not alter dosage without checking with your physician.

How taken

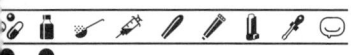

Tablets, slow-release capsules, oral liquid.

Frequency and timing of doses
Up to 3 x daily with meals.

Adult dosage range
1 – 15mg daily.

Onset of effect
1 hour.

Duration of action
6 – 12 hours.

Diet advice
None.

Storage
Keep in a closed container in a cool, dry place away from reach of children.

Missed dose
Take as soon as you remember. If your next dose is due within 2 hours, take a single dose now and skip the next.

Stopping the drug
Do not stop taking the drug without consulting your physician; symptoms may recur. A gradual reduction in dosage is usually necessary.

Exceeding the dose
An occasional unintentional extra dose is unlikely to cause problems. Large overdoses may cause an increase in heart rate and agitation. Notify your physician.

SPECIAL PRECAUTIONS

Be sure to tell your physician if:
▼ You have high blood pressure.
▼ You have had glaucoma.
▼ You have heart problems.
▼ You have had prostate trouble.
▼ You have impaired liver or kidney function.
▼ You are taking other medications.

Pregnancy
▼ Not usually prescribed. Safety in pregnancy not established. Discuss with your physician.

Breast feeding
▼ Unlikely to be required.

Infants and children
▼ Not recommended.

Over 60
▼ Sensitivity to this drug is likely to increase with age, requiring lower dosages. Regular monitoring is necessary.

Driving and hazardous work
▼ Avoid such activities until you have learned how the drug affects you; it can cause blurred vision and confusion.

Alcohol
▼ Avoid. Alcohol may increase the sedative effects of this drug.

POSSIBLE ADVERSE EFFECTS

Most of the adverse effects of this drug are the result of its anticholinergic action. The severity of such effects can sometimes be reduced by adjustment of dosage.

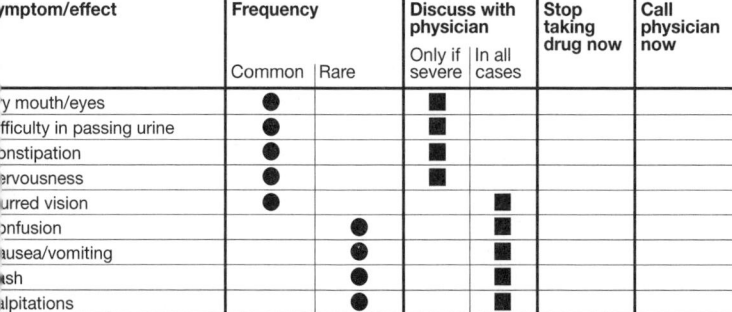

Symptom/effect	Frequency		Discuss with physician		Stop taking drug now	Call physician now
	Common	Rare	Only if severe	In all cases		
Dry mouth/eyes	●		■			
Difficulty in passing urine	●		■			
Constipation	●		■			
Nervousness	●		■			
Blurred vision	●			■		
Confusion		●		■		
Nausea/vomiting		●		■		
Rash		●		■		
Palpitations		●		■		

INTERACTIONS

Antihistamines and anticholinergic drugs The effects of such drugs are likely to be increased by trihexyphenidyl.

Phenothiazine antipsychotic drugs Trihexyphenidyl may increase some of the adverse effects of these drugs.

Alcohol The effects of alcohol are increased when taken with this drug.

Antacids and antidiarrheal drugs may reduce the effects of trihexyphenidyl. Do not take within 1 hour of taking trihexyphenidyl.

PROLONGED USE

Sensitivity to this drug can develop during prolonged use, especially in the elderly, and dosage may need to be reduced periodically. Occasionally, prolonged trihexyphenidyl treatment may cause abnormal movements of the face and limbs, or provoke the onset of glaucoma.

Monitoring Regular eye examinations are usually carried out to ensure that glaucoma is not developing.

TRIMEBUTINE

Brand name Modulon
Used in the following combined preparations None

GENERAL INFORMATION

Trimebutine is an *antispasmodic* drug that relieves painful abdominal cramps caused by spasms in the lower gastrointestinal tract. Used to treat irritable bowel syndrome (spastic colon), it is also used after abdominal surgery to hasten the return of normal bowel activity.

Trimebutine relieves symptoms, but does not cure the underlying condition. Additional treatments with other drugs and self-help measures may therefore be recommended by your physician.

QUICK REFERENCE

Drug group Drug for irritable bowel syndrome (p.122)

Overdose danger rating Low

Dependence rating Low

Prescription needed Yes

Multi-source suppliers No

INFORMATION FOR USERS

Your drug prescription is tailored for you. Do not alter dosage without checking with your physician.

How taken

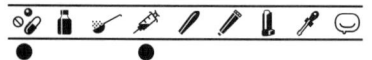

Tablets, injection.

Frequency and timing of doses
3 x daily, before meals.

Dosage range
300 – 600mg daily (tablets).

Onset of effect
Within 2 hours.

Duration of action
Approximately 6 – 8 hours.

Diet advice
None.

Storage
Keep in a closed container in a cool, dry place away from reach of children. Protect from light.

Missed dose
Do not take the missed dose. Take your next dose as usual.

Stopping the drug
Can be safely stopped as soon as you no longer need it.

Exceeding the dose
An occasional unintentional extra dose is unlikely to cause problems. But if you notice unusual symptoms, or if a large overdose has been taken, notify your physician.

POSSIBLE ADVERSE EFFECTS

Most adverse effects associated with trimebutine tablets are mild. They may improve after a few days of use (as your body adjusts to the drug) or they may be overcome by an adjustment of dosage. The most common adverse effects are drowsiness and gastrointestinal disorders (diarrhea, nausea, constipation, heartburn, and acid indigestion).

Symptom/effect	Frequency		Discuss with physician		Stop taking drug now	Call physician now
	Common	Rare	Only if severe	In all cases		
Fatigue/dizziness	●		■			
Gastrointestinal disorders	●		■			
Headache		●	■			
Rash/hives		●		■	▲	▮

INTERACTIONS

Sedatives All drugs, including alcohol, that have a sedative effect on the central nervous system are likely to increase the sedative effects of trimebutine.

SPECIAL PRECAUTIONS

Be sure to tell your physician if:
▼ You have urinary problems.
▼ You have any problems with your hearing.
▼ You have epilepsy.
▼ You are taking other medications.

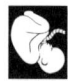

Pregnancy
▼ Not recommended.

Breast feeding
▼ Not recommended.

Infants and children
▼ Not recommended for children under 12 years.

Over 60
▼ Increased likelihood of adverse effects. Reduced dose may therefore be necessary.

Driving and hazardous work
▼ Avoid such activities until you have learned how the drug affects you; it can cause drowsiness and dizziness.

Alcohol
▼ Avoid. Alcohol may increase the sedative effects of this drug.

PROLONGED USE

No problems expected.

TRIMETHOPRIM

Brand name Proloprim
Used in the following combined preparations Apo-Sulfatrim, Bactrim, Coptin, Novo-Trimel, Polytrim, Septra

GENERAL INFORMATION

Trimethoprim, introduced in 1980, is an antibiotic prescribed for a wide variety of infections. On its own, trimethoprim is most commonly prescribed for the prevention and treatment of urinary tract infections. Trimethoprim is often prescribed in combined preparations with either sulfamethoxazole (a combination known as co-trimoxazole) or sulfadiazine (co-trimazine).

Trimethoprim alone has fewer adverse effects than co-trimoxazole or co-trimazine and is equally effective in many conditions. The most common *side effects* of trimethoprim are rash and itching.

If, however, the drug is taken for prolonged periods, tests to monitor blood composition are generally advised.

INFORMATION FOR USERS

Your drug prescription is tailored for you. Do not alter dosage without checking with your physician.

How taken

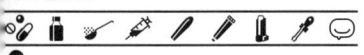

Tablets.

Frequency and timing of doses
1 – 2 x daily.

Adult dosage range
200mg daily.

Onset of effect
Symptoms usually improve within 1 – 2 days, depending on the condition.

Duration of action
12 hours.

Diet advice
None.

Storage
Keep in a closed container in a cool, dry place away from reach of children. Protect from light.

Missed dose
Take as soon as you remember.

Stopping the drug
Take the full course. Even if you feel better, the original infection may still be present and symptoms may recur if treatment is stopped too soon.

Exceeding the dose
An occasional unintentional extra dose is unlikely to be a cause for concern. But if you notice unusual symptoms, or if a large overdose has been taken, notify your physician.

SPECIAL PRECAUTIONS

Be sure to tell your physician if:
▼ You have impaired liver or kidney function.
▼ You have a blood disorder.
▼ You are taking other medications.

Pregnancy
▼ Safety in pregnancy not established. Discuss with your physician.

Breast feeding
▼ Not recommended. Discuss with your physician.

Infants and children
▼ Reduced dose necessary.

Over 60
▼ Increased likelihood of adverse effects, particularly when combined trimethoprim-diuretic therapy is given.

Driving and hazardous work
▼ No known problems.

Alcohol
▼ No known problems.

POSSIBLE ADVERSE EFFECTS

Trimethoprim taken on its own rarely causes side effects, the most common being rash and itching. However, additional adverse effects of the sulfonamides may occur when trimethoprim is taken in combination with these agents.

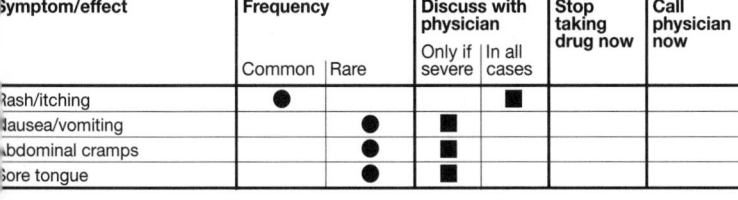

Symptom/effect	Frequency		Discuss with physician		Stop taking drug now	Call physician now
	Common	Rare	Only if severe	In all cases		
Rash/itching	●			■		
Nausea/vomiting		●	■			
Abdominal cramps		●	■			
Sore tongue		●	■			

INTERACTIONS

Phenytoin The antifolate effect of phenytoin may be enhanced by trimethoprim.

Warfarin The anticoagulant effect of warfarin may be increased by trimethoprim.

Pyrimethamine Co-administration of trimethoprim with pyrimethamine may lead to the development of megaloblastic anemia.

PROLONGED USE

Long-term use of this drug may lead to folate deficiency, which in turn may lead to blood abnormalities. Folate supplements may be prescribed.

Monitoring Periodic blood tests to monitor blood composition are usually required.

TRIMIPRAMINE

Brand names Surmontll, Apo-Trimip, Novo-Tripramine, Rhotrimine
Used in the following combined preparations None

GENERAL INFORMATION

Trimipramine belongs to a class of antidepressant drugs known as the tricyclics. It is mainly used in the long-term treatment of depression. It elevates mood, increases physical activity, improves appetite, and restores interest in everyday activities.

Trimipramine is more likely to cause drowsiness than many other tricyclics.

In overdose, it may cause coma, seizures, and dangerously abnormal heart rhythms, but in normal use, serious *side effects* are rare.

INFORMATION FOR USERS

Your drug prescription is tailored for you. Do not alter dosage without checking with your physician.

How taken

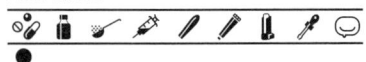

Tablets, capsules.

Frequency and timing of doses
Single dose at bedtime or 2 – 3 x daily.

Adult dosage range
75 – 300mg daily.

Onset of effect
Some benefits and effects may appear within hours, but full antidepressant effect may not be felt for 2 – 6 weeks.

Duration of action
Following prolonged treatment, antidepressant effect may persist for up to 6 weeks. Adverse effects may wear off within a few days.

Diet advice
None.

Storage
Keep in a closed container in a cool, dry place away from reach of children.

Missed dose
If taken once at bedtime, take next dose as usual. If taken 2 – 3 x daily and next dose is due within 3 hours, take single dose now and skip the next, otherwise take as soon as you remember.

Stopping the drug
Do not stop the drug without consulting your physician.

OVERDOSE ACTION

 Seek immediate medical advice in all cases. Take emergency action if palpitations are noticed or consciousness is lost.

See Drug poisoning emergency guide (p.574).

SPECIAL PRECAUTIONS

Be sure to tell your physician if:
▼ You have heart problems.
▼ You have had epileptic seizures.
▼ You have impaired liver or kidney function.
▼ You have had glaucoma.
▼ You have urinary difficulties.
▼ You have a blood disease.
▼ You have a thyroid disorder.
▼ You are taking other medications.

 **Pregnancy**
▼ Safety in pregnancy not established. Discuss with your physician.

 Breast feeding
▼ The drug passes into the breast milk and may affect the baby. Discuss with your physician.

 Infants and children
▼ Not usually prescribed.

 Over 60
▼ Increased likelihood of adverse effects. Reduced dose may therefore be necessary.

 Driving and hazardous work
▼ Avoid such activities until you have learned how the drug affects you; it can cause drowsiness and blurred vision.

 Alcohol
▼ Avoid. Alcohol may increase the sedative effects of this drug.

Surgery and general anesthetics
▼ Trimipramine treatment may need to be stopped before you have a general anesthetic. Discuss this with your physician or dentist before any surgery.

POSSIBLE ADVERSE EFFECTS

The possible adverse effects of this drug are mainly the result of its *anticholinergic* action and its blocking action on the transmission of signals in the heart. Some problems can be overcome by medically supervised adjustment of dosage.

Symptom/effect	Frequency		Discuss with physician		Stop taking drug now	Call physician now
	Common	Rare	Only if severe	In all cases		
Drowsiness	●		■			
Dry mouth	●		■			
Blurred vision	●			■		
Dizziness/fainting	●			■		
Rash		●		■	▲	
Urinary difficulties		●		■	▲	
Palpitations		●		■	▲	■

INTERACTIONS

Sedatives All drugs, including alcohol, that have a sedative effect are likely to increase the sedative effects of trimipramine.

Antihypertensive drugs Trimipramine may reduce the effect of some of these drugs, especially guanethidine and clonidine.

Monoamine oxidase inhibitors (MAOIs) Usually, trimipramine should not be given during or within 14 days of treatment with an MAOI. Serious reactions may occur. Such drugs are prescribed together only under strict medical supervision.

PROLONGED USE

No problems expected.

URSODIOL

Brand name Ursofalk
Used in the following combined preparations None

GENERAL INFORMATION

Ursodiol (ursodeoxycholic acid) is a chemical that occurs naturally in bile, where it has an important role in controlling the concentration of cholesterol in the blood. As an orally administered drug, it is prescribed as an alternative to surgery in the treatment of gallstones.

Ursodiol acts by reducing levels of cholesterol in the bile, helping gallstones that consist predominantly of cholesterol to dissolve. The drug is not effective with stones of a high calcium or bile acid content. Its benefits are increased by weight loss and a diet high in fiber and low in fat.

Ursodiol dissolves gallstones in 3 to 18 months. The progress of treatment is assessed regularly by ultrasound or by X ray. Drug treatment is continued for at least 3 months after the stones have disappeared in order to prevent a recurrence. Recurrence of gallstones still occurs in about 25 per cent of people within a year of stopping treatment. Renewed therapy may then be required.

INFORMATION FOR USERS

Your drug prescription is tailored for you. Do not alter dosage without checking with your physician.

How taken

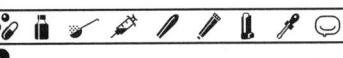

Capsules.

Frequency and timing of doses
x daily after food.

Adult dosage range
According to body weight.

Onset of effect
Within 30 minutes. Full beneficial effects may not be felt for up to 18 months.

Duration of action
Up to 12 hours.

Diet advice
A low cholesterol, high fiber diet is advisable since it enhances gallstone dissolution, prevents new stones forming, and reduces circulating cholesterol levels.

Storage
Keep in a closed container in a cool, dry place away from reach of children.

Missed dose
No cause for concern but take as soon as you remember. If your next dose is due within 2 hours, take a single dose now and skip the next.

Stopping the drug
Do not stop the drug without consulting your physician; symptoms may recur.

Exceeding the dose
An occasional unintentional extra dose is unlikely to be a cause for concern. But if you notice unusual symptoms or if a large overdose has been taken, notify your physician.

POSSIBLE ADVERSE EFFECTS

Adverse effects from ursodiol are rare.

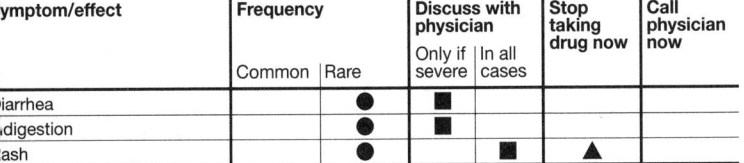

Symptom/effect	Frequency		Discuss with physician		Stop taking drug now	Call physician now
	Common	Rare	Only if severe	In all cases		
Diarrhea	●		■			
Indigestion	●		■			
Rash	●			■	▲	

INTERACTIONS

Cholestyramine, colestipol, and aluminum antacids These reduce the beneficial effect of ursodiol.

Estrogens, oral contraceptives, and lipid-lowering agents These may counter the beneficial effects of ursodiol.

SPECIAL PRECAUTIONS

Be sure to tell your physician if:
▼ You have impaired liver function.
▼ You are hypersensitive to bile acids.
▼ You are taking other medications.

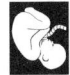
Pregnancy
▼ Not usually prescribed. The drug may affect the baby. Discuss with your physician.

Breast feeding
▼ Safety not established. Discuss with your physician.

Infants and children
▼ Safety and effectiveness not established.

Over 60
▼ No special problems.

Driving and hazardous work
▼ No known problems.

Alcohol
▼ No known problems.

PROLONGED USE

Safety of use of ursodiol beyond 24 months is not established.

Monitoring Ultrasound or X-ray examinations may be carried out to assess the progress of treatment.

VALPROIC ACID

Brand name Depakene
Used in the following combined preparations None

GENERAL INFORMATION

Valproic acid is a first-line drug used in the treatment of epilepsy. It can be used alone or in combination with other anticonvulsant drugs. Its action is similar to that of other anticonvulsant drugs (see p.98), reducing electrical discharges in the brain.

Drowsiness due to valproic acid is usually slight and temporary; this makes it particularly suitable for children who suffer from tonic-clonic (grand mal) seizures or absence seizures (during which a person seems to be daydreaming).

INFORMATION FOR USERS

Your drug prescription is tailored for you. Do not alter dosage without checking with your physician.

How taken

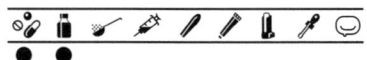

Capsules, oral liquid.

Frequency and timing of doses
1 – 3 x daily with food.

Dosage range
Dosage is calculated on an individual basis according to age and weight.

Onset of effect
Within 30 minutes.

Duration of action
12 hours or more.

Diet advice
None.

Storage
Keep in a tightly closed container in a cool, dry place away from reach of children.

Missed dose
Take as soon as you remember. If your next dose is due within 2 hours, take a single dose now and skip the next.

Stopping the drug
Do not stop the drug without consulting your physician; symptoms may recur.

Exceeding the dose
An occasional, unintentional extra dose is unlikely to cause problems. Large overdoses may lead to coma. Notify your physician.

SPECIAL PRECAUTIONS

Be sure to tell your physician if:
▼ You have impaired liver or kidney function.
▼ You have a blood disorder.
▼ You are taking other medications.

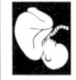

Pregnancy
▼ Not usually prescribed. May cause abnormalities in the unborn baby. Discuss with your physician.

Breast feeding
▼ Not recommended. The drug passes into the breast milk. Discuss with your physician.

Infants and children
▼ Reduced dose necessary.

Over 60
▼ Reduced dose may be necessary.

Driving and hazardous work
▼ Your underlying condition, as well as the possibility of reduced alertness while taking this drug, may make such activities inadvisable. Discuss with your physician.

Alcohol
▼ Avoid. Valproic acid may increase the depressant effects of alcohol.

Surgery and general anesthetics
▼ Be sure to tell your physician or dentist that you are taking valproic acid. This drug may prolong bleeding.

POSSIBLE ADVERSE EFFECTS

The most commonly reported adverse effects are nausea, vomiting, and indigestion. However, most serious adverse effects of valproic acid are rare. They include liver failure, and platelet and bleeding abnormalities.

Symptom/effect	Frequency		Discuss with physician		Stop taking drug now	Call physician now
	Common	Rare	Only if severe	In all cases		
Abdominal discomfort	●		■			
Nausea/vomiting	●			■		▮
Temporary loss of hair		●	■			
Weight gain		●	■			
Tremor		●		■		▮
Drowsiness/lethargy		●		■		▮
Jaundice		●		■	▲	▮
Rash		●		■	▲	▮

INTERACTIONS

Anticoagulant drugs Valproic acid can increase the effect of such drugs as warfarin and ASA. The dose of the anticoagulant drug may need to be reduced.

Other anticonvulsant drugs may reduce blood levels of valproic acid.

Monoamine oxidase inhibitors (MAOIs) may depress the central nervous system when taken with valproic acid. Dosage of the monoamine oxidase inhibitors should be adjusted accordingly.

PROLONGED USE

Use of this drug may cause liver damage, which is more likely in the first 6 months of use.

Monitoring Periodic checks on blood levels of the drug are usually required. Blood tests of liver function and blood composition and coagulation may also be carried out, especially in children.

VASOPRESSIN

Brand names Pitressin, Pressyn
Used in the following combined preparations None

GENERAL INFORMATION

Vasopressin, an antidiuretic hormone produced in the pituitary gland, controls the body's water balance. It acts on the kidneys to increase water reabsorption, thereby reducing the volume of urine produced.

Vasopressin was originally used for the treatment of diabetes insipidus, a disease caused by a deficiency of the natural antidiuretic hormone.

It has now been replaced in that use by desmopressin, an analogue of vasopressin.

Vasopressin is now used mainly to prevent or treat abdominal swelling after surgery and to prevent gas shadows in abdominal X rays.

QUICK REFERENCE

Drug group Drug for diabetes insipidus (p.154)

Overdose danger rating High

Dependence rating Low

Prescription needed Yes

Multi-source suppliers Yes

INFORMATION FOR USERS

Your drug prescription is tailored for you. Do not alter dosage without checking with your physician.

How taken

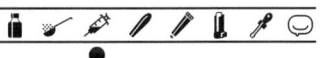

Injection.

Frequency and timing of doses
1 – 3 x daily or as prescribed.

Dosage range
Adults 0.25 – 0.5mL
Children Reduced dose necessary according to age and weight.

Onset of effect
Within a few minutes.

Duration of action
2 – 8 hours.

Diet advice
For diabetes insipidus, your physician may advise you to reduce fluid intake at the start of the treatment.

Storage
Keep in a closed container in a dry place away from reach of children.

Missed dose
Take as soon as you remember. Space your subsequent doses at equal intervals throughout the day.

Stopping the drug
Do not stop the drug without consulting your physician; symptoms may recur.

OVERDOSE ACTION

Seek immediate medical advice in all cases. Take emergency action if palpitations, vomiting, seizures, or loss of consciousness occurs.

See Drug poisoning emergency guide (p.574).

SPECIAL PRECAUTIONS

Be sure to tell your physician if:
▼ You have high blood pressure.
▼ You have heart problems.
▼ You have impaired kidney function.
▼ You have had seizures.
▼ You suffer from migraine.
▼ You suffer from asthma.
▼ You are taking other medications.

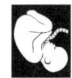

Pregnancy
▼ Safety in pregnancy not established. Discuss with your physician.

Breast feeding
▼ The drug may pass into the breast milk, but at normal doses adverse effects on the baby are unlikely. Discuss with your physician.

Infants and children
▼ Reduced dose necessary.

Over 60
▼ No special problems.

Driving and hazardous work
▼ No known problems.

Alcohol
▼ No known problems.

Surgery and general anesthetics
▼ Your treatment may need to be changed before you have a general anesthetic. Discuss this with your physician or dentist before any surgery.

POSSIBLE ADVERSE EFFECTS

The drug may stimulate contractions in the bowel wall, causing nausea, abdominal cramps, and an increased urge to defecate.

Headache, drowsiness, and confusion may be signs of water retention. Chest pain may be due to angina.

Symptom/effect	Frequency		Discuss with physician		Stop taking drug now	Call physician now
	Common	Rare	Only if severe	In all cases		
Pain at injection site	●			■		
Nausea/abdominal pain	●			■		
Urge to defecate		●		■		
Headache		●		■	▲	▮
Drowsiness/confusion		●		■	▲	▮
Chest pain		●		■	▲	▮

INTERACTIONS

None.

PROLONGED USE

Not usually prescribed for long-term treatment.

VENLAFAXINE

Brand name Effexor
Used in the following combined preparations None

GENERAL INFORMATION

Venlafaxine is a new antidepressant that has a chemical structure unlike any other available antidepressant agent. It possesses the therapeutic properties of both the tricyclics and selective serotonin reuptake inhibitors (SSRIs), without *anticholinergic* adverse effects.

As with other antidepressants, it elevates mood, increases physical activity, and restores interest in every-day activities.

Nausea, somnolence, insomnia, dizziness and restlessness are common adverse effects. Weight loss may occur due to decreased appetite. Venlafaxine can cause an elevation of blood pressure, which should be monitored during the course of treatment.

INFORMATION FOR USERS

Your drug prescription is tailored for you. Do not alter dosage without checking with your physician.

How taken

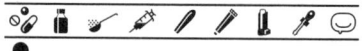

Tablets.

Frequency and timing of doses
2 – 3 x daily, taken with food.

Dosage range
75 – 225mg daily for outpatients; higher doses may be needed for severely depressed patients in hospital.

Onset of effect
Can appear within days, though full antidepressant effect may not be felt for 2 – 4 weeks, or longer.

Duration of action
About 8 – 12 hours. Following prolonged treatment, antidepressant effects may persist for up to 6 weeks.

Diet advice
None.

Storage
Keep in a closed container in a cool, dry place away from reach of children.

Missed dose
Do not make up for a missed dose. Just take your next regularly scheduled dose.

Stopping the drug
Do not stop the drug without consulting your physician, who may supervise a gradual reduction in dosage.

OVERDOSE ACTION

 Seek immediate medical advice in all cases. Take emergency action if slow or irregular pulse, seizures, and/or loss of consciousness occur.

See Drug poisoning emergency guide (p.574).

SPECIAL PRECAUTIONS

Be sure to tell your physician if:
▼ You have had an adverse reaction to any other antidepressants.
▼ You have impaired liver or kidney function.
▼ You have a heart problem or elevated blood pressure.
▼ You have had epileptic seizures.
▼ You have had problems with alcohol or drug misuse/abuse.
▼ You are taking other medications.

 Pregnancy
▼ Safety in pregnancy not established. Discuss with your physician.

 Breast feeding
▼ Not recommended as the effect on breast feeding is unknown. Discuss with your physician.

 Infants and children
▼ Not recommended in patients under 18 years.

 Over 60
▼ Increased likelihood of adverse effects. Reduced dose may therefore be necessary.

 Driving and hazardous work
▼ Avoid such activities until you have learned how the drug affects you; it can cause dizziness, drowsiness, and blurred vision.

 Alcohol
▼ Avoid. Alcohol may increase the sedative effects of this drug.

Surgery and general anesthetics
▼ Venlafaxine may need to be stopped before you have a general anesthetic. Discuss with your physician or dentist before any surgery.

POSSIBLE ADVERSE EFFECTS

The most common adverse effects are weakness, nausea, restlessness, and drowsiness. Some of these effects may wear off within a few days. Restlessness may include nervousness, anxiety, tremor, abnormal dreams, agitation, and confusion.

Symptom/effect	Frequency		Discuss with physician		Stop taking drug now	Call physician now
	Common	Rare	Only if severe	In all cases		
Nausea	●		■			
Restlessness/insomnia	●		■			
Weakness/blurred vision	●		■			
Drowsiness/dizziness	●		■			
Decreased appetite		●		■		
Sexual dysfunction		●		■	▲	
Rash/hives		●		■	▲	■

INTERACTIONS

Monoamine oxidase inhibitors (MAOIs) Venlafaxine may interact with these drugs to produce a dangerous rise in blood pressure; at least 14 days should elapse between stopping MAOIs and starting venlafaxine.

Sedatives All drugs that have a sedative effect are likely to increase the sedative effects of venlafaxine.

Antihypertensives Treatment with venlafaxine may reduce the effectiveness of these drugs.

PROLONGED USE

Because venlafaxine is a new drug, little is known of its long-term effects.

Monitoring Blood pressure should be measured periodically. Blood tests may be advised.

VERAPAMIL

Brand names Isoptin, Apo-Verap, Novo-Veramil, Verelan
Used in the following combined preparations None

GENERAL INFORMATION

Verapamil belongs to a group of drugs known as calcium channel blockers (p.113), which interfere with the conduction signals in the muscles of the heart and blood vessels. Used in treatment of hypertension and arrhythmias, verapamil is also frequently given for angina. It reduces the frequency of angina attacks but does not work quickly enough to help relieve pain while an attack is in progress. Verapamil increases your ability to tolerate physical exertion, and since it

does not affect breathing, it will not worsen asthma.

Because of its effects on the heart, verapamil is also prescribed for certain types of abnormal heart rhythm. For such disorders it can be given by injection as well as in tablet form.

It is not generally prescribed for people with low blood pressure, slow heartbeat, or heart failure, because it may make these conditions worse. The most frequent *side effects* are constipation, dizziness, and nausea.

INFORMATION FOR USERS

Your drug prescription is tailored for you. Do not alter dosage without checking with your physician.

How taken

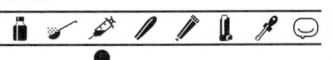

Tablets, slow-release tablets/capsules, injection.

Frequency and timing of doses
1 – 4 x daily. Slow-release preparations and tablets are taken 1 – 2 x daily with food.

Adult dosage range
0 – 480mg daily.

Onset of effect
1 – 2 hours (tablets); 2 – 3 minutes (injection).

Duration of action
6 – 8 hours (tablets). During prolonged treatment some beneficial effects may last for

up to 12 hours. Slow-release preparations act for 12 – 24 hours.

Diet advice
None.

Storage
Keep in a closed container in a cool, dry place away from reach of children.

Missed dose
Take regular tablets as soon as you remember. If your next dose is due within 3 hours, take a single dose now and skip the next. For slow-release preparations, consult your physician.

Stopping the drug
Do not stop the drug without consulting your physician; symptoms may recur.

Exceeding the dose
An occasional unintentional extra dose is unlikely to be a cause for concern. Large over-doses may cause dizziness. Notify your physician.

SPECIAL PRECAUTIONS

Be sure to tell your physician if:
▼ You have impaired liver or kidney function.
▼ You have heart failure.
▼ You are taking other medications.

Pregnancy
▼ Safety in pregnancy not established. Discuss with your physician.

Breast feeding
▼ The drug passes into the breast milk and may affect the baby. Discuss with your physician.

Infants and children
▼ Safety and effectiveness not established.

Over 60
▼ Increased likelihood of adverse effects. Reduced dose may therefore be necessary.

Driving and hazardous work
▼ Avoid such activities until you have learned how the drug affects you; it can cause dizziness.

Alcohol
▼ Avoid. Alcohol may further reduce blood pressure, causing dizziness or other symptoms.

PROLONGED USE

No problems expected.

POSSIBLE ADVERSE EFFECTS

Verapamil has fewer adverse effects than other calcium channel blockers, but it can still cause a variety of minor symptoms, such as nausea, constipation, and headache.

Symptom/effect	Frequency		Discuss with physician		Stop taking drug now	Call physician now
	Common	Rare	Only if severe	In all cases		
Constipation	●		■			
Headache	●		■			
Nausea	●		■			
Ankle swelling	●		■			
Dizziness	●				■	
Flushing		●		■		

INTERACTIONS

Beta blockers When verapamil is taken with these drugs, there is a slight risk of abnormal heartbeats and heart failure. If these drugs are prescribed together, reduced doses are necessary.

Carbamazepine Blood levels of carbamazepine may be raised by verapamil.

Digoxin The effects of this drug may be increased if it is taken with verapamil. The dosage of digoxin usually needs to be reduced.

Antihypertensive drugs Blood pressure may be further lowered when these drugs are taken with verapamil.

WARFARIN

Brand names Coumadin, Warfilone
Used in the following combined preparations None

GENERAL INFORMATION

Warfarin is an anticoagulant used to prevent blood clots, mainly in areas where the blood flow is at its slowest, particularly in the leg and pelvic veins. Such clots can break off and travel through the bloodstream to lodge in the lungs, where they cause pulmonary embolism. Warfarin is also used to reduce the risk of clots forming in the heart in people with atrial fibrillation or after the insertion of artificial heart valves. These clots may travel to the brain, where they could cause a stroke.

A widely used oral anticoagulant, warfarin requires regular monitoring to assure proper maintenance dosage. Because full beneficial effects of warfarin are not felt for 2 to 3 days, a faster-acting anticoagulant such as heparin is often used to complement the effects of warfarin at the start of treatment.

Its most serious adverse effect, as with all anticoagulants, is the risk of excessive bleeding, usually from overdosage.

QUICK REFERENCE

Drug group Anticoagulant drug (p.116)

Overdose danger rating High

Dependence rating Low

Prescription needed Yes

Multi-source suppliers Yes

INFORMATION FOR USERS

Your drug prescription is tailored for you. Do not alter dosage without checking with your physician.

How taken

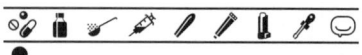

Tablets.

Frequency and timing of doses
Once daily, or less often.

Dosage range
Dose is individualized to produce the desired effect as assessed by blood tests. Maintenance is usually 2.5 – 7.5mg daily.

Onset of effect
Within 24 – 48 hours, with full effect after several days.

Duration of action
3 – 5 days.

Diet advice
None.

Storage
Keep in a closed container in a cool, dry place away from reach of children.

Missed dose
Take as soon as you remember and take the following dose on your original schedule.

Stopping the drug
Do not stop taking the drug without consulting your physician; stopping the drug may lead to worsening of the underlying condition.

OVERDOSE ACTION

Seek immediate medical advice in all cases. Take emergency action if severe bleeding or loss of consciousness occurs.

See Drug poisoning emergency guide (p.574).

SPECIAL PRECAUTIONS

Be sure to tell your physician if:
▼ You have impaired liver or kidney function
▼ You have high blood pressure.
▼ You have peptic ulcers.
▼ You bleed easily.
▼ You are taking other medications.

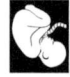

Pregnancy
▼ Not usually prescribed. Given in early pregnancy the drug can cause malformations in the unborn child. Taken near the time of delivery, it may cause the mother to bleed excessively. Discuss with your physician.

Breast feeding
▼ The drug passes into the breast milk and may affect the baby adversely. Discuss with your physician.

Infants and children
▼ Reduced dose necessary.

Over 60
▼ No special problems.

Driving and hazardous work
▼ Use caution. Even minor bumps can cause bad bruises and excessive bleeding.

Alcohol
▼ Avoid. Alcohol may increase or decrease the effects of this drug.

Surgery and general anesthetics
▼ Discuss the possibility of stopping warfarin with your physician or dentist before any surgery.

POSSIBLE ADVERSE EFFECTS

Hemorrhaging is the most common adverse effect with warfarin. Any bruising, dark stools, dark urine, or bleeding should be reported to your physician at once.

Symptom/effect	Frequency		Discuss with physician		Stop taking drug now	Call physician now
	Common	Rare	Only if severe	In all cases		
Loss of appetite	●		■			
Bleeding/bruising	●			■	▲	∎
Nausea/vomiting		●	■			
Abdominal pain/diarrhea		●		■		
Rash		●		■		
Hair loss		●		■		

INTERACTIONS

General note A wide variety of drugs interact with warfarin, either by increasing or decreasing the anticlotting effect. These include barbiturates, oral contraceptives, cimetidine, diuretics, certain laxatives, and certain antibiotics. Consult your pharmacist before purchasing over-the-counter medications.

ASA When taken with warfarin, ASA may significantly prolong or intensify its effect.

PROLONGED USE

No special problems.

Monitoring Blood tests are done regularly to assess anticoagulant effect.

XYLOMETAZOLINE

Brand name Otrivin
Used in the following combined preparation Ophtrivin-A

GENERAL INFORMATION

Xylometazoline is a *sympathomimetic* nasal decongestant that can be bought over the counter to relieve a stuffy nose caused by colds, hay fever, or sinusitis. It works by constricting the small blood vessels in the nose, thereby reducing inflammation and swelling.

Because the effect of xylometazoline may last for up to 10 hours, it needs to be used only two or three times daily.

Using the drug more often than this will increase the likelihood of adverse effects such as headache, palpitations, and drowsiness. Nor should xylometazoline be used for more than a few days at a time; this may cause "rebound" congestion, making nasal stuffiness worse.

INFORMATION FOR USERS

Follow instructions on the label. Call your physician if symptoms worsen.

How taken

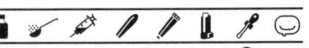

Nose drops, nasal spray.

Frequency and timing of doses
As needed up to 3 x daily.

Dosage range
Adults 2 – 3 drops or 1 – 2 sprays in each nostril (0.1 per cent solution).
Children under 6 years 1 drop or 1 spray in each nostril (0.05 per cent solution).
Children 6 years and over 2 – 3 drops or 1 – 2 sprays in each nostril (0.05 per cent solution).

Onset of effect
Within 10 minutes.

Duration of action
Up to 10 hours.

Diet advice
None.

Storage
Keep in a closed container in a cool, dry place away from reach of children. Protect from light.

Missed dose
No cause for concern. Take only if needed.

Stopping the drug
Can be safely stopped as soon as you no longer need it. Seek medical advice if symptoms persist for more than a few days.

Exceeding the dose
An occasional unintentional extra dose is unlikely to cause problems. Large overdoses or accidental poisoning may cause headaches, insomnia, and drowsiness. Notify your physician.

SPECIAL PRECAUTIONS

Be sure to consult your physician or pharmacist before using this drug if:
▼ You have glaucoma.
▼ You have heart problems.
▼ You have high blood pressure.
▼ You are taking other medications.

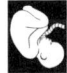

Pregnancy
▼ No evidence of risk if used sparingly. However, overuse can cause a rise in blood pressure that could harm the developing baby. Discuss with your physician.

Breast feeding
▼ The drug passes into the breast milk, but at normal doses adverse effects on the baby are unlikely. Discuss with your physician.

Infants and children
▼ Reduced dose is necessary.

Over 60
▼ Increased likelihood of adverse effects. Reduced dose may therefore be necessary.

Driving and hazardous work
▼ Exercise caution if blurred vision or drowsiness occurs.

Alcohol
▼ No special problems.

POSSIBLE ADVERSE EFFECTS

The adverse effects of xylometazoline are mild and infrequent when the medication is taken for short periods of time. When they do occur it is usually a signal that too much of the drug is being absorbed into the body, and this can be helped by reducing the dose.

Symptom/effect	Frequency		Discuss with physician		Stop taking drug now	Call physician now
	Common	Rare	Only if severe	In all cases		
Headache/lightheadedness		●	●	■		
Nasal discomfort		●	●	■		
Insomnia		●	●	■		
Blurred vision		●	●	■		
Excessive sneezing		●	●	■		
Drowsiness		●	●	■		
Palpitations		●			■	

INTERACTIONS

Sympathomimetic drugs There is an increased risk of adverse effects when drugs such as ephedrine, pseudo-ephedrine, and phenylpropanolamine are taken with xylometazoline.

Monoamine oxidase inhibitors (MAOIs) increase the risk of high blood pressure with xylometazoline, with potentially serious effects. Xylometazoline should not be taken during or within 14 days of MAOI treatment.

Antihypertensive drugs Xylometazoline may reduce the blood pressure-lowering effect of antihypertensive drugs such as methyldopa and guanethidine.

PROLONGED USE

Long-term use of this drug may lead to worsening of the condition. Also, it may lead to a rise in blood pressure. The drug increases the risk of lightheadedness, sleeplessness, and palpitations. Courses of longer than a few days are not recommended.

ZIDOVUDINE (AZT)

Brand names Retrovir, Apo-Zidovudine, Novo-AZT
Used in the following combined preparations None

GENERAL INFORMATION

Zidovudine, formerly known as azidothymidine (AZT), is an antiviral agent used in the treatment of AIDS (acquired immune deficiency syndrome).

Zidovudine is used for people with serious AIDS-related illnesses such as pneumocystis pneumonia and AIDS-virus infection of the brain. It reduces the frequency and severity of infections.

Currently, zidovudine is also being used in certain patients infected with HIV, but who have no symptoms of the disease. There is evidence that zidovudine delays the onset of severe symptoms.

The most common adverse effect of zidovudine is reduction in bone marrow activity, leading to serious blood disorders that may necessitate stopping the drug. For this reason, regular blood checks are performed.

Zidovudine has not provided a lasting cure for AIDS, but it has dramatically improved the prospects for many of those treated.

INFORMATION FOR USERS

Your drug prescription is tailored for you. Do not alter dosage without checking with your physician.

How taken

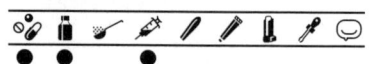

Capsules, syrup, injection.

Frequency and timing of doses
Every 4 hours.

Adult dosage range
0.5 – 1.2g daily (by mouth).

Onset of effect
Within 48 hours.

Duration of action
About 4 hours.

Diet advice
None.

Storage
Keep in a tightly closed container in a cool, dry place away from the reach of children. Protect from light.

Missed dose
Take as soon as you remember. If your next dose is due within 2 hours, take a single dose now and skip the next.

Stopping the drug
Do not stop the drug without consulting your physician; symptoms may recur.

Exceeding the dose
An occasional unintentional extra dose is unlikely to cause problems. Serious adverse effects from large overdoses are unusual, but notify your physician.

POSSIBLE ADVERSE EFFECTS

The most common adverse effect of zidovudine is anemia. Symptoms include pallor, fatigue, and shortness of breath; sore throat and fever are less frequent effects.

Restlessness, insomnia, and fever may occur with too high a dose. These effects may be overcome by reducing the frequency of doses.

Symptom/effect	Frequency		Discuss with physician		Stop taking drug now	Call physician now
	Common	Rare	Only if severe	In all cases		
Nausea/vomiting	●		■			
Headache	●		■			
Pallor/fatigue	●			■		
Breathlessness	●			■		▮
Loss of appetite	●		■			
Insomnia		●		■		
Aching muscles		●		■		
Sore throat/fever		●		■		

INTERACTIONS

General note A wide range of drugs may increase the risk of harmful effects with zidovudine. These include any drug that affects the bone marrow (such as anticancer drugs) and drugs that interfere with the breakdown and elimination of zidovudine (such as probenecid, co-trimoxazole, and acetaminophen). Obtain full information from your physician.

SPECIAL PRECAUTIONS

Be sure to tell your physician if:
▼ You have impaired liver or kidney function.
▼ You have had a previous allergic reaction to zidovudine.
▼ You have a history of blood disorders.
▼ You are taking other medications.

Pregnancy
▼ Safety in pregnancy not established. Discuss with your physician.

Breast feeding
▼ It is not known whether the drug passes into the breast milk. Discuss with your physician.

Infants and children
▼ Not recommended in infants less than 3 months old. Reduced dose necessary for older children.

Over 60
▼ Increased likelihood of adverse effects. Reduced dose may therefore be necessary.

Driving and hazardous work
▼ No special problems.

Alcohol
▼ No known problems.

PROLONGED USE

There is an increased risk of serious blood disorders with prolonged use of zidovudine.

Monitoring Regular blood checks are required during treatment.

ZOPICLONE

Brand name Imovane
Used in the following combined preparations None

GENERAL INFORMATION

Zopiclone is a hypnotic (sleeping drug) used for the short-term treatment of insomnia. Sleep problems can take the form of difficulty in falling asleep, frequent nighttime awakenings and/or early morning awakenings. Hypnotics are used only when non-drug measures prove ineffective.

Unlike benzodiazepine, zopiclone possesses no anti-anxiety properties. Therefore it may be suited for instances of insomnia not accompanied by anxiety, for example international travel or change in nighttime shift work.

Hypnotic medications are intended for occasional use only. *Dependence* can develop after as little as one week of continuous use.

QUICK REFERENCE

Drug group Sleeping drug (p.94)
Overdose danger rating Medium
Dependence rating Medium
Prescription needed Yes
Multi-source suppliers No

INFORMATION FOR USERS

Your drug prescription is tailored for you. Do not alter dosage without checking with your physician.

How taken

Tablets.

Frequency and timing of doses
Once daily at bedtime when required.

Dosage range
3.75 – 7.5mg.

Onset of effect
Within 30 minutes.

Duration of action
4 – 6 hours.

Diet advice
None.

Storage
Keep in a closed container in a cool, dry place away from reach of children. Protect from light.

Missed dose
If you fall asleep without having taken a dose and wake some hours later, do not take the missed dose.

Stopping the drug
If you have been taking the drug continuously for less than 1 week, it can be safely stopped as soon as you feel you no longer need it. However, if you have been taking the drug for longer, consult your physician.

Exceeding the dose
An occasional, unintentional extra dose is unlikely to cause problems. Large overdoses may cause prolonged sleep, drowsiness, lethargy, and poor muscular coordination and reflexes. Notify your physician immediately.

SPECIAL PRECAUTIONS

Be sure to tell your physician if:
▼ You have or have had any problems with alcohol or drug misuse/abuse.
▼ You have myasthenia gravis.
▼ You have had epileptic seizures.
▼ You have impaired liver or kidney function.
▼ You have glaucoma.
▼ You are taking other medications.

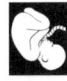

Pregnancy
▼ Not recommended.

Breast feeding
▼ Not recommended.

Infants and children
▼ Not recommended in patients under 18 years.

Over 60
▼ Increased likelihood of adverse effects. Reduced dose may therefore be necessary.

Driving and hazardous work
▼ Avoid such activities until you have learned how the drug affects you; it can cause drowsiness, reduced alertness, and slowed reactions.

Alcohol
▼ Avoid. Alcohol increases the sedative effects of this drug.

POSSIBLE ADVERSE EFFECTS

The most common adverse effects of zopiclone are drowsiness, which normally diminishes after the first few days of treatment, and a bitter taste left in the mouth. Morning drowsiness and/or impaired coordination are signs of excessive dose.

Symptom/effect	Frequency		Discuss with physician		Stop taking drug now	Call physician now
	Common	Rare	Only if severe	In all cases		
Bitter taste	●		■			
Daytime drowsiness/headache	●		■			
Dizziness/weakness	●		■			
Nausea/vomiting/diarrhea	●		■			
Amnesia/confusion		●		■	▲	▌
Rash		●		■	▲	▌

INTERACTIONS

Sedatives All drugs, including alcohol, that have a sedative effect on the central nervous system are likely to increase the sedative effects of zopiclone. Such drugs include other anti-anxiety and sleeping drugs, antihistamines, antidepressants, narcotic analgesics, and antipsychotics.

PROLONGED USE

Intended for occasional use only. Continuous use of zopiclone – or any other sleeping drug – for as little as one week may cause dependence.

A – Z OF VITAMINS AND MINERALS

This section on individual vitamins and minerals gives detailed information on the 24 major chemicals that are required by the body for good health – chemicals that are essential, but which the body is unable to manufacture itself. These include the main vitamins – A, C, D, E, K, H (biotin), and the six B vitamins, together with 12 essential minerals.

The section on Vitamins in Part 3 (p.161) describes in general terms the main sources of the major vitamins and minerals, their roles in the body, and their primary uses, while the following profiles discuss each vitamin and mineral in detail.

The following pages may be particularly useful as a guide for those who think their diet lacks sufficient amounts of a certain vitamin or mineral, and for those with disorders of the digestive tract or liver, who may need extra vitamins. If you think that you may be deficient in a particular vitamin or mineral, refer to the table on page 162 to check that your diet includes good sources of each vitamin and mineral.

The vitamin and mineral profiles

For ease of reference the vitamin and mineral profiles are arranged in alphabetical order and give information under standard headings. These include the different names by which each chemical is known; whether it is available over the counter or by prescription only; its role in body maintenance; specific foods in which it can be found; the recommended daily amounts; how to detect a deficiency; how and when to supplement your diet; and the risks of excessive intake of a particular vitamin or mineral.

Normal daily vitamin and mineral requirements are usually based on recommended nutrient intakes (RNIs) as set out in the Report of the Scientific Review Committee of Health and Welfare Canada in 1990.

HOW TO UNDERSTAND THE PROFILES

Each vitamin and mineral profile contains information arranged under standard headings to enable you to find the information you need.

Other names
Lists the chemical and non-chemical names by which the vitamin or mineral is also known.

Dietary and other natural sources
Tells you how the vitamin or mineral is obtained naturally.

When supplements are helpful
Suggests when a physician may recommend that you take supplements.

Dosage range for treating deficiency
Gives a usual recommended dosage of vitamin and mineral supplements.

Availability
Tells you whether the vitamin or mineral is available over the counter or by prescription only.

Actions on the body
Explains the role played by each vitamin and mineral in maintaining healthy body function.

Normal daily requirement
Gives you a guide to the recommended nutrient intake (RNI) of each vitamin and mineral.

Symptoms of deficiency
Describes the common symptoms of deficiency to watch for.

Symptoms and risks of excessive intake
Describes the risks that may accompany excessive intake of each vitamin or mineral and warning signs to watch for.

VITAMIN K

Other names Menadione, phytonadione, vitamin K₁, vitamin K₂, vitamin K₃

Availability
Vitamin K is available without prescription as a dietary supplement on its own and in several vitamin/mineral preparations. Injectable and oral preparations used to treat bleeding disorders are available only by prescription.

Actions on the body
Vitamin K is necessary for the formation in the liver of several substances that promote the formation of blood clots (blood clotting factors) including prothrombin (clotting factor II).

Dietary and other natural sources
The best dietary sources of vitamin K are green, leafy vegetables and root vegetables, fruits, seeds, cow's milk, and yogurt. Alfalfa is also an excellent source. In adults and children the intestinal bacteria manufacture a large part of the vitamin K that is required.

Normal daily requirement
A recommended nutrient intake (RNI) has not been determined, but an average intake of 300 – 500mcg is considered adequate.

When supplements are helpful
Vitamin K requirements are generally met adequately by dietary intake and by manufacture of the vitamin by bacteria that live in the intestine. Supplements are given routinely to newborn infants since they lack intestinal bacteria capable of producing the vitamin and are therefore more at risk of deficiency. In adults and children, additional vitamin K is usually necessary only on medical advice for deficiency associated with prolonged use of antibiotics or sulfonamide antibacterials that destroy bacteria in the intestine, or when absorption of nutrients from the intestine is impaired. These conditions include liver disease, obstruction of the bile duct, and intestinal disorders causing chronic diarrhea. Vitamin K may also be given to reduce blood loss during labor or after surgery in people who have been taking ASA or oral anticoagulants. Vitamin K also reverses the effect of an overdose of oral anticoagulants.

Symptoms of deficiency
Vitamin K deficiency leads to low levels of prothrombin (hypothrombinemia) and other clotting factors, resulting in delayed blood clotting and a tendency to bleed. This may cause oozing from wounds, nosebleeds, and bleeding from the gums, intestine, urinary tract, and, rarely, in the brain.

Dosage range for treating deficiency
Depends on the individual and on the nature and severity of the disorder.

Symptoms and risks of excessive intake
Excess dietary intake of vitamin K has no known harmful effects. Synthetic vitamin K (menadione) may cause liver damage or rupture of red blood cells (hemolysis) at large doses and in people with glucose-6-phosphate dehydrogenase (G6PD) deficiency. This may lead to reddish-brown urine, jaundice, and, in extreme cases, anemia. Adverse effects are extremely rare with vitamin K preparations taken by mouth.

530

ZINC

Other names Zinc amino acid chelate, zinc chloride, zinc sulfate, zinc gluconate

Availability
Zinc supplements are available without prescription in single-ingredient and vitamin/mineral preparations. Zinc chloride is an injectable preparation given only under medical supervision during intravenous feeding. Zinc is also one ingredient included in a variety of topical formulations used for the treatment of minor skin irritations, dandruff, and fungal infections.

Actions on the body
Zinc plays a vital role in the activities of over 100 enzymes. It is essential for the manufacture of proteins and nucleic acids (the genetic material of cells), and is involved in the function of the hormone insulin in the utilization of carbohydrates. It is necessary for a normal rate of growth, development of the reproductive organs, normal function of the prostate gland, and healing of wounds and burns.

Dietary and other natural sources
Zinc is present in small amounts in a wide variety of foods. Zinc from animal sources is better absorbed than that from plants. Protein-rich foods such as lean meat and seafood are the best sources of the mineral. Whole-grain breads and cereals and dried beans are good dietary sources.

Normal daily requirement
The recommended nutrient intake (RNI) for zinc is: 2mg (birth – 4 months); 3mg (5 – 12 months); 4mg (1 – 3 years); 5mg (4 – 6 years); 7mg (7 – 9 years); 9mg (10 – 12 years); 12mg (males 13 years or older); 9mg (females 10 years or older). In pregnancy and breast feeding, the RNI is increased by 6mg.

When supplements are helpful
A balanced diet containing natural, unprocessed foods usually provides adequate amounts of zinc. Dietary deficiency is rare in Canada and is likely only in people who are generally malnourished such as debilitated elderly people on poor diets. Supplements are usually recommended on medical advice for those with reduced absorption of the mineral due to certain intestinal disorders, such as cystic fibrosis, for those with increased zinc requirements due to sickle cell disease or major burns, and for people with liver damage (for example, as a result of excessive alcohol intake).

Symptoms of deficiency
Deficiency may cause loss of appetite and impair the sense of taste. In children, it may also lead to poor growth and, in severe cases, to delayed sexual development and dwarfism. Severe, prolonged lack of zinc may result in a rare skin disorder involving hair loss, rash, inflamed areas of skin with pustules, and inflammation of the mouth, tongue, eyelids, and around the fingernails.

Dosage range for treating deficiency
Depends on the individual and on the cause and severity of the deficiency. In general, 30 – 50mg daily is sufficient, usually in the form of zinc sulfate.

Symptoms and risks of excessive intake
The risk of harmful effects is low with excess zinc intake. However, prolonged intake of large doses may interfere with the absorption of iron and copper, leading to deficiency of these minerals, and may cause nausea, vomiting, headache, fever, malaise, and abdominal pain.

BIOTIN

Other names Coenzyme R, vitamin H

Availability
Biotin is available without a prescription, alone and in a wide variety of vitamin/mineral preparations.

Actions on the body
Biotin plays a vital role in the activities of several *enzymes*. It is essential for the breakdown of fatty acids and carbohydrates in the diet for conversion into energy, for the manufacture of fats, and for excretion of the products of protein breakdown.

Dietary and other natural sources
Traces of biotin are present in a wide variety of foods. Rich dietary sources include liver, nuts, beans, egg yolks, and cauliflower.

Normal daily requirement
A recommended nutrient intake (RNI) has not been established, but a daily intake of 100 – 200mcg meets the body's requirements.

When supplements are helpful
Most diets provide adequate amounts of biotin, and it is also manufactured in relatively large amounts by bacteria that live in the intestine. The need for supplements is rare. However, deficiency can occur with prolonged excessive consumption of raw egg whites (as in eggnogs), since these contain a protein – avidin – that prevents absorption of the vitamin in the intestine. The risk of deficiency is also increased during long-term treatment with antibiotics or sulfonamide antibacterial drugs, which may destroy the biotin-producing bacteria in the intestine. However, additional biotin is not usually necessary with a balanced diet.

Symptoms of deficiency
Symptoms of biotin deficiency include weakness, tiredness, poor appetite, hair loss, and depression. Severe deficiency may cause eczema of the face and body, and inflammation of the tongue.

Dosage range for treating deficiency
Depends on the individual and on the nature and severity of the disorder. In general, dietary deficiency is treated with 50 – 300mcg of biotin daily. Deficiency of biotin resulting from a genetic defect that limits use of the vitamin by body cells is treated with doses of 5mg given once or twice daily.

Symptoms and risks of excessive intake
None known.

CALCIUM

Other names Calcium amino acid chelate, calcium carbonate, calcium chloride, calcium citrate, calcium glubionate, calcium gluceptate, calcium gluconate, calcium lactate

Availability
Oral forms are available over the counter. Injectable forms of calcium should only be used under a physician's supervision.

Actions on the body
The most abundant mineral in the body, calcium makes up more than 90 per cent of the hard matter in bones and teeth. It is essential for the formation and maintenance of strong bones and healthy teeth, blood clotting, the transmission of nerve impulses, and the contraction of muscle.

Dietary and other natural sources
The main dietary sources of calcium are milk and other dairy products, sardines, dark green, leafy vegetables, dried beans, and nuts. Calcium may also be obtained by drinking water in hard-water areas.

Normal daily requirement
The recommended nutrient intake (RNI) of calcium is: 250mg (birth – 4 months); 400mg (5 months – 1 year); 500mg (1 year); 550mg (2 – 3 years); 600mg (4 – 6 years); 700mg (7 – 9 years); 900mg (males 10 – 12 years); 1,100mg (females 10 – 12 years); 1,100mg (males 13 – 15 years); 1,000mg (females 13 – 15 years); 900mg (males 16 – 18 years); 700mg (females 16 – 49 years); 800mg (males 19 years or older); 800mg (females 50 years or older). Daily requirements of calcium are increased by 500mg during pregnancy and breast feeding.

When supplements are helpful
Unless a sufficient amount of dairy products is consumed – a pint of milk contains approximately 600mg – the diet may not contain enough calcium, and supplements may be needed. Women are especially vulnerable to calcium deficiency because pregnancy and breast feeding demand large amounts of calcium, which may be extracted from the skeleton if intake is not adequate. Osteoporosis (fragile bones) has been linked to dietary calcium deficiency in some cases, but may not be helped by supplements in all women. Hormone replacement therapy may also be necessary (see Drugs for bone disorders, p.134).

Symptoms of deficiency
Symptoms of deficiency do not develop because when dietary intake is inadequate, the body obtains the calcium it needs from the skeleton. Chronic deficiency of calcium may lead to softening of the bones, which in children leads to abnormal bone development (rickets) and in adults to osteoporosis and osteomalacia, causing backache, muscle weakness, bone pain, and fractures of the long bones. Severe deficiency, resulting in low levels of calcium in the blood, causes abnormal stimulation of the nervous system, resulting in cramp-like spasms in the hands, feet, and face.

Dosage range for treating deficiency
Oral supplements of up to 800mg daily may be advised for children with rickets, and up to 1,000mg daily may be given for osteoporosis and osteomalacia. Severe deficiency is treated in the hospital by intravenous injection of calcium. Vitamin D is usually given together with calcium to increase its absorption from the intestine.

Symptoms and risks of excessive intake
Excessive intake of calcium may reduce the amount of iron and zinc absorbed and also may cause constipation and nausea. There is an increased risk of palpitations and, for susceptible persons, of calcium deposits in the kidneys leading to kidney stones and kidney damage. These symptoms do not usually develop unless calcium is taken with large amounts of vitamin D.

CHROMIUM

Other names Chromium amino acid chelate, glucose tolerance factor (GTF)

Availability
Chromium supplements are available without prescription.

Actions on the body
Chromium plays a vital role in the activities of several *enzymes*. It is involved in the breakdown of sugar for conversion into energy and in the manufacture of certain fats. It works together with insulin and is thus essential to the body's ability to use sugar. It may also be involved in the manufacture of proteins in the body.

Dietary and other natural sources
Traces of chromium are present in a wide variety of foods. Meat, dairy products, and whole-grain cereals are good sources of this mineral.

Normal daily requirement
Only minute quantities of chromium are required. A recommended nutrient intake (RNI) has not been determined, but 20 – 40 mcg is an average daily adult intake.

When supplements are helpful
Most people who eat a healthy diet containing plenty of fresh or unprocessed foods receive adequate amounts of chromium. However, supplements may be advised in malnourished children and elderly people (who retain less of the mineral). Diabetics and those with diabetes-like symptoms may also benefit from additional chromium. Supplements may also be helpful if symptoms show chromium deficiency.

Symptoms of deficiency
Although the usual dietary intakes of chromium in Canada are believed to fall within a safe range, it is not possible to estimate requirements. A diet of too many processed foods may contribute to chromium deficiency. Inadequate intake of chromium over a prolonged period may impair the body's ability to use sugar, leading to high blood sugar levels. However, in most cases, this is symptomless. In some people, there may be diabetes-like symptoms such as tiredness, mental confusion, and numbness or tingling of the hands and feet. Deficiency may worsen preexisting diabetes and may depress growth in children. Chromium deficiency may also contribute to the development of atherosclerosis (narrowing of the arteries).

Dosage range for treating deficiency
Severe chromium deficiency may be treated with daily doses of up to 5 – 10mcg.

Symptoms and risks of excessive intake
Chromium is poisonous in excess. Levels that produce symptoms are usually obtained from exposure to industrial waste in drinking water or the atmosphere, not from excessive dietary intake. Symptoms include inflammation of the skin and, if inhaled, damage to the nose. People who are repeatedly exposed to chromium fumes have a greater-than-average risk of developing lung cancer.

COPPER

Other names Copper amino acid chelate, cupric chloride, copper chloride dihydrate, copper gluconate, copper sulfate

Availability
Copper gluconate, copper sulfate, and copper amino acid chelate are available in oral preparations without a prescription. Copper chloride dihydrate is part of a multiple-ingredient preparation for hospital use.

Actions on the body
Copper is an essential constituent of several proteins and *enzymes*. It plays an important role in the development of red blood cells, helps to form the dark pigment that colors hair and skin, and helps the body to use vitamin C. It is essential for the formation of collagen and elastin – proteins found in ligaments, blood vessel walls, and the lungs – and for the proper formation and maintenance of strong bones. It is also required for central nervous system activity.

Dietary and other natural sources
Most unprocessed foods contain copper. Liver, shellfish, nuts, whole-grain cereals, and dried peas and beans are particularly rich sources.

Normal daily requirement
A recommended nutrient intake (RNI) has not been determined, but intakes of 0.3mg for infants, 1mg for children (3 – 10 years), and 2mg for older children and adults appear adequate.

When supplements are helpful
A diet that regularly includes a selection of the foods mentioned above provides sufficient copper. Supplements are rarely necessary. However, physicians may advise additional copper for malnourished children and infants.

Symptoms of deficiency
Copper deficiency is very rare. The major change is anemia due to failure of production of red blood cells, the main symptoms of which are pallor, fatigue, shortness of breath, and palpitations. In severe cases, abnormal bone changes may occur. An inherited copper deficiency disorder called Menke's syndrome (kinky hair disease) results in brain degeneration, retarded growth, sparse and brittle hair, and weak bones.

Dosage range for treating deficiency
This depends on the individual and on the nature and severity of the disorder.

Symptoms and risks of excessive intake
As little as 10 – 15mg of copper taken by mouth can produce toxic effects. Symptoms of poisoning include nausea, vomiting, abdominal pain, diarrhea, and general aches and pains. Large overdoses of copper may cause destruction of red blood cells (hemolytic anemia), and liver and kidney damage. Copper poisoning can occur in people who drink homemade alcohol distilled through copper tubing. In Wilson's disease, an inherited disorder, the patient cannot excrete copper and suffers from long-term copper poisoning. The disease is treated with *chelating agents* such as penicillamine, p.423.

FLUORIDE

Other names Calcium fluoride, sodium fluoride, sodium monofluorophosphate, stannous fluoride

Availability
Sodium fluoride is added to drinking water and is available in single or multiple ingredient preparations. Fluoride mouth rinses and toothpastes containing sodium fluoride, stannous fluoride, or sodium monofluorophosphate are available over the counter. Calcium fluoride is the naturally occurring form of the mineral.

Actions on the body
Fluoride helps to prevent tooth decay and contributes to the strength of the bone. It is thought to work on the teeth by strengthening the mineral composition of the tooth enamel, making it more resistant to attack by acid in the mouth. Fluoride is most effective when taken during the formation of teeth in childhood, since it is then incorporated into the tooth itself. It may also strengthen developing bones.

Dietary and other natural sources
Fluoride has been added to drinking water in many communities, and water is therefore a prime source of this mineral (fluoride levels in water vary from one part of the country to the next, and untreated water also contains a small amount of fluoride). Foods grown or prepared in areas with fluoride-treated water may also contribute fluoride.

Normal daily requirement
A recommended nutrient intake (RNI) has not been established, but intakes of 0.5mg, for infants and children, and 1.5mg, for adults, appear safe.

When supplements are helpful
Most diets typically provide 0.6 – 2.8mg of fluoride per day, depending on whether or not the water supply contains fluoride. Drinking water containing fluoride at 1 part per million (the recommended level is 0.7 – 1.2 ppm) provides an additional 1.4 – 1.8mg per day for adults and 0.4 – 0.8mg per day for young children. If the level is inadequate, children may be given fluoride drops or tablets. The use of supplements is currently under investigation for the prevention and treatment of osteoporosis (fragile bones).

Symptoms of deficiency
Fluoride deficiency increases the risk of tooth decay, especially in children.

Dosage range for treating deficiency
Dietary supplements may be given to children when the concentration of fluoride in the water supply is less than 0.7ppm. When fluoride is present at less than 0.3ppm, the recommended daily dose is: 0.25mg (6 months – 3 years); 0.5mg (3 – 6 years); and 1mg (6 – 16 years). When the fluoride concentration is 0.3 – 0.6ppm, supplements are not recommended for infants under 3, and the recommended daily dose for older children is 0.25mg (3 – 6 years) and 0.5mg (6 – 16 years).

Symptoms and risks of excessive intake
In large quantities, fluoride may cause slow poisoning — called fluorosis. Prolonged intake of water containing more than 2 parts per million may lead to mottled or brown discoloration of the enamel in developing teeth. Very high levels (over 8ppm) may also lead to bone disorders and degenerative changes in the kidneys, liver, adrenal glands, heart, central nervous system, and reproductive organs. Suggestions of a link between fluoridation of the water supply and cancer are without foundation. A child who has taken a number of fluoride tablets may vomit and lose consciousness. Give milk if the child is conscious, and seek immediate medical help.

FOLIC ACID

Other names Folacin, vitamin M, folate sodium, leucovorin calcium (folinate calcium, citrovorum factor), folates

Availability
Folic acid is available without prescription, alone and in a variety of vitamin/mineral preparations. Strengths of 1mg and over are available only by prescription.

Actions on the body
Folic acid is essential for the activities of several *enzymes*. It is required for the manufacture of nucleic acids – the genetic material of cells – and thus for the processes of growth and reproduction. It is vital for the formation of red blood cells by the bone marrow and the development and proper function of the central nervous system.

Dietary and other natural sources
The best sources are green, leafy vegetables, mushrooms, and liver. Root vegetables, oranges, nuts, dried beans and peas, and egg yolks are also rich sources.

Normal daily requirement
The recommended nutrient intake (RNI) for folic acid, as folate, is: 25mcg (birth – 4 months); 40mcg (5 months – 2 years); 50mcg (2 – 3 years); 70mcg (4 – 6 years); 90mcg (7 – 9 years); 120mcg (males 10 – 12 years); 130mcg (females 10 – 12 years); 175mcg (males 13 – 15 years); 170mcg (females 13 – 15 years); 220mcg (males 16 – 24 years); 190mcg (females 16 – 18 years); 180mcg (females 19 – 24 years); 230mcg (males 25 – 74 years); 185mcg (females 25 – 49 years); 195mcg (females 50 – 74 years); 215mcg (males 75 years or older); 200mcg (females 75 years or older). In pregnancy and breast feeding, RNIs are increased by 200mcg and 100mcg, respectively.

When supplements are helpful
A varied diet containing fresh fruit and vegetables usually provides adequate amounts. However, minor deficiencies can be corrected by the addition of one uncooked fruit or vegetable or a glass of fruit juice daily. Supplements are given routinely during pregnancy and breast feeding, and may also be needed in premature or low birth-weight infants and those fed on goat's milk (breast and cow's milk contain adequate amounts of the vitamin). Physicians may recommend additional folic acid for people on hemodialysis, those who have certain blood disorders or psoriasis, or are taking certain drugs that deplete folic acid, including anticonvulsants, antimalarial drugs, estrogen-containing contraceptives, certain analgesics, corticosteroids, and sulfonamide antibacterial drugs. It may also be recommended for certain conditions in which absorption of nutrients from the intestine is impaired, severe alcoholism, and liver disease. In women who are considering becoming pregnant, a supplement of folic acid is recommended in order to prevent neural tube defects. This special supplement is taken two months before conception and during the first three months of pregnancy.

Symptoms of deficiency
Folic acid deficiency leads to abnormally low numbers of red blood cells (anemia). The main symptoms include fatigue, loss of appetite, nausea, diarrhea, and hair loss. Mouth sores are common and the tongue is often sore. Deficiency may also cause poor growth in infants and children.

Dosage range for treating deficiency
Symptoms of anemia are usually treated with 1,000mcg of folic acid daily, together with vitamin B_{12}. Occasionally, doses of up to 1mg daily may be given if absorption of folic acid from the intestine is impaired. A maintenance dose of 100 – 400mcg daily may be substituted after symptoms subside.

Symptoms and risks of excessive intake
Excessive folic acid is not toxic. However, it may worsen the symptoms of a coexisting vitamin B_{12} deficiency and should never be taken to treat anemia without a full medical investigation of the cause of the anemia.

IODINE

Other names Calcium iodide, potassium iodide, sodium iodide

Availability
Iodine supplements are available without prescription as kelp tablets and in several vitamin/mineral preparations. Iodine skin preparations are also available without a prescription for antiseptic use. Treatments for thyroid suppression are available only by prescription.

Actions on the body
Iodine is essential for the formation of thyroid hormone which regulates the body's energy production, promotes growth and development, and helps burn excess fat.

Dietary and other natural sources
Seafood is the best source of iodine, but bread and dairy products are the main sources of this mineral in most diets. Iodized table salt is also a major source. Most diets contain adequate amounts of iodine, and use of iodized table salt can usually make up for any lack. Iodine may be inhaled from the atmosphere in coastal regions or from pollution produced by automobile exhaust fumes.

Normal daily requirement
The recommended nutrient intake (RNI) of iodine is: 30mcg (birth – 4 months); 40mcg (4 – 12 months); 55mcg (1 year); 65mcg (2 – 3 years); 85mcg (4 – 6 years); 110mcg (males 7 – 9 years); 95mcg (females 7 – 9 years); 125mcg (males 10 – 12 years); 110mcg (females 10 – 12 years); 160mcg (males and females 13 years or older). In pregnancy and breast feeding, the RNIs are increased by 25mcg and 50mcg, respectively.

When supplements are helpful
Supplements are rarely necessary except on medical advice. However, excessive intake of raw cabbage or nuts may reduce uptake of iodine into the thyroid gland and lead to deficiency if iodine intake is otherwise low. Kelp supplements may be helpful.

People exposed to radiation from radioactive iodine released into the environment may be given sodium iodide at 10 – 100mg per day (adults and children over 1 year) or 15mg per day (children under 1 year) for 3 – 10 days.

Symptoms of deficiency
Deficiency may result in a goiter (enlargement of the thyroid gland) and hypothyroidism (deficiency of thyroid hormone). Symptoms of hypothyroidism include tiredness, physical and mental slowness, weight gain, facial puffiness, and constipation. Babies born to iodine-deficient women are lethargic and difficult to feed. Left untreated, they develop cretinism, with poor growth and mental retardation.

Dosage range for treating deficiency
Deficiency may be treated with doses of 150mcg of iodine daily, often as iodized table salt (4g or 1 teaspoon daily).

Symptoms and risks of excessive intake
Iodine that occurs naturally in food is non-toxic, but iodine taken as a drug can be harmful in excess. Large overdoses of iodine may cause abdominal pain, vomiting, bloody diarrhea, and swelling of the thyroid and salivary glands. Prolonged use of 6mg or more daily may suppress the activity of the thyroid gland.

IRON

Other names Ferrous fumarate, ferrous gluconate, ferrous sulfate, iron sorbitol

Availability
Ferrous sulfate, ferrous fumarate, and ferrous gluconate are available without prescription, alone and in vitamin/mineral preparations. Iron sorbitol, an injectable product, is used only under a physician's direction.

Actions on the body
Iron has an important role in the formation of red blood cells and is a vital component of the oxygen-carrying pigment hemoglobin. It is involved in the formation of myoglobin, a pigment that stores oxygen in muscles for use during exercise. It is also an essential component of several *enzymes*, and is involved in the uptake of oxygen by the cells and the conversion of blood sugar to energy.

Dietary and other natural sources
Liver is the best dietary source of iron. Meat (especially organ meat), eggs, chicken, fish, green, leafy vegetables, dried fruit, enriched or whole-grain cereals, breads or pastas, nuts, and dried beans are also rich sources. Iron in meat, eggs, chicken and fish is better absorbed than that in vegetables.

Normal daily requirement
The recommended nutrient intake (RNI) of iron is: 0.3mg (birth – 4 months); 7mg (5 – 12 months); 6mg (1 – 3 years); 8mg (4 – 12 years); 10mg (males 13 – 18 years); 13mg (females 13 – 15 years); 12mg (females 16 – 18 years); 9mg (males 19 years or older); 13mg (females 19 – 49 years); 8mg (females 50 years or older). In pregnancy, the RNI is increased by 5mg and 10mg in the second and third trimesters, respectively.

When supplements are helpful
Most average diets supply adequate amounts of iron. However, larger amounts are necessary during pregnancy. Supplements are therefore given throughout pregnancy and for two to three months after childbirth to maintain and replenish adequate iron stores in the mother. Premature babies may be prescribed supplements soon after birth (breast-fed) or after 6 months of age (formula-fed) to prevent deficiency. Supplements may be helpful in young vegetarian women with heavy menstrual periods, and people with chronic blood loss due to disease.

Symptoms of deficiency
Iron deficiency causes *anemia*, symptoms of which are pallor, fatigue, shortness of breath, and palpitations. Apathy, irritability, and lowered resistance of the body to infection may also occur.

Dosage range for treating deficiency
Depends on the individual and the nature and severity of the condition. In adults, iron deficiency anemia is usually treated with 50 – 100mg of iron two or three times daily. In children the dose is reduced according to age and weight. Iron supplements are prescribed throughout pregnancy.

Symptoms and risks of excessive intake
Iron poisoning is extremely dangerous. Abdominal pain, nausea, and vomiting may be followed by fever, abdominal bloating, dehydration, and dangerously lowered blood pressure. Immediate medical attention is vital.

Excessive intake, especially when taken with large amounts of vitamin C, may cause iron to accumulate in organs, causing congestive heart failure, cirrhosis of the liver, and diabetes mellitus.

MAGNESIUM

Other names Magnesium amino acid chelate, magnesium gluconate, magnesium oxide, magnesium oxide dolomite, magnesium sulfate

Availability
Magnesium is available without prescription in a variety of vitamin/mineral preparations. Magnesium is also an ingredient of numerous over-the-counter antacid and laxative preparations, but it is not absorbed well from these sources.

Actions on the body
About 70 per cent of the body's magnesium is found in bones and teeth. It is essential for the formation of healthy bones and teeth, the transmission of nerve impulses, and the contraction of muscles. It activates several *enzymes*, and is important in the conversion of carbohydrates, fats, and proteins into energy. It also helps to regulate body temperature.

Dietary and other natural sources
The best dietary sources of magnesium are leafy, green vegetables. Nuts, whole grains, soybeans, and seafood are also rich in magnesium. Drinking water in hard-water areas may also be a source of this mineral.

Normal daily requirement
The recommended daily intake (RNI) of magnesium is: 20mg (birth – 4 months); 32mg (5 – 12 months); 40mg (1 year); 50mg (2 – 3 years); 65mg (4 – 6 years); 100mg (7 – 9 years); 130mg (males 10 – 12 years); 135mg (females 10 – 12 years); 185mg (males 13 – 15 years); 180mg (females 13 – 15 years); 230mg (males 16 – 18 years); 200mg (females 16 – 49 years); 240mg (males 19 – 24 years); 250mg (males 25 – 74 years); 270mg (females 50 years or older); 230mg (males 75 years or older). In pregnancy, the RNI is increased by 15mg in the first trimester, and 45mg in the second and third trimesters. In breast feeding, the RNI is increased by 65mg.

When supplements are helpful
A varied diet provides adequate amounts of magnesium, particularly in hard-water areas. Supplements are usually necessary only on medical advice for magnesium deficiency associated with certain conditions in which absorption from the intestine is impaired, which occurs in repeated vomiting or diarrhea, advanced kidney disease, severe alcoholism, or prolonged treatment with certain diuretic drugs.
Estrogens and estrogen-containing oral contraceptives may reduce blood magnesium levels, but women on adequate diets do not need supplements.

Symptoms of deficiency
Symptoms include anxiety, restlessness, tremors, confusion, palpitations, depression, irritability, and disorientation. Severe magnesium deficiency causes marked overstimulation of the nervous system, resulting in cramp-like spasms of the hands and feet and seizures. Inadequate intake may be a possible factor in the development of coronary heart disease, and may also lead to calcium deposits in the kidneys, resulting in kidney stones.

Dosage range for treating deficiency
This depends on the individual and on the nature and severity of the disorder. Severe deficiency is usually treated in the hospital by injection of magnesium sulfate.

Symptoms and risks of excessive intake
Magnesium toxicity (hypermagnesemia) is rare but can occur in people with impaired kidney function after prolonged intake of large amounts (more than 3,000mg daily) found in antacid or laxative preparations. Symptoms include nausea, vomiting, dizziness (due to a drop in blood pressure), and muscle weakness. Very large increases in magnesium in the blood may cause fatal respiratory failure or heart arrest.

NIACIN

Other names Niacinamide, nicotinamide, nicotinic acid, vitamin B_3, xanthinol niacinate

Availability
Niacin is available without prescription in a wide variety of single-ingredient and vitamin/mineral preparations. However, high doses of niacin should be taken only under a physician's direction.

Actions on the body
Niacin plays a vital role in the activities of many *enzymes*. It is important in the production of energy from carbohydrates, fats, and proteins, and in the manufacture of fats. Niacin is essential for the proper functioning of the nervous system, for a healthy skin and digestive system, and for the manufacture of sex hormones (estrogens, progesterone, and testosterone).

Dietary and other natural sources
Liver, lean meat, poultry, fish, whole-grain products, nuts, and dried beans are the best dietary sources of niacin.

Normal daily requirement
The recommended nutrient intake (RNI) for niacin, in niacin equivalents (1 niacin equivalent [NE] equals 1mg of niacin or 60mg of tryptophan) is: 4NE (birth – 4 months); 7NE (5 – 12 months); 8NE (1 year); 9NE (2 – 3 years); 13NE (4 – 6 years); 16NE (males 7 – 9 years); 14NE (females 7 – 9 years); 18NE (males 10 – 12 years); 16NE (females 10 – 12 years); 20NE (males 13 – 15 years); 16NE (females 13 – 15 years); 23NE (males 16 – 18 years); 15NE (females 16 – 24 years); 22NE (males 19 –24 years); 19NE (males 25 – 49 years); 14NE (females 25 years or older); 16NE (males 50 – 74 years); 14NE (males 75 years or older). In pregnancy, the RNI is increased by 1NE in the first trimester, and 2NE in the second and third trimesters. In breast feeding, the RNI is increased by 3NE.

When supplements are helpful
Most North American diets provide adequate amounts of niacin, and dietary deficiency is rare, except in areas where corn is the staple diet. Supplements are required for niacin deficiency associated with bowel disorders in which absorption from the intestine is impaired, and with liver disease and severe alcoholism. Niacin (nicotinic acid) in doses of 1.5 to 9g daily has been used to lower the levels of certain fats in the blood, including cholesterol, and is used in the treatment of hyperlipidemia (raised blood fat levels). There is no convincing medical evidence that niacin helps psychiatric disorders (except those associated with pellagra) or that it has a beneficial effect in peripheral vascular disease.

Symptoms of deficiency
Severe niacin deficiency causes pellagra (literally, rough skin). Symptoms include sore, red, cracked skin in areas exposed to sun, friction or pressure, inflammation of the mouth and tongue, abdominal pain and distension, nausea, diarrhea, and mental disturbances such as the anxiety, depression, and dementia that accompany pellagra.

Dosage range for treating deficiency
For severe pellagra, adults are usually treated with 100 – 500mg niacinamide daily by mouth, and children are usually given 100 – 300mg daily. For less severe deficiency, doses of 25 – 50mg are given.

Symptoms and risks of excessive intake
At doses of over 50mg, niacin may cause transient itching, flushing, tingling, or headache. However, niacinamide (nicotinamide) is free of these effects. Large doses of niacin may cause nausea and may aggravate a peptic ulcer. This can be prevented by taking the drug on a full stomach. At doses of over 2g daily (which have been used to treat hyperlipidemia), there is a risk of gout, liver damage, and high blood sugar levels, which lead to nervousness and extreme thirst.

PANTOTHENIC ACID

Other names Calcium pantothenate, panthenol, vitamin B_5

Availability
Pantothenic acid, calcium pantothenate, and panthenol are available without prescription in a variety of vitamin/mineral preparations. Pantothenic acid (as the calcium or sodium salt) is available alone in oral or intravenous preparations containing 5 to 100mg of the vitamin.

Actions on the body
Pantothenic acid plays a vital role in the activities of many *enzymes*. It is essential for the production of energy from sugars and fats, for the manufacture of fats, corticosteroids and sex hormones, for the utilization of other vitamins, for the proper function of the nervous system and the adrenal glands, and for normal growth and development.

Dietary and other natural sources
Pantothenic acid is present in almost all vegetables, cereals, and animal foods. Liver, kidney, heart, fish, and egg yolks are good dietary sources. Brewer's yeast, wheat germ, and royal jelly (the substance on which queen bees feed) are also rich in the vitamin.

Normal daily requirement
A recommended nutrient intake (RNI) for pantothenic acid has not been established, but daily intakes of 2mg for infants and 5 – 7mg for adults appear adequate.

When supplements are helpful
Most diets provide adequate amounts of pantothenic acid. Any deficiency is likely to occur together with other B vitamin deficiency diseases such as pellagra (see niacin), beriberi (see thiamine), or in alcoholism, and is treated with B complex supplements. There is no firm evidence that large doses help, as some believe, in the prevention of graying hair, nerve disorders in diabetes, or psychiatric illness. As with other B vitamins, the need for pantothenic acid is increased by injury, surgery, severe illness, and psychological stress.

Symptoms of deficiency
Pantothenic acid deficiency may cause low blood sugar levels, duodenal ulcers, respiratory infections, and general ill-health. Symptoms include fatigue, headache, nausea, abdominal pain, numbness and tingling in the limbs, muscle cramps, faintness, confusion, and lack of coordination.

Dosage range for treating deficiency
Usually 5 – 20mg per day.

Symptoms and risks of excessive intake
In tests, doses of 1,000mg or more of pantothenic acid have not caused toxic effects. The risk of toxicity is considered to be very low, since pantothenic acid is a water-soluble vitamin that does not accumulate in the tissues. Any excess is eliminated rapidly in the urine. Very high intakes of 10 – 20g can cause diarrhea.

POTASSIUM

Other names Potassium acetate, potassium amino acid, potassium chloride, potassium citrate, potassium gluconate

Availability
Potassium chloride, potassium gluconate, potassium phosphate, and potassium chloride-potassium bicarbonate complex are available without a prescription in a number of preparations. Potassium chloride and potassium gluconate are also available in sodium-free salt.

Actions on the body
Potassium works together with sodium in the control of the body's water balance, conduction of nerve impulses, contraction of muscle, and maintenance of a normal heart rhythm. It is essential for storage of carbohydrate and its breakdown for energy.

Dietary and other natural sources
The best dietary sources of potassium are green, leafy vegetables, oranges, potatoes, and bananas. Lean meat, beans, and milk are also rich in the mineral. Many methods of food processing may lower potassium levels found in fresh food.

Normal daily requirement
Recommended nutrient intake (RNI) for potassium has not been established, but intakes of about 800mg per day, for infants and children up to 3 years of age, and about 3g, for older children and adults, appear adequate.

When supplements are helpful
Most diets contain adequate amounts of potassium, and supplements are rarely required in normal circumstances. However, people who drink large amounts of coffee or alcohol or eat lots of salty foods may become marginally deficient. Diabetics may also be deficient in potassium. Supplements are usually advised only when symptoms suggest deficiency or in people at particular risk. Prolonged treatment with certain diuretics is the most common cause of deficiency; long-term use of corticosteroids may also deplete the body's potassium. Kidney disease, laxative abuse, prolonged vomiting, or diarrhea may also deplete potassium.

Symptoms of deficiency
Early symptoms of potassium deficiency may include muscle weakness, fatigue, dizziness, and mental confusion. Impairment of nerve and muscle function may progress to cause disturbances of the heart rhythm, paralysis of the skeletal muscles, and paralysis of the bowel, leading to constipation.

Dosage range for treating deficiency
Depends on the preparation, the individual, and the cause and severity of deficiency. In general, daily doses equivalent to 4 – 6g of potassium chloride are given to prevent deficiency (for example, in people treated with diuretics that deplete potassium). Doses equivalent to 3 – 7.2g of potassium chloride daily are used to treat deficiency.

Symptoms and risks of excessive intake
Blood potassium levels are normally regulated by the kidneys, and any excess is rapidly eliminated in the urine. Doses of over 18g may cause serious disturbances of the heart rhythm and muscular paralysis. In people with impaired kidney function, excess potassium may accumulate, increasing the risk of potassium poisoning. People on hemodialysis treatment should stay on a carefully controlled low-potassium diet.

PYRIDOXINE

Other names Pyridoxine hydrochloride, vitamin B_6

Availability
Pyridoxine and pyridoxine hydrochloride are available without prescription in a variety of single-ingredient and vitamin/mineral preparations.

Actions on the body
Pyridoxine plays a vital role in the activities of many *enzymes*. It is essential for the breakdown and utilization of proteins, carbohydrates, and fats from food for the release of carbohydrates stored in the liver and muscles for energy; and for the manufacture of niacin (vitamin B_3). It is needed for the production of red blood cells and *antibodies*, for healthy skin and for healthy digestion. It is also important for normal function of the central nervous system and the action of several hormones.

Dietary and other natural sources
Liver, chicken, fish, whole-grain cereals, wheat germ, and eggs are rich in this vitamin. Bananas, avocados, and potatoes are also good sources.

Normal daily requirement
Recommended nutrient intake (RNI) for pyridoxine has not been established, but intakes of 0.9 to 1.8mg per day for males, and 0.6 to 1.1mg per day for females, appear adequate.

When supplements are helpful
Most balanced diets contain adequate amounts of pyridoxine, and it is also manufactured in small amounts by bacteria that live in the intestine. However, breast-fed infants may require additional pyridoxine. Elderly adults may also require supplements. Supplements can be given on medical advice together with other B vitamins to people with certain conditions in which absorption from the intestine is impaired. Supplements may also be recommended to prevent or treat deficiency caused by alcoholism and treatment with drugs such as penicillamine and hydralazine. Supplements may also help relieve depression caused by a deficiency of the vitamin in women taking estrogen-containing oral contraceptives, and may help prevent morning sickness in pregnancy. Supplements may help relieve premenstrual depression, irritability, and breast tenderness.

Symptoms of deficiency
Pyridoxine deficiency may cause weakness, irritability, nervousness, depression, skin disorders, inflammation of the mouth and tongue, and cracked lips. In adults, it may cause anemia (abnormally low levels of red blood cells). Seizures may occur in infants.

Dosage range for treating deficiency
In cases of dietary deficiency, the dosage is 10 – 20mg daily for three weeks. Follow-up treatment is recommended daily for several weeks with an oral multivitamin preparation containing 2 – 5mg of pyridoxine. Deficiency resulting from genetic defects that prevent use of the vitamin is treated with doses of 2 – 15mg daily in infants and 10 – 250mg daily in adults and children. Daily doses of 50mg given with other B vitamins from day 10 of a menstrual cycle to day 3 of the following cycle may help relieve premenstrual syndrome.

Symptoms and risks of excessive intake
Daily doses of over 500mg taken over a prolonged period may damage the nervous system, resulting in unsteadiness, numbness, and awkwardness of the hands.

RIBOFLAVIN

Other names Vitamin B_2, vitamin G

Availability
Riboflavin is available without a prescription, alone and in a wide variety of vitamin/mineral preparations.

Actions on the body
Riboflavin plays a vital role in the activities of several *enzymes*. It is involved in the breakdown and utilization of carbohydrates, fats, and proteins and in the production of energy in cells using oxygen. It is needed for utilization of other B vitamins and for production of hormones by the adrenal glands.

Dietary and other natural sources
Riboflavin is found in most foods. Good dietary sources are liver, milk, cheese, eggs, leafy green vegetables, whole grains, and beans. Brewer's yeast is also a rich source of the vitamin.

Normal daily requirement
The recommended nutrient intake (RNI) of riboflavin is: 0.3mg (birth – 4 months); 0.5mg (5 – 12 months); 0.6mg (1 year); 0.7mg (2 – 3 years); 0.9mg (4 – 6 years); 1.1mg (males 7 – 9 years); 1mg (females 7 – 9 years); 1.3mg (males 10 – 12 years); 1.1mg (females 10 - 24 years); 1.4mg (males 13 – 15 years); 1.6mg (males 16 – 18 years); 1.5mg (males 19 – 24 years); 1.4mg (males 25 – 49 years); 1.2mg (males 50 – 74 years); 1mg (females 25 years or older; males 75 years or older). In pregnancy, the RNI is increased by 0.1mg in the first trimester, and by 0.3mg in the second and third trimesters. In breast feeding, the RNI is increased by 0.4mg.

When supplements are helpful
A balanced diet generally provides adequate amounts of riboflavin. Supplements may be beneficial in people on very low calorie diets. Requirements may also be increased by prolonged use of phenothiazine antipsychotics, tricyclic antidepressants, and estrogen-containing oral contraceptives. Supplements are required for riboflavin deficiency associated with certain conditions in which absorption of nutrients from the intestine is impaired. Riboflavin deficiency is also common among alcoholics. As with other B vitamins, the need for riboflavin is increased by injury, surgery, severe illness, and psychological stress. In all cases, treatment with supplements works best in a complete B-complex formulation.

Symptoms of deficiency
Prolonged deficiency may lead to chapped lips, cracks, and sores in the corners of the mouth, and a red, sore tongue. The eyes may itch, burn, and may become unusually sensitive to light. Twitching of the eyelids and blurred vision may also occur.

Dosage range for treating deficiency
Usually treated with 5 – 25mg daily in combination with other B vitamins.

Symptoms and risks of excessive intake
Excessive intake does not appear to have harmful effects. However, prolonged use of large doses of riboflavin alone may deplete other B vitamins; it is therefore best taken with other B vitamins.

SELENIUM

Other names Selenious acid, sodium selenite, selenium sulfide, selenium yeast

Availability
Selenium is available without prescription for oral administration. It is also available for addition to intravenous solutions given for total parenteral nutrition. Selenium sulfide is the active ingredient of several antidandruff shampoos.

Actions on the body
Selenium works in association with vitamin E to preserve elasticity in the tissues, thus slowing down the processes of aging. It also increases endurance by improving the supply of oxygen to the heart muscle. It is necessary for the formation of a group of substances called prostaglandins, which give protection against high blood pressure, help to prevent the abnormal blood clotting in arteries that may lead to a stroke or heart attack, and stimulate contractions of the uterus in labor.

Dietary and other natural sources
Meat, fish, whole grains, and dairy products are good dietary sources. The amount of selenium found in vegetables depends on the content of the mineral in the soil where they were grown.

Normal daily requirement
A recommended nutrient intake (RNI) has not been established, but the average intake is around 60 – 75mcg.

When supplements are helpful
Most normal diets provide adequate amounts of selenium, and supplements are, therefore, rarely necessary. At present, there is no conclusive medical evidence in support of some claims that selenium may provide protection against cancer or that it prolongs life. A daily intake of more than 150mcg is not recommended except on the advice of a physician.

Symptoms of deficiency
Long-term lack of selenium may result in loss of stamina and reduced elasticity of tissues, leading to premature aging. Severe deficiency may cause muscle pain and tenderness, and can eventually lead to fatal heart disease in children in areas where selenium levels in the diet are very low.

Dosage range for treating deficiency
Depends on the individual and on the nature and severity of the disorder. Severe selenium deficiency may be treated with doses of up to 200mcg daily.

Symptoms and risks of excessive intake
Selenium is the most poisonous of dietary minerals. Excessive intake may cause baldness, loss of nails and teeth, fatigue, nausea, vomiting, and sour-milk breath. A massive overdose of this mineral may be fatal.

SODIUM

Other names Sodium acetate, sodium bicarbonate, sodium chloride, sodium phosphate

Availability
Sodium is widely available in the form of common table salt (sodium chloride). Sodium acetate is used in intravenous feeding. Sodium phosphate is a laxative.

Actions on the body
Sodium works with potassium in controlling the water balance in the body, transmission of nerve impulses, contraction of muscle, and maintenance of a normal heart rhythm.

Dietary and other natural sources
Sodium is present in almost all foods as a natural ingredient, or as an extra ingredient added during processing. The main sources are table salt, processed foods, cheese, breads and cereals, and smoked, pickled, or cured meats and fish. High concentrations are found in pickles and snack foods, including potato chips and olives. Sodium is also present in water that has been treated with water softeners.

Normal daily requirement
A recommended nutrient intake (RNI) has not been established, but a daily intake of 1 – 3g appears adequate.

When supplements are helpful
Most North American diets contain amounts of sodium far exceeding requirements. The average consumption of sodium is 3 – 7g daily. The need for supplementation is rare in temperate climates, even with low-salt diets. In tropical climates, however, sodium supplements may help prevent heat stroke from occurring as a result of sodium loss caused by excessive perspiration during heavy work. Supplements may be given on medical advice to replace salt loss due to prolonged diarrhea and vomiting, particularly in infants, and to prevent or treat deficiency due to certain kidney disorders, cystic fibrosis, adrenal gland insufficiency, use of diuretics, or severe bleeding.

Symptoms of deficiency
Dietary sodium deficiency is rare. Most deficiency usually results from conditions that increase loss of sodium from the body, such as diarrhea, vomiting, and excessive perspiration. Early symptoms include lethargy, muscle cramps, and dizziness. In severe cases, there may be a marked drop in blood pressure leading to confusion, fainting, and palpitations.

Dosage range for treating deficiency
Depends on the individual and on the nature and severity of symptoms. In extreme cases, intravenous sodium chloride may be required.

Symptoms and risks of excessive intake
Excessive sodium intake is thought to contribute to the development of high blood pressure. In people whose blood pressure is already raised, it may increase the risk of heart disease, stroke, and kidney damage. Other adverse effects include abnormal fluid retention, leading to dizziness and swelling of the legs and face. Large overdoses, even of table salt, may cause seizures or coma and can be fatal.

THIAMINE

Other names Thiamine hydrochloride, thiamine mononitrate, vitamin B_1

Availability
Thiamine is available without prescription alone and in a variety of vitamin/mineral preparations.

Actions on the body
Thiamine plays a vital role in the activities of many *enzymes*. It is essential for the breakdown and utilization of carbohydrates. It is important for a healthy nervous system, healthy muscles, and normal heart function.

Dietary and other natural sources
Thiamine is present in all unrefined food. Good dietary sources include pork, whole-grain or enriched cereals and breads, brown rice, pasta, liver, kidneys, meat, fish, beans, nuts, eggs, and most vegetables. Wheat germ and bran are excellent sources.

Normal daily requirement
The recommended nutrient intake (RNI) for thiamine is: 0.3mg (birth – 4 months); 0.4mg (5 – 12 months); 0.5mg (1 year); 0.6mg (2 – 3 years); 0.7mg (4 – 6 years); 0.9mg (males 7 – 9 years); 0.8mg (females 7 – 9 years); 1mg (males 10 – 12 years); 0.9mg (females 10 – 15 years); 1.1mg (males 13 – 15 years); 1.3mg (males 16 – 18 years); 0.8mg (females 16 – 18 years); 1.2mg (males 19 – 24 years); 0.8mg (females 19 years or older); 1.1mg (males 25 – 49 years); 0.9mg (males 50 – 74 years); 0.8mg (males 75 years or older). In pregnancy and breast feeding, the RNIs are increased by 0.1mg and 0.2mg, respectively.

When supplements are helpful
A balanced diet generally provides adequate amounts of thiamine. However, supplements may be helpful in elderly people and in those with high energy requirements caused, for example, by overactivity of the thyroid or heavy manual work. As with other B vitamins, requirements of thiamine are increased during severe illness, surgery, serious injury, and prolonged psychological stress. Additional thiamine is usually necessary on medical advice for deficiency associated with conditions in which absorption of nutrients from the intestine is impaired, and for prolonged liver disease or severe alcoholism.

Symptoms of deficiency
Mild deficiency may cause fatigue, irritability, loss of appetite, and disturbed sleep. Severe deficiency may cause confusion, loss of memory, depression, abdominal pain, constipation, and beriberi, a disorder that affects the nerves, brain, and heart. Symptoms of beriberi include tingling or burning sensations in the legs, cramps and tenderness in the calf muscles, incoordination, palpitations, mental disturbances, and heart failure. In infants, beriberi can cause seizures, vomiting, and heart failure. In chronic alcoholics with malnutrition, vitamin B_1 deficiency may lead to a characteristic deterioration of central nervous system function known as Wernicke's syndrome, which results eventually in paralysis of the eye muscles, severe memory loss, and dementia, for which urgent treatment is needed.

Dosage range for treating deficiency
Depends on the individual and on the nature and severity of the disorder. The usual adult dose to treat deficiency is 5 to 30mg daily given as a single dose or in three divided doses. Injections of the vitamin are sometimes given in severe deficiency or when symptoms have appeared suddenly.

Symptoms and risks of excessive intake
The risk of adverse effects is very low, since any excess is rapidly eliminated in the urine. However, prolonged use of large doses of thiamine may deplete other B vitamins; it should therefore be taken in a vitamin B complex formulation. Allergic reactions have occurred in rare cases after intravenous injection of large doses of this vitamin.

VITAMIN A

Other names Acitretin, beta-carotene, carotenoids, etretinate, retinoids, retinoic acid, retinol, retinol palmitate, isotretinoin, tretinoin

Availability
Retinol, retinol palmitate, and beta-carotene are available without prescription in various single-ingredient and vitamin/mineral preparations. Acitretin, etretinate, tretinoin, and isotretinoin are related to vitamin A and are available only by prescription for skin disorders such as acne and psoriasis.

Actions on the body
Vitamin A is essential for normal growth and strong bones and teeth in children. It is necessary for normal vision and healthy cell structure. It helps keep skin healthy and protects the linings of the mouth, nose, throat, lungs, and digestive and urinary tracts against infection. Vitamin A is also necessary for fertility in both sexes.

Dietary and other natural sources
Liver, fish liver oils, eggs, dairy products, orange and yellow vegetables and fruits (carrots, squash, apricots, and peaches), and dark green, leafy vegetables (spinach, kale, and broccoli) are good dietary sources. Vitamin A is also added to margarine.

Normal daily requirement
The recommended nutrient intake (RNI) for vitamin A in retinol equivalents (RE) is: 400RE (birth – 3 years); 500RE (4 – 6 years); 700RE (7 – 9 years); 800RE (males 10 – 12 years, females 10 years or older); 900RE (males 13 – 15 years); 1,000RE (males 16 years or older). In breast feeding, the RNI is increased by 400RE.

When supplements are helpful
Most diets provide adequate amounts of vitamin A. However, diets exceptionally low in fat or protein can lead to deficiency. Supplements may be necessary for people with certain intestinal disorders, cystic fibrosis, obstruction of the bile ducts, diabetes mellitus, and overactivity of the thyroid gland, and for people on long-term treatment with lipid-lowering drugs, since these reduce absorption of the vitamin from the intestine.

Symptoms of deficiency
Night blindness (difficulty in seeing in dim light) is the earliest symptom of deficiency. Other symptoms include dry, rough skin, loss of appetite, and diarrhea. Resistance to infection is decreased. Eyes may become dry and inflamed. Severe deficiency may lead to corneal ulcers and weak bones and teeth.

Dosage range for treating deficiency
Severe deficiency in adults and children over age 8 is treated with 1,000 – 9,000RE (5,000 – 30,000 IU) until the amount of vitamin in the blood returns to normal.

Symptoms and risks of excessive intake
Prolonged excessive intake of 2,000RE (10,000 IU) in children and 7,500RE (25,000 IU) in adults can cause headache, nausea, diarrhea, dry, itchy skin, hair loss, and loss of appetite. Fatigue and irregular menstruation are also common. In extreme cases, bone pain and enlargement of the liver and spleen may occur. High doses of beta-carotene may turn the skin orange but are not dangerous. Excessive intake of vitamin A in pregnancy may lead to birth defects.

VITAMIN B12

Other names Cobalamin, cobalamins, cyanocobalamin, hydroxycobalamin

Availability
Vitamin B$_{12}$ is available without prescription in a wide variety of preparations. Hydroxycobalamin is given only by injection under medical supervision.

Actions on the body
Vitamin B$_{12}$ plays a vital role in the activities of several *enzymes*. It is essential for the manufacture of the genetic material of cells and thus for growth and development. The formation of red blood cells by the bone marrow is particularly dependent on this vitamin. It is also involved in the utilization of folic acid and carbohydrates in the diet, and is necessary for maintaining a healthy nervous system.

Dietary and other natural sources
Liver is the best dietary source of vitamin B$_{12}$. Kidney, lean meats, fish, chicken, eggs, and dairy products are also rich in the vitamin.

Normal daily requirement
The recommended nutrient intake (RNI) for vitamin B$_{12}$ is: 0.3mcg (birth – 4 months); 0.4mcg (5 – 12 months); 0.5mcg (1 year); 0.6mcg (2 – 3 years); 0.8mcg (4 – 6 years); 1mcg (7 years or older). In pregnancy and breast feeding, the RNI is increased by 0.2mcg.

When supplements are helpful
A balanced diet usually provides more than adequate amounts of the vitamin, and deficiency is generally due to impaired absorption from the intestine rather than a low dietary intake. However, a strict vegetarian or vegan diet lacking in eggs or dairy products is likely to be deficient in vitamin B$_{12}$ and supplements are usually needed. The most common cause of deficiency is pernicious anemia, in which absorption of the vitamin is impaired due to inability of the stomach to secrete a special substance – intrinsic factor – that normally combines with the vitamin so that it can be taken up in the intestine. Supplements are also prescribed on medical advice in certain bowel disorders such as celiac disease and steatorrhea, after surgery to the stomach or intestine, and in tapeworm infestation.

Symptoms of deficiency
Vitamin B$_{12}$ deficiency usually develops over months or years – the liver can store up to 6 years' supply. It leads to *anemia*. The mouth and tongue often become sore. Deficiency of the vitamin also affects the brain and spinal cord, leading to numbness and tingling of the limbs, memory loss, and depression.

Dosage range for treating deficiency
Pernicious anemia (due to impaired absorption of vitamin B$_{12}$) is treated in adults with 30mcg daily for 5 to 10 days, followed by 100mcg monthly, given by intramuscular or deep subcutaneous injection. Children are treated with a total of 1,000 – 5,000mcg given in divided doses of 100mcg each over two or more weeks; thereafter, 50 –100mcg every four weeks. Folic acid should be given early unless folic acid levels are adequate. Dietary deficiency is usually treated with oral supplements of 6mcg daily (2 – 3mcg in infants). Deficiency resulting from a genetic defect that prevents use of the vitamin is treated with 250mcg every three weeks throughout life.

Symptoms and risks of excessive intake
Harmful effects from high doses of vitamin B$_{12}$ are unknown. Allergic reactions may in rare cases occur with impure preparations given by injection.

VITAMIN C

Other names Ascorbic acid, ascorbate calcium, ascorbate sodium

Availability
Vitamin C is available without prescription in a wide variety of single-ingredient and vitamin/mineral preparations. Ascorbate sodium is given only by injection under medical supervision.

Actions on the body
Vitamin C plays an essential role in the activities of several *enzymes*. It is vital for the growth and maintenance of healthy bones, teeth, gums, ligaments, and blood vessels, and is an important component of all body organs. It is important for the manufacture of certain *neurotransmitters* and adrenal hormones. It is also required for the utilization of folic acid and absorption of iron. Vitamin C is also necessary for normal immune responses to infection and for wound healing.

Dietary and other natural sources
Vitamin C is found in most fresh fruits and vegetables. Citrus fruits, tomatoes, potatoes, and green, leafy vegetables are good dietary sources. Strawberries and cantaloupes are also rich in the vitamin.

Normal daily requirement
The recommended nutrient intake (RNI) for vitamin C is: 20mg (birth – 3 years); 25mg (4 – 12 years); 30mg (males 13 – 15 years, females 13 years or older); 40mg (males 16 years or older). In pregnancy, the RNI is increased by 10mg in the second and third trimesters. In breast feeding, the RNI is increased by 25mg.

When supplements are helpful
A healthy diet generally contains sufficient quantities of vitamin C. However, it is used up more rapidly after a serious injury, major surgery, burns, and in extremes of temperature. Because inhalation of carbon monoxide destroys the vitamin, city dwellers need more than people who live in the country, and smokers are likely to be deficient. Supplements may be necessary to prevent or treat deficiency in the elderly and chronically sick, and in severe alcoholism; women taking estrogen-containing contraceptives may also require supplements. There is no convincing evidence that vitamin C in large doses prevents colds, although it may reduce the severity of symptoms.

Symptoms of deficiency
Mild deficiency may cause weakness, aches, pains, swollen gums, and nosebleeds. Severe deficiency results in scurvy, the symptoms of which include inflamed, bleeding gums, excessive bruising, and internal bleeding. In adults, bones fracture easily and teeth become loose. In children there is abnormal bone and tooth development. Wounds fail to heal and become infected. Deficiency often leads to anemia (abnormally low levels of red blood cells), symptoms of which are pallor, fatigue, shortness of breath and palpitations. Untreated scurvy may cause seizures, coma, and death.

Dosage range for treating deficiency
For scurvy, 300mg of vitamin C is given daily for several weeks. Adding a daily source of vitamin C, such as a glass of orange juice, is also recommended.

Symptoms and risks of excessive intake
The risk of harmful effects is low, as excess vitamin C is excreted in the urine. However, doses of over 1g daily may cause diarrhea, nausea, and stomach cramps. Kidney stones may occasionally develop.

VITAMIN D

Other names Alfacalcidol, calcefediol, calciferol, calcitriol, cholecalciferol, ergocalciferol, vitamin D$_2$, vitamin D$_3$

Availability
Vitamin D is available without prescription in various single-ingredient and vitamin/mineral preparations. Injections are given only under medical supervision.

Actions on the body
Vitamin D (with parathyroid hormone) helps regulate the balance of calcium and phosphate in the body. It aids the absorption of calcium from the intestinal tract, and is essential for strong bones and teeth.

Dietary and other natural sources
Fortified milk is the best dietary source of vitamin D. Oily fish (sardines, herring, salmon, and tuna), liver, dairy products, and egg yolks are good, but not reliable, sources of this vitamin. It is also formed by the action of ultraviolet rays in sunlight on chemicals naturally present in the skin.

Normal daily requirement
The recommended nutrient intake (RNI) for vitamin D is: 10mcg (birth – 1 year); 5mcg (2 – 6 years); 2.5mcg (7 – 49 years); 5mcg (50 years or older). In pregnancy and breast feeding, the RNI is increased by 2.5mcg.

When supplements are helpful
Vitamin D requirements are small and usually adequately met by dietary sources and normal exposure to sunlight. However, a poor diet and inadequate sunlight may lead to deficiency; dark-skinned people (particularly those living in smoggy urban areas) and night-shift workers are more at risk. In areas of moderate sunshine, supplements may be given to infants. Premature infants, strict vegetarians, and the elderly may benefit from supplements. Supplements are usually necessary on medical advice to prevent and treat vitamin D deficiency-related bone disorders, and for conditions in which absorption from the intestine is impaired, deficiency due to liver disease, certain kidney disorders, prolonged use of certain drugs, and genetic defects. It is also used in treatment of hypoparathyroidism.

Symptoms of deficiency
Long-term deficiency leads to low blood levels of calcium and phosphate, which results in softening of the bones. In children, this causes abnormal bone development (rickets), and in adults, osteomalacia, causing backache, muscle weakness, bone pain, and fractures.

Dosage range for treating deficiency
Correction of vitamin D deficiency: 5,000 IU daily until a biochemical and radiographic response is apparent. Vitamin D resistant rickets: 12,000 – 500,000 IU daily. Hypoparathyroidism: 50,000 – 200,000 IU daily plus 4g of calcium lactate, administered 6 times per day.

Symptoms and risks of excessive intake
Doses of over 400 IU of vitamin D daily are not beneficial to most people and may increase the risk of adverse effects such as weakness, unusual thirst, increased urination, gastrointestinal disturbances, and depression. Prolonged excessive use disrupts the balance of calcium and phosphate in the body and may lead to abnormal calcium deposits in the soft tissues, blood vessel walls, and kidneys and retarded growth in children. Daily doses of over 25mcg (1,000 IU) in infants and 1.25mg (50,000 IU) in adults and children are considered excessive.

VITAMIN E

Other names Alpha-tocopherol acetate, tocopherol, tocopherols

Availability
Vitamin E is available without prescription in many single-ingredient and vitamin/mineral preparations. It is also included in skin creams. Alpha-tocopherol is the most powerful form.

Actions on the body
Vitamin E is vital for healthy cell structure, for slowing the effects of the aging process on cells, and for maintaining the activities of certain *enzymes*. Vitamin E protects the lungs and other tissues from damage by pollutants, and protects red blood cells against destruction by poisons in the bloodstream. It also helps to form red blood cells, and is involved in the production of energy in the heart and muscles.

Dietary and other natural sources
Vegetable oils are good sources. Other sources rich in this vitamin include green, leafy vegetables, whole-grain cereals, and wheat germ.

Normal daily requirement
The recommended nutrient intake (RNI) for vitamin E is: 3mg (birth – 1 year); 4mg (2 – 3 years); 5mg (4 – 6 years); 7mg (males 7 – 9 years); 6mg (females 7 – 9 years); 8mg (males 10 – 12 years); 7mg (females 10 – 24 years); 9mg (males 13 – 15 years); 10mg (males 16 – 24 years); 9mg (males 25 – 49 years); 6mg (females 25 – 74 years); 7mg (males 50 – 74 years); 6mg (males 75 years or older); 5mg (females 75 years or older). In pregnancy and breast feeding, the RNI is increased by 2mg and 3mg, respectively.

When supplements are helpful
A normal diet supplies adequate amounts of vitamin E, and supplements are rarely necessary. However, people consuming large amounts of polyunsaturated fats in vegetable oils, especially if used in cooking at high temperatures, may need supplements, as may people with impaired intestinal absorption, liver disease, or cystic fibrosis. Supplements of vitamin E are also recommended for premature infants.

Symptoms of deficiency
Vitamin E deficiency leads to destruction of red blood cells (hemolysis) and eventually anemia (abnormally low levels of red blood cells), symptoms of which are pallor, fatigue, shortness of breath, and palpitations. In infants, deficiency causes irritability and fluid retention.

Dosage range for treating deficiency
Doses are generally four to five times the recommended nutrient intake (RNI) in adults and children.

Symptoms and risks of excessive intake
Harmful effects are rare, but prolonged use of over 250mg daily may lead to nausea, abdominal pain, vomiting, and diarrhea. Large doses may also reduce the amounts of vitamin A, D, and K absorbed from the intestines.

VITAMIN K

Other names Menadione, phytonadione, vitamin K_1, vitamin K_2, vitamin K_3

Availability
Vitamin K is available without prescription as a dietary supplement on its own and in several vitamin/mineral preparations. Injectable and oral preparations used to treat bleeding disorders are available only by prescription.

Actions on the body
Vitamin K is necessary for the formation in the liver of several substances that promote the formation of blood clots (blood clotting factors) including prothrombin (clotting factor II).

Dietary and other natural sources
The best dietary sources of vitamin K are green, leafy vegetables and root vegetables, fruits, seeds, cow's milk, and yogurt. Alfalfa is also an excellent source. In adults and children the intestinal bacteria manufacture a large part of the vitamin K that is required.

Normal daily requirement
A recommended nutrient intake (RNI) has not been determined, but an average intake of 50 – 80mcg is considered adequate.

When supplements are helpful
Vitamin K requirements are generally met adequately by dietary intake and by manufacture of the vitamin by bacteria that live in the intestine. Supplements are given routinely to newborn infants, since they lack intestinal bacteria capable of producing the vitamin and are therefore more at risk of deficiency. In adults and children, additional vitamin K is usually necessary only on medical advice for deficiency associated with prolonged use of antibiotics or sulfonamide antibacterials that destroy bacteria in the intestine, or when absorption of nutrients from the intestine is impaired. These conditions include liver disease, obstruction of the bile duct, and intestinal disorders causing chronic diarrhea. Vitamin K may also be given to reduce blood loss during labor or after surgery in people who have been taking ASA or oral anticoagulants. Vitamin K also reverses the effect of an overdose of oral anticoagulants.

Symptoms of deficiency
Vitamin K deficiency leads to low levels of prothrombin (hypothrombinemia) and other clotting factors, resulting in delayed blood clotting and a tendency to bleed. This may cause oozing from wounds, nosebleeds, and bleeding from the gums, intestine, urinary tract, and, rarely, in the brain.

Dosage range for treating deficiency
Depends on the individual and on the nature and severity of the disorder.

Symptoms and risks of excessive intake
Excess dietary intake of vitamin K has no known harmful effects. Synthetic vitamin K (menadione) may cause liver damage or rupture of red blood cells (hemolysis) at large doses and in people with glucose-6-phosphate dehydrogenase (G6PD) deficiency. This may lead to reddish-brown urine, jaundice, and, in extreme cases, *anemia*. Adverse effects are extremely rare with vitamin K preparations taken by mouth.

ZINC

Other names Zinc amino acid chelate, zinc chloride, zinc gluconate, zinc oxide, zinc sulfate

Availability
Zinc supplements are available without prescription in single-ingredient and vitamin/mineral preparations. Zinc chloride is an injectable preparation given only under medical supervision during intravenous feeding. Zinc is also one ingredient included in a variety of topical formulations used for the treatment of minor skin irritations, dandruff, and fungal infections.

Actions on the body
Zinc plays a vital role in the activities of over 100 *enzymes*. It is essential for the manufacture of proteins and nucleic acids (the genetic material of cells), and is involved in the function of the hormone insulin in the utilization of carbohydrates. It is necessary for a normal rate of growth, development of the reproductive organs, normal function of the prostate gland, and healing of wounds and burns.

Dietary and other natural sources
Zinc is present in small amounts in a wide variety of foods. Zinc from animal sources is better absorbed than that from plants. Protein-rich foods such as lean meat and seafood are the best sources of the mineral. Whole-grain breads and cereals and dried beans are good dietary sources.

Normal daily requirement
The recommended nutrient intake (RNI) for zinc is: 2mg (birth – 4 months); 3mg (5 – 12 months); 4mg (1 – 3 years); 5mg (4 – 6 years); 7mg (7 – 9 years); 9mg (10 – 12 years); 12mg (males 13 years or older); 9mg (females 10 years or older). In pregnancy and breast feeding, the RNI is increased by 6mg.

When supplements are helpful
A balanced diet containing natural, unprocessed foods usually provides adequate amounts of zinc. Dietary deficiency is rare in Canada and is likely only in people who are generally malnourished such as debilitated elderly people on poor diets. Supplements are usually recommended on medical advice for those with reduced absorption of the mineral due to certain intestinal disorders, such as cystic fibrosis, for those with increased zinc requirements due to sickle cell disease or major burns, and for people with liver damage (for example, as a result of excessive alcohol intake).

Symptoms of deficiency
Deficiency may cause loss of appetite and impair the sense of taste. In children, it may also lead to poor growth and, in severe cases, to delayed sexual development and dwarfism. Severe, prolonged lack of zinc may result in a rare skin disorder involving hair loss, rash, inflamed areas of skin with pustules, and inflammation of the mouth, tongue, eyelids, and around the fingernails.

Dosage range for treating deficiency
Depends on the individual and on the cause and severity of the deficiency. In general, 30 – 50mg daily is sufficient, usually in the form of zinc sulfate.

Symptoms and risks of excessive intake
The risk of harmful effects is low with excess zinc intake. However, prolonged use of large doses may interfere with the absorption of iron and copper, leading to deficiency of these minerals, and may cause nausea, vomiting, headache, fever, malaise, and abdominal pain.

DRUGS OF ABUSE

The purpose of these pages is to clarify the medical facts concerning certain drugs (or classes of drugs) that are most commonly abused in Canada. Their physical and mental effects sometimes combined with habit-forming potential have led to their use outside a medical context. Some of the drugs listed here are illegal, others have legitimate medical uses – for example, sleeping drugs and anti-anxiety drugs – and are also discussed elsewhere in the book. Alcohol, caffeine, nicotine, and solvents, although not medical drugs, are all substances with drug-like effects and abuse potential.

The individual profiles are designed to instruct and inform the reader so that he or she may become more aware of the hazards of drug abuse, and be able to recognize signs of abuse in others.

Since a large proportion of drug abusers are young people, the following pages may serve as a useful source of reference for parents and teachers concerned that young people in their charge may be taking drugs.

The drugs of abuse profiles

The profiles are arranged in alphabetical order under their medical names, with street names, drug categories, and cross-references to other sections of the book where appropriate. Each profile contains information on that drug under standard headings. Topics covered include the various ways it is taken, its habit-forming potential, its legitimate medical uses, effects and risks, the signs of abuse, and interactions with other drugs.

HOW TO UNDERSTAND THE PROFILES

Each drug of abuse profile contains standard headings under which you will find information covering important aspects of the drug.

Drug category
Categorizes the drug according to its principal effects on the body, with cross-references to other parts of the book where relevant.

Other common names lists the various alternative and street names of each drug.

How taken tells you about the various forms in which each substance is taken.

Short-term effects tells you the immediate mental and physical effects of the drug.

Signs of abuse describes the outward effects of taking the drug, both short- and long-term, that concerned observers may notice.

AMPHETAMINES

Other common names Speed, uppers, bennies
Drug category Central nervous system stimulant (see p.100)

Habit-forming potential
Regular use of amphetamines and methamphetamine leads to the rapid development of tolerance, so that higher and higher doses are required to achieve the same effect. Users become psychologically and physically dependent on the effects of the drug.

How taken
Usually swallowed as tablets. Sometimes sniffed or mixed with water and injected.

Legitimate uses
In the 1950s and 1960s, amphetamines were widely prescribed as appetite suppressants. This use has largely been abandoned because of the risk of dependence and abuse. They are still prescribed for attention deficit disorders and narcolepsy (see also Nervous system stimulants, p.100). Amphetamines are classified under the Food and Drugs Act, Part III (Controlled Drugs – General). Possession is illegal without a prescription.

Short-term effects
In small doses, amphetamines increase mental alertness and physical energy. Breathing and heart rate speed up, the pupils dilate, appetite decreases, and dryness of the mouth is common. As these effects wear off, depression and fatigue may follow. At high doses, amphetamines may cause tremor, sweating, anxiety, headache, palpitations, and severe chest pain. Very large doses may cause delusions, hallucinations, delirium, seizures, and coma.

Long-term effects and risks
Regular use of amphetamine drugs frequently leads to weight loss and constipation. Regular users may also become emotionally unstable. Severe depression and suicide are associated with withdrawal. Heavy long-term use reduces resistance to infection and also carries a risk of damage to blood vessels and heart failure.
Use of amphetamines in early pregnancy may increase the risk of birth defects, especially in the heart. Taken throughout pregnancy, amphetamines lead to premature birth and low birth weight.

Signs of abuse
The amphetamine user may appear unusually energetic, cheerful, and excessively talkative while under the influence of the drug. Restlessness and agitation are also characteristic. There is a lack of interest in food and unusual sleeping patterns; regular users may use the drug to stay awake for two or three nights at a stretch, then sleep for up to 48 hours afterward. Mood swings are common.

Interactions
Amphetamines interact with a variety of drugs. They may lead to an increase in blood pressure, thus opposing the effect of antihypertensive drug treatments. Taken with monoamine oxidase inhibitors (MAOIs), they may lead to a dangerous rise in blood pressure. They also increase the risk of abnormal heart rhythms with digitalis drugs, levodopa, and certain anesthetics given by inhalation. Amphetamines tend to counteract the sedative effects of drugs that depress the central nervous system. This effect is particularly dangerous with barbiturates, since it can lead to an accidental, life-threatening overdose of the latter.

BARBITURATES

Other common names Downers, goofballs
Drug category Central nervous system depressant (see also Sleeping drugs, p.94), sedative

Habit-forming potential
Long-term, regular use of barbiturates can be habit-forming. Both physical and psychological dependence may occur.

How taken
By mouth in the form of capsules or tablets.

Legitimate uses
In the past, barbiturates were widely prescribed as sleeping drugs. Since the 1960s, however, they have been increasingly replaced by benzodiazepines, which may also be addictive but are less likely to cause death from overdose.
The widest use of barbiturates today is for epilepsy (phenobarbital).
Most barbiturates are listed under the Food and Drugs Act, Part III (Controlled Drugs – Special Schedule). Secobarbital is listed under Controlled Drugs (General).

Short-term effects
Short-term effects are similar to those of alcohol. A low dose produces relaxation, while larger amounts make the user more intoxicated and drowsy. Coordination is impaired and slurred speech, clumsiness, and confusion may occur. Increasingly large doses may produce loss of consciousness, coma, and death caused by depression of the breathing mechanism.

Long-term effects and risks
The greatest risk of long-term barbiturate use is physical dependence. In an addicted person, sudden withdrawal of the drug precipitates a withdrawal syndrome that varies in severity, depending partly on the type of barbiturate, its dose, and the duration of use, but primarily on the availability and administration of supportive treatment, including appropriate medication. Symptoms may include irritability, disturbed sleep, nightmares, nausea, vomiting, weakness, tremors, and extreme anxiety; abrupt withdrawal after several months of use may cause seizures, delirium, and coma lasting for up to one week. Long-term, heavy use of barbiturates increases the risk of accidental overdose, and also of chest infections, since these drugs suppress the cough reflex.
Taken in pregnancy, barbiturates may cause fetal abnormalities and, used regularly in the last three months, may lead to withdrawal symptoms in the newborn baby.

Signs of abuse
Signs of long-term heavy use include prolonged bouts of intoxication with memory lapses ("blackouts"), neglect of personal appearance and responsibilities, personality changes, and episodes of severe depression.

Interactions
Barbiturates interact with a wide variety of drugs and increase the risk of sedation with any drug that has a sedative effect on the central nervous system. These include anti-anxiety drugs, narcotic analgesics, antipsychotics, tricyclic antidepressants, and antihistamines. High doses taken with alcohol can lead to a fatal coma.
Barbiturates also increase the activity of certain enzymes in the liver, leading to an increase in the breakdown of certain drugs, thus reducing their effects. Anticoagulants and many other drugs are affected in this way.

Habit-forming potential
Explains to what extent the drug is likely to produce physical or psychological *dependence*.

Legitimate uses
Describes the accepted medical uses of the substance, if any.

Long-term effects and risks
Explains the serious long-term effects on health and the risks involved with regular use of the drug.

Interactions
Tells you about interactions that may occur with other drugs.

533

ALCOHOL (ETHYL)

Other common names Liquor, drink, booze, sauce, hooch
Drug category Central nervous system depressant, sedative

Habit-forming potential

Because individual responses vary so widely, it is difficult to measure the habit-forming potential of alcohol. But there is certainly a behavioral abnormality or "disease" called alcoholism, characterized by a person's inability to control intake. Regular drinking and heavy drinking do not cause alcoholism so much as indicate that it may be present. Alcoholism involves psychological and physical *dependence,* evidenced by large daily consumption, heavy weekend drinking, or long episodic binges.

How taken

By mouth, usually in the form of wines, beers, and a variety of liquors.

Legitimate uses

While there are no legal restrictions on the consumption of alcohol, there are on its sale – such as the restriction of the sale of alcoholic beverages to people over a specified age, 19 for example.

Medically, rubbing alcohol (which is isopropyl alcohol, or denatured ethyl alcohol) is widely used as an *antiseptic* before injections to minimize the risk of infection. It can be extremely harmful if ingested. Rubbing alcohol may be used to harden the skin and thus prevent pressure sores in bedridden people, and foot sores in hikers or runners.

Short-term effects

Alcohol acts as a central nervous system depressant, thus reducing anxiety, tension, and inhibitions. In moderate quantities, it gives the drinker a feeling of relaxation and confidence and may increase sociability and talkativeness. Moderate amounts also dilate small blood vessels, particularly those in the skin, leading to flushing and a feeling of warmth. With increasing amounts, concentration and judgment are progressively impaired and the body's reactions are increasingly slowed. Accidents, particularly driving accidents, are more likely. As blood alcohol levels rise, violent or aggressive behavior is possible. Speech is slurred, and the person becomes unsteady, staggers, and may experience double vision and loss of balance. Nausea and vomiting are frequent. Loss of consciousness may follow if blood alcohol levels continue to rise, and there is a risk of death from inhalation of vomit or cessation of breathing.

Long-term effects and risks

A large number of heavy drinkers develop liver diseases, including alcoholic hepatitis, fatty liver (excess fat deposits that may lead to cirrhosis), cirrhosis, or liver cancer. Coronary heart disease, high blood pressure, and strokes are also possible consequences of heavy drinking. Inflammation of the stomach (gastritis) and peptic ulcers are also more common. Alcoholics have an above-average risk of developing dementia (irreversible mental deterioration).

Long-term heavy drinking is usually associated with physical dependence. An alcoholic may appear to be sober, even after heavy drinking, because of built-up tolerance. In addition to health problems, alcohol dependence is associated with a range of personal and social problems. Alcohol-dependent persons may suffer from anxiety and depression, and since they often eat poorly, they are at risk of nutritional deficiency diseases, particularly thiamine deficiency (see p.527).

Drinking during pregnancy can cause fetal abnormalities and poor physical and mental development in infants; even taking moderate amounts of alcohol can lead to miscarriage, low birth weight, and mental retardation.

Signs of abuse

Signs that alcohol consumption is getting out of control include any or all of the following: changes in drinking pattern (for example, early morning drinking or a switch from beer to vodka); changes in drinking habits (such as drinking alone or having a drink before an appointment or interview); personality changes; neglect of personal appearance; poor eating habits; increasingly frequent or prolonged bouts of intoxication with memory lapses ("blackouts") about events that occurred during drinking episodes. Physical symptoms may include nausea, vomiting, or shaking in the morning, abdominal pain, cramps, weakness in the legs and hands, redness and enlarged blood vessels in the face, unsteadiness, poor memory, and incontinence. Sudden discontinuation of heavy drinking, if untreated, can lead to delirium tremens (marked confusion with hallucinations) beginning after two to four days of abstinence and lasting for up to three days.

Interactions

Alcohol interacts with a wide variety of drugs. In particular, it increases the risk of sedation with any drug that has a *sedative* effect on the central nervous system. These include anti-anxiety drugs, sleeping drugs, general anesthetics, narcotic analgesics, antipsychotics, tricyclic antidepressants, antihistamines, and certain antihypertensive drugs (methyl-dopa and clonidine). Taking alcohol with other depressant drugs of abuse, particularly narcotics, barbiturates, or solvents, can lead to coma and may be fatal.

Taken with ASA and similar analgesics, alcohol increases the risk of bleeding from the stomach, particularly in people who have had peptic ulcers.

People on a regimen of disulfiram (Antabuse), a drug used to help people stay in an alcohol-free state, will experience highly unpleasant reactions if they then take even a small amount of alcohol. The results include flushing of the face, throbbing headache, palpitations, nausea, and vomiting.

Alcohol may interact with some oral antidiabetic drugs and oral anticoagulants, and thus increase their effects.

Taken with monoamine oxidase inhibitors (MAOIs), alcohol, particularly in the form of red wine, may cause a dangerous rise in blood pressure.

Practical points

If you drink, know what your limits are and behave responsibly. Generally, the body can only break down about one drink (i.e., one shot of liquor, one glass of wine, or one bottle of beer) per hour. If you drink faster than this, your blood alcohol will rise above the "legal limit" for driving. If you are a woman and are pregnant, or are planning to have a baby soon, the safest course is abstinence. If you are planning to drive, don't drink. If you find that you are having trouble controlling your drinking, seek help and advice from your physician or from one of the treatment programs available in most parts of the country. And even if you don't have a control problem, don't drink heavily – remember that alcohol can have harmful effects on many parts of your body, including your brain.

AMPHETAMINES

Other common names Speed, uppers, bennies
Drug category Central nervous system stimulant
(see p.100)

Habit-forming potential
Regular use of amphetamines and methamphetamine leads
to the rapid development of *tolerance*, so that higher and
higher doses are required to achieve the same effect. Users
become psychologically and physically dependent on the
effects of the drug.

How taken
Usually swallowed as tablets. Sometimes sniffed or mixed
with water and injected.

Legitimate uses
In the 1950s and 1960s, amphetamines were widely prescribed as appetite suppressants. This use has largely been
abandoned because of the risk of *dependence* and abuse.
They are still prescribed for attention deficit disorders and
narcolepsy (see also Nervous system stimulants, p.100).
Amphetamines are classified under the Food and Drugs Act,
Part III (Controlled Drugs – General). Possession is illegal
without a prescription.

Short-term effects
In small doses, amphetamines increase mental alertness and
physical energy. Breathing and heart rate speed up, the pupils
dilate, appetite decreases, and dryness of the mouth is
common. As these effects wear off, depression and fatigue
may follow. At high doses, amphetamines may cause tremor,
sweating, anxiety, headache, palpitations, and severe chest
pain. Very large doses may cause delusions, hallucinations,
delirium, seizures, and coma.

Long-term effects and risks
Regular use of amphetamine drugs frequently leads to weight
loss and constipation. Regular users may also become
emotionally unstable. Severe depression and suicide are
associated with withdrawal. Heavy long-term use reduces
resistance to infection and also carries a risk of damage to
blood vessels and heart failure.

Use of amphetamines in early pregnancy may increase the
risk of birth defects, especially in the heart. Taken throughout
pregnancy, amphetamines lead to premature birth and low
birth weight.

Signs of abuse
The amphetamine user may appear unusually energetic,
cheerful, and excessively talkative while under the influence
of the drug. Restlessness and agitation are also characteristic. There is a lack of interest in food and unusual sleeping
patterns; regular users may use the drug to stay awake for
two or three nights at a stretch, then sleep for up to 48 hours
afterward. Mood swings are common.

Interactions
Amphetamines interact with a variety of drugs. They may lead
to an increase in blood pressure, thus opposing the effect of
antihypertensive drug treatments. Taken with monoamine
oxidase inhibitors (MAOIs), they may lead to a dangerous rise
in blood pressure. They also increase the risk of abnormal
heart rhythms with digitalis drugs, levodopa, and certain
anesthetics given by inhalation. Amphetamines tend to
counteract the *sedative* effects of drugs that depress the
central nervous system. This effect is particularly dangerous
with barbiturates, since it can lead to an accidental, life-
threatening overdose of the latter.

BARBITURATES

Other common names Downers, goofballs
Drug category Central nervous system depressant (see also
Sleeping drugs, p.94), sedative

Habit-forming potential
Long-term, regular use of barbiturates can be habit-forming.
Both physical and psychological *dependence* may occur.

How taken
By mouth in the form of capsules or tablets.

Legitimate uses
In the past, barbiturates were widely prescribed as sleeping
drugs. Since the 1960s, however, they have been increasingly
replaced by benzodiazepines, which may also be addictive
but are less likely to cause death from overdose.

The widest use of barbiturates today is for epilepsy
(phenobarbital).

Most barbiturates are listed under the Food and Drugs Act,
Part III (Controlled Drugs – Special Schedule). Secobarbital is
listed under Controlled Drugs (General).

Short-term effects
Short-term effects are similar to those of alcohol. A low dose
produces relaxation, while larger amounts make the user
more intoxicated and drowsy. Coordination is impaired and
slurred speech, clumsiness, and confusion may occur.
Increasingly large doses may produce loss of consciousness,
coma, and death caused by depression of the breathing
mechanism.

Long-term effects and risks
The greatest risk of long-term barbiturate use is physical
dependence. In an addicted person, sudden withdrawal of
the drug precipitates a withdrawal syndrome that varies in
severity, depending partly on the type of barbiturate, its dose,
and the duration of use, but primarily on the availability and
administration of supportive treatment, including appropriate
medication. Symptoms may include irritability, disturbed
sleep, nightmares, nausea, vomiting, weakness, tremors, and
extreme anxiety; abrupt withdrawal after several months of
use may cause seizures, delirium, and coma lasting for up to
one week. Long-term, heavy use of barbiturates increases the
risk of accidental overdose, and also of chest infections,
since these drugs suppress the cough reflex.

Taken in pregnancy, barbiturates may cause fetal
abnormalities and, used regularly in the last three months,
may lead to withdrawal symptoms in the newborn baby.

Signs of abuse
Signs of long-term heavy use include prolonged bouts of
intoxication with memory lapses ("blackouts"), neglect of
personal appearance and responsibilities, personality
changes, and episodes of severe depression.

Interactions
Barbiturates interact with a wide variety of drugs and increase
the risk of sedation with any drug that has a *sedative* effect
on the central nervous system. These include anti-anxiety
drugs, narcotic analgesics, antipsychotics, tricyclic antidepressants, and antihistamines. High doses taken with
alcohol can lead to a fatal coma.

Barbiturates also increase the activity of certain enzymes in
the liver, leading to an increase in the breakdown of certain
drugs, thus reducing their effects. Anticoagulants and many
other drugs are affected in this way.

BENZODIAZEPINES

Other common names Tranquilizers
Drug category Central nervous system depressants (see Sleeping drugs, p.94, and Anti-anxiety drugs, p.95)

Habit-forming potential
The addictive potential of benzodiazepines is much lower than that of some other central nervous system depressants such as barbiturates. However, regular long-term use of these drugs can lead to psychological and physical *dependence.*

How taken
By mouth as tablets or capsules, or by injection.

Legitimate uses
Benzodiazepines are among the most commonly prescribed drugs. They are used mainly for short-term treatment of anxiety and for relief of sleeplessness. They are also used in anesthesia both as *premedication* and for induction of general anesthesia. Other medical uses include the management of alcohol withdrawal, control of seizures, and relief of muscle spasms. Benzodiazepines are classified as Schedule F drugs under the Food and Drugs Act.

Short-term effects
Benzodiazepines can reduce mental activity along with anxiety. In moderate doses, they may also cause poor memory and unsteadiness, reduce alertness, and slow the body's reactions, thus impairing driving ability and increasing the risk of accidents. Any benzodiazepine in a high enough dose induces sleep. Very large overdoses may cause depression of the breathing mechanism.

Long-term effects and risks
Benzodiazepines tend to lose their *sedative* effect with long-term use. This may lead the user to increase the dose progressively, a manifestation of tolerance and physical dependence. Older people may become apathetic or confused when taking these drugs. On stopping the drug, the chronic user may develop *withdrawal symptoms* that may include anxiety, panic attacks, palpitations, shaking, insomnia, headaches, dizziness, aches and pains, nausea, loss of appetite, and clumsiness. Symptoms can last for days or weeks. Babies born to women who use high doses of benzodiazepines regularly may suffer withdrawal symptoms during the first week of life.

Signs of abuse
Abuse can occur, but it is uncommon. The typical abuser is a middle-aged or elderly person who may have been taking these drugs by prescription for months or years. He or she is usually unaware of the problem, and may freely admit to taking "nerve pills" in large quantities.

Interactions
Benzodiazepines increase the risk of sedation with any drug that has a sedative effect on the central nervous system. These include other anti-anxiety and sleeping drugs, alcohol, narcotic analgesics, antipsychotics, tricyclic antidepressants, and antihistamines.

Practical points
In general, most benzodiazepines should normally be used for courses of two weeks' duration or less. If these drugs have been taken for longer than two weeks, it is usually best to reduce the dose gradually to reduce the risk of withdrawal symptoms. If you have been taking benzodiazepines for many months or years, it is best to consult your physician to work out a dose reduction program. If possible, it will help to tell your family and friends and enlist their support.

COCAINE

Other common names Coke, crack, snow
Drug category Central nervous system stimulant and local anesthetic

Habit-forming potential
Taken regularly, cocaine is habit-forming. Users may become psychologically dependent on its physical and mental effects, and may step up their intake to maintain or increase these effects or to prevent the feelings of severe fatigue and depression that may occur after the drug is stopped. The risk of *dependence* is especially pronounced with the form of cocaine known as "freebase" or "crack" (see below).

How taken
Smoked, sniffed, or occasionally injected.

Legitimate uses
Cocaine was once widely used as a local anesthetic. It is still sometimes given for *topical* anesthesia in the mouth and throat prior to minor surgery or other procedures. Because of its side effects and potential for abuse, cocaine has now largely been replaced by safer local anesthetic drugs. Cocaine is classified under the Narcotic Control Act (Narcotics – General).

Short-term effects
Cocaine is a central nervous system stimulant. In moderate doses it overcomes fatigue and produces feelings of well-being and elation. Appetite is reduced. Physical effects include an increase in heart rate and blood pressure, dilation of the pupils, tremor, and increased sweating. Large doses can lead to agitation, anxiety, paranoia, and hallucinations. Paranoia may cause violent behavior. Very large doses may cause seizures and death due to heart attack or heart failure. (See "Crack," below.)

Long-term effects and risks
Heavy, regular use of cocaine can cause restlessness, anxiety, hyperexcitability, nausea, insomnia, and weight loss. Continued use may lead to increasing paranoia and psychosis. Repeated sniffing also damages the membranes lining the nose and may eventually lead to the destruction of the septum, the structure separating the nostrils.

People with heart disease and high blood pressure run the risk of heart problems.

Signs of abuse
The cocaine user may appear unusually energetic and exuberant under the influence of the drug and show little interest in food. Heavy, regular use may lead to disturbed eating and sleeping patterns. Agitation, mood swings, aggressive behavior, and suspiciousness of other people may also be signs of a heavy user.

Interactions
Cocaine can increase blood pressure, thus opposing the effect of antihypertensive drugs. Taken with monoamine oxidase inhibitors (MAOIs), it can cause a dangerous rise in blood pressure. It also increases the risk of adverse effects on the heart when taken with certain general anesthetics.

CRACK

This potent form of cocaine is taken in the form of "rocks" that are smoked. Highly addictive, it has more intense effects than other forms of cocaine and there is an increased risk of abnormal heart rhythms, high blood pressure, stroke, and death. Long-term consequences include coughing of black phlegm, wheezing, irreversible lung damage, hoarseness, and parched lips, tongue, and throat from inhaling the hot fumes. Mental deterioration, personality changes, social withdrawal, paranoia or violent behavior, and suicide attempts may occur.

HEROIN (NARCOTICS)

Other common names Horse, junk, smack, scag, H
Drug category Central nervous system depressant

Habit-forming potential
Narcotic analgesics include not only drugs that are derived from the opium poppy (opium, morphine) but also synthetic drugs whose medical actions are similar to those of morphine (meperidine, methadone, hydrocodone). Their frequent use leads to *tolerance*, and all have a potential for *dependence*. Among them, heroin is the most important because of its association with criminality.

After only a few weeks of use *withdrawal symptoms* may occur when the drug is stopped; fear of such withdrawal effects may be a strong inducement to go on using the drug. In heavy users, the drug habit is often coupled with a life-style revolving around its use.

How taken
A white or speckled brown powder, heroin is either sniffed or injected. Other narcotics may be taken by mouth.

Legitimate uses
Heroin is used exclusively for the management of severe forms of pain and is listed under the Narcotic Control Act (Narcotics – Specialized). Other narcotic analgesics such as morphine and meperidine are listed under Narcotics – General. Less potent codeine-containing combination brand-name products used as cough suppressants or analgesics are classified under either Narcotics – Verbal Prescription or Exempt Codeine Preparations.

Short-term effects
Strong narcotics induce a feeling of well-being and content-ment. Pain is dulled and the activity of the nervous system is depressed; breathing and heart rate are slowed and the cough reflex is inhibited. First-time users often feel nauseated and vomit. With higher doses, there is increasing drowsiness, sometimes leading to coma and, in rare cases, death from respiratory arrest.

Long-term effects and risks
Long-term regular use of narcotics leads to constipation, reduced sexual drive, disruption of menstrual periods, and poor eating habits. Poor nutrition and personal neglect may lead to general ill health.

Street drugs are often mixed ("cut") with other substances, such as caffeine, quinine, talcum powder, and flour, that can damage blood vessels and clog the lungs. There is also a risk of abscesses at the injection site. Dangerous infections, such as hepatitis and human immunodeficiency virus (HIV; AIDS), may be transmitted via unclean or shared needles.

After several weeks of regular use, sudden withdrawal of narcotics produces a flu-like withdrawal syndrome beginning 6 – 24 hours after the last dose. Symptoms may include runny nose and eyes, hot and cold sweats, sleeplessness, aches, tremor, anxiety, nausea, vomiting, diarrhea, muscle spasms, and abdominal cramps. These effects are at their worst 48 – 72 hours after withdrawal and fade after 7 –10 days.

Signs of abuse
Signs of abuse include apathy, neglect of personal appear-ance and hygiene, loss of appetite and weight, loss of interest in former hobbies and social activities, personality changes, and furtive behavior. Signs of intoxication include pinpoint pupils and a drowsy or drunken appearance.

Interactions
Narcotics dangerously increase the risk of sedation with any drug that has a sedative effect on the central nervous system, including barbiturates and alcohol.

LSD

Other common names Lysergic acid diethylamide, acid
Drug category Hallucinogen

Habit-forming potential
Although it is not physically addictive, LSD may cause psychological *dependence*. After several days of regular use, a person may develop *tolerance* or lessened effect.

How taken
By mouth, as tiny colored tablets, or absorbed onto small squares of paper (known as "microdots"), gelatin sheets, or sugar cubes.

Legitimate uses
None. Early interest of the medical profession in LSD focused on its possible use in psychotherapy, but additional studies suggested that it could lead to psychosis in susceptible people. LSD is listed under the Food and Drugs Act, Part IV (Restricted Drugs).

Short-term effects
The effects of usual doses of LSD last for about 12 hours, beginning almost immediately after taking the drug. Initial effects may include restlessness, dizziness, a feeling of coldness with shivering, and an uncontrollable desire to laugh. Subsequent effects include distortions in perception of sound and vision; true hallucinations are rare. Introspection is often increased and mystical, pseudoreligious experiences may occur. Unpleasant or terrifying hallucinations, loss of emotional control, and overwhelming feelings of anxiety, despair, or panic may occur. Suicide may be attempted. Driving and other hazardous tasks are extremely dangerous. Some people under the influence of this drug have fallen off high buildings, mistakenly believing they could fly.

Long-term effects and risks
Long-term LSD use increases the risk of mental disturbances, including severe depression. In those with existing psycho-logical difficulties, it may lead to lasting mental problems. In addition, some frequent users experience brief but vivid recurrences of LSD's effects ("flashbacks") for months or years after last taking the drug, causing anxiety and disorientation.

Signs of abuse
A person under the influence of LSD may feel strange but rarely shows outward signs of intoxication. Occasionally, a user drugged with LSD may seem overexcited, or appear withdrawn or confused.

Interactions
Interactions with other drugs acting in the brain, such as alcohol, can be expected.

MARIJUANA

Other common names Cannabis, grass, pot, dope, weed, hash
Drug category Central nervous system depressant, hallucinogen, anti-emetic

Habit-forming potential
There is evidence that regular users of marijuana can become physically and psychologically dependent on its effects.

How taken
Usually smoked. May be eaten, often in cakes or cookies, or brewed like tea and drunk.

Legitimate uses
Preparations of the leaves and resin of the cannabis plant (marijuana) have been in use for over 2,000 years. Introduced into Western medicine in the mid-19th century, marijuana was once taken for a wide variety of complaints, including anxiety, insomnia, rheumatic disorders, migraine, painful menstruation, strychnine poisoning, and opiate withdrawal. Today, marijuana derivatives such as nabilone can be prescribed with certain restrictions for the relief of nausea and vomiting caused by treatment with anticancer drugs. Marijuana itself is listed under the Food and Drugs Act, Part IV (Restricted Drugs).

Short-term effects
These partly depend on the effects expected by the user as well as on the amount and strength of the preparation used. Marijuana available today is arguably more potent than that of a few years ago. In small doses, it promotes a feeling of relaxation and well-being, enhances auditory and visual perception, and increases talkativeness. Appetite is usually increased. In some individuals the drug may have little or no effect.

Under the influence of the drug, short-term memory may be impaired and driving ability and coordination are disrupted. Loss of the sense of time, confusion, and emotional distress can result. At high doses, hallucinations may occur in rare cases. The effects last for one to three hours after smoking marijuana and for up to 12 hours or longer after it is eaten. Death from overdose is unknown.

Long-term effects and risks
Marijuana smoking, like tobacco smoking, probably increases the risk of bronchitis and other pulmonary disorders. Regular users may become apathetic and lethargic, and neglect their work or studies and personal appearance. In susceptible people, heavy use may trigger a temporary mental disorder. Marijuana is thought by some physicians to increase the likelihood of experimentation with other drugs.

Since marijuana may lower blood pressure and increase the heart rate, people with heart disorders may be at risk from adverse effects of this drug. Regular use of marijuana may reduce fertility in both men and women and, during pregnancy, may contribute to premature birth.

Signs of abuse
The marijuana user may appear unusually talkative or drunk under the influence of the drug. Appetite is increased.

Marijuana smoke has a distinct herbal smell that may linger in the hair and clothes of those who use it.

Interactions
Marijuana may increase the risk of sedation with any drugs that have a *sedative* effect on the central nervous system. These include anti-anxiety drugs, sleeping drugs, general anesthetics, narcotic analgesics, antipsychotics, tricyclic antidepressants, antihistamines, and alcohol.

MESCALINE

Other common names Peyote, cactus buttons
Drug category Hallucinogen

Habit-forming potential
Mescaline has a low habit-forming potential; it does not cause physical *dependence* and does not usually lead to psychological dependence.

How taken
By mouth as capsules or in the form of peyote cactus buttons, eaten fresh or dried, drunk as tea, or ground up and smoked with marijuana.

Legitimate uses
The peyote cactus has been used by Mexican Indians for over 2,000 years, both as a religious sacrament and as a herbal remedy for various ailments ranging from wounds and bronchitis to failing vision. It is still used legally in the Native American Church in North America, which was set up for North American Indians in 1918. Mescaline is classified under the Food and Drugs Act, Part IV (Restricted Drugs).

Short-term effects
Mescaline alters visual and auditory perception, although true hallucinations are rare. Appetite is reduced under the influence of this drug. There is also a risk of unpleasant mental effects, particularly in people who are anxious or depressed.

Peyote may have additional effects caused by several other active substances (beside mescaline) in the plant. Strychnine-like chemicals may cause nausea, vomiting, and, occasionally, tremors and sweating, which usually precede the perceptual effects of mescaline by up to two hours.

Long-term effects and risks
The long-term effects of mescaline have not been well studied. It may increase the risk of mental disturbances, particularly in people with existing psychological problems.

Signs of abuse
Signs of mescaline or peyote abuse may not be obvious. Users might sometimes appear withdrawn, disoriented, or confused.

Interactions
The combination of alcohol and peyote is recognized to be dangerous. There is a risk of temporary derangement, leading to disorientation, panic, and violent behavior. Vomiting may occur.

NICOTINE

Other common names None
Drug category Central nervous system stimulant

Habit-forming potential
The nicotine in tobacco is largely responsible for tobacco *addiction* in up to 5million Canadian cigarette smokers. Most are also probably psychologically *dependent* on the process of smoking. Most people who start to smoke go on to do so regularly, and most become physically dependent on nicotine. Stopping can produce *withdrawal symptoms* that include nausea, headache, diarrhea, hunger, drowsiness, fatigue, insomnia, irritability, inability to concentrate, depression, and craving for cigarettes.

How taken
Usually smoked in the form of cigarettes, cigars, and pipe tobacco. Sometimes chewed (chewing tobacco), sniffed (tobacco snuff), or held between cheek and gum and sucked (snuff dipping).

Legitimate uses
There are no legal restrictions on tobacco use. Age-related restrictions for its sale, however, may exist in certain municipalities. Nicotine chewing gum or slow-release patches may be prescribed on a temporary basis along with behavior modification therapy to help people who want to give up smoking.

Short-term effects
Nicotine stimulates the sympathetic nervous system (see p.91). In regular tobacco users, it increases concentration, relieves tension and fatigue, and counters boredom and monotony. These effects are short-lived, thus encouraging frequent use. Physical effects include narrowing of blood vessels, increase in heart rate and blood pressure, and reduction in urine output. First-time users often feel dizzy and nauseated, and may vomit.

Long-term effects and risks
Nicotine taken regularly may cause a rise in fatty acids in the bloodstream. This effect, combined with the effects of the drug on heart rhythm and blood vessel size, may increase the risk of diseases of the heart and circulation, including angina, high blood pressure, peripheral vascular disease, stroke, and coronary thrombosis. In addition, its stimulatory effects may lead to excess production of stomach acid, thereby increasing the risk of peptic ulcers.

    Other well-known risks of tobacco smoking, such as chronic lung diseases, adverse effects on pregnancy, and cancers of the lung, mouth, and throat, are likely to be due to other harmful ingredients in tobacco smoke, principally tar and carbon monoxide.

Signs of abuse
Regular smokers often have yellow, tobacco-stained fingers and teeth, and bad breath. The smell of tobacco may linger on hair and clothes. A smoker's cough or shortness of breath are early signs of lung damage or heart disease.

Interactions
Cigarette smoking reduces the blood levels of a variety of drugs and reduces their effects. Such drugs include theophylline, propranolol, benzodiazepines, and caffeine. Diabetics may require larger doses of insulin. The health risks involved in taking oral contraceptives are increased by smoking.

Practical points
▼ Don't start smoking; nicotine is highly addictive.
▼ If you smoke already, give up now even if you have not yet suffered adverse effects.
▼ Ask your physician for advice and support.
▼ Inquire about self-help groups for people trying to give up smoking.

NITRITES

Other common names Amyl nitrite, butyl nitrite, poppers, snappers
Drug category Vasodilators (see also p.110)

Habit-forming potential
Nitrites do not seem to cause physical *dependence*; major *withdrawal symptoms* have never been reported. However, users may become psychologically dependent on the stimulant effect of these drugs.

How taken
By inhalation, usually from small bottles with screw or plug tops or from small glass ampules that are broken.

Legitimate uses
Amyl nitrite was originally introduced as a treatment for angina but has now largely been replaced by safer, longer-acting drugs. It is still used as an *antidote* for cyanide poisoning. Butyl and isobutyl nitrites are not used medically.

Short-term effects
Nitrites increase the flow of blood by relaxing blood vessel walls. They give the user a rapid "high," felt as a strong rush of energy. Less pleasant effects include an increase in heart rate, intense flushing, dizziness, pounding headache, nausea, and coughing. High doses may cause fainting, and regular use may produce a blue discoloration of the skin due to alteration of hemoglobin in the red blood cells.

Long-term effects and risks
Nitrites are very quick-acting drugs. Their effects start within 30 seconds of inhalation and last for about 5 minutes. Regular users may become tolerant to these drugs, thus requiring higher doses to achieve the desired effects. Lasting physical damage, including cardiac problems, can result from chronic use of these drugs, and deaths have occurred.

    The risk of *toxic* effects is increased in those with low blood pressure. Nitrites may also precipitate the onset of glaucoma in susceptible people, by increasing pressure inside the eye.

Signs of abuse
Nitrites have a pungent, fruity odor. They evaporate quickly; the contents of a small bottle left uncapped in a room usually disappear within 2 hours. Unless someone is actually taking the drug or is suffering from an overdose, the only sign of abuse is a bluish skin discoloration.

Interactions
The blood pressure-lowering effects of these drugs may be increased by alcohol, beta blockers, calcium channel blockers, and tricyclic antidepressants, thus increasing the risk of dizziness and fainting.

PHENCYCLIDINE

Other common names PCP, angel dust, crystal, hog, monkey, tranq, goon, DOA, ozone, cyclone, T
Drug category Dissociative general anesthetic, hallucinogen

Habit-forming potential
There is little evidence that phencyclidine causes physical *dependence.* Some users become psychologically dependent on this drug and tolerant to its effects.

How taken
May be sniffed, used in smoking mixtures (in the form of angel dust), eaten (as tablets) or, rarely, injected.

Legitimate uses
Although it was once infrequently given as an anesthetic, it no longer has any medical use. Its only legal use now is in veterinary medicine.

Short-term effects
Phencyclidine taken in small amounts generally produces a "high" but sometimes leads to anxiety or depression. Co-ordination of speech and movement deteriorates and thinking and concentration are impaired. Hallucinations and violent behavior may occur. Other effects include increase in blood pressure and heart rate, dilation of the pupils, dryness of the mouth, tremor, and numbness and reduced sensitivity to pain, which may make it difficult to restrain a person who has become violent under the influence of the drug. Shivering, vomiting, muscle weakness, and rigidity may occur. Higher doses lead to coma or stupor. The recovery period is often prolonged, with alternate periods of sleep and waking, usually followed by memory blackout of the whole episode.

Long-term effects and risks
Repeated phencyclidine use may lead to paranoia, auditory hallucinations, violent behavior, anxiety, and severe depression. While depressed, the user may attempt suicide by overdosing on the drug. Heavy users may also develop brain damage, causing memory blackouts, disorientation, visual disturbances, and speech difficulties.

Deaths due to prolonged seizures, cardiac or respiratory arrest, and ruptured blood vessels in the brain have been reported. After high doses or prolonged coma, there is also a risk of mental derangement, which may be permanent.

Signs of abuse
The phencyclidine user may appear drunk while under the influence of the drug. Hostile or violent behavior and mood swings with bouts of depression may be more common with heavy use.

Interactions
Phencyclidine is a potent drug which may interact with many other drugs.

SOLVENTS

Other common names Inhalants, glue
Drug category Central nervous system depressant

Habit-forming potential
There is a moderate risk of physical *dependence* with solvent abuse, but regular users may become psychologically dependent. Young people with family and personality problems are particularly at risk of becoming habitual users.

How taken
By breathing in the fumes, usually from a plastic bag placed over the nose and/or mouth or from a cloth or handkerchief soaked in the solvent.

Legitimate uses
Solvents are used in a wide variety of industrial, domestic, and cosmetic products. They function as aerosol propellants for spray paints, hair lacquer, lighter fuel, and deodorants. They are used in adhesives, paints, paint stripper, lacquers, gasoline, kerosene, and cleaning fluids. There are no legal restrictions on the sale of solvents.

Short-term effects
The short-term effects of solvents include lightheadedness, dizziness, confusion, and progressive drowsiness and loss of coordination with increasing doses. Accidents of all types are more likely. Large doses can lead to disorientation, hallucinations, and loss of consciousness. Nausea, vomiting, and headaches may also occur.

Long-term effects and risks
One of the greatest risks of solvent abuse is accidental death or injury while intoxicated. Some products, particularly aerosol gases, butane gas, and cleaning fluids, may seriously disrupt heart rhythm or cause heart failure and sometimes death. Aerosols and butane gas can also cause suffocation by sudden cooling of the airways and are particularly dangerous if squirted into the mouth. Butane gas has been known to ignite in the mouth. Aerosol products such as deodorant and paint may suffocate the user by coating the lungs. People have also suffocated while sniffing solvents from plastic bags placed over their heads. There is also a risk of death from inhalation of vomit and depression of the breathing mechanism.

Long-term misuse of solvent-based cleaning fluids can cause permanent liver or kidney damage, while long-term exposure to benzene (found in plastic cements, lacquers, paint remover, gasoline, and cleaning fluid) may lead to blood and liver disorders. Hexane-based adhesives may cause nerve damage leading to numbness and tremor. Repeated sniffing of leaded gasoline may cause lead poisoning. Regular daily use of solvents can lead to pallor, fatigue, and forgetfulness. Heavy use may affect school performance and lead to weight loss, depression, and general deterioration of health.

Solvent abuse and gasoline sniffing share similar effects and risks.

Signs of abuse
The majority of abusers are adolescents between the ages of 12 and 17, although the average age for this type of drug abuse is thought to be falling.

Obvious signs of solvent abuse include a chemical smell on the breath and traces of glue or solvents on the body or clothes. Other signs include furtive behavior, uncharacteristic moodiness, unusual soreness or redness around the mouth, nose, or eyes, and a persistent cough.

Interactions
Sniffing solvents increases the risk of sedation with any drug that has a *sedative* effect on the central nervous system. Such drugs include anti-anxiety drugs, sleeping drugs, and alcohol.

FOOD ADDITIVES

Almost all of us consume a number of processed, packaged, or other types of convenience foods every day. These include canned, dried, and frozen foods, breads, candy, and preserves. In addition to their basic food ingredients, most of these products contain a number of additional substances – chemicals that are supposed to enhance the appearance, flavor, texture, or freshness of the food.

Chemicals added to foods for sale in Canada are subject to rigorous scrutiny; only after they have been certified as safe are they approved for use by federal regulatory authorities. Like other chemicals, food additives can be harmful if consumed in large quantities. But the amounts of additives allowed in foods have been regulated to prevent this possibility. Except in the small number of people with sensitivity to certain additives such as sulfites, adverse effects are not common. For most people, the benefits of food additives outweigh any risks. Besides enhancing the appeal of food, these chemicals often act as safeguards by preventing production of poisons from spoilage and by inhibiting growth of disease-producing bacteria, molds, and other organisms. Nevertheless, increasing concern about the effects of chemicals taken in the form of medication is paralleled by a growing interest in the chemicals that are added to our diet. People want to know the purpose and possible effects of the often mysterious-sounding substances included in the list of ingredients on the labels of food products.

This page contains descriptions of the major types of food additives, explaining why they are used. The most common food additives are described individually and listed alphabetically on the following pages.

MAJOR TYPES OF ADDITIVES

Anticaking agents

These help powdered food or food particles, such as confectioner's, sugar and dried milk, to flow freely, preventing lumps from forming. They do this by absorbing moisture, thereby preventing it from entering the food particles.

Humectants

Humectants have a function opposite to that of anticaking agents – they attract moisture from the atmosphere, not from the food. They pass it on to the food and thus prevent it from drying out or becoming brittle.

Chemical preservatives

Chemical preservatives prevent foods from spoiling and increase their shelf life. They fall into two groups – anti-oxidants and antimicrobials. Anti-oxidants prevent certain fats (and, to a lesser extent, the vitamins) in food from deteriorating when they combine with oxygen. Without anti-oxidants, oxygen in the air reacts with chemicals in food (a process called oxidation), to produce substances that taint the food and make it taste or smell unpleasant, or even make it harmful. Vegetable oils contain varying amounts of vitamin E (tocopherol, which is a natural anti-oxidant) but it is often lost during processing. It can be replaced by the addition of synthetic anti-oxidants such as BHA (butylated hydroxyanisole) or BHT (butylated hydroxytoluene). Because of increasing public concern about the safety of synthetic anti-oxidants, many manufacturers are replacing them with ascorbic acid (vitamin C) in moist foods such as meat, bakery products, and beer, and with vitamin E in foods with a high fat content.

Antimicrobials prevent the multiplication of microorganisms that cause foods to decay. Sulfur dioxide and benzoic acid act as antibacterials; sorbic acid is an antifungal agent and is more effective against molds and yeasts; propionic acid is a fatty acid produced by bacteria and is also an antifungal agent. Antimicrobials include nitrates and nitrites, which prevent the growth in meats of *Clostridium botulinum*, the bacterium responsible for botulism, a sometimes fatal disorder.

Emulsifying agents

Emulsifiers are substances that help to form a stable mixture between two substances that do not normally mix. In food, this is usually fat and water. As an example, when egg yolk is used to make mayonnaise, the lecithin in the egg yolk works as an emulsifier. Emulsifiers also reduce the amount of fat that is needed in foods to which emulsifiers are added.

Sequestrants

Traces of metal, especially copper and iron, present in some foods, can speed the oxidation of fats and oils. By making those metals chemically inactive, sequestrants prevent foodstuffs from spoiling.

Flavorings

Flavorings are a very complex group; any one natural flavor can be a mixture of up to several hundred chemical substances. Flavorings may be natural substances obtained from fruits, nuts, vegetables, herbs, or spices. They may also be factory-made chemical copies of the original, or synthetic flavors developed in a laboratory. Synthetic flavors form the largest group. Manufacturers generally prefer synthetics because they are less likely to break down under the rigorous extremes of food processing and are less costly than their natural or nature-identical counterparts.

Most flavorings are safe, although some are only safe in limited use. A few have harmful effects.

Flavor enhancers

Flavor enhancers are included in foods to heighten the taste of the ingredients. Monosodium glutamate (MSG) is a particularly interesting flavor enhancer that occurs naturally in some soups when a meat-bone or fish stock is combined with vegetable ingredients to create a unique taste. MSG added to processed foods can bring out the sometimes weak flavor of a natural ingredient or intensify that of small amounts of artificial flavors.

Stabilizers

Stabilizers may have the same basic function as emulsifiers, or they may thicken the fat or, more usually, the watery part of the emulsion. They may also make the emulsion stickier and prevent its components from separating or curdling. Stabilizers therefore have a second function as jelling, thickening, or suspending agents.

A—Z OF ADDITIVES continued

ACACIA
Also known as gum arabic, sudan gum, gum Hashab, or Kordofan gum

Use Emulsifier, stabilizer, and thickening agent.
Found in Candies, jellies, glazes, puddings, gelatin desserts, ice cream, salad dressing, sodas, beer, wine, and appetite-reducing agents.
Adverse effects or risks Acacia slightly reduces the level of cholesterol in the blood. A few people have allergic reactions to it, after either eating it or inhaling it.

ACETATES
Also known as acetic acid. Includes allyl phenoxyacetate and allyl phenylacetate

Use Flavoring to give foods a variety of different flavors from liquor, nut, coffee, vanilla, and cheese to honey or pineapple.
Found in Beverages, ice creams, sherbets, cakes, cookies, pastries, and candy.
Adverse effects or risks None with normal use. May be irritating to the stomach if consumed in large quantities.

AGAR-AGAR
Also known as agar or Japanese isinglass

Use Thickener, stabilizer, and jelling agent.
Found in Ice cream, sherbet, baked goods, icings, and beverages.
Adverse effects or risks None in normal use. Excessive consumption could have a laxative effect and produce temporary distension of the abdomen and/or flatulence.

ALLYL ISOTHIOCYANATE
Also known as volatile oil of mustard, redskin, and allyl isosulfocyanate

Use Meat and spice flavoring.
Found in Mustard, horseradish, and onion (occurs naturally), beverages, ice creams, sherbets, candy, relishes, sauces, meats, and pickles.
Adverse effects or risks Negligible in the amounts used in food.

ANTHRANILATES
Also known as ethylanthranilate

Use Synthetic flavoring that gives a citrus, aniseed, licorice, vanilla, or rum flavor.
Found in Beverages, ice creams, sherbets, cakes, cookies, pastries, and candy.
Adverse effects or risks None.

ASCORBIC ACID
Also known as vitamin C

Use Anti-oxidant preservative. Prevents browning of cut fruit and fixes meat color in sausages.
Found in Frozen fruit, beer and ale, apple juice, candy, frankfurters, and cured or pickled meats.
Adverse effects or risks Although ascorbic acid is essential for healthy growth and iron absorption, excessively large amounts can cause diarrhea and some other disorders (see p.528).

BENZOIC ACID
Includes sodium benzoate

Use Antifungal and antibacterial preservatives.
Found in Margarine and a wide variety of acid-based foods and drinks, including purées, syrups, pickles, preserves, and alcoholic and non-alcoholic beverages.
Adverse effects or risks May have a numbing effect on the mouth and may trigger an asthma attack in asthma sufferers. People sensitive to ASA may find that benzoic acid causes allergic symptoms, such as breathlessness and watering eyes. It may also cause skin rashes.

BUTYLATED HYDROXYANISOLE
Also known as BHA

Use Anti-oxidant preservative.
Found in Many packaged foods, shortening, dry breakfast cereals, potatoes, ice creams, baked goods, candies, and beverages. It is the most widely used of the anti-oxidants.
Adverse effects or risks Safe at normal levels of intake.

BUTYLATED HYDROXYTOLUENE
Also known as BHT

Use Anti-oxidant preservative.
Found in Packaged convenience foods and snack foods, dry breakfast cereals, enriched rice, shortening, and chewing gum.
Adverse effects or risks Can cause skin rashes in certain people, who are often also sensitive to ASA.

BUTYRATES
Includes butyraldehyde, 2-ethyl-butyraldehyde, 2-ethylbutyric acid, isobutyl butyrate, alpha-alpha dimethyl-phenylbutyrate, isopropyl butyrate, and many more

Use Butter, butterscotch, caramel, chocolate, and fruit flavorings.
Found in Coffee and strawberries (occurs naturally), sodas and alcoholic beverages, ice creams and sherbets, candy, baked goods, puddings, and icings.
Adverse effects or risks None known in food use, but may cause skin irritation in factory workers.

CAFFEINE
Also known as methyltheobromine, guaranine, or theine

Use Flavoring.
Found in Coffee, cola, cocoa, root beer, and tea (occurs naturally).
Adverse effects or risks Stimulates the central nervous system, the heartbeat, and respiration rate, and acts as a diuretic (see p.111). An excess may cause insomnia, nervousness, irregular heartbeat, and diarrhea.

CALCIUM ALGINATE
Includes sodium alginate and potassium alginate

Use Stabilizer, thickener, suspending and jelling agent. Also a solvent and vehicle for flavorings. Sodium alginate is by far the most common of the three.
Found in Ice cream, popsicles, soft and cottage cheeses, cheese snacks, dressings and spreads, fruit drinks, beverages, and instant desserts.
Adverse effects or risks None known.

CARAMEL
Also known as plain (spirit) caramel, caustic sulfite caramel, ammonia caramel, and sulfite ammonia caramel

Use Brown coloring. It is the most widely used food coloring.
Found in Beverages, especially cola and a wide range of candy, chocolates, cakes and pastries, ice cream, and soya products.
Adverse effects or risks Its safety has been questioned for some time, especially when taken in large quantities. Sulfite ammonia caramel tested on humans produced soft to liquid stools and increased the frequency of bowel movements.

CARNAUBA WAX

Use Glazing and polishing agent for candy.
Found in Chocolates and candy.
Adverse effects or risks Occasional reports of skin irritation from skin contact with this substance.

CARRAGEENAN

Also known as Irish moss and Chondrus extract

Use Stabilizer, emulsifier, thickener, and suspending and jelling agent, especially in dairy products.
Found in Evaporated, condensed, and chocolate milks; milk shakes; sterilized, sour, and aerosol cream; and milk-based alcoholic beverages, pudding and custard mixes, ice cream, yogurt, cheese spreads, and salad dressing.
Adverse effects or risks Evidence suggests that carrageenan is safe.

CITRIC ACID

Use Sequestrant (especially in wine). Also used to prevent browning of cut fruit, to firm vegetables, add flavor, set jam, assist brewing, and cure meat.
Found in Canned and frozen fruit and vegetables, beer, wine, and cider, breakfast cereals, cheese, and cream.
Adverse effects or risks None likely in normal use.

ERYTHORBIC ACID

Also known as isoascorbic acid. Includes sodium erythorbate

Use Anti-oxidant preservative, color fixative in meat.
Found in Cured meat products, baked goods, beverages, and pickled products.
Adverse effects or risks None.

ETHYLENEDIAMINE TETRA-ACETIC ACID (EDTA)

Includes calcium disodium salt of EDTA and disodium dihydrogen salt of EDTA

Use Sequestrant.
Found in Canned foods, including crab, lobster, clams, shrimp, potato salad, mayonnaise, sandwich spreads, soda, beer, and malt whisky.
Adverse effects or risks None likely in food use.

ETHYL VANILLIN

Also known as ethovan

Use Flavoring.
Found in Ice creams, beverages, cakes, pastries, and other desserts.
Adverse effects or risks Appears to be safe in quantities used in foods.

FD & C RED No. 3

Also known as erythrosine

Use Red coloring.
Found in Cherries in canned fruit salads, maraschino and glacé cherries, and cherry pie mixes.
Adverse effects or risks Contains iodine and has been shown to affect the thyroid glands of laboratory animals, but not of humans. Children who eat huge amounts of artificially colored cherries could be at risk.

GLYCERIN

Use Humectant, sweetening agent, solvent.
Found in Candy, beverages, baked goods, chewing gum, and in edible coatings for meat and cheese.
Adverse effects or risks Safe in normal amounts.

GUAR GUM

Also known as guar flour, jaguar gum, and cluster bean gum

Use Stabilizer and suspending agent, thickener, dietary bulking agent, and firming and binding agent.
Found in Bottled sauces and salad dressings, carbonated beverages, meats, candies, baked goods, cream cheese, cheese spread, ice cream, yogurt, frozen fruit, and fruit drinks.
Adverse effects or risks In excessive amounts may cause nausea, flatulence, or abdominal cramps.

LECITHIN

Use Emulsifier, anti-oxidant, defoaming agent in yeast and sugar beet processing, cocoa substitute in chocolate. Increases volume in bread, protects vitamin A in margarine, and keeps the water content in food products.
Found in Chocolate and bakery products, breakfast cereals, frozen desserts, powdered milk, and popcorn.
Adverse effects or risks None.

MAGNESIUM CARBONATE

Also known as magnesite

Use Anticaking agent, alkali, acidity regulator, antibleaching agent.
Found in Table salt, flour, blue cheese, sour cream, and ice cream.
Adverse effects or risks None likely in the small amounts present in food.

METHYLCELLULOSE

Also known as methocel and cologel

Use Thickener, emulsifier, stabilizer, bulking and binding agent, and clarifier to form edible films for food products.
Found in Vinegar, beverages, and imitation jellies or jams. Used in foods for people on low-calorie diets.
Adverse effects or risks In large amounts may cause flatulence, distension of the abdomen, or intestinal obstruction; may also affect the absorption of minerals or other drugs.

METHYL PARABEN

Also known as methyl p-hydroxy-benzoate. Includes propyl p-hydroxy-benzoate and propyl paraben

Use Antimicrobial preservative.
Found in Beer, soda and fruit drinks, flavoring syrups, dessert sauces, fruit pulp and pie fillings, baked goods, candy, artificially sweetened jellies and preserves, and pickles.
Adverse effects or risks Asthmatics and people who are sensitive to ASA may be sensitive to the parabens and develop skin rashes or irritation of the lining of the mouth.

MONOGLYCERIDES

Includes diglycerides, mono- and diglycerides of fatty acids, glyceryl monostearate, distearate, and mono-sodium glycerides of edible fats and oils

Use Emulsifiers.
Found in Baked goods, margarines and shortenings, beverages, ice cream, ice milk, whipped toppings, and chocolate.
Adverse effects or risks None recorded.

MONOSODIUM GLUTAMATE

Also known as MSG

Use Flavor enhancer.
Found in A variety of savory canned and packaged foods, candy, baked goods, condiments, and pickles. Used extensively in Chinese cooking.
Adverse effects or risks MSG has been implicated in the "Chinese restaurant syndrome" (which includes facial flushing and headaches), but links with this condition have recently been shown to be tenuous.

MYRISTIC ACID
Also known as myristicin

Use Natural flavorings.
Found in Coconut, mace, palm seed and sperm whale oils, most animal and vegetable fats (occurs naturally), butterscotch, cocoa and fruit flavorings for beverages, candy, ice cream, and desserts.
Adverse effects or risks In the amounts used in foods it is not harmful.

OILS
Includes almond oil, bergamot oil, sandalwood oil, and many others

Use Natural flavorings.
Found in Beverages, ice cream, cakes, cookies, pastries, candy, chewing gum, soups, syrups, sauces and relishes, liqueurs, pickles, and meats.
Adverse effects or risks Some oils increase the levels of cholesterol and triglycerides in the blood.

PAPAIN
Also known as carica papaya, benase, and tomasin

Use Meat tenderizer and clarifying agent for beverages.
Found in Meat and meat products, beverages, and enriched farina.
Adverse effects or risks None known in normal food use. Most known cases of allergic reactions to papain have occurred in factory workers who have inhaled the powder, which caused asthma and urticaria (hives).

PECTIN
Use Stabilizer, jelling and thickening agent. Pectin is sometimes prescribed for diarrhea but has also been used as a bulk laxative (see Laxatives, p.123).
Found in Jams, jellies, marmalades, puddings and desserts, ice cream and sherbet, beverages, and syrups.
Adverse effects or risks It may cause distension or flatulence.

POLYSORBATE 60
Also known as polyoxyethylene (20) sorbitan monostearate

Use Emulsifier, stabilizer, wetting and dispersing agent for powdered processed foods, and a foaming agent for beverage mixes. It is added to chocolate coatings to prevent cocoa butter substitutes from tasting greasy.
Found in Frozen and gelatin desserts, cakes, cake mixes, doughnuts and artificial chocolate coatings, nondairy whipped cream and creamers, powdered convenience foods, salad dressings made without egg yolks, and vitamin supplements.
Adverse effects or risks None in normal food use.

POLYSORBATE 80
Also known as polyoxyethylene (20) sorbitan mono-oleate

Use Emulsifier, stabilizer, and humectant. Prevents oil from separating in nondairy whipped cream and helps nondairy coffee whiteners to dissolve.
Found in Baked goods, nondairy whipped cream, coffee whiteners, ice cream, frozen custard, shortenings, and in vitamin and mineral supplements.
Adverse effects or risks None in normal use.

PROPIONIC ACID
Includes calcium propionate and sodium propionate

Use Antifungal preservative, especially against the mold known as "rope" that affects bread. Also used as a flavoring.
Found in Baked goods such as bread and rolls, dairy products, pizzas, and processed cheeses. Propionic acid is also used in butter, fruit flavoring for beverages, ice creams, and candy. Calcium propionate is also used in poultry stuffing, chocolate products, cakes, and cupcakes.
Adverse effect or risks May cause migraine in migraine sufferers and contact with the chemical may cause skin irritations in bakery workers.

PROPYLENE GLYCOL
Use Humectant, solvent, and inhibitor of mold growth.
Found in Cakes, cookies, pastries, candy, breads and bread products, ice cream, icings and toppings, shredded coconut, beverages, emulsifiers, and meat products.
Adverse effects or risks None in normal use.

PROPYL GALLATE
Also known as propyl 3,4,5 trihydroxy-benzoate

Use Anti-oxidant preservative, on its own or combined with butylated hydroxy-anisole or butylated hydroxytoluene. Also used as a flavoring.
Found in Margarines, oils and shortenings; packaged snack foods such as popcorn, soup bases, potato flakes, dehydrated mashed potatoes, and mayonnaise. Propyl gallate provides citrus or spice flavors to beverages, ice cream, candy, and baked goods.
Adverse effects or risks Can cause stomach or skin irritation, especially in people who suffer from asthma or are sensitive to ASA.

SODIUM CARBOXYMETHYL CELLULOSE
Also known as carboxymethylcellulose, sodium salt, and cellulose gum

Use Stabilizer, thickener, jelling agent, and non-nutritive bulking aid. Used to prevent water loss, make food opaque, and to enhance the texture of food.
Found in Cakes, cookies, pastries, candy, bread and bread products, cake mixes, powdered beverages, pie fillings, dips and spreads, salad dressings, ice cream, whipped toppings, whipped cream, batter coatings, and processed and cottage cheeses.
Adverse effects or risks Could cause digestive disturbances.

SODIUM CITRATE
Includes monosodium citrate and disodium citrate

Use Adds acidity to food. Also used as sequestrant.
Found in Candy, ice cream, processed cheeses, fruit juices, and carbonated beverages.
Adverse effects or risks None known.

SODIUM HEXAMETA-PHOSPHATE

Also known as sodium polymeta-phosphate. Includes calcium hexameta-phosphate

Use Emulsifier, texturizing agent used to cure hams and as a sequestrant; used in bottled drinking water to prevent corrosion and buildup of scale.
Found in Bottled beer, water, and other beverages; processed cheese; breakfast cereals, angel food cake, ice cream, reconstituted lemon juice, and preserves.
Adverse effects or risks Phosphorus is an essential nutrient taken in balance with other minerals in the diet, such as calcium and magnesium. Too much phosphorus in the form of phosphates can upset the balance.

SODIUM NITRATE

Includes potassium nitrate (saltpeter), sodium nitrite, and potassium nitrite

Use Color fixatives.
Found in Processed meat and fish products.
Adverse effects or risks May cause dizziness, headaches, or difficulty in breathing, especially in children. There is some danger of nitrites (and converted nitrates) forming carcinogenic substances (nitrosamines), resulting in stomach cancer. The risk may be reduced by taking additional amounts of vitamins C and E.

SODIUM SULFITE

Also known as sodium and potassium hydrogen sulfite, disodium, and potassium pyrosulfite. Includes sodium and potassium bisulfites and metabisulfites

Use Antimicrobial preservatives, anti-oxidants, antibrowning agents.
Found in An extensive range of foods and beverages, including beer, wine, cider, fruit juices, syrups and purées, peeled potatoes, and cut, dried, or frozen fruit.
Adverse effects or risks Foods and drinks containing sulfites may release sulfur dioxide. If this is inhaled by people who suffer from asthma it can trigger an asthmatic attack. Sulfites are known to cause stomach irritation, nausea, diarrhea, skin rash, or swelling in sulfite-sensitive people. Deaths have occurred when sulfite-sensitive people were unaware that the foods they consumed either contained or were prepared with sulfites. People whose kidneys or livers are impaired may not be able to produce the enzymes that break down sulfites in the body. Sulfites may destroy thiamine and consequently are not added to foods that are sources of this vitamin.

SORBIC ACID

Includes potassium sorbate, calcium sorbate, and sodium sorbate

Use Preservatives against yeasts, molds, and bacteria in acid foods.
Found in Yogurts, processed cheeses, pickles and sauces, fruit pies, cordials, juices, jams, and jellies.
Adverse effects or risks None known in food use, although sorbic acid applied to the skin is irritating.

SORBITOL

Also known as D-glucitol and L-glucitol

Use Sweetening agent, especially in diabetic foods, humectant, sequestrant, stabilizer, and texturizer. Reduces the tendency of sugar to form crystals. It is also a diluent for food colors, masks the bitter aftertaste of saccharin, and helps to maintain the texture of chewy candy.
Found in A variety of chocolate, cakes, cookies, pastries, candy, ice cream, vegetable oils, bacon, and sausages.
Adverse effects or risks In small amounts, sorbitol presents no problems. Large amounts (60g for adults, 30g for children) may have a laxative effect or cause distension of the abdomen or flatulence.

SULFUR DIOXIDE

Use Preservative. Used to prevent oxidation and browning.
Found in Wine, beverages, fruit pulp, juice, and flavors, dehydrated fruit and vegetables, corn and table syrup, soups, sauces, and relishes.
Adverse effects or risks Only residual amounts should be present in or on the food, but even small amounts may provoke asthma in susceptible people. Sulfur dioxide may destroy thiamine and so is not added to foods containing this vitamin.

TARTARIC ACID

Includes sodium tartrate and sodium potassium tartrate (Rochelle salts)

Use Sequestrant (especially in wine), emulsifier, and acid diluent for food colors, constituent of grape and artificial sour- or tart-tasting products.
Found in Grapes (occurs naturally), wine, canned sodas and colas, candy, preserves, baked goods, dried egg white, lemon meringue pie mix, pasteurized processed cheese, cheese food and cheese spread, and some types of baking powder.
Adverse effects or risks Large amounts may have a laxative effect.

TARTRAZINE

Also known as FD&C Yellow No. 5

Use Yellow coloring.
Found in Foods, beverages, cosmetics, toothpastes, mouthwashes, and medications.
Adverse effects or risks Has been shown to cause a spectrum of reactions in sensitive individuals including hives, runny nose, asthma (ranging from mild to severe), and *anaphylaxis*. It is estimated that one quarter to one third of individuals sensitive to ASA are also sensitive to tartrazine.

TRIBASIC CALCIUM PHOSPHATE

Also known as tricalcium diorthophosphate and tricalcium phosphate

Use Anticaking agent, calcium supplement in grain products.
Found in Packaged cake mixes, candy, baked goods, gelatin desserts, powdered beverage mixes, seasoning mixes, soup mixes, and sugar.
Adverse effects or risks Too much phosphorus in the form of phosphates from processed food can upset the body's mineral balance.

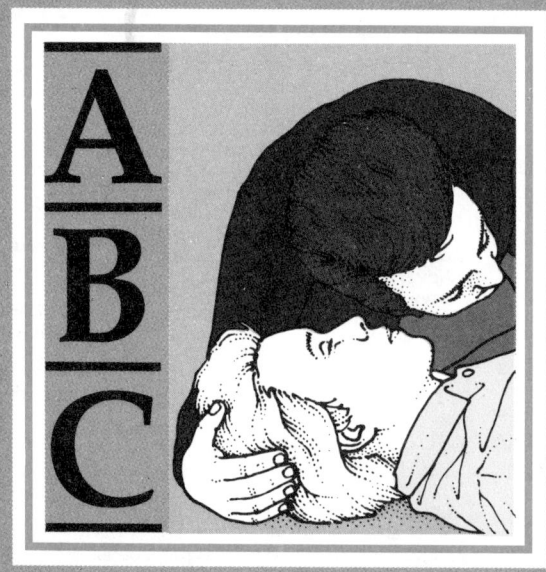

5

GLOSSARY
AND INDEX

GLOSSARY
GENERAL INDEX
DRUG POISONING EMERGENCY GUIDE

GLOSSARY

The following pages contain definitions of drug-related terms whose technical meanings are not explained in detail elsewhere in the book, or for which an easily located, precise explanation may be helpful. These are words that may not be familiar to the general reader or may have a meaning in the medical context that differs slightly from its ordinary meaning. Some of the terms included refer to particular drug actions or effects; others describe methods of drug administration.

A few medical conditions that may occur as a result of drug use are also defined. All words printed in italics within the main text are included as entries in this glossary.

The glossary is arranged in alphabetical order. Each entry has a bold heading. In order to avoid unnecessary repetition, entries include cross-references, where relevant, to another glossary term or to further information elsewhere in the book.

A

Addiction
An imprecise term that can cover anything from intense, habitual cravings for coffee, tea, or tobacco, to physical and psychological dependence on more potent agents such as narcotic drugs. See also *Dependence*.

Adjuvant
A drug that enhances the therapeutic effect of another, but does not necessarily have a beneficial effect alone. An example is aluminum, which is added to certain vaccines to augment the immune response, thereby enhancing the protection given by the vaccine.

Adrenergic
See *Sympathomimetic*.

Adverse reaction
An unexpected or unpredictable reaction to a drug, which is unrelated to the drug's usual effect. The cause may be an allergic reaction or the result of some genetic disorder, such as the lack of an enzyme that normally inactivates the drug. See also The effects of drugs (p.15).

Agonist
An agonist drug mimics the effect of a natural substance, such as a hormone, on a cell by binding to a cell's *receptor*, thereby stimulating a particular activity in that cell.

Amebacide
A drug that kills amebas (single-celled microorganisms). See also Antiprotozoal drugs (p.148).

Analeptic
Analeptic drugs cause excitation of the central nervous system. They are used in hospitals to stimulate breathing. See also Respiratory stimulants (p.100).

Analgesia
Relief of pain, usually by administration of drugs. See also Analgesics (p.92).

Anaphylaxis
A severe hypersensitivity reaction to an allergen, such as a drug or venom from a bee sting (see Allergy, p.135). Symptoms and signs may include rash, swelling, breathing difficulty and circulatory collapse. See also Dealing with anaphylactic shock (p.576).

Anemia
A condition of the blood in which the concentration of the oxygen-carrying pigment, hemoglobin, is below normal. Many different disorders may cause anemia; it may sometimes occur as a result of drug treatment. Severe anemia may cause fatigue, pallor and, occasionally, breathing difficulty.

Anesthetic, general
A drug or drug combination given to produce unconsciousness before and during surgery or potentially painful investigative procedures. General anesthesia is usually induced by an injection of a barbiturate drug, such as thiopental, and maintained by inhalation of a volatile liquid, such as halothane, or a gas, such as nitrous oxide mixed with oxygen. See also *Premedication*.

Anesthetic, local
A drug applied topically or injected to numb sensation in a small area. See also Local anesthetics (p.92).

Antagonist
An antagonist drug (often called a "blocker") blocks certain cellular activities by binding to a cell receptor, thereby preventing a normal substance or hormone from occupying that receptor. An antagonist does not stimulate any cellular activity.

Antibody
A protein manufactured by lymphocytes (one type of white blood cell) to neutralize foreign protein (an antigen) in the body. The formation of antibodies against an invading microorganism is part of the body's natural defense against infection.

Immunization is carried out to increase the body's resistance to a specific disease and involves either injection of specific antibodies or administration of vaccine that stimulates antibody production. See also Vaccines and immunization (p.146).

Anticholinergic
A drug that blocks the action of acetylcholine; anticholinergic drugs are also called *parasympatholytic* drugs. Acetylcholine is a *neurotransmitter* secreted by the endings of nerve cells that allows certain nerve impulses to be transmitted, including those that relax some involuntary muscles, tighten others and affect the release of saliva. Anticholinergic drugs are used to treat urinary incontinence because they relax the bladder's squeezing muscles while tightening those of the sphincter. Anticholinergic drugs also relax the muscles of the intestinal wall, helping to relieve irritable bowel syndrome (p.122). See also Autonomic nervous system (p.91).

Antidote
A substance that neutralizes or counteracts the effects of a poison. Very few poisons have a specific antidote.

Antineoplastic
An anticancer drug (p.166).

Antiperspirant
A substance applied to the skin to reduce excess sweating. Antiperspirants work by reducing the activity of the sweat glands or by blocking the ducts that carry sweat to the skin surface.

Antipyretic
A drug that reduces fever. The most commonly used antipyretic drugs are ASA and acetaminophen.

Antiseptic
A chemical that, when applied to the skin, destroys bacteria and prevents infection from spreading. See Anti-infective skin preparations (p.187).

Antispasmodic
A drug that reduces spasm (abnormally strong or inappropriate contractions) of the muscles of the gastrointestinal tract, airways, and blood vessels. Antispasmodic drugs are most commonly prescribed to relieve irritable bowel syndrome (p.122).

Antitussive
A drug that prevents or relieves a cough. See also Drugs to treat coughs (p.106).

Aperient
A mild laxative. See Laxatives (p.123).

Astringent
A substance that causes tissue to dry and shrink by reducing its ability to absorb water. Astringents are used in a number of *antiperspirants* and skin tonics because they remove excessive moisture from the skin surface. They are also used in ear drops for outer ear inflammation because they promote healing of the inflamed tissue.

B

Bactericidal
A term used to describe a drug that kills bacteria. See also Antibiotics (p.140) and antibacterial drugs (p.143).

Bacteriostatic
A term used to describe a drug that stops the growth or multiplication of bacteria. See also Antibiotics (p.140) and Antibacterial drugs (p.143).

Balm
A soothing or healing preparation applied to the skin.

Bioavailability
The amount of a drug that enters the bloodstream and thus reaches tissues throughout the body, usually expressed as a percentage of the dose given. The injection of a drug directly into a vein produces 100 per cent bioavailability. Drugs given by mouth generally have a much lower bioavailability because only a fraction of the drug can usually be absorbed through the digestive system. Also, some of the drug may be broken down in the liver before reaching the general circulation.

Body salts
Also known as electrolytes, these are compounds of various minerals that are present within cells and in such body fluids as blood, urine, and sweat. These salts play an important role in the regulation of water balance and acidity of the blood, conduction of nerve impulses, and muscle contraction. The balance between the various salts can be upset by such conditions as diarrhea and vomiting. The balance may also be altered by the action of drugs such as diuretics (p.111).

Brand name
See *Nonproprietary* name.

Bronchoconstrictor
A substance that causes the airways in the lungs to narrow, or constrict. An attack of asthma may be caused by the release of bronchoconstrictor substances such as histamine or certain prostaglandins.

Bronchodilator
A drug that widens the airways. See Bronchodilators (p.104).

C

Cathartic
A drug that stimulates bowel action to produce a soft or liquid bowel movement. See also Laxatives (p.123).

Chelating agent
A chemical used in the treatment of poisoning by metals such as iron, lead, arsenic, and mercury. It acts by combining with the metal to form a less poisonous substance and in some cases increases excretion in the urine. Penicillamine is a commonly used chelating agent.

Chemotherapy
The treatment of cancer or infections by drugs. *Cytotoxic* drugs (p.166) and antibiotics (p.140) are examples of drugs used in chemotherapy.

Cholinergic
A term used to describe a drug that stimulates the parasympathetic nervous system. A cholinergic drug is also known as a *parasympathomimetic* drug. See also Autonomic nervous system (p.91).

Coma
A state of unconsciousness and unresponsiveness to external stimuli such as noise and pain. Coma results from disturbance or damage to part of the brain. Drug overdose is a common cause.

Contraindication
A factor in a person's condition, medical history, or genetic make-up that may increase the risks of an adverse effect from a particular drug, to the extent that the drug should not be prescribed.

Counterirritant
Another term for *rubefacient*.

Cycloplegic
A term used to denote the action of paralyzing the ciliary muscle of the eye. Contraction of the ciliary muscle alters the shape of the lens, enabling the eye to focus on objects. A cycloplegic drug prevents this, and thus makes examination or surgery of the eye easier. See also Drugs affecting the pupil (p.182).

Cytotoxic
A term used to describe the ability to damage or kill cells. Cytotoxic drugs are most commonly used to treat cancer. They primarily affect abnormal cells but may also kill or damage healthy cells. See also Anticancer drugs (p.166).

D

Dependence
A term relating to physical or psychological dependence on a substance. Psychological dependence involves intense mental cravings if a drug is unavailable or withdrawn. Physical dependence produces physical signs and symptoms of withdrawal (sweating, shaking, abdominal pain, seizures, etc.) if the drug is not taken. Dependence also implies loss of control over intake. See also Drug dependence (p.23).

Depot injection
Injection of a drug that has been specially formulated to provide for a slow, steady absorption of its active ingredients into the bloodstream. The drug may be mixed with oil or wax. The release period can be made to last up to several weeks, depending on the formulation. See also Methods of administration (p.17).

Designer drugs
A group of unlicensed substances whose only purpose is to duplicate the effects of certain illegal drugs of abuse or to provide even stronger ones. Designer drugs differ chemically in some minor degree from the original drug, enabling the user and supplier to evade prosecution for possession of an illegal drug. They are extremely dangerous because they are often highly potent and may contain impurities.

Double-blind
A type of clinical trial commonly used to compare the effectiveness of a new drug or treatment with that of a *placebo* or an existing medication in which neither patients nor physicians know who is receiving what substance. Only after the test is complete and the patients' responses recorded is the identity of those who received the new drug or treatment revealed. Double-blind trials are carried out for almost all new drugs. See also Testing and approving new drugs (p.12).

Drip
A non-medical term for an *intravenous infusion*.

E

Electrolyte
See *Body salts*.

Elixir
A sweetened liquid often containing alcohol that forms a base for many medicines, such as those used to treat coughs.

Embrocation
An ointment rubbed on to the skin to relieve joint pain, muscle cramp, or muscle injury. An embrocation usually contains a *rubefacient*.

Emetic
Any substance that causes a person to vomit. An emetic may work by irritating the lining of the stomach or by stimulating the part of the brain that controls vomiting. An emetic, such as ipecac syrup, may be used in the treatment of drug overdose. See also Drug poisoning emergency guide (p.574).

Emollient
A substance that has a soothing, softening effect when applied to the skin. An emollient also has a moisturizing effect on dry skin, preventing loss of water from the skin surface by forming an oily film. See also Bases for skin preparations (p.187).

Emulsion
A combination of two substances that normally do not mix together properly but remain as particles of one suspended in the liquid form of the other. Many lotions are emulsions; they need to be shaken before use in case the constituent substances have separated.

Endorphins
A group of substances that occur naturally in the brain. Released in response to pain, they bind to specialized *receptors* and reduce perception of pain. Narcotic analgesics such as morphine work by mimicking the action of endorphins. See also Analgesics (p.92).

Enzyme
A protein that controls the rate of one or more chemical reactions in the body. There are thousands of active enzymes in the human body. Each type of body cell produces a specific range of enzymes. Cells in the liver contain enzymes that stimulate the breakdown of nutrients and drugs; cells in the digestive tract release enzymes that help digest food. Some drugs work by altering the activity of

enzymes – for example, certain anticancer drugs halt tumor growth by altering enzyme function in cancer cells.

Excitatory
A term meaning having a stimulating or enhancing effect. A chemical released from a nerve ending that causes muscle contraction has an excitatory effect. See also *Inhibitory*.

Expectorant
A type of cough remedy that enhances the production of sputum (phlegm) and is used in the treatment of a productive (sputum-producing) cough. See also Drugs to treat coughs (p.106).

FG

Formula, chemical
A way of expressing the constituents of a chemical in symbols and numbers. Every known chemical substance has a formula. Water, for instance, has the formula H_2O, indicating that it is composed of two hydrogen atoms (H_2) and one oxygen atom (O). Drugs have more complicated formulas.

Formulary
See *Pharmacopoeia*.

Generic name
A misnomer for *Nonproprietary name*.

H

Half-life
A term used in pharmacology for the time the body takes to eliminate half of the drug from the bloodstream. Knowledge of the half-life of a drug helps to determine frequency of dosage.

Hallucinogen
A drug that causes hallucinations (unreal perceptions of surroundings and objects). Common hallucinogens include the drugs of abuse LSD (p.535) and marijuana (p.536). Alcohol taken in large amounts may also have a hallucinogenic effect; hallucinations may also occur during alcohol withdrawal. Certain prescribed drugs may rarely cause hallucinations.

Hormone
A chemical released directly into the bloodstream by a gland or tissue. The body produces numerous hormones, each of which has a specific range of functions such as controlling the *metabolism* of cells, growth, sexual development, and the body's response to stress or illness. Hormone-producing glands make up the endocrine system (see Hormones and endocrine system,

p.152); the kidneys, intestine, and brain also release hormones.

I

Immunization
The process of inducing immunity (resistance to infection) as a preventive measure against the spread of infectious diseases. See Vaccines and immunization (p.146).

Infusion pump
A machine for administering a continuous controlled amount of a drug or other fluid through a needle inserted into a vein or under the skin. It consists of a small, battery-powered pump that controls the flow of fluid from a syringe into the attached needle. The pump is usually strapped to the patient and programmed to deliver the fluid at a constant rate. See also Methods of administration (p.17).

Inhaler
A device used for administering a drug in powder or vapor form into the lungs. Inhalers are used principally in the treatment of respiratory disorders such as asthma and chronic bronchitis. Among the medications administered in this way are corticosteroids and bronchodilator drugs. See also Methods of administration (p.17).

Inhibitory
A term meaning to have a blocking effect on cell activity. A chemical released from a nerve ending that prevents a muscle from contracting has an inhibitory effect. See also *Antagonist*.

Inoculation
Administration of microorganisms or other biological substances, usually by injection, to produce immunity to disease. See Vaccines and immunization (p.146).

Intramuscular injection
Injection of a drug into a muscle, usually into the upper arm or buttock. The drug is absorbed from the muscle into the bloodstream.

Intravenous infusion
Prolonged slow injection of fluid (often a solution of a drug) into a vein. The fluid flows at a controlled rate from a bag or bottle through a fine tube inserted into a needle placed in a vein. An intravenous infusion may also be administered via an *infusion pump*.

Intravenous injection
Direct injection of a drug into a vein, which puts the drug immediately into the circulation. Because it has a rapid effect, intravenous injection is useful in an emergency.

Investigational
A term used for a drug that is still being tested for efficacy and safety before approval for marketing is granted.

J

Jaundice
A condition in which the skin and whites of the eyes are yellowed. Jaundice is caused by an accumulation in the blood of the pigment bilirubin. Jaundice is a sign of excessive breakdown of red blood cells in the circulation, disorders of the liver, or blockage of the flow of bile to the digestive system. A drug may cause jaundice as an adverse effect either by damaging the liver or causing an increase in the breakdown of red blood cells.

LM

Lotion
A liquid preparation that may be applied to large areas of skin. See also Bases for skin preparations (p.187).

Medication
Any substance prescribed to treat illness.

Medicine
A term applied to a medication or drug that maintains, improves, or restores health. The practice of medicine is the diagnosis, assessment, treatment, and prevention of any disease, injury, dysfunction, disorder or other physical or mental condition.

Metabolism
The term for all chemical processes in the body that involve the formation of new substances or the breakdown of a substance to release energy. Metabolism provides energy required to keep the body functioning at rest – to maintain breathing, heartbeat, and body temperature. It also provides energy needed during exertion. Metabolism produces this energy from the breakdown of digested foods.

Miotic
A drug that constricts (narrows) the pupil. Opiate drugs such as morphine have a miotic effect, and someone who is taking one of these drugs characteristically has pinpoint pupils. The pupil is sometimes deliberately narrowed by other miotic drugs in the treatment of glaucoma. See also Drugs for glaucoma (p.180) and Drugs affecting the pupil (p.182).

Mucolytic
A drug that liquefies mucous secretions in the airways. See also Drugs to treat coughs (p.106).

Mydriatic
A term used to describe a drug that dilates (widens) the pupil. *Anticholinergic* drugs such as belladonna have this effect and may cause *photophobia* as a consequence. Mydriatic drugs may occasionally provoke the onset of glaucoma in susceptible people. See also Drugs affecting the pupil (p.182).

N

Narcotic
Stemming from the Greek word for numbness or stupor and once applied to drugs derived from the opium poppy, the word narcotic no longer has a precise medical meaning. Physicians today use the term narcotic analgesics to refer to opium-derived and synthetic drugs that have pain-relieving properties and other effects similar to those of morphine (see Analgesics p.92). See also Heroin (p.535).

Nebulizer
A method of administering a drug to the airways and lungs in aerosol form through a face mask. The apparatus includes an electric or hand-operated pump that sends a stream of air or oxygen through a length of tubing into a small canister containing the drug in liquid form. This inflow of gas causes the drug to be dispersed into a fine mist that is then carried through another tube into the face mask. Inhalation of this drug mist is much easier than inhaling from a pressurized aerosol (see also *Inhaler*).

Neuroleptic
A drug used to treat psychotic illness. See Antipsychotic drugs (p.97).

Neurotransmitter
A chemical released from a nerve ending after an electrical impulse arrives at the nerve ending. A neurotransmitter may carry a message from the nerve to another nerve so that the electrical impulse passes on to a muscle to stimulate contraction, or to a gland to stimulate secretion of a hormone. Acetylcholine and norepinephrine are examples of neurotransmitters. See also Brain and nervous system (p.90).

Nonproprietary name
A name (often called a generic name) applied to a single, therapeutically active drug not subject to trademark (proprietary) rights but recognized or recommended by government agencies (e.g., Health Protection Branch) and quasi-official organizations (e.g., World Health Organization, British Pharmacopoeia Commission) for public use. Example: diazepam is a nonproprietary name. Valium is a brand (proprietary) name product that contains diazepam.

O

Orphan drug
A drug that is effective for a rare condition, but that may not be marketed by a drug manufacturer because of the small sales and profit potential compared with the high cost of development, testing, and production.

OTC
The abbreviation for over-the-counter. OTC drug products can be purchased in pharmacies, or, in some cases, non-pharmacy outlets without a prescription from your physician.

P

Parasympatholytic
An *anticholinergic* drug that inhibits the parasympathetic nervous system by blocking the action of acetylcholine (see Autonomic nervous system, p.91).

Parasympathomimetic
A drug that stimulates the parasympathetic nervous system (see Autonomic nervous system, p.91). Parasympathomimetic (or *cholinergic*) drugs are used as *miotics* and to stimulate bladder contraction in urinary retention (see Drugs used for urinary disorders, p.178).

Parkinsonism
Neurological symptoms including tremor of the hands, muscle rigidity, and slowness of movements that resemble Parkinson's disease. Parkinsonism may be caused by prolonged treatment with an antipsychotic drug.

Pharmacist
A licensed, trained health professional who prepares and dispenses drugs. Pharmacists may advise on the correct use of non-prescription drugs and may answer many questions about the use of prescribed medications.

Pharmacokinetics
The term used to describe how the body deals with a drug, including how it is absorbed into the bloodstream, distributed to different tissues, broken down, and finally excreted from the body.

Pharmacologist
A scientist concerned with the study of drugs and their actions. Pharmacologists are responsible for research into new drugs. Clinical pharmacologists often may have an MD degree. They are primarily concerned with the actions of drugs in the treatment of specific disorders and with monitoring their

effects on patients in clinical trials and in medical practice.

Pharmacopoeia

A publication, also known as a formulary, that lists and describes drugs used in medicine. The term pharmacopoeia usually refers to an official national publication such as the British Pharmacopoeia (BP). Used as a reference book by physicians and pharmacists, a pharmacopoeia describes sources, preparations, doses, and tests that can be used to identify individual drugs and to determine their purity. It may also contain information about mechanisms of action, possible adverse effects, comments about the relative effectiveness and safety of a drug in treating a particular disorder, and price comparisons between similar drug products.

Pharmacy

The practice of pharmacy is the custody, compounding, and, upon the order of a practitioner legally qualified to order drugs, the dispensing of drugs, the provision of non-prescription drug products, health care aids and devices, and the provision of information related to the use of medications. The term pharmacy is also applied to the place where these activities are carried out.

Photophobia

Dislike of bright light. Photophobia may be induced by certain drugs.

Placebo

A substance, often in tablet or capsule form, that contains no medically active ingredient. Placebos are frequently used in clinical trials of new drugs (see *Double-blind*). A physician may administer a placebo because of the positive emotional or psychological benefit it may give to a patient convinced that his or her condition calls for some form of medication.

Poison

A substance that, in relatively small amounts, disrupts the structure or function of cells, causing harmful and sometimes fatal effects. Many drugs are poisonous if taken in overdose.

Premedication

The term applied to drugs given between one and two hours before an operation to prepare a person for surgery. Premedication usually contains a narcotic analgesic to help relieve pain and anxiety and to reduce the dose of anesthetic needed to produce unconsciousness (see also *Anesthetic, general*). An *anticholinergic* drug is sometimes included to reduce secretions in the airways.

Prescription

An instruction, usually in writing, from the physician or dentist to the pharmacist, giving the name of the drug or drug product to be dispensed, the dosage, how often it has to be taken, and other instructions as necessary. The prescription also carries the name and address of the patient for whom the medication is prescribed. The pharmacist keeps a record, often computerized, of all prescriptions dispensed. See also Managing your drug therapy (p.25).

Prophylactic

A term describing a drug, procedure, or piece of equipment used to prevent disease. For example, a course of drugs given to a traveler to prevent malarial infection is termed malaria prophylaxis.

Proprietary

A term now generally applied to the name of a drug product that is registered to a private manufacturer (i.e. a proprietor).

Purgative

A drug that helps eliminate feces from the body. See also *Cathartic*.

R

Receptor

A specific site on the surface of a cell with a characteristic chemical and physical structure. Natural body chemicals such as *neurotransmitters* bind to cell receptors to initiate a response in the cell. Many drugs also have an effect on cells by binding to a receptor. They may promote cell activity or may block it. See also *Agonist* and *Antagonist*.

Replication

The duplication of genetic material (DNA or RNA) within a cell as part of the process of cell division, which enables a tissue to grow or a virus to multiply.

Rubefacient

A preparation, also known as a counter-irritant, that, when applied to an area of skin, causes it to redden by increasing blood flow in vessels in that area. A rubefacient such as methyl salicylate may be included in an *embrocation*.

S

Sedative

A drug that dampens the activity of the central nervous system. Sleeping drugs (p.94) and anti-anxiety drugs (p.95) have a sedative effect, and many other drugs such as antihistamines (p.136) and antidepressants (p.96) can produce sedation as a side effect.

Side effect

A reaction to a drug that can be explain by the established effects of the drug itself. A side effect may be a predictable effect, such as dry mouth caused by an *anticholinergic* drug, or an exaggeration of the normal therapeutic effect, such as bleeding caused by an anticoagulant drug. The term is distinct from *adverse reaction*, which is an unpredictable effec

Subcutaneous injection

A method of administering a drug by which the drug is injected just beneath the skin. The drug is then slowly absorbed over a few hours into the surrounding blood vessels. Insulin is given in this way. See also Methods of administration (p.17).

Sublingual

A term meaning under the tongue. Som drugs are administered sublingually in tablet form. The drug is then very rapidl absorbed through the lining of the mout into the bloodstream within a few seconds. Nitrate drugs may be given thi way to provide rapid relief of an angina attack. See also Methods of administration (p.17).

Suppository

A bullet-shaped pellet usually containing a drug for insertion into the rectum or vagina. See also Methods of administration (p.17).

Sympatholytic

A term meaning blocking the effect of th sympathetic nervous system. Sympatho lytic drugs work either by reducing the release of the stimulatory *neurotrans-mitter* norepinephrine from nerve ending or by occupying the *receptors* to which the neurotransmitters epinephrine and norepinephrine normally bind, thereby preventing their normal actions. Beta blockers are examples of sympatholytic drugs. See also Autonomic nervous system (p.91).

Sympathomimetic

Having the same effect as stimulation o the sympathetic nervous system to cause, for example, an increase in the heart rate. A drug with a sympatho-mimetic action may work by causing the release of the stimulatory *neuro-transmitter* norepinephrine from nerve endings or by mimicking the action of stimulatory neurotransmitters. See also Autonomic nervous system (p.91).

Systemic

Having a generalized effect, causing physical or chemical changes in tissues throughout the body. For a drug to have systemic effect it must be absorbed into the bloodstream, usually via the digestiv tract, by injection or by rectal suppositc

T

Tardive dyskinesia
Abnormal, uncontrolled movements, mainly of the face, tongue, mouth, and neck, that may be caused by prolonged treatment with antipsychotic drugs. This condition is distinct from *parkinsonism*, which may also be caused by such drugs. See also Antipsychotic drugs (p.97).

Tolerance
The need to take a higher dosage of a specific drug to maintain the same physical or mental effect. Tolerance may occur during prolonged treatment with narcotic analgesics and benzodiazepines. See also Drug dependence (p.23).

Tonics
A diverse group of remedies prescribed or bought over the counter for relieving vague symptoms such as malaise, lethargy, and loss of appetite for which no obvious cause can be found. Tonics sometimes contain vitamins and minerals, but there is no scientific evidence that such ingredients have anything other than a *placebo* effect. Nevertheless, many individuals feel better after taking a tonic for a few weeks.

Topical
The term used to describe the application of a drug to the site where it is intended to have its effect. Disorders of the skin, eye, outer ear, nasal passages, and vagina are often treated with drugs applied topically.

Toxic reaction
Symptoms, which can sometimes be dangerous, caused by a drug as the result of either an overdose or an *adverse reaction*.

Toxin, toxic
A toxin is a poisonous substance such as a harmful chemical released by bacteria or created by a drug interaction. Drugs that are usually safe in normal doses may produce toxic effects when taken in overdose. An *adverse reaction* may also be produced by a toxin. See The effects of drugs (p.15).

Tranquilizer, major
A drug used to treat psychotic illnesses such as schizophrenia. See Antipsychotic drugs (p.97).

Tranquilizer, minor
A *sedative* drug used to treat anxiety and emotional tension. See Anti-anxiety drugs (p.95).

Transdermal patch
A method of administering a drug in which an adhesive patch impregnated with the drug is placed on the skin. The drug is slowly absorbed through the skin into the underlying blood vessels. Drugs administered in this way include scopolamine and estradiol. See also Methods of administration (p.17).

V

Vaccine
A substance administered to induce active immunity against a specific infectious disease (see Vaccines and immunization, p.146).

Vasoconstrictor
A drug that narrows blood vessels often prescribed to reduce nasal congestion. See Decongestants (p.105). Vasoconstrictors are also frequently given with injected local anesthetics (p.92). Pseudoephedrine is a commonly prescribed vasoconstrictor.

Vasodilator
A drug that widens blood vessels. See Vasodilators (p.110).

W

Withdrawal symptom
Any symptom caused by abrupt stopping of a drug. These symptoms occur as a result of physical *dependence* on a drug. Drugs that may cause withdrawal symptoms after prolonged use include narcotics, benzodiazepines, and nicotine. Withdrawal symptoms vary according to each drug, but common examples include sweating, shaking, anxiety, nausea, and abdominal pain. See also Drug dependence (p.23).

GENERAL INDEX

Use this index to look up specific drugs and medications or general topics such as drug groups, diseases, and conditions. In Part 2 there is a special Index of Medications where further information on individual drugs can be found (see pp.49–87). Many of the page numbers listed in this General Index refer to the drugs and other substances listed in the Index of Medications.

Entries for brand-name tablets and capsules that are shown in the Color Identification Guide contain italicized references to the appropriate page and grid letter.

References that consist of a page number followed by the letter g indicate terms that are defined in the glossary.

A

Abbokinase 49
Abenol see Acetaminophen 199
Acacia 540
Accupril see Quinapril 455
Accutane see Isotretinoin 352
Acebutolol 198
Acecainide 49
Aceclidine 49
ACE inhibitors 110, 114
Acetaminophen 199
Acetates 540; see also Acetic acid 49
Acetazolamide 49, 111, 181
Acetazone Forte 49
Acetazone Forte C8 49
Acetic acid 49; see also Acetates 540
Acetohexamide 49, 155
Acetone 49
Acetophenazine 49
Acetoxyl 49
Acetylcholine 49
Acetylcysteine 49
Acetylsalicylic acid 200
Achrocidin 49
Achromycin V see Tetracycline 489
Acid see LSD 535; see also Antacids 120; Anti-ulcer drugs 121
Acilac see Lactulose 356
Acitretin see Vitamin A 527
Aclarubicin 49
Acne, drugs for 189
Acnex 49
Acnomel 49
Acnomel Acne Mask 49
Acnomel B.P.5 see Benzoyl peroxide 224
Acrisorcin 49
Acritretin 49
Acrivastine 49
Acromegaly see Drugs for pituitary disorders 157
Acrosoxacin 49
ACTH see corticotropin 58
Acthar see corticotropin 58
Acti-B12 49
Actifed see Pseudoephedrine 450
Actifed DM 49

Actinac 50; see Chloramphenicol 249
Actiprofen see Ibuprofen 341
Activase see Tissue plasminogen activator 495
Activase rt-PA see Tissue plasminogen activator 495
Acular see Ketorolac 355
Acyclovir 201
Adalat see Nifedipine 404
Adalat PA 10 35M (illus.); see Nifedipine 404
Adalat PA 20 35J (illus.); see Nifedipine 404
Adalat XL 35K, 35L (illus.); see Nifedipine 404
Adasept Acne Gel 50
Adasept Cleanser 50
Addiction 546g; see Drug dependence 23-24
Addison's disease see Corticosteroids 153
Additives see Food additives 539-543
ADHD see Methylphenidate 385
Adjuvant 546g
Adrenalin see Epinephrine 300
Adrenergic 546g
Adrenocorticotropic hormone see Corticotropin 58
Adrucil see Fluorouracil 317
Adsorbent agents see Antidiarrheal drugs 122
Adverse reactions 15, 546g
Advil see Ibuprofen 341
Advil Cold & Sinus see Ibuprofen 341; pseudoephedrine 450
Aerosol inhalers 19
Aerosporin 50
Agar 50
Agar-agar 540
Agarol Plain 50
Agarol Tablets 50
Agarol Vanilla 50
Agonist 546g; action of 14
A-Hydrocort 50
AIDS, drugs for 169
AK-Cide see Sulfacetamide 473
Akineton 50
AK-Sulf see Sulfacetamide 473
Albalon Liquifilm 50
Albalon-A Liquifilm 50
Albert Glyburide 45M (illus.); see Glyburide 330

Albert Tiafen 41L (illus.); see Tiaprofenic acid 492
Albuterol see Salbutamol 461
Alcaine 50
Alcohol 532
Alcohol, rubbing 50; see also isopropyl alcohol 67
Alcometasone 50
Alcomicin see Gentamicin 328
Aldactazide see Hydrochlorothiazide 336; Spironolactone 469
Aldactone see Spironolactone 469
Aldomet see Methyldopa 384
Aldoril 50
Alfacalcidol see Vitamin D 529
Alfenta 50
Alfentanil 50
Algeldrate 50
Alginates see Antacids 120
Alginic acid 50
Alka-Seltzer 50
Alkeran 50
Alkylating agents 167
Allantoin 50
Allerdryl see Diphenhydramine 290
Allergy treatments 135-137 bronchodilator 104, 547g decongestant 105 See also Antihistamines
Allernix see Diphenhydramine 290
Allopurinol 202
Allylestrenol 50
Allyl isosulfocyanate see Allyl isothiocyanate 540
Allyl isothiocyanate 540
Allyl phenoxyacetate see Acetates 540
Allyl phenylacetate see Acetates 540
Almond oil see Oils 542
Aloin 50
Alomide 50
Alophen 50
Alpha-adrenergic blockers 178
Alpha-alpha Dimethylphenylbutyrate see Butyrates 540
Alpha-Baclofen see Baclofen 221
Alpha interferon 169
Alpha Keri 50
Alpha-Lac 50

Alphaprodine 50
Alpha-Tamoxifen see Tamoxifen 480
Alpha-tocopherol acetate see Vitamin E 529
Alphosyl 50
Alprazolam 44T (illus.); 203
Alprostadil 50
Alseroxylon 50
Altace 50
Alteplase see Tissue plasminogen activator 495
Altretamine 50
Aluminum acetate 50
Aluminum carbonate 50
Aluminum chloride 50
Aluminum hydroxide 204
Alupent see Orciprenaline 415
Alu-Tab see Aluminum hydroxide 204
Alverine 50
Amantadine 205
Amatine 50
Ambenonium 50
Ambenyl 50
Amcinonide 50
Amdinocillin 50
Amebacide 546g
Amebiasis 148
Amenorrhea see Drugs used to reduce prolactin levels 157; Drugs used to treat menstrual disorders 172
Amesec 50
Amethocaine 50
Amethopterin 50
Amicar 50
Amikacin 50
Amikin 50
Amiloride 206
Aminacrine 50
Aminoacetic acid 50
Aminobenzoate potassium 50
Aminobenzoic acid 51; see also Sunscreens 191
Aminocaproic acid 51
Aminoglutethimide 51
Aminoglycosides 141, 142
Aminophylline see Theophylline 490
Aminosalicylate sodium 51
5-aminosalicylic acid see Mesalamine 378
Aminothiadiazole 51
Amiodarone 207

amitriptyline 208
amlodipine 209
ammonia caramel see Caramel 540
ammoniated mercury 51
ammonium chloride 51
amobarbital 51
amodiaquine 51
amoxapine 51
amoxicillin 210
amoxil 47C, 47D (illus.); see Amoxicillin 210
amphetamines 533
amphojel see Aluminum hydroxide 204
amphojel 500 51
amphojel Plus 51
amphotericin B 211
ampicillin 212
ampicin see Ampicillin 212
amrinone 51
amsacrine 51
MSA-PD 51
amyl nitrite 51
amylobarbitone 51
amylocaine 51
amytal 51
anabolic steroids 158
anacin 51
anafranil see Clomipramine 264
anagrelide 51
ana-Kit 51
anal disorders, drugs for 125
analeptic 546g
analgesia 546g; see Analgesics 92-93
anandron 51
anaphylactic shock (anaphylaxis) 546g, 576
anapolon 50 51
anaprox 39K (illus.); see Naproxen 400
anbesol Gel 51
ancef 51
ancotil 51
ancrod 51
andriol see Testosterone 488
androcur 51
androgens 158
anectine 51
anemia 546g
anesthetic
  general 546g
  local 546g
  see Local anesthetics
anetholtrithione 51
anexate 51
angel dust see Phencyclidine 538
angina see Anti-angina drugs 113
angiotensin-converting enzyme inhibitors see ACE inhibitors 110, 114
anileridine 51
anisindione 51
ansaid see Flurbiprofen 321
ansamycin 51
antabuse see Disulfiram 294
antacids 120
antagonist 546g

Antazoline 51
Anthelmintic drugs 151
Anthraforte see Anthralin 213
Anthralin 213
Anthranilates 540
Anthranol see Anthralin 213
Anthrascalp see Anthralin 213
Anti-androgens 178
Anti-angina drugs 113
Anti-anxiety drugs 95
Anti-arrhythmic drugs 112
Antibacterial drugs 143
Antibiotics 140-142
  cytotoxic 167
Antibody 546g
Anticancer drugs 166-167
Anticholinergic 546g
  antiparkinsonism 99
  bronchodilator 104
  mydriatic 182
  in urinary disorders 178
Anticoagulant drugs 116-117
Anticonvulsant drugs 98
Antidepressant drugs 96
  as sleeping drugs 94
Antidiarrheal drugs 122
Antidote 546g
Anti-emetic drugs 102
Antifibrinolytic drugs 116, 117
Antifungal drugs 150
Antihemophilic factor 51
Antihistamines 136-137 and
  action of anti-ulcer drugs 121
  as anti-emetics 102
  as antipruritics 185
  interactions of 16
  as sleeping drugs 94
Antihypertensive drugs 114
Anti-infective skin preparations 187
Anti-inflammatory drugs, non-steroidal 128
Antimalarial drugs 149
Antimanic drugs 97
Antimetabolites 167
Antimicrobials see Chemical preservatives 539
Antimony-based agents 148
Antineoplastic 546g
Anti-oxidants see Chemical preservatives 539
Antiparkinsonism drugs 99
Antiperspirant 546g
Antiplatelet drugs 116, 117
Antiprotozoal drugs 148
Antipruritic medications 185
Antipsychotic drugs 97
Antipyretic 546g
Antipyrine 51
Antirheumatic drugs 129
Antiseptic 187, 546g
Antispasmodic 122, 547g
Antithymocyte globulin 168
Antithyroid drugs 156
Antituberculous drugs 144
Antitussive 547g; see Cough remedies 106
Anti-ulcer drugs 121
Antivert 51

Antiviral drugs 145
Anturan see Sulfinpyrazone 476
Anusol 51
Anusol-HC 51
Anusol Plus 51
Anuzinc 51
Anxiolytics see Anti-anxiety drugs 95
APAP 51
Aparkane see Trihexyphenidyl 505
APL see Human chorionic gonadotropin 334
Apo-Acetaminophen 41M, 41P (illus.); see Acetaminophen 199
Apo-Acetazolamide 51
Apo-Allopurinol 36P (illus.); see Allopurinol 202
Apo-Alpraz 36L, 44Q (illus.); see Alprazolam 203
Apo-Amilzide 36H (illus.); 51
Apo-Amitriptyline 38A, 39E, 40G (illus.); see Amitriptyline 208
Apo-Amoxi 47A, 47B (illus.); see Amoxicillin 210
Apo-Ampi see Ampicillin 212
Apo-ASA see ASA 200
Apo-Atenol 42H (illus.); see Atenolol 215
Apo-Benztropine 42S (illus.); see Benztropine 225
Apo-Bisacodyl see Bisacodyl 229
Apo-Bromocriptine see Bromocriptine 231
Apo-C 51
Apo-Cal 51
Apo-Capto 43R, 45T (illus.); see Captopril 239
Apo-Carbamazepine 42D (illus.); see Carbamazepine 240
Apo-Cephalex 36Q (illus.); see Cephalexin 245
Apo-Chlorax 52
Apo-Chlordiazepoxide see Chlordiazepoxide 250
Apo-Chlorpropamide see Chlorpropamide 253
Apo-Chlorthalidone see Chlorthalidone 254
Apo-Cimetidine see Cimetidine 257
Apo-Clomipramine see Clomipramine 264
Apo-Clonidine see Clonidine 266
Apo-Clorazepate see Clorazepate 267
Apo-Cloxi see Cloxacillin 269
Apo-Diazepam 38F, 39H (illus.); see Diazepam 282
Apo-Diclo 40K (illus.); see Diclofenac 283
Apo-Diflunisal see Diflunisal 285
Apo-Diltiaz 38J, 38O (illus.); see Diltiazem 287
Apo-Dimenhydrinate see Dimenhydrinate 288
Apo-Dipyridamole see Dipyridamole 292

Apo-Doxy 46I (illus.); see Doxycycline 297
Apo-Enalapril 37Q, 40D, 43S (illus.); see Enalapril 299
Apo-Erythro 52
Apo-Erythro-ES 52
Apo-Famotidine 40F (illus.); see Famotidine 309
Apo-Ferrous Gluconate 52
Apo-Ferrous Sulfate 52
Apo-Fluphenazine see Fluphenazine 319
Apo-Flurazepam 47J (illus.); see Flurazepam 320
Apo-Flurbiprofen see Flurbiprofen 321
Apo-Folic 52
Apo-Furosemide 38I, 43J (illus.); see Furosemide 325
Apo-Gain see Minoxidil 392
Apo-Gemfibrozil see Gemfibrozil 327
Apo-Glyburide 45P (illus.); see Glyburide 330
Apo-Guanethidine 52
Apo-Haloperidol see Haloperidol 332
Apo-Hydralazine see Hydralazine 335
Apo-Hydro 36B, 36C (illus.); see Hydrochlorothiazide 336
Apo-Hydroxyzine see Hydroxyzine 340
Apo-Ibuprofen 37F (illus.); see Ibuprofen 341
Apo-Imipramine see Imipramine 343
Apo-Indomethacin see Indomethacin 345
Apo-ISDN see Isosorbide dinitrate 351
Apo-K 37B (illus.); see potassium 524
Apo-Keto see Ketoprofen 354
Apo-Lorazepam 43K, 44N, 45R (illus.); see Lorazepam 367
Apo-Meprobamate see Meprobamate 377
Apo-Methazide 52
Apo-Methyldopa see Methyldopa 384
Apo-Metoclop see Metoclopramide 387
Apo-Metoprolol see Metoprolol 388
Apo-Metoprolol-L 35I (illus.); see Metoprolol 388
Apo-Metronidazole see Metronidazole 389
Apo-Nadol see Nadolol 398
Apo-Naproxen 36M, 38C (illus.); see Naproxen 400
Apo-Nifed see Nifedipine 404
Apo-Nitrofurantoin see Nitrofurantoin 407
Apo-Oxazepam 37N (illus.); see Oxazepam 417
Apo-Oxtriphylline 52

Apo-Pen VK *41S* (illus.); see
  Penicillin V 425
Apo-Perphenazine see
  Perphenazine 428
Apo-Phenylbutazone 52
Apo-Pindol see Pindolol 434
Apo-Piroxicam see Piroxicam 435
Apo-Prazo see Prazosin 438
Apo-Prednisone *43E* (illus.); see
  Prednisone 440
Apo-Primidone see Primidone
  441
Apo-Procainamide see
  Procainamide 443
Apo-Propranolol *38Q* (illus.); see
  Propranolol 448
Apo-Quinidine 52
Apo-Ranitidine *42C, 45F* (illus.);
  see Ranitidine 458
Apo-Salvent see Salbutamol 461
Apo-Spirozide see
  Spironolactone 469
Apo-Sulfamethoxazole see
  Sulfamethoxazole 474
Apo-Sulfatrim *41G* (illus.); 52
Apo-Sulfatrim DS *45C* (illus.); 52
Apo-Sulfatrim Pediatric 52
Apo-Sulfinpyrazone see
  Sulfinpyrazone 476
Apo-Sulfisoxazole see
  Sulfisoxazole 477
Apo-Sulin 52; see Sulindac 478
Apo-Tamoxifen see Tamoxifen
  480
Apo-Terfenadine see Terfenadine
  487
Apo-Tetra *47M* (illus.); see
  Tetracycline 489
Apo-Theo LA see Theophylline
  490
Apo-Thioridazine see Thioridazine
  491
Apo-Timol see Timolol 494
Apo-Timop see Timolol 494
Apo-Tolbutamide see
  Tolbutamide 497
Apo-Triazide *37J* (illus.); 52
Apo-Triazo *39J* (illus.); see
  Triazolam 503
Apo-Trifluoperazine see
  Trifluoperazine 504
Apo-Trihex see Trihexyphenidyl
  505
Apo-Trimip see Trimipramine 508
Apo-Verap see Verapamil 513
Apo-Zidovudine see Zidovudine
  516
Apraclonidine 52
Apresoline see Hydralazine 335
Aprindine 52
Aprotinin 52
Aquasol A 52
Aquasol A and D 52
Aquasol E 52
Arachis oil 52
Aralen 52
Aredia 52
Arfonad 52
Argipressin 52

Aristocort see Triamcinolone 501
Aristoform R 52
Aristospan see Triamcinolone 501
Arlidin 52
Arlidin Forte 52
Arnica 52
Arrhythmia see Anti-arrhythmic
  drugs 112
Artane see Trihexyphenidyl 505
Artemisinine 52
Arthritis, drugs for
  antirheumatic 129
  corticosteroid 130
  NSAID 128
Arthrotec *41Q* (illus.); 52
Articaine 52
Arvin 52
ASA 200
Asacol *40B* (illus.); see
  Mesalamine 378
Asaphen 53
Asasantine 53
Asbron see Theophylline 490
Ascariasis see Anthelmintic drugs
  151
Ascofer 53
Ascorbate calcium see Vitamin C
  528
Ascorbate sodium see Vitamin C
  528
Ascorbic acid see Vitamin C 528;
  A-Z of additives 540
Asendin 53
Asmavent see Salbutamol 461
Asparaginase 53
Aspercreme 53
Aspergum 53
Aspirin see ASA 200
Astemizole 214
Asthma, drugs for
  antihistamine 136-137
  bronchodilator 104
  corticosteroid 153
Astringent 547g
  in rectal and anal disorders 125
Atabrine 53
Atarax see Hydroxyzine 340
Atasol see Acetaminophen 199
Atasol-8 53
Atasol-15 53
Atasol-30 53
Atasol Forte 53
Atenolol 215
Atherosclerosis, drugs for
  Bezafibrate 228
  Lipid-lowering drugs 115
Athlete's foot see Antifungal
  drugs 150
Ativan *44P, 45S* (illus.); see
  Lorazepam 367
Ativan SL *38R* (illus.); see
  Lorazepam 367
Atovaquone 53
Atracurium 53
Atrial fibrillation see
  Anti-arrhythmic drugs 112
Atromid-S 53
Atropine 53
Atropisol 53

Atrovent see Ipratropium bromide
  348
Attapulgite 53
Attention-deficit hyperactivity
  disorder see ADHD
Auralgan 53
Auranofin 216
Aureomycin 53
Aurothioglucose 53
Autonomic nervous system 91
AVC 53
Aventyl see Nortriptyline 411
Avirax see Acyclovir 201
Avlosulfon 53
Avobenzone (Parsol 1789) 191
Axid *47S* (illus.); see Nizatidine
  409
Ayercillin see Penicillin G 424
Azacitidine 53
Azatadine 217
Azathioprine 218
Azidothymidine see Zidovudine
  516
Azithromycin 219
Azlocillin 53
Azmacort 53
Azo Gantrisin 53
Aztreonam 53
AZT see Zidovudine 516

B

Bacampicillin 53
Baciguent see Bacitracin 220
Bacitin see Bacitracin 220
Bacitracin 220
Baclofen 221
Bacterial infection see
  Antibacterial drugs 143
Bactericidal 547g
Bacteriostatic 547g
Bactigras 53
Bactine 53
Bactrim 53
Bactrim DS 53
Bactroban see Mupirocin 396
Balantidiasis 148
Baldness see Treatment for
  dandruff and hair loss 191
Balm 547g
Balminil Decongestant Syrup see
  Pseudoephedrine 450
Balminil DM see
  Dextromethorphan 281
Balminil Expectorant see
  Guaifenesin 331
Balnetar 53
Barbilixir see Phenobarbital 430
Barbiturates 533
Barriere 53
Barriere-HC 53
Basaljel see Aluminum hydroxide
  204
Bazalip see Bezafibrate 228

BCG vaccine 144
Beben 53
Beclodisk see Beclomethasone
  222
Becloforte see Beclomethasone
  222
Beclomethasone 222
Beclovent see Beclomethasone
  222
Beclovent Rotacaps 53
Beconase see Beclomethasone
  222
Bedsores, drugs for 187
Bedwetting see Drugs for urinary
  incontinence 178
Belladonna 53
Bellergal 53
Beminal 53
Beminal 500 53
Beminal Fortis Elixir 53
Beminal with C Fortis 53
Benadryl see Diphenhydramine
  290
Benadryl Decongestant 53
Benase see Papain 542
Benazepril 53
Bendroflumethiazide 53
Benemid see Probenecid 442
Ben Gay 53
Benign prostatic hyperplasia 178
Bennies see Amphetamines 533
Benoxinate 53
Benoxyl 53
Benserazide 54
Bentylol 54
Benuryl see Probenecid 442
Benylin Codeine-D-E 54
Benylin DM see
  Dextromethorphan 281
Benylin DM-D 54
Benylin DM-D-E 54
Benylin DM-E see Guaifenesin
  331
Benylin E see Guaifenesin 331
Benzac AC 54
Benzac W see Benzoyl peroxide
  224
Benzagel see Benzoyl peroxide
  224
Benzalkonium chloride 54; see
  also Artificial tear preparation
  182
Benzathine penicillin G 54
Benzethonium chloride 54
Benzhexol 54
Benznidazole 54
Benzocaine 223
Benzodiazepines 534
  as anti-anxiety drugs 95
  as anticonvulsants 98
  as sleeping drugs 94
Benzoic acid 54
Benzoin tincture 54
Benzophenone 191
Benzoyl peroxide 224
Benzquinamide 54
Benztropine 225
Benzydamine 226
Benzyl alcohol 54

enzyl benzoate 54
enzylpenicillin see Penicillin G 424
ephenium 54
ergamot oil see Oils 542
eriberi 527
erocca-C 54
erotec see Fenoterol 312
eta blockers 109
  as anti-angina drugs 113
  as anti-anxiety drugs 95
  as anti-arrhythmics 112
  as antihypertensives 114
  in glaucoma 181
eta-carotene see Vitamin A 527
etacort 54
etaderm 54
etadine 54
etahistine 54
etaloc see Metoprolol 388
etaloc Durules 54
etamethasone 227
etaxin 54
etaxolol 54
ethanechol 54
etnesol see Betamethasone 227
etnovate see Betamethasone 227
etoptic 54
evantolol 54
ewon 54
ezafibrate 228
ezalip 54
HA see Butylated hydroxyanisole 540; Chemical preservatives 539
HT see Butylated hydroxytoluene 540; Chemical preservatives 539
axin 38K (illus.); see Clarithromycin 260
carbonate see Sodium bicarbonate 120
cetonium 54
cillin see Penicillin G 424
CNU 54
le salts 54
oavailability 547g
oderm 54
onet 54
ct 519
penuen 54
quin see Quinidine 456
quin Durules 54
sacodyl 229
smed Liquid 54
smed Tablets 54
smuth 54
smuth subsalicylate 121
soprolol 54
thionol 54
tolterol 54
ackheads see Drugs used to treat acne 189
adder infection, drugs for 178
eeding see Blood clotting 116
enoxane 54
eomycin 54
ephamide 54

Bleph-10 54; see Sulfacetamide 473
Blocadren see Timolol 494
Blood
  circulation 107-117
  clotting, drugs affecting 116
  glucose monitoring 155
  pressure see Antihypertensive drugs 114
  vessels see Vasodilators 110
Body salts 547g
Bonamine see Meclizine 373
Bone
  cancer see Anticancer drugs 166-167
  disorders, drugs for 134
    antibiotics 141
Bonefos 54
Booze see Alcohol 532
Boric acid 54
Boropak 54
Bowel
  constipation see Laxatives 123
  inflammatory 124
  irritable 122
BPH, drugs for 178
Bradosol 54
Brain 90
  antibiotics and 141
  cancer see Anticancer drugs 166-167
  swelling see Dexamethasone 280
Brand name 547g
Breast cancer see Anticancer drugs 166-167
Breast-feeding 21
Breathing see Respiratory system
Breathlessness see Bronchodilators 104
Bretylate 54
Bretylium 54
Brevibloc 54
Brevicon 54
Bricanyl see Terbutaline 485
Brietal 54
Bromazepam 230
Bromides 54
Bromocriptine 231
Bromodiphenhydramine 54
Bromovinyldeoxyuridine 54
Brompheniramine 232
Bronalide see Flunisolide 315
Bronchitis, drugs for
  antibacterial 143
  antibiotic 140-142
  bronchodilator 104
Bronchoconstrictor 547g
Bronchodilators 104, 547g
Bronkaid see Epinephrine 300
Bronkaid Mistometer 55
Brucellosis see Tetracycline 489
Buccal tablets 17
Buclizine 55
Budesonide 233
Bufexamac 55
Bufferin 55
Bugs Bunny 55
Bulk-forming agents 122, 123

Bumetanide 234
Bupivacaine 55
Buprenorphine 55
Burinex see Bumetanide 234
Burn, drugs for
  anesthetic 92
  anti-infective 187
  See also Sunburn
Buro-Sol 55
Bursitis see Corticosteroids 130
Buscopan see Scopolamine 463
Buserelin 55
Buspar see Buspirone 235
Buspirone 235
Busulfan 55
Butabarbital 55
Butalbital 55
Butisol 55
Butoconazole 55
Butorphanol 236
Butoxyethyl nicotinate 55
Butyl aminobenzoate 55
Butylated hydroxyanisole 540; see also Chemical preservatives 539
Butylated hydroxytoluene 540; see also Chemical preservatives 539
Butyl nitrite see Nitrites 537
Butyraldehyde see Butyrates 540
Butyrates 540
Butyrophenones see Antipsychotic drugs 97

C

Cactus buttons see Mescaline 536
Cafergot 55
Cafergot-PB 55
Caffeine 55, 540
Caladryl 55
Calamine 55, 185
Calcefediol see Vitamin D 529
Calciferol see Vitamin D 529
Calcijex 55
Calcilean see Heparin 333
Calcimar 55
Calcipotriol 237
Calcite 500 55
Calcite D-500 55
Calcitonin 55
Calcitriol see Vitamin D 529
Calcium 38M (illus.); 134, 519
Calcium acetate see Calcium 519
Calcium alginate 540
Calcium amino acid chelate see Calcium 519
Calcium carbimide 55
Calcium carbonate 38M (illus.); 55
Calcium channel blockers
  as anti-angina drugs 113
  as anti-arrhythmics 112
  as antihypertensives 114
  as vasodilators 110

Calcium chloride see Calcium 519
Calcium citrate see Calcium 519
Calcium disodium salt of ethylenediamine tetra-acetic acid 541
  edetate disodium 62
Calcium fluoride see Fluoride 521
Calcium folinate see Folic acid 521
Calcium glubionate see Calcium 519
Calcium gluceptate see Calcium 519
Calcium gluconate see Calcium 519
Calcium hexametaphosphate see Sodium hexametaphosphate 543
Calcium iodide 55; see also Iodine 522
Calcium lactate see Calcium 519
Calcium leucovorin see Folic acid 521
Calcium pantothenate see Pantothenic acid 524
Calcium propionate see Propionic acid 542
Calcium-Sandoz 55
Calcium sorbate see Sorbic acid 543
Calcium undecylenate 55
Caldesene Medicated Baby Powder 55
Calmurid 55
Calmurid HC 55
Calmydone 55
Calmylin Expectorant see Guaifenesin 331
Calmylin #1 see Dextromethorphan 281
Calmylin with Codeine 55
Calsan 55
Caltine 55
Caltrate 55
Cambendazole 55
Camphor 55
Cancer 164-169; see Anticancer drugs 166-167
Candida infection see Antifungal drugs 150
Canesten see Clotrimazole 268
Cannabis see Marijuana 536
Canthacur 55
Canthacur-PS 55
Cantharidin 55
Cantharone 55
Cantharone Plus 55
Capastat Sulfate 55
Capoten 43Q (illus.); see Captopril 239
Capreomycin 55
Capsaicin 238
Capsule 19
  slow-release 18
Captopril 239
Caramel 540
Caramiphen 55
Carbachol 55

Carbamazepine 240
Carbamide 56
Carbamide peroxide 56
Carbaryl 56
Carbenicillin 56
Carbenoxolone 56
Carbetapentane 56
Carbidopa 56
Carbimide 56
Carbocaine 56
Carbocysteine 56
Carbohydrates 160
Carbol-fuchsin 56
Carbolith *46E* (illus.); see Lithium 364
Carbonic anhydrase inhibitor 181
Carboplatin 56
Carboxymethylcellulose see Laxatives 123
sodium carboxymethylcellulose 542
Cardene 56
Cardiac
compression 575
glycosides see Digitalis drugs 108
See also Heart disorders
Cardioquin see Quinidine 456
Cardioselective beta blockers 109
Cardizem see Diltiazem 287
Cardizem-CD *46F, 46H, 48G* (illus.); see Diltiazem 287
Cardizem-SR *48C, 48D, 48L* (illus.); see Diltiazem 287
Cardura 56
Carfecillin 56
Carica papaya see Papain 542
Carisoprodol 132
Carmustine 56
Carnauba wax 541
Carotenoids see Vitamin A 527
Carphenazine 56
Carrageenan 541
Casanthranol 56
Castellani's Paint 56
Castor oil 56
Catapres see Clonidine 266
Catarase 56
Cathartic 547g
Caustic sulfite caramel see Caramel 540
Ceclor *48J* (illus.); see Cefaclor 241
Cedocard-SR see Isosorbide dinitrate 351
CeeNU 56
Cefaclor 241
Cefadroxil 56
Cefamandole 56
Cefazolin 56
Cefixime 242
Cefizox 56
Cefonicid 56
Ceforanide 56
Cefotan 56
Cefotaxime 56
Cefotetan 56
Cefoxitin 243
Ceftazidime 56

Ceftin *45H* (illus.); see Cefuroxime 244
Ceftizoxime 56
Ceftriaxone 56
Cefuroxime 244
Celestoderm see Betamethasone 227
Celestoderm-V see Betamethasone 227
Celestone see Betamethasone 227
Celestone-S 56
Celestone Soluspan see Betamethasone 227
Celiac disease 528
Cellufresh 56
Cellulose gum see Sodium carboxymethylcellulose 542
Celluvisc 56
Celontin 56
Central nervous system see Nervous system
Centrum 56
Centrum Forte 56
Cephalexin 245
Cephalosporins see Classes of antibiotics 142
Cephradine 56
Cephulac see Lactulose 356
Ceptaz 56
Cerevon 56
Cerubidine 56
C.E.S. *35A* (illus.); see Conjugated estrogens 272
Cesamet 56
Cetamide see Sulfacetamide 473
Cetapred see Sulfacetamide 473
Cetirizine 246
Cetrimide 56
Cetylpyridinium 56
Ce-Vi-Sol 56
Chagas' disease see Trypanosomiasis 148
Charcoal 56
Charcodote 56
Chelating agent 547g
Chemical formula see Formula, chemical 548g
Chemical preservatives see Major types of additives 539
Chemotherapy 166-167, 547g
Chenodiol 56
Cheracol 56
Chickenpox, drugs for
antihistamine 136-137
antipruritic 185
antiviral 145
Childbirth see Pregnancy
Children, treatment of 20, 27
Chlamydia see Antibacterial drugs 143
Chlophedianol 56
Chloral hydrate 247
Chlorambucil 248
Chloramphenicol 249
Chlorbutanol 56
Chlorcyclizine 56
Chlordiazepoxide 250
Chlorhexidine 56

Chlormezanone 56
Chloroform 56
Chloroguanide 56
Chloromycetin see Chloramphenicol 249
Chlorophenothane see DDT 59
Chloroprocaine 56
Chloroptic see Chloramphenicol 249
Chloroquine
as antimalarial 149
as antirheumatic 129
Chlorothen 56
Chlorothiazide 57
Chlorotrianisene 57
Chloroxylenol 57
Chlorphenesin 57
Chlorpheniramine 251
Chlorpromazine 252
Chlorpropamide 253
Chlorprothixene 57
Chlortetracycline 57
Chlorthalidone 254
Chlor-Tripolon see Chlorpheniramine 251
Chlor-Tripolon Decongestant Syrup 57
Chlor-Tripolon Decongestant Tablets 57
Chlor-Tripolon N.D. 57
Chlorzoxazone 132
Cholecalciferol see Vitamin D 529
Choledyl 57
Choledyl Expectorant 57
Choledyl SA 57
Cholera see Tetracycline 489
Cholesterol 228
Lipid-lowering drugs 115
Drug treatment for gallstones 126
Cholestyramine 255
Cholinergic 547g
Choline magnesium trisalicylate 57
Choline salicylate 57
Choline theophyllinate 57
Choloxin 57
Chondrus extract see Carrageenan 541
Choriocarcinoma, drugs for 166
Methotrexate 381
Chorionic gonadotropin see HCG 334
Christmas disease 116
Chromium 520
Chronulac see Lactulose 356
Chymodiactin 57
Chymopapain 57
Chymotrypsin 57
Ciclopirox 256
Cidomycin see Gentamicin 328
Cigarettes see Drug abuse 24; Nicotine 537
Cilastatin-imipenem 57
Cilazapril 57
Ciloxan see Ciprofloxacin 258
Cimetidine 257
Cinchocaine 57
Cinchonism 112
Cinnamates 57

Cinnarizine 57
Cinoxacin 57
Cipro *41J, 45D* (illus.); see Ciprofloxacin 258
Ciprocinonide 57
Ciprofibrate 57
Ciprofloxacin 258
Circulation, drugs for 107-117
Cirrhosis see Diuretics 111
Cisapride 259
Cisplatin 57
Citanest-Forte 57
Citanest Plain 57
Citric acid 541
Citrocarbonate 57
Citro-Mag 57
Citrovorum factor see Folic acid 521
Cladribine 57
Claforan 57
Clarithromycin 260
Claritin *44R* (illus.); see Loratadine 366
Claritin Extra 57
Clavulanic acid see Potassium clavulanate 78
Clavulin-250 *44I* (illus.); 57
Clavulin-500 *44D* (illus.); 57
Clearasil BP Plus 57
Clear Eyes 57
Clemastine 57
Clidinium bromide 57
Climacteron 57
Clindamycin 261
Clinoril see Sulindac 478
Clioquinol 57
Clobazam 57
Clobetasol 153
Clobetasol propionate 262
Clobetasone butyrate 57
Clocortolone 57
Clodronate 57
Clofazimine 57
Clofibrate 115, 157
Clomid see Clomiphene 263
Clomiphene 263
Clomipramine 264
Clonazepam 265
Clonidine 266
Clorazepate 267
Clotrimaderm see Clotrimazole 268
Clotrimazole 268
Clotting of blood 116
Cloxacillin 269
Clozapine 57
Clozaril 57
Cluster bean gum see Guar gum 541
CoActifed 57
CoActifed Expectorant 57
Coal tar 57
Cobalamin see Vitamin B_{12} 528
Cobalt edetate 58
Cocaine 534
Codeine 270
in Non-prescription drugs 13
Cod liver oil 58

Coenzyme R see Biotin 519
Cogentin see Benztropine 225
Coke see Cocaine 534
Colace 58
Colaspase see Asparaginase 53
Colax-C 58
Colax-S 58
Colchicine 271
Cold remedies 105, 106
Cold sores see Antiviral drugs 145
Colestid 58
Colestipol 115
Colistin 58
Collagenase 58
Collodion 58
Colloidal oatmeal 58
Collyrium 58
Cologel see Methylcellulose 541
Colpermin 58
Colprone 58
Coly-Mycin M 58
Coly-Mycin Otic 58
Coma 547g
Comalose-R see Lactulose 356
Combantrin see Pyrantel 452
Combipres 58
Complamin 58
Compound W 58
Condyline 58
Congest see Conjugated
  estrogens 272
Conjugated estrogens 272
Conn's syndrome 469
Constipation see Laxatives 123
Contac Allergy Formula 58
Contac C 58
Contac C Cold Care Formula 58
Contac Sinus Pain 58
Contraceptives 173-175
Contraindication 547g
Controlled drugs 13
Convulsion, drugs for 98
Copper 520
Copper amino acid chelate see
  Copper 520
Copper chloride dihydrate see
  Copper 520
Copper gluconate see Copper 520
Copper sulfate see Copper 520
Coptin 58
Coradur see Isosorbide dinitrate
  351
Cordarone see Amiodarone 207
Corgard see Nadolol 398
Coricidin 58
Coricidin "D" 58
Coricidin "D" Long Acting 58
Coricidin "D" Non-Drowsy Sinus
  Formula 58
Coricidin Sinus Headache Tablets
  58
Coristex-DH 58
Coristine-DH 58
Cornebacterium parvum 58
Coronary
  arteries see Anti-angina drugs
    113
  thrombosis, drugs for 117
  See also Heart disorders

Coronex see Isosorbide dinitrate
  351
Corsym 58
Cortacet 58
Cortamed 58
Cortate see Hydrocortisone 338
Cortef see Hydrocortisone 338
Cortenema see Hydrocortisone
  338
Corticosteroids 153
  as antipruritics 185
  as antirheumatics 129
  as bronchodilators 104
  as immunosuppressants 168
  in inflammatory bowel disease
    124
  locally acting 130
  topical 186
Corticotropin 58
Corticreme 58
Cortifoam 58
Cortiment 58
Cortisol 58
Cortisone 153
Cortisporin 58
Cortoderm 58
Cortone 58
Cortosyn 58
Corzide 58
Cosmegen 58
CoSudafed 58
CoSudafed Expectorant 58
Cosyntropin 58
Cotazym 58
Cotridin 58
Co-Trimazine 58
Co-Trimoxazole 273
Cough remedies 106
Coumadin 36N, 38P, 39Q (illus.);
  see Warfarin 514
Counterirritant 547g
Coversyl 58
Cozaar 58
Crab lice, drugs for 188
Crack see Cocaine 534
Creams 19, 187
Creeping eruption see
  Anthelmintic drugs 151
Creon 58
Creo-Rectal 58
Cretinism see Drugs for thyroid
  disorders 156
Crohn's disease 124
Cromolyn sodium 274
Crotamiton 58
Cryptococcal meningitis 169; see
  Fluconazole 314
Crystal see Phencyclidine 538
Crystapen see Penicillin G 424
C2 with Codeine 58
Cuplex 58
Cupric chloride see Copper 520
Cuprimine see Penicillamine 423
Cutaneous larva migrans see
  Anthelmintic drugs 151
Cyanide poisoning see Nitrites
  537
Cyanocobalamin see Vitamin B$_{12}$
  528

Cyclacillin 58
Cyclamate 58
Cyclandelate 59
Cyclen 59
Cyclizine 59
Cyclobenzaprine 275
Cyclocort 59
Cyclogyl 59
Cyclomen see Danazol 278
Cyclomethicone 59
Cyclomethycaine 59
Cyclone see Phencyclidine 538
Cyclopentamine 59
Cyclopentolate 59
Cyclophosphamide 276
Cycloplegia 182
Cycloplegic 547g
Cycloserine 59
Cyclospasmol 59
Cyclosporine 277
Cyclothiazide 59
Cyklokapron 59
Cylert 59
Cyproheptadine 59
Cyproterone 59
Cystic fibrosis 530
Cystitis, drugs for 178
Cytadren 59
Cytarabine 59
Cytomel see Liothyronine 362
Cytosar 59
Cytosine arabinoside 59
Cytotec 43P (illus.); see
  Misoprostol 393
Cytotoxic 547g
  drugs 167
Cytovene 59
Cytoxan see Cyclophosphamide
  276

D

Dacarbazine 59
Dactinomycin 59
Dagenan 59
Dairyaid 59
Dalacin C see Clindamycin 261
Dalacin T see Clindamycin 261
Dalmane see Flurazepam 320
Danazol 278
Dandruff treatment 191
Dan-Gard 59
Danthron 59
Dantrium 59
Dantrolene 59
Dapsone 59
Daraprim see Pyrimethamine 454
Darvon-N see Propoxyphene 447
Darvon-N Compound 59
Darvon-N with ASA 59
Daunorubicin 59
DDAVP 59
ddC 59
DDS 59

DDT 59
Deadly nightshade see Where
  drugs come from 12
Debrisan 59
Decadron see Dexamethasone
  280
Deca-Durabolin see Nandrolone
  399.
Declomycin 59
Decongestants 105
Deferoxamine 59
Dehydral 59
Dehydrocholic acid 59
Dehydroemetine 59
Delatestryl see Testosterone 488
Delestrogen see Estradiol 304
Delfen 59
Delirium tremens 24
Delsym see Dextromethorphan
  281
Deltasone see Prednisone 440
Demdec 59
Demecarium 59
Demeclocycline 59
Dementia see Antipsychotic
  drugs 97
Demerol see Meperidine 376
Demulen 59
Denorex 59
Depakene see Valproic acid 510
Dependence 547g
Depen see Penicillamine 423
Depo-Medrol see
  Methylprednisolone 386
Depo-Medrol with Lidocaine 59
Depo-Provera see
  Medroxyprogesterone 374
Depo-Testosterone see
  Testosterone 488
Depot injection 547g
Deprenyl see Selegiline 464
Depression, drugs for 96
  manic 97
Dequadin 59
Dequalinium 59
Derma-Smoothe/FS see
  Fluocinolone 316
Dermasone see Clobetasol
  propionate 262
Dermatitis, drugs for 186
Dermoplast 59
Dermovate see Clobetasol
  propionate 262
Dermoxyl see Benzoyl peroxide
  224
DES 60
Desenex 60
Deserpidine 60
Desferal 60
Designer drugs 547g
Desipramine 279
Desmopressin 60
Desogestrel 60
Desonide 60
Desoximetasone 60
Desoxycorticosterone 60
Desquam-X see Benzoyl peroxide
  224
Desyrel see Trazodone 499

Detoxification 24
Dexamethasone 280
Dexasone see Dexamethasone 280
Dexbrompheniramine 60
Dexchlorpheniramine 60
Dexedrine 60
Dexpanthenol 60
Dexsone see Dexamethasone 280
Dextranomer 60
Dextroamphetamine 60
Dextromethorphan 281
Dextropropoxyphene see Propoxyphene 447
Dextrose 60
Dextrothyroxine 60
D-glucitol see Sorbitol 543
DHT see Vitamin D 529
DiaBeta 45L (illus.); see Glyburide 330
Diabetes, drugs for 154-155
  insipidus see Drugs for pituitary disorders 157
Diabinese see Chlorpropamide 253
Diacetylmorphine see Heroin 535
Diamicron 42N (illus.); see Gliclazide 329
Diamidine 60
Diamorphine see Heroin 535
Diamox 60
Diaper rash, drugs for 187
Diarrhea see Antidiarrheal drugs 122
Diazemuls see Diazepam 282
Diazepam 282
Diazoxide 60
Dibucaine 60
Dicetel 60
Dichloralphenazone 60
Dichlorphenamide 60
Diclectin 60
Diclofenac 283
Dicloxacillin 60
Dicyclomine 60
Didanosine 284
Didronel see Etidronate 307
Dienestrol 60
Dientamebiasis 148
Diet see Nutrition 160
Diethylamide see LSD 535
Diethylcarbamazine 60
Diethylpropion 60
Diethylstilbestrol 60
Diflorasone 60
Diflucan see Fluconazole 314
Diflucortolone 60
Diflunisal 285
Difluoromethylornithine 60
Digestive system see Gastrointestinal tract 118-126
Digitaline 60
Digitalis drugs 108
  as anti-arrhythmics 112
Digitoxin see Digitalis drugs 108
Diglycerides see Monoglycerides 541
Digoxin 286

Dihydrocodeine 60
Dihydroergotamine 60
Dihydrotachysterol see Vitamin D 529
Dihydroxyaluminum 60
Diiodohydroxyquin 60
Dilantin 47P (illus.); see Phenytoin 432
Dilantin with phenobarbital 60
Dilaudid see Hydromorphone 339
Dilaudid-HP see Hydromorphone 339
Diloxanide 60
Diltiazem 287
Dimelor 60
Dimenhydrinate 288
Dimercaprol 60
Dimercaptosuccinic acid 60
Dimetane see Brompheniramine 232
Dimetane Expectorant 60
Dimetane Expectorant-C 60
Dimetane Expectorant-DC 60
Dimetapp 60
Dimetapp-A Sinus 60
Dimetapp-C 61
Dimetapp-DM 61
Dimetapp Oral Infant Drops 61
Dimethicone 61
Dimethisoquin 61
Dimethothiazine 61
Dimethyl sulfoxide 61
Dimethyltryptamine 13
Dimethyltubocurarine see Metocurine 70
DIN number 13
Dinoprost 61
Dinoprostone 289
Diocaine 61
Diocarpine 61
Diochloram 61
Dioctyl calcium sulfosuccinate 61
Dioctyl sodium sulfosuccinate 61
Diodex 61
Diodoquin 61
Diogent see Gentamicin 328
Dionephrine see Phenylephrine 431
Diopred see Prednisolone 439
Dioptimyd 61
Diovol 61
Diovol Ex 61
Diovol Plus 61
Dipentum 61
Diperodon 61
Diphenhydramine 290
Diphenidol 61
Diphenoxylate 291
Diphenylhydantoin see Phenytoin 432
Diphenylpyraline 61
Diphtheria vaccine 147
Dipivalyl epinephrine see Dipivefrin 61
Dipivefrin 61
Diprogen 61
Diprolene see Betamethasone 227
Diprosalic 61

Diprosone see Betamethasone 227
Dipyridamole 292
Disalcid 61
Disinfectants, skin 187
Disipal see Orphenadrine 416
Diskhalers see Bronchodilators 104
Disodium see Sodium sulfite 543
Disodium citrate see Sodium citrate 542
Disodium dihydrogen salt of EDTA see Ethylenediamine tetra-acetic acid 541
Disodium edetate see Edetate disodium 62
Disopyramide 293
Distearate see Monoglycerides 541
Disulfiram 294
Dithranol see Anthralin 213
Ditropan 39C (illus.); see Oxybutynin 418
Diuretics 111
  as antihypertensives 114
  in menstrual disorders 172
Divalproex 61
Dixarit see Clonidine 266
DMSO see Dimethyl sulfoxide 61
DMT 13
DOA see Phencyclidine 538
Doan's Backache Pills 61
Dobutamine 61
Dobutrex see Dobutamine 61
Docusate calcium 61
Dolobid see Diflunisal 285
Domiphen 61
Domperidone 43D (illus.); 295
Donnagel 61
Donnagel-MB 61
Donnagel-PG 61
Donnatal 61
Dopamine 61
  dopamine-boosting drugs 99
Dope see Marijuana 536
Dopram see Doxapram 61
Doryx see Doxycycline 297
Doses 15
  ending therapy and 28
  exceeding 30
  in infants and children 20
  missed 28
  prescription terms and 26
Doss 61
Double-blind 547g; see Placebo response 15; Testing and clearing of new drugs 12
Dovonex see Calcipotriol 237
Downers see Barbiturates 533
Doxacurium 61
Doxapram 61
Doxate-C 61
Doxate-S 61
Doxazosin 61
Doxepin 296
Doxidan 61
Doxorubicin 167
Doxycin see Doxycycline 297

Doxycycline 297
Doxylamine 61
Drenison 61
Drink see Alcohol 532
Drip 548g
Drisdol 61
Dristan 61
Dristan Long Lasting Capsules 61
Dristan Long Lasting Nasal Mist/Spray 61
Dristan Nasal Mist 61
Dristan N.D. 61
Drixoral Day/Night Cold Relief System 61
Drixoral Nasal Solution 61
Drixoral N.D. 61
Drixoral Tablets 61
Drixtab 61
Dromostanolone 61
Dronabinol 62
Droperidol 62
Drugs
  abuse of 24, 531-538
  action of 14, 15
  classification of 13
  dangerous 576
  dependence on 23-24
  designer 547g
  forms of 19
    over-the-counter 25
    prescription 26
  poisoning 574-576
  therapy 25-33
    administration 17-18
    Do's and Don'ts 31
    exceeding dose 30
    interactions 16
    storing 29
    tolerance 23-24
DTIC see Dacarbazine 59
Dulcolax see Bisacodyl 229
Duofilm 62
Duoforte 27 62
Duogex see Testosterone 488
Duolube 62
Duonalc 62
Duonalc-E 62
Duoplant 62
Duovent UDV 62
Durabolin see Nandrolone 399
Duragesic 62
Duralith see Lithium 364
Duratears 62
Duratec 62
Duricef see Cefadroxil 56
Duvoid see Bethanechol 54
D-Vi-Sol see Vitamin D 529
Dwarfism, pituitary see Drugs for growth hormone disorders 157
Dyazide 37K (illus); 62
Dycholium 62
Dyphylline 62
Dyrenium see Triamterene 502
Dysentery, amebic see Amebiasis 148
Dysmenorrhea, drugs for 172
Dysne-Inhal see Epinephrine 300
Dystonia see Benztropine 225

E

Ear disorders, drugs for 183
  antibiotic 141
  ear drops 19
Echinococciasis see Hydatid
  disease 151
Echothiophate 62
Econazole 298
Ecostatin see Econazole 298
Ecotrin see ASA 200
Ectosone Mild see
  Betamethasone 227
Ectosone Regular see
  Betamethasone 227
Ectosone Scalp Lotion see
  Betamethasone 227
Eczema, drugs for 185, 186, 187
Edecrin see Ethacrynic acid 63
Edema see Diuretics 111
Edetate calcium disodium 62
Edetate disodium 62
  EDTA 541
Edrophonium chloride 62
EDTA 541
  edetate disodium 62
EES-600 see Erythromycin 302
Efamol see Evening primrose oil
  63
Effexor see Venlafaxine 512
Efudex see Fluorouracil 317
Elavil see Amitriptyline 208
Elavil Plus 62
Eldepryl see Selegiline 464
Elderly, drug treatment in 22
Eldisine 62
Eldopaque 62
Eldoquin 62
Electrolyte 548g
Elixir 19, 548g
Elocom 62
Eltor 120 62
Eltroxin 38B, 39L, 43F (illus.); see
  Levothyroxine 359
Embolism, drugs for 116, 117
Embrocation 548g
Emcyt 62
Emetic 548g
  anti-emetic drugs 102
Emetine 62
Emko 62
EMLA Cream/Patch 62
Emo-Cort see Hydrocortisone
  338
Emollient 548g
  antipruritics 185
Emphysema see Bronchodilators
  104
Empracet-30 36I (illus.); 62
Emtec-30 62
Emulsifying agents see Major
  types of additives 539
Emulsion 19, 548g
E-Mycin see Erythromycin 302
Enalapril 299
Encainide 62
Endantadine see Amantadine 205

Endocet 62
Endocrine system 152-159
Endodan 62
Endometrial cancer see
  Anticancer drugs 166-167
Endometriosis 172
Endorphins 548g
Enflurane 62
Enlon 62
Enoxaparin 62; see Injected
  coagulants 117
Entacyl 62
Enteric-coated ASA 92
Enterobiasis see Anthelmintic
  drugs 151
Entex LA 62
Entocort see Budesonide 233
Entozyme 62
Entrophen 39T (illus.); see ASA
  200
Enuresis see Drugs for urinary
  incontinence 178
Enviroxime 62
Enzyme 548g
  and effects of drugs 16
Ephedrine 62
Epidural anesthesia 92, 177
Epilepsy see Anticonvulsant
  drugs 98
E-Pilo 62
Epi-Lyt 62
Epimorph see Morphine 395
Epinephrine 300
Epinephryl borate 62
EpiPen see Epinephrine 300
Epirubicin 62
Epival see Divalproex 61
Epoprostenol 62
Eprex see Erythropoietin 303
Equagesic 62
Equanil see Meprobamate 377
Ergamisol 62
Ergocalciferol see Vitamin D
  529
Ergodryl 62
Ergoloid mesylates 62
Ergomar see Ergotamine 301
Ergometrine see Ergonovine 63
Ergonovine 63
Ergotamine 301
Ergotrate Maleate see Ergonovine
  63
Erybid see Erythromycin 302
ERYC 47N, 47O (illus.); see
  Erythromycin 302
Erysipelas, drugs for
  Penicillin G 424
  Penicillin V 425
Erythematosus see Systemic
  lupus erythematosus 168
Erythorbic acid 541
Erythrityl tetranitrate 63
Erythromid 35G (illus.); see
  Erythromycin 302
Erythromycin 302
Erythropoietin 303
Erythrosine see FD&C Red No. 3
  541
Esdepallethrin 63

Esmolol 63
Estar see Coal tar 57
Estazolam 63
Esterified estrogens 63
Estinyl see Ethinyl estradiol 306
Estrace see Estradiol 304
Estracomb 63
Estraderm see Estradiol 304
Estradiol 304
Estramustine 63
Estrogens 159
  for menstrual disorders 172
  in oral contraceptives 173-175
Estrone 63
Estropipate 305
Etafedrine 63
Ethacrynate sodium 63
Ethacrynic acid 63
Ethambutol 63
Ethamolin 63
Ethanolamine oleate 63
Ethchlorvynol 63
Ethinamide 63
Ethinyl estradiol 306
Ethionamide 63
Ethoheptazine 63
Ethopropazine 63
Ethosuximide 63
Ethotoin 63
Ethovan see Ethyl vanillin 541
Ethrane 63
Ethyl alcohol 532
Ethylanthranilate see
  Anthranilates 540
2-ethylbutyraldehyde see
  Butyrates 540
2-ethylbutyric acid see Butyrates
  540
Ethylenediamine tetra-acetic acid
  541
Ethylestrenol 63
2-ethylhexylsalicylate see
  Sunscreens 191
Ethyl vanillin 541
Ethynodiol 63
Ethynodiol diacetate 173
Etidocaine 63
Etidronate 307
Etodolac 63
Etofibrate 63
Etomidate 63
Etoposide 63
Etrafon 63
Etretinate 308; see also Vitamin A
  527
Eucalyptus oil 63
Eucatropine 63
Euflex 63
Euglucon see Glyburide 330
Eumovate 63
Eurax 63
Evening primrose oil 63
Excitatory 548g
Exdol-30 63
Ex-lax 63
Exophthalmos 156
Expectorant 106, 548g
Eye disorders, drugs for 179-182
  antibiotic 141
  eye drops 19

F

Famotidine 309
Famciclovir 63
Famvir 63
Fansidar 63
Fascioliasis see Anthelmintic
  drugs 151
Fastin 63
Fats 160
FD&C Red No. 3 541
FD&C Yellow No. 5 see Tartrazine
  543
Feen-A-Mint 63
Feldene see Piroxicam 435
Felodipine 310
Female sex hormones 159
Fenfluramine 63
Fenofibrate 311
Fenoprofen 63
Fenoterol 312
Fentanyl 63
Fer-In-Sol 63
Fermentol 63
Ferrous ascorbate see Iron 522
Ferrous fumarate see Iron 522
Ferrous gluconate see Iron 522
Ferrous succinate see Iron 522
Ferrous sulfate see Iron 522
Fertility 176
Fetus see Pregnancy
Feverfew 63
Fiber 160
Fibrates see Bezafibrate 228;
  Fenofibrate 311
Fibrepur see Psyllium 451
Fibrinolysin 63
Fibrinolytics see Thrombolytic
  drugs 117
Fibrocystic disease see Danazol
  278
Filariasis 139; see Anthelmintic
  drugs 151
Filgrastim 63
Finasteride 313
Fiorinal 41F (illus.); 63
Fiorinal-C 1/4 48H (illus.); 63
Fiorinal-C 1/2 48F (illus.); 64
First aid 575-576
Flagyl see Metronidazole 389
Flagystatin 64
Flamazine see Silver sulfadiazine
  466
Flamazine C 64
Flarex 64
Flavor enhancers see Major types
  of additives 539
Flavoxate 64
Flaxedil 64
Flecainide 64
Flexeril 37P (illus.); see
  Cyclobenzaprine 275
Flintstones 64
Floctafenine 64
Flonase see Fluticasone 322
Florinef 64
Florone 64

Flovent see Fluticasone 322
Floxin 64
Floxuridine 64
Fluanxol 64
Flubendazole 64
Fluclox 64
Fluconazole 314
Flucorolone 64
Flucytosine 64
Fludara see Fludarabine 167
Fludarabine 167
Fludrocortisone 64
Fluke infestation 139; see
  Anthelmintic drugs 151
Flumazenil 64
Flumethasone 64
Flunarizine 64
Flunisolide 315
Fluocinolone 316
Fluocinonide 64
Fluocortin 64
Fluoderm see Fluocinolone 316
Fluonide see Fluocinolone 316
Fluor-A-Day 64
Fluoride 521
Fluorometholone 64
Fluoroplex see Fluorouracil 317
Fluorosis 521
Fluorouracil 317
Fluothane 64
Fluotic 64
Fluoxetine 318
Fluoxymesterone 64
Flupenthixol 64
Fluphenazine 319
Flurandrenolide 64
Flurazepam 320
Flurbiprofen 321
Fluspirilene 64
Flutamide 64
Fluticasone 322
Flutone 64
Fluvastatin 64
Fluvoxamine 323
FML 64
FML Forte 64
FML-Neo 64
Folacin see Folic acid 521
Folate sodium see Folic acid
  521
Folates see Folic acid 521
Folic acid 521
Folinate calcium see Folic acid
  521
Folinic acid 64
Follicle-stimulating hormone see
  FSH 64
Folvite 64
Food
  additives 539-543
  allergy see Antihistamines
    136-137
  See also Nutrition 160-163
Forane 64
Formaldehyde 64
Formestane 64
Formula, chemical 548g
Formula 44 64
Formula 44 D 64

Formula 44 E 64
Formula 44 M (Adult) 64
Formula 44 M (Pediatric) 64
Formulary 548g
Fortamines 10 64
Fortaz 64
Fosinopril 324
Foxglove see Digitalis drugs 108
Framycetin 64
Freebase see Cocaine 534
Freezone 64
Frisium 64
Froben see Flurbiprofen 321
Frozen shoulder see Locally
  acting corticosteroids 130
FSH 64
Fucidin see Fusidic acid 326
FUDR see Floxuridine 64
Fulvicin P/G 64
Fulvicin U/F 64
Fungal infection see Antifungal
  drugs 150
Fungizone see Amphotericin B
  211
Furazolidone 148
Furosemide 325
Furoside see Furosemide 325
Fusidic acid 326

G

GABA 95, 100
Gabapentin 65
Galactorrhea see Drugs used to
  reduce prolactin levels 157
Gallamine 65
Gallstones, drugs for 126
Gamastan 65
Gamimune 65
Gamma-aminobutyric acid 95,
  100
Gamma benzene hexachloride
  65
Gammabulin Immuno 65
Gamma globulin 65
Ganciclovir 65
Garamycin see Gentamicin 328
Garasone 65
Garatec see Gentamicin 328
Gastrocote 65
Gastrointestinal tract 118-126
  infection 141
Gastrozepin 65
Gaviscon see Aluminum
  hydroxide 204
Gel "7" 65
Gelusil 65
Gemfibrozil 327
Gen-Clobetasol 65
Generic name 548g
Genetic engineering see Where
  drugs come from 12
Gen-Glybe 450 (illus.); see
  Glyburide 330

Genital tract infection, drugs for
  antibacterial 143
  antibiotic 140-142
  antiprotozoal 148
  antiviral 145
Gen-Minoxidil see Minoxidil
  392
Gen-Nifedipine see Nifedipine
  404
Gen-Salbutamol see Salbutamol
  461
Gentacidin see Gentamicin 328
Gentamicin 328
Gentian violet 65
Gen-Timolol see Timolol 494
Gen-Triazolam see Triazolam
  503
Geopen 65
German measles vaccine 147
Germicides 187
Giardiasis see Antiprotozoal
  drugs 148
Gigantism, pituitary, drugs for
  157
Gingivitis see Penicillin G 424;
  Penicillin V 425
Glaucoma, drugs for 180-181
Glibenclamide 65
Gliclazide 329
Glipizide 65
Glomerulonephritis see
  Corticosteroids 153
Glucagon 65
Glucophage 41B (illus.); see
  Metformin 379
Glucose
  G6PD deficiency 530
  GTF see Chromium 520
  monitoring 155
  See Drugs used in diabetes
    154-155
Glue see Solvents 538
Glutamic acid hydrochloride 65
Glutaral 65
Glutethimide 65
Glyburide 330
Glycerin 541
Glycerol see Glycerin 541
Glyceryl guaiacolate (Guaifenesin)
  331
Glyceryl monostearate see
  Monoglycerides 541
Glyceryl trinitrate see
  Nitroglycerin 408
Glycopyrrolate 65
Glycosides, cardiac see Digitalis
  drugs 108
Glysennid 65
Goiter 156
  iodine deficiency and 522
Gold-based drugs 129
Gold sodium thiomalate 65
GoLytely 65
Gonadotropin, human chorionic
  see HCG 334
Gonorrhea, drugs for
  Cefixime 242
  Cefuroxime 244
  See also Genital tract infection

Goodpasture's syndrome 168
Goofballs see Barbiturates 533
Goon see Phencyclidine 538
Goserelin 65
Gout, drugs for 131
Gramicidin 65, 187
Grass see Marijuana 536
Gravergol 65
Gravol see Dimenhydrinate 288
Griseofulvin 150
Grisovin-FP see Griseofulvin
  150
Growth hormone 65
  disorders, drugs for 157
G6PD deficiency 530
GTF see Chromium 520
Guaiacol 65
Guaiacolsulfonate 65
Guaifenesin 331
Guanabenz 65
Guanethidine 65
Guaranine see Caffeine 540
Guar flour see Guar gum 541
Guar gum 541
Gum arabic see Acacia 540
Gum Hashab see Acacia 540
Gyne Cure 65
Gynergen see Ergotamine 301

H

H see Heroin 535
H_1 blockers see Antihistamines
  136
H_2 blockers 121
H_2 oxyl see Benzoyl peroxide 22
Habitrol 65
Haemophilus influenzae vaccine
  147
Hair and scalp 65
Hair loss see Treatment for
  dandruff and hair loss 191
Halazepam 65
Halcinonide 65
Halcion see Triazolam 503
Haldol see Haloperidol 332
Haldol LA see Haloperidol 332
Half-life 548g
Hallucinogens 548g
Halobetasol 65
Halofantrine see Antimalarial
  drugs 149
Halofenate 65
Halog 65
Haloperidol 332
Haloprogin 65
Halotestin 65
Halothane 65
Hansen's disease 143
Hash see Marijuana 536
Hashimoto's disease 168
Hay fever 136
HCG 334
Heartburn see Antacids 120

Heart disorders, drugs for 107-117
  anti-angina 113
  anti-arrhythmic 112
  antibiotic 141
  antihypertensive 114
  beta blocker 109
  digitalis 108
  diuretic 111
  drugs that affect blood clotting 116
  immunosuppressant 168
  lipid-lowering 115
  thrombolytic 117
  vasodilator 110
Helminths see Anthelmintic drugs 151
Hemacort HC 65
Hemolysis 529, 530
Hemophilia, drugs for 116
Hemorrhoids, drugs for 125
Hemostatics see Antifibrinolytic drugs 116, 117
Hepalean see Heparin 333
Heparin 333
Hepatic see Liver
Hepatic encephalopathy see Lactulose 356
Hepatitis B vaccine 147
Herbalism see Where drugs come from 12
Heroin 535
Herpes infection see Antiviral drugs 145
Herplex see Idoxuridine 342
Herplex-D see Idoxuridine 342
Hetacillin 65
Hetrazan 66
Hexa-Betalin 66
Hexachlorophene 66
Hexadrol see Dexamethasone 280
Hexalen 66
Hexamethylmalamine 66
Hexetidine 66
Hexifoam 66
Hexit see Lindane 361
Hexocyclium 66
Hexylresorcinol 66
H-F Antidote Gel 66
Hibidil 66
Hibitane 66
Hip-Rex 66
Hismanal see Astemizole 214
Histamethazine see Meclizine 373
Histantil see Promethazine 446
HIV, drugs for 169
Hives, drugs for 185
Hivid 66
HMS Liquifilm 66
Hodgkin's disease 166
Hog see Phencyclidine 538
Homatropine 66
Homosalate 191
Honvol 66
Hooch see Alcohol 532
Hookworm see Anthelmintic drugs 151

Hormone 152-159, 548g
  deficiency 159
  hormone replacement therapy 159
  in infertility 176
  in menopause 159
  in menstrual disorders 172
  in pituitary disorders 157
  in thyroid disorders 156
  See also Anticancer drugs 167
Horse see Heroin 535
Human chorionic gonadotropin 334
Human immunodeficiency virus, drugs for 169
Human insulin 346
Humatrope 66
Humectants see Major types of additives 539
Humegon 66
Humulin see Insulin 346
Hyaluronidase 66
Hycanthone 66
Hycodan see Hydrocodone 337
Hycomine 66
Hydatid disease see Anthelmintic drugs 151
Hydergine 66
Hyderm see Hydrocortisone 338
Hydralazine 335
Hydrea 66
Hydrochlorothiazide 336
Hydrocodone 337
Hydrocortisone 338
HydroDiuril see Hydrochlorothiazide 336
Hydrogen peroxide 66
Hydromorphone 339
Hydrophilic ointment 66
Hydropres 66
Hydroquinone 66
Hydroxocobalamin see Vitamin B_{12} 528
Hydroxyamphetamine 66
Hydroxychloroquine 66
Hydroxycobalamin see Vitamin B_{12} 528
Hydroxydopamine 66
Hydroxyethylcellulose 66
Hydroxyprogesterone 66
Hydroxypropylcellulose 66
Hydroxypropylmethylcellulose 66
Hydroxyurea 66
Hydroxyzine 340
Hygeol 66
Hygroton see Chlorthalidone 254
Hygroton-Reserpine 66
Hyoscine see Scopolamine 463
Hyoscyamine 66
Hypertears Eye Ointment 66
Hyperglycemia, drugs for 154-155
Hyperlipidemia see Lipid-lowering drugs 115
Hypermagnesemia 523
Hyperstat 66
Hypertears Eye Ointment 66
Hypertears Liquid 66
Hypertension see Antihypertensive drugs 114

Hyperthyroidism, drugs for 156
Hypnotics see Sleeping drugs 94
Hypoglycemia 155
Hypogonadism see Female sex hormones 159
Hypokalemia see Diuretics 111
Hypoparathyroidism see Vitamin D 529
Hypothrombinemia see Vitamin K deficiency 530
Hypothyroidism, drugs for 156
Hytakerol 66
Hytrin see Terazosin 483

I

Ibuprofen *37E* (illus.); 341
Ichthammol 66
Ichthyosis see Etretinate 308
Idamycin 66
Idarac 66
Idarubicin 66
I.D.M. Solution 66
Idoxuridine 342
Iletin see Insulin 346
Ilosone see Erythromycin 302
Ilotycin see Erythromycin 302
IMAP 66
IMAP Forte 66
Imdur see Isosorbide dinitrate/mononitrate 351
Imipenem/cilastatin 66
Imipramine 343
Imitrex *35T* (illus.); see Sumatriptan 479
Immune
  disease 164-169
  globulins 146
  immunosuppressant drugs 168
Immune serum globulin 66
Immunization 146-147, 548g
Immunosuppressant drugs 168
  as antirheumatics 129
Imodium *39A* (illus.); see Loperamide 365
Imovane *39F* (illus.); see Zopiclone 517
Impetigo, drugs for 187
Implants 18
Impril see Imipramine 343
Imuran see Azathioprine 218
Inapsine 67
Incontinence, drugs for 178
Incremin with Iron 67
Indapamide 344
Inderal see Propranolol 448
Inderal-LA *46G* (illus.); see Propranolol 448
Inderide 67
Indigestion see Antacids 120
Indocid see Indomethacin 345
Indocid PDA see Indomethacin 345

Indocid SR *48A* (illus.); see Indomethacin 345
Indomethacin 345
Indoramin 67
Indotec see Indomethacin 345
Infantol 67
Infection
  drugs for 138-151
    antibacterial 143
    antibiotic 140-142
    antifungal 150
    anti-infective 187
    antiprotozoal 148
    antiviral 145
    transmission of 139
    vaccination against 146-147
Infertility, drugs for 176
Infestation, drugs for 138-151
  skin parasites 188
Inflamase see Prednisolone 439
Inflammation, drugs for
  analgesic 92-93
  corticosteroid 153
  locally acting 130
Inflammatory bowel disease, drugs for 124
Influenza see Antiviral drugs 145
  vaccine 147
Infusion
  intravenous 548g
  pump 548g
Inhalation 18
Inhalers 19, 548g
  abuse of see Solvents 538
  Bronchodilators 104
Inhibace 67
Inhibitory 548g
INH (isoniazid) 349
Injection 18, 19
  depot 547g
  intramuscular 548g
  intravenous 548g
  subcutaneous 550g
Innovar 67
Inocor 67
Inoculation 548g
Inosiplex 67
Insect bites and stings, drugs for
  antihistamine 136-137
  antipruritic medications 185
Insecticides see Drugs to treat skin parasites 188
Insomnia see Sleeping drugs 94
Insulin 346
  administration of 154
Intal see Cromolyn sodium 274
Interactions of drugs 16
Interferon 165, 347
Intramuscular injection 548g
  administration of 18
Intravenous
  infusion 548g
  injection 18, 548g
Intrinsic factor 67; see also Vitamin B_{12} 528
Intron-A see Interferon 347
Intropin 67
Investigational 549g
Iodinated glycerol 67

Iodine 156, 522
Iodochlorhydroxyquin 67
Iodoquinol 148
Iolasis see Anthelmintic drugs 151
Ionamin 67
Ionil 67
Ionil-T 67
Ionil-T Plus 67
Iopidine 67
Ipecac 67
Ipratropium bromide 348
Irish moss see Carrageenan 541
Iron 522
Iron sorbitol see Iron 522
Irritable bowel see Antidiarrheal drugs 122
Ismelin 67
Ismelin-Esidrix 67
ISMO see Isosorbide dinitrate 351
Isoascorbic acid see Erythorbic acid 541
Isobutyl butyrate see Butyrates 540
Isobutyl nitrites see Nitrites 537
Isocaine 67
Isoetharine 67
Isoflurane 67
Isomeprobamate 67
Isoniazid (INH) 349
Isoprenaline see Isoproterenol 350
Isoprinosine 67
Isopropamide 67
Isopropyl alcohol 67; see also alcohol, rubbing 50
Isopropyl butyrate see Butyrates 540
Isoproterenol 350
Isoptin see Verapamil 513
Isoptin SR 38L (illus.); see Verapamil 513
Isopto Atropine 67
Isopto Carbachol 67
Isopto Carpine see Pilocarpine 433
Isopto Homatropine 67
Isopto Tears 67
Isordil see Isosorbide dinitrate 351
Isordil 10 Titradose 42M (illus.); see Isosorbide dinitrate 351
Isordil 30 Titradose 42E (illus.); see Isosorbide dinitrate 351
Isosorbide dinitrate 351
Isotamine see Isoniazid 349
Isotamine B see Isoniazid 349
Isotretinoin 352; see Vitamin A 527
Isotrex see Isotretinoin 352
Isotrex Gel see Isotretinoin 352
Isoxsuprine 67
Isuprel see Isoproterenol 350
Itching, drugs for 185, 186, 188
Itraconazole 67
Iveegam 67
Ivermectin 67

J

Jaa Aminophylline see Theophylline 490
Jaguar gum see Guar gum 541
Japanese isinglass see Agar-agar 540
Jaundice 549g
Jectofer see Iron 522
Jock itch see Antifungal drugs 150
Joints
    infected 141
    inflamed, drugs for
        antirheumatic 129
        corticosteroid 130, 153
        NSAID 128
Junk see Heroin 535

K

Kalium Durules 67
Kanamycin 67
Kaochlor 67
Kaochlor-20 67
Kaolin 67
Kaon 67
Kaopectate 67
Kaposi's sarcoma see Drugs for AIDS and immune deficiency 169; Interferon 347
Karaya gum 67
Karidium 67
K-Dur 67
K-Dur 20 44S (illus.)
Keflex see Cephalexin 245
Kefurox see Cefuroxime 244
Kefzol 68
Kemadrin see Procyclidine 445
Kemsol 68
Kenacomb 68
Kenalog see Triamcinolone 501
Keralyt 68
Ketalar 68
Ketamine 68
Ketanserin 68
Ketazolam 68
Ketoconazole 353
Ketoprofen 354
Ketorolac 355
Ketotifen 68
Kidney disorders, drugs for 22
    antibiotic 141
    anticancer 166-167
    corticosteroid 153
    diuretic 111
    in transplant rejection see Immunosuppressant drugs 168
    See also Drugs for gout 131
Kidrolase 68
K-Lor 68

K-Lyte 68
K-Lyte/Cl 68
K-Med 68
K-Med 900 68
Koffex see Dextromethorphan 281
Koffex DM see Dextromethorphan 281
Kordofan gum see Acacia 540
K-10 68
Kwashiorkor 160
Kwellada see Lindane 361

L

Labetalol 68
Labor see Pregnancy
Lac-Hydrin 68
Lacril see Methylcellulose 541
Lacri-Lube 68
Lacrisert 68
Lactaid 68
Lactase 68
Lactic acid 68
Lactogenic hormone see Prolactin 157
Lactose 68
Lactrase see Lactase 68
Lactulax see Lactulose 356
Lactulose 356
Lambiasis see Antiprotozoal drugs 148
Lamictal 68
Lamisil 41K (illus.); see Terbinafine 484
Lamotrigine 68
Lanolin 68
Lanoxin 38G, 42T (illus.); see Digoxin 286
Lansoprazole 68
Lansoyl 68
Lanvis 68
Largactil see Chlorpromazine 252
Lariam 68
Larodopa see Levodopa 358
Lasix see Furosemide 325
Lasix Special see Furosemide 325
Latamoxef 68
Laxatives 123
Lecithin 541; see also Emulsifying agents 539
Lectopam 35D, 38T (illus.); see Bromazepam 230
Ledercillin VK 68
Legatrin see Quinine 457
Legionnaires' disease see Erythromycin 302; macrolide antibiotics 142
Leishmaniasis see Antiprotozoal drugs 148
Lenoltec with Codeine 68
Lentaron 68

Leprosy, drugs for 143
Leritine 68
Lescol 68
Leucovorin calcium see Folic acid 521
Leukemia see Anticancer drugs 166-167
Leukeran see Chlorambucil 248
Leuprolide 68
Leustatin 68
Levamisole 68
Levobunolol 68
Levocabastine 357
Levodopa 358
Levodopa-carbidopa 464
Levo-Dromoran 68
Levomepromazine see Methotrimeprazine 382
Levonorgestrel 68
Levophed 68
Levorphanol 68
Levothyroxine 359
Levsin 68
L-glucitol see Sorbitol 543
Librax 68
Librium see Chlordiazepoxide 250
Lice-Enz 68
Lice infestation, drugs for 139, 188
Lidecomb 68
Lidemol 68
Lidex 68
Lidocaine 360
Lidoflazine 68
Lidosporin Ear Drops 68
Lignocaine see Lidocaine 360
Lincocin 68
Lincomycin 68
Lincosamides 141, 142
Lindane 361
Lioresal see Baclofen 221
Liothyronine 362
Lipactin 68
Lipidil 48M (illus.); see Fenofibrate 311
Lipidil Micro see Fenofibrate 311
Lipid-lowering drugs 115
Liquid forms of drugs 19
Liquid paraffin, liquid petrolatum 68
Liquifilm Forte 69
Liquifilm Tears 69
Liquor see Alcohol 532
Lisinopril 363
Lithane see Lithium 364
Lithium 364
Lithizine see Lithium 364
Liver
    cancer see Anticancer drugs 166-167
    cirrhosis see Diuretics 111
    disease, drugs for 22
    transplant rejection see Immunosuppressant drugs 168
Livostin see Levocabastine 357
Locacorten 69

Locacorten-Vioform 69
Local anesthetics 92
   as antipruritics 185
   in rectal and anal disorders
      125
   see Anesthetic, local 546g;
      Epidural anesthesia 177
Locasalen 69
Lodoxamide 69
Loestrin 69
Loftran 69
Lomotil Liquid see Diphenoxylate
   291
Lomotil Tablets 69
Lomustine 69
Loniten see Minoxidil 392
Loop diuretics 111
Loperamide 365
Lopid 44G (illus.); see Gemfibrozil
   327
Lopresor see Metoprolol 388
Loprox see Ciclopirox 256
Loratadine 366
Lorazepam 367
Lorcainide 69
Lorelco 69
Loroxide see Benzoyl peroxide
   224
Losartan 69
Losec 48K (illus.); see
   Omeprazole 413
Lotensin 69
Lotions 19, 187, 549g
Lotriderm 69
Lovastatin 368
Lovenox 69
Loxapac see Loxapine 369
Loxapine 369
Lozide 35F (illus.); see
   Indapamide 344
LSD 535
Lubricant laxatives 123
Ludiomil see Maprotiline 371
Lugol's Solution 69
Lung
   cancer see Anticancer drugs
      166-167
   infection, drugs for
      antibacterial 143
      antifungal 150
      antiprotozoal 148
   See also Respiratory system
Lupron 69
Lupus erythematosus see
   Systemic lupus erythematosus
Luvox 42G (illus.); see
   Fluvoxamine 323
Lyderm 69
Lymphatic cancer see
   Anticancer drugs 166-167
Lymph nodes, cancer of see
   Anticancer drugs 166-167
Lymphoma see Anticancer
   drugs 166-167; Corticosteroids
   153
Lypressin 69
Lysatec rt-PA 69
Lysergic acid see LSD 535
Lysodren 69

M

Maalox 69
Maalox GRF 69
Maalox Plus 69
Maalox TC 69
Macrobid see Nitrofurantoin 407
Macrodantin see Nitrofurantoin
   407
Macrolides 141, 142
Mafenide 69
Magaldrate 69
Maglucate 69
Magnesite see Magnesium
   carbonate 541
Magnesium 523
Magnesium alginate 69
Magnesium carbonate 541
   as Antacid 120
Magnesium citrate 69
Magnesium gluconate 69
Magnesium hydroxide 370
   as Antacid 120
Magnesium oxide see
   Magnesium 523
Magnesium salicylate 69
Magnesium sulfate see
   Magnesium 523
Magnesium trisilicate 69
Magnolax 69
Majeptil 69
Malabsorption 160
Malaria see Antimalarial drugs
   149
Malathion 69
Male sex hormones 158
Malignant disease 164-169
Maltlevol 69
Maltlevol-M 69
Mandelamine 69
Mandol 69
Manerix see Moclobemide 394
Manic depression, drugs for 97
Mannitol 69
MAOIs 16, 96
Maprotiline 371
Marasmus 160
Marcaine 69
Marijuana 536
Marvelon 69
Marzine 69
Materna 69
Maxenal see Pseudoephedrine
   450
Maxeran see Metoclopramide
   387
Maxibolin 69
Maxidex see Dexamethasone 280
Maxitrol 69
Mazindol 69
MDA see Schedule H drugs 13
Measles vaccine 147
Mebendazole 372
Mechlorethamine 69
Meclizine 373
Medication 549g; see also Drugs
Medicine 549g; see also Drugs

Medihaler-Epi see Epinephrine
   300
Medihaler-Ergotamine see
   Ergotamine 301
Medipren see Ibuprofen 341
Meditran see Meprobamate 377
Medrogestone 70
Medrol see Methylprednisolone
   386
Medroxyprogesterone 374
Medrysone 70
Mefenamic acid 375
Mefloquine 149
Mefoxin see Cefoxitin 243
Megace 70
Megacillin see Penicillin G 424
Megestrol 70
Megral 70
Melarsoprol 148
Mellaril see Thioridazine 491
Melphalan 70
Menadiol see Vitamin K 530
Menadione see Vitamin K 530
Meniere's disease, drugs for 183
   anti-emetic 102
   Dimenhydrinate 288
   diuretic 111
   Promethazine 446
Meningitis, cryptococcal 169; see
   Fluconazole 314
Menke's syndrome 520
Menogaril 70
Menopause 159
Menorrhagia, drugs for 172
Menotropins 176
Menstrual cycle 159
Menstrual disorders, drugs for 172
Mental illness, drugs for 97
Menthol 70
Mepacrine 70
Meperidine 376
Mephenytoin 70
Mephobarbital 70
Mepivacaine 70
Meprobamate 377
Mepron 70
Meptazinol 70
Mepyramine 70
Mequitazine 70
Mercaptopurine 70
Mercodol with Decapryn 70; see
   Hydrocodone 337
Mercury 70
   ammoniated 51
Mersyndol with Codeine 70
Mesalamine 378
Mesasal see Mesalamine 378
Mescaline 536
M-Eslon see Morphine 395
Mesna 70
Mesoridazine 70
Mestinon see Pyridostigmine 453
Mestranol 173, 175; see also
   Female sex hormones 159
Metabolism 549g
Metamucil see Psyllium 451
Metandron testosterone 488
Metaproterenol see Orciprenaline
   415

Metastases see Anticancer drugs
   166-167
Metformin 379
Methadone 70
Methamphetamine 70
Methandrostenolone 70
Methaqualone 70
Methazolamide 70
Methdilazine 70
Methenamine 70
Methicillin 70
Methimazole 70
Methocarbamol 380
Methocel see Methylcellulose 541
Methohexital 70
Methotrexate 381
Methotrimeprazine 382
Methoxamine 70
Methoxsalen 383
Methsuximide 70
Methylbenzethonium 70
Methyl-CCNU 70
Methylcellulose 70, 541
Methylclothiazide 70
Methyldopa 384
Methylene blue 70
Methylenedioxyamphetamine see
   Schedule H drugs 13
Methylergonovine 70
Methylformamide 70
Methyl-glyoxalbis-
   guanylhydrazone 70
Methylparaben 70, 541
Methylphenidate 385
Methyl p-hydroxybenzoate see
   Methylparaben 541
Methylprednisolone 386
Methyl salicylate 70
Methylsulfoxide 70
Methyltestosterone 70
Methyltheobromine see Caffeine
   540
Methyprylon 70
Methysergide 70
Metimyd 70
Metoclopramide 387
Metocurine 70
Metolazone 70
Metopirone 70
Metoprolol 388
Metreton 70
Metrifonate 70
Metrodin 70
Metrogel see Metronidazole 389
Metronidazole 389
Metubine Iodide 71
Metyrapone 71
Metyrosine 71
Mevacor 39N (illus.); see
   Lovastatin 368
Mexiletine 71
Mexitil 71
Mezlocillin 71
Micatin see Miconazole 390
Miconazole 390
Micro-K Extencaps 46D (illus.); 70
Micro-K-10 Extencaps 71
Micronor 70, 173
Midamor see Amiloride 206

Midazolam 71
Midodrine 71
Migraine, drugs for 101
Milrinone 71
Mineral oil 71
Minerals 163, 518-530
Minestrin 1/20 71
Minipress see Prazosin 438
Minocin *46C* (illus.); see
    Minocycline 391
Minocycline 391
Min-Ovral 71
Minoxidil 392
Minoxigain see Minoxidil 392
Mintezol 71
Miocarpine see Pilocarpine 433
Miochol 71
Miosal 71
Miostat 71
Miotics 181, 182, 549g
Misoprostol 393
Mites, drugs for 188
Mitolactol 71
Mitomycin 71
Mitotane 71
Mitoxantrone 71
Mobenol see Tolbutamide 497
Mobiflex see Tenoxicam 482
Moclobemide 394
Modecate see Fluphenazine 319
Moditen see Fluphenazine 319
Modulon see Trimebutine 506
Moduret 71
Moduret 50 *36G* (illus.); 71
Mogadon *42O, 43H* (illus.); see
    Nitrazepam 406
Moisturel 71
Molindone 71
Molybdenum 71
Mometasone 186
Monistat see Miconazole 390
Monitan see Acebutolol 198
Monkey see Phencyclidine 538
Monoamine oxidase inhibitors 16,
    96
Monobenzone 71
Monoglycerides 541
Monopril *43T* (illus.); see
    Fosinopril 324
Monosodium citrate see Sodium
    citrate 542
Monosodium glutamate 541; see
    also Flavor enhancers 539
Monosodium glycerides see
    Monoglycerides 541
Monosulfiram 71
Moricizine 71
Morphine 395; see also
    Hydromorphone 339
Morphitec see Morphine 395
M.O.S. see Morphine 395
Motilium see Domperidone 295
Motion sickness see
    Dimenhydrinate 288;
    Diphenhydramine 290
Motrin see Ibuprofen 341
Mouth
    infection 141
    thrush see Antifungal drugs 150

Mouth-to-mouth resuscitation
    575
Moxalactam 71
MS Contin see Morphine 395
MSD E.C. ASA *40A* (illus.); see
    ASA 200
MSG see Monosodium glutamate
MS.IR see Morphine 395
Mucaine 71
Mucolytics 106, 549g
Mucomyst 71
Multipax see Hydroxyzine 340
Multiple myeloma 166
Multi-Tar Plus 71
Mumps vaccine 147
Mupirocin 396
Murine 71
Murine Ear Wax Removal System
    71
Murocel 71
Muromonab-CD3 71
Muscle 127-134
    injury see Analgesics 92-93;
    Locally acting corticosteroids
    130
    spasm see Muscle-relaxant
    drugs 132
    See also Drugs used for
    myasthenia gravis 133
Mustargen 71
Mutamycin 71
M.V.I.-100 71
Myambutol 71
Myasthenia gravis, drugs for 133
Mycifradin see Neomycin 402
Myciguent see Neomycin 402
Mycil 71
Myclo see Clotrimazole 268
Mycobutin 71
Mycoplasma pneumonia see
    Erythromycin 302
Mycostatin see Nystatin 412
Mydfrin 71
Mydriacyl 71
Mydriatic drugs 182, 549g
Mydrin see Phenylephrine 431
Myleran 71
Myochrysine 71
Myoflex 71
Myotonachol 71
Myristic acid 542
Myristicin see Myristic acid 542
Mysoline see Primidone 441

N

Nabilone 72
Nabumetone 397
Nadolol 398
Nadopen-V 500 *36K* (illus.); see
    Penicillin V 425
Nadostine see Nystatin 412
Nafarelin 72
Nafcillin 72

Naftifine 72
Nail infection see Antifungal
    drugs 150
Nalbuphine 72
Nalcrom see Cromolyn sodium
    274
Nalfon 72
Nalidixic acid 72
Naloxone 72
Naltrexone 72
Nandrolone 399
NAPAP see Acetaminophen 199
Naphazoline 72
Naphcon-A 72
Naphcon Forte 72
Naprosyn see Naproxen 400
Naprosyn E *45G, 45J* (illus.); see
    Naproxen 400
Naproxen 400
Narcan 72
Narcolepsy, drugs for 100
Narcotics 549g
    analgesics 92-93
    in labor 177
    antidiarrheals 122
    classification of 13
    cough suppressants 106
    interactions of 16
Narcotine 72
Nardil 72
Nasacort see Triamcinolone 501
Nasal drops/spray 19
Nasocort see Triamcinolone
    501
Natamycin 72
Natulan 72
Naturetin 72
Nausea see Anti-emetic drugs
    102
Navane 72
Naxen see Naproxen 400
Nebcin see Tobramycin 496
Nebulizer 549g; see
    Bronchodilators 104
Nedocromil 401
Nefazodone 72
NegGram 72
Nembutal 72
Neo-Bex 72
Neo-Codema see
    Hydrochlorothiazide 336
Neo-Cortef 72
NeoDecadron 72; see
    Dexamethasone 280
Neo-Estrone 72
Neo-Medrol 72
Neomycin 402
Neo-Pause 72
Neoral see Cyclosporine 277
Neosporin 72
Neostigmine 403
NeoStrata HQ 72
Neo-Synephrine see
    Phenylephrine 431
Neotopic 72
Nephrotic syndrome see Diuretics
    111
Neptazane 72
Nerisone 72

Nervous system 90-91
    antibiotics for 141
    depressants
        heroin 535
        marijuana 536
        solvents 538
    stimulants 100
        nicotine 537
Nesacaine 72
Netilmicin 72
Netromycin 72
Neuleptil 72
Neupogen 72
Neuroleptic 549g; see
    Antipsychotic drugs 97
Neurontin 72
Neurotransmitter 549g
Neutralca-S 72
Nevo-Mepro see Meprobamate
    377
Niacin 523
Niacinamide see Niacin 523
Nicardipine 72
Nicoderm see Nicotine 537
Nicorette see Nicotine 537
Nicorette Plus see Nicotine 537
Nicotinamide see Niacin 523
Nicotine 537
Nicotinic acid see Niacin 523
Nicotinyl alcohol tartrate see
    Niacin 523
Nicotrol see Nicotine 537
Nicoumalone 72
NidaGel see Metronidazole 389
Nifedipine 404
Nifurtimox 148
Night blindness 527
Nightshade see Deadly
    nightshade
Nikethamide 72
Nilstat see Nystatin 412
Nilutamide 405
Nimodipine 72
Nimotop 72
Nipent 72
Nipride 72
Niradazole 72
Nitrates
    as anti-angina drugs 113
    as chemical preservatives 539
    as vasodilators 110
Nitrazepam 406
Nitrites 537
    as chemical preservatives 539
Nitro-Dur see Nitroglycerin 408
Nitrofurantoin 407
Nitrofurazone 72
Nitrogard-SR see Nitroglycerin
    408
Nitrogen mustard 72
Nitroglycerin 408
Nitrol see Nitroglycerin 408
Nitrolingual Spray see
    Nitroglycerin 408
Nitrong see Nitroglycerin 408
Nitrong SR *40N* (illus.); see
    Nitroglycerin 408
Nitrostat *43M* (illus.); see
    Nitroglycerin 408

Nitrous oxide 72
Nits, drugs for 188
Nivea 72
Nix see Permethrin 427
Nizatidine 409
Nizoral see Ketoconazole 353
Nolvadex see Tamoxifen 480
Nolvadex-D see Tamoxifen 480
Non-cardioselective beta
    blockers 109
Non-narcotic
    analgesics 92
    cough suppressants 106
Nonoxynol-9 72
Non-prescription drugs 13; see
    also OTC drugs
Nonproprietary name 549g
Non-steroidal anti-inflammatory
    drugs 128
Noradrenaline 73
Norcuron 73
Norepinephrine 73
Norethindrone 73
Norethisterone 73
Norethynodrel 73
Norfemac 73
Norflex 42F (illus.); see
    Orphenadrine 416
Norfloxacin 410
Norgesic 73
Norgesic Forte 73
Norgestimate 73
Norgestrel 159
Norinyl 1/50 73
Norlutate 73
Noroxin 44J (illus.); see
    Norfloxacin 410
Noroxin Ophthalmic Solution see
    Norfloxacin 410
Norpace see Disopyramide 293
Norpace CR see Disopyramide
    293
Norpramin see Desipramine 279
Nortriptyline 411
Norvasc 44A (illus.); see
    Amlodipine 209
Noscapine 73
Nose see Decongestants 105;
    The uses of antibiotics 141
Novahistex C 73
Novahistex DH 73
Novahistex DH Expectorant 73
Novahistex DM Expectorant with
    Decongestant 73
Novahistex DM with
    Decongestant 73
Novahistex Expectorant with
    Decongestant 73
Novahistine Decongestant see
    Phenylephrine 431
Novahistine DH 73
Novahistine DM Expectorant with
    Decongestant 73
Novahistine DM with
    Decongestant 73
Novamilor 73
Novamoxin 47E, 47F (illus.); see
    Amoxicillin 210
Novantrone 73

Nova-Rectal 73
Novasen 37C, 39S (illus.); see
    ASA 200
Novo-Alprazol see Alprazolam
    203
Novo-Ampicillin see Ampicillin
    212
Novo-Atenol 42I (illus.); see
    Atenolol 215
Novo-AZT see Zidovudine 516
Novo-Butamide see Tolbutamide
    497
Novocain 73
Novo-Captoril see Captopril 239
Novo-Capto see Captopril 239
Novo-Carbamaz see
    Carbamazepine 240
Novo-Chlorhydrate 46J (illus.);
    see Chloral hydrate 247
Novo-Cimetine 38N (illus.); see
    Cimetidine 257
Novo-Clonidine see Clonidine
    266
Novo-Clopate see Clorazepate
    267
Novo-Cloxin 47Q, 47R (illus.); see
    Cloxacillin 269
Novo-Cromolyn see Cromolyn
    sodium 274
Novo-Cycloprine see
    Cyclobenzaprine 275
Novo-Difenac 40J (illus.); see
    Diclofenac 283
Novo-Diflunisal see Diflunisal 285
Novo-Diltazem see Diltiazem 287
Novo-Dimenate see
    Dimenhydrinate 288
Novo-Dipam 37T (illus.); see
    Diazepam 282
Novo-Dipiradol see Dipyridamole
    292
Novo-Doxepin see Doxepin 296
Novo-Doxylin see Doxycycline
    297
Novo-Famotidine 40E (illus.); see
    Famotidine 309
Novo-Flupam 47I (illus.); see
    Flurazepam 320
Novo-Flurazine see
    Trifluoperazine 504
Novo-Gesic 45B, 45I (illus.); see
    Acetaminophen 199
Novo-Gesic-C8 73
Novo-Gesic-C15 73
Novo-Gesic-C30 73
Novo-Glyburide 45N (illus.); see
    Glyburide 330
Novo-Hexidyl see Trihexyphenidyl
    505
Novo-Hydrazide 36E, 36F (illus.);
    see Hydrochlorothiazide 336
Novo-Hydroxyzin 46K (illus.); see
    Hydroxyzine 340
Novo-Hylazin see Hydralazine
    335
Novo-Keto-EC see Ketoprofen
    354
Novo-Lexin 36R, 36S (illus.); see
    Cephalexin 245

Novolin see Insulin 346
Novo-Lorazem 43L, 44O, 45Q
    (illus.); see Lorazepam 367
Novo-Medopa see Methyldopa
    384
Novo-Metformin 41C (illus.); see
    Metformin 379
Novo-Methacin SP.C 48I (illus.);
    see Indomethacin 345
Novo-Metoprol 35H (illus.); see
    Metoprolol 388
Novo-Mucilax see Psyllium 451
Novo-Naprox 36D, 38H (illus.);
    see Naproxen 400
Novo-Nidazol 41D (illus.); see
    Metronidazole 389
Novo-Nifedin see Nifedipine 404
Novo-Oxapam see Oxazepam
    417
Novo-Pen G see Penicillin G 424
Novo-Pen-VK-500 37G (illus.);
    see Penicillin V 425
Novo-Peridol see Haloperidol 332
Novo-Pheniram see
    Chlorpheniramine 251
Novo-Phenytoin see Phenytoin
    432
Novo-Pindol see Pindolol 434
Novo-Pirocam see Piroxicam 435
Novo-Pramine see Imipramine
    343
Novo-Pranol see Propranolol 448
Novo-Prazin see Prazosin 438
Novo-Prednisone 42R (illus.); see
    Prednisone 440
Novo-Profen 37D (illus.); see
    Ibuprofen 341
Novo-Propamide see
    Chlorpropamide 253
Novo-Propoxyn see
    Propoxyphene 447
Novo-Purol 37A (illus.); see
    Allopurinol 202
Novo-Pyrazone see
    Sulfinpyrazone 476
Novo-Ranidine 42A, 45E (illus.);
    see Ranitidine 458
Novo-Reserpine 73
Novo-Ridazine see Thioridazine
    491
Novo-Rythro Encap see
    Erythromycin 302
Novo-Salmol see Salbutamol 461
Novo-Selegiline see Selegiline
    464
Novo-Semide 38D, 43I (illus.); see
    Furosemide 325
Novo-Sorbide see Isosorbide
    dinitrate 351
Novo-Soxazole see Sulfisoxazole
    477
Novo-Spiroton see
    Spironolactone 469
Novo-Spirozine see
    Spironolactone 469
Novo-Spirozine-25 73
Novo-Sucralate see Sucralfate
    472
Novo-Sundac see Sulindac 478

Novo-Tamoxifen see Tamoxifen
    480
Novo-Terfenadine see
    Terfenadine 487
Novo-Tetra 47L (illus.); see
    Tetracycline 489
Novo-Timol see Timolol 494
Novo-Triamzide 37H (illus.); see
    Hydrochlorothiazide 336,
    Triamterene 502
Novo-Trimel 41E (illus.); see
    Sulfamethoxazole 474,
    Trimethoprim 507
Novo-Trimel DS 44F (illus.); see
    Sulfamethoxazole 474,
    Trimethoprim 507
Novo-Triolam see Triazolam 503
Novo-Tripamine see Trimipramine
    508
Novo-Triptyn 37O, 39G (illus.);
    see Amitriptyline 208
Novo-Veramil see Verapamil 513
Novoxapam 37L, 42Q (illus.); see
    Oxazepam 417
Nozinan see Methotrimeprazine
    382
NSAIDs 128
Nu-Alpraz see Alprazolam 203
Nu-Amilzide 74
Nu-Amoxi 47G (illus.); see
    Amoxicillin 210
Nu-Ampi see Ampicillin 212
Nu-Atenol see Atenolol 215
Nu-Cal 74
Nu-Capto see Captopril 239
Nu-Cephalex see Cephalexin 245
Nu-Cimet see Cimetidine 257
Nu-Clonidine see Clonidine 266
Nu-Cloxin see Cloxacillin 269
Nu-Cotrimox see Co-Trimoxazole
    273
Nu-Diclo see Diclofenac 283
Nu-Diflunisal see Diflunisal 285
Nu-Diltiaz see Diltiazem 287
Nu-Hydral see Hydralazine 335
Nu-Indo see Indomethacin 345
Nu-Loraz see Lorazepam 367
Nu-Medopa see Methyldopa 384
Nu-Metop see Metoprolol 388
Numorphan 74
Nu-Nifed see Nifedipine 404
Nupercainal 74
Nu-Pindol see Pindolol 434
Nu-Pirox see Piroxicam 435
Nu-Prazo see Prazosin 438
Nuprin see Ibuprofen 341
Nu-Prochlor see Prochlorperazine
    444
Nu-Ranit 41T (illus.); see
    Ranitidine 458
Nuromax 74
Nu-Tetra see Tetracycline 489
Nu-Triazide 37I (illus.); see
    Hydrochlorothiazide 336,
    Triamterene 502
Nu-Triazo see Triazolam 503
Nutrifer Plus 74
Nutrition 160-163
Nyaderm see Nystatin 412

Nylidrin 74
Nyquil Liquid Nighttime Colds Medicine 74
Nystatin 412
Nytol see Diphenhydramine 290

O

Obsessive-compulsive disorder see Fluvoxamine 323
Occlucort see Betamethasone 227
Occlusal 74
OCD see Fluvoxamine 323
Octoxynol 74
Octyl methoxycinnamate 191
Ocuclear see Oxymetazoline 420
Ocudex see Dexamethasone 280
Ocufen see Flurbiprofen 321
Ocugram see Gentamicin 328
Ocusert Pilo see Pilocarpine 433
Ocuvite 74
Oestradiol see Estradiol 304
Oestrilin 74
Ofloxacin 74
Ogen see Estropipate 305
Oils 542
Ointments 19, 187
Olsalazine 74
Omeprazole 413
Omni-Tuss 74
Onchocerciasis see Anthelmintic drugs 151
Oncovin 74
Ondansetron 414
One A Day Advance Adult 74
One A Day Advance Fem 74
One-Alpha 74
Onyvul 74
Opcon 74
Opcon-A 74
Ophthetic 74
Ophtho-Chloram see Chloramphenicol 249
Ophthocort 74
Ophtho-Sulf see Sulfacetamide 473
Ophtho-Tate see Prednisolone 439
Ophtrivin-A 74
Opiates see Narcotics
Opioids see Narcotics
Opium 74
Opticrom see Cromolyn sodium 274
Optimine see Azatadine 217
Oracort see Triamcinolone 501
Orajel see Benzocaine 223
Oral anticoagulants 16
Oral contraceptives 173-175
Oramorph SR see Morphine 395
Orap 74
Orbenin see Cloxacillin 269
Orciprenaline 415

Organ transplant rejection see Immunosuppressant drugs 168
Orifer-F 74
Orinase see Tolbutamide 497
Ornade 75
Ornade-A.F. 75
Ornade-DM 75
Ornade Expectorant 75
Ornidazole 75
Oro-Clense CHX 75
Orphan drug 549g
Orphenadrine 416
Ortho 0.5/35 75
Ortho 1/35 75
Ortho 7/7/7 75
Ortho 10/11 75
Ortho-Cept 75
Orthoclone OKT3 75
Ortho-Novum 1/50 75
Orudis see Ketoprofen 354
Orudis E see Ketoprofen 354
Oruvail see Ketoprofen 354
Os-Cal 75
Os-Cal-D 75
Osmitrol 75
Osmotic diuretics 111
Osmotic laxatives 123
Ostac 75
Osteoarthritis, drugs for
  corticosteroid 130
  NSAID 128
Osteomalacia, drugs for 134
Osteoporosis, drugs for 134
Ostoforte see Vitamin D 529
OTC drugs See Over-the-counter drugs
Otitis 183
Otrivin see Xylometazoline 515
Ouabain 75
Overdose 30; see also Doses
Over-the-counter drugs 25, 549g
  for children 27
  interacting with prescription drugs 16
  See also Non-prescription drugs 13
Ovol 75
Ovral 75
Oxacillin 75
Oxazepam 417
Oxethazaine 75
Oxilapine see Loxapine 369
Oxipor 75
Oxpam see Oxazepam 417
Oxprenolol 75
Oxsoralen see Methoxsalen 383
Oxsoralen-Ultra see Methoxsalen 383
Oxtriphylline 75
Oxybenzone 191
Oxybuprocaine 75
Oxybutynin 418
Oxychlorosene 75
Oxycocet 41A (illus.); 75
Oxycodan see ASA 200; Oxycodone 419
Oxycodone 419
Oxyderm see Benzoyl peroxide 224

Oxy 5 Vanishing Formula see Benzoyl peroxide 224
Oxymetazoline 420
Oxymetholone 75
Oxymorphone 75
Oxyphenbutazone 75
Oxyquinoline 75
Oxytocin 421
Ozone see Phencyclidine 538

P

PABA 75; see also Sunscreens 191
Paclitaxel 75, 167
Padimate O see Sunscreens 191
Paget's disease see Etidronate 307
Painkillers see Analgesics 92
Palafer 75
Palafer CF 75
Paludrine 75
Pamabrom 75
Pamergan 75
Pamidronate 75
Pamprin 75
Pancreas
  cancer of see Anticancer drugs 166-167
  disorders of 126
Pancrease 75
Pancreatin 75
Pancrelipase 75
Pancuronium 75
P & S Liquid Phenol 75
P & S Plus 75
P & S Shampoo 75
Panectyl 75
Panoxyl see Benzoyl peroxide 224
Panthenol see Pantothenic acid 524
Pantopon 75
Pantothenic acid 524
Papain 542
Papaverine 75
Papulex 75
Para-aminobenzoic acid see Sunscreens 191; see also Aminobenzoic acid 51
Paracetamol see Acetaminophen 199
Parafon Forte 75
Parafon Forte C8 75
Paraldehyde 76
Paramethadione 76
Paramettes Adults Complete 76
Paramettes 50+ Complete 76
Paramettes Teens 76
Paranoia, drugs for 97
Paraplatin 76
Parasites, skin, drugs for 188
Parasympathetic nervous system 91

Parasympatholytic 549g
Parasympathomimetic 549g
  in urinary disorders 178
Paregoric 76
Parkinsonism 549g
  caused by antipsychotics 97
  drugs for 99
Parkinson's disease 99; see also Parkinsonism
Parlodel see Bromocriptine 231
Paromomycin 148
Paroxetine 422
Parsitan 76
Parsol 1789 191
Parvolex 76
PAS 76
Pastes 187
Patch see Transdermal patch
Pavulon 76
Paxil 35E (illus.); see Paroxetine 422
PCE 40M (illus.); see Erythromycin 302
PCNU 76
PCP see Phencyclidine 538
PDF 76
Pectin 76, 542
Pediapred see Prednisolone 439
Pediatrix see Acetaminophen 199
Pediazole 76
Pedi-Dent 76
Pellagra 523
Pelvic infection, drugs for
  antibacterial 143
  antibiotic 140-142
Pemoline 76
Penbritin see Ampicillin 212
Penbutolol 76
Penfluridol 76
Penglobe 76
Penicillamine 423
Penicillin G 424
Penicillins see Antibiotics 142
Penicillin V 425
Penntuss 76
Penta/3B 76
Penta/3B+C 76
Penta/3B Plus 76
Pentacarinat 76
Pentaerythritol tetranitrate 76
Pentamidine 76
Pentamycetin see Chloramphenicol 249
Pentamycetin-HC 76
Pentasa see Mesalamine 378
Pentazocine 76
Pentetic acid 76
Pentobarbital 76
Pentostatin 76
Pentothal 76
Pentoxifylline 426
Pentrax 76
Pen-Vee see Penicillin V 425
Pepcid see Famotidine 309
Peppermint oil 76
Pepsin 76
Pepto-Bismol Liquid 76
Pepto-Bismol Tablets 76
Peptol see Cimetidine 257

Percocet 76
Percocet-Demi 76
Percodan 76
Percodan-Demi 76
Pergolide 76
Pergonal 76
Periactin 76
Peri-Colace 76
Pericyazine 76
Peridol see Haloperidol 332
Perindopril 76
Periods, menstrual see Menstrual
  cycle 159
Peripheral vascular disease see
  Vasodilators 110
Peritonitis see Antibacterial drugs
  143
Peritrate 76
Permax 76
Permethrin 427
Pernox 76
Peroxide see Benzoyl peroxide
  224
Perphenazine 428
Persantine see Dipyridamole 292
Persol see Benzoyl peroxide 224
Persol Forte see Benzoyl
  peroxide 224
Pertofrane see Desipramine 279
Pertussis vaccine 146-147
Peruvian balsam 76
Pethidine see Meperidine 376
PETN 76
Petrolatum see Mineral oil 71
Peyote see Mescaline 536
Pharmacal 500 76
Pharmacist 549g
Pharmacokinetics 549g
Pharmacologist 549g
Pharmacopoeia 550g
Pharmacy 550g
Pharmorubicin 76
Pharyngitis see Throat infection
  141
Phazyme 76
Phenacemide 76
Phenacetin 76
Phenaphen with Codeine 76
Phenazo see Phenazopyridine
  429
Phenazocine 76
Phenazopyridine 429
Phencyclidine 538
Phenelzine sulfate 76
Phenergan see Promethazine
  446
Phenergan Expectorant Plain 76
Phenergan Expectorant with
  Codeine 76
Phenergan VC Expectorant see
  Promethazine 446
Phenergan VC Expectorant Plain
  76
Phenergan VC Expectorant with
  Codeine 76
Pheniramine 77
Phenobarbital 430
Phenol 77
Phenolphthalein 77

Phenothiazines
  as anti-emetics 102
  as antipsychotics 97
Phenoxybenzamine 77
Phenoxymethylpenicillin 77
Phensuximide 77
Phentermine 77
Phentolamine 77
Phenylbutazone 77
Phenylephrine 431
Phenylpropanolamine 77
Phenyl salicylate 77
Phenyltoloxamine 77
Phenytoin 432
Phillips' Gelcaps 77
Phillips' Milk of Magnesia see
  Magnesium hydroxide 370
pHisoHex 77
Pholcodine 77
Phospholine Iodide 77
Phosphorus 77
Photophobia 550g
Phyllocontin see Theophylline 490
Physostigmine 77
Phytomenadione 77
Phytonadione 77, 116, 117; see
  Vitamin K 530
Piles see Hemorrhoids 125
Pilocarpine 433
Pilopine HS see Pilocarpine 433
Pimozide 77
Pinaverium 77
Pindolol 434
Pinworm see Anthelmintic drugs
  151
Pipenzepine 77
Piperacillin 77
Piperazine 77
Piperazine estrone sulfate 77
Piperonyl butoxide 188
Piportil L4 77
Pipotiazine 77
Pipracil 77
Pirmenol 77
Piroxicam 435
Pitressin see Vasopressin 511
Pitrex see Tolnaftate 498
Pituitary disorders, drugs for 157
Pivampicillin 436
Pivmecillinam 77
Pizotyline 77
Placebo 550g; see Placebo
  response 15
Placenta, cancer of see
  Choriocarcinoma
Placidyl 77
Plaquenil 77
Platelets see Antiplatelet drugs
  116
Platinol 77
Plendil 35R (illus.); see Felodipine
  310
Plicamycin 77
PMS-Amantadine see
  Amantadine 205
PMS-ASA see ASA 200
PMS-Baclofen see Baclofen 221
PMS-Benztropine see
  Benztropine 225

PMS-Cholestyramine see
  Cholestyramine 255
PMS-Clonazepam see
  Clonazepam 265
PMS Dimenhydrinate see
  Dimenhydrinate 288
PMS-Docusate Calcium 77
PMS-Docusate Sodium 77
PMS-Egozinc 77
PMS-Fluphenazine see
  Fluphenazine 319
PMS-Hydromorphone see
  Hydromorphone 339
PMS-Isoniazid see Isoniazid
  349
PMS-Ketoprofen see Ketoprofen
  354
PMS-Lactulose see Lactulose
  356
PMS-Levazine 77
PMS-Levothyroxine Sodium see
  Levothyroxine 359
PMS-Lindane see Lindane 361
PMS-Loperamide Hydrochloride
  see Loperamide 365
PMS-Methylphenidate see
  Methylphenidate 385
PMS-Nylidrin 77
PMS-Prochlorperazine see
  Prochlorperazine 444
PMS-Procyclidine see
  Procyclidine 445
PMS Promethazine see
  Promethazine 446
PMS-Promethazine Syrup see
  Promethazine 446
PMS-Propranolol see Propranolol
  448
PMS-Pyrazinamide 77
PMS-Sulfasalazine see
  Sulfasalazine 475
PMS-Testosterone Enanthate see
  Testosterone 488
PMS-Trazodone see Trazodone
  499
PMS-Trihexyphenidyl see
  Trihexyphenidyl 505
Pneumocystis pneumonia see
  Antiprotozoal drugs 148; see
  also Pneumocystis carinii
  pneumonia 169
Pneumonia
  chlamydial 143
  pneumocystis 148
    PCP 169
  walking see Erythromycin 302
  See also Antibiotics 140-142;
  Respiratory system 103-106
Podifilox 77
Podofilm 77
Podophyllin 77
Poison 550g
Poisoning 574-576
Polaramine 77
Polio vaccine 147
Polocaine 77
Polycarbophil calcium 77
Polyethylene glycol 77
Polymyxin B 77

Polyoxyethylene (20) sorbitan
  mono-oleate see Polysorbate
  80 542
Polyoxyethylene (20) sorbitan
  monostearate see Polysorbate
  60 542
Polysorbate 60 542
Polysorbate 80 542
Polysporin 77
Polysporin Burn Formula 77
Polytopic 77
Polytrim 77
Poly-Vi-Flor 77
Polyvinyl alcohol 77
Poly-Vi-Sol 78
Ponderal 78
Pondimin 78
Pondocillin 44H (illus.); see
  Pivampicillin 436
Ponstan 48B (illus.); see
  Mefenamic acid 375
Pontocaine 78
Poppers see Nitrites 537
Pork roundworm see Anthelmintic
  drugs 151
Pot see Marijuana 536
Potaba 78
Potassium 524
Potassium acetate see Potassium
  524
Potassium alginate see Calcium
  alginate 540
Potassium amino acid see
  Potassium 524
Potassium bicarbonate see
  Potassium 524
Potassium bisulfite see Sodium
  sulfite 543
Potassium chloride see
  Potassium 524
Potassium citrate see Potassium
  524
Potassium clavulanate 78; see
  also Clavulanate potassium
Potassium gluconate see
  Potassium 524
Potassium iodide 78; see Iodine
  522
Potassium metabisulfite see
  Sodium sulfite 543
Potassium nitrate see Sodium
  nitrate 543
Potassium nitrite see Sodium
  nitrate 543
Potassium permanganate 78
Potassium pyrosulfite see
  Sodium sulfite 543
Potassium-Sandoz 78
Potassium sorbate see Sorbic
  acid 543
Potassium-sparing diuretics 111
Povidone 78
Povidone-iodine 187
Pralidoxime 78
Pramox H.C. 78
Pramoxine 78
Pravachol 41O (illus.); see
  Pravastatin 437
Pravastatin 437

Prazepam 78
Praziquantel 78, 151, 167
Prazosin 438
Pred Forte see Prednisolone 439
Pred Mild see Prednisolone 439
Prednisolone 439
Prednisone *43G* (illus.); 440
Prefrin see Phenylephrine 431
Prefrin-A 78
Pregnancy
  hormone levels during 159
  infertility drugs 176
  oral contraceptives 173-175
  treatment during 21
  See also Drugs used in labor
    177; Drugs used to reduce
    prolactin levels 157
Premarin *35B, 37M, 38S, 39R*
  (illus.); see Conjugated
  estrogens 272
Premedication 550g
Premenstrual syndrome, drugs
  for 172
Prenalterol 78
Prenavite 78
Prenylamine 78
Prepidil Gel see Dinoprostone
  289
Prepulsid *42L, 43B* (illus.); see
  Cisapride 259
Prescription 550g
  drugs 26
    classification of 13
    interacting with OTC drugs 16
  See also Drugs
Preservatives see Major types of
  additives 539
Pressyn see Vasopressin 511
Prevacid 78
Prevex 78
Prevex B see Betamethasone 227
Prevex Baby Diaper Rash Cream
  78
Prevex HC see Hydrocortisone
  338
Prilocaine 78
Primaquine 149
Primaxim 78
Primidone 441
Primrose oil see Evening primrose
  oil 63
Prinivil *37R, 43O* (illus.); see
  Lisinopril 363
Prinzide 78
Priscoline 78
Privine 78
Pro-Air 78
Pro-Banthine 78
Probenecid 442
Probucol 115
Procainamide 443
Procaine 78
Procan SR see Procainamide 443
Procarbazine 167
Procaterol 78
Prochlorperazine 444
Procinonide 78
Proctofoam-HC 78
Proctosone 78

Procyclid see Procyclidine 445
Procyclidine 445
Procytox see Cyclophosphamide
  276
Prodiem Plain see Psyllium 451
Prodiem Plus 78
Profasi HP see HCG 334
Progestasert 78
Progesterone 159
Progestins 159
  for Menstrual disorders 172
  in Oral contraceptives 173-175
Proglycem 78
Proguanil 78
Prolactin 157
Prolopa 78
Proloprim see Trimethoprim 507
Promani 78
Promatussin DM 78
Promazine 78
Promethazine 446
Prometrium 78
Pronestyl see Procainamide 443
Pronestyl SR see Procainamide
  443
Propaderm see Beclomethasone
  222
Propafenone 78
Propantheline 78
Proparacaine 78
Prophylactic 550g
Propine 78
Propionic acid 542; see Chemical
  preservatives 539
Propoxyphene 447
Propranolol 448
Proprietary 550g
Propylene glycol 78, 542
Propyl gallate 542
Propyl p-hydroxybenzoate see
  Methylparaben 541
Propylparaben 78
Propylparaben see
  Methylparaben 541
Propylthiouracil 449
Propyl 3,4,5 trihydroxybenzoate
  see Propyl gallate 542
Propyl-Thyracil see
  Propylthiouracil 449
Proscar see Finasteride 313
Prosom 79
Prostaglandin E1 see Misoprostol
  393
Prostaglandin E2 see
  Dinoprostone 289
Prostaglandins 177
Prostate cancer see Anticancer
  drugs 166-167
Prostatitis see Co-Trimoxazole
  273
Prostigmin see Neostigmine 403
Prostin E2 see Dinoprostone 289
Prostin VR 79
Proteins 160
Protirelin 79
Protopam Chloride 79
Protozoa see Antimalarial drugs
  149; Antiprotozoal drugs 148
Protriptyline 79

Protropin 79
Provera *36J, 39I, 43C* (illus.); see
  Medroxyprogesterone 374
Proviodine 79
Prozac *48E* (illus.); see Fluoxetine
  318
Pruritus, drugs for 185
Pseudoephedrine 450
Psilocybin 13
Psoralens see Drugs for Psoriasis
  190
Psoriasis, drugs for 190
Psorigel 79
Psychotic disorders see
  Antipsychotic drugs 97
Psyllium 451
Puberty see Sex hormones 158,
  159
Pubic lice, drugs for 188
Puffers see Inhalers
Pulmicort see Budesonide 233
Pulmophylline see Theophylline
  490
Pulmorphan Expectorant 79
Pupil, drugs affecting 182
Purgative 550g
Purinethol 79
Purinol see Allopurinol 202
PUVA therapy 190
PVF K see Penicillin V 425
Pyopen 79
Pyrantel 452
Pyrazinamide 79
Pyrethrins 79
Pyribenzamine 79
Pyridium see Phenazopyridine
  429
Pyridostigmine 453
Pyridoxine 525
Pyrilamine 79
Pyrimethamine 454
Pyrvinium 79

R

Radiation therapy, nausea caused
  by see Anti-emetic drugs 102
Radioactive iodine 156
Radiostol see Vitamin D 529
Ramipril 79
R & C 79
Ranitidine *42B* (illus.); 458
RAS 95, 100
Rash see Antihistamines; Skin
Raubasine 79
Rauwolfia 79
Raynaud's disease see
  Vasodilators 110
Razoxane 79
Reactine *44C* (illus.); see
  Cetirizine 246
Receptor 550g
  effects of drugs 16
Recovery position 575
Rectal administration of drugs 18,
  19
Rectal disorders, drugs for 125
Rectocort see Hydrocortisone
  338
Rectovalone 79
Redoxon see Vitamin C 528
Redoxon-B 79
Redoxon-Cal 79
Redskin see Allyl isothiocyanate
  540
Refresh 79
Regional enteritis see Crohn's
  disease 124
Reglan see Metoclopramide 387
Regonol see Pyridostigmine 453
Regulex 79
Regulex-D 79
Reiter's syndrome see Sulindac
  478
Relafen see Nabumetone 397
Relefact TRH 79
Renacidin 79
Renedil *35Q* (illus.); see
  Felodipine 310
Replication 550g
Reproductive tract 170-178
Reserpine 79
Resorcinol 79
Respiratory system, drugs for
  103-106
    antibiotic 141
    respiratory stimulants 100
  See also Allergy treatments
Restoril *47H, 47K* (illus.); see
  Temazepam 481

Q

Q fever see Chloramphenicol
  249; Tetracycline 489
Quazepam 79
Quelicin Chloride 79
Questran see Cholestyramine 255
Questran Light see
  Cholestyramine 255
Quibron-T see Theophylline 490
Quibron-T/SR see Theophylline
  490
Quinacrine 148
Quinalbarbitone 79
Quinapril 455
Quinate see Quinidine 456
Quinestrol 79
Quinfamide 79
Quinidex see Quinidine 456
Quinidine 456
Quinine 457

Quinolones
  as antibacterials 143
  as antibiotics 142
  Ciprofloxacin 258
  uses of 141
Quintasq see Mesalamine 378

Resuscitation, mouth-to-mouth 575
Resyl see Guaifenesin 331
Reticular activating system 95, 100
Retin-A see Tretinoin 500
Retinoic acid see Vitamin A 527
Retinoids see Vitamin A 527
Retinol see Vitamin A 527
Retinol palmitate see Vitamin A 527
Retisol-A see Tretinoin 500
Retrovir see Zidovudine 516
Reversible inhibitors of monoamine oxidase A 394
Revimine 79
Revitalose-C-1000 see Vitamin C 528
Reye's syndrome 93, 200
Rheumatoid arthritis see Antirheumatic drugs 129
Rheumatrex see Methotrexate 381
Rhinalar see Flunisolide 315
Rhinaris F see Flunisolide 315
Rhinocort see Budesonide 233
Rhinocort Aqua see Budesonide 233
Rhinocort Turbuhaler see Budesonide 233
Rhodis see Ketoprofen 354
Rhoprolene see Betamethasone 227
Rhoprosone see Betamethasone 227
Rhotral see Acebutolol 198
Rhotrimine see Trimipramine 508
Ribavirin 80
Riboflavin 525
Rickets, drugs for 134
Ridaura see Auranofin 216
Rifabutin 143
Rifadin see Rifampin 459
Rifampicin see Rifampin 459
Rifampin 459
Rifater see Isoniazid 349; Rifampin 459
RIMA 394
Rimactane see Rifampin 459
Rimso-50 80
Ringworm see Antifungal drugs 150
Riopan 80
Riopan Extra Strength 80
Riopan Plus 80
Riopan Plus Extra Strength 80
Risperdal 80
Risperidone 80
Ritalin 39B (illus.); see Methylphenidate 385
Ritalin SR see Methylphenidate 385
Ritodrine 460
Rivotril 36T, 42P (illus.); see Clonazepam 265
R.O. Carpine see Pilocarpine 433
R.O.-Dexsone see Dexamethasone 280
R.O.-Dry Eyes 80

R.O.-Eye Drops 80
R.O.-Gentycin see Gentamicin 328
R.O.-Naphz 80
R.O.-Parcaine 80
R.O.-Predphate Forte see Prednisolone 439
R.O.-Tropamide 80
Robaxacet 80
Robaxacet-8 80
Robaxin see Methocarbamol 380
Robaxisal 80
Robaxisal-C 80
Robaxisal-C 1/2 80
Robaxisal-C 1/4 80
Robaxisal-C 1/8 80
Robidex see Dextromethorphan 281
Robidone see Hydrocodone 337
Robidrine see Pseudoephedrine 450
Robinul 80
Robinul Forte 80
Robitussin see Guaifenesin 331
Robitussin A-C 80
Robitussin CF 80
Robitussin DM 80; see Dextromethorphan 281
Robitussin-DM see Guaifenesin 331
Robitussin PE 80
Robitussin with Codeine 80
Rocaltrol 529
Rocephin 80
Rochelle salts see Tartaric acid 543
Rocky Mountain spotted fever see Chloramphenicol 249; Tetracycline 489
Rofact see Rifampin 459
Roferon-A see Interferon 347
Rogaine see Minoxidil 392
Rogitine 80
Roniacol 80
Rotohalers see Bronchodilators 104
Roubac 80
Roundworm infestation 139; see Anthelmintic drugs 151
Rovamycine 80
Roxicet 80
Roychlor 80
Royflex 80
Rubbing alcohol see Alcohol, rubbing 50; isopropyl alcohol 67
Rubefacient 550g
Rubella vaccine 147
Rubramin 80
Rynacrom see Cromolyn sodium 274
Rythmodan see Disopyramide 293
Rythmodan-LA see Disopyramide 293
Rythmol 80

S

Sabril 80
Salac 80
Salazopyrin see Sulfasalazine 475
Salazosulfapyridine see Sulfasalazine 475
Salbutamol 461
Salcatonin 80
Salicylamide 80
Salicylazosulfapyridine see Sulfasalazine 475
Salicylic acid 80
Salicylsalicylic acid 80
Saline from Otrivin 80
Saline laxatives 123
Salinex 80
Salinol 80
Salmeterol 462
Salofalk see Mesalamine 378
Salsalate 128
Saltpeter see Sodium nitrate 543
Sandalwood oil see Oils 542
Sandimmune see Cyclosporine 277
Sandomigran 80
Sandomigran DS 80
Sanorex 80
Sans-Acne 80
Sansert 80
Santyl 80
Sarna HC see Hydrocortisone 338
Sarna-P 80
SAS-500 see Sulfasalazine 475
Sastid 80
Sauce see Alcohol 532
Savlodil 80
Savlon Hospital Concentrate 80
Scabene 80
Scabies infestation 139, 188
Scag see Heroin 535
Scalp ringworm see Antifungal drugs 150
Scarlet fever see Penicillin G 424; Penicillin V 425
Schamberg's Lotion 81
Schedule F, G, H drugs 13
Schizophrenia, drugs for 97
Scopolamine 463
Scurvy 528
Sebcur 81
Sebcur/T 81
Sebulex 81
Sebulon 81
Sebutone 81
Secaris 81
Secobarbital 24
Seconal see Secobarbital 24
Sectral 39D, 43N (illus.); see Acebutolol 198

Sedative 550g
Seizure 576
drugs for 98
Selax 81
Seldane see Terfenadine 487
Selective serotonin reuptake inhibitors 96
Selegiline 464
Selenious acid see Selenium 526
Selenium 526
Selenium sulfide 81
Selexid 81
Selsun 81
Semustine 81
Senna see Laxatives 123
Senokot 40O (illus.); see Senna 123
Senokot/S 81
Septra 81
Septra DS 44E (illus.); 81
Sequestrants see Major types of additives 539
Ser-Ap-Es 81
Serax see Oxazepam 417
Serc see Oxazepam 417
Serentil 81
Serevent see Salmeterol 462
Seromycin 81
Serophene see Clomiphene 263
Serotonin 96
Serpasil 81
Serpasil-Esidrix 81
Sertraline 465
Serzone 81
Sevin 81
Sex hormones 158, 159
Sexually transmitted diseases genital herpes see Antiviral drugs 145
gonorrhea see Cefixime 242; Cefuroxime 244
See also Genital tract infection
Shepard's Skin Cream 81
Shock, anaphylactic 576
Sialor 81
Sibelium 81
Side effects 15, 550g
ending therapy and 28
Silicone 81
Silon 81
Silver nitrate 81
Silver sulfadiazine 466
Simethicone 81
Simvastatin 467
Sinemet 81
Sinemet CR 81
Sinequan see Doxepin 296
Sintrom 81
Sinutab N.D. Daytime Formula 81
Sinutab Nighttime Formula 81
Sinutab No Drowsiness 81
Sinutab Regular 81
Sinutab SA 81
Sinutab with Codeine 81
642 Tablets see Propoxyphene 447
692 Tablets 81
Sjögren's syndrome see Artificial tear preparations 182

Skin 184-191
cancer see Anticancer drugs
166-167
infection 141, 187
itchy see Antipruritic
medications 185
niacin deficiency and 523
parasites, drugs for 188
ringworm see Antifungal drugs
150
Sleep-Eze D see
Diphenhydramine 290
Sleep-Eze D Extra Strength see
Diphenhydramine 290
Sleeping drugs 94
Sleeping sickness see
Trypanosomiasis 148
Slim Mint 81
Slo-Bid see Theophylline 490
Slow-Fe 81
Slow-Fe-Folic 81
Slow-K 40H (illus.); 81
Slow-release preparations 18
Slow-Trasicor 81
Smack see Heroin 535
Snappers see Nitrites 537
Sniffing solvents see Solvents 538
Snow see Cocaine 534
Sodium 526
Sodium acetate see Sodium 526
Sodium alginate see Calcium
alginate 540
Sodium ascorbate see Vitamin C
528
Sodium benzoate see Benzoic
acid 540
Sodium bicarbonate 120
Sodium biphosphate 81
Sodium bisulfite see Sodium
sulfite 543
Sodium borate 81
Sodium carboxymethylcellulose
542
Sodium cellulose phosphate 81
Sodium chloride see Sodium 526
Sodium citrate 120, 542
Sodium cromoglycate see
Cromolyn sodium 274
Sodium erythorbate see
Erythorbic acid 541
Sodium fluoride see Fluoride 521
Sodium fusidate see Fusidic acid
326
Sodium hexametaphosphate 543
Sodium hypochlorite 81
Sodium iodide 81
Sodium metabisulfite see Sodium
sulfite 543
Sodium monofluorophosphate
see Fluoride 521
Sodium nitrate 81
Sodium nitrite 543; see also
Sodium nitrate 81
Sodium nitroprusside 81
Sodium phosphate see Sodium
526
Sodium polymetaphosphate see
Sodium hexametaphosphate
543

Sodium potassium tartrate see
Tartaric acid 543
Sodium propionate see Propionic
acid 542
Sodium salicylate 81
Sodium salt see Sodium
carboxymethylcellulose 542
Sodium selenite see Selenium
526
Sodium sorbate see Sorbic acid
543
Sodium Sulamyd see
Sulfacetamide 473
Sodium sulfite 543
Sodium tartrate see Tartaric acid
543
Sodium thiosulfate 81
Soflax 46A (illus.); 82
Sofracort 82
Soframycin Eye Drops/Ointment
82
Soframycin Nasal Spray 82
Soframycin Ointment 82
Sofra-Tulle 82
Soft tissue
cancer see Anticancer drugs
166-167
infection 141
injury see NSAIDs 128
Solaquin 82
Solaquin Forte 82
Solar keratoses see Fluorouracil
317
Solium see Chlordiazepoxide 250
Solu-Cortef see Hydrocortisone
338
Solugel see Benzoyl peroxide 224
Solu-Medrol see
Methylprednisolone 386
Soluver 82
Solvents 538
Soma 82
Somatrem see Growth hormone
157
Somatropin see Growth hormone
157
Somnol see Flurazepam 320
Somophyllin-12 see Theophylline
490
Sonacide 82
Sopamycetin see
Chloramphenicol 249
Sopamycetin-HC 82
Sorbic acid 543; see Chemical
preservatives 539
Sorbitol 543
Soriatane 82
Sotacor 39O (illus.); see Sotalol
468
Sotalol 468
Spasticity see Muscle-relaxant
drugs 132
Specific serotonin reuptake
inhibitors see Fluoxetine 318;
Fluvoxamine 323
Spectinomycin 82
Spectro Gram "2" 82
Spectro Tar Antiseptic Shampoo
82

Spectro Tar Skin Wash 82
Speed see Amphetamines 533
Spermicides 173
Spersacarpine see Pilocarpine
433
Spersadex see Dexamethasone
280
SPF see Sunscreens 191
Spiramycin 148
Spironolactone 469
Sporanox 82
SSD see Silver sulfadiazine 466
SSRIs 96
Stabilizers see Major types of
additives 539
Stadol NS see Butorphanol 236
Stannous fluoride see Fluoride
521
Statex see Morphine 395
Staticin see Erythromycin 302
Statin drugs 115
Status epilepticus 98
Steatorrhea 528
Stelabid 82
Stelazine see Trifluoperazine 504
Stemetil see Prochlorperazine 444
Steri/Sol 82
Steroids see Anabolic steroids
158
Stibocaptate 82
Stibogluconate 82
StieVA-A see Tretinoin 500
Stievamycin see Erythromycin
302; Tretinoin 500
Stilboestrol 82
Stimulants
laxative 123
nervous system 100
respiratory 100
uterine 177
Streptase see Streptokinase 470
Streptokinase 470
Streptomycin 471
Streptozocin 82
Strongyloidiasis see Anthelmintic
drugs 151
Subcutaneous injection 550g
administration of 18
Sublimaze 82
Sublingual 17, 550g
Sucaryl 82
Succinylcholine 82
Sucralfate 472
Sucrets 82
Sudafed see Pseudoephedrine
450
Sudafed Cough and Cold Extra
Strength 82
Sudafed DM 82
Sudafed Expectorant 82
Sudafed Sinus Extra Strength 82
Sudan gum see Acacia 540
Sufenta 82
Sufentanil 82
Sulcrate 45A (illus.); see
Sucralfate 472
Sulcrate Suspension Plus see
Sucralfate 472

Sulfabenzamide 82
Sulfacetamide 473
Sulfacet-R 82
Sulfacytine 82
Sulfadiazine 82
Sulfadoxine 82
Sulfa drugs 143
Sulfaguanidine 82
Sulfamerazine 82
Sulfamethazine 82
Sulfamethoxazole 474
Sulfanilamide 82
Sulfasalazine 475
Sulfathiazole 82
Sulfex see Sulfacetamide 473
Sulfex 10% see Sulfacetamide
473
Sulfinpyrazone 476
Sulfisoxazole 477
Sulfite ammonia caramel see
Caramel 540
Sulfizole see Sulfisoxazole 477
Sulfonamides 141
as antibacterials 143
as antibiotics 142
Sulfonylurea drugs 154-155
Sulfoxyl see Benzoyl peroxide 224
Sulfur 82
Sulfur dioxide 543; see Chemical
preservatives 539
Sulindac 478
Sultrin 82
Sumatriptan 479
Sunburn see Benzocaine 223;
Sunscreens 191
Sunscreens 191
Supeudol see Oxycodone 419
Suplevit 82
Suppository 19, 550g
administration of 18
Supracaine 82
Supraventricular tachycardia see
Anti-arrhythmic drugs 112
Suprax see Cefixime 242
Suprefact 82
Supres 82; see Methyldopa 384
Suramin 82
Surbex-500 82
Surbex-500 Plus Iron 82
Surbex-500 Plus Zinc 82
Surfak 83
Surgam see Tiaprofenic acid 492
Surgam SR 41H (illus.); see
Tiaprofenic acid 492
Surmontil see Trimipramine 508
Sus-Phrine see Epinephrine 300
Sutilains 83
Suxamethonium 83
Swelling see Inflammation
Swiss One 83
Symmetrel see Amantadine 205
Sympathetic nervous system 91
Sympatholytics 550g
as antihypertensives 114
as vasodilators 110
Sympathomimetics 550g
as bronchodilators 104
mydriatic 182
in urinary disorders 178

Synacthen-Depot 83
Synalar see Fluocinolone 316
Synalar Bi-Otic 83
Synamol see Fluocinolone 316
Synarel 83
Syn-Captopril see Captopril 239
Syn-Diltiazem see Diltiazem 287
Synflex 83
Syn-Flunisolide see Flunisolide 315
Syn-Nadolol see Nadolol 398
Synphasic 83
Syn-Pindolol see Pindolol 434
Synthroid 38E, 39M, 39P, 40L, 43A (illus.); see Levothyroxine 359
Syn-Trazodone see Trazodone 499
Syrup 19
Systemic 550g
Systemic lupus erythematosus 168; see Corticosteroids 153

T

T see Phencyclidine 538
Tablet 19
Tachycardia see Anti-arrhythmic drugs 112
Tagamet see Cimetidine 257
Talampicillin 83
Talwin 83
Tambocor 83
Tamofen see Tamoxifen 480
Tamone see Tamoxifen 480
Tamoxifen 480
Tanacet 125 83
Tannic acid 83
Tantaphen see Acetaminophen 199
Tantum see Benzydamine 226
Tapazole 83
Tapeworm infestation 139
vitamin B$_{12}$ for 528
See Anthelmintic drugs 151
Tardan 83
Tardive dyskinesia 551g
due to antipsychotics 97
Target 83
Taro-Sone see Betamethasone 227
Tartaric acid 543
Tartrazine 543
Tavist 83
Taxol 83
Tazidime 83
Tazobactam 83
Tazocin 83
Teardrops 83
Tears Naturale 83
Tears Plus 83
Tebrazid 83
Tecnal 83
Tecnal C 83

Tedral 83
Teejel 83
Tegafur 83
Tegison see Etretinate 308
Tegopen see Cloxacillin 269
Tegretol see Carbamazepine 240
Tegretol CR 40I (illus.); see Carbamazepine 240
Temazepam 481
Temposil 83
Tempra see Acetaminophen 199
Tendinitis 130
Teniposide 83
Tennis elbow 130
Tenoretic see Atenolol 215; Chlorthalidone 254
Tenormin 42J (illus.); see Atenolol 215
Tenoxicam 482
Tensilon 83
Tenuate 83
Terazol see Terconazole 486
Terazosin 483
Terbinafine 484
Terbutaline 485
Terconazole 486
Terfenadine 487
Terfluzine see Trifluoperazine 504
Terpin hydrate 83
Tersac 83
Tersaseptic 83
Tersa-Tar 83
Tersa-Tar Mild 83
Testosterone 488
Tetanus vaccine 147
Tetrabenazene 83
Tetracaine 185
Tetrachloroethylene 83
Tetracycline 489
as antibiotic 142
uses of 141
Tetracyn see Tetracycline 489
Tetrahydrozoline 83
Texacort see Hydrocortisone 338
T/Gel 83
Theine see Caffeine 540
Theo-Bronc see Theophylline 490
Theochron see Theophylline 490
Theo-Dur 44L, 45K (illus.); see Theophylline 490
Theolair see Theophylline 490
Theolair-SR see Theophylline 490
Theolixir see Theophylline 490
Theophylline 490
Theophylline KI see Theophylline 490
Theo-SR see Theophylline 490
Thiabendazole 151
Thiamine 527
Thiamine mononitrate see Thiamine 527
Thiamylal 84
Thiazides see Diuretics 111
Thiazine see Spironolactone 469
Thiethylperazine 84
Thimerosal 84; see also Artificial tear preparations 182
Thioguanine 84
Thiopental 84

Thioproperazine 84
Thioridazine 491
Thiotepa 84
Thiothixene 84
Threadworm see Anthelmintic drugs 151
Throat infection 141
Thrombocytopenia, drugs for Prednisone 440
Triamcinolone 501
Thrombolytic drugs 117
Thrush see Antifungal drugs 150
Thymoxamine 84
Thyro-Block 84
Thyroid disorders, drugs for 156
Thyrotoxicosis, drugs for 156
Thyroxine see Levothyroxine 359
Tiaprofenic acid 492
Ticar 84
Ticarcillin 84
Ticlid 44K (illus.); see Ticlopidine 493
Ticlopidine 493
Tilade see Nedocromil 401
Timentin 84
Timolide 84
Timolol 494
Timoptic see Timolol 494
Timpilo see Pilocarpine 433; Timolol 494
Tinactin see Tolnaftate 498
Tinea infection see Antifungal drugs 150
Tinidazole 84
Tioconazole 84
Tissue plasminogen activator 495
Titanium dioxide 191
Tixocortal 84
Tobacco see Drug abuse 24; Nicotine 537
Tobradex see Dexamethasone 280; Tobramycin 496
Tobramycin 496
Tobrex Ophthalmic see Tobramycin 496
Tocainide 84
Tocopherol see Vitamin E 529
Tocopheryl acetate 84
Today Sponge 84
Toesen see Oxytocin 421
Tofranil see Imipramine 343
Tolazoline 84
Tolbutamide 497
Tolectin 84
Tolerance 551g
Tolmetin 84
Tolnaftate 498
Tomasin see Papain 542
Tonics 551g
Tonocard 84
Tonsillitis see Throat infection 141
Toothache see Analgesics 92-93
Topicaine see Benzocaine 223
Topical 551g
application 18
corticosteroids 186, 190
skin preparations 19
Topicort 84
Topilene see Betamethasone 227

Topisone see Betamethasone 227
Topsyn 84
Toradol 42K (illus.); see Ketorolac 355
Torecan 84
Totopherols see Vitamin E 529
Tourette's syndrome see Haloperidol 332
Toxic megacolon see Diphenoxylate 291
Toxic reaction 551g
Toxin, toxic 551g
Toxocariasis see Anthelmintic drugs 151
Toxoplasmosis see Antiprotozoal drugs 148; Pyrimethamine 454
tPA see Tissue plasminogen activator 495
Tracrium 84
Trandate 84
Tranexamic acid 84
Tranq see Phencyclidine 538
Tranquilizer
major 551g
minor 551g
See Anti-anxiety drugs 95; Antipsychotic drugs 97; Benzodiazepines 534
Transdermal patch 551g
administration of 18
Transderm-Nitro see Nitroglycerin 408
Transderm-V see Scopolamine 463
Transplant see Organ transplant rejection
Trans-Plantar 84
Trans-Ver-Sal 84
Tranxene see Clorazepate 267
Trasicor 84
Trasylol 84
Travase 84
Travel Aid see Dimenhydrinate 288
Travel Tabs see Dimenhydrinate 288
Trazodone 499
Trental 35C (illus.); see Pentoxifylline 426
Tretinoin 500 see Vitamin A 527
Triacomb 84
Triadapin see Doxepin 296
Triaderm see Triamcinolone 501
Triamcinolone 501
Triaminic-DM Expectorant 84
Triaminic-DM Nighttime 84
Triaminic Expectorant 84
Triaminic Expectorant DH 84
Triaminicin 84
Triaminicol DM 84
Triaminic Tablets 84
Triamterene 502
Triavil see Amitriptyline 208; Perphenazine 428
Triazolam 503
Tribasic calcium phosphate 543
Tricalcium diorthophosphate see Tribasic calcium phosphate 543

Tricalcium phosphate see Tribasic calcium phosphate 543
Trichinosis see Anthelmintic drugs 151
Trichloracetic acid 84
Trichomoniasis see Antiprotozoal drugs 148
Trichuriasis see Anthelmintic drugs 151
Triclocarban 84
Triclosan 84
Tri-Cyclen 84, 173
Tricyclic antidepressants 96
Tridesilon 84
Tridil see Nitroglycerin 408
Trientine 84
Triethanolamine salicylate 85
Triethylenetetramine 85
Trifluoperazine 504
Trifluridine 145
Trihexyphenidyl 505
Triiodothyronine see Liothyronine 362
Trikacide see Metronidazole 389
Trilafon see Perphenazine 428
Trilisate 85
Trilostane 85
Trimazosin 85
Trimebutine 506
Trimeprazine 85
Trimethaphan 85
Trimethoprim 507
Trimipramine 508
Trinalin see Azatadine 217; Pseudoephedrine 450
Trinsicon 85
Trioxsalen 85
Tripelennamine 85
Triphasil 85, 173
Triprolidine 85
Triptil 85
Triquilar 85, 173
Trisoralen 85
Trisulfaminic 85
Trisyn 85
Tri-Vi-Flor 85
Tri-Vi-Sol 85
Tri-Vi-Sol with Fluoride 85
Trobicin 85
Tropicamide 182
Trosyd AF 85
Trypanosomiasis 148
Trypsin 85
Tryptan 85
Tryptophan 85
T-Stat see Erythromycin 302
Tubarine 85
Tuberculosis see Antituberculous drugs 144
Tubocurarine 85
Tuinal 85
Tumor see Cancer
Tums 85
Turbuhalers see Bronchodilators 104
Tussaminic C 85
Tussaminic DH 85
Tussionex 85
282 MEP 83

282 Tablets 83
292 Tablets 83
217 Strong Tablets 83
217 Tablets 83
222 AF see Acetaminophen 199
222 Forte Tablets 83
Tylenol see Acetaminophen 199; Codeine 270
Tylenol Allergy Sinus Medication 85
Tylenol Cold Medication 85
Tylenol No.2 41N (illus.); see Acetaminophen 199
Tylenol No.3 see Acetaminophen 199
Tylenol Sinus Medication 85
Tylenol with Codeine No.2 41N (illus.); 85
Tylenol with Codeine No.3 41I (illus.); 85

U

Ulcer see Anti-ulcer drugs 121
Ulcerative colitis 124
Ulone 85
Ultradol 85
Ultra Mide 25 85
Ultra MOP see Methoxsalen 383
Ultraquin 85
Ultravate 85
Ultraviolet light treatment 190
Uncinariasis see Anthelmintic drugs 151
Undecylenic acid 85
Unipen 85
Uniphyl see Theophylline 490
Univol 85
Uppers see Amphetamines 533
Urea 85
Urecholine 85
Uremol 85
Uremol-HC 85
Urethritis, drugs for 178
Uricosuric drugs 131
Uridon see Chlorthalidone 254
Urinary disorders, drugs for 178
antibiotic 141
Urisec 85
Urispas 85
Uritol see Furosemide 325
Urofollitropin 176
Urokinase 85
Uromitexan 85
Urozide see Hydrochlorothiazide 336
Ursodeoxycholic acid see Ursodiol 509
Ursodiol 509
Ursofalk see Ursodiol 509
Urticaria, drugs for 185
Uterine muscle relaxants, stimulants 177
Uveitis see Drugs affecting the pupil 182

V

Vaccine 146-147, 551g
action of 14
Valisone see Betamethasone 227
Valisone-G 86
Valium see Diazepam 282
Valproic acid 510
Vancenase see Beclomethasone 222
Vanceril see Beclomethasone 222
Vancocin 86
Vancomycin 86
Vanoxide-HC 86
Vanquin 86
Vaponefrin see Epinephrine 300
Vaseline Petroleum Jelly 86
Vaseretic see Enalapril 299; Hydrochlorothiazide 336
Vasocidin 86
Vasocon 86
Vasocon-A 86
Vasoconstrictor 551g
Vasodilator 110, 551g
Vasopressin 511
Vasosulf see Phenylephrine 431; Sulfacetamide 473
Vasotec 37S, 40C, 44B (illus.); see Enalapril 299
Vasoxyl 86
V-Cillin K see Penicillin V 425
Vecuronium 86
Velbe 86
Velosulin see Insulin 346
Velvelan 86
Venlafaxine 512
as SSRI 96
Ventodisk see Salbutamol 461
Ventolin see Salbutamol 461
Ventolin Rotocaps see Salbutamol 461
Ventricular tachycardia see Anti-arrhythmic drugs 112
Vepesid 86
Verapamil 513
Verelan see Verapamil 513
Vermox see Mebendazole 372
Versed 86
Versel 86
Vertigo see Anti-emetic drugs 102
Viaderm-K.C. 86
Vibramycin see Doxycycline 297
Vibra-Tabs see Doxycycline 297
Vicks Vaporub 86
Vidarabine 86, 145
Videx see Didanosine 284
Vigabatrin 86
Viloxazine 86
Vinblastine 166
Vincent's gingivitis see Penicillin G 424; Penicillin V 425
Vincristine 167
Vindesine 166
Vioform 86
Vioform-Hydrocortisone 86
Viokase 86
Viprynium 86

Vira-A 86
Viral infection see Antiviral drugs 145
vaccination against 146-147
Virazole 86
Viroptic 86
Visceral larva migrans see Toxocariasis 151
Viskazide 86
Visken see Pindolol 434
Vistacrom see Cromolyn sodium 274
Vitaday Forte 86
Vitamin 161-163, 518-530
daily requirements of 163
food sources of 162
Vitamin A 527
Vitamin A Acid see Tretinoin 500
Vitamin B_1 see Thiamine 527
Vitamin B_2 see Riboflavin 525
Vitamin B_3 see Niacin 523
Vitamin B_5 see Pantothenic acid 524
Vitamin B_6 see Pyridoxine 525
Vitamin B_{12} 528
Vitamin C 528
Vitamin D 529; see Calcipotriol 237
Vitamin D_2 see Vitamin D 529
Vitamin D_3 see Vitamin D 529
Vitamin E 529
Vitamin G see Riboflavin 525
Vitamin H see Biotin 519
Vitamin K 530
Vitamin K_1 see Vitamin K 530
Vitamin K_2 see Vitamin K 530
Vitamin K_3 see Vitamin K 530
Vitamin M see Folic acid 521
Vitiligo see Methoxsalen 383
Vivol see Diazepam 282
Volatile oil of mustard see Allyl isothiocyanate 540
Volmax see Salbutamol 461
Voltaren see Diclofenac 283
Voltaren Ophtha see Diclofenac 283
Voltaren Rapide see Diclofenac 283
Voltaren SR 35N, 35S (illus.); see Diclofenac 283
Vomiting see Anti-emetic drugs 102
how to induce 576
Vosol HC 86
Vumon 86

W

Warfarin 514
Warfilone see Warfarin 514
Weed see Marijuana 536
Wellferon see Interferon 347
Wernicke's syndrome 527

Westcort see Hydrocortisone 338
Whipworm see Anthelmintic
  drugs 151
Whooping cough vaccine
  146-147
Wigraine 86
Wilms' tumor 166
Wilson's disease see
  Penicillamine 423
Winpred see Prednisone 440
Witch hazel 86
Withdrawal symptoms 24, 551g
Worm infestation 139; see
  Anthelmintic drugs 151
Wounds, infected see
  Anti-infective skin preparations
  187
Wycillin see Penicillin G 424
Wydase 86

X

Xanax 36O, 44M (illus.); see
  Alprazolam 203
Xanthine bronchodilators 104
Xanthinol niacinate see Niacin
  523
X-Prep 87
X-Seb 87
X-Seb Plus 87
X-Seb T 87
X-Seb T Plus 87
Xylocaine see Lidocaine 360
Xylocaine Test Dose 87
Xylocard see Lidocaine 360
Xylometazoline 515

Y

Yeast infection see Antifungal
  drugs 150
Yocon 87
Yohimbine 87
Yutopar see Ritodrine 460

Z

Zaditen 87
Zalcitabine 169
Zanosar 87
Zantac 41R (illus.); see Ranitidine
  458
Zarontin 87
Zaroxolyn 87

Zedsorb AF see Tolnaftate 498
Zephiran 87
Zestoretic 87
Zestril 35O, 35P (illus.); see
  Lisinopril 363
Zetar 87
Zidovudine 516
Zilactin 87
Zinacef see Cefuroxime 244
Zinaderm 87
Zinc 530
Zinc amino acid chelate see Zinc
  530
Zinc chloride see Zinc 530
Zincfrin 87
Zincfrin-A 87
Zinc gluconate see Zinc 530
Zincofax 87
Zinc oxide 87
Zinc pyrithione 87
Zinc sulfate see Zinc 530
Zithromax see Azithromycin 219
ZNP 87
Zocor 36A (illus.); see Simvastatin
  467
Zofran see Ondansetron 414
Zoladex 87
Zoloft 46B, 47T (illus.); see
  Sertraline 465
Zonalon see Doxepin 296
Zopiclone 517
Zostrix see Capsaicin 238
Zostrix H.P. see Capsaicin 238
Zovirax see Acyclovir 201
Z-Plus 87
Zyloprim see Allopurinol 202

DRUG POISONING EMERGENCY GUIDE

The information on the following pages is intended to give practical advice for dealing with a known or suspected drug poisoning emergency. Although many of the first-aid techniques described can be used in a number of different types of emergency, instructions apply only to drug overdose or poisoning.

Emergency action is necessary in any of the following circumstances:

● If a person has taken an overdose of any of the high-danger drugs listed in the box on p.576.
● If a person has taken an overdose of a less dangerous drug, but has one or more of the danger symptoms listed below.
● If a person has taken, or is suspected of having taken, an overdose of an unknown drug.
● If a child has swallowed, or is suspected of having swallowed, any prescription or non-prescription drug.

What to do

If you are faced with a drug poisoning emergency, it is important to carry out first aid and arrange immediate medical help in the right order. The Priority Action Decision Chart, below, will help you to assess the situation and to determine your priorities. The following information should help you to remain calm in an emergency if you ever need to deal with a case of drug poisoning.

DANGER SYMPTOMS

Take emergency action if the person has one or more of the following symptoms:
● Drowsiness or unconsciousness
● Shallow, irregular, or stopped breathing
● Vomiting
● Seizures or convulsions

PRIORITY ACTION DECISION CHART

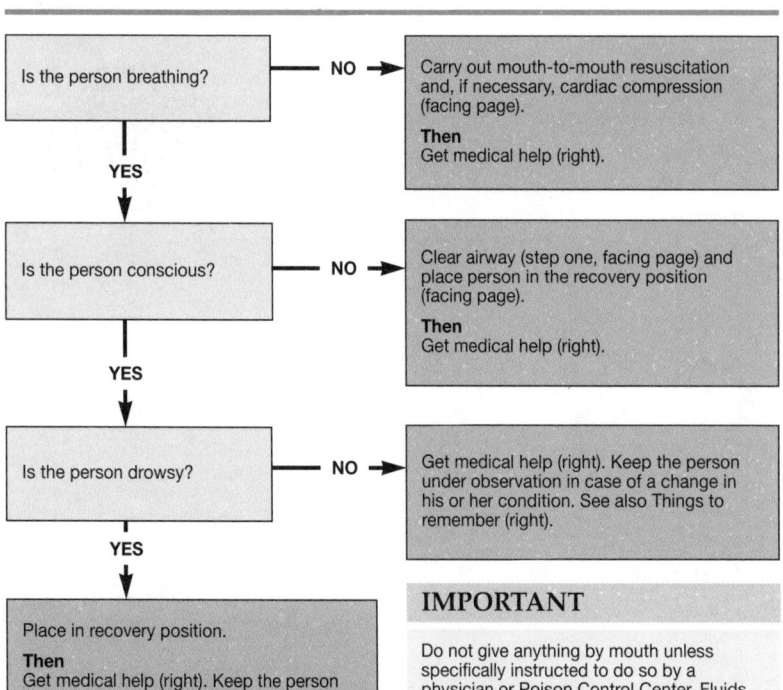

| Is the person breathing? | **NO** → | Carry out mouth-to-mouth resuscitation and, if necessary, cardiac compression (facing page).
Then
Get medical help (right). |

YES ↓

| Is the person conscious? | **NO** → | Clear airway (step one, facing page) and place person in the recovery position (facing page).
Then
Get medical help (right). |

YES ↓

| Is the person drowsy? | **NO** → | Get medical help (right). Keep the person under observation in case of a change in his or her condition. See also Things to remember (right). |

YES ↓

Place in recovery position.
Then
Get medical help (right). Keep the person under observation in case his or her condition changes. See also Things to remember (right).

IMPORTANT

Do not give anything by mouth unless specifically instructed to do so by a physician or Poison Control Center. Fluids may hasten absorption of the drug, thereby increasing the danger to the overdose victim.

GETTING MEDICAL HELP

In an emergency, a calm person who is competent in first aid should stay with the victim while others summon help. However, if you have to deal with a drug poisoning emergency on your own, use first aid (see the Priority Action Decision Chart) before getting help.

Call the emergency medical service (911 in many areas) for an ambulance. Then call a Poison Control Center or your physician for advice. If possible, tell what drug has been taken, how much has been taken, and the age of the victim. Follow instructions precisely, especially with regard to vomiting.

THINGS TO REMEMBER

Effective treatment of drug poisoning depends on the physician making a rapid assessment of the type and amount of drug taken. Collecting evidence that will assist the diagnosis will help. After you have carried out first aid, look for empty or opened medicine containers. Keep any of the drug that is left together with its container (or syringe), and give these to the physician. Save any vomit for analysis.

ESSENTIAL FIRST AID

MOUTH-TO-MOUTH RESUSCITATION

When there is no rise and fall of the chest and you can feel no movement of exhaled air, immediately commence mouth-to-mouth resuscitation.

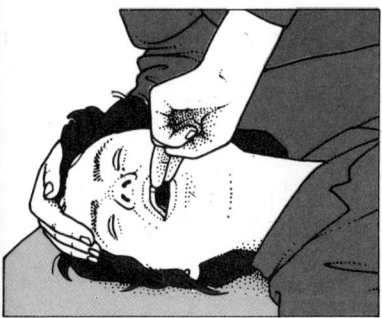

1 Lay the victim on his or her back on a firm surface. Clear the mouth of vomit or any other foreign material that might otherwise block the airways, and remove false teeth.

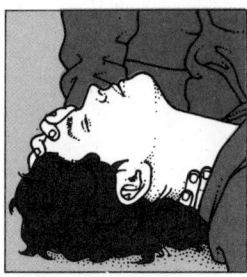

2 Place one hand under the neck and lift gently to tip the head back and raise the chin, while pressing down on the forehead. This should allow the mouth to drop open.

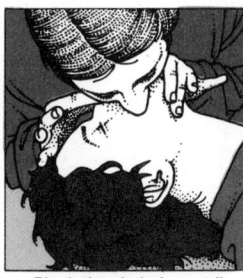

3 Pinch the victim's nostrils closed with the hand that is placed on the forehead and use the other to grip his or her chin firmly to keep the mouth open. Take a deep breath, seal your mouth over that of the victim, and give two quick breaths. Continue to give further breaths every 5 seconds.

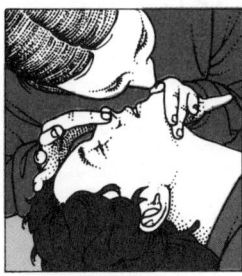

4 After each breath, turn to watch the chest falling while you listen for the sound of air leaving the victim's mouth. Continue until the victim starts to breathe regularly on his or her own, or until medical help arrives.

CARDIAC COMPRESSION

This is a technique used in conjunction with mouth-to-mouth resuscitation to restart a stopped heartbeat. It is a procedure that should normally be undertaken only by someone who has received training.

Cardiac compression involves putting repeated, strong pressure on the center of the chest with the heels of both hands, at a rate of 80 compressions per minute for adults (right). After every 15 compressions, two breaths should be given using mouth-to-mouth resuscitation (above).

CHECKING PULSE

If the victim does not start breathing after two breaths of mouth-to-mouth resuscitation, check the pulse in the neck. If there is no pulse, start cardiac compression if you have been trained in this technique.

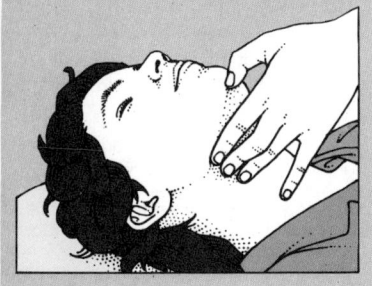

This sequence should be continued until breathing restarts.

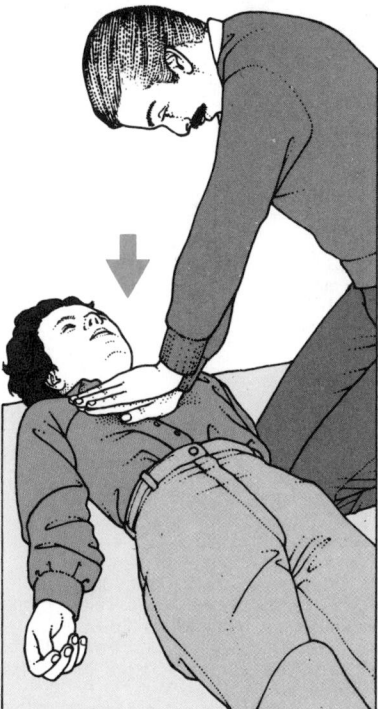

THE RECOVERY POSITION

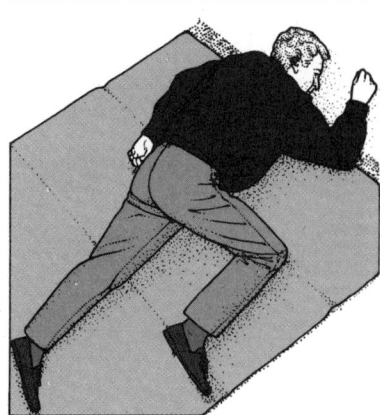

The recovery position is the safest position for an unconscious or a drowsy person. It allows the person to breathe easily and will help to prevent choking if vomiting occurs. A victim of drug poisoning should be placed in the recovery position after more urgent first aid, such as mouth-to-mouth resuscitation, has been carried out and when shock (p.576) is not suspected. Place the victim on his or her stomach with one leg bent and the arm on that side raised. Turn the head to the same side. Tilt the head back so that the chin juts forward. Cover the person with a blanket for warmth.

DEALING WITH A SEIZURE

Certain types of drug poisoning may provoke seizures. These may occur whether the person is conscious or not. The victim usually falls to the ground twitching or making uncontrolled movements of limbs and body. If you witness a seizure, remember the following points:

● Do not try to hold the person down.

● Do not put anything into the person's mouth.

● Remove any objects or furniture on which the victim could be injured.

● Once the seizure is over, place the person in the recovery position (p.575).

HIGH-DANGER DRUGS

The following is a list of drugs given a high overdose rating in the drug profiles. If you suspect that someone has taken an overdose of one of these drugs, immediate medical attention must be sought.

Acebutolol	Desipramine	Hydrocodone
Acetaminophen	Digoxin	Hydromorphone
Amitriptyline	Disopyramide	
ASA	Doxepin	Imipramine
Atenolol		Insulin
	Epinephrine	Isoniazid
Butorphanol		Isoproterenol
	Fluoxetine	
Chloral hydrate	Fluvoxamine	Lithium
Chlorpropamide		Loxapine
Clomipramine	Gliclazide	
Codeine	Glyburide	Maprotiline
Colchicine		Meperidine
Cyclobenzaprine	Heparin	Meprobamate
	Hydralazine	Metformin
		Methotrexate
		Methylphenidate
		Metoprolol
		Minoxidil
		Misoprostol
		Morphine

Nadolol	Theophylline
Neostigmine	Timolol
Nilutamide	Tolbutamide
Nortriptyline	Trimipramine
Orphenadrine	Vasopressin
Oxycodone	Venlafaxine
Phenobarbital	Warfarin
Pindolol	
Primidone	
Procyclidine	
Propoxyphene	
Propranolol	
Pseudoephedrine	
Pyridostigmine	
Quinidine	
Quinine	
Selegiline	
Sotalol	

DEALING WITH ANAPHYLACTIC SHOCK

Anaphylactic shock occurs as the result of a severe allergic reaction to a drug or insect sting or bite. Blood pressure drops dramatically and the airways may become narrowed. The reaction usually occurs within minutes of taking the drug. The main symptoms are:

● Pallor
● Tightness in the chest
● Breathing difficulty
● Rash
● Facial swelling
● Collapse

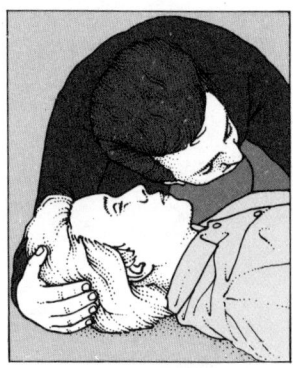

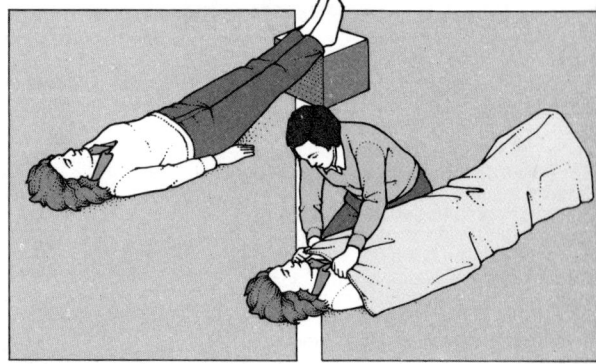

1 First ensure that the person is breathing. If breathing has stopped, immediate mouth-to-mouth resuscitation should be carried out as described on p.575.

2 If the person is breathing normally, lay him or her down, face up, with legs raised above the level of the heart to ensure the adequate circulation of the blood. Use a footstool, carton, or a similar item to support the feet.

3 Cover the person with a blanket or articles of clothing and phone for medical help. Do not attempt to administer anything by mouth.

HOW TO INDUCE VOMITING

In certain circumstances you may be advised to make a person vomit in order to expel a drug from the stomach, thus preventing the drug from being absorbed. This should be attempted only when specifically advised by your physician or Poison Control Center. Never induce vomiting when the person is unconscious. The simplest method of inducing vomiting is to give ipecac syrup, a medication that should be kept among your regular medical supplies. Recommended dosages are: 6 – 12 months of age 5 – 10mL plus 15mL of clear fluids per kilogram body weight; 12 months – 12 years of age 15mL plus 240mL of clear fluids; over 12 years of age 30mL plus 240 – 480mL of clear fluids. This normally stimulates vomiting within 20 – 30 minutes. Do not push fingers down the throat. When vomiting occurs, remember the following:

1 Ensure that the victim leans well forward to avoid choking or inhaling vomit.

2 Keep the vomit for later analysis (see Things to remember, p.574).

3 Give water to rinse the mouth. This should be spat out, not swallowed.